BMA

British Medical Association

A-Z FAMILY MEDICAL ENCYCLOPEDIA

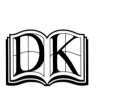

LONDON, NEW YORK, MUNICH,
MELBOURNE, DELHI

First UK edition published in 1990 as the *British Medical Association Complete Family Health Encyclopedia*. Second UK edition published in 1995. Third UK edition published in 1999 and then reprinted in 2000 as the *British Medical Association A-Z Family Health Encyclopedia*. Fourth edition published in 2004.

This fifth edition published in 2008 in the United Kingdom by
Dorling Kindersley Limited, 80 Strand, London WCR 0RL
A Penguin Company

2 4 6 8 10 9 7 5 3 1

A CIP catalogue record for this book is available from the British Library.

ISBN 978 1 4053 2987 3

Printed and bound in Singapore by Star Standard Industries

Discover more at
www.dk.com

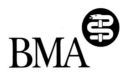

BMA
British Medical Association

A-Z FAMILY MEDICAL ENCYCLOPEDIA

BMA CONSULTING MEDICAL EDITOR
Dr. Michael Peters

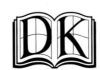

BRITISH MEDICAL ASSOCIATION

Chairman of the Council Dr. Hamish Meldrum
Treasurer Dr. David Pickersgill
Chairman of Representative Body Dr. Peter Bennie

BMA CONSULTING MEDICAL EDITOR

Dr. Michael Peters MB BS

DORLING KINDERSLEY

Managing Editor Julie Oughton
Managing Art Editor Louise Dick
Production Editors Phil Sergeant, Lucy Baker
Production Controller Hema Gohil
Publisher Jonathan Metcalf
Art Director Bryn Walls

Edited for Dorling Kindersley by Martyn Page
Child Health Reviewer Ann Peters RGN HV

PREVIOUS EDITIONS
DORLING KINDERSLEY

Senior Managing Editor Martyn Page • **Managing Editor** Ruth Midgley • **Editors** Andrea Bagg, Ann Baggaley, Joanna Benwell, Dr. Stephen Carroll, Robert Dinwiddie, Dawn Henderson, Katie John, Alyson Lacewing, Gail Lawther, Mary Lindsay, Maugan Lloyd, Richenda Milton-Thompson, Ricki Ostrov, Teresa Pritlove, Nikki Sims, Jillian Somerscales, Tony Whitehorn • **Additional editorial assistance** Maria Adams, Simon Adams, Donald Berwick, Deirdre Clark, Jean Cooke, Mike Darton, Elizabeth Galfalvi, Claire Isaac, Ann Kramer, Cathy Meeus, Terence Monaighan, Theodore Rowland-Entwistle, Ruth Swan, Rena Taylor, Pat White, Kathryn Wilkinson, Kay Wright • **Indexer** Kay Wright • **Managing Art Editors** Denise Brown, Louise Dick, Marianne Markham, Chez Picthall • **Art Editors** Melissa Gray, Caroline Murray, Anne Renel, Ian Spick • **Designers** Sandra Archer, Peter Cross, Tina Hill, Gail Jones, Phillip Lord, Andrew O'Brien, Sarah Ponder, Tracy Timson, Lydia Umney • **Design assistants** Iona Hoyle, Francis Wong • **Additional design assistance** Peter Blake, Carol Briggs, Thomas Keenes, Chris Scollens • **Illustrators** Karen Cochrane, Paul Cooper, Sandra Doyle, Tony Graham, Will Giles, Brian Hewson, Chris Jenkins, Kevin Jones, Janos Marffy, Kevin Marks, Coral Muller, Patrick Mulrey, Frazer Newman, Andrew O'Brien, Nick Oxloby, Lynda Payne, Sandra Ponder, Patricia Sempron, Mark Surridge, John Temperton, Richard Tibbits, John Woodcock • **DTP Design** Julian Dams, Jason Little • **Picture Research** Carolyn Clerkin, Diana Morris, Sandra Schneider, Sharon Southren • **Production** Elizabeth Cherry, Eunice Paterson, Wendy Penn, Kirsti Rippon, Hilary Stephens, Michelle Thomas • **Editorial Directors** Amy Carroll, Jackie Douglas • **Art Director** Bryn Walls • **Category Publisher** Corinne Roberts

DORLING KINDERSLEY INDIA

Managing Editor Ira Pande • **Editors** Sudhanshu Gupta, K. J. Ravi, Ranjana Saklani • **Managing Art Editors** Shuka Jain, Aparna Sharma • **Illustrations Project Co-ordinator** Malavika Talukder **Illustrations** Umesh Aggarwal, Rajesh Chhibber, Vinod Harish, Nain Singh Rawat, Pankaj Sharma, Sunil Sharma, Balwant Singh, Ashwani Tyagi • **DTP Co-ordinator** Pankaj Sharma • **DTP Design** Ajay Verma

PREVIOUS EDITIONS

BMA Consulting Medical Editor Dr. Michael Peters MB BS
Medical Editor Dr. Tony Smith MA BM BCh

MEDICAL REVIEWERS

Dr. Wendy Abrams MB BS MRCGP DRCOG, Mr. John Ballantyne CBE FRCS, Dr. Ian Beider BDS (U.Lond), Professor Arnold E. Bender DSc PhD, Dr. Brendan M. Buckley DPhil FRCP(I), Professor James Calnan FRCS FRCP, Dr. Sue Davidson MB BS MRCP MRCGP DRCOG, Dr. Dewi Davies MD FRCP, Dr. A.K. Dixon MD FRCR, Dr. James Owen Drife MD FRCS(Ed), Mr. Edgar Gordon MSc DDS, Professor Terry J. Hamblin DM FRCP, Dr. Anthony John Holland MPhil MRCP, Dr. Helen M. Kingston MD MRCP, Professor W.R. Lee MD FRCP, Dr. E.B. Lewis MB FFARCS, Mr. C.D.R. Lightowler FRCS, Dr. G. Keith Morris MD FRCP, Dr. Graham Peter Mulley DM FRCP, Dr. R.T.D. Oliver MD FRCP, Dr. Alex Paton MD FRCP, Ann Peters RGN HV, Dr. Penny Preston MB ChB MRCGP, Dr. T. Richards MRCP, MRCGP, Dr. J.A. Savin MD, FRCP, Dr. Leonard Sinclair FRCP, DCH, Dr. R.N.T. Thin MD, FRCP, Mr. Patrick D. Trevor-Roper MD, FRCS, Mr. Robert H. Whitaker MD, FRCS, Dr. Frances Williams MA MBBChir MRCP MRCPCH DTM&H, Dr. George Bernard Wyatt FRCP, DCH

CONTRIBUTORS

Vivienne Owen Ankrett MRCGP DRCOG, Igor Anrep LRCP MRCS, Ann Ashworth PhD, Alan Bailey MB MRCP, Julian Barth MB MRCP, Margaret A. Barrie FRCP DRCOG, R.J. Berry FRCP FRCR, A.K. Bhalla MD MRCP, Charles Eric Blank PhD MB, Geoffrey Blundell, Susan Bosanko, Arthur William Boylston MD MRCPath, Amanda Bridges, Peter Bromwich MB MRCOG, W.B.J. Broom MB, N.F. Burnett Hodd FBCO DCLP, E.P. Cameron MCh FRCS, Rosalind Carr MB DRCOG, Nicola Jane Carroll, N.R. Carroll BDS LDSRCS, Simon StC. Carter MB FRCS, Michael D. Chard MB MRCP, Lyn Cheater, Julian Chomet MSc, Neil Citron MChir FRCS, A.M. de Lacy Costello MB MRCP, Richard Dawood FRCR DTM&H, J.J. Dawson MS FRCS, Jonathan H. Dean, Jane Deverson, John H. Dubois, Andrew Duncombe MB MRCP, Patrick Durston FASI REMT, Adrian Eddleston DM FRCP, Martin Brian Edwards BDS FDSRCS, Anne Eldred MB MRCGP, Christopher John Ellis FRCP DTM&H, M.G. Falcon FRCS FCOphth, Ivor L. Felstein MB, P.H. Fentem MB MRCP, Colin Ferguson MB FRCS, Loraine Fergusson, Richard E. Field FRCSE, Michael W. Flowers MB FRCS, Michael D. Flynn MB MRCP, John Foley MD FRCP, T.J. Fowler DM FRCP, Roger Gabriel MB FRCP, Ruth Garland, Michael Glasspool FRCS DO, Max Glatt FRCP FRCPsych, J. Graham MB MRCGP, Roger F. Gray MB FRCS, Brian Glenville MB FRCS, Alison Hadley SRN HV, John W. Harcup SBStJ MRCGP, Richard Harding AFOM RCP DAv Med, David Haslam MRCGP DObstRCOG, Roderick J. Hay DM FRCP, Kenneth W. Heaton MD FRCP, John A. Henry MB FRCP, Anthony David Heyes PhD, Ann Hill PhD, K.E.F. Hobbs ChM FRCS, David Honeybourne MD MRCP, Judith Hooper DObstRCOG MRCGP, Graham Robert Vivian Hughes MD FRCP, Alex T. Inglis BDS FDSRCS, J. Jenner MD MRCP, Lydia Jones MB MRCP, Jack Joseph MD FRCOG, Adrian D. Joyce MB FRCS, Patricia A. Judd PhD SRD, Arthur Kaufman MSc ABPsS, Patrick Kesteven FRCAP FRCPA, R.B. Kinder MB FRCS, Ronald L. Kleinman MB DObstRCOG, J.D.E. Knox FRCPE FRCGP, Paul W. Lambden FDS RCS MB, Richard Lamerton MRCS LRCP, R.S. Ledward FRCS FRCOG, Colin John Leonard FRCGP DCH, S.G. Lim BDS, E.S. Lin FFARCS, Peter C. Lindsay MA MB, Jane MacDougall MB MRCOG, Shelia Macey, Norma MacMillan, T.E. Martin MB, John A. Matthews MD FRCP, Francis Matthey MB MRCP, J.Q. Matthias MD FRCP, Kenneth A. McLean MB MRCP, P.W.D. Meerstadt MRCP DCH, Debbie Mills, P.J.A. Molitor MB FRCS, Alex J. Munro, MSc MRCP, Nabil M. Mustapha MB FRCS, Paul Myers MRCGP DObstRCOG, David S. Nairn MB FRCS, Margaret Nanson MA MB, C.G.H. Newman FRCP DCH, Kenneth Arthur Newton FRCP FRCR, A.N. Nicolaides MS FRCS, Mark Noble PhD, N.P. Norwell DA MRCGP, P.M. Owens MB, Malcolm Padwick MB MRCOG, A.M. Peters MD MRCPath, Michael Peter Powell MB FRCS, W.D.W. Rees MD MRCP, Anthony John Richards FRCP DPhysMed, M.B. Richter FRACP PhD, Amanda Jane Roberts MB, M. Rogers BPharm MRPharmS DipInfSc MIInfSc, N.D. Rothnie MB FRCS, Rosalind J.D. Rothnie MB DObstRCOG, Robert Royston, Quentin Sattentau PhD, Peter Saul MRCGP DCH, Glenis K. Scadding MD MRCP, D.F. Scott FRCP DPM, Christina M. Scott-Moncrieff MB MFHom, Mike Seymour MB FRCS, Sarah-Jane Seymour MB, J.F.L. Shaw ChM FRCS, Caroline M. Shreeve MB, Valerie Sinason, Albert Singer DPhil FRCOG, T.M. Skerry BVetMed MRCVS, Arlene Sobel, Michael Spira MB, Venetia Stent MB MRCGP, Richard Stern MD FRCPsych, Susan Sturrock, Paul Sweny MD FRCP, M.F. Sturridge MS FRCS, Margaret Elizabeth Taylor BDS MB, A. Theodossi MD MRCP, Malcolm Keith Thompson DObstRCOG FRCGP, Michael Townend MB, G.D.W. Towse, Trevor H. Turner MB MRCPsych, H.A. Waldron MD FFOM, Rae Ward, Michael Anthony Waugh MB DipVen, Moya de Wet, Saffron Ann Whitehead PhD, Marcia Wilkinson DM FRCP, Ian Williams MRCGP DRCOG, Pamela Wood, W. Keith Yeates MD FRCS, Robert M. Youngson DTM&H, FCOphth

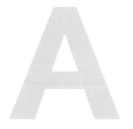

A

abdomen

The region of the body between the chest and the pelvis. The abdominal cavity is bounded by the ribs and diaphragm above, and by the pelvis below, with the spine and abdominal muscles forming the back, side, and front walls. The abdominal cavity contains the liver, stomach, intestines, spleen, pancreas, and kidneys. In the lower abdomen, enclosed by the pelvis, are the bladder, rectum, and, in women, the uterus and ovaries.

STRUCTURE
The spine, pelvis, and ribs provide attachments for the layers of muscle that make up the abdominal walls. There is a layer of fat between these muscles and the skin. The inner surface of the abdominal muscles is covered by a thin membrane, the peritoneum, which also covers the organs, such as the pancreas and kidneys, that are fixed to the back wall. Folds of peritoneum also cover the mobile organs, such as the stomach and intestines.

abdomen, acute

The medical term for persistent, severe abdominal pain, of sudden onset, that is usually associated with spasm of the abdominal muscles, vomiting, and fever.

CAUSES
The most common cause of an acute abdomen is *peritonitis* (inflammation of the membrane that lines the abdomen); underlying causes include *appendicitis*, abdominal injury, or perforation of an internal organ as a result of disorders such as *diverticular disease* (the presence of small, protruding pouches in the intestinal wall) or *peptic ulcer*.

SYMPTOMS
Acute abdomen commonly begins as a vague pain in the centre of the abdomen that gradually localizes to a particular region of the body, depending on the condition. For example, pain is felt on the right side of the body in appendicitis.

DIAGNOSIS AND TREATMENT
An acute abdomen requires urgent medical investigation usually comprising detailed questioning about the condition, a physical examination, laboratory tests, and imaging procedures such as *ultrasound scanning*. The investigation may also involve a *laparoscopy* (internal examination using a rigid or flexible viewing tube) or a *laparotomy* (surgical exploration of the abdomen). Treatment depends on the underlying cause.

abdominal

Relating to the *abdomen*.

abdominal hysterectomy

The surgical removal of the uterus (womb) through an incision in the abdomen (see *hysterectomy*).

abdominal pain

Discomfort in the abdominal cavity. Symptoms accompanying abdominal pain may include belching, nausea, vomiting, rumbling and gurgling noises, and flatulence (wind).

CAUSES
Mild abdominal pain is common and is often due to excessive alcohol intake, eating unwisely, wind, an attack of *diarrhoea*, or irritable bowel syndrome. Pain in the lower abdomen is common during menstruation but may occasionally be due to a gynaecological disorder such as *endometriosis* (in which fragments of uterine lining are present in abnormal sites in the abdomen). *Cystitis* is another common cause of pain or discomfort in the lower abdomen. Bladder distension due to urinary obstruction may also cause abdominal pain.

Abdominal colic is the term used for pain that occurs every few minutes as one of the internal organs goes into muscular spasm. Colic is an attempt by the body to overcome an obstruction such as a stone or an area of inflammation. The attacks of colic may become more severe and may be associated with vomiting (see *abdomen, acute*).

A *peptic ulcer*, which is associated with an increase in the amount of acid formed in the stomach, often produces recurrent gnawing pain. Other possible causes of abdominal pain are infection, such as *pyelonephritis* (infection of the kidneys) and *pelvic inflammatory disease* (infection of the internal female reproductive organs), and *ischaemia* (a lack of blood supply), as occurs when a *volvulus* (twisting of the intestine) obstructs blood vessels. Tumours affecting an abdominal organ can cause pain. Abdominal pain may also have a psychological cause, such as anxiety.

LOCATION OF THE **ABDOMEN**

The *abdomen* is bounded by the lower rips at the top and the pelvis below. The illustration shows the position of the abdominal organs in an adult woman.

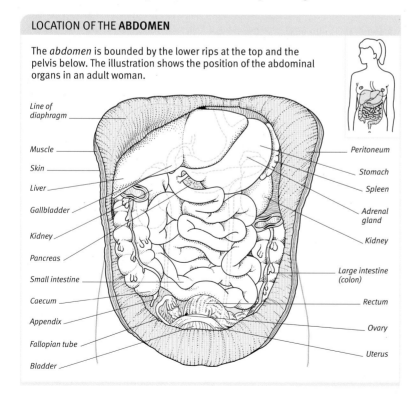

Line of diaphragm
Muscle
Skin
Liver
Gallbladder
Kidney
Pancreas
Small intestine
Caecum
Appendix
Fallopian tube
Bladder

Peritoneum
Stomach
Spleen
Adrenal gland
Kidney
Large intestine (colon)
Rectum
Ovary
Uterus

TREATMENT

For mild abdominal pain, self-treatment measures, such as a wrapped hot-water bottle or a milky drink, are often effective. Pain due to peptic ulcer can be temporarily relieved by consuming food or by taking *antacid drugs*.

Abdominal pain that is not relieved by vomiting, persists for more than six hours, or is associated with sweating or fainting requires urgent medical attention. Urgent attention is also necessary if pain is accompanied by persistent vomiting, vomiting of blood, or passing of bloodstained or black faeces. Abdominal pain that is accompanied by unexplained weight loss or changes in bowel habits should always be investigated by a doctor.

INVESTIGATION AND DIAGNOSIS

The doctor makes a diagnosis of abdominal pain based on a physical examination and a detailed description of the patient's symptoms. Investigation of severe abdominal pain may also include *blood tests*, imaging tests such as *ultrasound scanning*, and endoscopy (examination of a body cavity using a flexible viewing tube) in the form of *laparoscopy* (viewing the abdominal cavity), *gastroscopy* (viewing the stomach and duodenum), or *colonoscopy* (viewing the large intestine).

abdominal swelling

Enlargement of the abdomen, which may be due to a variety of causes. Abdominal swelling is a natural result of *obesity* and enlargement of the uterus during pregnancy.

Some causes of abdominal swelling are harmless. Wind in the stomach or intestine may cause uncomfortable, bloating distension. Distension as a result of temporary water retention may occur in some women just before *menstruation*. Other causes may be more serious. For instance, *ascites* (fluid accumulation in the abdominal cavity) may be a symptom of cancer or disease of the heart, kidneys, or liver; swelling may also be due to intestinal obstruction (see *intestine, obstruction of*) or an *ovarian cyst*.

INVESTIGATION

Diagnosis of the underlying cause may involve X-rays (see *abdominal X-ray*), *ultrasound scanning, laparotomy* (surgical exploration of the abdomen) or *laparoscopy* (examination of the inside of the abdomen using a rigid or flexible viewing tube). In ascites, some of the fluid in the abdomen may be drained for detailed examination.

abdominal thrust

Also known as the Heimlich manoeuvre, a first-aid technique for treating severe *choking* in older children and adults (the corresponding technique for babies is the chest thrust). It involves applying sharp upward and inward pressure to the upper abdomen, just below the ribcage, to clear an airway obstruction.

abdominal X-ray

An *X-ray* examination of the abdominal contents. An abdominal X-ray is often one of the first steps in the investigation of acute abdominal disease.

X-rays do not reveal the internal structure of organs, but they do show their outlines. X-rays can therefore show whether any organ is enlarged and can detect swallowed foreign bodies in the digestive tract. X-rays also show accumulations of fluid and gas: distended loops of bowel containing collections of fluid indicate the presence of an obstruction (see *intestine, obstruction of*); gas outside the intestine indicates intestinal *perforation*.

Calcium, which is opaque to X-rays, is present in most kidney stones (see *calculus, urinary tract*) and in some *gallstones* and aortic *aneurysms*; these can sometimes be detected on an abdominal X-ray.

Abdominal X-rays may need to be followed by investigative procedures that provide more information, such as *ultrasound scanning, barium X-ray examinations* (use of a contrast medium to detect disorders of the gastrointestinal tract), *laparoscopy* (internal examination of the abdomen using a viewing instrument), *CT scanning* or *MRI* (magnetic resonance imaging).

abducent nerve

The sixth *cranial nerve*. The abducent nerve supplies the lateral rectus muscle of each eye, which is responsible for moving the eyeball outwards. The abducent nerve originates in the pons (part of the *brainstem*) and passes along the

---

DIAGNOSING **ABDOMINAL PAIN**

The doctor conducts a physical examination and listens to the patient's description of the pain. More investigations, such as blood tests, X-rays, or imaging tests (including ultrasound scanning), may be carried out. If the diagnosis is still in doubt, endoscopic inspection of the stomach and duodenum (gastroscopy), large intestine (colonoscopy), or abdominal cavity (laparoscopy) may be performed.

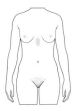
Oesophageal reflux
A burning pain in the chest that is accompanied by regurgitation of stomach acid and is often worse after meals or when lying down at night.

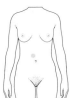
Duodenal ulcer pain
This pain often occurs in the same small area and may be temporarily relieved by eating or taking antacids.

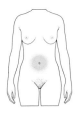
Wind
Excess wind in the digestive system affects a large area of the abdomen and can cause an uncomfortable, distended feeling.

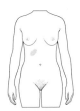
Gallbladder pain
A cramplike or steady pain under the right ribs that is often accompanied by vomiting and fever.

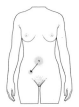
Appendicitis pain
This pain starts around the navel before finally settling in the lower right side of the abdomen.

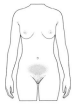
Pelvic organ inflammation
A constant diffuse pain, usually accompanied by vaginal discharge or fever, that extends over the lower abdomen.

base of the skull, entering the back of the eye socket through a gap between the skull bones.

The abducent nerve may be damaged in fractures of the base of the skull, or by disorders, such as tumours, that distort the brain. Such damage may give rise to *double vision* or a *squint*.

abduction

Movement of a limb away from the central line of the body, or of a digit away from the axis of a limb. Muscles that carry out this movement are called abductors. (See also *adduction*.)

abductor

Any one of the muscles that carry out the movement of *abduction*.

aberrant

A term meaning abnormal; in medical usage the word is often applied to a blood vessel or nerve that deviates from its normal route.

abetalipoproteinaemia

A rare, inherited *genetic disorder* of *lipoprotein* (a protein that combines with fats or other lipids) metabolism. It is inherited in an autosomal recessive manner and is characterized by *malabsorption* of fats, acanthocytosis (distorted red blood cells), *retinopathy* (disease of the retina), *ataxia* (incoordination and clumsiness), slurred speech, muscle weakness, curvature of the spine, *neuropathy* (peripheral nerve disease), fatty stools, diarrhoea, and *failure to thrive* in infancy.

Treatment with high doses of fat soluble vitamins (*vitamin A*, *vitamin D*, *vitamin E*, and *vitamin K*) may slow the progression of certain abetalipoproteinaemia-related problems such as retinal degeneration.

ablation

The removal or destruction of diseased tissue by excision (cutting away), *cryosurgery*, *radiotherapy*, *diathermy*, *laser treatment* or *radiofrequency ablation*.

ablepharia

A *birth defect* in which the eyelids fail to develop normally, leaving the eyeball completely covered over.

abnormality

A physical deformity or malformation, behavioural or mental problem, or variation from normal in the structure or function of a body cell, tissue, or organ.

ABO blood groups

See *blood groups*.

abort

A term meaning to terminate a pregnancy, either spontaneously (see *miscarriage*) or through medical intervention (see *abortion, induced*).

abortifacient

An agent that causes *abortion*. In medical practice, abortion is induced using *prostaglandin drugs*, often given as vaginal pessaries. These cause softening and widening of the cervix and muscular contractions of the uterus.

abortion

In medical usage, a term denoting either spontaneous abortion (see *miscarriage*) or medically induced termination (see *abortion, induced*) of pregnancy. (See also *complete miscarriage*; *habitual miscarriage*; *incomplete miscarriage*; *septic abortion*.)

abortion, induced

Medically induced termination of pregnancy (also sometimes known as TOP). In the UK, abortion can legally be performed up to the end of the 23rd week of pregnancy (a week of pregnancy is measured from the first day of the last normal menstrual period). Legally, abortion may be performed if continuation of the pregnancy would constitute a greater risk to the woman's life than the termination, if the mental or physical health of the woman or her existing children is at risk, or if there is a substantial risk of serious handicap to the baby.

MEDICAL REASONS FOR ABORTION

A doctor may recommend an abortion if the woman suffers from a life-threatening condition, such as severe heart disease, chronic kidney disease, or cancer, especially of the breast or cervix.

If a serious fetal abnormality is discovered, for example, severe developmental defects (such as *anencephaly*) or chromosomal abnormalities (such as *Down's syndrome*), the parents may be offered the option of a termination. Abortion may also be recommended if the mother contracts *rubella* (German measles) during early pregnancy.

HOW IT IS DONE

Abortion may be performed by various methods, the choice of which depends on how long the woman has been pregnant, her personal preferences, and whether there are any medical reasons for or against a specific method.

Early medical abortion This procedure can be carried out up to the ninth week of pregnancy. It involves taking two drugs to cause an early miscarriage. First, oral *mifepristone* is given, then one to three days later a *prostaglandin drug* (*misoprostol*) is also given, usually as a vaginal pessary. These end the pregnancy by inducing the uterus to contract and expel the embryo and placenta, usually within a few hours.

Medical abortion This procedure may be carried out between the ninth and 20th weeks of pregnancy. It is similar to an early medical abortion: an initial dose of oral mifepristone is given, and one to three days later misoprostol is also given. However, several doses of misoprostol are given (up to five), at intervals of about three hours. In most cases, the embryo and placenta are expelled within a few hours of treatment with misoprostol. However, if this does not occur, misoprostol treatment can be repeated after a 12-hour interval.

Medical induction abortion This procedure may be carried out between the 19th and end of the 23rd week of pregnancy. It involves giving drugs to stimulate an early labour and is usually carried out under sedation. First, a hollow needle is inserted into the abdomen to withdraw fluid from the uterus, then drugs to induce contractions are administered through the needle. These contractions cause the uterine contents to be expelled, as in a normal labour.

Suction termination This procedure may be carried out between the seventh and 12th weeks of pregnancy, although it may sometimes be used before the seventh week and up to the 15th week. It may be carried out under local or general anaesthesia. Before the procedure the cervix may be softened by administering medication (for example, a misoprostol pessary inserted into the vagina). During the procedure the cervix is dilated and the contents of the uterus are removed with a suction device.

Surgical dilatation and evacuation This procedure may be carried out between the 15th and end of the 23rd week of pregnancy. It is usually performed under general anaesthesia. During the procedure, the cervix is dilated and the contents of the uterus are removed with forceps; any remaining uterine contents are then removed with a suction device.

AFTER THE PROCEDURE

There will probably be some bleeding, discomfort, and pain afterwards, which may last for a few days, and the woman will therefore be offered appropriate *analgesic drug*s (painkillers). However, if the bleeding or pain is severe, or if the woman develops a fever or has an unusual vaginal discharge, she may have an infection and should consult a doctor. It is safe to start using contraception (including having an *IUD* or *IUS* fitted) immediately after an abortion.

COMPLICATIONS

If termination is performed by a qualified gynaecologist in a well-equipped clinic or hospital, complications are rare. Infection, resulting in a condition called *septic abortion*, or serious bleeding occasionally occur. Repeated terminations may increase the risk of miscarriage occurring in subsequent pregnancies; but a single termination is unlikely to affect future fertility. (See also *complete miscarriage*; *habitual miscarriage*; *incomplete miscarriage*.)

abrasion

Also called a graze, a *wound* on the surface of the skin that is caused by scraping or rubbing.

abrasion, dental

The wearing away of tooth enamel, which is often accompanied by the erosion of dentine (the layer beneath the enamel) and cementum (the bonelike tissue that covers the tooth root). Dental abrasion is usually a result of brushing the teeth too vigorously.

Abraded areas are often sensitive to hot, cold, or sweet food and drink; a desensitizing toothpaste and/or protection with a bonding agent (see *bonding, dental*) or filling (see *filling, dental*) may be necessary.

abrasive

A substance that is used in dentistry for polishing and cleaning the teeth. (See also *dentifrice*.)

abreaction

In *psychoanalysis*, the process of becoming consciously aware of painful feelings and memories that have previously been repressed (buried). The emotional discharge of such experiences is believed to have therapeutic benefits. The concept of abreaction originates in Freudian psychoanalytical theory, in which the process ideally occurs as a result of *catharsis* (the open expression of emotions that are associated with forgotten memories).

abruption

The medical term for the separation of one structure from another. (See also *placental abruption*.)

abruptio placentae

The medical term for the premature separation of the placenta from the wall of the uterus (see *placental abruption*) during pregnancy.

abscess

A collection of *pus* caused by infection by microorganisms, usually bacteria. Pus is formed from destroyed tissue cells, leukocytes (a type of white blood cell) that have been carried to the area to fight infection, and dead and live microorganisms. A lining (called a pyogenic membrane) often forms around the abscess.

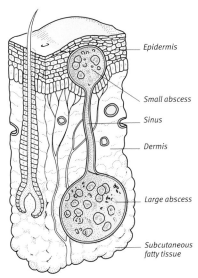

Epidermis

Small abscess

Sinus

Dermis

Large abscess

Subcutaneous fatty tissue

Cross section of a collar-stud abscess
A small cavity in the epidermis, just beneath the skin's surface, connects, via a sinus (channel), to a larger cavity in deeper, subcutaneous tissue.

TYPES

An abscess may develop in any organ, and in the soft tissues beneath the skin, sometimes as a collar-stud abscess, a small cavity that connects to a larger cavity in deeper tissues. Common sites of abscesses include the armpit, breast (see *breast abscess*), groin, and gums (see *abscess, dental*). Rarer sites include the liver (see *liver abscess*) and brain (see *brain abscess*).

CAUSES AND INCIDENCE

Common bacteria, such as staphylococci, are the usual cause of abscesses, although fungal infections are another cause. Amoebae (single-celled micro-

organisms) are an important cause of liver abscesses (see *amoebiasis*). Infectious organisms reach internal organs via the bloodstream or penetrate to tissues under the skin through an infected wound or bite.

People with impaired immunity, such as those who are taking *immuno-suppressant drugs* and those with *HIV* infection or *AIDS*, are especially susceptible to abscesses.

SYMPTOMS

An abscess may cause pain, depending on where it occurs. Most larger abscesses cause fever (sometimes with chills), sweating, and malaise. Abscesses may produce a sensation of intense pressure and those close to the skin may cause redness and swelling.

TREATMENT

Antibiotic drugs are usually prescribed to treat bacterial infections, *antifungal drugs* are used to treat fungal infections, and amoebicides are used for amoebiasis. Most abscesses need to be drained by making a cut in the lining of the abscess cavity to allow the pus to escape; a tube may be left in place to allow continuous drainage (see *drain, surgical*). Some abscesses burst and drain spontaneously.

OUTLOOK

Many abscesses subside following drainage alone; others subside after a combination of drainage and drug treatment. Occasionally the presence of an abscess within a vital organ damages enough surrounding tissue to cause permanent loss of normal function, or even death. (See also *appendix abscess*; *Bartholin's abscess*; *bone abscess*; *caseous abscess*; *cold abscess*; *hot abscess*; *metastatic abscess*; *pelvic abscess*; *periodontal abscess*; *peritonsillar abscess*; *sterile abscess*; *subphrenic abscess*; *tubercular abscess*.)

abscess, dental

Also called a periapical abscess, a pus-filled sac in the tissue around the end of the root of a tooth, usually caused by bacterial infection.

CAUSE

A periapical abscess may occur when bacteria invade the pulp (the tissues in the central cavity of a tooth), causing the pulp to die. This commonly happens as a result of dental caries (see *caries, dental*), as the tooth's enamel and dentine are destroyed, allowing bacteria to reach the pulp. Bacteria can also gain access to the pulp when a tooth is injured. The infection in the pulp then spreads into the surrounding tissue to form an abscess.

An abscess that occurs when bacteria accumulate in pockets that form between the teeth and gums is called a periodontal abscess. This type of abscess indicates chronic *periodontal disease*, in which the periodontal membrane (attachment of tooth to bone) is damaged and, in severe cases, the supporting bone eroded.

SYMPTOMS
The affected tooth aches or throbs, and biting or chewing is often painful. The gum around the tooth is tender and may be red and swollen. An untreated abscess may eventually erode a sinus (a channel) through the jawbone to the gum surface, where it forms a gumboil (a swelling). If the gumboil bursts, pus is discharged into the mouth, and the pain usually lessens. As the abscess spreads through the surrounding tissues and bones, glands in the neck and face may become swollen and symptoms of infection, such as headache and fever, may develop.

TREATMENT
A periapical abscess may be drained by drilling through the crown of the tooth into the pulp cavity in order to allow the pus to escape, followed by *root-canal treatment* (filling of the pulp cavity with dental cement). In some cases, extraction of the tooth (see *extraction, dental*) is necessary. *Antibiotic drugs* are prescribed if the infection has spread.

A periodontal abscess can usually be treated by careful scraping away of the infected material by the dentist.

absence

In medical usage, a temporary loss or impairment of consciousness that occurs in some forms of *epilepsy*, typically generalized absence (petit mal) seizures in childhood.

absorption

The process by which fluids or other substances are taken up by body tissues. The term absorption is commonly applied to the uptake of nutrients (from digested food) into the blood and lymph from the digestive tract.

The major site of absorption is the small intestine, which is lined with millions of microscopic fingerlike projections known as villi (see *villus*). The villi greatly increase the surface area of the intestine, thereby increasing the rate of absorption.

abuse

Maltreatment of a person or misuse of a substance. (See also *child abuse*; *drug abuse*; *heroin abuse*; *sexual abuse*; *solvent abuse*; *substance abuse*.)

acamprosate

A drug used to help those who are dependent on alcohol (see *alcohol dependence*) maintain abstinence. Possible side effects include diarrhoea, nausea, and abdominal pain. Acamprosate is not generally advised for those with kidney or sever liver damage.

acanthoma

A noncancerous tumour composed of cells of the outer layer of skin. There are various types of acanthoma. They are most likely to occur on the face, where they develop in hair follicles, or on the legs. (See also *keratoacanthoma*.)

acanthosis nigricans

A rare, untreatable condition in which thickened dark patches of skin appear in the groin, armpits, neck, and other skin folds. Acanthosis nigricans may occur in young people as a genetic disorder or as the result of an endocrine disorder such as *Cushing's syndrome*. The condition also occurs in people with cancerous tumours of the lung and other organs.

Pseudoacanthosis nigricans is a much more common condition that is usually seen in dark-complexioned people who are overweight. In this form, the skin in fold areas is both thicker and darker than the surrounding skin, and excessive sweating usually occurs in affected areas. Pseudoacanthosis nigricans may improve with weight loss.

acarbose

A drug that is used in the treatment of type 2 *diabetes mellitus*. Acarbose acts on enzymes in the intestines, inhibiting the digestion of starch and therefore slowing the rise in *blood glucose* levels after a carbohydrate meal.

accessory nerve

The 11th *cranial nerve*. Unlike the other cranial nerves, most of the accessory nerve originates from the spinal cord.

The small part of the accessory nerve that originates from the brain supplies many muscles of the palate, pharynx (throat), and larynx (voicebox). If this part of the nerve is damaged, the result may be *dysphonia* (difficulty in speaking) and/or dysphagia (difficulty in swallowing).

The spinal part of the accessory nerve supplies large muscles in the neck and back, most notably the sternomastoid (which runs from the breastbone to the side of the skull) and trapezius (the large, triangular muscle of the upper back, shoulder, and neck). Damage to the spinal fibres of the accessory nerve paralyses these muscles.

THE MECHANISM OF **ACCOMMODATION**

In a normal, healthy eye, light reflected from a near object is brought into focus on the retina by a process called accommodation. Focusing is achieved by an automatic change in lens shape.

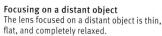

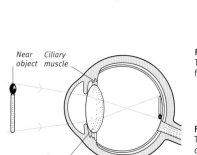

Focusing on a distant object
The lens focused on a distant object is thin, flat, and completely relaxed.

Focusing on a near object
To bring a near object into sharp focus, the ciliary muscles contract and the lens becomes more convex in shape.

accidental death

Death that occurs as a direct result of an accident. A high proportion of deaths in young adults, particularly among males, are accidental. Many of these deaths are as a result of road traffic accidents, drowning, or drug overdose; and alcohol is a significant contributory factor.

Falls in the home, and burning or asphyxiation as a result of fires, are common causes of accidental death in the elderly. Important causes of accidental death in infants are choking on food, smothering by bedclothes or other materials such as plastic bags, and *sudden infant death syndrome* (SIDS). Fatal accidents at work have become less common with the introduction of effective safety measures.

acclimatization

Physical and/or psychological adjustment to a different environment (for example, high altitude), climate, or situation. (See also *heat disorders*; *mountain sickness*.)

accommodation

Adjustment, especially the process by which the eye adjusts itself to focus on near objects. At rest, the eye is focused for distant vision, when its lens is thin and flat. To focus on a nearer object, the ciliary muscle of the eye contracts, which reduces the pull on the outer rim of the lens, allowing it to become thicker and more convex.

With increasing age, the lens gradually becomes less elastic. This makes accommodation increasingly difficult and results in a form of longsightedness called *presbyopia*.

accretion

A manner of growth involving the accumulation of additional material of the same type as that already present. The term accretion is used in dentistry to refer to the collection of foreign material, such as plaque (see *plaque, dental*), on the surface of a tooth or in a dental cavity.

acebutolol

A *beta-blocker drug* that is used to treat *hypertension* (high blood pressure), *angina pectoris* (chest pain caused by impaired blood supply to the heart muscle), and certain types of *arrhythmia* (abnormal heart rhythm) in which the heart beats too rapidly.

ACE inhibitor drugs

COMMON DRUGS

- Captopril • Cilazapril • Enalapril • Fosinopril
- Lisinopril • Moexipril • Perindopril
- Quinapril • Ramipril • Trandolapril

A group of drugs used to treat *heart failure* (reduced pumping efficiency of the heart), *hypertension* (high blood pressure), and kidney problems associated with *diabetes mellitus*. ACE (*angiotensin-converting enzyme*) inhibitors may be given alone or in combination with other *antihypertensive drugs*.

HOW THEY WORK
ACE inhibitors block the action of an *enzyme* responsible for converting *angiotensin* (a protein in blood) from inactive angiotensin I to angiotensin II. Angiotensin II encourages blood vessels to constrict; its absence permits them to dilate, thus reducing blood pressure. In diabetic nephropathy, ACE inhibitors slow the progress of the disorder and reduce the loss of *albumin* in the urine.

SIDE EFFECTS
Possible side effects include nausea, loss of taste, headache, dizziness, and a dry cough. The first dose may dramatically reduce blood pressure.

acellular

A term meaning "without cells" that is generally used to describe pertussis (whooping cough) *vaccines* that contain only certain parts, rather than the whole, of the pertussis bacteria cell.

acetabulum

A cuplike hollow in the pelvis into which the head of the femur (thigh bone) fits to form the *hip* joint.

acetaminophen

An *analgesic drug* that is more commonly known as *paracetamol*.

acetazolamide

A drug that is used in the treatment of *glaucoma* (raised pressure in the eyeball) and, occasionally, to prevent or treat symptoms of *mountain sickness*.

Possible side effects of acetazolamide include lethargy, nausea, diarrhoea, and reduced libido.

acetic acid

The colourless, pungent, organic acid that gives vinegar its sour taste. In medicine, acetic acid is an ingredient of preparations that are used to treat certain ear infections.

acetone

A chemical produced naturally when the body enters a state known as *ketosis*, in which fats are broken down to produce energy. This can occur as the result of metabolic changes caused by *diabetes mellitus* or, sometimes, as the result of extreme dieting.

Pharmaceutical preparations containing acetone are used as antiseptics and solvents. Acetone is also used in cosmetics such as nail varnish remover. (See also *solvent abuse*.)

acetylcholine

A type of *neurotransmitter* (a chemical that transmits messages between nerve cells or between nerve and muscle cells). Acetylcholine is the neurotransmitter found at all nerve-muscle junctions and at many other sites in the nervous system. The actions of acetylcholine are called cholinergic actions, and these can be blocked by *anticholinergic drugs*.

acetylcholinesterase inhibitors

COMMON DRUGS

- Donepezil • Rivastigmine

A group of drugs used in the treatment of mild to moderate *dementia* due to *Alzheimer's disease*, or occurring in *Parkinson's disease*. In Alzheimer's and parkinsonian dementia there is a deficiency of *acetylcholine* in the brain.

HOW THEY WORK
Acetylcholinesterase inhibitors work by blocking the action of acetylcholinesterase, an enzyme in the brain that breaks down acetylcholine. This raises acetylcholine levels, and, in up to half of all patients, the drugs slow the rate of progression of dementia. However, they have no effect on dementia due to other causes, such as stroke or head injury.

SIDE EFFECTS
Common side effects include nausea, dizziness, and headache. Rarely, difficulty in passing urine may occur.

acetylcysteine

A drug used in the treatment of *paracetamol* overdose. As eye-drops, it is also used as a *mucolytic* drug to treat deficiency of tear production. To be effective as an antidote to paracetamol poisoning, acetylcysteine must be given by injection within a few hours of the overdose. The drug reduces the amount of toxic substances produced during the breakdown of paracetamol, thereby reducing the risk

A

of liver damage. When acetylcysteine is taken in large doses, vomiting, rash, or breathing difficulties may occur as rare side effects.

achalasia

A rare condition, of unknown cause, in which the muscles at the lower end of the *oesophagus* and the sphincter (valve) between the oesophagus and the stomach fail to relax to allow food into the stomach after swallowing. As a result, the lowest part of the oesophagus is narrowed and becomes blocked with food, while the part above widens.

SYMPTOMS AND SIGNS

Symptoms include difficulty and pain in swallowing, and pain in the lower chest and upper abdomen. A foul taste in the mouth and bad breath may arise due to the regurgitation of food. The ability to swallow gradually deteriorates until the swallowing of liquids is also impeded.

DIAGNOSIS AND TREATMENT

A barium swallow (a type of *barium X-ray examination*) and *gastroscopy* (in which a narrow viewing tube is passed down the oesophagus) may be performed in order to investigate achalasia.

Drug treatment is rarely successful. It is possible to widen the oesophagus for prolonged periods by *oesophageal dilatation* (passing a rod or a *balloon catheter* down the oesophagus). Surgery to cut muscles at the stomach entrance may be needed to widen the passageway for food.

LOCATION OF THE ACHILLES TENDON

The tendon runs from the base of the calf to the calcaneus.

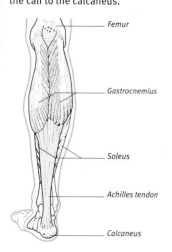

Femur

Gastrocnemius

Soleus

Achilles tendon

Calcaneus

ache

A continuous, fixed, and often dull pain that is distinct from twinges. (See also *bone pain*; *earache*; *headache*; *stomachache*; *toothache*.)

Achilles tendon

The tendon that raises the heel. The Achilles tendon is formed from the calf muscles (the gastrocnemius, soleus, and plantaris muscles) and is attached to the *calcaneus* (the heel bone). The Achilles tendon is named after Achilles, the legendary Greek hero who was vulnerable only in his heel.

Minor injuries to the Achilles tendon are common. They are usually provoked by too much exercise, faulty running technique, or the wearing of unsuitable footwear. All of these injuries can result in inflammation of the tendon (*tendinitis*) and tearing of the tendon fibres. In most cases, these conditions clear up with rest and physiotherapy.

Violent stretching of the Achilles tendon can cause it to rupture, producing pain, swelling, and impaired movement of the affected part. Surgical repair may be needed, but immobilization of the ankle in a plaster cast may be sufficient.

achlorhydria

Absence of stomach acid secretions. This may be due to chronic atrophic *gastritis* or to an absence or malfunction of acid-producing parietal cells in the stomach lining.

Achlorhydria may not produce symptoms and is not in itself a cause for concern. However, it is sometimes associated with *stomach cancer* and is also a feature of pernicious anaemia, a blood disorder caused by defective absorption of vitamin B_{12} from the stomach (see *anaemia, megaloblastic*).

achondroplasia

A rare genetic disorder of bone growth that leads to *short stature*. Individuals with achondroplasia have short limbs, a well-developed trunk, and a head of normal size, except for a protruding forehead.

The condition is caused by a defect of a dominant gene (see *genetic disorders*) but often arises as a new *mutation*, rather than being inherited from a parent. The long bones of the arms and legs are affected mainly. The cartilage that links each bone to its epiphysis (the growing area at its tip) is converted to bone too early, thereby preventing further limb growth.

Achondroplasia is usually obvious at birth or during the first year of life and no treatment is available to alter the outlook. Intelligence and sexual development are not affected, and lifespan is close to normal.

aciclovir

An *antiviral drug* that can be taken orally in tablet or liquid form, applied to the skin as a cream, taken as eye-drops, or given intravenously for viral infections including *herpes simplex* (cold sores), *herpes zoster* (shingles), and varicella zoster (*chickenpox*) in adults.

Aciclovir can be used as a life-saving treatment for *encephalitis* (inflammation of the brain). When it is used to treat *cold sores* or recurrent genital herpes, for which an ointment is available over the counter, aciclovir does not provide a cure but does reduce the severity of attacks.

Side effects of aciclovir are uncommon, but they can include nausea, vomiting, and fatigue. Local reactions commonly occur after topical use.

acid

A substance that is defined as a donor of hydrogen ions (hydrogen atoms with positive electrical charges). In water, acid molecules split up to release their constituent ions; all acids release hydrogen as the positive ion (positive ions are known as cations; and negative ions are called anions).

Examples of acids in the body include hydrochloric acid (a mineral acid produced by the stomach lining), and many organic acids, such as lactic acid, carbonic acid, ascorbic acid (vitamin C), and pyruvic acid. (See also *acid–base balance; alkali.*)

acid–base balance

A combination of mechanisms that ensures that the body's fluids are neither too *acid* nor too alkaline (*alkalis* are also called bases). The body functions normally only when its fluids are close to chemical neutrality.

Metabolic processes cause fluctuations in the acidity and alkalinity of the blood and other body fluids. The body has three mechanisms for maintaining the normal acid–base balance: buffers, breathing, and the activities of the kidneys. Buffers are substances in the blood that neutralize acid or alkaline wastes. Rapid breathing increases the rate at which carbon dioxide is eliminated from the blood, resulting in the blood becoming less acidic; slow breathing has the opposite effect. The kidneys help to maintain a constant acidity level in the blood by regulating the amounts of acid or alkaline wastes in the urine.

Disturbances of the body's acid–base balance result in either *acidosis* (excessive blood acidity) or *alkalosis* (excessive blood alkalinity).

acidosis

A disturbance of the body's *acid–base balance* in which there is an accumulation of acid or loss of *alkali* (base). There are two types of acidosis: metabolic and respiratory.

In metabolic acidosis, increased acid is produced by metabolic processes. One form of metabolic acidosis is ketoacidosis, which occurs in uncontrolled *diabetes mellitus* and starvation. Metabolic acidosis may also be caused by loss of bicarbonate (an alkali) due to severe diarrhoea. In *kidney failure*, insufficient acid is excreted in the urine.

Respiratory acidosis occurs when breathing fails to remove enough carbon dioxide from the lungs. Impaired breathing leading to respiratory acidosis may be caused by chronic obstructive pulmonary disease (see *pulmonary disease, chronic obstructive*), bronchial *asthma*, or *airway obstruction*.

acid reflux

Regurgitation of acidic fluid from the stomach into the *oesophagus*. The condition is now generally known as *gastro-oesophageal reflux disease*.

acitretin

A retinoid drug (see *vitamin A*) used to treat severe *psoriasis* and rare skin conditions such as *ichthyosis*. Possible side effects include headaches, skin problems such as blistering and *dermatitis*, and kidney damage. Acitretin should not be used during pregnancy because of the risk of damage to the fetus. Women should avoid becoming pregnant for at least a month before starting acitretin, while taking the drug, and for at least two years after stopping it

acne

A chronic skin disorder in which there is inflammation of the *sebaceous glands* at the base of hair follicles in the skin.
TYPES
The most common type of acne is sometimes known as acne vulgaris, which almost always develops during puberty, although it can occur at any age. Chemical acne is caused by exposure of the skin to certain chemicals and oils. This results in the development of acne in areas where the chemical has come into contact with the skin. Certain prescribed drugs, such as *corticosteroid drugs*, can also cause acne.
CAUSE
Acne spots are caused by the obstruction of hair follicles by excess sebum (the oily substance that is secreted by

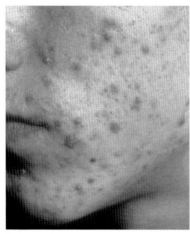

Acne
The spots on this boy's face are typical of acne; the darker marks are healed spots, which fade gradually. Severe acne may leave pits in the skin.

the sebaceous glands). Bacteria multiply in the follicle, causing inflammation. Hormonal changes at puberty, including increased levels of *androgen hormones* (male sex hormones) in both males and females, stimulate the production of sebum. There may also be a genetic predisposition to acne.
SYMPTOMS
Acne develops in areas in which there is a high concentration of sebaceous glands, mainly the face, centre of the chest, upper back, shoulders, and around the neck. Milia (whiteheads), comedones (blackheads), nodules (firm swellings under the skin), and cysts (larger, fluid-filled swellings) are the most common types of spot. Some, particularly cystic spots, leave scars after they heal, which may cause emotional distress.
TREATMENT AND OUTLOOK
There is no instant cure for acne, although washing the affected areas at least twice a day with a mild soap may help to keep it under control. Over-the-counter topical drug treatments such as benzoyl peroxide or azelaic acid are often effective. Prescribed topical *antibiotic drugs*, such as clindamycin, or retinoic acid (a derivative of *vitamin A*) may be used to treat moderate acne. An alternative treatment is with oral antibiotics, often *tetracycline drugs*. In very severe cases of acne, *isotretinoin* may be given under hospital supervision. In all cases, exposure to ultraviolet light (either natural or artificial) may also be beneficial. However, it is important not to burn the skin.

Acne improves slowly over time, and it often clears up by the end of the teenage years.

acoustic nerve

The part of the *vestibulocochlear nerve* (the eighth cranial nerve) concerned with hearing. The acoustic nerve is also called the auditory or cochlear nerve.

acoustic neuroma

A rare, noncancerous tumour arising from supporting cells that surround the *vestibulocochlear nerve*, usually within the internal auditory meatus (the canal in the skull through which the nerve passes from the inner ear to the brain).
CAUSE AND INCIDENCE
Acoustic neuromas most commonly occur in people between the ages of 40 and 60 and are slightly more common in women than in men.

Usually, the cause of an acoustic neuroma is unknown. However, tumours that affect the nerves on both sides of the head simultaneously may be part of a widespread *neurofibromatosis* (a disease characterized by changes in the nervous system, skin, and bones).
SYMPTOMS
An acoustic neuroma can cause *deafness*, *tinnitus* (noises in the ear), loss of balance, and pain in the face and the affected ear. As the tumour enlarges, it may lead to additional complications, such as *ataxia* (loss of coordination) due to the compression of the brainstem and cerebellum.
DIAGNOSIS AND TREATMENT
Diagnosis is made by *hearing tests* followed by an *MRI* (magnetic resonance imaging) scan.

If the tumour is small, regular monitoring with MRI may be all that is required. A large tumour may need to be removed by *microsurgery*, although *radiotherapy* to shrink the tumour may also be effective. Follow-up MRI scans are usually also performed to check for any recurrence of the tumour.

acquired

A term relating to a condition that occurs after birth rather than being attributable to heredity. Acquired contrasts with *congenital*, which means present from birth.

acquired immunity

A form of *immunity* that develops after birth through exposure to microorganisms or through *immunization*.

acrocyanosis

A circulatory disorder in which the hands and feet turn blue, may become cold, and sweat excessively. Acrocyanosis is caused by spasm of the small blood vessels and is often aggravated by cold weather.

Acrocyanosis is related to *Raynaud's disease*, in which the skin of the fingers and toes may be damaged by reduced blood flow.

acrodermatitis

Inflammation of the skin, principally on the hands or feet. *Acrodermatitis enteropathica* is a chronic (long-term), inherited variety of the condition.

acrodermatitis enteropathica

A rare, inherited disorder in which areas of the skin (most commonly of the fingers, toes, scalp, and the areas around the anus and mouth) are reddened, ulcerated, and covered with *pustules* (pus-filled spots).

Acrodermatitis enteropathica is inherited in an autosomal recessive manner (see *genetic disorders*) and is due to the inability to absorb sufficient zinc from food. Zinc supplements usually bring about a rapid improvement.

acromegaly

A rare disease that is characterized by abnormal enlargement of the skull, the jaw, the hands and feet, and also of the internal organs.

CAUSE

Acromegaly is caused by excessive secretion of *growth hormone* from the anterior *pituitary gland* at the base of the brain and is the result of a noncancerous *pituitary tumour*.

If such a tumour develops before puberty, the result is *gigantism* (in which growth is accelerated) instead of acromegaly. More commonly, however, the tumour develops after growth in the long bones of the limbs has stopped. This leads to acromegaly, although it

may take several years for the symptoms and signs of the condition to appear.

SYMPTOMS AND SIGNS

Symptoms and signs of acromegaly include enlargement of the hands, feet, ears, and nose; a jutting lower jaw; and a long face. There may also be deepening or huskiness of the voice. Symptoms common to any brain tumour, such as headache and visual disturbances, are also possible.

DIAGNOSIS AND TREATMENT

Acromegaly is diagnosed by the measurement of blood levels of growth hormone before and after a quantity of glucose has been administered. Glucose usually suppresses the secretion of growth hormone; if the glucose has no effect on the blood level of the hormone, uncontrolled secretion of growth hormone by the pituitary gland can be confirmed. *CT scanning* or *MRI* (techniques that produce cross-sectional or three-dimensional images of body structures) may be carried out to reveal a tumour or overgrowth of the pituitary gland.

A tumour of the pituitary gland may be removed surgically or treated by *radiotherapy*. The drug *octreotide* prevents growth hormone production and may be used to control symptoms by a person awaiting surgery or until the effects of radiotherapy are felt. *Bromocriptine* sometimes causes the tumour to become smaller.

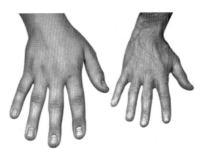

Appearance of acromegaly
Enlargement of the hands is a typical feature of acromegaly. The condition is apparent when the acromegalic hand, on the left, is compared to a normal hand.

acromioclavicular joint

The joint that lies between the outer end of the *clavicle* (collarbone) and the acromion (the bony prominence at the top of the shoulderblade).

INJURIES TO THE JOINT

Injuries to the acromioclavicular joint are rare. They are usually caused by a fall on to the shoulder and may result

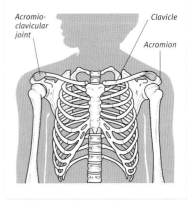

LOCATION OF THE ACROMIOCLAVICULAR JOINT

The joint lies at the junction of the outer end of the clavicle and the acromion.

Acromioclavicular joint

Clavicle

Acromion

in subluxation (incomplete dislocation with the bones still in contact) or, rarely, *dislocation* (complete displacement of the bones so that they are no longer in contact).

In subluxation, the synovium (joint lining) and the ligaments around it are stretched and bruised, the joint is swollen, and the bones feel slightly out of alignment. In dislocation, the ligaments are torn, the swelling is greater, and the bone deformity is more pronounced. In both cases, the joint is painful and tender, and movement of the shoulder is restricted.

TREATMENT

Treatment for subluxation is by resting the arm and shoulder in a sling. If the pain and tenderness persist, injection of a *corticosteroid drug* and a local anaesthetic (see *anaesthesia, local*) into the joint may help.

Dislocation of the acromioclavicular joint requires strapping around the clavicle and elbow, for about three weeks, to pull the outer end of the clavicle back into position. Surgical correction may occasionally be required.

acromion

The bony prominence at the top of the *scapula* (shoulderblade) that articulates with the end of the *clavicle* (collarbone) to form the *acromioclavicular joint*.

acroparaesthesia

A medical term for tingling sensations that occur in the fingers or toes (see *pins-and-needles*).

ACTH

The common abbreviation for adrenocorticotrophic hormone (also called corticotrophin). ACTH is produced by the anterior part of the *pituitary gland* (at the base of the brain) and stimulates the adrenal cortex (the outer layer of the *adrenal glands*, situated on the top of the kidneys) to release various *corticosteroid hormones*. ACTH is also necessary for the growth and maintenance of the cells of the adrenal cortex.

ACTIONS

The most important function of ACTH is to stimulate the adrenal cortex to increase its production of *hydrocortisone* (cortisol). ACTH also causes the adrenal cortex to release *aldosterone* and *androgen hormones*.

The production of ACTH is controlled by a feedback mechanism that involves both the *hypothalamus* (an area in the centre of the brain) and the level of hydrocortisone in the blood. When ACTH levels are high, the production of hydrocortisone increases, which in turn suppresses the release of ACTH from the pituitary gland. If ACTH levels are low, hydrocortisone production falls and the hypothalamus releases factors that stimulate the pituitary gland to increase production of ACTH.

ACTH levels increase in response to stress, emotion, injury, burns, infection, surgery, and decreased blood pressure. Cancerous tumours, particularly those of the lung, can sometimes produce a chemical that is similar to ACTH and which causes symptoms.

DISORDERS OF ACTH PRODUCTION

A tumour of the pituitary gland can cause excessive production of ACTH, which, in turn, leads to overproduction of hydrocortisone by the adrenal cortex, resulting in *Cushing's syndrome* (a hormonal disorder). Insufficient ACTH production results in decreased production of hydrocortisone, causing *hypotension* (low blood pressure).

MEDICAL USES

Synthetic ACTH was once given in the treatment of *arthritis* or to treat *allergy*, but it is now rarely used.

actin

A *protein* component of *muscle* fibres that, together with myosin (another protein), provides the mechanism for muscles to contract. The microscopic filaments of actin and myosin slide in between each other to make the muscle fibres shorter.

acting out

Impulsive actions that may reflect an individual's unconscious wishes. The term is most often used by psychotherapists to describe behaviour during analysis when the patient "acts out", rather than reports, his or her fantasies, wishes, or beliefs. Acting out can also occur as a reaction to frustrations encountered in everyday life, often taking the form of antisocial, aggressive behaviour that may be directed against oneself or others.

actinic

Relating to changes caused by the ultraviolet rays in sunlight, as in actinic *dermatitis* (inflammation of the skin) and actinic *keratosis* (roughness and thickening of the skin). Both are caused by overexposure to solar radiation.

actinomycosis

An infection caused by *ACTINOMYCES ISRAELII* or related actinomycete bacteria. These bacteria resemble fungi and cause diseases of the mouth, jaw, chest, and pelvis.

TYPES AND CAUSES

The most common form of actinomycosis affects the jaw area. A painful swelling appears and pus and characteristic yellow granules discharge through small openings that develop in the skin. Poor oral hygiene may contribute to this form of the infection.

Another form of actinomycosis affects the pelvis in women, causing lower abdominal pain and bleeding between menstrual periods. This form was associated mainly with a type of *IUD*, no longer in use, that did not contain copper. Rarely, forms of the disorder affect the appendix or lung.

Actinomycosis is usually treated successfully with *antibiotic drugs*.

acuity, visual

See *visual acuity*.

acupressure

A derivative of *acupuncture* in which pressure is applied instead of needles.

acupuncture

A branch of *Chinese medicine* in which needles are inserted into a patient's skin as therapy for various disorders, to relieve pain or to induce *anaesthesia*.

Traditional Chinese medicine maintains that the chi (life-force) flows through the body along channels known as meridians. A blockage in one or more of these meridians is thought to cause ill health. Acupuncturists aim to restore health by inserting needles at appropriate sites, known as acupuncture points, along the affected meridians.

HOW IT WORKS AND WHY IT IS DONE

Research suggests that acupuncture provokes the release within the central nervous system of *endorphins* (substances resembling morphine), which act as natural analgesics (painkillers).

The disorder that is being treated and degree of anaesthesia required determine the needle temperature, place of insertion, whether the needles are stimulated by rotation or electric current, and the length of time the needles remain in position.

Acupuncture may be used as an anaesthetic for surgical procedures as well as to provide pain relief following operations and for chronic conditions such as chronic back pain. Acupuncture is also claimed to help in the treatment of addiction, depression, and anxiety.

SIDE EFFECTS

After treatment with acupuncture, some people experience temporarily exacerbated symptoms. Other people may feel lightheaded, drowsy, or exhilarated for a short while.

It is important that acupuncture is performed by a fully qualified acupuncturist because the use of inadequately sterilized needles could result in the transmission of a variety of infections, including *hepatitis B* and *HIV*.

acute

A term often used to describe a disorder or symptom that develops suddenly. Acute conditions may or may not be severe, and they are usually of short duration. (See also *chronic*.)

acute heart failure

See *heart failure, acute*.

acyanotic

A diagnostic term meaning without *cyanosis*, a bluish coloration of the skin that is seen when blood *oxygen* levels are abnormally low. The term is commonly used in relation to the classification of congenital (present from birth) heart disease (see *heart disease, congenital*).

Adam's apple

The projection at the front of the neck, just beneath the skin, that is formed by a prominence on the thyroid

This projection at the front of the
neck, beneath the skin, is formed by
a prominence on the thyroid cartilage.

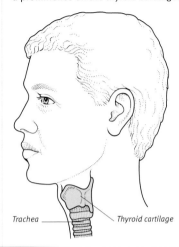

Trachea   Thyroid cartilage

cartilage, which is part of the *larynx*
(voicebox). The Adam's apple enlarges
in males at puberty.

ADD

The abbreviation for attention deficit
disorder, more commonly known as
attention deficit hyperactivity disorder.

addiction

Dependence on, and craving for, a particular drug, such as alcohol, diazepam
(a tranquillizer), or heroin. Reducing or
stopping intake of the drug may lead to
characteristic physiological and/or psychological symptoms (see *withdrawal
syndrome*), such as tremor or anxiety.
The term addiction may also be used in
relation to compulsive behaviour, such
as gambling. (See also *alcohol dependence*; *drug dependence*.)

Addison's disease

A rare chronic disorder in which there
is deficiency of the corticosteroid hormones *hydrocortisone* and *aldosterone*,
which are normally produced by the
adrenal cortex (the outer parts of the
adrenal glands, which are situated on
the top of the kidneys). In addition,
excessive amounts of the hormone *ACTH*
are secreted by the pituitary gland (at
the base of the brain) in an attempt to
increase output of the corticosteroid
hormones. The secretion and activity of

another hormone, melanocyte stimulating hormone (MSH), also increase,
which leads to increased synthesis of
melanin pigment in the skin.

CAUSES

Addison's disease can be caused by any
disease that destroys the adrenal cortices. The most common cause is an
autoimmune disorder in which the
immune system produces antibodies
that attack the adrenal glands.

SYMPTOMS

Symptoms of the disease generally
develop gradually over months or years
and include tiredness, weakness,
abdominal pain, and weight loss. Excess
MSH may cause darkening of the skin in
the creases of the palms, pressure areas
of the body, and the mouth.

Acute episodes, called Addisonian crises, brought on by infection, injury, or
other stresses, can also occur. The symptoms of these are mainly due to
aldosterone deficiency and include
extreme muscle weakness, dehydration,
hypotension (low blood pressure), confusion, and coma. *Hypoglycaemia* (low
blood glucose) also occurs due to a
deficiency of hydrocortisone.

DIAGNOSIS AND TREATMENT

Diagnosis of Addison's disease is generally made if the patient fails to respond
to an injection of ACTH, which normally stimulates hydrocortisone secretion.

Lifelong *corticosteroid drug* treatment
is needed to replace the deficient hormones. Treatment of Addisonian crises
involves rapid infusion of saline and
glucose and supplementary doses of
corticosteroid hormones.

additives

See *food additives*.

adduction

Movement of a limb towards the central
line of the body, or of a digit towards
the axis of a limb. Muscles that carry out
this movement are often called adductors. (See also *abduction*.)

adductor

Any one of the muscles that carry out
the movement of *adduction*.

adenitis

Inflammation of *lymph nodes*. Cervical
adenitis (swelling and tenderness of the
lymph nodes in the neck) occurs in certain bacterial infections, especially
tonsillitis, and the viral infection glandular fever (see *mononucleosis, infectious*).

Mesenteric lymphadenitis is inflammation
of the lymph nodes inside the abdomen
and is usually caused by a viral infection.

In many cases of adenitis, treatment
is not necessary. When it occurs as the
result of a bacterial infection, treatment
of the infection with *antibiotic drugs* will
generally also result in an improvement
in the condition of the lymph nodes.

adenocarcinoma

The technical name for a *cancer* of a
gland or glandular tissue, or for a cancer in which the cells form glandlike
structures. An adenocarcinoma arises
from epithelium (the layer of cells that
lines organs).

Cancers of the colon (see *colon, cancer
of*) breast (see *breast cancer*), pancreas,
and kidney are usually adenocarcinomas,
as are some cancers of the cervix,
oesophagus, salivary glands, and various
other organs. (See also *intestine, cancer
of*; *kidney cancer*; *pancreas, cancer of.*)

adenoidectomy

Surgical removal of the *adenoids*. An
adenoidectomy is usually performed on
a child with abnormally large adenoids
that are causing recurrent infections of
the middle ear or air sinuses. The operation may be performed together with
tonsillectomy.

There are few after-effects, and the
patient can generally begin to eat normally the following day.

These swellings of glandular tissue
are found at the back of the nasal
passage above the tonsils. Enlarged
adenoids are sometimes implicated
in sleep apnoea.

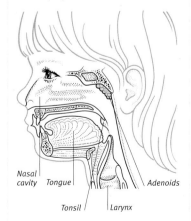

Nasal
cavity   Tongue   Adenoids

Tonsil   Larynx

adenoids

A mass of glandular tissue at the back of the nasal passage above the tonsils. The adenoids are made up of *lymph nodes*, which form part of the body's defences against upper respiratory tract infections. They tend to enlarge during early childhood, a time when such infections are common.

DISORDERS

In most children, the adenoids shrink after the age of about five years, and disappear altogether by puberty. In some children, however, they enlarge, obstructing the passage from the nose to the throat and causing snoring, breathing through the mouth, and a characteristically nasal voice. The eustachian tubes, which connect the middle ear to the throat, may also become blocked, resulting in recurrent middle ear infections and deafness.

Obstruction to the flow of secretions behind the nose can result in *rhinitis* (inflammation of the nose), which may spread to the middle ear (see *otitis media*) and to the air sinuses behind the nose (see *sinusitis*).

TREATMENT

Infections usually become less frequent as the child grows. If they do not, adenoidectomy (surgical removal of the adenoids) may be recommended.

adenoma

A noncancerous tumour or cyst that resembles glandular tissue and arises from the epithelium (the layer of cells that lines organs).

Adenomas of *endocrine glands* (such as the pituitary gland, thyroid gland adrenal glands, and pancreas) can result in excessive hormone production, leading to disease. For example, an adenoma of the pituitary gland can result in *acromegaly* or *Cushing's syndrome*.

adenomatosis

An abnormal condition of glands in which they are affected either by *hyperplasia* (overgrowth) or by numerous *adenomas* (noncancerous tumours).

Adenomatosis may simultaneously affect two or more different *endocrine glands*, such as the adrenal glands, pituitary gland, and pancreas.

adenosine diphosphate

See *ADP*.

adenosine triphosphate

See *ATP*.

ADH

The abbreviation for antidiuretic hormone (also called vasopressin), which is released from the posterior part of the *pituitary gland* and acts on the kidneys to increase their reabsorption of water into the blood.

ACTIONS

Water is continually being taken into the body in food and drink and is also produced by the chemical reactions in cells. Conversely, water is also continually being lost in urine, sweat, faeces, and in the breath as water vapour. ADH reduces the amount of water lost in the urine and helps to maintain the body's overall water balance.

ADH production is controlled by the *hypothalamus* (an area in the centre of the brain), which detects changes in blood concentration and volume. If the blood concentration increases (in other words, the blood contains less water), the hypothalamus stimulates the pituitary gland to release more ADH. If the blood is too dilute, less ADH is produced; as a result, more water is lost from the body in the urine.

DISORDERS OF ADH PRODUCTION

Various factors can affect ADH production and thus disturb the body's water balance. For example, alcohol reduces ADH production by direct action on the brain, resulting in a temporary increase in the production of urine. Urine production is also increased in the disorder *diabetes insipidus*, in which there is either insufficient production of ADH by the pituitary gland or, more rarely, failure of the kidneys to respond to the ADH produced.

The reverse effect, water retention, may result from temporarily increased ADH production after a major operation. Water retention may also be caused by the secretion of ADH by some tumours, especially of the lung.

MEDICAL USES

Synthetic ADH is used in the treatment of a variety of conditions, such as diabetes insipidus. Side effects of the drug may include abdominal cramps, nausea, headache, drowsiness, and confusion.

ADHD

The abbreviation for *attention deficit hyperactivity disorder*.

adhesion

The joining of normally unconnected parts of the body by bands of fibrous tissue. Adhesions are sometimes congenital (present from birth), but they most often develop as a result of scarring after inflammation.

Adhesions are most common in the abdomen, where they often form after *peritonitis* (inflammation of the abdominal lining) or surgery. Sometimes, loops of intestine are bound together by adhesions, causing intestinal obstruction (see *intestine, obstruction of*). In such cases, surgery is usually required to cut the bands of tissue.

adipose tissue

A layer of fat cells lying just beneath the surface of the skin and around various internal organs.

Adipose tissue is made up of fat stored within adipocytes (fat cells). Fat is deposited as a result of excess food intake, thus acting as an energy store; excessive amounts of fat stored within the adipose tissue is a feature of *obesity*. The tissue insulates against loss of body heat and helps to absorb shock in areas subject to sudden or frequent pressure, such as the buttocks, palms of the hands or soles of the feet. Another function of adipose tissue is to cushion organs such as the heart, kidneys, and eyeballs.

After puberty, the distribution of superficial adipose tissue differs in males and females. In men, superficial adipose tissue tends to accumulate around the shoulders, waist, and abdomen; in women, it occurs more commonly on the breasts, hips, and thighs. Adipose tissue tends to make up a larger proportion of the total body weight of women than of men. In obesity, central distribution of body fat around the waist is associated with a greater risk of *cardiovascular disease* and *diabetes*. This may be because fat in this area tends to result in raised blood lipid levels. (See also *brown fat*.)

adjuvant

A substance that enhances the action of another substance in the body. The term is used to describe an ingredient added to a *vaccine* to increase the production of antibodies by the immune system, thus enhancing the vaccine's effect. (See also *adjuvant therapy*.)

adjuvant therapy

Treatment for *cancer*, usually with anticancer drugs, that is given once all the evidence of the original tumour has been removed. The aim of adjuvant therapy is to destroy any microscopic deposits of malignant cells that may exist, which reduces the risk of recurrence of the cancer and increases survival times.

Adlerian theory

The psychoanalytical ideas set forth by the Austrian psychiatrist Alfred Adler (1870–1937). Also known as individual psychology, Adler's theories were based on the idea that everyone is born with natural feelings of inferiority. Life is seen as a constant struggle to overcome these feelings; and failure to do so leads to neurosis. (See also *psychoanalytic theory*.)

adnexa

An anatomical term meaning the structures that are adjacent to an organ. Most commonly, the word adnexa is used to refer to the various appendages of the *uterus*: the ovaries, fallopian tubes, and ligaments.

adolescence

The period between childhood and adulthood, which broadly corresponds to the teenage years. Adolescence is a complex stage of psychological development. It commences at and overlaps with, but is not the same as, *puberty*.

Common patterns of adolescent behaviour include moodiness, a general lack of interest, and fluctuating academic performance. Adolescents often worry about their changing body shape and physical appearance. They may lack self-confidence, feel nervous and shy and be unsure of their personal identity.

Adolescents experiment with their appearance, with views and opinions, with allegiances to peer groups, and with political movements or other role models. Gender identity and sexuality may be questioned. Adolescents may also experiment with drugs and alcohol; those who do so to relieve anxiety or depression are more likely to become dependent than those who experiment due to peer-group pressure. Sexual activity is common during adolescence and may result in unwanted pregnancies and *sexually transmitted infections*.

Some adolescents are assertive and strive for independence. Rebellion against parents is common but conflicts with the emotional and financial support that adolescents still require. Aggression and delinquency usually constitute a transient phase. However, a teenager who remains too dependent may not develop sufficiently to make his or her own decisions or to form new relationships outside the family.

Most behavioural problems resolve themselves over time. Maintaining open lines of communication between parents and children is important in easing this process. The most valuable support parents can offer is to encourage self-confidence and responsibility and thus prepare their children for adult life. Parents should also ensure that their children are informed about issues such as *contraception* and safer sex.

ADP

The abbreviation for adenosine diphosphate, the chemical that takes up energy released during biochemical reactions to form *ATP* (adenosine triphosphate), the body's main energy-carrying chemical. When ATP releases its energy ADP is re-formed. (See also *metabolism*.)

adrenal failure

Insufficient production of hormones by the adrenal cortex (the outer part of the *adrenal glands*, situated on the top of the kidneys). Adrenal failure can be acute (of sudden onset) or chronic (of gradual onset). The condition may be caused by a disorder of the adrenal glands, in which case it is called *Addison's disease*, or by reduced stimulation of the adrenal cortex by *ACTH*, a hormone produced by the *pituitary gland*. (See also *adrenal glands* disorders box, p.20.)

adrenal glands

A pair of small, triangular *endocrine glands* (glands that secrete hormones directly into the bloodstream) that are located on the top of the kidneys. Each adrenal gland has two distinct parts: the outer adrenal cortex and the smaller, inner adrenal medulla.

ADRENAL CORTEX

The adrenal cortex secretes *aldosterone*, which, by inhibiting the amount of sodium excreted in the urine, helps to maintain blood volume and blood pressure. The cortex also secretes *hydrocortisone* and corticosterone, as well as small amounts of *androgen hormones*. Hydrocortisone controls the body's use of fats, proteins, and carbohydrates and is also important in helping the body to cope with stress. Hydrocortisone and corticosterone also suppress inflammatory reactions and some activities of the immune system.

Hormone production by the adrenal cortex is governed by other hormones, such as *ACTH*, that are produced in the *hypothalamus*, in the centre of the brain, and the *pituitary gland* beneath it (see *feedback mechanism* box).

ADRENAL MEDULLA

The adrenal medulla is part of the sympathetic division of the *autonomic nervous system*, which is the body's first line of defence against physical and emotional stress. The medulla secretes the hormones *adrenaline* (epinephrine) and *noradrenaline* (norepinephrine) in

---

ANATOMY OF THE **ADRENAL GLANDS**

Also sometimes called the suprarenal glands, the adrenal glands are situated on top of the kidneys. Each gland is divided into two regions: the adrenal cortex (which secretes hormones that affect the metabolism) and the adrenal medulla (which is part of the sympathetic nervous system).

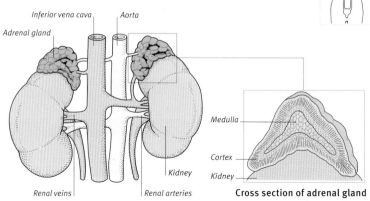

Inferior vena cava · Aorta
Adrenal gland
Renal veins · Renal arteries · Kidney
Medulla · Cortex · Kidney

Cross section of adrenal gland

FEEDBACK MECHANISM

The rate at which many glands produce hormones is influenced by other hormones, especially those secreted by the pituitary gland and the hypothalamus. If the amount of hormone produced is increased, negative feedback mechanisms act on the hypothalamus and pituitary so that they produce less of their stimulating hormones, thus reducing the target gland's activity. If the amount of hormone produced is decreased, the feedback weakens, causing increased production of stimulating hormones.

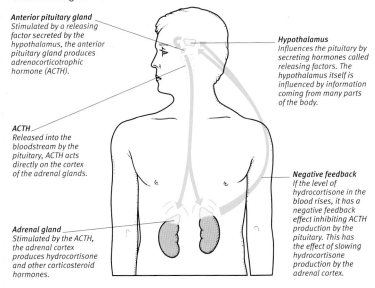

Anterior pituitary gland
Stimulated by a releasing factor secreted by the hypothalamus, the anterior pituitary gland produces adrenocorticotrophic hormone (ACTH).

ACTH
Released into the bloodstream by the pituitary, ACTH acts directly on the cortex of the adrenal glands.

Adrenal gland
Stimulated by the ACTH, the adrenal cortex produces hydrocortisone and other corticosteroid hormones.

Hypothalamus
Influences the pituitary by secreting hormones called releasing factors. The hypothalamus itself is influenced by information coming from many parts of the body.

Negative feedback
If the level of hydrocortisone in the blood rises, it has a negative feedback effect inhibiting ACTH production by the pituitary. This has the effect of slowing hydrocortisone production by the adrenal cortex.

response to stimulation by sympathetic nerves. These nerves are most active during times of stress.

The release of these hormones into the circulation produces effects similar to sympathetic nerve stimulation. The heart rate and force of contraction of the heart muscle increase so that more blood is pumped around the body and the airways are widened to ease breathing. The hormones constrict blood vessels in the intestines, kidneys, and liver, and widen blood vessels supplying the skeletal muscles. Consequently, more blood is supplied to the active muscles and less to the internal organs.

adrenal hyperplasia, congenital

A rare *genetic disorder*, present from birth, in which an *enzyme* (a protein that acts as a catalyst) defect blocks the production of corticosteroid hormones (*hydrocortisone* and *aldosterone*) from the adrenal glands.

SYMPTOMS

The enzyme block results in production of excessive amounts of *androgens* (male sex hormones), which can cause abnormal genital development in an affected fetus. In females, these androgens cause enlargement of the clitoris and some fusion of the outer lips of the vulva, resulting in genital ambiguity (see *sex determination*). Some affected males have an enlarged penis, which may either be evident at birth or may develop later.

Other effects of the enzyme defect include *hypotension* (low blood pressure), *hypoglycaemia* (low blood sugar levels), weight loss, and dehydration. *Hyperplasia* (enlargement) of the adrenal gland occurs due to excessive secretion of the hormone *ACTH*, which is a result of insufficient production of hydrocortisone. Excessive skin pigmentation may occur in skin creases and around the nipples.

In severe cases, congenital adrenal hyperplasia is apparent soon after birth. In milder cases, symptoms appear later, sometimes producing premature puberty in boys and delayed menstruation, *hirsutism* (excessive hairiness), and potential infertility in girls.

DIAGNOSIS AND TREATMENT

A diagnosis is confirmed by measuring corticosteroid hormones in the blood and urine. *Ultrasound scanning* may be carried out to verify that there is no tumour of the adrenal glands.

Treatment of congenital adrenal hyperplasia is with hormone replacement. If the treatment is started early, normal sexual development and fertility generally follow.

adrenaline

Also called epinephrine, a hormone released by the adrenal glands in response to signals from the sympathetic nervous system, part of the *autonomic nervous system*. These signals are triggered by stress, exercise, or emotions such as fear.

Adrenaline increases the speed and force of the heartbeat. It widens the airways to improve breathing and narrows blood vessels in the skin and intestine so that an increased flow of blood reaches the muscles.

Synthetic adrenaline is sometimes given by injection as emergency treatment of *anaphylactic shock* (a severe allergic reaction) and *cardiac arrest* (a halt in the heart's pumping action). Eye-drops containing dipivefrine (a drug that passes quickly into the tissues and converts to adrenaline), may be used to treat acute (closed-angle) *glaucoma*. Regular use can cause a burning pain and, occasionally, blurred vision or pigment deposits on the eye surface. (See also *noradrenaline*.)

adrenal tumours

Rare cancerous or noncancerous tumours in the *adrenal glands*, usually causing excess secretion of hormones.

Tumours of the adrenal cortex may secrete *aldosterone*, causing primary *aldosteronism* (also called Conn's syndrome), or hydrocortisone, causing *Cushing's syndrome*.

Tumours of the adrenal medulla may cause excessive secretion of *adrenaline* (epinephrine) and *noradrenaline* (norepinephrine). Two types of tumour affect the medulla: *phaeochromocytoma* and *neuroblastoma*, which affects children. These tumours may cause intermittent *hypertension* (high blood pressure) and sweating attacks.

Surgical removal of a tumour or an adrenal gland usually cures noncancerous tumours. Cancerous tumours may require additional treatment with *radiotherapy* and/or *chemotherapy*. (See also *adrenal glands* disorders box, overleaf.)

adrenocorticotrophic hormone

See *ACTH*.

A

DISORDERS OF THE **ADRENAL GLANDS**

Adrenal gland disorders are a range of uncommon but sometimes serious conditions that result from deficient or excessive production of hormones by one or both of the adrenal glands.

Congenital defects

A genetic defect causes congenital *adrenal hyperplasia*, in which the adrenal cortex is unable to make sufficient hydrocortisone and *aldosterone*. As a side effect of the reduced hydrocortisone production, the glands are stimulated into producing excess androgens (male sex hormones); this can cause masculinization of female babies.

Autoimmune disorders

Deficient production of hormones by the adrenal cortex is called *adrenal failure*; if the deficiency is due to disease of the adrenal glands themselves, it is called *Addison's disease*. The most common cause of Addison's disease is an autoimmune process (in which the body's immune system attacks its own tissues). Addison's disease can take a chronic course characterized by weakness, weight loss, and skin darkening, or an acute form (Addisonian crisis or acute adrenal failure), in which the patient may become confused and comatose.

Infection

Destruction of the adrenal glands by *tuberculosis* was once a major cause of Addison's disease but is now uncommon. The onset of an infection or other acute illness in someone with Addison's disease can precipitate acute adrenal failure.

Impaired blood supply

Loss or obstruction of the blood supply to the adrenal glands, sometimes as a result of arterial disease, is another possible cause of Addison's disease or acute adrenal failure.

Tumours

Cancerous or noncancerous growths in the adrenal glands are rare but generally lead to excess secretion of hormones. A tumour of the adrenal cortex can secrete aldosterone, causing primary *aldosteronism* (also called Conn's syndrome), a condition that is characterized by thirst and high blood pressure. A tumour can also secrete hydrocortisone, causing *Cushing's syndrome*, which has various features including muscle wasting and obesity of the trunk. Androgens may also be produced in excess, causing masculinization in females.

Two types of tumour affect the adrenal medulla, *phaeochromocytoma* and *neuroblastoma*, which affects children. These tumours may cause excess secretion of adrenaline (epinephrine) and noradrenaline (norepinephrine).

Other disorders

In many cases, disturbed activity of the adrenals is caused, not by disease of the glands themselves, but by an increase or decrease in the blood level of hormones that influence the activity of the glands.

Hydrocortisone production by the adrenal cortex is controlled by the secretion of ACTH (adrenocorticotrophic hormone) by the pituitary gland.

A tumour or other pituitary gland disorder, or tumours in the lung, breast, and elsewhere, can cause excess ACTH secretion, leading to excess production of hydrocortisone by the adrenals and, hence, to Cushing's syndrome. Pituitary disease is a cause of Cushing's syndrome.

INVESTIGATION

Blood and/or urine tests can detect the high levels of adrenal hormones that occur with adrenal tumours. They can also detect the high levels of natural corticosteroids that occur in Cushing's syndrome, and the low levels that occur in congenital adrenal hyperplasia. Blood tests are used to measure salt and potassium levels if Addison's disease is suspected; further blood tests may be carried out to measure corticosteroid hormone levels. Diagnosis of Addison's disease can be confirmed by the response to an injection of ACTH, which, under normal circumstances, will stimulate the adrenal glands. MRI or CT scanning can detect abnormalities of the adrenal glands and can confirm the presence of an adrenal tumour. They can also distinguish between raised hormone levels due to an adrenal tumour, or those due to a pituitary tumour. Ultrasound scanning can rule out an adrenal tumour as the cause of congenital adrenal hyperplasia.

adrenogenital syndrome

See *adrenal hyperplasia, congenital*.

advanced life support

Treatment of *cardiac arrest* (a halt in the heart's pumping action) by medical or paramedical professionals when *basic life support*, (which may be performed by a first-aider) has failed to restore a normal heartbeat and spontaneous breathing. Advanced life support involves the use of drugs and medical equipment.

An *ECG* monitor is used to record the electrical activity of the heart muscle. *Ventilation* delivers oxygen by way of an *endotracheal tube* inserted, via the mouth, into the trachea (windpipe). A *cannula* (a thin plastic tube inserted into a vein) allows administration of drugs such as *adrenaline* (epinephrine). In the event of *ventricular fibrillation* (rapid uncoordinated contractions of the heart), *defibrillation* (a brief electric shock to the heart using two paddles placed on the chest) may be used.

adverse reaction

See *side effect*.

Aedes

A genus of disease-transmitting mosquitoes. Many species of AEDES are responsible for spreading important viral infections; AEDES AEGYPTI is the main vector of *dengue* and *yellow fever*. (See also *mosquito bites*.)

aerobic

A term that refers to anything that requires oxygen to live, function, and grow. Humans and many other forms of life are dependent on oxygen for "burning" foods in order to produce energy (see *metabolism*). Because of this dependence, they are described as obligate aerobes.

In contrast, many bacteria have fundamentally different metabolisms and thrive without oxygen (some are even killed by exposure to oxygen); such microorganisms are described as *anaerobic*. There are also certain bacteria and yeasts, known as facultative aerobes, that flourish in oxygen but can also live without it. (See also *aerobics*.)

aerobics

Exercises, such as swimming, jogging, and cycling, that allow muscles to work at a steady rate with a constant, adequate supply of oxygen-carrying blood that allows them to be sustained for long periods. Oxygen is needed to release energy from the body's stores. To fuel aerobic exercise, the muscles use fatty acid, burning it completely to produce energy, carbon dioxide, and water.

Anaerobic exercise relies on a different series of biochemical reactions to obtain energy from the muscles' stores of fat and sugar. The waste products of anaerobic exercise are acidic and, as they accumulate in muscles, cause muscle fatigue; high-intensity exercises, which are anaerobic, can be performed only for relatively short periods.

BENEFITS OF AEROBIC EXERCISE

When performed regularly, aerobic exercise improves stamina and endurance. It encourages the growth of capillaries (small blood vessels), thereby improving blood supply to the cells. It improves the body cells' capacity to use oxygen and increases the amount of oxygen that the body can use in a given time.

As the body becomes fitter, the condition of the heart also improves: the heart rate becomes slower, both at rest and during exercise; the heart muscle becomes thicker and stronger; and the amount of blood pumped with each beat (the stroke volume) increases. The overall result is that the heart needs to do less work to achieve the same level of efficiency in pumping blood around the body. (See also *exercise*; *fitness*.)

aerodontalgia

Sudden pain in a tooth brought on by a change in surrounding air pressure. Flying at high altitudes in lowered atmospheric pressure can cause a pocket of air in the dental pulp to expand and irritate the nerve in the root. Aerodontalgia is more likely with improperly fitted fillings or poorly filled root canals.

aerophagy

Excessive swallowing of air, which may occur during rapid eating or drinking or may be caused by anxiety. After *laryngectomy* (surgical removal of the larynx), voluntary aerophagy is used to produce oesophageal speech.

aerosol

A suspension of minute liquid or solid particles in the air, producing a fine mist. Some drugs are prescribed in this form for use in an *inhaler* or in a *vaporizer*. (See also *solvent abuse*.)

aetiology

The cause of, or the study of the various factors involved in causing, a disease.

For some cases of a particular disorder, a specific aetiology can be identified. For example, laboratory studies may show that an attack of diarrhoea is the result of a particular type of virus or bacterium. Other disorders have a multifactorial aetiology: the causative factors of degenerative arthritis, for example, include genetic susceptibility, repeated joint injuries, and excess weight. On the other hand, many disorders, such as schizophrenia, are of unknown aetiology.

afebrile

A medical term meaning without *fever*. (See also *febrile*.)

affect

A term used to describe a person's mood. The two extremes of affect are elation and depression. A person who has extreme moods or changes in moods may have an *affective disorder*. Shallow or reduced affect (in which responses to events seem flat) may be a sign of *schizophrenia* or of an organic *brain syndrome*.

affective disorders

Mental illnesses that are characterized predominantly by marked changes in *affect* (mood). Mood may vary over a period of time between *mania* (extreme elation) and severe *depression*. (See also *bipolar disorder*.)

afferent

A term meaning carrying towards. Afferent is used mainly to describe blood vessels that supply organs, or nerves that carry impulses from peripheral sense *receptors* to the brain and spinal cord.

affinity

A term used to describe the attraction between chemicals that causes them to bind together, as, for example, between an antigen and an antibody (see *immune response*). In microbiology, affinity describes the physical similarity between organisms (viruses, for example). In psychology, the term refers to attraction between two people.

aflatoxin

A poisonous substance produced by *ASPERGILLUS FLAVUS* moulds, which contaminate stored foods, especially peanuts, grains, and cassava. Aflatoxin is believed to be one of the factors responsible for the high incidence of *liver cancer* in tropical Africa.

afterbirth

The common name for the tissues that are expelled from the uterus following the delivery of a baby (see *childbirth*). The afterbirth consists of the *placenta* and the membranes that surrounded the fetus.

aftercare

The medical care of a patient following treatment, particularly after *surgery*.

afterpains

Contractions of the uterus that continue after *childbirth*. Afterpains are normal, indicating that the uterus is shrinking as it should, and are experienced by many women, especially during breast-feeding. Afterpains usually disappear a few days after the birth, but *analgesic drugs* (painkillers) may be needed.

agammaglobulinaemia

A type of *immunodeficiency disorder* in which there is an almost complete absence of *B-lymphocytes* (a type of white blood cell) and *immunoglobulins* (also known as antibodies, proteins that play a key role in the body's immune response) in the blood.

agar

An extract of certain seaweeds that has similar properties to gelatine. Agar is also used as a gelling agent in media for growing bacterial *cultures*.

age

A person's age is usually measured chronologically but can also be measured in terms of physical, mental, or developmental maturity. Age may be of medical significance in diagnosis and in deciding treatment.

PHYSICAL AGE

The age of a fetus is known as gestational age, which can be calculated from the date of the mother's last menstrual period. Alternatively, it can be assessed by *ultrasound scanning*, which is more accurate. The estimation of gestational age is important in neonatal paediatrics for identification of babies who are too small and who may subsequently have problems as a result of their low birthweight.

In children, bone age (the degree of bone maturity as seen on an *X-ray*) can be a useful measure of physical development because all healthy individuals reach the same adult level of skeletal maturity and each bone passes through the same sequence of growth. Assessment of bone age is useful in the investigation of delayed *puberty* or *short stature* in children. A prediction of the final adult height can be made if the chronological age, bone age, and current height are known.

Dental age, which is another measure of physical maturity, can be assessed by the number of teeth that have erupted (see *eruption of teeth*) or by the amount of dental calcification (see *calcification, dental*), as seen on an X-ray, compared with standard values.

In adults, physical age is difficult to assess other than by physical appearance. It can be estimated after death by the state of certain organs, particularly by the amount of atheroma (fatty deposits) lining the arteries.

MENTAL AND DEVELOPMENTAL AGE

Mental age can be assessed by the comparison of scores achieved in *intelligence tests* with standard scores for different chronological ages.

A young child's age can be expressed in terms of his or her level of developmental skills, manual dexterity, social skills, and language when compared to those of other children. Patterns of development in these fields have been described for children up to the age of five. (See also *child development*.)

agenesis

The complete absence, at birth, of an organ or a component of the body. Agenesis is caused by developmental failure in the embryo.

agent

Any substance or force capable of bringing about a biological, chemical, or physical change. (See also *reagent*.)

Agent Orange

A herbicide and defoliant of which the major constituent (50 per cent by volume) is the phenoxy acid herbicide 2,4,5 T. The highly toxic contaminant TCDD, commonly known as dioxin, may be added to this substance during manufacture (see *defoliant poisoning*).

age spots

Blemishes that appear on the skin with increasing age. The most common type are brown or yellow slightly raised spots called seborrhoeic *keratoses*, which can occur at any site. Also common in elderly people are freckles, solar keratoses (small scaly patches, often appearing on the backs of the hands, that are a result of overexposure to the sun), and *De Morgan's spots*, which are red, pinpoint blemishes on the trunk.

THE PRACTICAL EFFECTS OF **AGING**

In the body, aging is associated with loss of elasticity in the skin, blood vessels, and tendons. There is also progressive decline in the functioning of organs such as the lungs, kidneys, and liver. Mechanical wear and tear causes cumulative damage to certain organ systems. Brain cells, specialized kidney units, and many other body structures are never replaced after they have reached maturity.

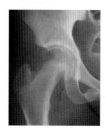

Hip joint in a young person
The X-ray shows the rounded head of the thigh-bone (femur) separated by cartilage from the surrounding hip socket.

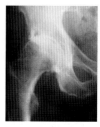

Hip joint in an elderly person
This X-ray of an osteoarthritic hip shows almost complete degeneration and disappearance of the cartilage in the joint.

EFFECTS OF AGING

Organ or tissue	Natural effects	Accelerated by
Skin	Loss of elastic tissue causes skin to sag and wrinkle. Weakened blood capillaries cause skin to bruise more easily.	Exposure to sun; smoking.
Brain and nervous system	Loss of nerve cells leads to reduction in ability to memorize or to learn new skills. Reaction time of nerves increases, making responses slower.	Excessive consumption of alcohol and other drugs; repeated head trauma (for example from boxing).
Senses	Some loss of acuity in all senses, mainly due to loss of nerve cells.	Loud noise (hearing); smoking (smell/taste).
Lungs	Loss of elasticity with age, so that breathing is less efficient.	Air pollution; smoking; lack of exercise.
Heart	Becomes less efficient at pumping, causing reduced tolerance to exercise.	Excessive use of alcohol and cigarettes; a fatty diet.
Circulation	Arteries harden, causing poor blood circulation and higher blood pressure.	Lack of exercise; smoking; poor diet.
Joints	Pressure on intervertebral discs causes height loss; wear on hip and knee joints reduces mobility.	Athletic injuries; being overweight.
Muscles	Loss of muscle bulk and strength.	Lack of exercise; starvation.
Liver	Becomes less efficient in processing toxic substances in the blood.	Damage from alcohol consumption and virus infections.

Treatment is usually unnecessary for any of these age spots, apart from solar keratoses, which may eventually progress to a form of skin cancer. Freezing the keratoses with liquid nitrogen or applying a cream containing a *cytotoxic drug* is the usual treatment. They may also be removed surgically under a local anaesthetic (see *anaesthesia, local*).

ageusia

The lack of, or an impairment of, the sense of taste (see *taste, loss of*).

agglutination

See *clumping*.

aggregation, platelet

The clumping together of platelets (small, sticky blood particles). Aggregation takes place when a blood vessel is damaged. It is the first stage of *blood clotting*, helping to plug injured vessels.

Inappropriate aggregation can have adverse effects; if it occurs in an artery, for example, *thrombosis* (a blood clot forming in an undamaged blood vessel) may result. Many drugs, including *aspirin* and *clopidogrel*, help to reduce platelet aggregation.

aggression

A general term for a wide variety of acts of hostility. A number of factors, including human evolutionary survival strategies, are thought to be involved.

CAUSES
Androgen hormones (male sex hormones) seem to promote aggression, whereas *oestrogen hormones* (the female sex hormones) may suppress it. Age is another factor; aggression is more common in teenagers and young adults, and some people believe that it can result from frustration or lack of affection as a child. Sometimes a brain tumour or head injury may lead to aggression.

Psychiatric conditions associated with aggressive outbursts are *schizophrenia*, *antisocial personality disorder*, *mania*, and abuse of alcohol or amphetamine drugs. *Temporal lobe epilepsy*, *hypoglycaemia*, and *confusion* due to physical illnesses are other, less common, medical causes.

aging

Aging is the physical and mental changes that occur with the passing of time and is associated with degenerative changes in various organs and tissues, such as loss of elasticity in the skin and a progressive decline in organ function.

Wear and tear causes cumulative damage to the joints, and the muscles lose bulk and strength. Wound healing and resistance to infection also decline. Gradual loss of nerve cells can lead to reduced sensory acuity and difficulties with learning and memory. However, *dementia* occurs in only a minority of elderly people.

Heredity is an important determinant of life expectancy, but physical degeneration may be accelerated by factors such as smoking, excessive alcohol intake, poor diet, and insufficient exercise. With advances in medical science, life expectancy in the developed world has risen dramatically over the last century.

agitation

Restlessness and the inability to keep still, usually as a result of anxiety or tension. People who are agitated engage in aimless, repetitive behaviour, such as pacing up and down or wringing their hands, and they often start tasks and fail to complete them.

Persistent agitation is seen in *anxiety disorders*, especially if there is an underlying physical cause such as alcohol withdrawal. *Depression* may also be accompanied by agitation.

agnathia

A developmental defect in the fetus in which the lower jaw is only partially formed or may be entirely absent. (See also *birth defects*.)

agnosia

The inability to recognize objects, despite adequate sensory information about them reaching the brain via the eyes or ears or through touch. In order for an object to be recognized, the sensory information it provides must be interpreted, which involves the recall of memorized information about similar objects. Agnosia is caused by damage to areas of the brain involved in interpretative and recall functions. The most common causes of this kind of damage are *stroke* or *head injury*.

TYPES
Agnosia is usually associated with just one of the senses of vision, hearing, or touch and is described as visual, auditory, or tactile respectively. For example, an object may be completely recognizable by hearing and touch, but it cannot be recognized by sight, despite the sense of vision being perfectly normal (an example of visual agnosia).

Some people, after suffering a stroke that damages the right cerebral hemisphere, seem unaware of any disability in the affected left limbs. This is called anosognosia or sensory inattention.

OUTLOOK
There is no specific treatment for agnosia, but some of the lost interpretative ability may eventually return.

agonist

A term that means to have a stimulating effect. In pharmacology, an agonist drug, which is sometimes known as an activator, is a drug that binds to a specific area on the surface of a cell (a *receptor*) and triggers or increases a particular activity in that cell.

agoraphobia

Fear of going into open spaces or public places. Agoraphobia may sometimes overlap with *claustrophobia* (a fear of enclosed spaces). Agoraphobic individuals who do venture out may have a *panic attack*, further restricting their activities, and may eventually be housebound. Treatment with *behaviour therapy* is often successful; *antidepressant drugs* may also help.

agranulocytosis

A potentially life-threatening disorder in which there is a severe acute lack of neutrophils (white blood cells that seek and destroy infective microorganisms). This deficiency seriously weakens the body's defences against infection.

In agranulocytosis, the bone marrow fails to produce adequate neutrophils. This may occur as an adverse effect of a drug such as *carbimazole* (used to treat thyroid diseases) or as an effect of *chemotherapy*. Fever and mouth ulcers are common symptoms.

Treatment involves stopping the causative drug. *Antibiotic drugs* may be used to treat any specific infection, and a drug to stimulate production of neutrophils in the bone marrow may also be given.

agraphia

Loss of or impaired ability to write, despite normal functioning of the hand and arm muscles. It can result from damage to parts of the *cerebrum* (main mass of the brain) concerned with writing.

CAUSES
Writing depends on a complex sequence of mental processes, including the selection of words and recall from memory of how words are spelled, formulation

and execution of the required hand movements, and visual checking that written words match their representation in the brain. These processes may take place in a number of connected regions of the brain. Agraphia may be caused by damage to any of these regions (commonly as a result of a *head injury*, *stroke*, or *brain tumour*) and can therefore be of different types and degrees of severity.

Agraphia is often accompanied by *alexia* (loss of reading ability) or may be part of an expressive *aphasia* (a general disturbance in expression of language).

OUTLOOK
There is no specific treatment for agraphia, but some of the lost writing skills may return in time.

AIDS

The abbreviation for acquired immune deficiency syndrome, a deficiency of the *immune system* due to infection with the human immunodeficiency virus (see *HIV*). The interval between infection and the development of AIDS is highly variable. Without treatment, around half of those individuals infected will develop AIDS within eight to nine years. In about one in ten cases, however, progression to AIDS is very slow, taking up to 20 years or longer. Illness and death from AIDS is a major health problem worldwide, and there is, as yet, no cure or vaccine.

METHODS OF TRANSMISSION
HIV is transmitted in body fluids such as semen, blood, vaginal secretions, and breast milk. Major methods of transmission are sexual contact (vaginal, anal, or oral), blood-to-blood (via transfusions, or needle-sharing in drug users), and mother-to-fetus. HIV has also been transmitted through blood products given to treat *haemophilia*, kidney transplants, and artificial insemination by donated semen; but improved screening has greatly reduced these risks. HIV is not spread by everyday contact, such as hugging or sharing crockery.

EFFECTS OF THE VIRUS
The virus enters the bloodstream and infects cells with a particular receptor, called the CD4 receptor, on their surface. These cells include a type of white blood cell called a CD4 lymphocyte (a T-lymphocyte with a CD4 receptor), that is responsible for fighting infection, and cells in other tissues such as the brain. The virus reproduces within the infected cells, which then die, releasing more virus particles into the blood. If the infection is left untreated, the number of CD4 lymphocytes falls, resulting in greater susceptibility to certain infections and some types of cancer.

SYMPTOMS AND SIGNS
Some people experience a short-lived illness similar to infectious *mononucleosis* when they are first infected with HIV. Many individuals have no obvious symptoms but are, nevertheless, infectious. After the initial illness, many people remain well. Some may suffer from enlarged lymph nodes, muscle pain, and excessive sweating. Severe bacterial infections, such as pneumonia, are common. Later, vague complaints, such as weight loss, fevers, sweats, or unexplained diarrhoea (known as AIDS-related complex) may herald the development of AIDS.

Other features of infection with HIV include skin disorders such as seborrhoeic *dermatitis*, and a variety of viral, fungal and bacterial infections, such as persistent *herpes simplex* infections, oral *candidiasis* (thrush), *tuberculosis*, and *shigellosis*. HIV may also affect the brain, causing a variety of neurological disorders, including *dementia*.

Certain conditions, known as AIDS-defining illnesses, mark the development of full-blown AIDS. These include cancers (*Kaposi's sarcoma* and lymphoma of the brain), and various infections (*pneumocystis pneumonia*, tuberculosis, *human papillomavirus*, *cytomegalovirus* infection, *toxoplasmosis*, diarrhoea due to CRYPTOSPORIDIUM or ISOSPORA, candidiasis, disseminated *strongyloidiasis*, and *cryptococcosis*), many of which are described as *opportunistic infections*.

DIAGNOSIS
Confirmation of HIV infection involves testing a blood sample for the presence of antibodies to HIV (see *HIV test*), which may not develop for three months after initial infection. The condition is monitored using blood tests that measure the number of CD4 lymphocytes in the blood or by measuring viral load (the amount of virus detectable in the blood). Diagnosis of full-blown AIDS is based on a positive HIV test along with the presence of an AIDS-defining illness. Sometimes people only become aware that they have HIV when they develop an AIDS-defining illness and then have an HIV test.

TREATMENT AND OUTLOOK
The treatment of HIV infection can be divided into treatment for the HIV infection itself and treatment of the conditions and complications that are associated with HIV/AIDS.

Treatment of the infection with a combination of *antiretroviral drugs* can slow progress of the disease and may prevent the development of full-blown AIDS by reducing the amount of virus in the bloodstream. The two main types of antiretroviral drugs are *reverse transcriptase inhibitors,* such as zidovudine, and *protease inhibitors*, such as indinavir. Both groups of drugs work by disrupting replication of HIV inside cells. Several drugs are usually used in combination in a regimen known as highly active antiretroviral therapy, or HAART. The emergence of resistant strains of HIV has led to the development of a new group of drugs called *fusion inhibitors* (such as enfuvirtide), which work by interfering with the entry of the virus into cells. The mainstay of treatment for HIV/AIDS-related illnesses consists of antibiotics, antifungals, and other antimicrobial drugs to treat specific infections as they develop.

Since the introduction of combination drug therapy, deaths from AIDS in the developed world have fallen dramatically. However, such therapy is not a cure and HIV-infected people are still infectious even when the infection is being controlled successfully with drug treatment. Therefore, the most effective strategy for defeating HIV/AIDS remains prevention of infection

PREVENTION OF INFECTION
The risk of infection can be reduced by practising *safer sex*. and by intravenous drug users not sharing needles. There is a small risk to health workers handling infected needles (see *needlestick injury*) or blood products, but this can be minimized by the adoption of safe practices in the workplace.

AIDS-related complex

A combination of symptoms including weight loss, fever, neurological problems, and recurrent infections in an individual who has been infected with *HIV* (the virus that causes *AIDS*) but has not yet developed AIDS. Many people with AIDS-related complex will eventually develop the features of AIDS.

air

The colourless, odourless mixture of gases that forms the Earth's atmosphere. Air consists of 78 per cent *nitrogen*, 21 per cent *oxygen*, small quantities of *carbon dioxide* and other gases, and some water vapour.

CAUSES AND PREVENTION OF **AIDS**

AIDS is caused by the human immunodeficiency virus (HIV) (right), which consists of some nucleic acid (genetic material) inside two protective shells and an outer envelope. Full-blown AIDS develops in only some people infected with HIV.

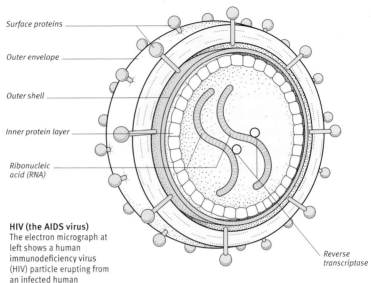

Surface proteins

Outer envelope

Outer shell

Inner protein layer

Ribonucleic acid (RNA)

Reverse transcriptase

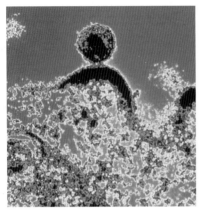

HIV (the AIDS virus)
The electron micrograph at left shows a human immunodeficiency virus (HIV) particle erupting from an infected human lymphocyte (cell of the immune system).

HOW HIV AFFECTS THE IMMUNE SYSTEM

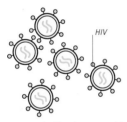

HIV

1 HIV enters the bloodstream and infects cells that have CD4 receptors on their surface, particularly CD4 lymphocytes, which are responsible for fighting infection.

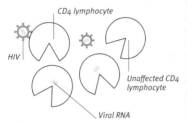

CD4 lymphocyte

HIV

Unaffected CD4 lymphocyte

Viral RNA

2 The virus attaches to and enters the CD4 lymphocytes. It then loses its protective shell, releasing its RNA and reverse transcriptase (an enzyme).

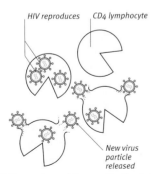

HIV reproduces

CD4 lymphocyte

New virus particle released

3 Reverse transcriptase enables the viral RNA to use the host CD4-lymphocyte's genetic material to reproduce itself. The new virus particles are released into the blood, killing the infected CD4-lymphocyte.

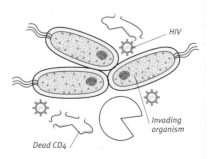

HIV

Invading organism

Dead CD4

4 When disease organisms invade, immune responses may fail, due to a shortage of CD4-lymphocytes. The disease organism may then overwhelm the immune system and lead to the features of AIDS.

RECOMMENDATIONS FOR PREVENTING THE SPREAD OF AIDS

- Do not have sexual intercourse with many partners, and especially not with people known to have HIV, without using a condom.

- Do not use intravenous (IV) drugs. If you use IV drugs, do not share needles or syringes.

- Do not have sex with people who use IV drugs.

- People with AIDS or who are HIV-positive may pass the disease on to others and should not donate blood, plasma, body organs, other tissues, or sperm. They should not exchange body fluids during sexual activity. HIV-positive mothers may pass on the virus through their breast milk.

- There is a risk of infecting (or being infected by) others through sexual intercourse, sharing needles, and, possibly, exposure to saliva through oral-genital contact or "wet" kissing. Condoms substantially reduce the risk of infection.

- Toothbrushes, razors, or other items that could become contaminated with blood should not be shared.

The balance of atmospheric gases is maintained largely by the mutual needs of plants and animals. Plants use carbon dioxide and release oxygen in a process called photosynthesis; animals use oxygen during respiration, and produce carbon dioxide as a waste product; However, the level of carbon dioxide in the atmosphere is increasing as a result of large-scale deforestation and the burning of fossil fuels, which is leading to global warming.

air conditioning

A system that controls the temperature, humidity, and purity, of the air in a building. Contaminated air-conditioning systems may cause *legionnaires' disease* (a type of pneumonia) and humidifier fever (a lung disease causing coughing and breathing difficulties). Air conditioning is also thought to be a factor in some cases of *sick building syndrome*, which produces headache, irritability, and loss of energy.

air embolism

The blockage of a small artery by an air bubble in the blood. Air embolism is rare. In most cases, it is caused by air entering the circulation through a vein, either as a result of injury or following surgery. Air embolism can also occur during scuba-diving or air-travel accidents, in which lung tissue ruptures, releasing air into the bloodstream.

air swallowing

See *aerophagy.*

air travel

See *aviation medicine*; *barotrauma.*

airway

A collective term for the passages through which air enters and leaves the lungs (see *respiratory system*). The airway is made up of the nasal passages, the oral cavity, the upper part of the pharynx (throat), the larynx (voicebox), the trachea (windpipe), the bronchi (the main air passages to the lungs), and the bronchioles (the smaller air passages in the lungs that branch off from the bronchi).

The term airway is also applied to a tube that is inserted into the mouth of an unconscious person to prevent the tongue from obstructing breathing. Preservation of the airway can also be achieved by inserting an *endotracheal tube* into the trachea, either through the

mouth or nose or via an incision in the neck, as in a *tracheostomy* operation. (See also *respiratory system*.)

airway obstruction

Narrowing or blockage of the respiratory passages. The obstruction may be due to a foreign body, such as a piece of food, that becomes lodged in part of the upper airway and may result in *choking*. Certain diseases and disorders, such as *diphtheria* and *lung cancer*, can cause obstruction. Additionally, spasm of the muscular walls of the airway, as occurs in *bronchospasm* (a feature of *asthma* and *bronchitis*), results in *breathing difficulty*. (See also *rescue breathing*; *lung* disorders box.)

akathisia

The inability to sit still. It may occur as a side effect of an *antipsychotic drug* or a complication of *Parkinson's disease.*

akinesia

Complete or almost complete loss of movement. Akinesia may result from damage to part of the brain due, for example, to a *stroke* or *Parkinson's disease.*

albinism

A rare, inherited disorder that is characterized by a lack of the pigment *melanin*, which gives colour to the skin, hair, and eyes.

Oculocutaneous albinism (the most common type) is transmitted as an autosomal recessive trait (see *genetic disorders*). The genetic defect results in deficiency of a specific *enzyme*, and this deficiency interferes with the production of melanin in the affected tissues.

In oculocutaneous albinism, the hair, skin, and eyes are all affected. The skin cannot tan and ages prematurely. In addition, *skin cancers* may develop on areas of skin exposed to the sun. Less often, only the eyes are affected. There may be visual problems, including *photophobia* (intolerance to bright light), *nystagmus* (abnormal flickering movements), *myopia* (shortsightedness), and *squint.*

Glasses are usually needed from an early age, and tinted glasses help to reduce photophobia. If the skin is affected, it should be protected from the sun.

albumin

The most abundant protein in the *blood* plasma. Albumin is made in the liver from *amino acids* that have been absorbed from digested protein.

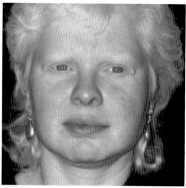

Appearance of albinism
Albinism is characterized by the lack of melanin pigment in the skin, hair, and eyes.

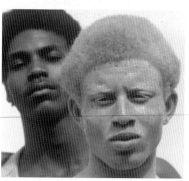

Albinism in an African boy
The condition occurs only rarely, but it is found in people of all ethnic groups.

Albumin helps to retain substances (such as calcium, some hormones, and certain drugs) in the circulation by binding to them to prevent them from being filtered out by the kidneys and excreted in the urine. Albumin also regulates the movement of water between tissues and the bloodstream by *osmosis*. (See also *albuminuria*.)

albuminuria

The presence of the protein *albumin* in the urine; a type of *proteinuria*. Normally, the glomeruli (filtering units of the kidneys) do not allow albumin to pass into the urine. Albuminuria therefore usually indicates that there is damage to the kidneys' filtering mechanisms. Such damage may be due to a kidney disorder, such as *glomerulonephritis* or *nephrotic syndrome*, or it may be a sign that the kidneys have been affected by *hypertension*. In *diabetes mellitus*, the presence of even small amounts of albumin in the urine (known as microalbuminuria) is an early indicator of kidney damage. Albuminuria can be detected by a simple urine test.

alcohol

A colourless liquid produced from the fermentation of carbohydrates by yeast. Also known as ethanol or ethyl alcohol, alcohol is the active constituent of alcoholic drinks such as beer, wine, and spirits. In medicine, alcohol is used as an antiseptic and a solvent. *Methanol*, also known as methyl alcohol, is a related, highly toxic, substance.

MENTAL EFFECTS

Alcohol is a drug and produces a wide range of mental and physical effects. The effect of alcohol on the *central nervous system* (brain and spinal cord) is as a depressant, decreasing its activity and thereby reducing anxiety, tension, and inhibitions. In moderate amounts, alcohol produces a feeling of relaxation, confidence, and sociability. However, alcohol slows reactions, and the more that is drunk, the greater the impairment of concentration and judgment. Excessive consumption results in poisoning or *alcohol intoxication*, with effects ranging from euphoria to unconsciousness.

PHYSICAL EFFECTS

Short-term physical effects include peripheral *vasodilation* (widening of small blood vessels), causing flushing and increased flow of gastric juices, which stimulates the appetite. Alcohol increases sexual confidence, but high levels can cause *erectile dysfunction*. Alcohol also acts as a diuretic, increasing urine output.

In the long term, regular excessive consumption of alcohol can cause *gastritis* (inflammation and ulceration of the stomach lining) and can lead to *alcohol-related disorders*. Binge drinking can cause similar problems. Heavy drinking in the long term may also lead to *alcohol dependence*. However, individuals who drink regular, small amounts of alcohol, (1–2 units per day; see *alcohol, unit of*) seem to have lower rates of *coronary artery disease* and *stroke* than those who abstain totally.

The consumption of alcohol during pregnancy may result in *fetal alcohol syndrome*, *miscarriage*, or a disruption in normal fetal development.

alcohol dependence

An illness characterized by habitual, compulsive, long-term, heavy alcohol consumption and the development of withdrawal symptoms when drinking is stopped suddenly.

CAUSES

Causative factors that interact in the development of alcohol dependence include personality, environment, and the addictive nature of alcohol. People with an inadequate, insecure, or immature personality are at greater risk. Environmental factors are important, especially the ready availability, affordability, and widespread social acceptance of alcohol. Genetic factors may play a part in causing alcohol dependence in some cases, but it is now widely believed that anyone, irrespective of personality, environment, or genetic background, is capable of becoming dependent. Stress is often a major factor in precipitating heavy drinking.

DEVELOPMENT OF DEPENDENCE

Alcohol dependence usually develops in four main stages that occur over a number of years and merge imperceptibly. In the first phase, tolerance (being able to drink more alcohol before experiencing its effects) develops in the heavy social drinker. In the second phase, the drinker experiences memory lapses relating to events during the drinking episodes. In the third phase, there is loss of control over alcohol consumption. The final phase is characterized by prolonged binges of intoxication, and mental or physical complications.

SYMPTOMS AND EFFECTS

Behavioural symptoms are varied. They can include grandiose, aggressive, or furtive behaviour; personality changes (such as irritability, jealousy, or uncontrolled anger); neglect of food intake and personal appearance; and lengthy periods of intoxication.

Physical symptoms may include nausea, vomiting, or shaking in the morning; abdominal pain; cramps; numbness or tingling; weakness in the legs and hands; enlarged blood vessels in the face; irregular pulse; unsteadiness; confusion; memory lapses; and incontinence. Sudden withdrawal from alcohol may lead to *delirium tremens* (severe shakes, hallucinations, and convulsions).

Alcohol-dependent persons are more susceptible than others to a variety of physical and mental disorders (see *alcohol-related disorders*).

TREATMENT

Many problem drinkers require medical help in overcoming their physical withdrawal symptoms (detoxification) when they stop drinking alcohol, followed by long-term treatment. There are different treatments, which may be combined.

Psychological treatments for alcohol dependence involve *psychotherapy*, such as *cognitive-behavioural therapy*, and are commonly carried out as *group therapy*. Social treatments may offer practical help, such as with problems at work, and tend to involve family members in the process. Physical treatment generally includes the use of *disulfiram*, a drug that sensitizes the drinker to alcohol so that he or she experiences unpleasant side effects when drinking. Other treatments may include *benzodiazepine drugs* to help control withdrawal symptoms and vitamins to treat any deficiency. *Acamprosate* may also be given to help maintain abstinence. *Alcoholics Anonymous* and other self-help organizations can provide support and advice.

Alcoholics Anonymous

A worldwide, independent, self-help organization to help people overcome *alcohol dependence*. Regular group meetings are held in which members are encouraged to help each other stay sober by offering support and advice.

ALCOHOL AND PREGNANCY

Drinking alcohol during pregnancy increases the risk of *fetal alcohol syndrome* and the risk of miscarriage. A proportion of the alcohol consumed by the mother reaches the fetus and there is a risk that even small amounts may disrupt normal fetal development and may also cause low birthweight. Therefore pregnant women are advised to abstain from alcohol entirely. However, if they do choose to drink, they should have a maximum of one or two units of alcohol (see *alcohol, unit of*) no more than once or twice a week; they should not binge drink nor should they get drunk.

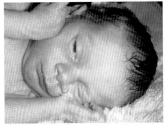

Fetal alcohol syndrome
An affected baby is abnormally small, with small eyes and a small jaw. He or she may also suffer from heart defects or a cleft lip and palate, may suckle poorly, sleep badly, and be irritable.

A

ALCOHOL AND THE BODY

Alcohol is a drug and, even in small amounts, its effects on the body are noticeable. Problems arise when people fail to take into account the effects of alcohol on tasks requiring coordination (such as driving) when they become intoxicated or when they become dependent on the drug. Alcohol dependence can cause early death and is a major factor in crime, marital breakdown, child abuse, accidents, and absenteeism.

Prolonged heavy drinking that stops just short of dependence still may cause a wide variety of diseases, such as cardiomyopathy and cirrhosis of the liver.

The table below highlights the effects of alcohol on the occasional social drinker. These effects occur with higher concentrations as alcohol tolerance increases.

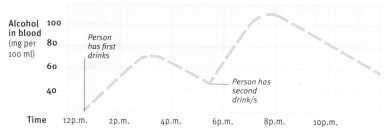

Cumulative effects of alcohol
The body takes some time to eliminate even small amounts of alcohol. If a person has two drinks at lunchtime, and then has one or two early in the evening, the cumulative blood alcohol level could be over the legal limit for driving, even after several hours.

Alcohol levels in different drinks
A unit is the measure used to define the amount of alcohol in an alcoholic drink. One unit constitutes 10 ml of pure alcohol. The number of units per drink is calculated by the volume of the drink and the percentage of alcohol by volume. The drinks shown here each contain approximately one unit of pure alcohol.

Beer (250 ml) (4 per cent by volume) **Wine (100 ml)** (10 per cent by volume) **Sherry (50ml)** (20 per cent by volume) **Whisky (25ml)** (40 per cent by volume)

EFFECTS OF INCREASING BLOOD ALCOHOL LEVELS

Concentration (milligrams per 100 millilitres)	Observable effects
30-50	Flushed face, euphoria, talkativeness, increased social confidence
50-150	Disturbed thinking and coordination, irritability, reduced self-control, irresponsible talk and behaviour
150-250	Marked confusion, unsteady gait, slurred speech, unpredictable shows of emotion and aggression
250-400	Extreme confusion and disorientation, difficulty remaining upright, drowsiness, delayed or incoherent reaction to questions progressing to coma (a state of deep unconsciousness from which the person cannot be aroused)
400-500	Risk of death due to arrest of breathing (although habitual drinkers may survive even such high levels) and choking on vomit

LONG TERM EFFECTS ON THE BODY

Persistent heavy drinking eventually damages body tissues; the main effects are shown below.

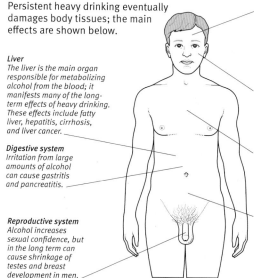

Liver
The liver is the main organ responsible for metabolizing alcohol from the blood; it manifests many of the long-term effects of heavy drinking. These effects include fatty liver, hepatitis, cirrhosis, and liver cancer.

Digestive system
Irritation from large amounts of alcohol can cause gastritis and pancreatitis.

Reproductive system
Alcohol increases sexual confidence, but in the long term can cause shrinkage of testes and breast development in men.

Brain and nervous
Alcohol depresses the central nervous system. Prolonged alcohol abuse permanently impairs brain function and damages peripheral nerves.

Skin
Alcohol causes facial flushing, which becomes constant in heavy drinkers.

Heart and circulation
Prolonged heavy drinking can cause heart failure, hypertension, and stroke.

Urinary system
Alcohol acts as a diuretic, increasing urine output.

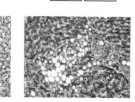

Cirrhosis of the liver
This condition is commonly caused by heavy drinking. When compared to a normal liver (far left), the cirrhotic liver clearly shows the formation of bands of scar tissue, which impair its function.

alcohol intoxication

The condition that results from consuming an excessive amount of *alcohol*, often over a relatively short period.

EFFECTS

The effects of high intake alcohol depend on many factors, including mental and physical state, body size, social situation, and acquired tolerance; but the important factor is the blood alcohol level. Mild intoxication promotes relaxation and increases social confidence.

However, alcohol causes acute poisoning if it is consumed in sufficiently large amounts. It depresses the activity of the *central nervous system*, (brain and spinal cord), leading to loss of normal mental and physical control. In extreme cases, consumption of a large amount of alcohol over a short time may lead to loss of consciousness and even death.

TREATMENT

In most cases, recovery from alcohol intoxication occurs naturally as the alcohol is broken down in the liver. Medical attention is required if the intoxication has resulted in *coma*. For a the effects of long-term heavy drinking, see *alcohol dependence* and *alcohol-related disorders*.

alcoholism

See *alcohol dependence*.

alcohol-related disorders

A wide variety of physical and mental disorders associated with heavy, prolonged consumption of alcohol.

High alcohol consumption increases the risk of cancer of the mouth, tongue, pharynx (throat), larynx (voicebox), and oesophagus (gullet), especially if combined with smoking. Incidence of liver diseases, such as *liver cancer*, alcoholic *hepatitis* and *cirrhosis*, is higher in alcohol-dependent persons. High consumption of alcohol increases the risk of *cardiomyopathy* (disease of heart muscle), *hypertension* (high blood pressure), and *stroke*. Alcohol irritates the digestive tract and may cause *gastritis*. Heavy drinking during pregnancy increases the risk of miscarriage and *fetal alcohol syndrome*. Problem drinkers are more likely to suffer from *anxiety* and *depression* and to develop *dementia*.

Many problem drinkers have a poor diet and are prone to diseases caused by nutritional deficiency, particularly of thiamine (see *vitamin B complex*). Severe thiamine deficiency (see *beriberi*) disturbs nerve function, causing cramps, numbness, and weakness in the legs and hands. Its effects on the brain can cause confusion, disturbances of speech and gait, and eventual coma (see *Wernicke–Korsakoff syndrome*). Severe deficiency can also cause *heart failure*.

A prolonged high level of alcohol in the body can disturb the metabolism, resulting in *hypoglycaemia* (low blood glucose levels) and *hyperlipidaemia* (high blood fat levels). These may damage the heart, liver, blood vessels, and brain; irreversible damage may cause premature death.

alcohol, unit of

A measure commonly used to define the amount of *alcohol* in a single alcoholic drink. A unit is defined as 10 millilitres of pure alcohol. The number of units in one drink is calculated by multiplying the alcohol content of that drink with its volume, then dividing by 1000. As a rough guide, half a pint (or a bottle) of beer, lager, or cider has one unit; a single measure (25 ml) of spirits has one unit; and a small glass of wine has one unit.

In the UK, the Department of Health has defined the safe maximum alcohol intake for men as three to four units per day (or less) and for women as two to three units per day (or less). In addition, one or two alcohol-free days per week are usually recommended.

Pregnant women are advised not to drink at all but if they chose to do so, to drink a maximum of one or two units no more than once or twice a week; they should not binge drink nor get drunk. The same recommended limits apply to women who are breast-feeding.

aldosterone

A hormone secreted by the adrenal cortex (outer part of the *adrenal glands*). Aldosterone plays an important role in the control of blood pressure and regulation of sodium and potassium concentrations in the blood and tissues.

Aldosterone acts on the kidneys to decrease the amount of sodium lost in the urine; the sodium is reabsorbed into the blood from urine before it leaves the kidneys and is replaced in the urine by potassium. The sodium draws water back into the blood with it, thereby increasing the blood volume and raising the blood pressure.

Aldosterone production is stimulated mainly by the action of *angiotensin* II, a chemical produced by a series of reactions involving the enzymes *renin* and *angiotensin-converting enzyme*. Production of aldosterone is also stimulated by the action of the hormone *ACTH*, which is produced by the pituitary gland.

aldosteronism

A disorder that results from excessive production of the hormone *aldosterone* from one or both of the *adrenal glands*. Aldosteronism caused by an *adrenal tumour* is known as Conn's syndrome. Aldosteronism may also be due to disorders, such as *heart failure* or liver damage, that reduce blood flow through the kidneys. This reduction in blood flow leads to overproduction of *renin* and *angiotensin*, which, in turn, leads to excessive aldosterone production.

SYMPTOMS AND SIGNS

Symptoms are directly related to the actions of aldosterone. Excess sodium is retained in the body, leading to a rise in blood pressure, and excess potassium is lost in the urine. Low levels of potassium cause tiredness and muscle weakness and impair kidney function, leading to thirst and overproduction of urine.

TREATMENT

Treatment includes restriction of salt in the diet and use of the diuretic drug *spironolactone*. This drug blocks the action of aldosterone on the kidneys, leading to increased loss of sodium from the body, lowered blood pressure, and reduced potassium loss. If the cause of aldosteronism is an adrenal tumour, this may be surgically removed.

alendronate sodium

See *alendronic acid*.

alendronic acid

A *bisphosphonate drug* that is used in the treatment of *osteoporosis* and *Paget's disease* of bone. The most common side effect of the drug is inflammation of the oesophagus, which causes heartburn or difficulty in swallowing. Other side effects may include headache, abdominal pain and distension, and diarrhoea or constipation.

Alexander technique

A therapy that aims to improve health by teaching people to stand and move more efficiently.

Developed in the 1920s by F. Mathias Alexander, the technique is based on the belief that bad patterns of body movement interfere with the proper functioning of the body and therefore contribute to the development of disease. By releasing unnecessary muscle

A

ALCOHOL-RELATED DISORDERS

Cancer

High alcohol consumption increases the risk of breast cancer in women and cancers of the mouth, tongue, pharynx (back of the throat), larynx (voicebox), and oesophagus, probably due to irritant action. In each of these cancers, alcohol intake, along with smoking, produces a much higher total risk of cancer than the sum of their separate risks. The risk of *liver cancer*, along with most types of liver disease, is also higher among problem drinkers.

Liver damage and disease

Liver diseases caused by a high alcohol consumption include fatty liver, alcoholic *hepatitis*, cirrhosis, and liver cancer. They develop in sequence over a period of years. It is thought that a breakdown product of alcohol (acetaldehyde) has a toxic effect on liver cells and is the main cause of these diseases, although nutritional deficiency may also play some part. The risk of alcoholic hepatitis and cirrhosis developing increases in proportion to the amount of alcohol consumed and the number of years of high consumption; liver cancer develops in about one in five sufferers of cirrhosis.

Nervous system disorders

Thiamine (vitamin B1) deficiency, also known as beriberi (which disturbs nerve functioning), may develop in problem drinkers. The effect of severe deficiency on the brain produces Wernicke's encephalopathy, with symptoms such as confusion, disturbances of speech and gait, and eventual coma. Korsakoff's psychosis may also occur (see *Wernicke–Korsakoff syndrome*). The effect on the peripheral nervous system (nerve pathways outside the brain and spinal cord) produces polyneuropathy, with symptoms such as pain, cramps, numbness, tingling, and weakness in the legs and hand. Excessive consumption of alcohol can also cause *dementia*.

Psychiatric illness

Problem drinkers are more likely than others to suffer from anxiety and depression (frequently with related financial, work , or family problems) and from paranoia. They are also more likely to develop dementia (irreversible mental deterioration). The incidence of suicide attempts and actual suicide is also higher among problem drinkers.

Heart and circulatory disorders

Severe deficiency of thiamine in problem drinkers can result in heart failure (reduced pumping efficiency), which is usually combined with oedema (the collection of fluid in tissues). A high consumption of alcohol also increases the risk of hypertension (high blood pressure), cerebral haemorrhage, and *cardiomyopathy*. One type of stroke is also associated with excessive consumption of alcohol.

Genito-urinary system disorders

High consumption of alcohol can lead to fertility problems in women and to erectile dysfunction in men. Heavy drinking during pregnancy carries the risk of spontaneous abortion and of the baby being born with *fetal alcohol syndrome*.

Other medical disorders

Other physical diseases and disorders that are associated with high intake of alcohol include *gastritis* and acute and chronic *pancreatitis*, (all of which are probably linked to an irritant action of alcohol), *osteoporosis* (thinning of the bones), and damage to the skeletal muscles and those of the genito-urinary tract.

tensions, the Alexander technique aims to eliminate or reduce the severity of many disorders, including back pain, asthma, and stammering.

alexia

Word blindness; the inability to recognize and name written words. Alexia results from damage to part of the cerebrum (the main mass of the brain) by, for example, a *stroke*. The condition severely disrupts the reading ability of an individual who was previously literate. (See also *dyslexia*.)

alfacalcidol

A synthetic form of *vitamin D*.

alginates

Substances used in certain types of *antacid drugs*. Alginates float on top of the stomach contents, forming a raft, which reduces regurgitation of stomach acid into the oesophagus.

alienation

Feeling like a stranger, even when among familiar people or places, and being unable to identify with family, a culture, or a peer group. Alienation is common in adolescents, and it also occurs in individuals who are isolated by cultural or language differences. In some people, alienation may be an early symptom of *schizophrenia* or a *personality disorder*.

alignment, dental

The movement of teeth by the use of either fixed or removable *orthodontic appliances* (braces) to correct *malocclusion* (an incorrect bite).

alimemazine

An *antihistamine drug* that is used mainly to relieve the itching that occurs in allergic conditions such as *urticaria* and atopic *eczema*. Alimemazine frequently causes drowsiness.

alimentary tract

Also known as the alimentary canal, the tubelike structure that extends from the mouth to the anus (see *digestive system*).

alkali

Also called a base, an alkali is chemically defined as a donor of hydroxyl ions (each of which comprises an atom of hydrogen linked to an atom of oxygen and has an overall negative electrical charge). *Antacid drugs*, such as sodium bicarbonate (bicarbonate of soda), are examples of alkalis. Some alkalis, such as sodium hydroxide (caustic soda), are corrosive and cause burns. (See also *acid*; *acid–base balance*.)

alkaloids

A group of nitrogen-containing substances that are obtained from plants. *Morphine*, *codeine*, *nicotine*, and strychnine (see *strychnine poisoning*) are examples of alkaloids.

alkalosis

A disturbance of the body's *acid–base balance* in which there is an accumulation of alkali (base) or a loss of acid. There are two types of alkalosis: metabolic and respiratory.

In metabolic alkalosis, the increase in alkalinity may be caused by taking too much of an *antacid drug* or by losing a large amount of stomach acid as a result of severe vomiting.

In respiratory alkalosis, there is a reduction in the blood level of carbonic acid (derived from carbon dioxide). This reduction is a consequence of *hyperventilation* (overbreathing), which may occur during a panic attack or at high altitudes due to lack of oxygen. (See also *acidosis*.)

Alka-Seltzer

A brand-name analgesic and antacid containing *aspirin*, *sodium bicarbonate*, and citric acid. Alka-Seltzer is used to treat headaches and stomach upsets.

alkylating agents

A class of *anticancer drugs*.

allele

One of two or more different forms of a *gene* that occupies a specific position on a *chromosome*. (See also *inheritance*.)

allergen

A normally harmless substance that causes an allergic reaction (see *allergy*) in people who have become sensitized to it. Allergens can include foods (for example, nuts, eggs, and shellfish); inhaled substances (such as pollen, house dust, and fur); and some drugs.

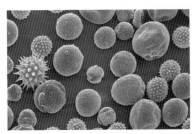

Electron micrograph of various pollen grains
Pollen is a common example of an allergen. The airborne pollen grains from plants (such as grasses and trees) can trigger an allergic reaction, the most common of which is allergic rhinitis (hay fever).

allergic alveolitis, extrinsic

See *extrinsic allergic alveolitis*.

allergic rhinitis

See *rhinitis, allergic*.

allergy

Various conditions caused by inappropriate or exaggerated reactions of the *immune system* to a wide variety of substances known as *allergens*. Many common illnesses, such as *asthma* and hay fever (see *rhinitis, allergic*), are caused by allergic reactions to substances that, in the majority of people, cause no symptoms.

Allergic reactions occur only on second or subsequent exposure to the allergen, after first contact has sensitized the body. It is unclear why only certain

ALLERGY AND THE BODY

An allergy is an inappropriate immune system response (causing symptoms) to substances that, in most people, cause no response. The response is mainly to harmless substances that come in contact with the respiratory airways, skin, or eye surface. Common *allergens* are pollen, spores, house-dust mites, and animal *dander*. Certain drugs, and some foods, most commonly dairy products, seafood, strawberries, and cereals, can also cause allergies. In diagnosing an allergy, the individual's medical history is important. The doctor needs to know if the symptoms vary according to the time of the day or the season, and if there are pets or other likely sources of allergens in the home.

THE ORIGIN OF AN ALLERGY

The immune system is sensitized once it has been exposed to an allergen (steps 1 to 3). Symptoms occur when the allergen is met again (step 4).

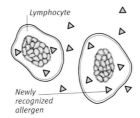

1 An allergen enters the body and is recognized by lymphocytes (blood cells that form part of the body's immune system).

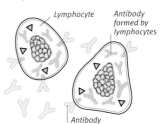

2 A few days to weeks later, the lymphocytes produce antibodies that are specific to the allergens.

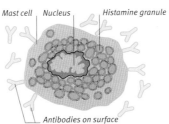

3 The antibodies attach to cells in the tissues called mast cells, which contain granules of histamine.

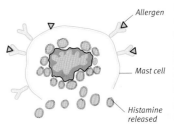

4 Binding of allergens to antibodies on the surface of mast cells leads to the release of histamine and to the symptoms of allergy.

DIAGNOSING SKIN ALLERGY

One type of skin allergy, also known as allergic contact dermatitis, develops slowly. Tests are performed to identify specific reactions to allergens. Small amounts of various substances are applied to the skin to see whether or not a reaction occurs.

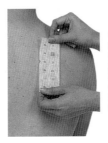

1 Tiny samples of allergens are placed on small discs and stuck to the skin with inert tape. The discs are removed after two days.

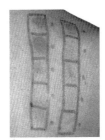

2 A reddened area of skin where a disc had been in contact denotes a positive reaction. Some reactions may take longer to appear.

people develop allergies, but about one person in eight seems to have an inherited predisposition to them (see *atopy*).

TYPES AND CAUSES

The function of the immune system is to recognize *antigens* (foreign proteins) on the surfaces of microorganisms and to form *antibodies* (also called immunoglobulins) and sensitized *lymphocytes* (white blood cells). When the immune system next encounters these antigens, the antibodies and sensitized lymphocytes interact with them, leading to the destruction of the microorganisms.

A similar immune response occurs in allergies, except that the immune system forms antibodies or sensitized lymphocytes against harmless substances because these allergens are misidentified as potentially harmful antigens.

The inappropriate or exaggerated reactions that are seen in allergies are known as *hypersensitivity* reactions and can have any of four different mechanisms (which are termed Types I to IV hypersensitivity reactions).

TYPE I HYPERSENSITIVITY REACTIONS

Most well known allergies are caused by Type I (also known as anaphylactic or immediate) hypersensitivity, in which allergens cause immediate symptoms by provoking the immune system into producing specific antibodies, belonging to a type called immunoglobulin E (IgE), which coat cells (known as mast cells or basophils) that are present in the skin and the lining of the stomach, lungs, and upper respiratory airways. When the allergen is encountered for the second time, it binds to the IgE antibodies and causes the granules in mast cells to release various chemicals, which are responsible for the symptoms of the allergy.

Among the chemicals released is *histamine*, which causes widening of blood vessels, leakage of fluid into tissues, and contraction of muscles, especially in the airways of the lung. Symptoms can include itching, swelling, sneezing, and wheezing. Particular conditions associated with Type I reactions include asthma, hay fever, *urticaria* (nettle rash), *angioedema*, *anaphylactic shock* (a severe, generalized allergic reaction), possibly atopic *eczema*, and some food allergies.

TYPES II TO IV HYPERSENSITIVITY REACTIONS

Because Types II to IV hypersensitivity reactions have different mechanisms to Type I reactions, they are less often implicated in allergies. However, contact allergic dermatitis, in which the skin reacts to prolonged contact with substances such as nickel, is the result of a Type IV hypersensitivity reaction.

TREATMENT

Whenever possible, the most effective treatment for allergy of any kind is avoidance of the relevant allergen.

Drug treatment for allergic reactions includes the use of *antihistamine drugs*, which relieve the symptoms. Some antihistamines have a sedative effect, which is useful, for example, in treating itching at night due to eczema; many do not cause drowsiness, making them more suitable for daytime use. Drugs such as *sodium cromoglicate*, montelukast, and *corticosteroids* can be used regularly to prevent symptoms from developing.

Hyposensitization can be valuable for a minority of people who suffer allergic reactions to specific allergens such as bee stings. Treatment involves gradually increasing doses of the allergen to promote formation of antibodies that will block future reactions. Hyposensitization must be carried out under close supervision because a severe allergic reaction can result. (See also *delayed allergy*.)

allograft

Sometimes referred to as a homograft, tissue or an organ transplanted from one person to another. (See also *grafting*.)

allopathy

The practice of conventional medicine. (See also *homeopathy*.)

allopurinol

A drug used in the long-term prevention of *gout* attacks. Allopurinol works by decreasing production of *uric acid* in the body, thereby preventing the formation of uric acid crystals in the joints.

Possible adverse effects of allopurinol include itching, rashes, and nausea. The drug cannot relieve the pain of an acute gout attack and may even precipitate one at the start of treatment. Such attacks can be prevented by taking a combination of allopurinol and a *nonsteroidal antiinflammatory drug* (NSAID) or *colchicine*.

almond oil

An oil prepared from the seeds of the bitter almond tree (PRUNUS AMYGDALUS). Almond oil is a common ingredient of *emollient* skin preparations.

almotriptan

A *serotonin agonist* drug that is used in the treatment of acute migraine attacks.

aloe

The juice of leaves from various plants of the ALOE genus. Aloe may be added to compound benzoin tincture, an aromatic *inhalation* for relieving *sinusitis* and *nasal congestion*.

alopecia

Loss or absence of *hair*, which may occur at any hair-bearing site on the body but which is usually noticeable only on the scalp.

TYPES

Male-pattern baldness, the most common form of alopecia, is hereditary and most commonly affects men. Normal hair is lost, initially from the temples and crown, and is replaced by fine, downy hair; the affected area gradually widens. Other hereditary forms of alopecia are rare and may be due to absence of hair roots or abnormalities of the hair shaft.

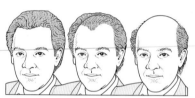

Stages in male pattern baldness
In this common form of alopecia, the man first loses hair from the temples and the crown, then the bald area gradually widens.

In generalized alopecia, the hair falls out in large amounts. Such hair loss occurs when all the hairs simultaneously enter the resting phase; they then fall out about three months later. Causes include surgery, prolonged illness, or childbirth. In such cases, the hair will regrow without treatment. Many *anticancer drugs* cause temporary alopecia. The hair usually regrows when the treatment is completed.

Localized alopecia may be the result of permanent skin damage (for example, following burns or *radiotherapy*) or of trauma to the hair roots by styling or, rarely, *trichotillomania* (a disorder in which sufferers pull out their hair). The most common type of localized hair loss is alopecia areata, an *autoimmune disorder* (in which the immune system attacks the body's own tissues). There is no specific treatment for alopecia areata, but the hair usually regrows within a few months. Alopecia universalis is a rare, permanent form of alopecia areata that causes loss of all hair on the scalp and body, including the eyelashes and eyebrows. Skin diseases such as scalp ringworm (see *tinea*), *lichen planus*, *lupus erythematosus*, and *skin tumours* may also cause localized hair loss.

TREATMENT

Treatments for male-pattern baldness include *hair transplants* or drug treatments with *minoxidil* or *finasteride*. Generalized alopecia often resolves without treatment. Treatment of localized alopecia depends on the cause.

alpha₁-antitrypsin deficiency

A rare *genetic disorder* in which a person is missing the enzyme alpha₁-antitrypsin, which protects the body from damage by other enzymes. The disease mainly affects tissues in the lungs, resulting in *emphysema*, and the liver, causing *cirrhosis*. The effects of alpha₁-antitrypsin deficiency may not become apparent until after the age of 30. There is no cure, but symptoms can be relieved by drug treatment. In severe cases, a *liver transplant* may be a possibility.

alpha-blocker drugs

COMMON DRUGS

• Alfuzosin • Doxazosin • Indoramin • Prazosin
• Tamsulosin • Terazosin

A group of drugs used to treat *hypertension* (high blood pressure) and urinary symptoms resulting from an enlarged prostate gland (see *prostate, enlarged*).

Alpha-blocker drugs interfere with the nerve signals that govern the contraction of blood vessels. This causes the vessels to widen (vasodilation), thereby reducing the blood pressure. In the treatment of an enlarged prostate gland, alpha-blockers relax the ring of muscles at the bladder outlet, which improves the outflow of urine.

Side effects may include dizziness (caused by a drop in blood pressure on standing up) and fatigue, drowsiness, headache, nausea, and a dry mouth.

alpha-fetoprotein

A protein that is produced in the liver and gastrointestinal tract of the fetus and by some abnormal tissues in adults.

ALPHA-FETOPROTEIN IN PREGNANCY

Alpha-fetoprotein (AFP) is excreted in the fetal urine into the amniotic fluid; the fluid is swallowed by the fetus, which introduces AFP into the fetal digestive system. Most of the AFP is broken down in the fetal intestine, but some of it passes into the mother's circulation. AFP can be measured in the maternal blood from the latter part of the first trimester of pregnancy, and its concentration rises between the 15th and 20th weeks.

Raised levels of AFP are associated with fetal *neural tube defects*, such as *spina bifida* or *anencephaly*, and certain kidney abnormalities. High levels of AFP also occur in multiple pregnancies (see *pregnancy, multiple*) and threatened or actual *miscarriage*.

AFP levels may be unusually low if the fetus has *Down's syndrome*. For this reason, measurement of blood AFP is included in blood tests that are used to screen pregnant women for increased risk of Down's syndrome.

ALPHA-FETOPROTEIN IN ADULTS

AFP levels are commonly raised in adults with hepatoma (see *liver cancer*), cancerous *teratoma* of the testes or ovaries, or cancer of the pancreas, stomach, or lung. For this reason, AFP is known as a "tumour marker".

AFP levels can be used to monitor results of treatment of such cancers; increasing levels after chemotherapy or surgery may indicate recurrence. However, AFP levels are also raised in some noncancerous conditions such as viral and alcoholic *hepatitis* and *cirrhosis*.

alprazolam

A *benzodiazepine drug* that is used in the treatment of *anxiety*, *panic attacks*, and *phobias*.

alprostadil

A *prostaglandin drug* used to minimize the effects of congenital heart defects in newborn babies prior to corrective surgery; it is usually administered in hospital. Alprostadil is also used as treatment for erectile dysfunction. To produce an erection, it is self-administered, either by injection into the penis or as a gel introduced into the *urethra*.

alternative medicine

Also called *complementary medicine*, any medical system based on a theory of disease or method of treatment other than orthodox Western medicine.

altitude sickness

See *mountain sickness*.

aluminium

A light, metallic element that is found in bauxite and various other minerals. Aluminium compounds are used in *antacid drugs* and in *antiperspirants*.

Most of the aluminium taken into the body is excreted. Excessive amounts are toxic and are stored in the lungs, brain, liver, and thyroid gland, where they may result in organ damage.

Certain industrial processes give off fumes containing aluminium into the air. Inhalation of these fumes can cause *fibrosis* of lung tissue. Drugs that contain aluminium interfere with the absorption and excretion of a number of other drugs and should not, therefore, be taken simultaneously.

alveolectomy

See *alveoloplasty*.

alveolitis

Inflammation and thickening of the walls of the alveoli (the tiny air sacs in the lungs). Alveolitis reduces the elasticity of the lungs during breathing and reduces the efficiency of the transfer of gas between the lungs and the surrounding blood vessels.

CAUSES

Alveolitis is commonly caused by an allergic reaction to inhaled dust of animal or plant origin, as in *farmer's lung* (caused by spores from mouldy hay), *bagassosis* (caused by spores from mouldy sugar-cane residue), and pigeon fancier's lung (caused by particles from bird droppings). This type of alveolitis is known as extrinsic allergic alveolitis.

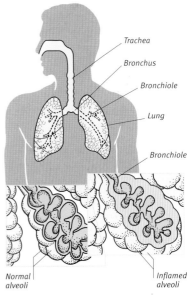

Trachea
Bronchus
Bronchiole
Lung
Bronchiole

Normal alveoli   *Inflamed alveoli*

Effects of alveolitis
The alveoli become inflamed and their walls thicken, causing the lungs to become less elastic and less able to transfer oxygen.

Fibrosing alveolitis is an *autoimmune disorder* (in which the immune system attacks the body's own tissues). In some cases, it occurs with other autoimmune disorders, such as *rheumatoid arthritis* or systemic *lupus erythematosus*.

Radiation alveolitis is caused by irradiation of the lungs and may occur as a rare complication of *radiotherapy* for lung or breast cancer.

SYMPTOMS AND DIAGNOSIS
Alveolitis usually causes a dry cough and breathing difficulty on exertion.

A *chest X-ray* of a person suffering from alveolitis usually shows mottled shadowing across the lungs. *Blood tests* may be performed to look for specific antibodies (proteins manufactured by the immune system: see *antibody*) to an allergen. They may also be performed to look for evidence of an autoimmune disorder (in which the immune system attacks the body's own tissues). *Pulmonary function tests* show reduced lung capacity without obstruction to air flow through the bronchi (air passages to the lungs). A lung *biopsy* (removal of a sample of tissue for microscopic analysis) may be the only way to make a conclusive diagnosis of alveolitis.

TREATMENT AND OUTLOOK
For most types of alveolitis, a short course of *corticosteroid drugs* relieves symptoms, but for fibrosing alveolitis the drugs may need to be taken indefinitely. If the cause of allergic alveolitis is recognized and avoided before lung damage occurs, the effects are not permanent. In fibrosing alveolitis, the damage progresses despite treatment, causing increasing breathing difficulty and, sometimes, *respiratory failure*.

alveoloplasty
Dental surgery that is carried out to remove protuberances and to smooth out other uneven areas from bone in the jaw. Alveoplasty is performed either under a general anaesthetic (see *anaesthesia, dental*) or, more usually, under local anaesthetic. The procedure is usually carried out to facilitate the fitting of dentures on people whose alveolar ridge, underlying the gums, would not otherwise be smooth and even enough for dentures to be fitted easily or to be worn comfortably.

An incision is made in the gum, which is then peeled back to expose the uneven bone. The bone is then either reshaped with large forceps or filed down to the required shape. Finally, the gum is drawn back over the bone and stitched together. Some bruising and swelling of the mouth may occur, but the gum usually heals within two weeks.

alveolus, dental
The bony cavity or socket supporting each tooth in the jaw.

alveolus, pulmonary
One of millions of tiny, balloonlike sacs at the end of a bronchiole (one of the many small air passages in the lungs) where gases are exchanged during *respiration*. In each lung, there are approximately 300 million alveoli that are arranged in groups resembling bunches of grapes.

ANATOMY OF THE **ALVEOLI**

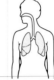

These tiny sacs contain capillaries in their thin walls that allow oxygen to be absorbed into the blood.

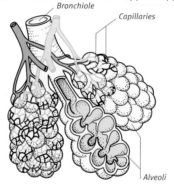

Bronchiole

Capillaries

Alveoli

Alzheimer's disease
A progressive condition in which nerve cells in the brain degenerate and the brain shrinks. Alzheimer's disease is the most common cause of *dementia* (a general decline in all areas of mental ability). Its onset is uncommon before the age of 60, but incidence increases steadily with age thereafter.

CAUSES
In most cases, Alzheimer's disease occurs without an identifiable cause. However, early-onset Alzheimer's disease, in which symptoms develop before age 60, may rarely be inherited as a *dominant* disorder, and late-onset Alzheimer's disease is sometimes associated with various genes, including three that are responsible for the production of the blood protein *apolipoprotein* E. These genes also result in the deposition of a protein called beta amyloid in the brain. Other chemical abnormalities may include deficiency of the *neurotransmitter* acetylcholine.

SYMPTOMS AND SIGNS
The features of Alzheimer's disease vary, but there are three broad stages. At first, the affected individual becomes increasingly forgetful; and problems with memory may cause *anxiety* and *depression*. Some deterioration in memory is a feature of normal *aging*, and this alone is not evidence of dementia.

In the second stage, loss of memory, particularly for recent events, gradually becomes more severe, and there may be disorientation as to time or place. The person's concentration and numerical ability decline, and there is noticeable *dysphasia* (inability to find the right word). Anxiety increases, mood changes unpredictably, and personality changes may occur. If the person is left unsupervised, he or she may repeatedly wander off.

Finally, confusion becomes profound. There may be symptoms of *psychosis*, such as *hallucinations* and *delusions*. Signs of nervous system disease, such as abnormal *reflexes* and faecal or urinary *incontinence*, begin to develop.

DIAGNOSIS
Alzheimer's disease is usually diagnosed from the symptoms, but tests including blood tests and *CT scanning* or *MRI* (techniques that produce cross-sectional or three-dimensional images) of the brain may be needed to exclude treatable causes of dementia.

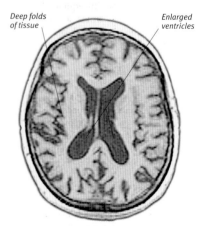

Deep folds of tissue

Enlarged ventricles

MRI of the brain in Alzheimer's disease
The volume of the brain substance has shrunk markedly, resulting in deep folding of the tissue and enlargement of the fluid-filled brain ventricles.

TREATMENT

There is no cure for Alzheimer's disease. The most important aspect of treatment is the provision of suitable nursing and social care for sufferers and support for their relatives. *Tranquillizer drugs* can often improve difficult behaviour and may help with sleep. Treatment with *acetylcholinesterase inhibitors*, such as rivastigmine and donepezil, may slow the progress of the disease for a time. Side effects such as nausea and dizziness may occur.

amalgam, dental

A material, consisting of an alloy of mercury with other metals, that is used as fillings for teeth. Amalgam is soft enough to be easily workable by the dentist but sets rapidly into a hard, strong solid (see *filling, dental*).

amantadine

An *antiviral drug* that is used in the prevention and treatment of *influenza* A. Amantadine is also used to help relieve symptoms of *Parkinson's disease*.

amaurosis fugax

Brief loss of vision, lasting for seconds or minutes, usually affecting one eye only and caused by the temporary blockage of a small blood vessel in the eye by an *embolus* (a particle of solid matter such as cholesterol or clotted blood). These emboli are carried in the bloodstream from diseased arteries in the neck or, rarely, the heart. Sufferers typically experience a loss or dimming of vision, in one eye only, rather like a shade being pulled down or up.

Attacks may be infrequent, or they may occur many times a day, which indicates an increased risk of *stroke* and requires medical investigation.

ambidexterity

The ability to perform manual skills, such as writing or using cutlery, equally well with either hand because there is no definite *handedness* (preference for the use of one hand in particular). Ambidexterity is an uncommon and often familial trait.

amblyopia

A permanent defect of visual acuity in which there is usually no structural abnormality in the eye. In many cases, there is a disturbance of the visual pathway between the *retina* and the brain. The term amblyopia is also some-times applied to toxic or nutritional causes of decreased visual acuity, as in tobacco–alcohol amblyopia.

If normal vision is to develop during infancy and childhood, it is essential that clear, corresponding visual images are formed on both retinas so that compatible nerve impulses pass from the eyes to the brain. If no images are received, normal vision cannot develop. If the images from each eye differ markedly, one will be suppressed to avoid double vision.

CAUSES

The most common cause of amblyopia is *squint* (a deviation of one eye relative to the other) in young children. Failure to form normal retinal images may also result from congenital (present from birth) *cataract* (opacity of the lens of the eye), and severe, or unequal, focusing errors, such as when one eye is normal and there is an uncorrected large degree of *astigmatism* in the other. Toxic and nutritional amblyopia may be the result of damage to the retina and/or the optic nerve.

TREATMENT AND OUTLOOK

The usual treatment for amblyopia due to squint is patching (covering up the good eye to force the deviating eye to function properly). Surgery to place the deviating eye in the correct position may be necessary. Glasses may be needed to correct severe focusing errors. Cataracts may be removed surgically. After the age of eight, amblyopia cannot usually be remedied.

ambulance

A vehicle for transporting sick, injured, or disabled people, usually to hospital, that is staffed by trained personnel who can provide emergency treatment during the journey.

ambulatory ECG

In ambulatory *ECG* (electrocardiography), a wearable device called a *Holter monitor* is used to record the electrical activity of the heart by means of electrodes attached to the chest. The monitor is usually worn for at least 24 hours and detects intermittent *arrhythmias* (abnormal heart rates and rhythms). It is also used to assess the programming of a cardiac pacemaker. The wearer presses a button on the monitor to mark the recording whenever symptoms occur. The recording can be analysed later to determine whether the periods of arrhythmia coincide with the symptoms. In some cases, the patient can send the recording over the telephone by means of *telecardiography* (transmission of an impulse to a site that is remote from the patient).

amelioration

In medical usage, improvement in the medical condition of a patient.

amelogenesis imperfecta

An inherited condition of the teeth in which the enamel is either abnormally thin or is deficient in calcium. The teeth of affected individuals may be pitted and discoloured (see *discoloured teeth*) and more susceptible to dental *caries* (tooth decay) and wear.

amenorrhoea

The absence of menstrual periods. Primary amenorrhoea is defined as failure to start menstruating by the age of 16. Secondary amenorrhoea is the temporary or permanent cessation of periods in a woman who has menstruated regularly in the past.

PRIMARY AMENORRHOEA

The main cause of primary amenorrhoea is the delayed onset of *puberty*. The delay may not indicate a disorder but, rarely, may result from a disorder of the *endocrine system*, such as a *pituitary tumour*, *hypothyroidism* (underactivity of the thyroid gland), an *adrenal tumour*, or *adrenal hyperplasia*. Another rare cause of delayed puberty is *Turner's syndrome*, in which one female sex chromosome is missing. In some cases, menstruation fails to take place because the vagina or uterus has been absent from birth. It may also fail to occur because there is no perforation in the hymen (the membrane across the opening of the vagina) to allow blood to escape.

SECONDARY AMENORRHOEA

The most common cause of temporary secondary amenorrhoea is *pregnancy*. Secondary amenorrhoea may also be caused by hormonal changes that occur as a result of stress, *depression*, *anorexia nervosa*, certain drugs, or a pituitary or thyroid disorder. Another possible cause is a disorder of the ovary, such as polycystic ovary (see *ovary, polycystic*) or an ovarian tumour. Amenorrhoea occurs permanently after the *menopause* or following a *hysterectomy* (a surgical operation to remove the uterus).

INVESTIGATION AND TREATMENT

Investigation of amenorrhoea usually involves a physical examination and

A

blood tests to measure hormone levels. *CT scanning* or *MRI* (techniques that produce three-dimensional or cross-sectional images) of the skull may be carried out to exclude the possibility of a pituitary tumour and *ultrasound scanning* of the abdomen and pelvis to exclude a tumour of the adrenal glands or ovaries. In some cases, *laparoscopy* (examination of the inside of the abdomen using a rigid or flexible viewing tube) may be required to inspect the ovaries.

Treatment of amenorrhoea, if found to be necessary, is of the underlying cause. (See also *dietary amenorrhoea*.)

amfebutamone

Also known as bupropion, a drug used, along with self-help measures, as an aid to stopping smoking. Side effects include a dry mouth and gastrointestinal disturbances. It is not usually prescribed for people with a history of seizures or who are at increased risk of seizures, nor for those who have an eating disorder.

amfetamine

An alternative spelling for amphetamine (see *amphetamine drugs*). (See also *controlled drugs*.)

amiloride

A potassium-sparing *diuretic drug*, amiloride is used in combination with loop or thiazide diuretics in the treatment of *hypertension* (high blood pressure) and the oedema (fluid retention) that results from *heart failure* (reduced pumping efficiency of the heart) or liver *cirrhosis*.

amino acids

A group of chemical compounds that form the basic structural units of all *proteins*. Each amino acid molecule consists of amino and carboxyl groups of atoms that are linked to a variable chain or ring of carbon atoms.

Individual amino acid molecules are linked together by chemical bonds (called *peptide* bonds) to form short chains of molecules called *polypeptides*. Hundreds of polypeptides are, in turn, linked together (also by peptide bonds) to form a protein molecule. What differentiates one protein from another is the sequence of the amino acids.

There are 20 different amino acids that make up all the proteins in the body. Of these, 12 can be made by the body; they are known as nonessential amino acids because they do not need

to be obtained from the diet. The other eight, the essential amino acids, cannot be made by the body and must be obtained in the diet.

The 20 amino acids that make up proteins also occur free within cells and in body fluids. In addition, there are more than 200 other amino acids that are not found in proteins but play an important role in chemical reactions within cells.

aminoglycoside drugs

Aminoglycosides, a type of *antibiotic drug*, are given by injection and, because their use can damage the inner ear or kidneys, are generally reserved for the treatment of serious infections. Important examples of these drugs are *gentamicin* and *streptomycin*, which are also used topically for eye and ear infections.

aminophylline

A *bronchodilator drug* used to treat *asthma* and chronic obstructive pulmonary disease (see *pulmonary disease, chronic obstructive*). Aminophylline relieves breathing difficulty by widening the bronchi (main air passages to the lungs).

Possible side effects of aminophylline include nausea, vomiting, headache, dizziness, and palpitations.

amiodarone

An *antiarrhythmic drug* used in the treatment of various types of *arrhythmia* (irregular heart rate or rhythm). Long-term use of amiodarone may result in inflammation of the liver, thyroid problems, and damage to the eyes and lungs. For this reason, amiodarone is usually given only when other drugs have failed to be effective.

amitriptyline

A tricyclic *antidepressant drug* with a sedative effect. Amitriptyline is useful in the treatment of *depression* accompanied by *anxiety* or *insomnia*. Possible adverse effects include blurred vision, dizziness, and drowsiness.

amlodipine

A *calcium channel blocker* drug that is used to prevent *angina* and to treat *hypertension* (high blood pressure). Possible side effects of amlodipine include headaches and dizziness.

ammonia

A colourless, pungent gas that dissolves in water to form ammonium hydroxide,

an alkaline solution (see *alkali*). Ammonia consists of one nitrogen atom linked to three hydrogen atoms. Ammonia is produced in the body and helps to maintain the *acid–base balance*.

In severe liver damage, the capacity of the liver to convert ammonia to *urea* is diminished. This leads to a high concentration of ammonia in the blood, which is thought to be a major cause of the impaired consciousness that occurs in *liver failure*.

amnesia

Loss of the ability to memorize information and/or recall information stored in *memory*. Amnesic conditions affect mainly long-term memory (where information is retained indefinitely) rather than short-term memory (where it is only retained for seconds or minutes).

Many people with amnesia have a memory gap that extends back for some time before the onset of the disorder. This condition, known as retrograde amnesia, is principally a deficit of recall. In the majority of cases, the memory gap gradually shrinks over time.

Some people with amnesia are unable to store new information in the period following the onset of the illness. The resultant gap in memory, known as anterograde amnesia, extends from the moment of onset of the amnesia to the time when the long-term memory resumes (if at all). This memory gap is usually permanent.

CAUSES
Amnesia is the result of damage to, or disease of, regions in the brain that are concerned with memory function. Possible causes of such damage are *head injury*; degenerative disorders such as *Alzheimer's disease* and other forms of *dementia*; infections such as *encephalitis*; thiamine deficiency in problem drinkers, which leads to *Wernicke–Korsakoff syndrome*; *brain tumours*; *strokes*; and *subarachnoid haemorrhage*. Amnesia can also occur in some forms of psychiatric illness (in which there is no apparent physical damage to the brain). Some deterioration of memory is a common feature of *aging*.

amniocentesis

A diagnostic procedure in which a small amount of *amniotic fluid* is withdrawn, using a syringe guided by *ultrasound scanning*, from the *amniotic sac* (the membrane that surrounds the *fetus* in the *uterus*).

WHY IT IS DONE

The amniotic fluid contains fetal cells, which can be subjected to *chromosome analysis* in order to identify or exclude various chromosomal defects, such as *Down's syndrome*, or genetic analysis to look for *genetic disorders* such as *haemophilia*, *cystic fibrosis*, and *Tay–Sachs disease*.

The amniotic fluid also contains various chemicals; and analysis of the fluid can help to diagnose or exclude developmental abnormalities such as *spina bifida* (a neural tube defect). The severity of *rhesus incompatibility* and the maturity of the fetal lungs can also be checked by amniocentesis.

HOW IT IS DONE

Amniocentesis is usually performed between the 15th and 20th weeks of pregnancy. It may be performed earlier, but it is technically more difficult at this early stage.

The skin of the abdomen is cleaned and a needle is inserted into the amniotic sac; in all cases, ultrasound scanning is used to avoid contact with the fetus and placenta. An attached syringe removes some fluid for analysis.

COMPLICATIONS

Amniocentesis slightly increases the risk of *miscarriage* or early rupture of the membranes, and the procedure is therefore recommended only when the fetus is thought to be at increased risk of an abnormality. (See also *antenatal care*; *chorionic villus sampling*.)

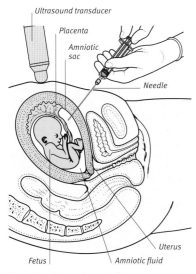

Procedure for amniocentesis
A needle, guided by ultrasound, is introduced through the uterine wall into the amniotic sac; a sample of amniotic fluid is then withdrawn.

amnion

One of the membranes that surrounds the *fetus* in the *uterus*. The outside of the amnion is covered by another membrane called the *chorion*.

amniotic fluid

The clear, watery fluid (popularly called the "waters") that surrounds the *fetus* in the *uterus* and is contained within the *amniotic sac* (a thin, membranous bag). Amniotic fluid cushions the fetus against pressure from the mother's internal organs, allowing movement.

Amniotic fluid is produced by cells that line the amniotic sac and is constantly circulated. The fetus swallows the fluid, which is absorbed into the fetal bloodstream and then excreted by the kidneys as urine. The fluid is 99 per cent water. The remainder consists of dilute concentrations of the substances found in *blood* plasma, along with cells and *lipids* (fats) from the fetus.

Amniotic fluid appears during the first week following conception, and it gradually increases in volume until the tenth week, when it increases very rapidly. After approximately 35 weeks' gestation, the volume of fluid slowly starts to decline.

In a small number of pregnancies, *polyhydramnios* (the formation of excessive amounts of amniotic fluid) occurs; less frequently, *oligohydramnios* (the formation of insufficient fluid) occurs.

amniotic sac

The membranous bag that surrounds the *fetus* and is filled with *amniotic fluid* as pregnancy advances. The sac is made up of two membranes, the inner *amnion* and the outer *chorion*.

amniotomy

Artificial rupture of the amniotic membranes. Amniotomy, which is popularly known as "breaking of the waters", is performed for *induction of labour*.

amoeba

A type of protozoon (see *protozoa*). An amoeba is a microscopic single-celled organism with an irregular, changeable shape. Amoebae live in moist environments such as fresh water and soil. Some types are parasites of humans, causing diseases such as *amoebiasis*.

amoebiasis

An infection caused by the amoeba ENTAMOEBA HISTOLYTICA, a tiny single-celled parasite that lives in the human large intestine. Amoebiasis is spread through eating food or drinking water contaminated by human excreta containing cysts of the amoeba.

Once the cysts are swallowed, the cyst walls break down, and the amoebae hatch out to parasitize the large intestine. In the intestine, the amoebae multiply and develop protective capsules, forming new cysts. These cysts are passed out of the body in the faeces and can survive for long periods before the next person acquires them.

SYMPTOMS

Some individuals carry the ENTAMOEBA HISTOLYTICA parasite in their intestines and excrete cysts without having symptoms. However, some strains of the amoebae invade and ulcerate the intestinal wall, causing diarrhoea and abdominal pain, which may develop into full-blown *dysentery*.

The amoebae may spread through the bloodstream to the liver or, rarely, to the brain or lung, where they cause abscesses. Symptoms of an amoebic liver abscess include weight loss, chills, fever, and painful liver enlargement. Liver abscesses may also sometimes occur in the absence of symptoms.

PREVENTION AND TREATMENT

Travellers to countries where sanitary standards are low can reduce their risk of acquiring amoebiasis by drinking only bottled or thoroughly boiled water and by not eating uncooked vegetables or unpeeled fruit.

Treatment of all forms of amoebiasis is with drugs such as *metronidazole* or diloxanide. These drugs kill the parasite within a few weeks, leading to complete recovery.

amoebic dysentery

See *amoebiasis*.

amoebicides

A group of drugs that are used to treat *amoebiasis*. Examples of amoebicides are diloxanide and *metronidazole*. The drugs work by killing amoebae (see *amoeba*) in the intestine and in other body tissues.

amoxicillin

A *penicillin drug* commonly used to treat a variety of infections, including *cystitis*, *bronchitis*, and ear and skin infections. Allergy to it causes a blotchy rash and, rarely, fever, swollen mouth and tongue, itching, and breathing difficulty.

Amoxil

A brand name for the antibiotic drug *amoxicillin*.

amoxycillin

See *amoxicillin*.

amphetamine drugs

COMMON DRUGS

• Dexamfetamine

A group of *stimulant drugs* used mainly in the treatment of *narcolepsy* (a rare disorder that is characterized by excessive sleepiness).

HOW THEY WORK

Amphetamine drugs stimulate secretion of *neurotransmitters* (chemicals released by nerve endings), such as *noradrenaline* (norepinephrine), which increase nerve activity in the brain and make a person wakeful and alert.

SIDE EFFECTS

In high doses, amphetamines can cause tremor, sweating, anxiety, and sleeping problems. Delusions, hallucinations, high blood pressure, and seizures may also occur. Prolonged use may produce *tolerance* and *drug dependence*.

ABUSE

Amphetamines may be abused for their stimulant and appetite suppressant effects, and for these reasons they are *controlled drugs*.

amphotericin

An antifungal drug used to treat *candidiasis* of the mouth or intestine. The drug is taken as tablets but is also given by intravenous infusion to treat life-threatening systemic (generalized) fungal infections such as *cryptococcosis* and *histoplasmosis*.

Side effects, which include vomiting, fever, headache, and, rarely, seizures, may occur with intravenous infusion.

ampicillin

A *penicillin drug* commonly used to treat *cystitis*, *bronchitis*, and ear infections. Diarrhoea is a common adverse effect. Some people are allergic to ampicillin and suffer from rash, fever, swelling of the mouth and tongue, itching, and breathing difficulty.

ampoule

A small glass or plastic vessel that can be hermetically sealed to hold liquid substances, in a sterile condition, for *injection*. Each ampoule usually contains a single dose of a drug.

ampulla

An enlarged, flask-shaped area at the end of a tubular structure or canal. There are several ampullae in the body, including those at the end of each fallopian tube, on each of the three semicircular canals of the inner ear, and at the opening of the bile duct leading into the intestine.

amputation

The surgical removal of part or all of a limb. Amputation may be needed if the blood supply to the limb has been permanently lost. It may also be necessary in some instances of cancer. The operation is now quite rarely performed.

WHY IT IS DONE

Amputation is necessary if *peripheral vascular disease*, as a result of *atherosclerosis* or *diabetes mellitus*, has destroyed the blood supply to a limb. If the blood supply cannot be restored, amputation is carried out to prevent the development of *gangrene* (tissue death).

Amputation may also occasionally be performed to prevent the spread of a *bone cancer* or malignant melanoma (see *melanoma, malignant*), a type of skin cancer. If a limb has been irreparably damaged in an accident, a decision may also be taken to amputate.

HOW IT IS DONE

During the operation, skin and muscle are cut below the level at which the bone is to be severed to create flaps that will later provide a fleshy stump. The blood vessels are tied off, the bone is sawn through, the area is washed with saline (salt solution), and the flaps of skin and muscle are stitched over the sawn end of bone to form a smooth and rounded stump.

If a prosthesis (see *limb, artificial*) is to be fitted, the surgeon tries to ensure that nerves are severed well above the stump in order to reduce the risk of pressure pain. In an amputation at the ankle (Syme's amputation), the tough skin of the heel pad is retained to cover the stump, reducing the need for a prosthetic foot.

RECOVERY AND OUTLOOK

The stump is usually swollen for about six weeks after the operation. For some time after amputation, there may also be an unpleasant sensation that the limb is still present. This phenomenon is known as "phantom limb". A prosthesis will usually be fitted, if necessary, once the stump has healed and the swelling has gone down.

amputation, congenital

The separation of a body part (usually a limb, finger, or toe) from the rest of the body, as a result of the blood supply to the part being blocked, in the uterus, by a band of *amnion* (fetal membrane). At birth, the affected part may be either completely separated, or it may show the marks of the "amniotic band". (See also *limb defects*.)

amputation, traumatic

Loss of a finger, toe, or limb through injury. (See also *microsurgery*.)

amylase

An *enzyme* that is found in *saliva* and pancreatic secretions (see *pancreas*). Amylase helps the body to digest dietary starch, breaking it down into smaller components, such as the sugars *glucose* and maltose.

Amsler chart

A diagnostic tool used by ophthalmologists to detect changes in the retina, particularly those changes that indicate *macular degeneration*. A typical Amsler chart consists of a grid of black lines on a white background. In an individual with retinal changes, the lines may appear distorted.

amyl nitrite

A *nitrate drug* that was once prescribed to relieve *angina pectoris*. It frequently caused adverse effects and is no longer legally available; it has been superseded by other drugs such as *glyceryl trinitrate* and *isosorbide*. Amyl nitrite is sometimes abused for its effect of intensifying pleasure during orgasm.

amyloidosis

An uncommon disease in which a substance called amyloid, composed of fibrous protein, accumulates in tissues and organs, including the liver, kidneys, tongue, spleen, and heart.

CAUSES

Amyloidosis may occur for no known reason, in which case it is known as primary amyloidosis; more commonly, however, it is a complication of some other disease, and in such cases it is known as secondary amyloidosis.

Conditions that may lead to amyloidosis include *multiple myeloma* (a cancer of bone marrow), *rheumatoid arthritis*, *familial Mediterranean fever*, *tuberculosis*, and other longstanding infections such as chronic *osteomyelitis* (bone infection). Amyloid is also deposited in the brain in *Alzheimer's disease*. Small deposits of amyloid are a normal feature of *aging*.

SYMPTOMS AND SIGNS

The symptoms of amyloidosis vary, depending on the organs affected and the duration of the condition. Affected organs typically become enlarged. An accumulation of amyloid in the heart may result in *arrhythmias* (disturbances of the heart rate or rhythm) and *heart failure* (reduced pumping efficiency of the heart). If the stomach and intestines are affected, symptoms such as diarrhoea may develop, and the lining of these organs may become ulcerated. Primary amyloidosis is often characterized by deposits of amyloid in the skin, which appear as slightly raised, waxy spots. Deposits of amyloid in the kidneys may cause *kidney failure*, which can be fatal.

TREATMENT

There is no treatment for the removal of amyloid deposits. However, it is possible to halt the progression of secondary amyloidosis by treatment of the underlying disorder.

amyotrophic lateral sclerosis

See *motor neuron disease*.

amyotrophy

Shrinkage or wasting away of a muscle, caused by a reduction in the size of its fibres, leading to weakness. Amyotrophy is usually the result of poor nutrition, reduced use of the muscle (as occurs when a limb is immobilized for a long period), or disruption of the blood or nerve supply to the muscle (as can occur in *poliomyelitis* or *diabetes mellitus*). (See also *atrophy*.)

anabolic steroids

See *steroids, anabolic*.

anabolism

The manufacture of complex molecules such as *fats* and *proteins* from simpler molecules by metabolic (chemical and physical) processes in living cells. (See also *catabolism*; *metabolism*.)

anaemia

A condition in which the concentration of the oxygen-carrying pigment *haemoglobin* in the blood is below normal. Haemoglobin molecules are carried inside red *blood cells* and transport oxygen from the lungs to the tissues. Normally, stable haemoglobin concen-

trations in the blood are maintained by a balance between red-cell production in the bone marrow and red-cell destruction in the spleen. Anaemia may result if this balance is upset.

TYPES AND CAUSES

Anaemia is not a disease in itself but a feature of many different disorders. There are various types, which can be classified into those due to decreased or defective red blood cell production by bone marrow (see *anaemia, aplastic*; *anaemia, megaloblastic*; *anaemia, iron-deficiency*) and those due to decreased survival of the red cells in the blood (see *anaemia, haemolytic*). The illustrated box shows the main types of anaemia.

SYMPTOMS

The symptoms common to all forms of anaemia result from the reduced oxygen-carrying capacity of the blood, and the severity of symptoms depends on how low the haemoglobin concentration has become. Slightly reduced levels can cause tiredness, and lethargy. Severely reduced levels can cause breathing difficulty on exercise, dizziness due to reduced oxygen reaching the brain, *angina pectoris* (chest pain due to insufficient oxygen reaching the heart), and palpitations as the heart works harder to compensate. General symptoms include pallor, particularly of the skin creases, lining of the mouth, and inside of the eyelids.

TYPES AND CAUSES OF **ANAEMIA**

Anaemia results either from reduced or defective production or an excessively high rate of destruction of oxygen-carrying red blood cells. Four of the main types are shown below, but anaemia can have many other causes (such as various forms of leukaemia).

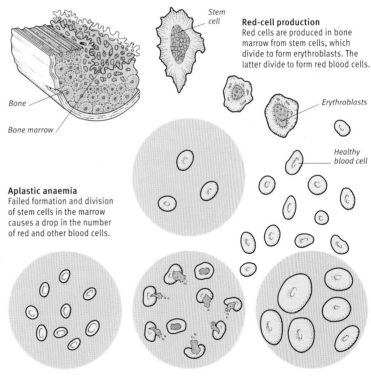

Stem cell

Red-cell production
Red cells are produced in bone marrow from stem cells, which divide to form erythroblasts. The latter divide to form red blood cells.

Bone

Bone marrow

Erythroblasts

Healthy blood cell

Aplastic anaemia
Failed formation and division of stem cells in the marrow causes a drop in the number of red and other blood cells.

Iron-deficiency anaemia
Lack of iron prevents the bone marrow from making sufficient haemoglobin for the red cells. The cells produced are small and pale and have a reduced oxygen-carrying capacity.

Haemolytic anaemia
This type includes all anaemias in which the rate of red-cell production is normal or high but in which the cells are destroyed at a much faster rate than normal.

Megaloblastic anaemia
A deficient supply of certain vitamins causes the bone marrow to produce red cells that are larger than normal; they also have a reduced oxygen-carrying capacity.

A

Other features may occur with particular forms of anaemia. For example, some degree of *jaundice* occurs in most types of haemolytic anaemia because the high rate of destruction of red blood cells leads to an increased level of the yellow pigment bilirubin (produced by the breakdown of the haemoglobin in red cells) in the blood.

DIAGNOSIS
Anaemia is diagnosed from the patient's symptoms and by blood tests (see *blood count*). A *bone marrow biopsy* (removal of a small sample of bone marrow for analysis) may be required to determine whether or not red blood cell production is defective.

anaemia, aplastic
A rare but serious type of *anaemia* (a reduced level of the oxygen-carrying pigment *haemoglobin* in the blood). In aplastic anaemia, the red cells, white cells, and platelets in the blood are all reduced in number. The condition is caused by a failure of the *bone marrow* to produce stem cells, the initial form of all blood cells.

CAUSES
Treatment of cancer with *radiotherapy* or *anticancer drugs* can temporarily interfere with the cell-producing ability of bone marrow, as can certain viral infections and other drugs. Long-term exposure to toxic chemicals may cause more persistent aplastic anaemia; and another recognized cause is a moderate to high dose of nuclear radiation. An *autoimmune disorder* (in which the immune system attacks the body's own tissues) is responsible in some cases. Aplastic anaemia sometimes develops for no known reason.

SYMPTOMS
A low level of red blood cells may cause symptoms, such as fatigue and breathlessness, that are common to all types of anaemia. Deficiency of white cells increases susceptibility to infection, resulting in frequent or severe infections; platelet deficiency may lead to a tendency to bruise easily, bleeding gums, and nosebleeds.

DIAGNOSIS AND TREATMENT
Aplastic anaemia is usually suspected from results of a blood test, particularly a *blood count*, and is confirmed by a *bone marrow biopsy* (removal of a sample of bone marrow for microscopic analysis).

Blood and platelet transfusions can control symptoms. Immunosuppression (therapy to suppress the immune system) is used to treat aplastic anaemia due to an autoimmune process. Severe persistent aplastic anaemia may be fatal without a *bone marrow transplant* or a *stem cell* transplant.

anaemia, deficiency
Forms of *anaemia* (a reduced level of the oxygen-carrying pigment *haemoglobin* in the blood) caused by lack of one or more substance that are essential for normal haemoglobin synthesis and maintenance. Deficiency anaemia may arise by various means, such as by *malabsorption* or insufficient dietary intake of a particular nutrient. *Iron-deficiency anaemia* and *megaloblastic anaemia* are examples of deficiency anaemias.

anaemia, haemolytic
A form of *anaemia* (a reduced level of the oxygen-carrying pigment *haemoglobin* in the blood) caused by premature destruction of red blood cells in the bloodstream (see *haemolysis*). The bone marrow has the capacity to increase its red cell production approximately sixfold over normal rates. Haemolytic anaemia will result only if the shortening of the lifespan of red blood cells is sufficiently severe to overcome the reserve capacity of the bone marrow.

TYPES AND CAUSES
Haemolytic anaemias can be classified in two ways: if the cause of the haemolysis is an abnormality of the red cells themselves, the condition is usually inherited; if the cause of the haemolysis is outside the cells, the condition is usually acquired later in life.

When haemolysis is due to a defect in the red cells, the underlying problem may be abnormal rigidity of the cell membrane. This causes the cells to become trapped, at an early stage of their lifespan, in the small blood vessels of the spleen, where they are destroyed by macrophages (cells that ingest foreign particles). Abnormal rigidity may result from an inherited defect of the cell membrane (as in hereditary *spherocytosis*), a defect of the *haemoglobin* in the cell (as in *sickle-cell anaemia*), or a defect of a cell *enzyme*. An inherited deficiency of the glucose-6-phosphate dehydrogenase enzyme (see *G6PD deficiency*) may result in episodes of haemolytic anaemia since the red cells are prone to damage by infectious illness or certain drugs or foods. One variety of G6PD deficiency is most common in Mediterranean countries (see *favism*).

Haemolytic anaemias due to defects outside the red cells fall into three main groups. First are disorders in which red cells are destroyed by buffeting (by artificial surfaces such as replacement heart valves, abnormal blood-vessel linings, or a blood clot in a vessel, for example). In the second group, the red cells are destroyed by the *immune system*. Immune haemolytic anaemias may occur if foreign blood cells enter the bloodstream, as occurs in an incompatible blood transfusion, or they may be due to an *autoimmune disorder* (in which the immune system attacks the body's own tissues). In *haemolytic disease of the newborn*, the baby's red cells are destroyed by antibodies, produced by the mother, crossing the placenta. Thirdly, the red cells may be destroyed by microorganisms in the blood; the most common cause is *malaria*.

SYMPTOMS
People with haemolytic anaemia may have symptoms common to all types of anaemia, such as fatigue and breathlessness, or symptoms that are specifically due to haemolysis, such as *jaundice* (caused by an excessive concentration in the blood of bile pigments formed from the destruction of red blood cells).

DIAGNOSIS AND TREATMENT
Diagnosis is confirmed by microscopic examination of the blood (see *blood film*). Treatment depends on the cause. Some inherited anaemias can be controlled by removing the spleen (see *splenectomy*). Others, such as G6PD deficiency and favism, can be prevented by avoiding the drugs or foods that precipitate haemolysis. Anaemias due to immune processes can often be controlled by *immunosuppressant drugs*. Transfusions of red cells are sometimes needed for emergency treatment of life-threatening anaemia.

anaemia, iron-deficiency
The most common form of *anaemia* (a reduced level of the oxygen-carrying pigment *haemoglobin* in the blood). Iron-deficiency anaemia is caused by a deficiency of iron, an essential constituent of haemoglobin.

CAUSES
The commonest cause of iron-deficiency anaemia is iron loss due to heavy or persistent bleeding; the most common cause in women of childbearing age is particularly heavy periods (see *menorrhagia*). Pregnancy stops menstrual losses, but the baby is an even greater

drain on maternal iron stores. Other causes include blood loss from the digestive tract due to disorders such as erosive *gastritis*, *peptic ulcer*, *stomach cancer*, *inflammatory bowel disease*, *haemorrhoids*, and bowel tumours (see *colon, cancer of*). Prolonged use of aspirin and other *nonsteroidal anti-inflammatory drugs* (NSAIDs) can cause gastrointestinal bleeding. In some countries, *hookworm infestation* of the digestive tract is an important cause of anaemia. Rarely, bleeding may also occur as a result of disorders of the urinary tract (such as *kidney tumours* or *bladder tumours*).

Iron deficiency may also be caused or worsened by lack of iron in, or its poor absorption from, the diet. Malabsorption of iron may have various causes, including the removal of part or all of the stomach (see *gastrectomy*) or *coeliac disease* (a disorder that impairs digestion).

SYMPTOMS
The symptoms of iron-deficiency anaemia are those of the underlying cause, along with a sore mouth or tongue; and those that are common to all forms of anaemia, such as fatigue, headaches, and breathlessness.

DIAGNOSIS AND TREATMENT
Diagnosis is made from a *blood count* that reveals the red blood cells to be microcytic (abnormally small). Measurement of the iron levels in the blood confirms the diagnosis but further investigation will be needed to establish the underlying cause. Treatment is given for the underlying cause, along with a course of iron tablets or, very rarely, iron injections to build up the depleted iron stores.

anaemia, megaloblastic

A major type of *anaemia* (a reduced level of the oxygen-carrying pigment haemoglobin in the blood). Megaloblastic anaemia is caused by deficiency of vitamin B_{12} or another vitamin, folic acid. Either of these deficiencies seriously interferes with the production of red blood cells in the bone marrow. An excess of cells known as megaloblasts (abnormal immature red cells) appears in the marrow. Megaloblasts give rise to enlarged and deformed red blood cells known as macrocytes.

CAUSES
Vitamin B_{12} deficiency Vitamin B_{12} is found only in foods of animal origin, such as meat and dairy products. It is absorbed from the small intestine by first combining with intrinsic factor, a chemical produced by the stomach lin-

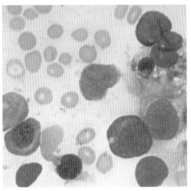

Bone marrow in megaloblastic anaemia
In this microscopic view, some of the large cells are abnormal red-cell precursors (megaloblasts).

ing. The most common cause of vitamin B_{12} deficiency is *pernicious anaemia* in which the stomach lining fails to produce intrinsic factor, usually as a result of an *autoimmune disorder* (in which the immune system attacks the body's own tissues). Total gastrectomy (removal of the stomach) also prevents the production of intrinsic factor, and removal of part of the small intestine prevents B_{12} absorption, as does the intestinal disorder *Crohn's disease*. In a minority of cases, vitamin B_{12} deficiency is due to a vegan diet (which excludes all foods of animal origin).

Folic acid deficiency Folic acid is found mainly in green vegetables and liver. The usual cause of deficiency is a poor diet. It can also be caused by anything that interferes with absorption of folic acid from the small intestine (Crohn's disease or *coeliac disease*, for example). Folic acid is required by rapidly dividing cells, as in the fetus. Women are advised to take the recommended dose of folic acid supplements before conception and in early pregnancy, although this is to reduce the risk of the fetus having a *neural tube defect* rather than to prevent anaemia.

SYMPTOMS
Many people with mild megaloblastic anaemia have no symptoms. Others may experience tiredness, a sore mouth and tongue, weight loss, and mild *jaundice*. If B_{12} deficiency continues for a long time, additional symptoms as a result of nerve damage, including numbness and tingling in the feet, may develop.

DIAGNOSIS AND TREATMENT
Megaloblastic anaemia is diagnosed by *blood tests* and confirmed if a *bone marrow biopsy* (removal of a sample of marrow for microscopic analysis) reveals the presence of numerous megaloblasts.

Megaloblastic anaemia caused by poor diet can be remedied with a short course of vitamin B_{12} injections or folic acid tablets and the introduction of a normal diet. A lifelong course of vitamin B_{12} injections or folic acid tablets is required if the underlying cause of malabsorption is incurable.

anaemia, pernicious

See *pernicious anaemia*.

anaemia, sickle cell

See *sickle cell anaemia*.

anaerobic

Capable of living, functioning, and growing without oxygen. Many bacteria are anaerobes and thrive in the intestinal canal or in tissue that has a poor supply of oxygenated blood.

Some human body cells are capable of limited anaerobic activity. When muscular exertion is so strenuous that oxygen is used faster than the blood circulation can supply it (during sprinting, for example), the muscle cells can temporarily work anaerobically. When this happens, lactic acid is produced as a waste product (instead of the carbon dioxide that is produced from *aerobic* activity). This acid buildup can cause muscle fatigue and pain, thereby limiting the time for which anaerobic activity can be carried out. Compensation for this anaerobic activity requires oxygen to convert the lactic acid to glucose or to carbon dioxide, which explains the need to continue to breathe rapidly following vigorous exertion. The deficit of oxygen that builds up in the muscles during exercise is known as the oxygen debt.

anaesthesia

The absence of all sensation; insensibility. The term most commonly refers to anaesthesia that is induced artificially for medical purposes.

Two types of anaesthesia may be used: local (see *anaesthesia, local*) and general (see *anaesthesia, general*). A patient given a local anaesthetic remains conscious, and sensation is abolished in only a specific part of the body. A patient under general anaesthesia is rendered unconscious and maintained in this state with a combination of drugs that are either injected into a vein or inhaled.

Damage to nerve tissues by injury or disease can produce anaesthesia in a localized area.

A

anaesthesia, dental

Reversible loss of sensation induced in a patient to prevent pain during dental treatment. Topical anaesthetics (usually using the drug lidocaine (lignocaine) as a cream or spray) are often used on the surface of the gums before injection of a local anaesthetic (see *anaesthesia, local*).

For minor procedures, a local anaesthetic is injected either into the gum at the site being treated or around the nerve a short distance away (a procedure known as a peripheral *nerve block*). For more complicated procedures, such as periodontal (gum) surgery and multiple tooth extractions, general anaesthesia (see *anaesthesia, general*) is carried out.

anaesthesia, epidural

See *epidural anaesthesia*.

anaesthesia, general

Reversible loss of sensation and consciousness induced to prevent the perception of pain throughout the body during surgery. General anaesthesia is also used to abolish muscle tone and cardiovascular reflexes in the patient.

The state of general anaesthesia is produced and maintained by an anaesthetist, who gives combinations of drugs by injection, inhalation, or both. The anaesthetist is also responsible for the pre-anaesthetic assessment and medication of patients, their safety during surgery, and their recovery during the post-anaesthetic period.

HOW IT IS DONE

General anaesthesia is usually induced by intravenous injection of propofol or a *barbiturate drug*, usually via a *cannula* (a blunt-ended tube), which is left in place in case further drugs need to be given. Anaesthesia is maintained by the inhalation of anaesthetic gases such as isoflurane or nitrous oxide, which may be introduced into the lungs via a face mask or an *endotracheal tube* (a flexible tube passed into the *trachea* through the nose or mouth). During the anaesthetic, blood pressure, pulse, oxygen saturation (see *oximeter*), and other vital signs are monitored continuously. The principal stages in administering, maintaining, and reversing general anaesthesia are shown in the illustrated box.

POSSIBLE COMPLICATIONS

General anaesthetics have become much safer and serious complications are now rare. However, the presence of severe pre-existing diseases, such as lung or heart disorders, increase the risks of the

procedure. Minor after-effects, such as nausea and vomiting, are usually controlled effectively with *antiemetic drugs*.

anaesthesia, local

Reversible loss of sensation induced in a limited region of the body to prevent pain during diagnostic or treatment procedures, examinations, and surgery. Local anaesthesia is produced by administration of drugs that temporarily interrupt the action of pain-carrying nerve fibres.

HOW IT IS DONE

Local anaesthetics may be applied topically, before injections or blood tests, as sprays, skin creams, and ointments. These are often used for children. The throat, larynx (voicebox), and respiratory passages can be sprayed with an anaesthetic before *bronchoscopy* (examination of the bronchi, the main airways of the lungs, using a rigid or flexible viewing tube) and the urethra can be numbed with a gel before *cystoscopy* (examination of the urethra and bladder using a rigid or flexible viewing tube).

For minor surgical procedures, such as stitching of small wounds, local anaesthesia is usually produced by dir-

ect injection into the area to be treated. To anaesthetize a large area, or when a local injection would not penetrate deeply enough into body tissues, a *nerve block* (in which the local anaesthetic is injected around nerves at a point remote from the area to be treated) may be used. Nerve impulses can also be blocked where they branch off from the spinal cord, as in *epidural anaesthesia*, which is used in childbirth or caudal block, and *spinal anaesthesia*, which is used for surgery on the lower limbs and abdomen.

POSSIBLE COMPLICATIONS

Serious reactions are uncommon, but repeated use of topical preparations may cause local allergic rashes.

anaesthesia, spinal

See *spinal anaesthesia*.

anaesthetics

A term for the group of drugs that produce *anaesthesia* and for the medical discipline that is concerned with their administration.

An anaesthetist is a specialist who administers anaesthetics. Before a patient goes to the operating theatre, the anaesthetist assesses the condition of the

LOCAL **ANAESTHETICS**

Drug	Common uses	How given
Tetracaine (amethocaine)	Prior to taking a blood sample or inserting a cannula	Gel
Benzocaine	To treat painful conditions of the mouth and throat, painful anal conditions (e.g. haemorrhoids), skin wounds	Lozenges, suppositories, spray, cream, ointment
Bupivacaine	As nerve block (e.g. epidural anaesthesia and caudal block)	Injection
Cocaine	For surgery on the nose, throat and larynx	Spray, liquid
Lidocaine (lignocaine)	For relief of pain during dental treatment; for spinal anaesthesia, nerve blocks (e.g. epidural anaesthesia), eye surgery, and before taking blood samples in children; for urethra prior to catheterization and larynx prior to laryngoscopy	Injection, gel, spray, cream, ointment, liquid, eye-drops, suppositories
Prilocaine	As nerve block (e.g. epidural anaesthesia and caudal block)	Injection

TECHNIQUES FOR **GENERAL ANAESTHESIA**

The main phases in the administration of a general anaesthetic are induction (bringing about unconsciousness), maintenance (of unconsciousness), and emergence (returning the patient to consciousness). Some of the main stages are shown below. Often, to allow surgical manipulation, a muscle relaxant must be given in addition to anaesthetic gases or injections. Because the relaxant temporarily paralyses the breathing muscles, the patient's lungs must be ventilated artificially. Modern general anaesthetics have few side effects, and recovery is usually prompt.

DRUGS USED IN GENERAL ANAESTHESIA

Type	Action	Examples
Drugs given as premedication	Relax patient, relieve anxiety; some reduce saliva and mucus formation	Atropine, diazepam, hyoscine, lorazepam, temazepam
Induction agents	Induce unconsciousness	Etomidate, ketamine, propofol, thiopental sodium
Anaesthetic gases and volatile agents	Induce and/or maintain unconsciousness	Isoflurane, nitrous oxide, desflurane, sevoflurane
Analgesics	Abolish pain	Fentanyl, ketoprofen, morphine
Muscle relaxants	Relax (paralyse) muscles	Pancuronium, vecuronium
Reversal agents	Reverse muscle relaxation	Neostigmine

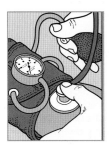

1 Before the operation, the anaesthetist talks to and examines the patient to assess his or her fitness for anaesthesia and surgery. He or she also answers any questions the patient may have.

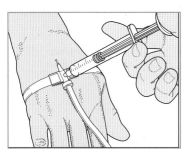

2 The induction agent is usually given via a cannula inserted into a vein. The cannula is left in position so that other drugs can be given rapidly if needed.

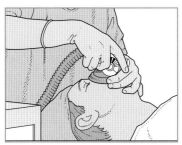

3 Sometimes, anaesthesia is induced or maintained with gases delivered by mask. If no muscle relaxant is used, the patient may be able to continue breathing naturally.

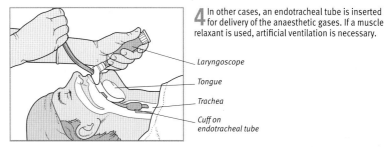

4 In other cases, an endotracheal tube is inserted for delivery of the anaesthetic gases. If a muscle relaxant is used, artificial ventilation is necessary.

Laryngoscope
Tongue
Trachea
Cuff on endotracheal tube

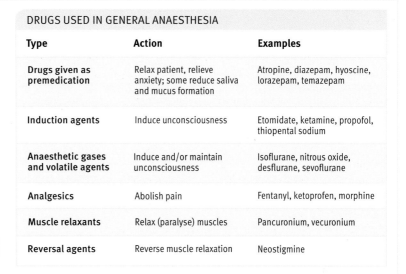

Monitor
Anaesthetic machine
Endotracheal tube
Anaesthetist
ECG leads connected to monitor

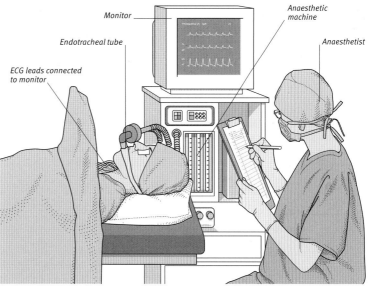

5 During surgery, the patient is kept at a level of anaesthesia deep enough for him or her to be unaware of the operation. The composition of the gas mixture, and the patient's heart rate, breathing, blood pressure, temperature, blood oxygenation, and exhaled carbon dioxide are monitored. After surgery, anaesthesia is stopped, and reversal agents are given if necessary.

patient's heart, lungs, and circulation. He or she decides the type and amount of drugs needed to induce and maintain anaesthesia, determines the patient's position on the operating table, watches for problems, and decides on the action to be taken if an emergency develops. The anaesthetist is also responsible for monitoring the progress of the waking patient, and watching for and treating any post-anaesthetic complications.

anal dilatation

A procedure in which the anus is stretched. Anal dilatation is used to treat conditions in which the anus becomes too tight, such as *anal stenosis* and *anal fissure*. It is also used to treat *haemorrhoids*. Anal dilatation is usually performed under general anaesthesia (see *anaesthesia, general*).

Reflex anal dilatation, in which the anus dilates in response to local contact, may occur in certain anal disorders or after repeated anal penetration.

anal discharge

The loss of mucus, pus, or blood from the anus. *Haemorrhoids*, *anal fissures* (tears), and *proctitis* (inflammation of the rectum) can all cause anal discharge. Rarely, cancer may be a cause.

analeptic drugs

Drugs that stimulate breathing. Replaced by *ventilation*, analeptic drugs are now seldom used.

anal fissure

A common disorder of the anus that is caused by an elongated ulcer or tear that extends upwards into the anal canal from the anal sphincter (the ring of muscle that surrounds the anal orifice). An anal fissure may be caused by the passage of hard, dry faeces.

There is usually pain during defaecation, and the muscles of the anus may go into spasm. There may also be a small amount of bright red blood on faeces or toilet paper.

The tear often heals naturally over a few days, although spasm of the anal muscles may delay healing. Treatment of recurrent or persistent fissures is usually by *anal dilatation* (a procedure to enlarge the anus) and a high-fibre diet, including whole-grain products, fruit and vegetables, and plenty of fluids, to help soften the faeces. Sometimes minor surgery is necessary to cure a chronic anal fissure.

anal fistula

An abnormal channel connecting the inside of the anal canal with the skin surrounding the anus.

An anal fistula may be an indication of *Crohn's disease*, *colitis*, or cancer of the colon or rectum (see *colon, cancer of*; *rectum, cancer of*). In most cases, it is the result of an *abscess* that develops for unknown reasons in the anal wall. The abscess discharges pus into the anus and out on to the surrounding skin.

An anal fistula is treated surgically by opening the abnormal channel and removing the lining. The operation is performed under a general anaesthetic (see *anaesthesia, general*). The wound is then left to heal naturally.

analgesia

The loss of or reduction in pain sensation. Analgesia differs from *anaesthesia* (loss of all sensation) in that sensitivity to touch is still preserved. Analgesia can be induced by the use of *analgesic drugs*.

analgesic drugs

COMMON DRUGS

OPIOIDS • Co-codamol • Co-codaprin • Codeine • Co-dydramol • Diamorphine • Dihydrocodeine • Fentanyl • Methadone • Morphine • Pentazocine • Pethidine • Tramadol

NSAIDS • Aspirin • Celecoxib • Diclofenac • Diflunisal • Etodolac • Fenbufen • Fenoprofen • Flurbiprofen • Ibuprofen • Indometacin • Ketoprofen • Mefenamic acid • Naproxen • Piroxicam

OTHER NONOPIOIDS • Nefopam • Paracetamol

Drugs used to relieve pain. The two main types are nonopioid and *opioid* analgesics. Nonopioid analgesics are useful for treating mild to moderate pain. They include *paracetamol* for headache or toothache and nonsteroidal anti-inflammatory drugs (NSAIDs), such as *aspirin* and *ibuprofen*, which can help to relieve mild pain and stiffness in arthritic conditions, such as *osteoarthritis*. Combinations of a weak opioid (such as *codeine*) with a nonopioid analgesic (such as paracetamol) can help to relieve more severe pain. Potent opioids such as *morphine* can produce *tolerance* and *drug dependence* and are used only when other analgesic preparations are ineffective.

HOW THEY WORK

When body tissues are damaged, they produce *prostaglandins* (chemicals that trigger the transmission of pain signals to the brain). Except for paracetamol, nonopioid analgesics work by preventing the production of prostaglandin; paracetamol works by blocking the pain impulses within the brain itself, preventing the perception of pain. Opioid analgesics act in a similar way to *endorphins* (pain-relieving substances formed naturally by the body) by blocking pain impulses at specific sites in the brain and spinal cord.

SIDE EFFECTS

Side effects are uncommon with paracetamol; aspirin and most NSAIDs may irritate the stomach lining and cause nausea, abdominal pain, and, rarely, a *peptic ulcer*. Nausea, drowsiness, constipation, and breathing difficulties may occur with opioid analgesics. The euphoric effect produced by some opioid analgesics have led to their abuse.

WARNING

Over-the-counter (nonopioid) analgesic drugs should not be taken for longer than 48 hours, after which time medical advice should be sought. If pain persists, becomes more severe, recurs, or differs from pain previously experienced, a doctor should be consulted. For precautions on specific drugs, see the individual drug entries.

anal phase

A term used in *psychoanalytic theory* to refer to a stage of a person's psychosexual development. The anal phase begins at around 18 months of age and lasts for up to two years. (See also *genital phase*; *oral phase*.)

anal stenosis

Tightness of the anus, sometimes known as anal stricture. Anal stenosis prevents normal passage of faeces, causing constipation and pain during defaecation.

Anal stenosis may be congenital (present from birth), or it may be caused by a number of conditions in which scarring has occurred, such as *anal fissure*, *colitis*, or cancer of the anus. The condition sometimes occurs following surgery on the anus (for example, to treat *haemorrhoids*).

Anal stenosis is treated by *anal dilatation* (a procedure that expands or enlarges the anus).

anal stricture

See *anal stenosis*.

anal tag

A type of *skin tag*.

analysis, chemical

Determination of the identity of a substance or of the individual chemical constituents of a mixture. Analysis may be qualitative (as in determining whether or not a particular substance is present), or it may be quantitative (that is, measuring the amount or concentration of one or more constituents). (See also *assay*.)

analysis, psychological

See *psychoanalysis*.

anaphylactic shock

A rare, life-threatening allergic reaction. Anaphylactic shock is a Type I hypersensitivity reaction (see *allergy*) that occurs in people with extreme sensitivity to a particular substance (known as an *allergen*), most commonly insect venom or certain foods (such as peanuts) or drugs.

When the allergen enters the bloodstream, massive amounts of *histamine* and other chemicals are released, causing sudden, severe lowering of blood pressure (which results in faintness or unconsciousness) and constriction of the airways (resulting in breathing difficulty). Other symptoms of anaphylactic shock may include abdominal pain, diarrhoea, swelling of the tongue and throat, and an itchy rash. In severe cases, anaphylactic shock may be fatal without treatment.

Anaphylactic shock requires emergency medical treatment. An injection of *adrenaline* (epinephrine) may be life-saving; a person known to be at risk of anaphylactic shock may be prescribed a preloaded syringe of adrenaline (epinephrine) by his or her doctor for use in emergencies. If the person's breathing or heartbeat has stopped, *cardiopulmonary resuscitation* should be performed; *antihistamine drugs* and *corticosteroid drugs* may also be given. (See also *hyposensitization*.)

anastomosis

A natural or artificial communication between two blood vessels or between tubular cavities that may or may not normally be joined.

Natural anastomoses usually occur when small *arteries* are attached directly to *veins* without passing through capillaries. Anastomoses occur in the skin where they are used to help control temperature regulation.

A surgical anastomosis is used to create a bypass around a blockage in an artery or in the intestine. They are also used to rejoin cut ends of the bowel or blood vessels. (See also *bypass surgery*.)

anastrozole

An *anticancer drug* that is used to treat certain types of *breast cancer* in postmenopausal women.

anatomical snuffbox

A depression on the back of the wrist that is formed between the tendons of the thumb when the thumb is stretched outwards. The anatomical snuffbox is of significance because tenderness in this area is a feature of a fracture of the *scaphoid* bone.

anatomy

The structure of the body of any living thing, and its scientific study. Human anatomy, together with *physiology* (the study of the functioning of the body), dates back to ancient Egyptian times and forms the foundation of all medical science. The dissection of human corpses has provided the primary source of information for anatomists.

Anatomy as a scientific study today is subdivided into many branches. These include comparative anatomy (the study of the differences between human and animal bodies), surgical anatomy (the practical knowledge required by surgeons), *embryology* (the study of structural changes that occur during the development of the embryo and fetus), systematic anatomy (the study of the structure of particular body systems), and *cytology* and *histology* (the microscopic study of cells and tissues respectively).

Every anatomical structure is scientifically named in Latin, but today anatomists prefer to use simpler terms,

---

HOW **ANALGESICS** WORK

When tissue is damaged (for example, by injury, inflammation, or infection) the body produces prostaglandins. These substances combine with receptors (specific sites on the surface of cells in the brain and spinal cord). As a result, a signal is passed along a series of nerve cells to the brain, where the signal is interpreted as pain by brain cells. Analgesics (except for paracetamol) work either by preventing the production of prostaglandins at the site of damage or by blocking pain impulses in the brain and spinal cord. Paracetamol works by blocking prostaglandin production in the brain, which prevents pain impulses from being transmitted in the brain.

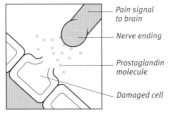

Action of opioids
When tissue damage occurs, the body produces prostaglandins, chemicals that trigger the transmission of pain signals (above). Normally, the pain signal is transmitted between brain cells, but opioid drugs (below) combine with opiate receptors to prevent the signals from being transmitted.

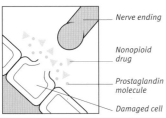

Action of NSAIDs
Nonopioid drugs block the production of prostaglandins (chemicals released in response to tissue damage). This action prevents stimulation of the nerve endings, so that no pain signal passes on to the brain. As a result, these drugs provide pain relief.

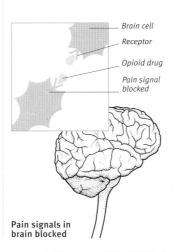

Pain signals in brain blocked

DESCRIPTIVE TERMS IN **ANATOMY**

The relative positions and movements of body parts are conventionally described with reference to the "anatomical position" (that is, an upright posture with the eyes and palms facing forwards). In this position, the parts of the body can be described in relation to various geometrical planes.

In radiology, body imaging pictures (such as CT scans and MRI) are often taken in a series of transverse planes through part of the body.

Joint movements
Extension is straightening, and flexion is bending; abduction is moving away from, adduction is moving towards, the midline of the body. Other movements are forms of rotation around an axis.

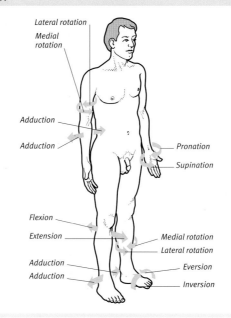

Lateral rotation
Medial rotation
Adduction
Adduction
Pronation
Supination
Flexion
Extension
Medial rotation
Lateral rotation
Adduction
Adduction
Eversion
Inversion

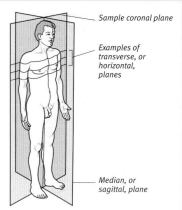

Sample coronal plane
Examples of transverse, or horizontal, planes
Median, or sagittal, plane

Planes through the body
The median plane divides the body into right and left halves. Coronal planes are vertical planes at right angles to the median plane; the coronal plane most often referred to divides the body into front and back halves. Transverse planes are horizontal slices through the body.

where they exist, as alternatives. For example, the main blood vessel in the femur (thigh bone) is usually referred to as the femoral artery rather than the arteria femoralis. For further information on the descriptive terms used in anatomy, see the illustrated box.

ancylostomiasis

Infestation of the small intestine by the ANCYLOSTOMA hookworm species. (See also *hookworm infestation*.)

androblastoma

See *arrhenoblastoma*.

androgen drugs

Natural or synthetic *androgen hormones* (male sex hormones) that are used as drugs, of which one of the most important is *testosterone*. Androgen drugs are used in the treatment of male *hypogonadism* (underactivity of the testes) to stimulate the development of male sexual characteristics.

Androgen drugs are very occasionally used to treat certain types of *breast cancer*. They have also been used by athletes and bodybuilders wishing to increase their muscle bulk and strength, which can be dangerous to health (see *steroids, anabolic*).

Possible side effects include fluid retention, weight gain, increased blood cholesterol, and, rarely, liver damage.

When taken by women, the drugs can lead to the development of male characteristics, such as facial hair.

androgen hormones

A group of hormones (the male sex hormones) that stimulate *virilization* (the development of male secondary sexual characteristics such as growth of facial hair, deepening of the voice, and increased muscle bulk).

FORMATION

Androgens are produced by specialized cells in the *testes* in males and the adrenal glands in both sexes. The ovaries secrete very small quantities of androgens until the menopause. The most active androgen is *testosterone* (produced in the testes). Androgen production by the testes is controlled by certain pituitary hormones called *gonadotrophins*. Adrenal androgens are controlled by *ACTH*, another pituitary hormone.

EFFECTS

Androgens stimulate the appearance, at *puberty*, of male secondary sexual characteristics such as deepening of the voice and the growth of facial hair. They have an anabolic effect (they raise the rate of protein synthesis and lower the rate at which it is broken down), which increases muscle bulk and accelerates growth. At the end of puberty, androgens cause the long bones to stop growing. They also stimulate the secretion of

sebum, which, if excessive, causes *acne*. In early adult life, androgens promote male-pattern baldness.

DEFICIENCY

Androgen deficiency may occur if the testes are diseased or the pituitary gland fails to secrete gonadotrophins. Typical effects include high-pitched voice, decreased body and facial hair, underdeveloped genitalia, reduced sexual drive, and poor muscle development.

EXCESS

Overproduction of androgens may be the result of adrenal disorders such as *adrenal tumours*, congenital adrenal hyperplasia (see *adrenal hyperplasia, congenital*), testicular tumours (see *testis, cancer of*), or, rarely, androgen-secreting ovarian tumours (see *ovary, cancer of*).

In men, excess androgens accentuate male physical characteristics; in boys, they cause premature sexual development. In women, excess androgens cause virilization, features of which include increased body hair, deepening of the voice, enlarged *clitoris*, and *amenorrhoea* (the absence of menstruation).

anencephaly

Absence of the brain and cranial vault (top of the skull) at birth. Most infants with anencephaly are stillborn or survive for only a few hours. Anencephaly is detectable early in pregnancy by measurement of the maternal *alpha-fetoprotein*,

TYPES OF **ANEURYSM**

An aneurysm forms when pressure from the blood flow causes a weakened artery wall to distend or forces blood through a fissure. Aneurysms can form anywhere in the body, although the most common sites are the aorta and the arteries supplying the brain.

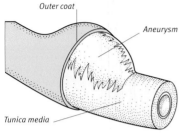

Common aneurysm
This type forms when the tunica media, the artery's middle wall, is weakened; the strong force of the blood flow distends the wall of the artery.

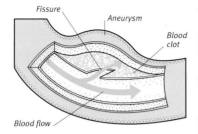

Dissecting aneurysm
In this type, blood is forced through a fissure in the internal wall of the artery. The internal lining is stripped away, forming a false channel.

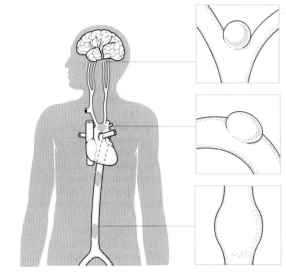

Cerebral (or berry) aneurysm
A swelling where arteries branch, often at the base of the brain, usually caused by congenital weakness.

Saccular aneurysm
A balloon-shaped distension of part of the wall of an artery, often seen in aortic aneurysms just above the heart.

Fusiform aneurysm
A spindle-shaped distension around the circumference of an artery, often seen in lower aortic aneurysms.

arterial wall can also be weakened by inflammation, as occurs in *polyarteritis nodosa*. A dissecting aneurysm is one in which the inner layer of the artery wall ruptures, allowing blood to track along the length of the artery and block any branching arteries. Ventricular aneurysms are aneurysms that sometimes develop in the heart wall due to weakening of an area of heart muscle as a result of a heart attack (see *myocardial infarction*).

Some of the common types, sites, and shapes of aneurysm are shown in the illustrated box.

SYMPTOMS AND SIGNS

Most aneurysms are symptomless and remain undetected. However, if the aneurysm expands rapidly and causes pain, or is very large, the symptoms are due to pressure on nearby structures. Aneurysms may eventually rupture, cause fatal blood loss, or, in the case of a cerebral aneurysm, loss of consciousness (see *subarachnoid haemorrhage*). A *dissecting aneurysm* usually causes severe pain, and there is a high risk of the vessel rupturing. Ventricular aneurysms seldom rupture, but they interfere with the pumping action of the heart.

DIAGNOSIS AND TREATMENT

Aneurysms of the aorta may be detected by *ultrasound scanning*, and cerebral aneurysms by *CT scanning* or *MRI*. Angiography can provide more detailed information on all types of aneurysm. A ruptured or enlarged aneurysm requires immediate *arterial reconstructive surgery*. (See also *microaneurysm*.)

angina

A strangling or constrictive pain. The term angina has become synonymous with the heart disorder *angina pectoris*. Other types of angina include abdominal angina (abdominal pain after eating caused by poor blood supply to the intestines) and Vincent's angina, which is pain caused by inflammation of the mouth (see *Vincent's disease*).

angina pectoris

Pain in the chest that is the result of insufficient oxygen being carried to the heart muscle in the blood. The pain of angina pectoris usually occurs when the heart is working harder and requires more oxygen, such as during exercise or at times of stress.

CAUSES

Inadequate blood supply to the heart is usually due to *coronary artery disease*, in which the coronary arteries are

by *ultrasound scanning*, by *amniocentesis*, or by *fetoscopy*; if anencephaly is detected, termination of the pregnancy may be considered (see *abortion, induced*).

Anencephaly is caused by a failure in the development of the neural tube, which is the nerve tissue in the embryo that normally develops into the spinal cord and brain (see *neural tube defects*).

aneurysm

Abnormal dilation (ballooning) of an *artery* caused by the pressure of blood flowing through a weakened area. The weakening may be due to disease, injury, or a congenital (present from birth) defect of the arterial wall.

Aneurysms most commonly affect the *aorta* and arteries supplying the brain.

TYPES AND CAUSES

The most common cause of an aneurysm is *atherosclerosis*, a condition in which fatty deposits weaken the artery wall. The aorta is the usual site of atherosclerotic aneurysms.

Less commonly, aneurysms may be due to a congenital (present from birth) weakness of the artery walls. Most cerebral aneurysms, known as *berry aneurysms* because of their appearance, are congenital. *Marfan syndrome*, an inherited disorder in which the wall of the aorta is defective, is often associated with aneurysms just above the heart. The

A

narrowed by *atherosclerosis* (fat deposits on the artery walls). Other causes include coronary artery spasm, in which the blood vessels narrow suddenly for a short time, *aortic stenosis*, in which the heart's aortic valve is narrowed, and cardiac *arrhythmias* (abnormal heart rhythms).

The pain of angina pectoris is brought on by exertion and is relieved by rest. If the pain continues, it may be due to a heart attack (see *myocardial infarction*). Rarer causes of the pain include severe *anaemia*, which reduces the blood's oxygen-carrying efficiency, and *polycythaemia*, which thickens the blood and causes its flow through the heart muscle to slow down.

SYMPTOMS

The chest pain of angina varies from mild to severe and is often described as a sensation of pressure on the chest. The pain usually starts in the centre of the chest but can spread to the throat, upper jaw, back, and arms (usually the left), or between the shoulderblades. If it develops during sleep or without provocation, it is called unstable angina.

Other possible symptoms of angina pectoris include nausea, sweating, dizziness, and breathing difficulty.

DIAGNOSIS AND TREATMENT

Diagnostic tests usually include an *ECG* (measurement of the electrical activity of the heart), which may register normal between attacks, and a *cardiac stress test* (an ECG undertaken while the patient is exercising). Blood tests and coronary *angiography* (*X-ray* examination of the blood vessels) may also be performed to look for an underlying cause of the angina.

Preventive measures include controlling high blood pressure (see *hypertension*) and reducing raised blood cholesterol levels. To help to control the symptoms of angina pectoris, it is important for the person to stop smoking and to lose weight if necessary. Attacks may be prevented and treated by *nitrate drugs*, which increase blood flow through the heart muscle. *Beta-blocker drugs*, *potassium channel activators*, *calcium channel blockers*, *lipid-lowering drugs*, and *antiplatelet drugs* may also be prescribed.

Drug treatment can control the symptoms for many years but cannot cure the disorder. If attacks become more severe or more frequent, despite treatment, *coronary artery bypass* surgery or *angioplasty* may be necessary.

angina, Prinzmetal's

A type of unstable angina pectoris (see *angina, unstable*) in which the attacks of chest pain occur while the body is at rest and are not brought on by exertion.

angina, unstable

A type of *angina pectoris* (chest pain due to impaired blood supply to the heart muscle) that occurs during sleep or without provocation (such as exertion).

angioedema

A type of reaction caused by *allergy*. Angioedema is similar to urticaria (hives) and is characterized by large, well-defined swellings, of sudden onset, in the skin, larynx (voicebox), and other areas. If they are left untreated, the swellings may last a number of days.

CAUSES

The most common cause of angioedema is a sudden allergic reaction to a food. Less commonly, the condition may be due to a drug allergy (such as to *penicillin*), a reaction to an insect bite or sting, or it may occur as a result of infection, emotional stress, or exposure to animals, moulds, pollens, or cold conditions. There is also a hereditary form of angioedema.

SYMPTOMS

Angioedema may cause sudden difficulty in breathing, swallowing, and speaking, accompanied by swelling of the lips, face, and neck, depending on the area of the body affected.

Angioedema that affects the throat and the larynx is potentially life-threatening because the swelling can block the airway, causing asphyxia (suffocation).

TREATMENT

Severe cases are treated with injections of *adrenaline* (epinephrine) and may require intubation (a breathing tube inserted via the mouth into the windpipe) or *tracheostomy* (surgical creation of a hole in the windpipe) to prevent suffocation. *Corticosteroid drugs* may also be given. In less severe cases, *antihistamine drugs* may relieve symptoms.

angiogenesis

The growth of new blood vessels. Angiogenesis is the process that enables tumours to grow: cancerous cells produce chemicals (called *growth factors*) that stimulate new blood vessels to form near the tumour, supplying it with nutrients and oxygen.

angiography

An imaging procedure that enables blood vessels to be seen clearly on X-rays after injection of a *contrast medium* (a substance that is opaque to *X-rays*). Digital subtraction angiography uses computer processing of images to remove unwanted background information. Magnetic resonance angiography (MRA) can produce images of blood vessels without the use of a contrast medium.

WHY IT IS DONE

Angiography is used to detect conditions that alter the appearance of blood vessels, such as an *aneurysm* (ballooning of an artery) and narrowing or blockage of blood vessels by *atherosclerosis* (fatty deposits lining artery walls), a *thrombus* (abnormal clot), or an *embolus* (fragment of a clot that is carried in the blood). Angiography is also used to

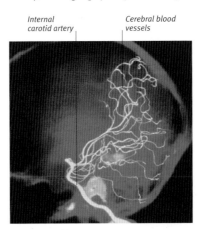

Angiogram of brain
Contrast medium is passed through a catheter into the arteries at the back of the brain, and a series of X-rays is taken.

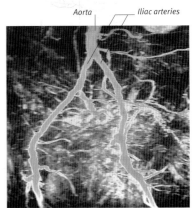

Magnetic resonance angiogram of groin
This MRA provides a clear image of the arteries of the groin area without the need for X-rays or the injection of radio-opaque dye.

detect changes in the pattern of blood vessels that supply organs injured or affected by a tumour.

Carotid angiography (angiography of the arteries in the neck) may be used to investigate *transient ischaemic attacks* (symptoms of *stroke* lasting for less than 24 hours). Cerebral angiography can be used to detect an aneurysm in the brain or to pinpoint the position of a brain tumour. Coronary angiography, often combined with cardiac *catheterization*, can identify sites of narrowing or blockage in *coronary artery disease*.

During angiography, some types of treatment, such as balloon angioplasty (see *angioplasty, balloon*) and *embolization*, that sometimes eliminate a previous need for surgery may be carried out. (See also *aortography*.)

angioma

A noncancerous tumour made up of blood vessels (see *haemangioma*) or lymph vessels (see *lymphangioma*).

angioplasty, balloon

A technique for widening a narrowed or blocked section of blood vessel by the introduction of a balloon-tipped catheter (flexible tube) into the constricted area of the vessel.

The balloon is inflated to widen the narrowed area, deflated, then removed. Balloon angioplasty is used to increase or restore blood flow in a significantly narrowed artery in *peripheral vascular disease* and *coronary artery disease*.

Balloon angioplasty is usually successful but narrowing of the affected vessel may recur, requiring repeat treat-

ment. Angioplasty of peripheral vessels is most successful in treating the femoral and iliac arteries in the legs. In some cases, *thrombolytic drugs* may be used to reduce the risk of arterial renarrowing.

In coronary angioplasty, a *stent* (rigid tube) is usually inserted into the affected artery during the procedure to reduce the likelihood of arterial renarrowing. Stents that are coated with slow-release drugs have been developed, which further reduce the risk of arterial renarrowing.

angiotensin

The name of two related proteins involved in regulating blood pressure. The first, angiotensin I, is inactive and is formed when renin, which is produced by the kidneys, acts on the substance angiotensinogen. Angiotensin I is then converted to the second, active, form, angiotensin II, by angiotensin-converting enzyme.

Angiotensin II causes narrowing of the small blood vessels in tissues, resulting in increased blood pressure. It also stimulates release (from the adrenal cortex, the outer part of each *adrenal gland*) of the hormone *aldosterone,* which also increases blood pressure.

Certain kidney disorders can increase the production of angiotensin II, resulting in *hypertension* (high blood pressure). Hypertension can be treated with *ACE inhibitor drugs*, which reduce the formation of angiotensin II, or with angiotensin II antagonists.

angiotensin-converting enzyme

A substance that converts angiotensin I to its active form, angiotensin II. Drugs that reduce the action of angiotensin-converting enzyme are known as *ACE inhibitor drugs* and are used in the treatment of *hypertension* (high blood pressure) and *heart failure* (reduced pumping efficiency of the heart).

angiotensin-II antagonists

COMMON DRUGS

- Candesartan • Irbesartan • Losartan
- Valsartan

A group of drugs used in the treatment of *hypertension* (high blood pressure). Angiotensin-II antagonists have a similar action to *ACE inhibitor drugs* (in that they block the action of *angiotensin* II) but do not cause the persistent dry cough that is a common side effect of treatment with ACE inhibitors.

PROCEDURE FOR BALLOON **ANGIOPLASTY**

A blockage or narrowing of a blood vessel may be treated by introducing a balloon catheter into the area and then inflating the balloon to stretch the constricted part. A stent may sometimes be inserted to keep the affected part open, then the catheter is withdrawn. The procedure is carried out using a local anaesthetic.

BALLOON CATHETER

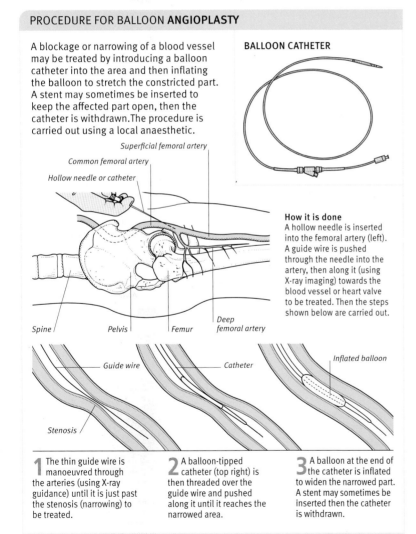

How it is done
A hollow needle is inserted into the femoral artery (left). A guide wire is pushed through the needle into the artery, then along it (using X-ray imaging) towards the blood vessel or heart valve to be treated. Then the steps shown below are carried out.

Superficial femoral artery
Common femoral artery
Hollow needle or catheter
Spine / *Pelvis* / *Femur* / *Deep femoral artery*
Guide wire / *Catheter* / *Inflated balloon*
Stenosis

1 The thin guide wire is manoeuvred through the arteries (using X-ray guidance) until it is just past the stenosis (narrowing) to be treated.

2 A balloon-tipped catheter (top right) is then threaded over the guide wire and pushed along it until it reaches the narrowed area.

3 A balloon at the end of the catheter is inflated to widen the narrowed part. A stent may sometimes be inserted then the catheter is withdrawn.

anhedonia

Total loss of the feeling of pleasure from activities that would normally give pleasure. Anhedonia is often one of the common symptoms of *depression*.

anhidrosis

Complete absence of sweating. (See also *hypohidrosis*.)

animal experimentation

The use of live animals in research and safety testing. In medicine, it has contributed to the development of drugs and surgical techniques but, due to ethical concerns, alternative methods are now used whenever possible.

animals, diseases from

See *zoonosis*.

anion

An *ion* of negative charge, such as a chloride ion. (See also *electrolyte*.)

anisometropia

Unequal focusing power in the two eyes, usually due to a difference in size and/or shape of the eyes, that causes visual discomfort. For example, one eye may be normal and the other affected by *myopia* (shortsightedness), *hypermetropia* (longsightedness), or *astigmatism*. Glasses or contact lenses usually correct the problem.

ankle joint

The hinge joint between the foot and the leg. The talus (uppermost bone in the foot) fits between the two bony protuberances formed by the lower ends of the tibia (shinbone) and the fibula (outer bone of the lower leg). Strong ligaments on either side of the ankle joint give it support. The ankle joint allows for up-and-down movement of the foot.

DISORDERS

An ankle *sprain* is one of the most common injuries. It is usually caused by twisting of the foot over on to its outside edge, which causes overstretching and bruising of the ligaments. Severe sprains can result in tearing of the ligaments, which may need to be repaired surgically.

Violent twisting of the ankle can result in a combined fracture and dislocation, known as *Pott's fracture*, in which the fibula breaks above the ankle and either the tibia breaks or the ligaments tear, resulting in dislocation of the ankle.

ankylosing spondylitis

An uncommon inflammatory disease affecting joints between the vertebrae of the spine and the sacroiliac joints (the joints between the spine and the pelvis). Ankylosing spondylitis may also affect other large joints, such as those in the hips.

CAUSES AND INCIDENCE

The cause of ankylosing spondylitis is usually unknown, but in some cases the disease may be associated with *colitis* (inflammation of the colon) or *psoriasis* (a skin disease). Ankylosing spondylitis may run in families; and about 90 per cent of people with the condition have the genetically determined *histocompatibility antigen* (HLA-B27).

SYMPTOMS

Ankylosing spondylitis usually starts with pain and stiffness in the hips and lower back that are worse after resting and are especially noticeable in the early morning. Other, less common, symptoms include chest pain, painful heels due to additional bone formation, and redness and pain in the eyes due to *iritis* (inflammation of the iris). In time, inflammation in the spine can lead to *ankylosis* (permanent stiffness and limited movement) and *kyphosis* (curvature of the spine).

DIAGNOSIS AND TREATMENT

Ankylosing spondylitis can be diagnosed by *X-rays* and *blood tests*. There is no cure, but treatment with a programme of exercise and physiotherapy and *anti-inflammatory drugs* can reduce the pain and limitation of movement. In some cases, DMARDs (see *disease-modifying antirheumatic drugs*) are also prescribed. To prevent curvature of the spine, patients are taught breathing exercises and exercises to improve posture.

ankylosis

Complete loss of movement in a joint that results from fusion of the bony surfaces. Ankylosis may be caused by degeneration as a result of inflammation, infection, or injury. The condition can also be produced surgically by an operation to fuse a diseased joint to correct deformity or to alleviate persistent pain (see *arthrodesis*). (See also *ankylosing spondylitis*.)

annular

A term meaning shaped like a ring. Annular is a description applied to certain body structures, such as ligaments, and, in dermatology, to the appearance of skin rashes, such as ringworm. The term may also be applied to a cancer that encircles an organ.

anodontia

Failure of some or all of the teeth to develop. Anodontia, which can be partial or total, may be due to the absence of tooth buds at birth, or it may be the result of damage to developing tooth buds by infection or other widespread disease. Both primary and permanent teeth may be affected. Partial anodontia is far more common than total.

If only a few teeth are missing, a dental *bridge* (false teeth that are attached to natural teeth on either side of the gap) can be fitted. If all the teeth are missing, a *denture* is required. Recently, however, dental implants (see *implant, dental*) have become the treatment of choice in selected cases (in which the individual has the correct anatomy and bone density).

anomaly

A deviation from what is accepted as normal, especially a birth defect such as a limb malformation.

Anopheles

A genus of disease-transmitting mosquitoes, many species of which are carriers of *malaria*. (See also *mosquito bites*.)

anorexia

The medical term for loss of appetite (see *appetite, loss of*).

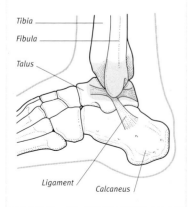

LOCATION OF THE **ANKLE JOINT**

The hinge joint is formed where the top of the talus fits in between the lower ends of the tibia and fibula.

Tibia
Fibula
Talus
Ligament
Calcaneus

COMMON FEATURES OF ANOREXIA NERVOSA

- Weight loss
- Overactivity and obsessive exercising
- Tiredness and weakness
- Lanugo (babylike) hair on body, thinning of hair on head
- Extreme choosiness over food
- Binge eating
- Induced vomiting
- Use of laxatives and/or diuretics to promote weight loss

anorexia nervosa

An eating disorder that is characterized by severe weight loss and altered self-image that leads sufferers to believe that they are fat even when they are, in fact, dangerously underweight.

CAUSES AND INCIDENCE

The causes of anorexia are unclear, but the condition may be linked to a lack of self-worth that leads to excessive concern over physical appearance. Sufferers may feel that they can have some control over their lives by controlling their eating. Normal dieting may develop into starvation.

The incidence of anorexia nervosa is not known. However, it most commonly affects teenage girls and young women, although it may also occur in older women and in men (particularly young men).

SYMPTOMS AND SIGNS

In the early stages, sufferers may be overactive and may exercise excessively. They are obsessed with food, and often make complicated meals for others, but are reluctant to eat socially and avoid eating the meals themselves. As their weight loss continues, they become tired and weak, the skin becomes dry, lanugo hair (fine, downy hair) grows on the body, and normal hair becomes thinner. Starvation leads to *amenorrhoea* (the absence of menstrual periods) in many women. *Osteoporosis* (brittle bones), caused by low levels of calcium, may also develop.

Some sufferers of anorexia nervosa have food binges and then make themselves vomit (see *bulimia*), or take *laxative drugs* and/or *diuretic drugs*, to promote weight loss. Chemical imbalances as a result of starvation, with or without vomiting, can cause potentially fatal cardiac *arrhythmias*.

TREATMENT AND OUTLOOK

The aim of treatment is to encourage healthy eating habits and weight gain to achieve a normal weight for the person's age and height. In most cases, treatment is on an outpatient basis and consists of dietary advice and psychotherapy, such as *cognitive-behavioural therapy* or interpersonal therapy. For some people, *antidepressant drugs* may also be helpful. In some cases, inpatient treatment is necessary to provide a controlled feeding programme, together with close physical monitoring and psychotherapy. Many sufferers relapse after treatment, and long-term psychotherapy is required. In about 10 to 20 per cent of cases, anorexia nervosa leads to death.

anorgasmia

Inability to achieve orgasm (see *orgasm, lack of*).

anosmia

Loss of the sense of *smell*.

anovulatory menstruation

The occurrence of a menstrual cycle during which there is no *ovulation* (release of an egg from the ovary). Anovulatory menstruation is often the result of reduced production of the hormone *oestrogen* and occurs most commonly at the beginning and end of reproductive life, in which case it is normal. However, it may also be a sign of a hormonal abnormality. (See also *fertility*; *menstruation*.)

anoxia

The total absence of oxygen within a body tissue such as the brain or a muscle. Anoxia causes disruption of cell *metabolism* (chemical activity) and results in cell death unless it is corrected within a few minutes.

Anoxia is rare, occurring during cardiopulmonary arrest or asphyxiation. It will cause permanent organ damage or even death if not corrected. *Hypoxia* (the reduction of oxygen supply to a tissue) is a more common problem.

Antabuse

A brand name for *disulfiram*, a drug used to treat *alcohol dependence*. Antabuse is a powerful deterrent, which, if taken with even a small amount of alcohol, produces extremely unpleasant side effects such as nausea, headache, dizziness, and *palpitations*.

antacid drugs

COMMON DRUGS
- Aluminium hydroxide • Calcium carbonate
- Hydrotalcite • Magnesium hydroxide
- Sodium alginate

Drugs taken to relieve the symptoms of *indigestion*, *heartburn*, *gastro-oesophragal reflux disease* (regurgitation of stomach acid into the oesophagus), *oesophagitis* (inflammation of the oesophagus), and *peptic ulcer*.

HOW THEY WORK

Antacids usually contain compounds of *magnesium* or *aluminium*, which neutralize stomach acid. Some also contain alginates, which protect the oesophagus by reducing acid reflux, or dimeticone, an antifoaming agent, which helps to relieve flatulence.

SIDE EFFECTS

Aluminium may cause constipation, and magnesium may cause diarrhoea. These effects can be avoided, however, if a preparation contains both ingredients. Antacids interfere with the absorption of many drugs and should therefore not be taken at the same time as other medications.

WARNING

Antacids should not be taken regularly except under medical supervision because they may suppress the symptoms of a more serious disorder or provoke serious complications.

antagonist

Having an opposing effect. For example, antagonist drugs counteract the effects of naturally occurring chemicals in the body. (See also *agonist*.)

antenatal care

The care of a pregnant woman and her unborn baby throughout pregnancy to ensure that both are healthy at delivery. Antenatal care involves regular visits to a doctor or midwife, who performs blood and urine tests and abdominal examinations and also monitors blood pressure and fetal growth in order to detect disease or potential problems (see the antenatal screening procedures chart, overleaf).

High-risk pregnancies, in which, for example, the woman suffers from *hypertension* (high blood pressure) or diabetes

A

ANTENATAL SCREENING PROCEDURES

When performed	Procedure	Reason for procedure
First visits (before 12 weeks)	Medical history and examination	To look for pre-existing risk factors, such as long-term illnesses.
	Urine tests	To check the urine for glucose, which may indicate diabetes developing in pregnancy and for protein, which may indicate pre-existing kidney disease.
	Blood test	To determine the woman's blood type and to check for anaemia; antibodies to rubella; hepatitis B virus; Down's syndrome; sickle cell anaemia; thalassaemia; and, after discussion, HIV infection which might be transmitted to the baby. Genetic counselling may be offered to couples with a family history of inherited disease or from ethnic groups at high risk.
	Weight and blood pressure	To provide initial measurements against which later ones can be compared.
Between 12 and 20 weeks	Ultrasound scans (one or more)	To check the age of the fetus and to look for fetal abnormalities.
Follow-up visits at regular intervals from 12 weeks to delivery	Weight (not routine in women of normal weight) and examination	To assess the growth of the fetus and to see which way it is lying in the uterus.
	Urine tests	To detect diabetes, pre-eclampsia, or urine infection.
	Blood pressure	To detect developing pre-eclampsia.
	Blood tests (at some visits only)	To look for anaemia and, in combination with ultrasound scanning, to assess the risk of fetal abnormalities such as neural tube defects or Down's syndrome. A test to screen for diabetes mellitus in the mother may also be necessary.
	Fetal heartbeat check	To assess whether the fetus's heart is beating normally.

(see *diabetic pregnancy*), require more frequent antenatal visits. In some cases, the woman may be admitted to hospital for closer observation.

Ultrasound scanning is carried out to assess the age of the fetus and to identify any abnormalities. *Amniocentesis* or *chorionic villus sampling* may be performed if the fetus is thought to be at increased risk of a *chromosomal abnormality* (such as *Down's syndrome*) or a *genetic disorder*. Electronic fetal monitoring may be carried out, in order to check the fetal heartbeat, in pregnancies that are high-risk or overdue.

The woman is also advised on general aspects of pregnancy, such as diet, exercise, and techniques to help her with childbirth. (See also *childbirth, natural*.)

antepartum haemorrhage

Bleeding from the vagina after the 28th week of pregnancy.

Antepartum haemorrhage is most commonly due to a problem with the placenta (the organ in the uterus that sustains the developing fetus), such as *placenta praevia* (in which the placenta is positioned too close to the birth canal) or *placental abruption* (detachment of part of the placenta from the wall of the uterus). Bleeding can also be caused by *cervical ectopy* or other disorders of the cervix or vagina.

SYMPTOMS

The bleeding is often painless but may be accompanied by abdominal pain if the placenta becomes partly separated from the uterus.

Investigation and treatment requires hospital admission. *Ultrasound scanning* is used to diagnose problems with the placenta. In some cases, it is necessary only to keep a careful watch on the condition of the woman and her baby. If the bleeding is severe, the woman is given a *blood transfusion*; the baby may be delivered immediately by *caesarean section*.

anterior

Relating to the front of the body. In human anatomy, the term is synonymous with *ventral*.

anterior knee pain syndrome

See *chondromalacia patellae*.

anterior compartment syndrome

See *compartment syndrome; shin splints*.

anthelmintic drugs

COMMON DRUGS

- Albendazole • Diethylcarbamazine
- Ivermectin • Levamisole • Mebendazole
- Niclosamide • Piperazine • Praziquantel
- Tiabendazole

A group of drugs used to eradicate *worm infestation* of the body. Anthelmintic drugs kill or paralyse worms in the intestines, preventing them from gripping the intestinal wall, and causing them to pass out of the body in the *faeces*.

Possible side effects of anthelmintic drugs include nausea, abdominal pain, rash, headache, and dizziness.

anthrax

A serious bacterial infection of livestock that occasionally spreads to humans. The most common form of the infection in humans is cutaneous anthrax, which affects the skin. Another form, pulmonary anthrax, affects the lungs and is potentially fatal.

CAUSES

Anthrax is caused by BACILLUS ANTHRACIS. This bacterium produces spores that can remain dormant for years in soil and animal products and can be reactivated.

Animals become infected by grazing on contaminated land. Infection can occur in humans via a scratch or a sore if materials from infected animals are handled. Pulmonary anthrax occurs as a result of inhaling spores from infected animal fibres.

SYMPTOMS AND TREATMENT

In cutaneous anthrax, a raised, itchy, area develops at the site of entry of the spores, progressing to a large blister and finally a black scab, with swelling of the surrounding tissues. Cutaneous anthrax is treatable in its early stages with *antibiotic drugs*. Without treatment, infection may spread to lymph nodes and the bloodstream and may be fatal.

Pulmonary anthrax causes severe breathing difficulty and may be fatal despite intensive treatment.

antiallergy drugs

Drugs used to treat or prevent allergic reactions (see *allergy*). There are several types of antiallergy drug, including *antihistamine drugs*, *leukotriene receptor antagonists*, *sodium cromoglicate*, and *corticosteroid drugs*.

antianxiety drugs

A group of drugs used to relieve symptoms of *anxiety*. *Benzodiazepine drugs*, buspirone, and *beta-blocker drugs* are the three main types of antianxiety drug, although *antidepressant drugs* are often used. In most cases, the underlying disorder is best treated by counselling, psychotherapy, or other forms of therapy.

Benzodiazepine drugs promote mental and physical relaxation by reducing nerve activity in the brain; they can also be used to treat insomnia but their use for this purpose is avoided because they are addictive; buspirone is less addictive. Beta-blockers reduce only the physical symptoms of anxiety, such as shaking and palpitations, and are not addictive.

antiarrhythmic drugs

A group of drugs used to prevent or treat different types of *arrhythmia* (irregular heartbeat).

A number of drugs are used to prevent intermittent arrhythmias or slow the rate if an arrhythmia is persistent. These include *beta-blocker drugs*, *calcium channel blockers*, *digoxin*, *amiodarone*, *disopyramide*, flecainide, *lidocaine* (lignocaine), mexiletine, and *procainamide*. Some antiarrhythmic drugs, such as adenosine and bretyllium, may only be used in hospital. They may be given intravenously to treat arrhythmias that are causing symptoms such as breathlessness or chest pain.

HOW THEY WORK
The heart's pumping action is governed by electrical impulses. Some antiarrhythmic drugs alter these impulses within, or on their way to, the heart; others affect the heart muscle's response to the impulses received.

SIDE EFFECTS
Side effects of antiarrhythmic drugs are common, and they often include nausea and a rash. Some antiarrhythmics can also cause tiredness or breathlessness because they reduce the pumping ability of the heart.

antibacterial drugs

A group of drugs that are used to treat infections caused by *bacteria*. The term "antibacterial" was once used to describe only those *antibiotic drugs* that had been produced synthetically rather than naturally. However, the two terms are now used interchangeably.

antibiotic drugs

COMMON DRUGS
AMINOGLYCOSIDES •Amikacin •Gentamicin •Neomycin •Netilmicin •Streptomycin •Tobramycin

CEPHALOSPORINS •Cefaclor •Cefadroxil •Cefalexin •Cefixime •Cefotaxime •Cefpodoxime •Cefradine •Ceftazidime

MACROLIDES •Azithromycin •Clarithromycin •Erythromycin

PENICILLINS •Amoxicillin •Ampicillin •Benzylpenicillin •Co-amoxiclav •Co-fluampicil •Flucloxacillin •Phenoxymethylpenicillin

TETRACYCLINES •Doxycycline •Lymecycline •Oxytetracycline •Tetracycline

OTHERS •Chloramphenicol •Ciprofloxacin •Colistin •Fusidic acid •Metronidazole •Rifampicin •Teicoplanin •Trimethoprim •Vancomycin

A group of drugs used to treat infections caused by *bacteria* and to prevent bacterial infection in individuals who are *immunocompromised* (for example, people who are taking immunosuppressant drugs). Most of the commonly used antibiotic drugs belong to one of the following classes: *aminoglycosides*, *cephalosporins*, *macrolides*, *penicillins*, and *tetracyclines*. Some antibiotics are effective against only certain types of bacteria; others, which are known as broad-spectrum antibiotics, are effective against a wide range.

ANTIBIOTIC RESISTANCE
Some bacteria develop resistance to a previously effective antibiotic drug. This resistance is most likely to occur during long-term treatment. Some alternative antibiotics are available to treat bacteria that have become resistant to the more commonly prescribed drugs.

SIDE EFFECTS
Most antibiotic drugs can cause nausea, diarrhoea, or a rash. Antibiotics may disturb the normal balance of "good" bacteria in the body. This can cause problems such as *candidiasis* (thrush), in which there is excess growth of a fungus. Some individuals experience a severe allergic reaction to the drugs, resulting in facial swelling, itching, or breathing difficulty.

WARNING
Patients should inform their doctor of any previous allergic reaction that they have had to an antibiotic drug.

HOW **ANTIBIOTICS** WORK

Antibiotic drugs are either bactericidal or bacteriostatic. Bactericidal antibiotics, such as penicillins and cephalosporins, kill bacteria directly. Bacteriostatic antibiotics, such as erythromycin, halt growth and multiplication of the bacteria, allowing the immune system to cope with the infection.

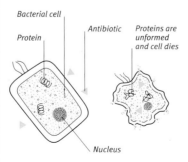

Bacteriostatic antibiotics
These drugs prevent the production of proteins that the bacterial cell needs in order to grow and multiply, and the cell eventually dies.

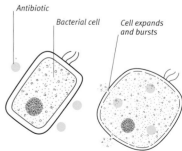

Bactericidal antibiotics
These kill bacteria directly by causing the cell wall to disintegrate; water is taken into the cell, which expands and then bursts.

A

antibody

A protein that is made by certain lymphocytes (white blood cells) to neutralize an *antigen* (foreign protein) in the body. Bacteria, viruses, and other microorganisms contain a number of antigens; antibodies that are formed against these antigens help the body to neutralize or destroy the invading microorganisms. Antibodies may also be formed in response to *vaccines*, thereby giving immunity against certain infections. Antibodies are also known as *immunoglobulins*.

Inappropriate or excessive formation of antibodies may lead to illness, as in an *allergy*. Antibodies against antigens in organ transplants may result in rejection of the transplanted organ. In some disorders, antibodies are formed against the body's own tissues, resulting in an *autoimmune disorder*.

antibody, monoclonal

An artificially produced *antibody* that neutralizes only one specific *antigen* (foreign protein).

Monoclonal antibodies are produced in a laboratory by stimulating the growth of large numbers of antibody-producing cells that are genetically identical. In effect, this process enables antibodies to be tailor-made to react with a particular antigen.

Monoclonal antibodies are used in the study of human cells, hormones, microorganisms, and in the development of vaccines. They are also being used in the diagnosis and treatment of some forms of cancer, such as *lymphoma*. Genetically engineered monoclonal antibodies are designed to bind to the proteins on the surface of certain cancer cells, marking them out for destruction. The immune system can then recognize these marked cells and destroy them.

anticancer drugs

COMMON DRUGS

ALKYLATING AGENTS • Chlorambucil • Cyclophosphamide • Melphalan
ANTIMETABOLITES • Cytarabine • Fluorouracil • Mercaptopurine • Methotrexate
CYTOTOXIC ANTIBIOTICS • Doxorubicin • Epirubicin
HORMONE TREATMENTS • Anastrozole • Bicalutamide • Cyproterone acetate • Flutamide • Goserelin • Letrozole • Leuprorelin • Medroxyprogesterone • Megestrol • Tamoxifen
CYTOKINES • Interferon alfa • Interleukin 2
TAXANES • Docetaxel • Paclitaxel
OTHERS • Carboplatin • Cisplatin • Etoposide • Irinotecan • Rituximab • Trastuzumab

Drugs that are used to treat many forms of *cancer*. Some tumours respond to drug treatment better than others. Anticancer drugs are particularly useful in the treatment of *lymphomas*, *leukaemias*, *breast cancer*, cancer of the testis (see *testis, cancer of*), and *prostate cancer*.

HOW THEY WORK

Most anticancer drugs are cytotoxic (they kill or damage cells or prevent them from dividing). Cytotoxic drugs fall into several classes, including alkylating agents, antimetabolites, cytotoxic antibiotics, and taxanes. *Cytokines* (proteins released by cells in response to the presence of harmful organisms) such as interferon alpha bind to other cells, activating the immune response (see *immune system*).

In some cases, drug treatment is used alone, but it is often combined with surgery or *radiotherapy*. Anticancer drugs are often given in combination to maximize their effects. Treatment with cytotoxic drugs is commonly given by injection in short courses repeated at intervals.

SIDE EFFECTS

Some cytotoxic drugs cause nausea and vomiting and may cause hair loss and increased susceptibility to infection. Others (such as tamoxifen for breast cancer) are given continuously by mouth for months or years and cause few side effects.

anticholinergic drugs

COMMON DRUGS

AS BRONCHODILATORS • Ipratropium bromide • Tiotropium
FOR IRRITABLE BOWEL SYNDROME • Atropine • Dicycloverine • Hyoscine • Propantheline
FOR PARKINSONISM • Benztropine • Biperiden • Orphenadrine • Procyclidine • Trihexyphenidyl (Benzhexol)
FOR URINARY INCONTINENCE • Flavoxate • Oxybutynin • Propiverine • Tolterodine • Trospium

A group of drugs, also called antimuscarinics, that are used in the treatment of *irritable bowel syndrome*, urinary incontinence (see *incontinence, urinary*), chronic obstructive pulmonary disease (COPD; see *pulmonary disease, chronic obstructive*), *Parkinson's disease*, and *bradycardia* (an abnormally slow heartbeat). Anticholinergic drugs are used to dilate the pupil before eye examination or surgery. They may also be used as *premedication* before general anaesthesia (see *anaesthesia, general*) and to treat *motion sickness*.

HOW THEY WORK

Anticholinergics block the effects of *acetylcholine*, a chemical released from nerve endings in the parasympathetic *autonomic nervous system*. Acetylcholine triggers activity in a number of cells. For example, it stimulates muscle contraction, slows the heartbeat, and increases secretions in the mouth and lungs.

SIDE EFFECTS

Possible side effects of anticholinergics may include dry mouth, blurred vision, urinary retention, and confusion.

HOW **ANTICHOLINERGICS** WORK

Acetylcholine combines with a receptor on the cell's surface. This interaction stimulates activity in that cell (e.g. contraction of a muscle fibre or secretion of a fluid). Anticholinergic drugs block the stimulatory action of acetylcholine by combining with the acetylcholine receptors. This action produces, for example, muscle relaxation (e.g. in the bladder, intestine, and bronchi) and dries up secretions in the mouth and lungs. Anticholinergic drugs are used to treat COPD and other conditions.

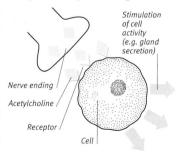

Nerve ending
Acetylcholine
Receptor
Cell
Stimulation of cell activity (e.g. gland secretion)

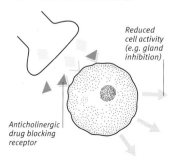

Anticholinergic drug blocking receptor
Reduced cell activity (e.g. gland inhibition)

anticoagulant drugs

COMMON DRUGS

- Dalteparin • Enoxaparin • Heparin
- Nicoumalone • Tinzaparin • Warfarin

A group of drugs used to treat and prevent abnormal *blood clotting*, to treat *thrombosis*, and, occasionally, to prevent and treat *stroke* and *transient ischaemic attack* (symptoms of stroke lasting less than 24 hours). Anticoagulant drugs are also given long-term to prevent abnormal blood clotting after major surgery (especially heart-valve replacement) or during haemodialysis (see *dialysis*).

The most common anticoagulants are *heparin* and the newer heparin-derived drugs, such as tinzaparin, all of which have to be given by injection, and *warfarin*, which is taken orally. Heparin is usually given initially and is then withdrawn when warfarin therapy has become effective.

HOW THEY WORK

Anticoagulant drugs reduce the activity of certain enzymes, known as blood clotting factors, that are needed for the blood to clot. Anticoagulants do not dissolve clots that have already formed, which can be treated with *thrombolytic drugs*, however they may help to stabilize an existing clot so that it does not break away causing an *embolism* (blockage of an artery by a blood clot).

SIDE EFFECTS

Excessive doses of warfarin or its use with other drugs, such as aspirin and alcohol, may increase the risk of unwanted bleeding. Regular monitoring with *blood-clotting tests* is required.

WARNING

A doctor should always be consulted before any other drug is taken during anticoagulant treatment.

anticonvulsant drugs

COMMON DRUGS

- Carbamazepine • Clobazam • Clonazepam
- Diazepam • Ethosuximide • Gabapentin
- Lamotrigine • Lorazepam • Phenobarbital
- Phenytoin • Piracetam • Primidone
- Sodium valproate • Tiagabine
- Topiramate • Vigabatrin

A group of drugs that are used to treat or prevent seizures. Anticonvulsant drugs are used mainly in the treatment of *epilepsy*, but they are also prescribed to prevent seizures following serious *head injury* or some types of brain surgery. They may be needed to control seizures in children with a high fever

(see *convulsions, febrile*). Different anticonvulsant drugs are effective at treating different types of seizure.

HOW THEY WORK

Seizures are caused by an abnormally high level of electrical activity in the brain. Anticonvulsant drugs have an inhibitory effect that suppresses this excessive electrical activity, thereby preventing its spread throughout areas of the brain. If seizures continue following treatment with an anticonvulsant, two drugs may be used in combination.

SIDE EFFECTS

Anticonvulsants may produce various side effects, including impaired memory, reduced concentration, poor coordination, and fatigue. If the side effects are troublesome, an alternative anticonvulsant can be tried. The dose of an anticonvulsant drug may need to be monitored using *blood tests*.

WARNING

The dosage of anticonvulsants should not be reduced or the treatment stopped without a doctor being consulted first; the doctor will supervise a gradual reduction in dosage. Stopping the drugs abruptly could cause withdrawal symptoms and a recurrence of the original problem.

antidepressant drugs

COMMON DRUGS

SELECTIVE SEROTONIN REUPTAKE INHIBITORS (SSRIS) • Citalopram • Escitalopram
- Fluoxetine • Fluvoxamine • Paroxetine
- Sertraline

TRICYCLICS (TCAS) • Amitriptyline
- Clomipramine • Dosulepin • Imipramine
- Lofepramine • Nortriptyline • Trimipramine

MONOAMINE OXIDASE INHIBITORS (MAOIS)
- Isocarboxazid • Moclobemide • Phenelzine

OTHERS • Flupentixol • Mianserin
- Mirtazapine • Reboxetine • Trazodone
- Venlafaxine

Drugs used in the treatment of *depression*. Most of the commonly used antidepressant drugs belong to one of the following groups: *tricyclic antidepressants* (TCAs), *selective serotonin reuptake inhibitors* (SSRIs), and *monoamine oxidase inhibitors* (MAOIs).

HOW THEY WORK

Normally, brain cells release enough *neurotransmitters* (chemical messengers) in the brain to stimulate nearby brain cells. Neurotransmitters are constantly being reabsorbed into the brain cells by another chemical, monoamine oxidase. Depression is thought to be due to a

reduction in the release of neurotransmitters. TCAs increase the level of the neurotransmitters noradrenaline (norepinephrine) and serotonin by preventing their reabsorption. MAOIs work by blocking the action of monoamine oxidase, which increases neurotransmitter levels. SSRIs only prevent the reabsorption of serotonin.

Antidepressants usually relieve the symptoms of depression, but it often takes two to three weeks for any beneficial effects to be felt. Treatment usually lasts for at least six months; and the dosage is reduced gradually before being stopped altogether.

SIDE EFFECTS

TCAs may cause constipation, dry mouth, drowsiness, blurred vision, urinary difficulty, and irregular heartbeat. SSRIs may cause nausea, indigestion, loss of appetite, insomnia, agitation, or sexual difficulties but are less dangerous in overdose than other antidepressants; they are not generally prescribed to anyone under the age of 18. MAOIs may cause dangerous interactions with some foods and drugs, although *moclobemide* is less likely to cause problems.

Antidepressants are not addictive, but abrupt withdrawal of some types can result in physical symptoms and should therefore be avoided.

WARNING

Food and drink containing tyramine (for example, cheese and red wine) and other drugs may cause a dangerous rise in blood pressure when taken during treatment with an MAOI. Always tell your doctor if you are taking an MAOI.

antidiabetic drugs

COMMON DRUGS

SULPHONYLUREA DRUGS • Chlorpropamide
- Glibenclamide • Gliclazide • Glimepiride
- Glipizide • Tolbutamide

OTHERS • Acarbose • Glucagon • Insulin
- Metformin • Repaglinide
- Rosiglitazone

A group of drugs used to treat *diabetes mellitus*, in which a lack of *insulin*, or resistance to its actions, results in *hyperglycaemia* (high levels of glucose in the blood). A wide range of antidiabetics are used to keep the blood glucose level as close to normal as possible, thereby reducing the risk of complications. Antidiabetic drugs include insulin, which must be administered by injection, and oral hypoglycaemics (see *hypoglycaemics, oral*) such as *glibenclamide* and *metformin*.

A

A

HOW THEY WORK

Most antidiabetic drugs promote the uptake of glucose into the body tissues, helping to prevent an excessive rise in blood glucose levels. However, different antidiabetics work in different ways. For example, *acarbose* reduces or slows the absorption of carbohydrate from the intestines after meals. *Repaglinide* stimulates release of insulin from the pancreas. *Rosiglitazone* reduces resistance to the effects of insulin in the tissues and may be used together with other hypoglycaemics.

SIDE EFFECTS

Certain antidiabetics may lower the blood glucose level too much, leading to *hypoglycaemia* (low blood glucose levels). Rarely, these drugs may also cause a decreased blood cell count, a rash, or intestinal or liver disturbances.

Metformin does not cause hypoglycaemia, although treatment with this drug may result in nausea, appetite loss, abdominal distension, and diarrhoea. It should not be taken by people with liver, kidney, or heart problems.

antidiarrhoeal drugs

COMMON DRUGS

ANTISPASMODICS • Atropine • Dicycloverine
• Hyoscine
OPIOIDS • Codeine • Diphenoxylate
• Loperamide
BULK-FORMING AGENTS AND ADSORBENTS
• Ispaghula • Kaolin • Methylcellulose

Drugs that are used to reduce or stop diarrhoea and to help regulate bowel action in people who have had a *colostomy* or *ileostomy*. In most acute (of sudden onset) cases of diarrhoea, the only treatment recommended is *oral rehydration therapy*. Antidiarrhoeal drugs are not suitable for children.

HOW THEY WORK

Antidiarrhoeal drugs include adsorbents (such as kaolin), which can absorb the toxic substances that cause diarrhoea; bulk-forming agents (such as ispaghula), which absorb water from the faeces thereby making them firmer; and antimotility drugs (including the opioid drug *codeine*, and loperamide, which is chemically similar to opioids but does not have an opioid effect), which slow movement through the intestine.

SIDE EFFECTS

Antidiarrhoeal drugs may cause constipation. In cases of diarrhoea that has resulted from an infection, antidiarrhoeals may delay recovery by slowing down the elimination of the causative microorganisms. Bulk-forming agents may cause intestinal obstruction if taken without sufficient drinking water or if the bowel is narrowed. Prolonged use of opioid antidiarrhoeals may lead to physical dependence (see *drug dependence*), producing nausea, abdominal pain, and diarrhoea if the drug is stopped suddenly.

WARNING

Antidiarrhoeals should not be taken regularly except on medical advice since they may mask a serious underlying disorder.

antidiuretic hormone

See *ADH*.

antidote

A substance that neutralizes or counteracts the effects of a poison.

anti-D(Rh₀) immunoglobulin

An *antiserum* that contains antibodies (see *antibody*), proteins that are manufactured by the immune system against Rhesus (Rh) D factor, a substance present on the red blood cells of people with Rh-positive blood.

Anti-D(Rh₀) immunoglobulin is given to all Rh-negative women routinely at intervals during normal pregnancy and at delivery. A dose is also given after an *amniocentesis*, miscarriage, or any event in which the baby's blood may enter the mother's circulation. The injected antibodies destroy any red blood cells from the fetus that have entered the woman's bloodstream. This helps to prevent the woman from forming her own antibodies against Rh-positive blood, which might adversely affect a subsequent pregnancy. (See also *haemolytic disease of the newborn*; *Rhesus incompatibility*.)

antiemetic drugs

COMMON DRUGS

ANTICHOLINERGICS • Hyoscine hydrobromide
ANTIHISTAMINES • Cinnarizine • Cyclizine
• Promethazine
BUTYROPHENONES • Haloperidol
PHENOTHIAZINES • Chlorpromazine
• Perphenazine • Prochlorperazine
SEROTONIN ANTAGONISTS • Granisetron
• Ondansetron • Tropisetron
MOTILITY STIMULANTS • Domperidone
• Metoclopramide
OTHERS • Betahistine • Nabilone

A group of drugs used in the treatment of the *nausea* and *vomiting* that are associated with *motion sickness*, *vertigo*, *Ménière's disease*, *radiotherapy*, and certain drugs. Antiemetics are not normally used in the treatment of food poisoning because the body needs to rid itself of harmful substances.

HOW THEY WORK

Antihistamines and *anticholinergic drugs* reduce vomiting associated with vertigo by suppressing the vomiting reflex (in which the stomach muscles contract to expel the stomach contents), which is triggered by nerve activity in the balance centre of the inner ear. *Motility stimulants* work by increasing movement through the gastrointestinal tract. The most powerful antiemetics are used to control nausea and vomiting associated with radiotherapy or *anticancer drugs* and include *serotonin antagonists*, such as *ondansetron*, and *nabilone*. These drugs act on *neurotransmitters* in the brain.

SIDE EFFECTS

Many antiemetic drugs can cause drowsiness. Only certain antiemetics are used to treat vomiting in early pregnancy because some can damage the developing fetus.

WARNING

Antiemetic drugs should not be taken regularly, except on medical advice, because they may mask a serious underlying disorder.

antifreeze poisoning

Most antifreeze in the UK contains ethylene glycol, which is poisonous. Most cases of antifreeze poisoning, which is extremely rare, occur as a result of accidental swallowing.

SYMPTOMS

Drinking antifreeze initially produces effects similar to *alcohol intoxication*, but vomiting, stupor, seizures, unconsciousness, and coma may follow; acute *kidney failure* may occur within 24 to 36 hours of having drunk antifreeze. With delayed or no treatment, antifreeze poisoning may be fatal.

TREATMENT

Any person who is believed to have drunk antifreeze requires immediate medical attention.

Hospital treatment may include removing the antifreeze from the stomach using a stomach pump (see *lavage, gastric*) and giving activated charcoal, intravenous bicarbonate to correct excess acidity in the body fluids, and medications to slow the formation of toxins. In severe cases, *dialysis* may be required to treat kidney failure.

antifungal drugs

COMMON DRUGS

- Amorolfine • Amphotericin • Benzoyl
peroxide • Clotrimazole • Econazole
- Fenticonazole • Fluconazole • Griseofulvin
- Itraconazole • Ketoconazole • Miconazole
- Nystatin • Sulconazole • Terbinafine
- Tioconazole

A group of drugs used to treat infections caused by *fungi*. Antifungals are commonly used to treat different types of *tinea* (including *athlete's foot* and scalp ringworm); *candidiasis* (thrush) and rare infections, such as *cryptococcosis*, that affect internal organs. Antifungals are available in various forms, including tablets, injection, creams, and pessaries.

HOW THEY WORK

Antifungal drugs work by damaging the cell walls of fungi, causing chemicals essential for normal cell function and growth to escape. The fungal cells are unable to survive without these chemicals.

SIDE EFFECTS

Topical antifungals rarely cause side effects but may occasionally increase skin irritation. Prolonged treatment, by mouth or injection, of serious fungal infections can result in side effects including liver or kidney damage.

antigen

A substance that can trigger an *immune response*, resulting in production of an *antibody* as part of the body's defence against infection and disease. Many antigens are foreign proteins such as parts of microorganisms and toxins or tissues from another person that have been used in organ transplants. Sometimes, harmless substances (such as pollen) are misidentified by the immune system as potentially harmful antigens, which results in an allergic response (see *allergy*).

antihistamine drugs

COMMON DRUGS

NON-SEDATING • Acrivastine • Cetirizine
- Desloratadine • Fexofenadine • Loratadine
- Mizolastine

SEDATING • Alimemazine (trimeprazine)
- Chlorphenamine • Clemastine
- Promethazine

A group of drugs that block the effects of *histamine*, a chemical released during allergic reactions (see *allergy*).

Antihistamines are used to treat rashes such as *urticaria* (hives) and to relieve sneezing and a runny nose in allergic *rhinitis*. They are also sometimes included in *cough remedies* and *cold remedies*, and they are used as *antiemetic drugs* because they suppress the vomiting reflex. Antihistamines are usually taken by mouth but may be given by injection for *anaphylactic shock*.

HOW THEY WORK

Antihistamine drugs block the effect of histamine on tissues such as the skin, eyes, and nose. Without drug treatment, histamine dilates small *blood vessels*, resulting in *inflammation* of the surrounding tissue due to leakage of fluid from the circulation. Antihistamines also prevent histamine from irritating nerve fibres, which causes itching.

SIDE EFFECTS

Many antihistamines cause drowsiness, but newer drugs have little sedative effect. Other uncommon side effects include loss of appetite, nausea, dry mouth, blurred vision, and difficulty in passing urine.

WARNING

A person should not drive or operate potentially dangerous machinery while taking an antihistamine drug unless he or she is certain that the treatment is not causing dizziness, drowsiness, or impaired concentration.

antihypertensive drugs

COMMON DRUGS

ACE INHIBITORS • Captopril • Cilazapril
- Enalapril • Fosinopril • Lisinopril • Moexipril
- Perindopril • Quinapril • Ramipril
- Trandolapril

ALPHA-BLOCKERS • Doxazosin • Prazosin
- Terazosin

ANGIOTENSIN-II ANTAGONISTS • Candesartan
- Irbesartan • Losartan • Valsartan

BETA-BLOCKERS • Acebutolol • Atenolol
- Bisoprolol • Carvedilol • Celiprolol
- Labetalol • Metoprolol • Nadolol • Pindolol
- Propranolol • Sotalol • Timolol

CALCIUM CHANNEL BLOCKERS • Amlodipine
- Diltiazem • Nicardipine • Nifedipine

CENTRALLY ACTING HYPERTENSIVES • Clonidine
- Methyldopa • Moxonidine

DIURETICS • Amiloride • Bendroflumethiazide
- Bumetanide • Chlortalidone
- Cyclopenthiazide • Furosemide
- Hydrochlorothiazide
- Hydroflumethiazide • Indapamide
- Metolazone • Spironolactone
- Torasemide • Triamterene • Xipamide

A group of drugs that are used in the treatment of *hypertension* (high blood pressure) to prevent complications such as *stroke*, *heart failure* (reduced pumping efficiency of the heart), *myocardial infarc-*tion (heart attack), and kidney damage. There are several types of antihypertensive drug, each working in a different way to lower the blood pressure.

HOW THEY WORK

Antihypertensive drugs work in a variety of ways to lower blood pressure. ACE inhibitors and angiotensin-II antagonists act on enzymes in the blood to dilate blood vessels; alpha-blockers block nerve signals that trigger the constriction of blood vessels; beta-blockers reduce the force of the heartbeat, thereby lowering the pressure of blood flow; diuretics increase the amount of salts and water excreted in the *urine*, thereby reducing blood volume; calcium channel blockers and ACE inhibitors control the size of blood vessels by preventing constriction of arterial wall muscles; and centrally acting hypertensives act on the mechanism in the brain that controls the size of blood vessels.

SIDE EFFECTS

Side effects depend on the type of antihypertensive used, but all types can cause dizziness if the blood pressure falls excessively.

WARNING

The dosage of antihypertensives should not be reduced or the treatment stopped without first consulting a doctor, who will supervise a gradual reduction in dosage. Abrupt cessation of the drug could cause a dangerous rise in blood pressure.

anti-inflammatory drugs

Drugs that reduce *inflammation*. The main groups of these drugs are *corticosteroid drugs* and *nonsteroidal anti-inflammatory drugs* (NSAIDs). (See also *analgesic drugs*.)

antimalarial drugs

Drugs used to treat *malaria*. One antimalarial drug, *chloroquine*, also works as a *disease-modifying antirheumatic drug* and may be used to treat *rheumatoid arthritis* and systemic *lupus erythematosus*.

antimotility drugs

See *antidiarrhoeal drugs*.

antimuscarinic drugs

See *anticholinergic drugs*.

antiobesity drugs

A group of drugs that includes *appetite suppressants* and *orlistat*, a drug that acts on the gastrointestinal tract to prevent the digestion of fats.

anti-oestrogen drugs

A group of drugs that oppose the action of the hormone *oestrogen*. The most important of these drugs is *tamoxifen*, which is used in the treatment of certain breast cancers.

antioxidant

A type of chemical that neutralizes potentially damaging oxidizing molecules known as *free radicals* (molecules that bind to and destroy body cells). Some antioxidants occur naturally in the body; others (vitamin C, vitamin E, and beta-carotene, for example) are obtained from food or dietary supplements.

antiperspirant

COMMON DRUGS
• Aluminium chloride

A substance applied to the skin in the form of a lotion, cream, or spray in order to reduce sweating. High concentrations are sometimes used to treat *hyperhidrosis* (abnormally heavy sweating).

HOW IT WORKS
An antiperspirant reduces the production of sweat by the *sweat glands* and blocks the ducts that drain sweat on to the surface of the skin.

SIDE EFFECTS
Antiperspirants may cause skin irritation, particularly if they are used on broken skin. (See also *deodorants*.)

antiplatelet drugs

COMMON DRUGS
• Abciximab • Aspirin • Clopigogrel
• Dipyridamole • Tirofiban

Drugs that reduce the tendency of *platelets* to stick together to form blood clots (see *blood clotting*) when blood flow in the arteries is disrupted. Antiplatelet drugs reduce the risk of *thromboembolism* (in which a clot breaks off and is carried in the bloodstream to lodge elsewhere in the body), which can cause potentially fatal disorders such as a *myocardial infarction* (heart attack) or *stroke*.

antipruritic drugs

COMMON DRUGS
ANTIHISTAMINES • Antazoline • Trimeprazine
CORTICOSTEROIDS • Hydrocortisone
LOCAL ANAESTHETICS • Benzocaine • Lignocaine
• Tetracaine (amethocaine)
EMOLLIENT AND COOLING PREPARATIONS
• Aqueous cream • Calamine lotion
• Emulsifying ointment
OTHERS • Colestyramine • Doxepin

Drugs that are used to relieve persistent itching (*pruritus*), including pruritus that occurs as a result of a specific condition. For example, colestyramine (a *lipid-lowering drug*) is used to relieve pruritus associated with primary *biliary cirrhosis*. Antipruritic drugs can be applied as creams and *emollients* and may contain *corticosteroid drugs*, *antihistamine drugs*, or *local anaesthetics*. Oral antihistamines may also be used to relieve itching.

HOW THEY WORK
Irritation of the skin causes the release of substances, such as histamine, that cause the blood vessels to dilate and fluid to accumulate under the skin, which results in inflammation and itching. Antipruritic drugs work either by reducing inflammation, and therefore itching, or by numbing the nerve impulses that transmit sensation to the brain.

SIDE EFFECTS
Prolonged or heavy use of any antipruritic, especially antihistamine and local anaesthetic creams, may lead to further skin irritation. Oral antihistamines may cause drowsiness. Prolonged use of potent topical corticosteroids may result in permanent skin changes, most commonly thinning of the skin.

antipsychotic drugs

COMMON DRUGS
PHENOTHIAZINES • Chlorpromazine
• Fluphenazine • Levomepromazine
(methotrimeprazine) • Pericyazine
• Perphenazine • Pipotiazine
• Trifluoperazine
BUTYROPHENONES • Benperidol
• Haloperidol
OTHERS • Amisulpride • Clozapine
• Flupentixol • Olanzapine • Pimozide
• Quetiapine • Risperidone • Zotepine
• Zuclopenthixol

A group of drugs used to treat *psychoses* (mental disorders involving loss of contact with reality), particularly *schizophrenia* and *mania* (abnormal elation and overactivity) in manic-depressive illness (see *bipolar disorder*). Antipsychotic drugs may also be used to sedate people who are suffering from other mental disorders (such as *dementia*) and who are very agitated or aggressive.

HOW THEY WORK
Most antipsychotic drugs block the action of *dopamine*, a chemical that stimulates nerve activity in the brain. Antipsychotic drugs include *pheno-*thiazine drugs, butyrophenones such as *haloperidol*, and several newer drugs, including risperidone.

SIDE EFFECTS
Antipsychotic drugs can cause drowsiness, lethargy, *dyskinesia* (abnormal muscular movements), and *parkinsonism*. Other possible side effects include dry mouth, blurred vision, and difficulty in passing urine. However, newer drugs may have fewer side effects when used long term.

antipyretic drugs

Drugs that reduce fever. Examples of antipyretic drugs include *paracetamol*, *aspirin*, and other *nonsteroidal anti-inflammatory drugs*.

antiretroviral drugs

COMMON DRUGS
NUCLEOSIDE REVERSE TRANSCRIPTASE INHIBITORS
• Didanosine • Lamivudine • Stavudine
• Zidovudine (AZT)
NON-NUCLEOSIDE REVERSE TRANSCRIPTASE INHIBITORS
• Efavirenz • Nevirapine
NUCLEOTIDE REVERSE TRANSCRIPTASE INHIBITORS
• Tenofovir
PROTEASE INHIBITORS • Indinavir • Nelfinavir
• Ritonavir • Saquinavir
FUSION INHIBITORS
• Enfuvirtide

Drugs that are used to slow or halt the spread of viruses (see *retrovirus*) in people who have HIV infection and *AIDS*. There are two main types of antiretroviral drug: reverse transcriptase inhibitors (which are subdivided according to their chemical structure into nucleoside, non-nucleoside, and nucleotide reverse transcriptase inhibitors) and protease inhibitors. A combination of antiretroviral drugs from different groups is often used. The emergence of resistant strains of HIV has led to the development of a new group of drugs called *fusion inhibitors*.

HOW THEY WORK
Reverse transcriptase inhibitors and protease inhibitors work by interfering with the action of enzymes used by the virus to produce genetic material. Fusion inhibitors work by interfering with the entry of the virus into cells.

SIDE EFFECTS
Antiretroviral drugs can have a range of side effects, including nausea, vomiting, diarrhoea, tiredness, and various effects on blood chemistry, particularly involving fats. (See also *antiviral drugs*.)

antirheumatic drugs

COMMON DRUGS

IMMUNOSUPPRESSANTS •Azathioprine
•Cyclophosphamide •Ciclosporin
•Methotrexate

GOLD-BASED DRUGS •Auranofin •Sodium
aurothiomalate

OTHERS •Chloroquine •Corticosteroids
•Cytokine inhibitors •Hydroxychloroquine
•NSAIDs •Penicillamine •Sulfasalazine

A group of drugs used to treat *rheumatoid arthritis* and other types of arthritis that are the result of other *autoimmune disorders*, such as systemic *lupus erythematosus*.

Antirheumatic drugs modify the disease process by affecting the body's immune response and may therefore limit joint damage. The principal antirheumatic drugs are *immunosuppressant drugs*, gold-based drugs (see *gold*), *chloroquine*, hydroxychloroquine, *penicillamine*, and *sulfasalazine*. Collectively, these drugs are known as *disease-modifying anti-rheumatic drugs* (DMARDs).

A new group of antirheumatic drugs, called *cytokine inhibitors*, may also occasionally be prescribed for active rheumatoid arthritis if DMARDs are unsuitable or have failed to work. Cytokine inhibitors, which include etanercept, infliximab, and adalimumab, also slow down the disease and help to prevent joint damage.

Nonsteroidal ant-inflammatory drugs (NSAIDs) and *corticosteroids* may also be used to reduce the pain and inflammation of rheumatic disorders but do not affect the disease process itself.

SIDE EFFECTS

Many antirheumatic drugs can have serious side effects, and treatment, other than with NSAIDs and/or corticosteroids, is therefore given only under specialist medical supervision.

antiseptics

Chemicals that are applied to the skin in order to destroy bacteria and other microorganisms, thereby preventing sepsis (infection). Antisepsis (the use of antiseptics to prevent infection) is not the same as asepsis, which is the creation of a germ-free environment (see *aseptic technique*). Antiseptics are milder than *disinfectants*, which decontaminate inanimate objects but are too strong to be used on the body.

Antiseptic fluids are generally used for bathing wounds; antiseptic creams are applied to wounds before they are dressed. Common antiseptics are *chlorhexidine*, *cetrimide*, and compounds containing *iodine*.

antiserum

A preparation containing antibodies (proteins manufactured by the immune system, see *antibody*) that combine with specific *antigens* (foreign proteins), usually components of microorganisms, leading to the deactivation or destruction of the microorganisms.

Antiserum is usually used, along with *immunization*, as an emergency treatment when an individual has been exposed to a dangerous infection, such as *rabies*, and has not previously been immunized against it. The antiserum helps to provide some immediate protection against the infective microorganisms while full immunity is developing. Such measures are not as effective in preventing disease as earlier (pre-exposure) immunization, however.

antisocial personality disorder

Impulsive, destructive behaviour that often disregards the feelings and rights of others. People who have an antisocial personality lack a sense of guilt and cannot tolerate frustration. They may have problems with relationships and are frequently in trouble with the law.

Behaviour therapy and various forms of *psychotherapy* may help to improve social integration. In general, the effects of the condition decrease with age.

antispasmodic drugs

COMMON DRUGS

•Atropine •Dicycloverine •Hyoscine
•Mebeverine

A group of drugs that relax spasm in smooth (involuntary) muscle in the wall of the intestine or bladder. Antispasmodic drugs are used in the treatment of irritable bowel syndrome and irritable bladder.

HOW THEY WORK

Some antispasmodic drugs have an anticholinergic action (that is, they work by blocking the action of *acetylcholine*, a neurotransmitter chemical released from nerve endings that stimulates muscle contraction). Others work by direct action on smooth muscle.

SIDE EFFECTS

Possible side effects of antispasmodic drugs include a dry mouth, blurred vision, and difficulty in passing urine. (See also *anticholinergic drugs*.)

antithyroid drugs

COMMON DRUGS

•Carbimazole •Iodine •Propylthiouracil

A group of drugs that are used to treat *hyperthyroidism*, in which the thyroid gland is overactive. They may be used as the sole treatment for hyperthyroidism or may be given prior to thyroid surgery.

HOW THEY WORK

Carbimazole and *propylthiouracil* work primarily by interfering with production of thyroid hormones by the thyroid gland. Radioactive iodine works by destroying part of the thyroid tissue in people with hormone-secreting thyroid nodules.

SIDE EFFECTS

Side effects of carbimazole and propylthiouracil include nausea, headaches, mild gastrointestinal disturbances, dizziness, joint pain, itching, and rash. Carbimazole can suppress white blood cell production. Iodine can cause hypersensitivity reactions resembling coryza (nasal symptoms of the common cold).

antitoxin

Any of a variety of commercially prepared substances containing *antibodies* (proteins manufactured by the *immune system*) that can combine with and neutralize the effect of a specific *toxin* that has been released into the bloodstream by particular bacteria (such as those that cause *tetanus* and *diphtheria*).

Antitoxins are usually given by injection into a muscle. Occasionally, an antitoxin may cause an allergic reaction (see *allergy*); rarely, it may cause *anaphylactic shock* (a severe allergic reaction requiring emergency treatment).

antitussive drugs

Drugs that suppress or relieve a *cough* (see *cough remedies*).

antivenom

A specific treatment for bites or stings inflicted by venomous animals such as snakes, spiders, and scorpions.

Antivenom is prepared by the inoculation of animals, such as horses, with venom from a particular poisonous animal, thereby provoking the production of *antibodies* (proteins manufactured by the *immune system*) that neutralize the poisons in the venom. A preparation of these antibodies can be produced from samples of the animal's blood.

Antivenoms are given by intravenous injection and may cause allergic reactions (see *allergy*).

antiviral drugs

COMMON DRUGS

ANTIRETROVIRALS •Didanosine •Efavirenz •Indinavir •Lamivudine •Nelfinavir •Nevirapine •Ritonavir •Saquinavir •Stavudine •Zidovudine

OTHERS •Aciclovir •Amantadine •Cidofovir •Famciclovir •Foscarnet •Ganciclovir •Idoxuridine •Inosine pranobex •Interferon •Oseltamivir •Penciclovir •Ribavirin •Valaciclovir •Zanamivir

Drugs used in the treatment of infection by *viruses*. No drugs have been developed that can eradicate viruses completely, and at present *immunization* is the most effective way of preventing serious viral infections. However, antiviral drugs can reduce the severity of some viral infections (most notably *herpes*, *influenza*, viral *hepatitis*, and *cytomegalovirus* infections), particularly in people who have reduced immunity. Advances have also been made in the treatment of HIV infection (see *antiretroviral drugs*).

HOW THEY WORK

Most antiviral drugs destroy viruses by disrupting the chemical processes necessary for the virus to grow and multiply within a cell. Some antivirals actually prevent viruses penetrating the cells.

SIDE EFFECTS

Side effects of antiviral drugs used in the treatment of HIV infection and AIDS may include nausea, diarrhoea, and tiredness. These drugs may also affect blood chemistry, leading to conditions such as *anaemia* (a reduced level of the oxygen-carrying pigment *haemoglobin* in the blood).

Most other antivirals rarely cause side effects. Antiviral creams may cause skin irritation and those given by mouth or injection may lead to nausea, dizziness, and rarely, in prolonged treatment, to kidney damage.

antral irrigation

Irrigation (flushing out) of the maxillary antrum, one of the nasal sinuses. More commonly known as a sinus washout, antral irrigation is used to treat persistent *sinusitis*. The procedure is performed less often nowadays since the introduction of nasal *endoscopy*, (examination of the nasal cavity using a flexible viewing tube).

anuria

Complete cessation of urine output. Anuria may be caused by a severe mal-function of the kidneys, but a much more common cause is a complete blockage of the flow of urine as a result of enlargement of the prostate gland (see *prostate, enlarged*), a *bladder tumour*, or a bladder or kidney stone in the (see *calculus, urinary tract*). Failure of the kidneys to produce urine may be due to oxygen depletion as a result of reduced blood flow through the kidneys, as occurs in *shock*, or to severe kidney damage caused by a disease such as *glomerulonephritis*.

Anuria requires urgent investigation to establish the cause and to allow treatment (such as rehydration or removal of the blockage) to begin. Treatment of the cause may restore urine production, but any delay can result in permanent kidney damage, leading to *uraemia* (excess urea and other waste products in the blood).

anus

The end of the alimentary tract through which faeces are expelled from the body. The anus is an extension of the rectum as it passes downwards and backwards through the pelvic floor.

The orifice at the end of the anal canal is open only during defaecation; at other times it is kept closed by the muscles of the anal sphincter. These muscles are arranged in two layers: the internal sphincter, which cannot be controlled voluntarily, and the external sphincter, which can be relaxed at will for defaecation. Disorders of the anus include anal cancer (see *anus, cancer of*) and imperforate anus (see *anus, imperforate*). (See also *digestive system*.)

anus, cancer of

A rare cancer of the skin of the anus. Possible early signs of anal cancer are the development of swelling or an ulcer at the anus, accompanied by bleeding and discomfort. Treatment is by surgical removal and/or *radiotherapy*.

anus, imperforate

A rare congenital (present from birth) abnormality in which the anal opening is missing or covered over. The severity of the condition varies from complete absence of the anal canal to only a layer of skin covering the anal opening.

Treatment is with surgery. In severe cases, a *colostomy* may be needed initially before definitive surgery to construct an anus. Where surgery simply involves removal of a layer of skin over the anal

STRUCTURE OF THE ANUS

The anus is a canal at the end of the alimentary tract, with internal and external sphincters to open and close the orifice.

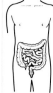

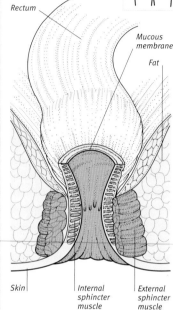

Rectum

Mucous membrane

Fat

Skin

Internal sphincter muscle

External sphincter muscle

opening, *anal dilation* (a procedure to enlarge the anus) may be required for several months afterwards.

anxiety

An unpleasant emotional state that ranges from mild unease to intense fear. Anxiety is a normal response to stressful situations and prepares the mind and body to respond effectively. However, anxiety that occurs without reason may be a symptom of an *anxiety disorder* or another psychological disorder such as *depression*.

SYMPTOMS

A variety of physical symptoms are associated with anxiety. The most common include palpitations (a more forceful or faster heartbeat), chest pains, a feeling of tightness in the chest, and a tendency to overbreathe (see *hyperventilation*). Muscle tension leads to headaches and back pains.

Gastrointestinal symptoms of anxiety include dry mouth (see *mouth, dry*), bloating, diarrhoea, nausea, and difficulty in swallowing. Other symptoms

DISORDERS OF THE **ANUS**

Most anal disorders are minor but may cause considerable discomfort and concern. Many are aggravated by constipation and may be helped by regular toilet habits, an increased intake of fluids, wholemeal products, fruits, and vegetables to soften the faeces, and the use of glycerine suppositories, if necessary.

Congenital defects

Imperforate anus is an uncommon birth defect in which the anus is sealed (see *anus, imperforate*).

In *anal stenosis*, the anus is too narrow to allow the normal passage of faeces. This is sometimes a congenital abnormality, but it can also result from scarring following surgery to treat another disorder.

Injury

Anal fissures originate from small tears in the lining of the anus, usually as a result of straining to pass hard, dry faeces.

Tumours

Cancer of the skin around the anus is rare (see *anus, cancer of*).

Other disorders

Haemorrhoids are enlarged blood vessels under the lining of the anus and may cause bleeding during defaecation, itching, and pain.

An *anal fistula* is an abnormal tunnel connecting the inside of the anal canal with the skin surrounding the anus. These fistulas usually result from an abscess in the wall of the anus.

Itching of the anus (pruritus ani) may be a direct result of another disorder, such as an anal fistula, haemorrhoids or *threadworm* infestation.

Anal warts (see *warts, genital*) are transmitted by sexual contact and are caused by a papillomavirus.

INVESTIGATION

Investigation of anal disorders is usually by visual inspection, sometimes involving *proctoscopy* (use of a rigid internal viewing tube) and digital examination (feeling with a finger). Sometimes a *biopsy* (small sample of tissue removed for microscopic analysis) or *swab* may be taken for bacteriological culture.

include lightheadedness, sweating, pallor, blushing, and a frequent need to urinate or defaecate.

People with anxiety may have a constant feeling that something bad is going to happen. They may fear illness or worry about the health and safety of family and friends. Fear of losing control is also common. Anxiety often leads to increasing dependence on others, irritability, a sense of fatigue, and frustration. Inability to relax may lead to difficulty in sleeping.

TREATMENT
People suffering from anxiety may be helped by *counselling* or *psychotherapy*. If there is an underlying disorder, such as depression, treatment with *antidepressant drugs* can help. Antianxiety drugs are occasionally used for short-term control of symptoms but are avoided for long-term treatment because they are addictive.

anxiety disorders

A group of mental illnesses, including several specific syndromes, in which symptoms of *anxiety* are the principal feature. Anxiety disorders are common and mainly affect young adults.

TYPES
In *generalized anxiety disorder*, the affected individual suffers from persistent tension and apprehension that has no specific focus or cause, together with physical or psychological symptoms that disrupt normal activity. *Panic disorder* is characterized by sudden and recurrent attacks of extreme, unreasonable fear and anxiety. *Phobias* are irrational fears, such as the fear of open spaces or of spiders, that lead to avoidance of certain situations or objects. *Post-traumatic stress disorder* is a form of anxiety that develops following a stressful or traumatic event and *obsessive–compulsive disorder* is a condition in which a person's obsessions and fears lead them to carry out repetitive, ritualized acts.

TREATMENT
Counselling, *psychotherapy*, group therapy, or *cognitive–behavioural therapy* are used to treat anxiety disorders. *Antidepressant drugs* may be used, and

antianxiety drugs (especially *benzodiazepine drugs*) may be given for short-term treatment but are addictive.

anxiolytics

See *antianxiety drugs*.

aorta

The main *artery* of the body, which supplies oxygenated blood to all other parts. The aorta arises from the left ventricle (the main pumping chamber of the *heart*) and arches up over the heart before descending, behind it, through the chest cavity. It terminates in the abdomen by dividing into the two common iliac arteries of the legs. The aorta is thick-walled and has a large diameter to cope with the high pressure and large volume of blood passing through it.

DISORDERS
The aorta, like other arteries, can become narrowed as a result of *atherosclerosis* (fat deposits on its walls), which may cause *hypertension* (high blood pressure). *Coarctation of the aorta* (in which the aorta is abnormally narrow at birth) and *aortitis* (inflammation of the aorta wall) are examples of aorta-specific disorders. Both aortitis and atherosclerosis may result in an aortic *aneurysm* (ballooning of the aorta wall), which may require surgery. (See also *arteries, disorders of*; *circulatory system*.)

aortic incompetence

Leakage of blood through the aortic valve (one of the *heart valves*), resulting in a backflow of blood from the aorta into the left ventricle (the heart's main pumping chamber).

CAUSES
Failure of the aortic valve to close properly may be due to a *congenital* (present from birth) abnormality in which the valve has two leaflets (flaps) rather than three. The valve leaflets can be destroyed by infective *endocarditis* (inflammation of the membrane lining the heart). Long-term *hypertension* can sometimes cause the root of the aorta to stretch so that the valve does not close properly.

Aortic incompetence is also associated with *ankylosing spondylitis* (a disorder that affects the spine), and *Marfan syndrome*, a congenital disorder of connective tissues. *Rheumatic fever*, which is now rare, may damage the valve, causing a combination of *aortic stenosis* (narrowing of the aortic valve) and incompetence. In addition, aortic incompetence may occur in untreated *syphilis*.

A

LOCATION AND STRUCTURE OF THE **AORTA**

From its origin at the left ventricle, the aorta passes upwards, curves behind the heart, and runs downwards, passing through the thorax (chest) and into the abdomen, where it terminates by dividing into two common iliac arteries. The aorta is thick-walled and large in diameter (about 2.5 cm at its origin) to cope with the high pressure and large volume of blood that passes through it. The thick walls of the aorta have an elastic quality that helps to even out the peaks and troughs of pressure that occur with each heartbeat.

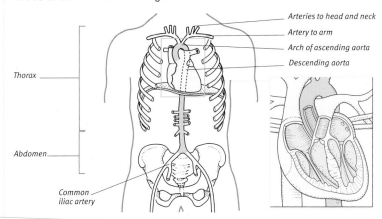

Arteries to head and neck
Artery to arm
Arch of ascending aorta
Descending aorta

Thorax

Abdomen

Common iliac artery

SYMPTOMS AND SIGNS

Aortic incompetence may not cause symptoms; it is sometimes found during a routine medical examination when the doctor hears a murmur (abnormal heart sound) over the front of the chest wall to the left of the sternum (breastbone).

The heart compensates for the backflow of blood into the left ventricle by working harder, until the combination of hypertrophy (muscle thickening) and dilatation (ballooning) of the left ventricle wall eventually leads to *heart failure* (reduced pumping efficiency of the heart); this causes breathing difficulty and *oedema* (a buildup of fluid).

DIAGNOSIS AND TREATMENT

A *chest X-ray*, *ECG* (measurement of the electrical activity of the heart), and *echocardiography* (imaging of the heart structures by measuring the pattern of reflection of sound waves from them) may be carried out to diagnose aortic incompetence. A cardiac catheter (flexible tube inserted into the heart via blood vessels) is sometimes used to assess the degree of incompetence (see *catheterization, cardiac*).

Heart failure resulting from aortic incompetence can be treated with *diuretic drugs* or other drugs to remove retained fluid from the lungs. *Heart-valve surgery* to replace the damaged valve may eventually be necessary.

aortic stenosis

Narrowing of the opening of the aortic valve (one of the *heart valves*), causing obstruction of blood flow into the circulation. Aortic stenosis makes the heart work harder and causes the muscle in the wall of the left ventricle (the main pumping chamber of the heart) to thicken. Narrowing of the valve also reduces the amount of blood flowing into the *coronary arteries* (the main arteries that supply the tissues of the heart with oxygen-rich blood).

CAUSES

The most common cause of aortic stenosis is deposition of calcium on the aortic valve. This deposition is usually associated with *atherosclerosis* (fatty deposits). Aortic stenosis may also be the result of a *congenital* (present from birth) abnormality.

SYMPTOMS AND SIGNS

Aortic stenosis may not cause any symptoms; it is sometimes found during a routine medical examination when the doctor hears a murmur (an abnormal heart sound) over the front of the chest wall to the right of the sternum (breastbone) and sometimes up into the neck. Symptoms, when they do occur, include fainting, lack of energy, chest pain on exertion as a result of *angina pectoris*, and breathing difficulties. Other features, which occur at a late stage, include a weak pulse and *cardiomegaly*, (enlargement of the heart).

DIAGNOSIS AND TREATMENT

A *chest X-ray*, an *ECG* (measurement of the electrical activity of the heart), and *echocardiography* (imaging of the heart structures by measuring the pattern of reflection of sound waves from them) may be carried out to diagnose aortic incompetence. A cardiac catheter (flexible tube that is inserted into the heart via blood vessels) can be used to assess the degree of stenosis (see *catheterization, cardiac*).

Heart-valve surgery may be needed to widen or replace the damaged valve.

aortitis

Inflammation of the *aorta* (the main artery of the body). Aortitis is a rare condition that occurs in people with *arteritis* (inflammation of the arteries) or untreated *syphilis* and in some people with *ankylosing spondylitis* (a disorder affecting the spine).

Aortitis may cause part of the aorta to widen and its walls to become thinner. This may lead to an *aneurysm* (ballooning of the artery), which may burst and cause severe, sometimes fatal, blood loss. Aortitis may also damage the ring around the aortic valve in the heart, leading to *aortic incompetence* (a condition which allows the backflow of blood into the heart), which may eventually result in *heart failure* (reduced pumping efficiency of the heart).

aortography

An imaging technique that enables the *aorta* (the main artery of the body) and its branches to be seen clearly on *X-ray* film following injection of a *contrast medium* (a substance that is opaque to X-rays) into the aorta.

HOW AND WHY IT IS DONE

The contrast medium is usually injected into the aorta through a fine catheter (a flexible plastic tube) that is inserted either into the femoral artery at the groin, the brachial artery on the inside of the elbow, or directly into the aorta within the lower abdomen.

Aortography is used if surgery is needed to treat an *aneurysm* (ballooning of the aorta).

apathy

The absence of feelings that is often associated with a lack of energy. Healthy people may be described as apathetic, but true apathy is a feature of certain

APGAR SCORE CHART

Sign	0	1	2
Colour	Blue, pale	Body pink; extremities blue	Completely pink
Respiratory effort	Absent	Weak cry; irregular breathing	Good strong cry; regular breathing
Muscle tone	Limp	Bending of some limbs	Active motion; limbs well-flexed
Reflex irritability	No response	Grimace (on nasal stimulation)	Cry
Heart rate	Absent	Slow (below 100 beats per minute)	Over 100 beats per minute

mental illnesses, such as *schizophrenia*. An affected person fails to take interest in everyday activities and tends to be inactive and lacking in volition (drive).

aperient

A mild *laxative drug*.

apex

The tip or uppermost surface of an organ or structure, such as the lungs or the heart. The apex of a tooth is the tip of its root.

apex beat

A normal heartbeat felt through the chest wall. As the heart contracts, its tip hits the chest wall and the beat can be felt between the fifth and sixth ribs on the left side of the chest. The apex beat is displaced when the heart is enlarged.

Apgar score

A system devised by Virginia Apgar, an American anaesthetist, to assess the condition of a newborn baby and help to direct appropriate care. Five features (breathing, heart rate, colour, muscle tone, and response to stimulation) are scored one minute, and again five minutes, after birth.

aphakia

The absence of the *lens* from the eye. Aphakia may be congenital (present from birth), may result from surgery (for example, *cataract surgery*), or may be due to a penetrating injury.

Aphakia causes severe loss of focusing in the affected eye and requires correction by implanting a lens or with contact lenses or glasses.

aphasia

Complete absence of previously acquired language skills caused by a brain disorder that affects the ability to speak and write, and/or comprehend and read. Related disabilities that may occur as a feature of aphasia are *alexia* (word blindness) and *agraphia* (writing difficulty).

CAUSES

Language function in the brain lies in the dominant cerebral hemisphere (see *cerebrum*). Two particular areas in this hemisphere, Broca's and Wernicke's areas, and the pathways connecting the two, are important in language skills. Damage to these areas, which most commonly occurs as a result of *stroke* or *head injury*, can lead to aphasia.

TYPES AND SYMPTOMS

Broca's aphasia causes difficulty in expressing language. Speech is laboured and normal rhythm is lost, but the few words uttered tend to be meaningful. Writing may also be impaired.

Wernicke's aphasia causes difficulty in language comprehension. Speech is fluent but its content is disturbed, with errors in word selection and grammar. Writing is also impaired, and spoken and/or written language may not be understood.

In *associative aphasia*, comprehension is normal, and the affected individual can write and speak. However, he or she is unable to repeat what has been heard and cannot read aloud.

Global aphasia comprises the total, or near total, inability to speak, write, or understand language.

Nominal aphasia is restricted to difficulty in naming objects or in finding words, although the sufferer may be able to choose the correct word from several offered.

In *jargon aphasia*, an affected individual cannot form grammatical sentences and utters meaningless phrases composed of jumbled words or neologisms.

TREATMENT AND OUTLOOK

Some recovery from aphasia is usual following a stroke or head injury, but the more severe the aphasia, the less the chances of recovery. *Speech therapy* is the main treatment. (See also *aphonia*; *dysarthria*; *dysphasia*; *dysphonia*; *speech*; *speech disorders*.)

apheresis

A procedure in which blood is withdrawn from a donor or patient and reinfused after one or more selected components have been separated and removed. For example, in *plasmapheresis*, *antibodies* (proteins manufactured by the *immune system*) that are causing a disease (such as *Guillain–Barré syndrome* or *Goodpasture's syndrome*) are removed; in leukapheresis, white blood cells (see *lymphocyte*) are removed either to reduce their number or to harvest them for use in a *blood transfusion*.

aphonia

Complete loss of the voice, which may result from surgery to the *larynx* (voice-box) or may be temporary, sudden in onset, and due to emotional stress. In aphonia, the vocal cords fail to meet as normal when an individual tries to speak, although they may come together when the person coughs.

There is no particular treatment for aphonia, but in the temporary form of the condition, the sufferer's voice usually returns as suddenly as it disappeared. (See also *dysphonia*.)

aphrodisiac

Any substance that is thought to stimulate erotic desire and enhance sexual performance. Aphrodisiacs are named after Aphrodite, the Greek goddess of love, beauty, and fertility.

For centuries, various substances (most notably oysters and rhinoceros horn) have been used as aphrodisiacs. In fact, there is no substance that has a proven aphrodisiac effect.

aphthous ulcer

See *ulcer, aphthous.*

apical

A term used to describe the position of structures that are found at the *apex* (tip) of particular organs and structures, including the lungs and heart.

apicectomy

The surgical removal of the tip of a tooth root in order physically to eliminate an infection or an infected cyst at the root tip. The procedure was once performed as part of *root-canal treatment* but is now used less often because root-canal treatment alone usually achieves the desired result.

aplasia

Absent or severely reduced growth and development of any organ or tissue. For example, in bone marrow aplasia, the rate of cell division in the bone marrow is reduced, leading to insufficient blood-cell production (see *anaemia, aplastic*). Some birth defects, such as stunted limbs (see *phocomelia*), occur as a result of incomplete tissue formation during prenatal development.

aplastic anaemia

See *anaemia, aplastic.*

apnoea

Cessation of breathing that can occur either temporarily (for a few seconds or up to a minute or two) or for a prolonged period.

CAUSES

Breathing is an automatic process that is controlled by the respiratory centre in the *brainstem* (a stalk of nerve tissue linking the brain to the spinal cord). The respiratory centre sends nerve impulses that regulate contraction of the diaphragm and muscles in the chest wall, thereby controlling the rate and depth of breathing. Failure of this centre to maintain normal breathing is known as central apnoea. The condition may occur in babies, particularly those who are premature, and can be detected by an apnoea alarm. Central apnoea can also be the result of damage to the brainstem (following a *stroke* or *head injury*, for example).

In obstructive apnoea, breathing is prevented by a blockage in the airway. The most common type is *sleep apnoea*, in which blockage of the upper airway occurs repeatedly during sleep.

Deliberate temporary apnoea occurs in *breath-holding attacks*. Another type of apnoea occurs in *Cheyne–Stokes respiration*, in which cycles of deep, rapid breathing alternate with episodes of breathing stoppage.

TREATMENT

Treatment depends on the cause; in newborn babies, apnoea resolves itself as they mature. In cases of stroke or head injury, artificial ventilation may be necessary, temporarily, until recovery occurs.

apocrine gland

A gland that discharges cellular material in addition to the fluid that it secretes. The term apocrine is usually applied to the type of *sweat glands* that appear in hairy areas of the body after puberty. (See also *eccrine gland.*)

apocrinitis

Inflammation of the *apocrine glands*, which are located in the armpit, groin, and perineum.

apolipoprotein

Any of a group of proteins that are constituents of *lipoproteins*, the carriers of fat in the bloodstream. Apolipoproteins are also involved in the growth and repair of nerve tissues.

apomorphine

A drug that is used in the treatment of *Parkinson's* disease. Nausea and vomiting are common side effects of apomorphine at the start of treatment.

aponeurosis

A wide sheet of tough, fibrous tissue that acts as a tendon by attaching a muscle to a bone or a joint.

apophysis

An outgrowth of bone at the site of attachment of a tendon to bone. Inflammation may occur, as in *Osgood–Schlatter disease.*

apoplexy

An outdated term for a *stroke.*

apoptosis

The natural process of programmed cell death. Apoptosis occurs in embryonic development, when the shaping of body parts is taking place, and continues throughout life in the constant cycle of death and renewal of body cells. Failure of apoptosis is implicated in the development of cancers.

apothecary

An outdated term for a *pharmacist.*

LAPAROSCOPIC APPENDICECTOMY

Surgery to remove the appendix can be carried out, under general anaesthesia, either conventionally or laparoscopically.

Laparoscopic appendicectomy takes approximately an hour, which is three times as long as conventional surgery, but recovery is quicker.

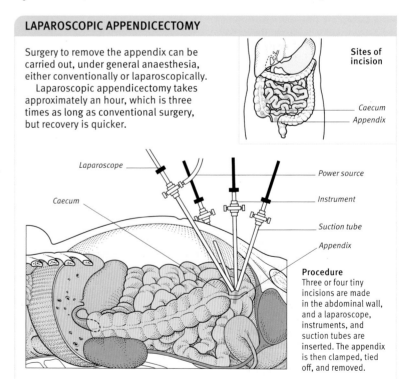

Sites of incision

Caecum
Appendix

Laparoscope

Power source

Instrument

Suction tube

Caecum

Appendix

Procedure

Three or four tiny incisions are made in the abdominal wall, and a laparoscope, instruments, and suction tubes are inserted. The appendix is then clamped, tied off, and removed.

appendage

An additional piece of *tissue* that is attached to a main structure. An auricular appendage is a small tag of tissue attached near the ear that may be present from birth.

appendicectomy

Surgical removal of the appendix to treat acute *appendicitis* (inflammation of the appendix).

WHY IT IS DONE

Appendicectomy is performed to prevent an inflamed appendix bursting and causing *peritonitis* (inflammation of the peritoneum, the lining of the abdominal cavity) or an abdominal abscess.

HOW IT IS DONE

The two methods of appendicectomy are conventional appendicectomy and *minimally invasive surgery*. Conventional surgery involves making a hole in the abdominal wall that is large enough for the surgeon's instruments and fingertips to be introduced. In minimally invasive surgery, three or four small holes are made in the abdominal wall; a laparoscope (viewing instrument) that incorporates a video camera is inserted into one of the openings, and instruments and suction tubes into the others. In both types of operation, the appendix is identified, clamped, tied off at its base, and removed.

If the appendix has burst, the infected area of the abdominal cavity is washed out with saline and drained via a tube inserted into one of the incisions. Antibiotic drugs may also be given to prevent peritonitis.

COMPLICATIONS AND OUTLOOK

Possible complications are infection of the incision wound, an abscess at the site from which the appendix was removed, or localized peritonitis.

In the absence of complications, normal physical activities can usually be resumed within two to three weeks.

appendicitis

Acute inflammation of the *appendix* (a narrow, finger-shaped tube that branches off the large intestine), which is a common cause of abdominal pain and *peritonitis* (inflammation of the lining of the abdominal cavity).

CAUSE AND SYMPTOMS

The cause of appendicitis is usually not known, but the condition is sometimes caused by obstruction of the appendix by a lump of faeces. The closed end of the appendix beyond the obstruction

LOCATION OF THE **APPENDIX**

In the lower right-hand side of the abdomen, the appendix may lie behind the caecum, or in front of or behind the ileum.

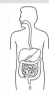

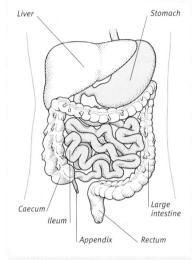

Liver · Stomach · Caecum · Ileum · Appendix · Rectum · Large intestine

becomes inflamed, swollen, and infected. This may lead to *gangrene* (tissue death) in the appendix wall, which may perforate (burst).

The first symptom is usually vague discomfort around the navel. Within a few hours, this develops into severe, more localized pain, which is usually most intense in the lower right-hand side of the abdomen. Symptoms may differ if the appendix is not in the most common position. For example, if the appendix impinges on the ureter, the urine may become bloodstained.

DIAGNOSIS AND TREATMENT

Diagnosis may be difficult because the symptoms of appendicitis are similar to those of many other abdominal disorders. Sometimes a *laparotomy* (surgical investigation of the abdomen) is necessary in order to confirm or exclude a diagnosis of appendicitis.

The usual treatment for appendicitis is *appendicectomy*, which is often performed endoscopically (see *minimally invasive surgery*).

COMPLICATIONS

If treatment is delayed, an inflamed appendix may burst, releasing its contents into the abdomen. At this point, the pain ceases abruptly, but the perforation leads to peritonitis. In some

cases, the omentum (fold of peritoneum that covers the intestines) envelops the inflamed appendix; this prevents the spread of infection but may result in a localized *abscess* around the appendix.

appendix

A small, narrow tube that projects out of the caecum (the first part of the colon) at the lower right-hand side of the abdomen. The appendix may lie behind or below the caecum, or in front of or behind the ileum (part of the small intestine).

The appendix has no known function, but it contains a large amount of lymphoid tissue, which provides a defence against localized infection. The position of an person's appendix partly determines the symptoms produced by acute *appendicitis* (inflammation of the appendix).

appendix abscess

An *abscess* (a collection of pus) that may form after the rupture of an inflamed appendix (see *appendicitis*).

appetite

A desire for food; a pleasant sensation that is felt in anticipation of eating. Appetite is distinct from *hunger*, which is a disagreeable feeling caused by the need for food.

Appetite, which is regulated by two parts of the *brain* (the *hypothalamus* and cerebral cortex), is learned by enjoying a variety of foods that smell, taste, and look good. It combines with *hunger* to ensure that the right amount of a wide range of foods is eaten in order to stay healthy. (See also *appetite, loss of*.)

appetite, loss of

Loss of appetite, known medically as anorexia, is usually temporary and due to an emotional upset or minor illness. Persistent loss of appetite may be a symptom of a more serious underlying physical or psychological disorder and requires investigation by a doctor.

CAUSES

In adolescents and young adults, loss of appetite may be due to *anorexia nervosa* (an eating disorder) or to *drug abuse*, particularly of *amphetamine drugs*. Depression or anxiety may result in loss of appetite at any age.

Possible physical causes of appetite loss include a *stroke* (damage to part of the brain caused by an interruption to its blood supply), a *brain tumour*, or a

A

head injury that has damaged the *hypothalamus* or cerebral cortex (the parts of the brain that control appetite). Other physical causes include intestinal disorders, such as *gastritis* (inflammation of the stomach lining, which is common in problem drinkers), *stomach cancer*, a *gastric ulcer*, and liver disorders such as *hepatitis*. Many infectious diseases, such as *influenza*, can also lead to loss of appetite.

Between the ages of about two and four, some children go through a period of refusing food. If there are no other symptoms, this phase should be regarded as a normal part of a child's development.

For an otherwise healthy person, a period of two or three days without food is not harmful, provided that plenty of nonalcoholic fluids are drunk. A doctor should always be consulted, however, if there are other health problems (particularly *diabetes mellitus*) or if regular medication is being taken.

All cases of appetite loss that last for more than a few days should be investigated by a doctor. Appetite generally returns to normal once any underlying illness has been treated. (See also *appetite stimulants*.)

appetite stimulants

Various tonics and remedies that have been traditionally prescribed to stimulate the appetite. None are proven to be effective. Some drugs, such as *corticosteroid drugs*, may stimulate the appetite when used to treat unrelated disorders.

appetite suppressants

A group of drugs that reduce the desire to eat and are used in the treatment of severe *obesity*, along with dieting and exercise. Sibutramine and rimonabant are the main appetite suppressants.

HOW THEY WORK

Sibutramine works by inhibiting the reuptake of *noradrenaline* (norepinephrine) and serotonin. Rimonabant acts by blocking the action of natural chemicals in the brain called cannabinoids, which are involved in regulating hunger and appetite, particularly for sweet and fatty foods.

SIDE EFFECTS

Common side effects of sibutramine include constipation, a dry mouth, insomnia, nausea, palpitations, *hypertension* (high blood pressure), headache, anxiety, sweating, and taste disturbances. The use of sibutramine is limited to a maximum of one year.

Adverse effects of rimonabant are usually mild and transient. They include nausea, digestive disturbances, vomiting, dry mouth, sleep disturbances, back or muscle pain, memory loss, irritability, and anxiety. Some people also develop depression and therefore rimonabant is not generally recommended for people who are depressed or have a history of depression.

apraxia

The inability to carry out purposeful movements despite normal muscle power and coordination. Apraxia is caused by damage to nerve tracts in the *cerebrum* (the main mass of the brain) that translate the idea for a movement into an actual movement. People with apraxia usually know what they want to do but are unable to recall from memory the sequence of actions necessary to achieve the movement. Damage to the cerebrum that results in apraxia may be caused by a *head injury*, an infection, a *stroke* (damage to part of the brain caused by interruption to its blood supply), or a *brain tumour*.

TYPES

Apraxia takes various forms, and each is related to damage in different parts of the brain. Ideomotor apraxia is the inability to carry out a spoken command to make a certain movement, but to make the same movement unconsciously at other times. In sensory apraxia, a person may not be able to use an object due to loss of ability to recognize its purpose.

Agraphia (difficulty in writing) and *aphasia* (severe difficulty in expressing language) are special forms of apraxia.

OUTLOOK

Recovery from apraxia is highly variable and is dependent on the cause. Lost skills may need to be relearned.

APUD cell tumour

A growth composed of cells that produce various hormones. APUD (amine precursor uptake and decarboxylation) cells occur in different parts of the body.

Some tumours of the thyroid gland, pancreas, and lungs are APUD cell tumours, as are carcinoid tumours (tumours of the intestine or lung, see *carcinoid syndrome*) and *phaeochromocytoma* (a type of adrenal tumour).

aqueous cream

An *emollient* preparation that is commonly used to treat dry, scaly, or itchy skin in conditions such as *eczema*.

aqueous humour

A watery fluid that fills the front chamber of the *eye*, behind the *cornea* (the transparent front part of the eyeball).

arachidonic acid

One of the fatty acids in the body that are essential for growth.

arachis oil

Peanut or ground-nut oil. Arachis oil is used in *enemas* to lubricate and soften impacted faeces and to make bowel movements easier. It can also be applied to the scalp, followed by shampooing, in the treatment of *cradle cap*.

arachnodactyly

A term for long, thin, spiderlike fingers and toes. Arachnodactyly sometimes occurs spontaneously but is also characteristic of *Marfan syndrome*, an inherited connective tissue disease.

arachnoiditis

A rare condition that is characterized by chronic inflammation and thickening of the arachnoid mater, which is the middle of the three *meninges* (membranes) that cover the brain and spinal cord.

The cause of arachnoiditis is often unknown. However, the condition may develop following an episode of *meningitis* (inflammation of the meninges) or a *subarachnoid haemorrhage* (a type of brain haemorrhage). Arachnoiditis may also be a feature of *syphilis* or *ankylosing spondylitis* (a disorder affecting the spine). It may also result from injury or certain medical procedures.

Symptoms of arachnoiditis may include headache, epileptic seizures, blindness, or difficulty with movements due to increased muscle tension. There is no effective treatment for the condition.

arachnoid mater

The middle of the three layers of membrane (see *meninges*) that cover the *brain* and spinal cord.

arbovirus

Any of the many viruses transmitted by a member of the arthropod group of animals, including insects, mites, and ticks. (See also *insects and disease; mites and disease; ticks and disease*).

ARC

An abbreviation for *AIDS-related complex*. (See also *AIDS*.)

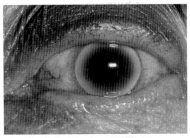

Arcus senilis
The arcus senilis is the lighter ring that overlies the edge of the iris (the coloured part of the eye).

arcus senilis

A grey-white ring near the edge of the *cornea* (the transparent front part of the eyeball) overlying the iris (the coloured part of the eye).

Arcus senilis, which is caused by degeneration of fatty material in the cornea, develops gradually during adult life. The ring never spreads to the centre and does not affect eyesight. The development of the condition in early adulthood may be associated with an abnormally high level of fats in the blood (see *hyperlipidaemia*).

areola

The pigmented circular area surrounding the *nipple*. The term is also used to describe an inflamed area around a pimple (see *pustule*).

Aricept

A brand name for donepezil, an *acetylcholinesterase inhibitor* used to treat *Alzheimer's disease*.

aromatherapy

A form of *complementary medicine* that uses aromatic oils extracted from plants to treat a wide range of disorders. Practitioners claim that aromatherapy is particularly effective in treating stress-related and *psychosomatic* conditions.

The oil is applied in small quantities through massage; it may also be inhaled, incorporated into creams or lotions, or, very occasionally, taken internally. There is no conclusive scientific evidence of the benefits.

arousal

The awakening of a person from unconsciousness or semiconsciousness. The term is also used to describe any state of heightened awareness, such as that caused by sexual stimulation or fear. Arousal is regulated by the reticular formation in the *brainstem*.

arrhenoblastoma

A rare tumour of the ovary that occurs in young women. The tumour is noncancerous, but it secretes *androgen hormones* (male sex hormones) that cause *virilization* (development of male characteristics). Treatment of arrhenoblastoma is by surgical removal of the affected ovary.

arrhythmia, cardiac

An abnormality of the rhythm or the rate of the *heartbeat*. Arrhythmias are the result of a disturbance in the electrical impulses within the *heart* (see *Cardiac arrhythmia* box, below). Any isolated irregular beat is known as an *ectopic heartbeat*. Ectopic beats do not necessarily indicate the presence of an abnormality, however.

TYPES
Arrhythmias can be divided into two main groups: tachycardias, in which the rate of the heartbeat is faster than normal, and bradycardias, in which the rate is slower. The rhythm may be regular, with each beat of the atria (upper chambers, see *atrium*) being followed by one beat of the *ventricles* (lower chambers).

Tachycardias In sinus tachycardia, the rate is raised, the rhythm is regular, and the beat originates in the sinoatrial node (see *pacemaker*). *Supraventricular tachycardia* is faster and the rhythm is regular. It may be caused by an abnormal electrical pathway that allows an impulse to circulate continuously in the heart and take over from the sinoatrial node. A rapid, irregular beat that originates in the ventricles is known as a *ventricular tachycardia*. In *atrial flutter*, the atria beat regularly and very rapidly, but not every impulse reaches the ventricles, which beat at a slower rate. Uncoordinated, fast beating of the atria is known as *atrial fibrillation* and produces totally irregular ventricular beats. *Ventricular fibrillation* is a form of *cardiac arrest* in which the heart does not pump blood because the ventricles are twitching very rapidly in a disorganized manner.

CARDIAC ARRHYTHMIA

Any disorder that interferes with the generation or transmission of impulses through the heart's electrical conducting system (below) can lead to a disturbance of cardiac rate or rhythm. These ECG recordings show two kinds of arrhythmia: sinus bradycardia and atrial fibrillation.

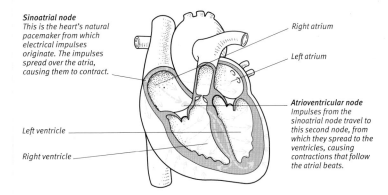

Sinoatrial node
This is the heart's natural pacemaker from which electrical impulses originate. The impulses spread over the atria, causing them to contract.

Right atrium

Left atrium

Atrioventricular node
Impulses from the sinoatrial node travel to this second node, from which they spread to the ventricles, causing contractions that follow the atrial beats.

Left ventricle

Right ventricle

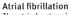

Sinus bradycardia
The heart rate is slow, but the rhythm normal, with each atrial beat (small rise) followed by a ventricular beat (spike). Sinus bradycardia is common in athletes but can also be caused by hypothyroidism.

Atrial fibrillation
The atria beat rapidly and irregularly. Ventricular beats (spikes) do not follow each atrial beat and are irregularly spaced. This arrhythmia is common in the elderly and in people with hyperthyroidism.

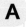

A

Bradycardias *Sinus bradycardia* is a slow, regular beat. In *heart block*, the conduction of electrical impulses through the heart muscle is either partially or completely blocked, leading to a slow, irregular heartbeat. Periods of bradycardia may alternate with periods of tachycardia due to a fault in impulse generation (see *sick sinus syndrome*).

CAUSES
A common cause of arrhythmia is *coronary artery disease*, in which the coronary arteries are narrowed by *atherosclerosis* (fat deposits on the artery walls), particularly when following *myocardial infarction* (heart attack). Some tachycardias are the result of a *congenital* (present from birth) defect in the heart's conducting system.

Caffeine can cause tachycardia in some people. *Amitriptyline* and some other *antidepressant drugs* can cause serious cardiac arrhythmias if they are taken in high doses.

SYMPTOMS
An arrhythmia may be felt as palpitations, in which the individual becomes aware of an abnormally rapid heartbeat. However, in some cases, arrhythmias cause fainting and dizziness as a result of reduced blood flow to the brain, or chest pain and breathlessness if there is a reduction in blood flow to the lungs. These may be the first symptoms.

DIAGNOSIS
Arrhythmias are diagnosed by an *ECG*, which shows the pattern of electrical activity within heart muscle. If the arrhythmia is intermittent, a continuous recording may need to be made using an *ambulatory ECG*. If an arrhythmia is present, other tests, such as *echocardiography*, may be performed.

TREATMENT
Treatments for arrhythmias include *antiarrhythmic drugs*, which prevent or slow tachycardias. With an arrhythmia that has developed suddenly, it may be possible to restore normal heart rhythm by using an electric shock to the heart (see *defibrillation*).

Repeated attacks of tachycardia can sometimes be treated by *radiofrequency ablation* (the removal of dead or diseased tissue) of the heart's abnormal conduction pathway. This may be carried out during cardiac catheterization (see *catheterization, cardiac*). In some cases, a *pacemaker* is be fitted to restore normal heartbeat by overriding the heart's abnormal rhythm.

arsenic

A poisonous metallic element that occurs naturally in its pure form and various compounds. Arsenic poisoning, now rare, once occurred as a result of continuous industrial or pesticide exposure.

arterial reconstructive surgery

An operation to repair *arteries* that are narrowed, blocked, or weakened.

WHY IT IS DONE
Arterial reconstructive surgery is most often performed to repair arteries that have been narrowed by *atherosclerosis* (fatty deposits on artery walls). It is also used to repair *aneurysms* (ballooning of arteries) and arteries damaged as a result of injury.

HOW IT IS DONE
A narrowed or blocked section of artery, particularly a coronary artery, can be bypassed by sewing in a length of vein above and below the constricted area. Elsewhere in the body, the affected section is commonly replaced using an artificial tube or a section of vein. (See also *angioplasty, balloon*; *coronary artery bypass*; *endarterectomy*.)

arteries, disorders of

Disorders of the arteries may take the form of abnormal narrowing (which reduces blood flow and may cause tissue damage), complete obstruction (which may cause tissue death), or abnormal widening and thinning of an artery wall (which may cause rupture of the blood vessel).

TYPES
Atherosclerosis, in which fat deposits build up on the lining of artery walls, is the most common arterial disease. It can involve arteries throughout the body, including the brain (see *cerebrovascular disease*), heart (see *coronary artery disease*), and legs (see *peripheral vascular disease*). Atherosclerosis is the main type of *arteriosclerosis*, a group of disorders that cause thickening and loss of elasticity of artery walls.

Hypertension (high blood pressure) is another common cause of thickening and narrowing of arteries. Hypertension predisposes people to coronary artery disease and increases the risk of a *stroke* or *kidney failure*.

Arteritis is inflammation of artery walls that causes narrowing and sometimes blockage.

Aneurysm is ballooning of an artery wall caused by the pressure of blood flowing through a weakened area.

Thrombosis occurs when a thrombus (blood clot) forms in a blood vessel, causing obstruction of the blood flow.

An *embolism* is blockage of an artery by a fragment of blood clot or other material travelling in the circulation.

Raynaud's disease is a disorder in which there is intermittent spasm of small arteries in the hands and feet, usually precipitated by the cold.

arteriography

An alternative name for *angiography*, an X-ray technique for imaging arteries.

arteriole

A blood vessel that is a branch from an *artery* and which branches further to form *capillaries*. Arterioles have muscular walls and a nerve supply, enabling them to narrowed or widened to meet the blood-flow needs of tissues they supply.

arteriopathy

Any disorder of an artery (see *arteries, disorders of*).

arterioplasty

Surgical repair of an artery (see *arterial reconstructive surgery*).

arteriosclerosis

A group of disorders that cause thickening and loss of elasticity of artery walls. *Atherosclerosis* is the most common type of arteriosclerosis, and the two terms are often used synonymously.

Other types are medial arteriosclerosis (in which muscle and elastic fibres in larger arteries are replaced by fibrous tissue) and Monckeberg's arteriosclerosis (in which there are calcium deposits in the arterial lining).

arteriovenous fistula

An abnormal communication directly between an artery and a vein. An arteriovenous fistula may be present at birth or may result from injury. A fistula can also be created surgically for easy access to the bloodstream, as occurs in *dialysis*.

If a fistula is close to the skin surface it may cause a small, pulsating swelling. If there are several in the lungs, uptake of oxygen into the blood may be impaired, resulting in *cyanosis* (blue skin colour) and breathing difficulty on exertion.

An isolated fistula that is causing symptoms can often be cut away and the ends of the blood vessels stitched closed. However, if there are many fistulas, surgery is not practicable.

arteritis

Inflammation of an artery wall, which causes narrowing or complete blockage of the affected artery, reduced blood flow, and, in some cases, *thrombosis* (formation of a blood clot in the affected artery) and tissue damage.

TYPES

There are several types of arteritis. *Buerger's disease* is an arteritis that affects the limbs, causing pain, numbness, and, in severe cases, *gangrene*. *Polyarteritis nodosa*, a serious *autoimmune disorder* (in which the immune system attacks the body's own tissues), can affect arteries in any part of the body, especially the heart and kidneys. *Temporal arteritis* affects arteries in the scalp over the temples and may also affect the retinal artery in the eye. Takayasu's arteritis is thought to be an autoimmune disorder. It is a rare type of arteritis that usually affects young women and involves the arteries that branch from the *aorta* (the body's main artery) into the neck and arms.

STRUCTURE OF AN **ARTERY**

The walls of an artery consist of three layers: a smooth inner lining, a thick, muscular, elastic middle layer, and a tough, fibrous outer covering. Veins have thinner walls, and most of them contain valves.

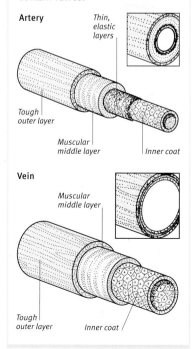

Artery

Thin, elastic layers

Tough outer layer

Muscular middle layer

Inner coat

Vein

Muscular middle layer

Tough outer layer

Inner coat

artery

A blood vessel that carries blood away from the *heart*. Systemic arteries carry blood that has been pumped from the left ventricle (lower chamber) of the heart to all other parts of the body except the lungs. The largest systemic artery is the *aorta*, which emerges from the left ventricle; other major systemic arteries branch off from the aorta. The pulmonary arteries carry blood from the right ventricle to the lungs.

STRUCTURE

Arteries are tubes with thick, elastic, muscular walls able to withstand the high blood pressure to which they are subjected at each heartbeat. The structure of arteries helps to even out the peaks and troughs of blood pressure caused by the heartbeat, so that the blood is flowing at a relatively constant pressure by the time it reaches the smaller blood vessels (*arterioles*, which branch directly off the arteries and connect to the even smaller *capillaries*). The pulmonary arteries are thinner-walled than systemic arteries and contain blood at a lower pressure. (See also *arteries, disorders of.*)

arthralgia

Pain in the joints or in a single joint. (See also *arthritis*; *joint.*)

arthritis

Inflammation of one or more joints that is characterized by pain, swelling, and stiffness. Arthritis can vary in severity from a mild ache and joint stiffness to severe pain and, subsequently, deformity of the joints.

TYPES AND CAUSES

There are several different types of arthritis, each having different characteristics. The most common type is *osteoarthritis*, which most often involves the knees, hips, and hands. It usually affects middle-aged and older people because it results principally from wear and tear on the joints. *Cervical osteoarthritis* is a form of osteoarthritis that affects the joints in the neck.

Rheumatoid arthritis is a damaging *autoimmune disorder* (in which the immune system attacks the body's own tissues) that causes inflammation in the joints and other body tissues such as the pericardium (the membrane covering the heart), the lungs, and the eyes. The disorder has different effects in children (see *juvenile chronic arthritis*).

Ankylosing spondylitis is another persistent type of arthritis that initially

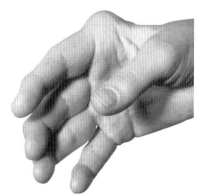

Arthritis in the hands
The joints in the hands of a person suffering from rheumatoid arthritis are painful, swollen, and stiff. in severe cases, the joints become deformed.

affects the spine and the joints between the base of the spine and the pelvis. Other tissues, such as the eyes, may also be affected. Eventually, the disorder may cause the vertebrae (the bones of the spine) to fuse.

Reactive arthritis typically develops in susceptible people following an infection, most commonly of the genital tract or intestines.

Gout and *pseudogout* are types of arthritis in which crystals are deposited in a joint, causing swelling and pain.

Septic arthritis is a relatively rare condition that can develop when infection enters a joint, either through a wound or from the bloodstream.

DIAGNOSIS

Diagnosis of particular types of arthritis is made from *blood tests* and, in some cases, microscopic examination of fluid from the affected joint. *X-rays* or *MRI* (a technique that produces cross-sectional or three-dimensional images of body structures) can indicate the type and extent of joint damage.

TREATMENT

Physiotherapy and exercises can help to minimize the effects of arthritis, and *nonsteroidal anti-inflammatory drugs* and *corticosteroids* may be used to relieve pain and inflammation.

There are also specific treatments for particular types of arthritis; for example, *antibiotic drugs* may be used for treating septic arthritis and *disease-modifying antirheumatic drugs* (DMARDs) for rheumatoid arthritis.

In severe cases, one or more of the diseased joints may require *arthroplasty* (replacement of a joint with an artificial substitute) or *arthrodesis* (fusion of the bones in a joint).

A

arthrodesis

A surgical procedure in which the bones in a diseased joint are fused to prevent the joint from moving, which relieves pain in the affected area.

HOW AND WHY IT IS DONE

Arthrodesis is performed if a joint is painful or unstable and other treatments, such as drugs or *arthroplasty* (replacement of the joint with an artificial substitute), have failed or are inappropriate.

Arthrodesis of a small joint, such as a finger joint, may be carried out under local anaesthesia (see *anaesthesia, local*). Otherwise, a general anaesthetic (see *anaesthesia, general*) is used. In most cases, cartilage (smooth, shock-absorbing tissue) is removed from the ends of the two bones, along with a surface layer of bone from each. The two ends are then joined so that they will fuse when fresh bone cells grow. The bones may need to be kept in position with plates, rods, or screws; a *bone graft* may also be carried out in some cases.

In arthrodesis of the knee or ankle joints, additional immobilization of the joint (by transfixing it with pins inserted through the skin) may be necessary to keep the area stable until healing is complete.

RECOVERY AND OUTLOOK

Complete union of the bones can take up to six months but may be much quicker. In some cases the bones fail to fuse, but fibrous tissue usually fills the gap between them and is strong enough to provide the same effect and strength as bone fusion.

Following arthrodesis, no movement can take place in the affected joint, unlike after arthroplasty. However, the advantage of arthrodesis over arthroplasty is that, once it has been performed, it requires no regular surveillance or further care; and the patient can be reasonably confident that the problem with the joint has been resolved permanently.

arthrography

A diagnostic technique in which the interior of a damaged joint is imaged using contrast *X-rays* or *MRI* (magnetic resonance imaging). *Ultrasound scanning* and *arthroscopy* may also be used.

arthrogryposis

See *contracture*.

arthropathy

A medical term for any disease or disorder that involves the *joints*. (See also *diabetic arthropathy*.)

arthroplasty

Replacement of a joint or part of a joint by metal or plastic components. A *hip replacement* is one of the most common operations of this type, as is a *knee-joint replacement*. Replacement of other joints, such as the finger (see *finger-joint replacement*), shoulder, and elbow, is also common.

arthroscopy

A surgical procedure in which an arthroscope, a type of *endoscope* (viewing tube) is used to diagnose and/or treat problems inside a joint.

WHY IT IS DONE

Arthroscopy is most often used to investigate disorders of the knee joint but can also be used in other joints such as the shoulder, hip, or wrist. It allows the surgeon to see the surface of the bones, the ligaments, the cartilages, and the synovial membrane. Specimens can be taken for examination, and instruments attached to the arthroscope enable various surgical procedures to be performed, such as removing loose or damaged cartilage, repairing damaged ligaments, and shaving the patella (kneecap).

Arthrotec

The brand name of an *antirheumatic drug* containing *diclofenac* and *misoprostol*.

articulation

The junction point of two or more bones (see *joint*).

artificial feeding

See *feeding, artificial*.

artificial heart

See *heart, artificial*.

artificial insemination

A form of assisted conception in which semen is introduced artificially into the uterus, instead of by sexual intercourse, with the aim of inducing conception and pregnancy.

HOW **ARTHROSCOPY** IS DONE

The procedure is usually performed under general anaesthesia. The joint is distended by injecting air or a saline solution, and the arthroscope and a probe are inserted into it through small skin incisions. While watching the monitor, the surgeon can repair or remove tissue, such as damaged cartilage, or drill or shave the surface of the patella (kneecap).

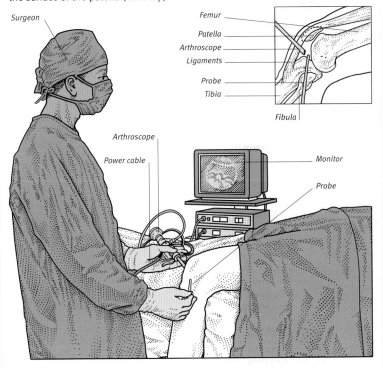

Surgeon

Femur
Patella
Arthroscope
Ligaments
Probe
Tibia

Fibula

Arthroscope
Power cable

Monitor
Probe

TYPES
There are two types of artificial insemination: AIH, artificial insemination with the semen of the woman's male partner; and DI, donor insemination (formerly known as AID). AIH is usually used for couples who are unable to have intercourse, or if the man has a low sperm count or a low volume of ejaculate. It is also used when a man's semen has been stored prior to his having treatment (such as chemotherapy) that has made him sterile. DI is available to couples if the man is infertile or a carrier of a genetic disease. It may also be used by a woman who wants children but has no male partner.

HOW IT IS DONE
Artificial insemination is carried out at centres that are specially staffed and equipped to obtain, test, and store semen, to carry out the insemination, and to give counselling before and after the procedure. Semen donors are screened for a wide variety of physical and mental disorders.

Insemination is performed by injecting a sample of semen into the woman's cervix using a small syringe. The procedure is timed to coincide with her natural ovulation (the development and release of an egg from the ovary), or it may be combined with treatment to stimulate ovulation.

artificial kidney

The common name for the machine used in *dialysis*.

artificial limb

See *prosthesis*.

artificial respiration

See *rescue breathing*.

artificial rupture of membranes

See *amniotomy*.

artificial saliva

A preparation used to relieve a persistently dry mouth, which may be a side effect of certain drugs or *radiotherapy* or may be due to *Sjögren's syndrome* (an autoimmune disorder in which the immune system attacks the body's own tissues). Artificial saliva, as a spray, gel, or pastilles, is formulated to resemble natural saliva as closely as possible.

artificial sweeteners

Synthetic substitutes for sugar that are used by people on slimming diets and by the food industry; examples include aspartame and saccharin. Sorbitol is an artificial sweetener that is useful for people with diabetes mellitus but it can cause diarrhoea and bloating when consumed in large quantities.

artificial tears

Preparations that are used to supplement tear production in disorders, such as *keratoconjunctivitis sicca*, that cause dry eye and to relieve irritation.

arytenoid

One of two pyramid-shaped cartilages that form part of the *larynx* (voicebox).

asbestos-related diseases

A variety of diseases that are caused by inhalation of asbestos fibres. Asbestos is a fibrous mineral formerly used as a heat- and fire-resistant insulating material. There are three main types of asbestos fibre: white, which is widely used, blue, and brown. Blue and brown are the most dangerous types of asbestos. The use of all types is now carefully controlled.

TYPES
In asbestosis, widespread fine scarring occurs in the lungs. The disease causes breathlessness and a dry cough, eventually leading to severe disability and death. Asbestosis develops mostly in industrial workers who have been heavily exposed to asbestos. The period from initial exposure to development of the disease is usually at least 20 years. Diagnosis is by *chest X-ray*. Asbestosis increases the risk of developing *lung cancer*.

Mesothelioma is a cancerous tumour of the *pleura* (the membrane surrounding the lungs) or the *peritoneum* (the membrane lining the abdominal cavity). In the pleura, mesotheliomas cause pain and breathlessness; in the peritoneum they cause enlargement of the abdomen and intestinal obstruction. The condition cannot be treated and usually leads to death within one or two years. The average interval between initial exposure to asbestos and death is between 20 and 30 years. Mesothelioma affects people who have been exposed to blue or brown asbestos.

Diffuse pleural thickening is a condition in which the outer and inner layers of the pleura become thickened, and excess fluid may accumulate in the cavity between them. This combination restricts the ability of the lungs to expand, resulting in shortness of breath. The condition may develop even after short exposure to asbestos.

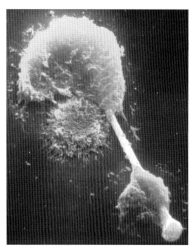

Electron micrograph of asbestos fibre in lung
An inhaled asbestos fibre impales and kills a macrophage (a scavenger cell that would normally engulf and destroy foreign particles in the lungs).

asbestosis

See *asbestos-related diseases*.

ascariasis

Infestation with the roundworm ASCARIS LUMBRICOIDES, which lives in the small intestine of its human host. Ascariasis is common worldwide, especially in the tropics. One or several worms may be present, but symptoms usually only occur with heavy infestation.

CAUSES
The parasite that causes ascariasis is a pale, cylindrical, tapered roundworm, which reaches between 15 and 35 cm in length in its adult form.

Ascariasis is spread by ingestion of worm eggs, usually from food grown in soil that has been contaminated by human faeces. In some dry, windy climates, airborne eggs may be swallowed after being blown into the mouth.

SYMPTOMS
Light infestation may cause no symptoms, although mild nausea, abdominal pain, and irregular bowel movements may occur. A worm may be passed via the rectum, or it may be vomited. A large number of worms may compete with the host for food, leading to malnutrition and *anaemia*, which, in children, can retard growth.

TREATMENT
The worm infestation is treated with *anthelmintic drugs*, such as levamisole, which usually bring about complete recovery. The worms are passed out of the body via the rectum some days after the drug is taken.

A

LIFE CYCLE OF THE **ASCARIS WORM**

The person becomes infested by swallowing the eggs, which hatch into larvae in the intestine. The larvae travel in the blood through the wall of the intestine to the lungs, up the windpipe, and are swallowed back into the small intestine. There they become adult worms.

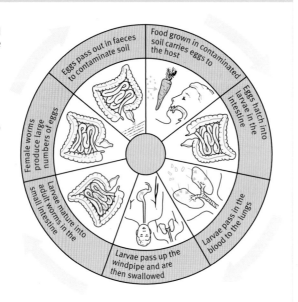

ascites

Excess fluid in the peritoneal cavity, the space between the two layers of the peritoneum (the membranes that line the inside of the abdominal wall and cover the abdominal organs).

CAUSES

Ascites may occur in any condition that causes generalized *oedema* (excessive accumulation of fluid in the body tissues), such as in congestive *heart failure*, *nephrotic syndrome*, and *cirrhosis* of the liver. Ascites may occur in *cancer* if metastases (secondary growths) from a cancer elsewhere in the body develop in the peritoneum. The condition also occurs if *tuberculosis* affects the abdomen.

SYMPTOMS

Ascites causes abdominal swelling and discomfort. Additionally, it may cause breathing difficulty as a result of pressure on, and the immobilization of, the diaphragm, the sheet of muscle that separates the thorax (the chest) from the abdomen.

DIAGNOSIS

The doctor diagnoses the cause of ascites by removing and analysing a sample of ascitic fluid via a sterile needle inserted through the abdominal wall.

TREATMENT

The underlying cause is treated if it is possible. *Diuretic drugs*, particularly *spironolactone*, are often used to treat ascites associated with cirrhosis. If the

ascites is causing discomfort or breathing difficulty, fluid can be drained from the peritoneal cavity.

ascorbic acid

The chemical name for *vitamin C*.

ASD

The abbreviation for *atrial septal defect*.

aseptic necrosis

Death of an area of bone tissue in the absence of infection. The cause of aseptic necrosis is almost always damage to the blood supply to bone, often as a result of a fracture. In some cases, the condition is associated with treatment with *corticosteroid drugs*.

Aseptic necrosis often results in chronic (long-term) pain and may cause stiffness in adjacent joints. Early treatment of fractures reduces the risk of the condition developing.

The head of the *femur* (thigh-bone) and the *scaphoid* (a bone in the wrist) are particularly likely to be affected. Aseptic necrosis may be diagnosed from *X-rays*; the affected area of bone appears denser than the surrounding bone.

aseptic technique

The creation of a germ-free environment to protect a patient from infection. Aseptic technique is used during surgery and other minor procedures, such

as the insertion of a urinary catheter. It is also used during the care of people who are suffering from diseases in which the *immune system* is suppressed, such as *leukaemia*.

All people who come in contact with the patient must scrub their hands and wear disposable gloves and masks and pre-sterilized gowns. Surgical instruments are sterilized in an *autoclave*. The patient's skin is cleaned with *antiseptic* solutions. In operating theatres, special ventilation systems purify the air. (See also *barrier nursing*; *isolation*.)

aspartame

An *artificial sweetener* used in some foods and drugs.

Asperger's syndrome

A developmental disorder that is usually first recognized in childhood because of difficulties with social interactions and very specialized interests. It is more common in boys than girls, and intelligence is normal or high.

Asperger's syndrome is one of a group of conditions known as pervasive developmental disorders; it is considered to be an *autism spectrum disorder*. For individuals with Asperger's syndrome, special educational support may be necessary, although this is often possible within mainstream education. Asperger's syndrome is a lifelong condition.

aspergillosis

An infection caused by inhalation of spores of aspergillus, a fungus that grows in decaying vegetation. Aspergillus is harmless to healthy people but may proliferate in the lungs of people with *tuberculosis*. It can also worsen the symptoms of *asthma* and may produce serious, even fatal, infection in people with reduced immunity, such as those taking *immunosuppressant drugs*.

aspermia

See *azoospermia*.

asphyxia

The medical term for suffocation. Asphyxia may be caused by the obstruction of a large airway, usually by a foreign body (see *choking*), by insufficient oxygen in the surrounding air (as occurs when, for example, a closed plastic bag is put over the head), or by poisoning with a gas, such as carbon monoxide, that interferes with the uptake of oxygen into the blood.

The person initially breathes more rapidly and strongly to try to overcome the lack of oxygen in the blood. There is also an increase in heart rate and blood pressure.

First-aid treatment is by clearing the airway of obstruction followed by *rescue breathing*. Untreated asphyxia leads to death within a few minutes.

aspiration

The withdrawal of fluid or cells from the body by suction. The term also refers to the act of accidentally inhaling a foreign body, usually food or drink. If consciousness is impaired, for example by a head injury or excess alcohol intake, aspiration of the stomach contents is common.

Aspiration *biopsy* is the removal of cells or fluid, using a needle attached to a syringe, for examination. Aspiration biopsy is commonly used to obtain cells from a fluid-filled cavity (such as a *breast cyst*). The procedure is also used to obtain cells from the bone marrow (see *bone marrow biopsy*), or from internal organs, when a fine needle is guided to the site of the biopsy by *CT scanning* or *ultrasound scanning*. (See also *aspiration pneumonia*.)

aspiration pneumonia

A form of pneumonia that results from accidental inhalation of vomit. Aspiration pneumonia usually occurs in people whose cough reflex is not functioning, such as those who have drunk excessive amounts of alcohol, taken certain illegal drugs, or suffered a head injury.

aspirin

A nonopioid *analgesic drug* (painkiller) that may be given in tablet or suppository form to treat disorders such as headache, menstrual pain, and muscle discomfort. Aspirin has an *anti-inflammatory* action. It also reduces fever and is included in some *cold remedies*.

In small doses, aspirin reduces the stickiness of platelets (blood particles involved in clotting). This has led to its use in preventing *thrombosis* (abnormal blood clots) in people at risk of developing *stroke* or *myocardial infarction* (heart attack) and as an initial treatment of chest pain that may be due to myocardial infarction.

In children, aspirin can cause *Reye's syndrome*, a rare but serious brain and liver disorder. For this reason, it should not be given to children under the age of 16 years, except on the advice of a doctor. Aspirin should also not be used by women who are breast-feeding because it can pass into the breast milk.

Aspirin may cause irritation of the stomach lining, resulting in indigestion or nausea. Prolonged use may cause bleeding from the stomach due to *gastric erosion* (disruption of the stomach lining) or *peptic ulcer*. Aspirin should be avoided in pregnancy because it may affect the fetus or cause bleeding problems in the mother.

Aspro

A brand name for *aspirin*.

assay

The analysis or measurement of a substance to determine its presence or effects. A qualitative assay determines only whether or not a substance is present, whereas a quantitative assay determines the actual amount present.

Biological assays (known as bioassays) measure the response of an animal or organ to particular substances. Assays can be used, for example, to assess the effects of a drug or to measure hormone levels. (See also *immunoassay*; *radioimmunoassay*.)

assisted conception

Treatment for *infertility* involving techniques that assist the fertilization and implantation of eggs.

association area

One of a number of areas in the cortex (outer layer) of the *brain* that are concerned with higher levels of mental activity. Association areas interpret information received from sensory areas and prompt appropriate responses, such as voluntary movement.

associative aphasia

Also known as conductive aphasia, a form of *aphasia* (loss of language skills, including comprehension and/or speech production) in which comprehension is normal, and the affected individual can write and speak, but he or she is unable to repeat what has been heard and cannot read aloud. Associative aphasia is caused by damage to a localized area in the brain, often as a result of a *stroke*.

astereognosis

The inability to recognize objects by touch when they are placed in the hand, even though there is no defect of sensation in the fingers or difficulty in holding the object. Astereognosis is either left- or right-sided; tactile recognition is normal on the other side. If both sides are affected, the condition is called tactile *agnosia*.

Astereognosis and tactile agnosia are caused by damage to parts of the *cerebrum* (the main mass of the brain) that are involved in recognition by touch. The conditions may occur as a result of a *stroke* or a *head injury*.

asthma

A lung disease in which there is intermittent narrowing of the *bronchi* (airways), which causes shortness of breath, wheezing, and a cough. The illness often starts in childhood, although it can develop at any age. At least one child in seven suffers from asthma, and the number affected has increased dramatically in recent years. However, childhood asthma may be outgrown in about half of all cases.

During an asthma attack, the muscle in the walls of the airways contracts, causing narrowing. The lining of the airways also becomes swollen and inflamed, producing excess mucus that can block the smaller airways.

TYPES AND CAUSES

In some people, an allergic response triggers the swelling and inflammation in the airways. This allergic type of asthma tends to occur in childhood, and it may develop in association with the allergic skin condition, *eczema* or certain other allergic conditions such as hay fever (see *rhinitis*, *allergic*). Susceptibility to these conditions frequently runs in families.

Some substances are known to trigger attacks of allergic asthma (see *allergens*). These include pollen, house-dust mites, mould, feathers, and dander (tiny scales) and saliva from furry animals such as cats and dogs. Rarely, certain foods, such as milk, eggs, nuts, wheat, and shellfish, provoke an allergic asthmatic reaction. Some people with asthma are sensitive to *aspirin*, and taking it may trigger an attack.

When asthma starts in adulthood, there are usually no identifiable allergic triggers. The first attack is sometimes brought on by a respiratory tract infection, stress, or anxiety.

In some cases, a substance that is inhaled regularly in the work environment can result in the development of asthma in a person who was previously healthy. This is known as occupational

THE CAUSE OF ASTHMA

Breathlessness and wheezing in asthma are caused by narrowing of the bronchioles (small airways in the lungs). Asthma can be triggered by a wide variety of stimuli, including exercise, infection, pollen, and dust, which would have no effect on non-asthmatic people.

Inflammation of the linings of these bronchioles results in increased production of sputum (phlegm), which makes the obstruction worse. A dry cough often develops as the sufferer attempts to clear the airways.

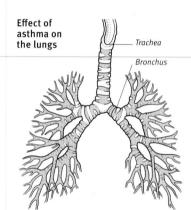

Effect of asthma on the lungs

Trachea

Bronchus

TREATMENT OF AN ASTHMA ATTACK

Attacks are treated by inhalation of a bronchodilator drug from an inhaler. For a severe attack, a nebulizer can be used to dispense the drug as fine mist through a face mask or mouthpiece. Babies, young children, or any adults who are unable to coordinate their breathing, require a spacer.

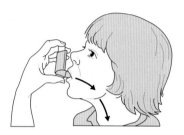

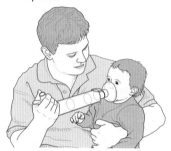

Using an inhaler
To use the inhaler correctly, exhale first then tilt the head back. Take in a slow, deep breath while releasing the drug by depressing the canister. Two puffs should increase air flow within 15 minutes.

Using a spacer
The inhaler, fitted with a spacer and face mask, is placed over the baby's nose and mouth. This allows the baby to inhale the drug while breathing normally.

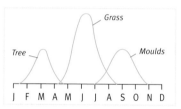

Healthy bronchiole
Inhalation of the bronchodilator widens the bronchiole and improves airflow.

Obstructed bronchiole
Before treatment, the airflow is obstructed by a narrowing of the bronchiole.

Grass

Tree

Moulds

J F M A M J J A S O N D

Seasonal asthma
When symptoms occur only during a few months, the cause is likely to be allergy to pollen or spores.

asthma, and it is one of the few occupational lung diseases that are still increasing in incidence.

There are currently about 200 substances used in the workplace that are known to trigger symptoms of asthma, including glues, resins, latex, and some chemicals, especially isocyanate chemicals used in spray painting. However, occupational asthma can be difficult to diagnose because a person may be regularly exposed to a particular trigger substance for weeks, months, or even years before the symptoms of asthma begin to appear.

Factors that can provoke attacks in a person with asthma include cold air, exercise, smoke, and occasionally emotional factors such as stress and anxiety. Although industrial pollution and exhaust emission from motor vehicles do not normally cause asthma, they do appear to worsen symptoms in people who already have the disorder. Pollution in the atmosphere may also trigger asthma in susceptible people.

SYMPTOMS

Asthma attacks can vary in severity from mild breathlessness to *respiratory failure*. The main symptoms are wheezing, breathlessness, dry cough, and a tightness in the chest. In a severe attack, breathing and talking become increasingly difficult. The impaired breathing results in a low level of oxygen in the blood. This causes *cyanosis* (a bluish discoloration) of the face, particularly of the lips. Left untreated, such attacks can be fatal.

TREATMENT

There is no cure for asthma, but attacks can be prevented to a large extent if a particular allergen can be identified and consequently avoided.

If symptoms occur only occasionally, treatment usually consists of inhaled *bronchodilator drugs* (known as relievers) to widen the airways, thereby relieving symptoms. When symptoms occur frequently or are severe, inhaled *corticosteroids* are also prescribed. These drugs (known as preventers) are used continuously to prevent attacks by reducing inflammation in the airways.

If the asthma is not fully controlled with relievers and preventers, additional, long-acting bronchodilators may be prescribed. Other treatments include *sodium cromoglicate* and nedocromil sodium, both of which are useful in the prevention of exercise-induced asthma. The use of a *leukotriene receptor antagonist* in combination with a corticosteroid drug may enable the required dose of corticosteroid to be reduced. *Theophylline* or the inhaled *anticholinergic drug* ipratropium bromide may also be used as bronchodilators. An asthma attack that has not responded to treatment with a bronchodilator needs immediate medical attention.

asthma, cardiac

Breathing difficulty in which *bronchospasm* (narrowing of the airways) and wheezing occur as a result of fluid accumulation in the lungs (*pulmonary oedema*). Cardiac asthma is usually due to reduced pumping efficiency of the left side of the heart (see *heart failure*) and is not true asthma. Treatment is with *diuretic drugs* or other drugs for heart failure.

astigmatism

A condition in which the front of the *cornea* does not conform to the normal "spherical" curve, even though the eye is perfectly healthy. Because the cornea is unevenly curved, it refracts (bends) light rays to differing degrees. The *lens* is then unable to bring all the rays into focus on the *retina*. A minor degree of astigmatism is normal and does not require correction. More severe astigmatism causes blurring of lines at a certain angle and does require correction.

TREATMENT

Correction may be achieved by using special "cylindrical" glasses that can be framed at a precise angle; contact lenses that can give an even spherical surface for focusing; or by undergoing *laser treatment* on the cornea.

astringents

COMMON DRUGS

• Aluminium acetate • Potassium permanganate • Silver nitrate • Zinc sulphate

Substances that causes tissue to dry and shrink by reducing its ability to absorb water. Astringents are widely used in *antiperspirants* and to promote healing of broken or inflamed skin. They are also used in some eye or ear preparations. Astringents may cause burning or stinging when applied.

astrocytoma

A type of cancerous *brain tumour*. Astrocytomas are the most common type of *glioma*, a tumour that arises from the glial (supporting) cells within the nervous system.

Astrocytomas most commonly develop in the cerebrum (the main mass of the brain) and are classified in four grades (I to IV) according to their rate of growth and malignancy. A grade I astrocytoma is a slow-growing tumour that may spread widely throughout the brain but may be present for many years before causing symptoms. The most severe and fast-growing type is called *glioblastoma multiforme* (a grade IV astrocytoma).

Symptoms are similar to those of other types of brain tumour. Diagnostic tests include *CT scanning* or *MRI*. Treatment is with surgery as well as, in some cases, *radiotherapy* and/or *chemotherapy*.

asymptomatic

A medical term meaning without *symptoms* (indications of illness noticed only by the patient). For example, *hypertension* (high blood pressure) is often asymptomatic and is usually discovered during a routine blood pressure test and *diabetes mellitus* is often diagnosed from a routine blood or urine test.

Most disorders have no symptoms in their early stages. In the case of *cancer*, much effort has been made to devise screening tests for the detection of tumours at their early, asymptomatic, stage. (See also *sign*.)

asystole

A term meaning absence of the heartbeat (see *cardiac arrest*).

ataxia

Incoordination and clumsiness that may affect balance and gait (see *walking*), limb and eye movements, and/or speech.

CAUSES

Ataxia may be the result of damage to the *cerebellum* (the part of the brain concerned with coordination) or to nerve pathways in the *brainstem* (a stalk of nerve tissue linking the brain to the *spinal cord*) and/or spinal cord.

Possible causes of ataxia include injury to the brain or spinal cord. In adults, ataxia may be caused by *alcohol intoxication*; a *stroke* or *brain tumour* affecting the cerebellum or brainstem; a disease of the balance organ in the ear; or *multiple sclerosis* or other types of nerve degeneration. In children, causes of ataxia include acute infection, brain tumours, and the inherited condition *Friedreich's ataxia*.

SYMPTOMS

Symptoms of ataxia depend on the site of damage within the nervous system, although a lurching, unsteady gait is common to most forms. In addition, damage to certain parts of the brain may cause *nystagmus* (jerky eye movements) and slurred speech.

DIAGNOSIS AND TREATMENT

CT scanning or *MRI* (techniques that produce cross-sectional or three-dimensional images of body structures) may be used to determine the cause of ataxia. Treatment of the condition depends on the cause.

atelectasis

Collapse of part or all of a *lung* caused by obstruction of the bronchus (the main air passage through the lung) or the bronchioles (smaller air passages). When obstruction occurs, air already in the lung cannot be breathed out and is therefore absorbed into the blood, leading to the collapse of all or part of the lung. After collapsing, the lung loses its elasticity and cannot take in air; consequently, the blood passing through it can no longer absorb oxygen or dispose of carbon dioxide.

In an adult, atelectasis is not normally life-threatening because unaffected parts of the lung and/or the other lung can compensate for the loss of function in the collapsed area. However, when a newborn baby's lung collapses, the baby's life is at risk.

CAUSES

Obstruction of a bronchus or bronchiole may be caused by the accumulation of mucus. This buildup of mucus most commonly occurs in a baby at birth; in people with asthma; following an abdominal or chest operation that has made coughing difficult because of pain; in certain infections such as *pertussis* (whooping cough) in children or chronic *bronchitis* (inflammation of the bronchi) in adults.

Obstruction may also result from an accidentally inhaled foreign body, a tumour in the lung, or enlarged *lymph nodes* (which occur in *tuberculosis*, some other lung infections, or certain forms of *cancer*) exerting pressure on the airway. The collapsed lung may become infected.

SYMPTOMS

The main symptom of atelectasis is shortness of breath. There may also be a cough and chest pain, depending on the underlying cause.

DIAGNOSIS AND TREATMENT

Atelectasis can be diagnosed by *chest X-ray*, and treatment is aimed at removing the cause of the blockage. The treatment may include *physiotherapy* or *broncho-*

scopy, a procedure that involves removal of the blockage using a rigid or flexible viewing tube (see *endoscope*). If the obstruction can be removed, the lung should reinflate normally.

atenolol

A *beta-blocker drug* that is used to treat *hypertension* (high blood pressure), *angina pectoris* (chest pain caused by an impaired blood supply to the heart muscle), and certain types of *arrhythmia* (irregular heartbeat) in which the heart beats too rapidly.

atheroma

Fatty deposits on the inner lining of an artery that occur in *atherosclerosis* and restrict blood flow. The deposits are also known as atheromatous plaques.

atherosclerosis

The accumulation of *cholesterol* and other fatty substances (lipids) in the walls of arteries, causing the arteries to narrow. Atherosclerosis can affect arteries in any area of the body and is a major cause of *stroke*, heart attack (see *myocardial infarction*), and poor circulation in the legs.

The arteries become narrowed when fatty substances carried in the blood accumulate on the inside lining of the arteries and form yellow deposits known as atheromatous plaques. These deposits restrict the blood flow through the arteries. In addition, the muscle layer of the artery wall becomes thickened, which narrows the artery even further. Platelets (tiny blood cells that are responsible for blood clotting) may collect in clumps on the surface of the deposits and initiate the formation of blood clots. A large clot may completely block the artery, resulting in the organ it supplies being deprived of oxygen. A complete blockage in a coronary artery can cause a sudden, often fatal, heart attack.

CAUSES

Major risk factors for developing atherosclerosis are *hypertension* (high blood pressure) and raised blood lipid levels. Atherosclerosis is more common in developed countries, where most people eat a diet high in fat. Some disorders such as *diabetes mellitus* can be associated with a high cholesterol level, regardless of diet.

SYMPTOMS

Atherosclerosis usually produces no symptoms in its early stages. As the condition progresses, symptoms occur as a result of reduced, or total absence of, blood supply to the organs supplied by the affected arteries.

Partial blockage of the coronary arteries (which supply the heart muscle) may produce symptoms such as the chest pain of *angina pectoris*. Narrowing of the arteries supplying blood to the brain may cause *transient ischaemic attacks* (symptoms and signs of a *stroke* that last for less than 24 hours) and episodes of dizziness.

Intermittent *claudication* (a cramplike pain on walking) is often the first symptom of atherosclerosis in the leg arteries. If the condition is associated with an inherited lipid disorder (see *hyperlipidaemias*), fatty deposits may develop on tendons or as visible lumps under the skin.

DIAGNOSIS AND TREATMENT

Blood flow through an artery can be investigated by *angiography* (X-rays of arteries taken after injection of a *radiopaque* substance). Thallium *radionuclide scanning*, *echocardiography* (ultrasound scanning of the heart), and *ECG* (electrocardiography) may be used to investigate suspected atherosclerosis of the coronary arteries.

The best treatment for atherosclerosis is to prevent it from progressing by the maintenance of a healthy lifestyle. This includes adoption of a low-fat diet, not smoking, regular exercise, and maintenance of the recommended weight for height. These measures lead to a reduced risk of developing significant atherosclerosis.

Those individuals found to have high blood cholesterol levels but who are otherwise in good health will be

---

ARTERIAL DEGENERATION IN **ATHEROSCLEROSIS**

Atherosclerosis is narrowing of the arteries due to plaques of atheroma on their inner linings. The plaques consist mainly of fats deposited from the blood. Men are affected earlier than women because premenopausal women are protected by natural oestrogen hormones; after the menopause, the risk for women increases.

RISK FACTORS

- Cigarette smoking
- Hypertension
- High blood cholesterol
- Obesity
- Physical inactivity
- Diabetes mellitus
- Heredity
- Male gender

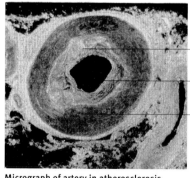

Micrograph of artery in atherosclerosis
The artery shown here has an atheromatous (fibrous and fatty) plaque deposit on its inner wall. The lumen (central channel) has been narrowed, disrupting blood flow.

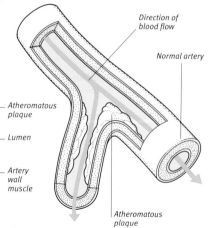

Direction of blood flow

Normal artery

Atheromatous plaque

Lumen

Artery wall muscle

Atheromatous plaque

Atherosclerotic artery
A deposit of atheromatous plaque disrupts normal blood flow through the artery at the point where it branches. This occurs because of the greater level of turbulence in this area.

advised to adopt a low-fat diet. They may also be given drugs that decrease blood cholesterol levels (see *lipid-lowering drugs*). For people who have had a heart attack, research has shown that there may be a benefit in lowering blood cholesterol levels, even if the level is within the average range for healthy people. For people with hypertension, reducing their blood pressure to within recommended limits can help reduce the risk of atherosclerosis. People with diabetes mellitus can help reduce their risk by careful control of their blood glucose levels.

People with atherosclerosis and those at risk may be prescribed a drug such as *aspirin* in order to reduce the likelihood of blood clots forming on the damaged artery lining.

Surgical treatment of atherosclerosis, such as coronary angioplasty (see *angioplasty, balloon*), may be recommended for those people thought to be at high risk of severe complications. In some cases, a *stent* (rigid tube) may be also inserted into an affected artery to help prevent it from renarrowing. If blood flow to the heart is severely obstructed, a *coronary artery bypass* may be carried out to restore blood flow.

athetosis

A disorder of the nervous system that is characterized by involuntary slow, writhing movements, most often of the face, head, neck, and limbs. These movements commonly include facial grimacing, with contortions of the mouth. There may also be difficulty in balancing and walking.

Athetosis tends to be combined with *chorea* (involuntary irregular, jerky movements). Both athetosis and chorea arise from damage to the *basal ganglia*, clusters of nerve cells in the brain that control movement.

Causes of athetosis include brain damage prior to or at birth (see *cerebral palsy*), *encephalitis* (brain infection), degenerative disorders such as *Huntington's disease*, or as a side effect of *phenothiazine drugs* or *levodopa*. If drug treatment is the cause of the condition, the abnormal movements may stop when the drug is withdrawn.

athlete's foot

A common condition in which the skin between the toes becomes itchy and sore and may crack, peel, or blister. Athlete's foot is usually the result of a fungal infection known medically as tinea pedis, although the condition may also be caused by bacteria.

Because the fungi thrive in humid conditions, athlete's foot is more common in people with particularly sweaty feet and those who wear shoes and socks made from synthetic fibres, which do not absorb sweat.

TREATMENT
Self-treatment with topical *antifungal drugs* is usually effective and should be combined with careful washing and drying of the feet.

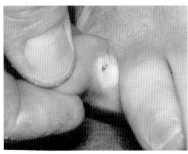

Athlete's foot
The typical appearance of athlete's foot is of fissuring in the cleft between the fourth and fifth toes. There is usually an annoying itch.

atlas

The topmost cervical *vertebra* in the *spine*. The atlas is attached to and supports the skull. A pivot joint connecting the atlas to the second cervical vertebra, the *axis*, allows the atlas to rotate, turning the head from side to side.

atony

Loss of tension in a muscle, so that it is completely flaccid. Atony can occur in some nervous system disorders or after injury to nerves. For example, the arm muscles may become atonic after injury to the *brachial plexus* (nerve roots in the neck passing into the arm).

atopic eczema

Atopic *eczema* is the most common form of eczema (an inflammatory skin condition). It usually begins in infancy but may flare up during adolescence and adulthood. The cause of atopic eczema is unknown, but people with *atopy* (a predisposition to allergic reactions) are more susceptible.

atopy

A predisposition to various allergic reactions (see *allergy*). Atopic individuals have a tendency to suffer from one or more allergic disorders, such as *asthma*, *eczema*, *urticaria* (nettle rash), and allergic *rhinitis* (hay fever).

The mechanism that underlies the predisposition is unclear, but atopy seems to run in families.

ATP

An abbreviation for the compound adenosine triphosphate, the principal energy-carrying chemical in the body. (See also *ADP*; *metabolism*.)

atresia

Congenital (present from birth) absence or severe narrowing of a body opening or tubular organ due to a failure of development in the uterus. Examples are *biliary atresia*, in which the bile ducts between the liver and duodenum are absent; *oesophageal atresia*, in which the oesophagus comes to a blind end; and anal atresia (see *anus, imperforate*), in which the anal canal is shut off. Most forms of atresia require surgical correction early in life.

atrial fibrillation

A type of abnormality of the heartbeat (see *arrhythmia, cardiac*) in which the atria (see *atrium*), the upper chambers of the heart, beat irregularly and very rapidly. The *ventricles* (the heart's lower chambers) also beat irregularly but at a slower rate. As a result, the pumping ability of the heart is reduced.

CAUSES
Atrial fibrillation can occur in almost any longstanding heart disease, but is often associated with *coronary artery disease* or *heart-valve* disorders. Atrial fibrillation may also be associated with *hypertension* (high blood pressure), *hyperthyroidism* (overactivity of the thyroid gland), or excessive intake of alcohol or caffeine.

SYMPTOMS AND SIGNS
Sudden onset of atrial fibrillation can cause *palpitations* (awareness of a fast, irregular heartbeat), *angina pectoris* (chest pain due to impaired blood supply to the heart muscle), breathlessness, or dizziness. The inefficient pumping action of the heart reduces the output of blood into the circulation. Blood clots may form in the atria and may enter the bloodstream and lodge in an artery (see *embolism*).

DIAGNOSIS AND TREATMENT
Diagnosis of atrial fibrillation is confirmed by an *ECG*, which shows the electrical activity of the heart.

Treatment of atrial fibrillation depends on the underlying cause but may include *anti-arrhythmic drugs* such as *digoxin*, *beta-blocker drugs*, and *calcium channel blockers*.

Atrial fibrillation of recent onset may be treated by *cardioversion* (restoration of a normal heart rhythm by applying an electric shock). In some cases, *radiofrequency ablation* (in which the heart tissue that triggers the abnormal rhythms is destroyed) may be recommended or an artificial *pacemaker* may be inserted to regulate heart rhythm. In most cases, *anticoagulant drugs* or *aspirin* are also given to reduce the risk of an embolism occurring.

atrial flutter

A type of abnormality of the heartbeat (see *arrhythmia, cardiac*) in which the atria (see *atrium*), the heart's upper chambers beat regularly but very rapidly. Symptoms and treatment of atrial flutter are the same as for *atrial fibrillation*.

atrial natriuretic peptide

A substance that is produced in special cells in the muscular wall of the atria (see *atrium*), the upper chambers of the heart. Atrial natriuretic peptide is released into the bloodstream in response to swelling of the atrial muscle due, for example, to *heart failure* or *hypertension* (high blood pressure).

Atrial natriuretic peptide increases the amount of sodium that is excreted in the urine. The excreted sodium draws water out with it, which decreases the volume of the blood and thereby reduces the blood pressure.

Children who have congenital (present from birth) heart disorders that result in heart disease (see *heart disease, congenital*) possess high levels of atrial natriuretic peptide. Following successful surgery to correct the congenital heart abnormality, the levels of atrial natriuretic peptide fall.

atrial septal defect (ASD)

A congenital (present from birth) heart abnormality (see *heart disease, congenital*) in which there is a hole in the dividing wall (see *septal defect*) between the heart's two upper chambers, or atria (see *atrium*). An atrial septal defect is usually repaired surgically if it causes symptoms or complications develop.

atrioventricular block

A type of *heart block*.

atrioventricular node

A small knot of specialized muscle cells in the right *atrium* (upper chamber) of the *heart*. Electrical impulses from the *sinoatrial node* (a cluster of muscle cells that act as the heart's natural pacemaker) pass through the atrioventricular node and along conducting fibres to the *ventricles* (the lower chambers of the heart), causing them to contract and pump blood around the body.

atrium

Also known as an auricle, either of the two (right and left) upper chambers of the *heart*. The atria open directly into the *ventricles* (lower chambers of the heart). Deoxygenated blood from the body enters the right atrium through the two *venae cavae*. Oxygenated blood from the lungs enters the left atrium through the *pulmonary veins*.

ANATOMY OF THE **ATRIUM**

Deoxygenated blood flows into the right atrium through the venae cavae; oxygenated blood flows into the left atrium via the pulmonary veins.

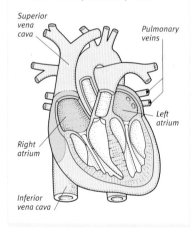

Superior vena cava

Pulmonary veins

Left atrium

Right atrium

Inferior vena cava

atrophy

The wasting away or shrinkage of a normally developed tissue or organ that results from a reduction in the size or number of its cells.

Atrophy is commonly caused by disuse (such as when a limb has been immobilized in a plaster cast) or inadequate cell nutrition as a result of poor blood circulation. Atrophy may also occur during prolonged illness, when the body needs to use up the protein reserves in the muscles. In some circumstances, atrophy is a normal process

(as in ovarian atrophy, for example, which occurs in women who have passed the *menopause*).

atropine

An *anticholinergic drug* that is derived from the deadly nightshade plant (see *belladonna*). Atropine is used to dilate the pupil in eye conditions such as *iritis* (inflammation of the iris) and *corneal ulcer*. It is also used in young children, in the form of eye-drops, to dilate (widen) the *pupil* for examination.

Atropine may rarely be used as a *premedication* before a general anaesthetic (see *anaesthesia, general*). It is used as emergency treatment for *bradycardia* (abnormally slow heartbeat) and is also sometimes combined with an *antidiarrhoeal drug* to relieve the abdominal cramps that accompany diarrhoea.

Side effects include dry mouth, blurred vision, retention of urine, and, in the elderly, confusion. Atropine eye-drops are rarely given to adults because they cause disturbance of vision that lasts for two to three weeks and may precipitate acute *glaucoma* in susceptible people.

attachment

An affectionate bond between individuals, especially between a parent and child (see *bonding*) or between a person and an object, such as a young child and a security blanket.

The term attachment is also used to refer to the site at which a muscle or tendon is attached to a bone.

attention deficit hyperactivity disorder (ADHD)

A behavioural disorder in which a child has a consistently high level of activity and/or difficulty in attending to tasks. Attention deficit hyperactivity, or hyperkinetic, disorder affects up to five per cent of children in the UK.

The disorder, which is more common in boys, should not be confused with the normal boisterous conduct of a healthy child. Children with ADHD show abnormal patterns of behaviour over a period of time. An affected child is likely to be constantly restless, unable to sit still for more than a few moments, inattentive, and impulsive.

CAUSES
The causes of ADHD are not fully understood, but the disorder often runs in families, which suggests that genetic factors may be involved. ADHD is not a result of poor parenting or abuse.

SYMPTOMS AND SIGNS

Symptoms of the condition develop in early childhood, usually between the ages of three and seven, and may include the inability to finish tasks; inability to concentrate in class; a short attention span; difficulty in following instructions; a tendency to talk excessively, frequently interrupting other people; difficulty in waiting or taking turns; inability to play alone, quietly; and physical impulsiveness.

Children with ADHD may have difficulty in forming friendships. Self-esteem is often low because an affected child is frequently scolded and criticized.

TREATMENT AND OUTLOOK

Treatment of ADHD includes behaviour modification techniques, both at home and at school. In some children, avoidance of certain foods or food additives seems to reduce symptoms.

In severe cases of ADHD, *stimulant drugs*, usually *methylphenidate*, may be prescribed; other medications that may be prescribed include atomoxetine and *amphetamine drugs*. If prescribed, these drugs should be part of a treatment programme that includes behaviour modification techniques.

The condition may improve by adolescence but it may be followed by antisocial behaviour, *drug abuse*, or *substance abuse*. In a significant number of cases, treatment needs to be continued into adolescence and may sometimes need to be continued into adulthood.

attenuated

A term used to refer to microorganisms that have been treated to reduce their ability to cause disease. Attenuated organisms are used in some *vaccines*, for example, the *BCG* vaccine.

atypical

A term used to describe something that is not the usual type or that does not fit into the usual pattern. The atypical presentation of a disease or disorder is one in which the early symptoms and signs differ from those that normally occur, which may make diagnosis of the condition more difficult.

audiogram

A graph that is produced as a result of *audiometry* (measurement of the sense of hearing). An audiogram shows the hearing threshold (the minimum audible decibel level) for each of a range of sound frequencies.

audiology

The study of hearing, especially impaired hearing.

audiometry

Measurement of the sense of hearing. The term audiometry often refers to *hearing tests* in which a machine is used to produce sounds of a defined intensity (loudness) and frequency (pitch), and in which the hearing in each ear is measured over the full range of normally audible sounds. (See also *impedance audiometry*.)

auditory nerve

The part of the *vestibulocochlear nerve* (the eighth *cranial nerve*) concerned with hearing. The auditory nerve is also known as the acoustic nerve.

aura

A peculiar "warning" sensation that precedes or marks the onset of a *migraine* attack or a seizure in *epilepsy*.

A migraine attack may be preceded by a feeling of elation, excessive energy, or drowsiness; thirst or a craving for sweet foods may develop. A migraine may also be heralded by flashing lights before the eyes, blurred or tunnel vision, or difficulty in speaking. There may also be weakness, numbness, or tingling in one half of the body. As these symptoms subside, the migraine headache begins.

An epileptic aura may occur in the form of a distorted perception, such as a hallucinatory smell or sound or a sensation of movement in a part of the body. One type of epileptic attack (in people who have *temporal lobe epilepsy*) is often preceded by a vague feeling of discomfort in the upper abdomen, which is sometimes followed by borborygmi (rumbling or gurgling bowel sounds) and by a sensation of fullness in the head.

auranofin

A *gold* preparation used as a *disease-modifying antirheumatic drug* in the treatment of active, progressive *rheumatoid arthritis*. Unlike other gold preparations, auranofin can be taken by mouth.

auricle

Another name for the pinna, the external flap of the *ear*. The term is also used to describe the earlike appendages of the atria (the upper chambers of the heart, see *atrium*).

auriscope

Also called an *otoscope*, an instrument for examining the ear.

auscultation

A procedure that involves listening to sounds within the body, using a *stethoscope*, to assess the functioning of an organ or to detect disease.

AUSCULTATION OF THE HEART

To listen to the heart, the doctor places the stethoscope on the chest at four points which correspond to the location of the heart valves. With the patient either sitting up, lying in a semi-reclining position, or lying on his or her left side, the doctor listens for any abnormality in the rate and rhythm of the heartbeat and for a heart *murmur* or other abnormal *heart sound* that may indicate a heart defect.

AUSCULTATION OF THE LUNGS

When listening to the lungs, the doctor places the stethoscope on numerous areas of the chest and back. The patient breathes normally, and then takes deep breaths, so that the doctor can compare the sounds on the right and left sides. Abnormal breath sounds may indicate *pneumonia*, *bronchitis*, and *pneumothorax* (in which air enters the space between the *pleura*, the membranes lining the outside of the lungs and the inside of the chest cavity). Cracking or bubbling sounds (known as crepitations) are caused by fluid in the lungs; wheezing sounds result from spasm of the airways, usually as a result of *asthma*. *Pleurisy* (inflammation of the pleura) causes a scratching sound as inflamed areas of the lung rub together.

The doctor may also test for vocal resonance by asking the patient to whisper something. The sound is louder if there is pus in the lung due to a condition such as pneumonia.

AUSCULTATION OF THE BLOOD VESSELS

Blood vessels near the skin surface (usually the carotid artery in the neck, the abdominal aorta, or the renal artery) may be listened to for bruits (sounds made by turbulent or abnormally fast blood circulation). Bruits occur when blood vessels are narrowed (for example by fatty deposits in *atherosclerosis*) or widened (by an *aneurysm*, for example). They may also be present if heart valves have been narrowed or damaged (for example by *endocarditis*).

AUSCULTATION OF THE ABDOMEN

The abdomen is auscultated for borborygmi (loud rumbling, gurgling sounds

PROCEDURE FOR **AUSCULTATION**

A doctor's examination often includes auscultation (listening to sounds within the body using a stethoscope). Some sounds, such as movement of fluid through the stomach and intestine, opening and closing of heart valves, the flow of blood through vessels near the skin surface, and flow of air through the lungs and airways, are made during normal functioning of the body. If there are abnormal sounds, that is usually an indication of a disorder.

STETHOSCOPE

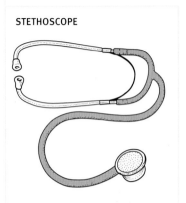

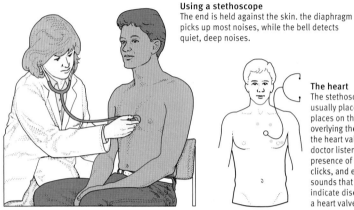

Using a stethoscope
The end is held against the skin. the diaphragm picks up most noises, while the bell detects quiet, deep noises.

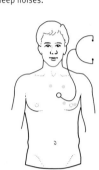

The heart
The stethoscope is usually placed at four places on the chest overlying the sites of the heart valves. The doctor listens for the presence of murmurs, clicks, and extra heart sounds that may indicate disease of a heart valve.

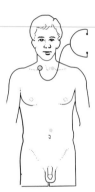

Carotid artery and abdominal aorta
The doctor may listen to the flow of blood through a blood vessel that passes just beneath the skin. The presence of bruits (sounds of turbulence) usually indicates abnormal narrowing or widening of an artery.

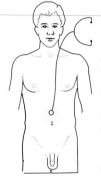

The abdomen
The doctor may listen to the abdomen for the sounds made by the movement of fluid through the intestine. A disorder of the intestine may cause these sounds to be absent, abnormal, or very loud.

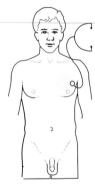

The lungs
The doctor places the stethoscope over several different areas of the chest and back to listen to the sounds made during breathing. The presence of crackles and dry or moist wheezes indicates various types of lung disease.

that are made by the movement of air and fluid in the intestine), and also for abnormal bowel sounds that may indicate intestinal obstruction (see *intestine, obstruction of*).

autism

A condition in which there is difficulty with social relationships, language, and communication; poor imagination, and repetitive patterns of behaviour. Autism is more common in boys. The condition is, by definition, evident before the age of 30 months and is usually apparent in the first year of life. The precise causes of autism are unknown.

SYMPTOMS AND SIGNS

Autistic children often seem normal for the first few months of life, before becoming increasingly unresponsive to parents or other stimuli. The child fails to form relationships, avoids eye contact, and has a preference for playing alone. Extreme resistance to change of any kind is an important feature of the condition, which can make it very difficult to teach an autistic child new skills.

Rituals develop in play, and there is often attachment to unusual objects or obsession with one particular idea. Delay in speaking is common and most autistic children have a low *IQ*. Other behavioural abnormalities may include walking on tip-toe, rocking, self-injury, screaming fits, and *hyperactivity*.

Appearance and coordination are normal. Some autistic people have an isolated special skill, such as musical ability or an outstanding rote memory.

TREATMENT AND OUTLOOK

There is no cure for autism, which is a lifelong condition. Special schooling, support and *counselling* for the families, and, in some cases, *behaviour therapy* (for example, to reduce violent self-injury) can be helpful. Medication is useful only for specific problems, such as hyperactivity.

The outlook depends on the intelligence and language ability of the individual. The majority of autistic people need special care.

autism spectrum disorders

A range of developmental disorders that are characterized by obsessive behaviour and impaired communication and social skills (see *Asperger's syndrome; autism*). Autism spectrum disorders are usually diagnosed during childhood.

autoantibody

An *antibody* (a protein that is manufactured by the immune system) that reacts against the body's own cells (see *autoimmune disorders*).

autoclave

A device that produces steam at high pressure in a sealed chamber to destroy microorganisms. Autoclaving is used in hospitals for *sterilization*.

autograft

Tissue that has been transplanted from one part of an individual's body to another (see *grafting*). Autografting is often used to treat severe burns.

autoimmune disorders

Any of a number of disorders caused by a reaction of the body's *immune system* against its own cells and tissues. Such disease-producing processes, known as *hypersensitivity* reactions, are similar to the reactions that occur in *allergy*, except that in autoimmune disorders the hypersensitivity response is to the body itself rather than to an external substance.

CAUSES

The immune system normally distinguishes "self" from "nonself". Some *lymphocytes* (a type of white blood cell) are capable of reacting against self, but these lymphocytes are generally suppressed. Autoimmune disorders occur when there is interruption of the normal control process, allowing such lymphocytes

AUTOIMMUNE DISORDERS

Specific (organs or cells affected)

- Addison's disease (adrenal glands)
- Autoimmune haemolytic anaemia (red blood cells)
- Autoimmune chronic active hepatitis (liver)
- Autoimmune infertility (sperm or ovary)
- Diabetes mellitus type 1 (pancreas)
- Goodpasture's syndrome (lung and kidney)
- Graves' disease (thyroid gland)
- Hashimoto's thyroiditis (thyroid gland)
- Idiopathic thrombocytopenic purpura (platelets)
- Myasthenia gravis (muscle receptors)
- Pernicious anaemia (stomach lining)
- Vitiligo (melanocytes)

Nonspecific

- Behcet's syndrome
- Rheumatoid arthritis
- Sjogren's syndrome
- Systemic lupus erythematosus

to escape from suppression, or when there is alteration in a particular body tissue meaning that it is no longer recognized as self and is attacked.

Bacteria, viruses, and drugs may play a role in initiating an autoimmune disorder in someone who already has a genetic (inherited) predisposition, but in most cases the trigger is unknown.

TYPES

Autoimmune processes can have various results, such as the destruction of a particular type of cell or tissue, stimulation of an organ into excessive growth, or interference in an organ's function.

Autoimmune disorders are classified into organ-specific and non-organ-specific types. In organ-specific disorders, the autoimmune process is directed mainly against one organ. Examples include *Hashimoto's thyroiditis* (thyroid gland), pernicious *anaemia* (stomach), *Addison's disease* (adrenal glands), and type 1 *diabetes mellitus* (pancreas).

In non-organ-specific disorders, autoimmune activity is towards a tissue, such as connective tissue, that is widespread in the body. Examples of such disorders are systemic *lupus erythematosus* and *rheumatoid arthritis*.

TREATMENT

Initial treatment for any autoimmune disorder is to reduce the effects of the disease by, for example, replacing any hormones that are not being produced.

In cases in which the disease is having widespread effects, treatment is also directed at diminishing the activity of the immune system while maintaining the body's ability to fight disease. *Corticosteroid drugs* are most commonly used for this purpose but may be combined with other *immunosuppressant drugs*.

autologous blood transfusion

See *blood transfusion, autologous*.

automatism

A state in which behaviour is not controlled by the conscious mind. An individual carries out activities without being aware of doing so, and later he or she has no clear memory of what happened. Episodes of automatism start abruptly and are usually no more than a few minutes in duration.

Automatism is uncommon and may be a symptom of *temporal lobe epilepsy*, *dissociative disorders* (psychological illnesses in which a particular mental function is lost), drug or *alcohol intoxication*, or *hypoglycaemia* (low blood sugar.

autonomic nervous system

Also called the involuntary nervous system, the part of the *nervous system* that controls the involuntary activities of a variety of body tissues, including blood vessels, organs, and glands. The autonomic nervous system consists of a network of nerves divided into the sympathetic and parasympathetic nervous systems.

The two systems act in conjunction and normally balance each other. However, during exercise or at times of stress, the activity of the sympathetic system predominates, while during sleep the parasympathetic system exerts greater control.

SYMPATHETIC NERVOUS SYSTEM

The sympathetic nervous system comprises two chains of nerves that pass from the spinal cord throughout the body tissues. Into these tissues, the nerve endings release the *neurotransmitters* (chemical messengers) *adrenaline* (epinephrine) and *noradrenaline* (norepinephrine). The sympathetic nervous system also stimulates the release of adrenaline from the adrenal glands.

In general, the actions of the sympathetic nervous system heighten activity in the body. This activity is known as the *fight-or-flight response*. Among the most important effects produced are the acceleration and strengthening of the heartbeat, widening of the airways, widening of the blood vessels in muscles and narrowing of those in the skin and abdominal organs (in order to increase the blood flow through the muscles), and the inducement of sweating. In addition, the activity of the digestive system is decreased and the pupils are dilated.

PARASYMPATHETIC NERVOUS SYSTEM

The parasympathetic nervous system is composed of a chain of nerves that passes from the brain and another that leaves the lower spinal cord. The nerves are distributed to the same tissues that are supplied by the sympathetic nerves. The parasympathetic nerves release the neurotransmitter *acetylcholine*, which has the opposite effect to those of adrenaline and noradrenaline.

The parasympathetic system is concerned mainly with everyday functions such as digestion and excretion.

EFFECT OF DRUGS

Certain disorders can be treated by administration of drugs that affect the autonomic nervous system. *Anticholinergic drugs*, for example, block the effect

A

FUNCTIONS OF THE **AUTONOMIC NERVOUS SYSTEM**

The autonomic nervous system (also known as the involuntary nervous system) is responsible for controlling the involuntary body functions, such as sweating, digestion, and heart rate.

The system affects smooth muscles, such as those of the airways and the intestine, rather than the striated muscles, which are under the body's voluntary control.

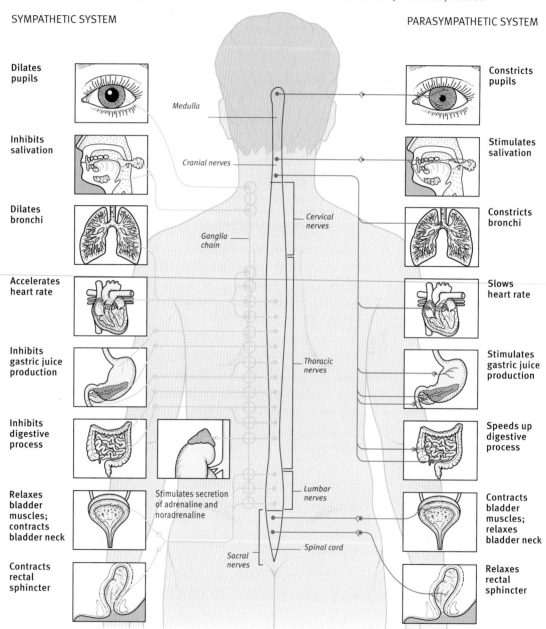

SYMPATHETIC SYSTEM

PARASYMPATHETIC SYSTEM

Dilates pupils

Inhibits salivation

Dilates bronchi

Accelerates heart rate

Inhibits gastric juice production

Inhibits digestive process

Relaxes bladder muscles; contracts bladder neck

Stimulates secretion of adrenaline and noradrenaline

Contracts rectal sphincter

Medulla

Cranial nerves

Ganglia chain

Cervical nerves

Thoracic nerves

Lumbar nerves

Sacral nerves

Spinal cord

Constricts pupils

Stimulates salivation

Constricts bronchi

Slows heart rate

Stimulates gastric juice production

Speeds up digestive process

Contracts bladder muscles; relaxes bladder neck

Relaxes rectal sphincter

The autonomic nervous system

The autonomic nervous system is divided into two separate systems: the sympathetic nervous system and the parasympathetic nervous system. The sympathetic system is primarily concerned with preparing the body for action; it predominates at times of stress or excitement. The sympathetic system stimulates functions such as heart rate and sweating and dilates the blood vessels to the muscles so that more blood is diverted to them. Simultaneously, it subdues the activity of the digestive system. In contrast, the parasympathetic nervous system is concerned mainly with the body's everyday functions such as digestion and the excretion of waste products; this system dominates during sleep. The parasympathetic system slows the heart rate and stimulates the organs of the digestive tract. Most of the time, activity is balanced between the two systems, with neither dominating. Both of the systems play an important part in sexual arousal and orgasm in both men and women.

of acetylcholine, which can reduce muscle spasms in the intestine. *Beta-blocker drugs* block the action of adrenaline (epinephrine) and noradrenaline (norepinephrine) on the heart, thus slowing the rate and force of the heartbeat.

autopsy

A postmortem examination of the body, including the internal organs, usually undertaken to determine the precise cause of death. In certain circumstances, an autopsy is required by law.

autoregulation

Processes in the body that maintain ideal conditions for normal function, such as maintaining the balance of the body's salt and water content.

autosomal disorders

See *genetic disorders*.

autosome

Any *chromosome* that is not a sex chromosome. Of the 23 pairs of chromosomes in each human cell, 22 pairs are autosomes.

avascular

A term meaning without blood vessels.

avascular necrosis

Cell death in body tissues due to damage to blood vessels that supply the area.

aversion therapy

An outdated form of *behaviour therapy* in which unpleasant stimuli, such as electric shocks, are administered at the same time as an unwanted behaviour in an attempt to alter behaviour patterns.

avian influenza

Commonly known as bird flu, avian influenza is a highly infectious disease of birds, especially poultry, that can sometimes be transmitted to people who are in close contact with infected birds. There are many strains of avian influenza but the strain caused by the H5N1 virus is particularly virulent. People infected with this strain may develop symptoms including fever, sore throat, muscle aches, headaches, breathing problems, and chest pains. In some cases, infection with H5N1 may be fatal. There is concern that this strain may develop the ability to pass from person to person, instead of only from birds to birds and birds to human. If this occurs, there is the possibility of a pandemic (global epidemic).

Normal influenza vaccines do not protect against the H5N1 virus, although drugs such as *oseltamivir* may be effective.

aviation medicine

The medical speciality concerned with the physiological effects of air travel, such as the effects of reduced oxygen, pressure changes, and accelerative forces, as well as with the causes and treatment of medical problems that may occur during a flight.

Aviation medicine includes assessment of the fitness of the aircrew, and sometimes of passengers, to fly, the management of medical emergencies in the air, the consequences of special types of flights (such as in helicopters and spacecraft), and the investigation of aircraft accidents.

AIR TRAVEL-RELATED PROBLEMS

Increasing altitude causes a fall in air pressure and with it a fall in the pressure of oxygen. *Hypoxia* (a seriously reduced oxygen level in the blood and tissues) is a threat to anyone who flies at altitude. Aviator's *decompression sickness* has the same causes as the related condition that affects scuba divers but it is not normally a risk for passengers on regular flights. Rapid decompression (a sudden drop in air pressure) in civil aircraft is extremely rare, but passengers and crew are provided with oxygen masks for use in emergencies while the aircraft descends to a safe altitude.

Hypoxia or, more commonly, anxiety can lead to *hyperventilation* (overbreathing), in which increased breathing results in excess loss of carbon dioxide. This loss alters the body's acidity and gives rise to symptoms such as tingling around the mouth, muscle spasms, and

SOME CONDITIONS AFFECTING SUITABILITY FOR **AIR TRAVEL**

Conditions	Comments
Respiratory conditions (such as asthma, chronic bronchitis, emphysema, chronic obstructive pulmonary disease, recent collapsed lung)	Asthma that is stable and controlled should not affect fitness to fly. People who have had a collapsed lung should not fly for at least a week after it has cleared up and must contact the PCMU (passenger medical clearance unit) before flying. For other respiratory conditions, flying may be possible but may require supplementary oxygen in some cases; consult your doctor and the PMCU.
Heart conditions (such as angina pectoris, recent heart attack)	Usually no restrictions for mild to moderate angina sufferers. For severe angina and other heart conditions, consult your doctor and/or the PMCU. You may need to wait before flying.
Recent chest, heart, cranial, eye, middle or inner ear, or abdominal surgery (including appendicectomy); tonsillectomy; angioplasty	Seek advice from your doctor and/or the PCMU. You may need to wait before flying.
Recent stroke	Consult your doctor and the PCMU. You may need to wait before flying.
Infectious disease	People with infectious diseases are prohibited from flying while they are contagious. Consult your doctor and/or the PMCU.
Pregnancy	No flying after 32 to 36 weeks on most airlines. Doctor's certificate may be needed after 28 weeks.
Newborn baby	An infant should not fly until at least 48 hours old.

lightheadedness. If such symptoms develop, the treatment is to rebreathe air from a paper bag held over the nose and mouth, which reduces the loss of carbon dioxide.

The changes in altitude or cabin pressure during a flight affect the body's gas-containing cavities, principally the middle ears, the facial sinuses, the lungs, and the intestines. When pressure drops during ascent, the volume of gas in these cavities increases and usually escapes freely. On descent, the gas volume decreases as pressure outside the body rises. Unless preventive measures are taken, this may cause pain and, rarely, damage (see *barotrauma*).

There is increasing concern about the risk of developing deep vein thrombosis (see *thrombosis, deep vein*) during air travel. The condition may be caused by long periods of sitting in one position or compression of the tissues, both of which occur during long-haul flights.

The accelerative forces experienced by civil aircraft passengers are mild, even during take-off and landing, and no medical precautions are necessary. Military aircraft pilots, on the other hand, may experience severe accelerations and must wear special suits and use a reclined seat to prevent pooling of blood in the feet, which would cause immediate loss of consciousness.

Motion sickness usually causes fewer problems during air travel than during road or sea travel. However, passengers who are prone to motion sickness may benefit from taking an anti-motion sickness preparation.

Air travel allows the rapid crossing of several time zones within a short period of time, which can affect sleep-waking cycles, causing *jet-lag*.

AVIATION MEDICINE SPECIALISTS
Most large airlines have doctors who are specially trained in aviation medicine who are responsible for the healthcare of the airline staff. The doctors also give advice on transporting sick passengers, training and equipment to deal with illness during flight, and the maintenance of airline hygiene. In addition, the passenger medical clearance unit (PMCU) gives advice to passengers with medical conditions about flying. Anybody who is in any doubt about their medical suitablity for flying should consult their doctor, the airline, and/or the PMCU.

avitaminosis

See *hypovitaminosis*.

avulsed tooth

A tooth that has become completely dislodged from its socket following an injury. If the tooth is kept clean and moist (ideally by being stored in milk, saliva, or contact-lens solution), is not otherwise washed, and treatment is sought immediately, reimplantation (see *reimplantation, dental*) may be possible.

avulsion

The tearing away of a body structure from its point of attachment. Avulsion may be due to an injury, for example excessive contraction of a *tendon* may avulse a small piece of bone at its attachment point. Avulsion may also be performed as part of a surgical procedure, as in the surgical removal of *varicose veins*.

axilla

The medical name for the armpit.

axis

The second cervical *vertebra* in the human *spine*. The axis is attached by a pivot joint to the *atlas*, the topmost vertebra, which in turn is attached to the base of the skull. The pivot joint allows the head to turn to either side.

axon

The thin, elongated part of a *neuron* (nerve cell) that conducts nerve impulses. Many axons in the body are covered with a fatty *myelin* sheath.

Ayurvedism

See *Indian medicine*.

azathioprine

A *disease-modifying antirheumatic drug* and *immunosuppressant drug* used to treat active, progressive *rheumatoid arthritis* and other *autoimmune disorders* (in which the *immune system* attacks the body's own tissues). It is also used to prevent organ rejection after *transplant surgery*. Side effects include increased susceptibility to infection.

azelaic acid

A *topical* (applied to the skin) drug that is used to treat mild to moderate *acne*.

azithromycin

A macrolide *antibiotic drug* used to treat infections of the skin, chest, throat, and ears. Azithromycin is also used to treat genital infections due to chlamydia (see *chlamydial infections*).

azoospermia

The absence of sperm from semen, causing *infertility* in males. Azoospermia may be caused either by a congenital (present from birth) disorder or by one that develops later in life. It can also occur following a *vasectomy*.

CAUSES
Congenital azoospermia may be due to a *chromosomal abnormality* such as *Klinefelter's syndrome* (the presence of an extra sex chromosome); failure of the testes to descend into the scrotum; absence of the vasa deferentia (ducts that carry sperm from the testes to the seminal vesicles, where it is stored prior to ejaculation); or *cystic fibrosis* (a genetic disease of the lungs and pancreas that may also cause defects of the vasa deferentia).

In some males, azoospermia may be the result of hormonal disorders affecting the onset of puberty. Another cause is blockage of the vasa deferentia, which may follow a *sexually transmitted infection*, *tuberculosis*, or surgery on the groin.

Azoospermia can also be the result of damage to the testes. This can follow *radiotherapy*, treatment with certain drugs (for example, *anticancer drugs*), prolonged exposure to heat, or the effects of occupational exposure to toxic chemicals. In some cases, production of sperm ceases permanently for no known reason.

TREATMENT AND OUTLOOK
If the cause is treatable (with hormones to bring on puberty or surgery to unblock ducts closed by infection, for example), sperm production may restart. However, in some cases the testes will have been permanently damaged.

AZT

The abbreviation for azidothymidine, the former name for *zidovudine*.

aztreonam

An *antibiotic drug* used to treat some types of *meningitis* and infections by certain types of bacteria, including *PSEUDOMONAS*.

azygous

A term meaning not paired. Azygous describes a structure such as the heart, which does not have a twin organ on the opposite side of the body. The azygous vein drains blood from the abdomen and chest and travels along the right side of the spine.

B

babesiosis

A tick-borne disease caused by the BABESIA genus of *protozoa* (single-celled parasites). Babesiosis is mainly a disease of animals; it may affect sheep, cattle, horses, and other domestic animals. However, babesiosis can be transmitted from animals to humans by tick bites, producing symptoms similar to those of *malaria*.

Treatment is with the antimalarial drug *quinine* and an *antibiotic drug*. (See also *ticks and disease*.)

Babinski's sign

A *reflex* movement in which the big toe bends upwards when the outer edge of the sole of the foot is scratched. In babies, Babinski's sign is a normal reflex action. In adults, Babinski's sign is an indication of damage to, or disease of, the *brain* or the *spinal cord*.

baby blues

A common name for a mild form of depression that sometimes occurs in women after childbirth. The baby blues almost always disappear without treatment but can occasionally develop into a more serious depressive illness (see *postnatal depression*).

baby teeth

Also known as milk teeth, an alternative term for the first teeth (see *primary teeth*).

bacillary dysentery

A type of *dysentery* (infection of the intestinal tract) caused by bacteria of the SHIGELLA genus (see *shigellosis*).

bacille Calmette-Guérin

See *BCG vaccination*.

bacilli

Rod-shaped *bacteria*. Bacilli (singular: bacillus) are responsible for causing a variety of diseases, including *infectious diseases* such as tuberculosis, tetanus, typhoid fever, pertussis (whooping cough), and diphtheria.

bacitracin

A type of *antibiotic drug* used in combination with other drugs to treat infections of the eyes and skin. Bacitracin is most commonly applied as an external skin preparation or as eye-drops.

back

The area between the shoulders and buttocks. The back is supported by the spinal column (see *spine*), which is bound together by *ligaments* (bands of tough, fibrous tissue) and supported by muscles that also help to control posture and movement.

DISORDERS

Back problems are numerous and may be the result of a variety of factors affecting the spine. They can be related to disorders of bones, muscles, ligaments, tendons, nerves, and joints in the spine, all of which can cause back pain. (See also *spine* disorders box.)

background radiation

The small amounts of natural *radiation* that emanate from such sources as rocks and the soil.

back pain

Most people suffer from back pain at some time in their lives. In many cases, no exact diagnosis is made because the pain gets better within a few weeks and because analgesic drugs (painkillers) are used before any tests, such as X-rays, are carried out. In such cases, doctors may use the term "nonspecific back pain" to describe the condition.

CAUSES

Nonspecific back pain is one of the largest single causes of working days lost through illness in the UK. The people most likely to suffer from back pain are those whose jobs involve a lot of heavy lifting and carrying or those who spend long periods sitting in one position or bending awkwardly. Overweight people are also more prone to back pain – their backs carry a heavier load and they tend to have weaker abdominal muscles, which usually help to provide support to the back.

Nonspecific back pain is thought to be caused by a mechanical disorder affecting one or more structures in the back. This may be a ligament strain, a muscle tear, damage to a spinal facet joint, or *disc prolapse* (slipped disc).

In addition to pain from a damaged structure, spasm of surrounding muscles will cause pain and tenderness over a wider area. This can result in temporary *scoliosis* (an abnormal sideways curvature of the spine).

Abnormalities of a facet joint and prolapse of an intervertebral disc can both cause *sciatica* (pain in the buttock and down the back of the leg into the foot). This condition is the result of pressure on a sciatic nerve root as it leaves the spinal cord. Coughing, sneezing, or straining increase the pain. Pressure on the sciatic nerve can also cause a *pins-and-needles* sensation in that leg as well as weakness in muscles activated by the nerve. Rarely, pain may radiate down the femoral nerve at the front of the thigh.

Osteoarthritis in the joints of the spine can cause persistent back pain. *Ankylosing spondylitis* (an inflammatory disorder in which arthritis affects the spine) causes back pain and stiffness with loss of back mobility. *Coccydynia* (pain and tenderness at the base of the spine) may occur after a fall in which the coccyx has struck the ground, during pregnancy, or spontaneously for unknown reasons.

Pyelonephritis can cause back pain as well as pain and tenderness in the loin, fever, chills, and pain when passing urine. Cancer in the spine can cause persistent back pain that disturbs sleep and is not relieved by rest.

SELF-HELP

People with back pain and sciatica are usually advised to remain as mobile as possible. Sleeping on a firm mattress and taking analgesic drugs can help to relieve pain. In most cases, back pain eventually clears up with such self-help measures.

INVESTIGATION

In most cases tests are not needed. However, if back pain persists, is severe, is associated with a back injury or with weakness in a leg or bladder control problems, immediate medical advice should be sought. Examination of the back may show tenderness in specific areas or loss of back mobility. Weakness or loss of sensation in the legs implies pressure on a nerve root, which needs prompt investigation.

X-rays of the spine may reveal narrowing between the intervertebral discs; osteoarthritis; *osteoporosis*; ankylosing spondylitis; compression fracture; stress fracture; *bone cancer*; or *spondylolisthesis* (displacement of vertebrae). X-rays will not reveal ligament, muscle, facet joint, or disc damage. To detect pressure on a nerve root (due to disc prolapse, for example), *myelography*, *CT scanning*, or *MRI* is performed.

BACK PAIN

Most people experience back pain at some time in their lives, but in most cases it is not serious and the problem corrects itself before investigation takes place. However, some kinds of back pain can be related to a specific disorder. The most common sites affected by back pain are shown in this diagram.

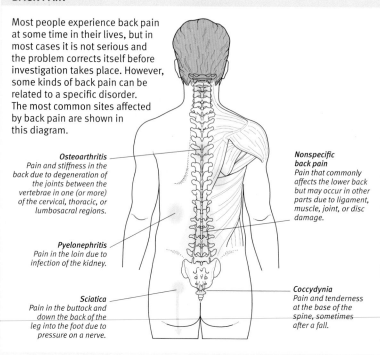

Osteoarthritis
Pain and stiffness in the back due to degeneration of the joints between the vertebrae in one (or more) of the cervical, thoracic, or lumbosacral regions.

Pyelonephritis
Pain in the loin due to infection of the kidney.

Sciatica
Pain in the buttock and down the back of the leg into the foot due to pressure on a nerve.

Nonspecific back pain
Pain that commonly affects the lower back but may occur in other parts due to ligament, muscle, joint, or disc damage.

Coccydynia
Pain and tenderness at the base of the spine, sometimes after a fall.

TREATMENT

If a specific cause is found for the back pain, treatment will be for that cause. Research has shown that acute nonspecific back pain is best treated by staying as active as possible, helped by analgesic drugs if necessary. Bed rest should not be continued for more than two days. *Physiotherapy, osteopathy, chiropractic, acupuncture*, or exercise may also be helpful.

Chronic nonspecific back pain is often more difficult to treat. Treatment may include the use of *nonsteroidal anti-inflammatory drugs, muscle-relaxant drugs*, or spinal injection. Use of a *TENS* machine may relieve pain in some people. Alternatively, the Alexander technique may be beneficial; this teaches how to amend posture and movement in order to relieve muscular tension. Very rarely, spinal surgery may be necessary to treat chronic back pain.

baclofen

A *muscle-relaxant drug* that blocks nerve activity in the spinal cord. Baclofen is used to relieve muscle *spasm* and stiffness caused by injury to either the brain or spinal cord, by neurological disorders such as *multiple sclerosis*, or by a *stroke*. The drug does not cure the underlying disorder but helps to facilitate movement and allows *physiotherapy* to be more effective. The drug is taken in either tablet or liquid form.

Side effects of baclofen may include drowsiness and muscle weakness. These effects can be reduced if the dose of the drug is increased gradually under medical supervision until the desired degree of relaxation is achieved.

bacteraemia

The presence of *bacteria* in the bloodstream. Bacteraemia commonly occurs for a few hours following minor surgical operations and dental treatment and may also occur in infections such as tonsillitis. The *immune system*, the body's natural defence mechanism, usually prevents the bacteria from multiplying and causing damage. However, in people with abnormal heart valves (due to conditions such as a congenital defect or scarring from rheumatic fever), the bacteria may cause *endocarditis* (inflammation of the heart lining and valves).

If bacteraemia affects a person whose immune system is weakened (for example, by illness, major surgery, or immunosuppressant drugs) *septicaemia* (a potentially serious infection of the blood) may develop.

bacteria

Single-celled *microorganisms* that are invisible to the naked eye. The singular form of the term is bacterium. Abundant in the air, soil, and water, most bacteria are harmless to humans. Some, such as those that live in the intestine, are beneficial and help to break down food for digestion.

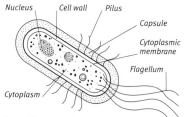

Nucleus Cell wall Pilus
Capsule
Cytoplasmic membrane
Flagellum
Cytoplasm

Magnified bacterium
A typical bacterial cell enlarged to approximately 20,000 times its normal size.

DISEASE-CAUSING TYPES

Disease-causing bacteria are known as pathogens and are classified, according to shape, into three main groups: *cocci* (spherical); *bacilli* (rod-shaped); and *spirochaetes* or spirilla (spiral-shaped).

Among the wide range of diseases caused by cocci are pneumonia, tonsillitis, bacterial endocarditis (inflammation of the lining inside the heart), meningitis (inflammation of the membranes surrounding the brain and spinal cord), toxic shock syndrome, and various disorders of the skin.

Diseases that are caused by bacilli include tuberculosis, pertussis (whooping cough), typhoid fever, diphtheria, tetanus, salmonellosis, shigellosis (bacillary dysentery), legionnaires' disease, and botulism.

Bacteria from the third, and smallest, group, the spirochaetes, are responsible for causing syphilis, yaws, leptospirosis, and Lyme disease.

GROWTH AND MOVEMENT

The bacteria that colonize the human body thrive in warm, moist conditions.

Common types of bacteria

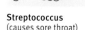

Staphylococcus
(causes boils)

Streptococcus
(causes sore throat)

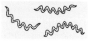

Salmonella typhi
(causes typhoid fever)

Spirochaete
(causes syphilis)

Some of these bacteria are aerobic (they need oxygen to grow and multiply) and are therefore most commonly found on the skin or within the respiratory system. Others are anaerobic, thriving where there is no oxygen, deep within tissue or wounds.

Some types of bacteria are naturally static; if they move around the body at all, they do so only when carried in currents of air or fluid. However, there are also highly motile types of bacteria, such as salmonella, which move through fluids by lashing with their whiplike tails (known as flagella) and can anchor themselves to other cells with filamentous threads called pili.

REPRODUCTION

Bacteria reproduce by simple cell division, which can occur every few minutes in ideal conditions (exactly the right temperature and sufficient nourishment for all cells). Some bacteria multiply by each producing a spore (a single new bacterium). Spores, which are protected by a tough membrane, can survive high temperatures, dry conditions, and lack of nourishment.

HOW BACTERIA ENTER THE BODY

Bacteria can enter the body through the lungs if they are inhaled in infected droplets spread by coughs and sneezes. The digestive tract may become infected if contaminated food is eaten. Some bacteria cause diseases, such as sexually transmitted infections, by entering the genitourinary system.

Bacteria can also penetrate the skin in various ways: through hair follicles; by way of superficial cuts and abrasions; through burns; and via deep, penetrating wounds.

HOW BACTERIA CAUSE DISEASE

Some bacteria release poisons (toxins) that are harmful to human cells. The toxins either destroy the cell or disrupt its chemical processes. Less commonly, certain types of bacteria directly enter, and multiply within, body cells, causing tissue damage as they spread.

THE BODY'S DEFENCES

The body's first defences against disease-causing bacteria are the skin and the *mucous membranes* lining the respiratory tract, the digestive tract, and the genitourinary system. The eyes are protected by an *enzyme* in tears and the stomach secretes hydrochloric acid, which kills many of the bacteria found in food and water.

If bacteria pass through these barriers, the body's *immune system* responds by

CULTURING AND TESTING BACTERIA

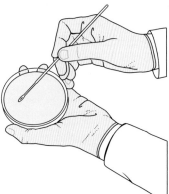

1 The bacteria are introduced on to a nutrient plate (i.e. agar or blood agar) and placed in an incubator at body temperature.

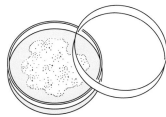

2 Any bacteria present multiply rapidly to form visible colonies that can be studied under the microscope and identified by different patterns of growth.

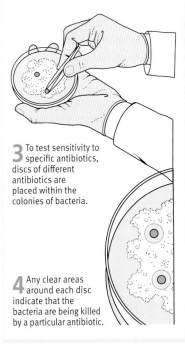

3 To test sensitivity to specific antibiotics, discs of different antibiotics are placed within the colonies of bacteria.

4 Any clear areas around each disc indicate that the bacteria are being killed by a particular antibiotic.

sending various types of white blood cell to seek and destroy the bacteria.

Immunity can also be generated by *immunization*. This involves injecting a weakened form of the bacterium or its poison into the body to stimulate an immune response. Immunization is now routine for a number of conditions, including *diphtheria*, *tetanus*, and some forms of *meningitis*.

TREATMENT OF BACTERIAL DISEASES

The immune response is sometimes enough to bring about recovery, and mild bacterial infections may not need any treatment. However, *antibiotic drugs* are the main form of treatment for more severe infections. Superficial infected wounds may be treated with *antiseptics*.

Some bacteria, such as *MRSA*, are now becoming resistant to treatment with antibiotics. In these circumstances, bacterial infections can be difficult or even impossible to treat and may be life-threatening. (See also *infectious disease*.)

bacterial endocarditis

See *endocarditis*.

bacterial food poisoning

See *food poisoning*.

bacterial vaginosis

An infection of the *vagina* that causes a greyish-white discharge and itching. The disorder is due to excessive growth of *bacteria* that normally live in the vagina. Bacterial vaginosis occurs most commonly in sexually active women and is treated with *antibiotic drugs*.

bactericidal

A term that is used to describe any substance that kills bacteria. (See also *antibiotic drugs*; *bacteriostatic*.)

bacteriology

The study of *bacteria*, particularly of the types that cause disease. Bacteriology includes techniques used to isolate and identify bacteria from specimens such as a throat swab or urine. Bacteria are identified by their appearance under a microscope, including their response to stains (see *Gram's stain*; *staining*), and by the use of *culture*. Testing for sensitivity to *antibiotic drugs* may be performed.

bacteriostatic

A term used to describe a substance that stops the growth or multiplication of *bacteria* but does not kill them. (See also *antibiotic drugs*; *bactericidal*.)

B

bacteriuria

The presence of *bacteria* in the urine. It is common for small, harmless numbers of bacteria to be found in the urine of healthy people. Bacteriuria is of significance only if more than 100,000 bacteria are present in each millilitre of urine, or if 100 white blood cells (pus cells) per millilitre of urine are present (which is an indication of the body's response to the infection).

Bacteroides

A genus of *anaerobic* (capable of living without oxygen) bacilli (rod-shaped *bacteria*) that normally inhabit the intestines. One particular type, BACTEROIDES FRAGILIS, is commonly found in abdominal wound infections and in the blood when the intestines are diseased.

bad breath

See *halitosis*.

bagassosis

An occupational disease affecting the lungs of workers who handle mouldy bagasse (the fibrous residue of sugarcane after juice extraction). Bagassosis is one cause of allergic *alveolitis*, a reaction of the lungs to inhaled dust containing fungal spores. Symptoms develop four to five hours after inhalation of the dust and may include shortness of breath, wheezing, fever, headache, and cough; typically, they last for about 24 hours. Repeated exposure to dust may lead to permanent lung damage. Protective measures taken by industry have made the disease rare.

Baker's cyst

A firm, fluid-filled lump behind the knee. A Baker's cyst occurs as a result of increased pressure in the knee joint due to a buildup of fluid. Such a buildup is a feature of disorders such as *rheumatoid arthritis*. The cyst is created by a backward ballooning-out of the synovial membrane covering the knee joint.

Most Baker's cysts are painless, and some disappear spontaneously, sometimes after many months. Occasionally, a cyst may rupture, causing fluid to seep down between the layers of the calf muscles. This can produce pain and swelling in the calf that may mimic a deep vein thrombosis (see *thrombosis, deep vein*).

Diagnosis of a Baker's cyst is confirmed by *ultrasound scanning*. Treatment is rarely needed, but in a few cases surgery may be performed.

balance

The ability to remain upright and move without falling over. Keeping one's balance is a complex process that relies on a constant flow of information to the brain about body position. The integration of all of this information, and continual instructions from the brain, enable the body to make the changes needed to maintain balance.

The brain receives data on body position from various sources: the eyes; the sensory organs (called proprioceptors) in the skin, muscles, and joints; and the three semicircular canals of the labyrinth of the inner *ear*. The part of the brain called the *cerebellum* collates this information and sends instructions to muscles to contract or relax to maintain balance.

DISORDERS

Balance can be affected by various disorders, particularly inner-ear disorders such as *labyrinthitis* (inflammation of the ear's labyrinth) and *Ménière's disease* (an abnormally high pressure of fluid in the labyrinth). Less commonly, *otitis media* (a disorder of the middle ear) may disturb balance.

Damage to nerve tracts in the spinal cord that carry information from position sensors in the joints and muscles to the brain can also impair balance. This damage to the nerves may result from spinal tumours, circulatory disorders, nerve degeneration due to deficiency of vitamin B_{12}, or, rarely, tabes dorsalis (a complication of *syphilis*). A tumour or *stroke* that affects the cerebellum in the brain may cause clumsiness of the arms and legs as well as other features of impaired muscular coordination.

balanitis

Inflammation of the foreskin and the glans (head) of the penis. Balanitis results in pain and/or itchiness, and the entire area may be red and moist. Causes of balanitis include bacterial or fungal infection, *phimosis* (tightness of the foreskin), or chemical irritation by contraceptive creams (see *contraception*) or laundry products.

Treatment is usually with *antibiotic drugs* or *antifungal drugs* (either applied to the skin as cream or taken orally) and careful washing of the penis and foreskin. If balanitis recurs frequently, or is due to phimosis, *circumcision* (surgical removal of the foreskin) may be recommended.

baldness

See *alopecia*.

ball-and-socket joint

A highly mobile *joint*, such as the shoulder or hip.

ballismus

Violent jerking and twitching of the limbs that is caused by brain damage within the area below the *thalamus* (a structure that relays sensory information). In most cases, only one side of the body is affected, in which case the condition is known as hemiballismus.

balloon angioplasty

See *angioplasty, balloon*.

ballottement

A technique occasionally used during a physical examination (see *examination, physical*) to check the position of an organ, particularly in a fluid-filled area of the body. It involves flicking or tapping the area with the fingers, causing the organ to move up and down. The technique was once widely used to confirm pregnancy; when the wall of the uterus is tapped, the fetus moves away and floats back with a responding tap.

balloon catheter

A flexible tube with a balloon at its tip, which, when inflated, keeps the tube in place or applies pressure to an organ or vessel. One type of balloon catheter is

BALLOON CATHETER

Sterile water tube to inflate balloon

Irrigation tube for fluid to wash out bladder

Tube to drain urine from bladder

Inflatable balloon filled with water

Hole through which urine enters

URINARY CATHETER

used to drain urine from the bladder (see *catheterization, urinary*). Balloon catheters are sometimes used to expand narrowed arteries (see *angioplasty, balloon*). They may also be used to control bleeding from widened veins in the lower part of the oesophagus (known as *oesophageal varices*) before surgery.

balm

A soothing or healing medicine applied to the skin.

balsam

An aromatic oily liquid that is obtained from various evergreen trees. Balsam is an *antiseptic* substance and was once also widely used in remedies for respiratory disorders.

bambuterol

A *bronchodilator drug* that is converted to *terbutaline* in the liver. Bambuterol can only be taken orally.

bandage

A strip or tube of fabric used to keep *dressings* in position, to apply pressure, to control bleeding, or to support a sprain or strain. Roller and tubular bandages are the type most widely used. Tubular gauze bandages require a special applicator and are used mainly for areas that are awkward to bandage, such as a finger. Triangular bandages are used to make *slings*. (See also *wounds*.)

banding

A procedure for treating *haemorrhoids* (piles) that are large or are causing particular discomfort. Using a special instrument, a doctor places a rubber band around the base of the haemorrhoid, which causes it to shrink and, eventually, to fall off. Banding is a virtually painless procedure.

barber's itch

See *sycosis barbae*.

barbiturate drugs

COMMON DRUGS

• Amobarbital • Butobarbital • Phenobarbital
• Secobarbital • Thiopental

A group of sedative drugs that work by depressing activity within the brain. Barbiturate drugs include thiopental, which is very short-acting and is used to induce anaesthesia (see *anaesthesia, general*), and phenobarbital, which is long-acting and is sometimes used as

an *anticonvulsant drug* in the treatment of epilepsy. In the past, barbiturates were widely used as *sleeping drugs*. They are now rarely used, and have been replaced by *benzodiazepine drugs* and other nonbarbiturates. Because barbiturates are readily habit-forming and are abused for their sedative effect, they are classified as *controlled drugs*.

HOW THEY WORK
The sedative action of barbiturate drugs is produced by the drug molecules blocking the conduction of stimulatory chemical signals between the nerve cells of the brain and reducing the ability of the cells to respond. Barbiturates, especially phenobarbital, also reduce the sensitivity of brain cells to abnormal electrical activity.

POSSIBLE SIDE EFFECTS
The possible adverse effects of barbiturate drugs include excessive drowsiness, staggering gait, and, in some cases, excitability. An overdose of barbiturates can be fatal, particularly when taken in combination with alcohol, which dangerously increases their depressant effect on the brain (including suppression of the respiratory centre).

Barbiturates readily produce dependence if used for more than a week or two, and withdrawal effects, such as sleeplessness and twitching, may then occur when treatment is stopped.

Bardet–Biedl syndrome

A very rare *genetic disorder* characterized by *learning difficulties*, *retinopathy* (an eye defect), *obesity*, *polydactyly* (the presence of extra fingers or toes) and *hypogonadism* (underactivity of the testes or ovaries).

barium sulphate

A salt that is used in solution as a *contrast medium* in X-ray examinations of the intestinal tract (see *barium X-ray examinations*). Barium is opaque to X-rays and is used to view the outline of hollow internal organs that would otherwise not be visible.

barium X-ray examinations

Procedures used to detect and follow the progress of some disorders of the gastrointestinal tract. Because barium (a metallic element) is opaque to X-rays, it is used to outline organs, such as the stomach, which are not normally visible on an X-ray image. Barium sulphate mixed with water is passed into the part of the tract requiring examination before X-rays are taken. In some cases,

barium X-ray examination is used as an alternative to *endoscopy* (internal examination using a flexible or rigid viewing tube), although endoscopy is often the preferred form of investigation.

Barium X-rays may be single- or double-contrast. Single-contrast X-rays use barium sulphate alone. The barium fills the section of the tract under examination and provides an outline image that shows up any prominent abnormalities. In double-contrast barium X-rays, the barium forms a thin film over the inner surface of the tract and the tract is subsequently filled with air so that any small surface abnormalities can be seen.

TYPES OF EXAMINATION
Various types of barium X-ray examination are used to investigate different parts of the gastrointestinal tract. A barium swallow involves drinking a solution of barium; this procedure is used to investigate the swallowing mechanism or the oesophagus. A barium meal is carried out to look at the lower oesophagus, stomach, and duodenum.

A barium follow-through examination can be used to investigate disorders of the small intestine; after barium has been swallowed, a series of X-rays are taken at intervals as the barium travels down the oesophagus to the intestine. A barium enema can be used to investigate disorders of the large intestine and the rectum; the barium is introduced into the body through a tube inserted in the rectum.

Any barium that remains in the intestine may be a cause of constipation. For this reason, it is important to ensure that a patient has a high-fibre diet and drinks plenty of water following a barium examination, until all the barium has passed through. (See also *Barium X-ray procedures* box, overleaf.)

barotrauma

Damage or pain, mainly affecting the middle *ear* and the facial *sinuses*, that is caused by changes in surrounding air pressure. Air travellers are at the greatest risk of barotrauma, but scuba divers face similar problems.

CAUSE
Aircraft cabin pressure decreases as the plane ascends and increases as it descends. As the aircraft ascends, the ears may seem to "pop" as the air in the middle ear expands and is expelled via the eustachian tubes, which connect the middle ear to the back of the throat. On descent, the higher pressure may push the eardrum inwards and cause pain.

BARIUM X-RAY PROCEDURES

Barium X-ray examinations are used to reveal abnormalities or disorders within the upper and lower gastrointestinal tract. Barium swallows are used to investigate the oesophagus, and barium meals are used for the examination of areas such as the stomach and duodenum. The large intestine is examined by means of a barium enema.

BARIUM SWALLOW/MEAL

Barium swallows and meals are used to investigate the upper gastrointestinal tract. No food or drink is permitted for six to nine hours beforehand. At the examination, the patient swallows a glass of barium mixed with a flavoured liquid, or is given a piece of bread or a biscuit soaked in barium if a disorder of the swallowing mechanism is being investigated.

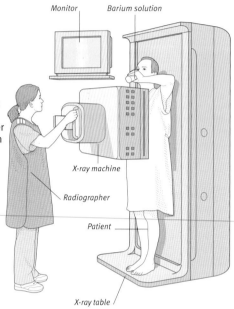

Monitor   Barium solution

X-ray machine

Radiographer

Patient

X-ray table

Taking the X-ray
The radiographer takes X-ray pictures while the patient swallows. For a barium swallow, the patient stands; for a barium meal, the patient lies on the table in different positions; for a barium follow-through, the patient lies on the right side and X-rays are taken at intervals until the barium has progressed through the small intestine.

Barium swallow result
This contrast X-ray has revealed a narrowed area, known as an oesophageal stricture, in the lower section of the oesophagus.

Narrowed oesophagus

Spinal column

Spine   Stomach

Stomach   Outline
outlet   of tumour

Barium meal result
In this X-ray, a thin film of barium has outlined the stomach lining. The introduction of air into the stomach has revealed the presence of a large tumour.

BARIUM ENEMA

A barium enema is carried out for examination of the large intestine and rectum. In order for an examination to be successful, the large intestine needs to be as empty and clean as possible because faeces can obscure or simulate a polyp or tumour. For this reason, the patient's intake of food and fluids is sometimes restricted for a few days before the examination, and laxatives are given to make sure that the bowel is empty prior to the procedure.

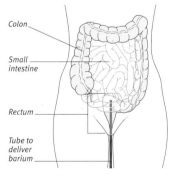

Colon

Small intestine

Rectum

Tube to deliver barium

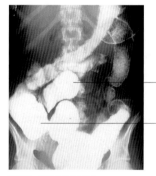

Small intestine

Colon filled with liquid barium

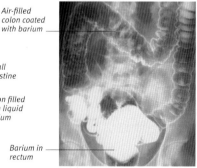

Air-filled colon coated with barium

Small intestine

Barium in rectum

The procedure
The radiographer or radiologist introduces the barium into the patient's intestine via a tube inserted into the rectum. The patient lies on his or her left side while the barium is infused. He or she then turns on to the other side, front, and back, and X-rays are taken.

Single-contrast result
In single-contrast barium enemas, the section of intestine to be examined is filled with liquid barium. Because barium is opaque to X-rays, it provides an outline image that shows up prominent abnormalities such as narrowing.

Double-contrast result
In double-contrast, barium and air are introduced into the tract. The barium forms a film on the tract's inner surface only, providing an image of small surface abnormalities that would not be visible using single-contrast.

SYMPTOMS
Minor pressure damage in the middle ear may cause pain, hearing loss, and *tinnitus* (ringing in the ears) for a few days; damage in the facial sinuses may also cause pain, and possibly a discharge of mucus or blood. Symptoms usually wear off within hours or days, but treatment may be needed if they worsen or persist. Large changes in pressure can rupture the eardrum (see *eardrum, perforated*).

PREVENTION
Barotrauma can be avoided by vigorous swallowing or by forcibly breathing out with the mouth closed and the nose pinched, which is known as the Valsalva manoeuvre. This action serves to equalize the internal and external pressures in the middle ear and sinuses.

If the eustachian tubes are blocked, as commonly occurs with a cold, use of a nasal spray containing a *decongestant drug* is recommended shortly before the descent of the aircraft. Anyone with a severe head cold should avoid air travel if possible. Infants should be breast- or bottle-fed during descent to encourage swallowing. (See also *aviation medicine*; *scuba-diving medicine*.)

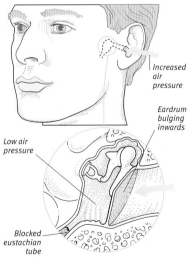

Mechanism of barotrauma
The diagram above shows the location of the middle ear and the pressure changes that occur when the eustachian tube is blocked and there is an increase in surrounding air pressure.

barrel chest
A prominent, rounded chest that is sometimes the result of lung distension in people with longstanding *emphysema* (enlarged air sacs in the lungs). Lung distention leads to an increase in distance between the front and back of the chest, thereby resulting in a change in the shape of the chest wall. (See also *pulmonary disease, chronic obstructive*.)

Barrett's oesophagus
A complication of long-term *gastro-oesophageal reflux* in which the cells that line the lower part of the oesophagus are replaced by cells that are normally found in the stomach. People with Barrett's oesophagus are at increased risk of developing an ulcer in the oesophagus, *oesophageal stricture*, and oesophageal cancer (see *oesophagus, cancer of*). The condition may be monitored regularly by *endoscopy* (internal examination using a viewing instrument) and *biopsy* (removal of a sample of tissue for analysis) of the oesophagus.

barrier cream
A cream that is used to protect the skin against the effects of irritant substances and excessive exposure to water. (See also *sunscreens*.)

barrier method
A method of preventing pregnancy by blocking the passage of sperm to the uterus (see *contraception, barrier methods of*). An example of a barrier method is the use of a condom or a diaphragm.

barrier nursing
The nursing technique by which a patient with an infectious disease is prevented from infecting other people (see *isolation*). In reverse barrier nursing, a patient with reduced ability to fight infection is protected against outside infection. (See also *aseptic technique*.)

bartholinitis
An infection of the *Bartholin's glands* at the entrance to the *vagina*. The disorder, which may be due to a *sexually transmitted infection* such as *gonorrhoea* or chlamydia (see *chlamydial infections*), causes an intensely painful red swelling at the opening of the gland ducts. Treatment is with *antibiotic drugs*, *analgesic drugs*, and warm baths.

Bartholinitis sometimes leads to the formation of an abscess (see *Bartholin's abscess*) or a painless cyst, known as a Bartholin's cyst, which may become infected. Abscesses are drained under general anaesthesia (see *anaesthesia, general*). Recurrent abscesses or infected cysts may require surgery to convert the duct into an open pouch (see *marsupialization*) or remove the gland completely.

Bartholin's abscess
The formation of pus in one or both of the *Bartholin's glands*, which are located on either side of the vulva (the folds of flesh that surround the opening of the vagina). Bartholin's abscesses develop as a result of bacterial infection of the glands (see *bartholinitis*).

Bartholin's glands
A pair of oval, pea-sized glands whose ducts open into the vulva (the folds of flesh that surround the opening of the vagina). During sexual arousal, the Bartholin's glands secrete a fluid that lubricates the vulval region. Infection of these glands causes *bartholinitis* or the development of a *Bartholin's abscess*.

BARTHOLIN'S GLANDS

These glands are located on each side of the entrance to the vagina.

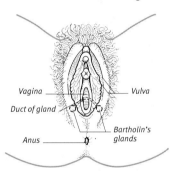

basal cell carcinoma
The commonest type of skin cancer, also known as a rodent ulcer or BCC. It occurs most frequently on the face or neck, but can affect any part of the body. The cells of the tumour closely resemble, and are possibly derived from, cells in the basal (innermost) skin layer.

Basal cell carcinoma is caused by skin damage from the ultraviolet radiation in sunlight. Fair-skinned people over the age of 50 are most commonly affected by this form of cancer; dark-skinned people are protected by the larger amount of *melanin* (a pigment that absorbs ultraviolet radiation) in their skin. The incidence of basal cell carcinoma is much higher among people living in sunny climates, especially those who have outdoor occupations; in parts of the US and Australia, over half the white population has had a basal cell carcinoma by the age of 75.

SYMPTOMS

The majority of basal cell carcinomas occur on the face, often at the side of an eye or on the nose. It starts as a small, flat nodule and grows slowly, eventually breaking down at the centre to form a shallow ulcer with raised edges.

Diagnosis is confirmed through a biopsy (removal of a small sample of cells for microscopic analysis). Without treatment, the tumour gradually invades and destroys the surrounding tissues, but it virtually never spreads to other parts of the body.

TREATMENT

Treatment of basal cell carcinoma is usually by surgical removal, *radiotherapy*, or *cryotherapy* (freezing). In some cases, *plastic surgery* may also be required, depending on the size and site of the tumour.

PREVENTION

The risk of developing this form of skin cancer can be reduced by avoiding overexposure to strong sunlight, by using *sunscreens*, and by wearing protective clothing such as sun hats. People who have previously had a basal cell carcinoma may develop further tumours and should be especially alert to any new changes in their skin. (See also *melanoma, malignant*; *squamous cell carcinoma*; *sunlight, adverse effects of*.)

basal ganglia

Paired nerve cell clusters deep within the cerebrum (the main mass of the *brain*) and the upper part of the brainstem. The basal ganglia play a vital part in producing smooth, continuous muscle actions and in stopping and starting movement. Any disease or degeneration affecting the basal ganglia and their connections may lead to the appearance of involuntary movements, trembling, and weakness, as occur in *Parkinson's disease*.

basal metabolic rate (BMR)

The rate at which energy is used by the body just to maintain vital functions. Such vital functions include breathing, circulation, and digestion. (See also *energy requirements*; *metabolism*).

base

See *alkali*.

basement membrane

The thin membrane that lies directly beneath the *epithelium* (the layer of cells that covers surfaces of the body and lines most hollow structures within it). The basement membrane is composed of protein fibres and carbohydrates.

base pair

Part of a *DNA* molecule comprising two chemicals known as nucleotide bases that are linked together by means of hydrogen bonds. A base pair forms one "rung" of the DNA "ladder". There are only two possible pairings of the four bases: guanine always pairs with cytosine and adenine with thymine. The sequence of base pairs in each DNA chain provides the code for the activities of the cell (see *genetic code*). (See also *nucleic acids*.)

basic life support

Resuscitation techniques that may be performed by a first aider (see *rescue breathing*; *cardiopulmonary resuscitation*). If basic life support measures fail to restore a normal heartbeat and spontaneous breathing, *advanced life support* must then be administered by trained medical personnel.

basilar membrane

A membrane within the cochlea (the inner *ear* structure containing the receptor for hearing). Sound waves cause the basilar membrane to vibrate, stimulating sensory hair cells to send electrical signals to the brain.

basophil

A type of *white blood cell* that plays a part in inflammatory and allergic reactions.

Batten's disease

One of a group of hereditary metabolic diseases (see *metabolism, inborn errors of*) to which *Tay–Sachs disease* also belongs. In Batten's disease, abnormal fatty substances accumulate in the cells of the *nervous system*, causing progressive dementia, worsening seizures, and loss of vision. Symptoms of the condition usually first appear during early childhood.

There is no known treatment for Batten's disease, which is generally fatal during childhood.

Bazin's disease

A rare disorder, mainly affecting young women, in which tender swellings develop under the skin in the calves. In most cases no cause can be found, although Bazin's disease may sometimes be linked to *tuberculosis*.

B-cell

See *B-lymphocyte*.

BCG vaccination

A vaccine that gives immunity against *tuberculosis*. The BCG vaccine is prepared from an artificially weakened strain of tubercle bacilli, the rod-shaped *bacteria* that are responsible for causing tuberculosis. The letters BCG stand for "bacille Calmette–Guérin", after the two men who developed the tuberculosis vaccine.

WHY IT IS DONE

The BCG vaccine is given to people who are at risk of tuberculosis and for whom a tuberculin test is negative, indicating that they are likely to have no immunity to the disease. People at risk include health workers, contacts of people with tuberculosis, and immigrants (including infants and children) from countries where there is a high rate of tuberculosis. Infants born to immigrants in this category are immunized, without having a tuberculin test, within a few days of birth, as are infants living in areas of the UK where there is a high incidence of tuberculosis.

HOW IT IS DONE

The vaccine is usually injected into the upper arm. About four weeks later, a small pustule appears. This normally heals completely, leaving a small scar, but can occasionally develop into a chronic *ulcer* (open sore).

Becker's muscular dystrophy

A type of *muscular dystrophy*.

beclometasone

A *corticosteroid drug* that is used in the treatment of *asthma*, hay fever (see *rhinitis, allergic*), and *eczema*.

Prescribed as a nasal spray, beclometasone controls the symptoms of hay fever by reducing inflammation and production of mucus in the lining of the nose. It also helps to reduce chest symptoms, such as wheezing and coughing.

Prescribed as an inhaler for the treatment of asthma, beclometasone reduces inflammation of the airways. However, the drug is slow to take full effect so it is used as a preventer to reduce the frequency and severity of attacks. Once an attack has started, the drug does not relieve symptoms. Beclometasone is usually used with *bronchodilator drugs* to manage asthma that has not responded to bronchodilators alone.

Possible adverse effects of beclometasone include hoarseness, throat irritation, and, on rare occasions, fungal infections in the mouth; but these can be minimized by rinsing the mouth with water and gargling after each inhalation.

Beclometasone is also prescribed in the form of a cream or as an ointment to treat inflammation of the skin resulting from *eczema*.

beclomethasone
The former name for the corticosteroid drug *beclometasone*.

Beconase
A brand name for a nasal spray that contains the corticosteroid drug *beclometasone*. Beconase is used to treat hay fever (see *rhinitis, allergic*) and also some other nasal allergies.

becquerel
A unit of radioactivity (see *radiation units*).

bed bath
A method of washing a bedridden person. A small area is washed and dried at a time, while the rest of the body is kept covered to prevent chilling.

bedbug
A flat, wingless, brown insect that is about 5 mm long and 3 mm wide. Bedbugs live in furniture and furnishings, especially in beds and carpets, emerging at night to feed on humans by sucking their blood. Bedbugs are not known to transmit disease, but their bites are itchy and they may develop into sores that become infected.

bedpan
A metal, plastic, or fibre container into which a patient can defaecate or urinate without getting out of bed.

bed rest
A term used to describe periods spent in bed. Bed rest is sometimes part of the treatment for certain illnesses, such as *rheumatic fever*, and for some types of injury, such as a fractured vertebra.

Prolonged bed rest carries risks such as muscle wasting, *bedsores*, and development of blood clots in the legs (see *thrombosis, deep vein*). Bed rest was once considered an essential part of the treatment of many common conditions, but is now avoided when possible. Patients are usually encouraged to be mobile as soon as possible after illness or surgery.

PREVENTING **BEDSORES**

Once a bedsore has developed it will heal only if pressure on it is minimized, so good nursing care of a bedridden or immobile patient is crucial. The patient's position should be changed at least every two hours; and it is important to wash and dry pressure areas carefully, especially if there is incontinence. Barrier creams can be used for additional protection.

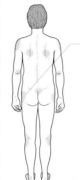
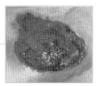

Common sites
These include the shoulders, elbows, lower back, hips and buttocks, knees, ankles, and heels.

bedridden
A term used to describe a person who is unable to leave bed due to illness or injury. People most likely to be bedridden are the very elderly, the terminally ill, and those paralysed as the result of an accident.

bedsore
Also known as a decubitus ulcer or pressure sore, an ulcer that forms on the skin of patients who are unconscious or immobile. Common sites for bedsores include the shoulders, elbows, lower back, hips, buttocks, ankles, and heels.

CAUSES
Bedsores may develop following a *stroke* or *spinal injuries* that result in loss of sensation. Incontinence (see *incontinence, urinary*), if it results in constantly wet skin, may also be a causative factor.

SYMPTOMS
Bedsores start as red, painful areas that become purple before the skin starts to break down, producing open sores. At this stage, the sores may become infected and take a long time to heal.

TREATMENT AND PREVENTION
Deep, chronic *ulcers* may require treatment with *antibiotic drugs* and, in some cases, *plastic surgery*. Good nursing care, including changing the patient's position regularly, skin care, protection of

vulnerable areas, and use of cushions and special mattresses, should prevent bedsores from developing in most cases.

bedwetting
The common name for poor bladder control at night (see *enuresis, nocturnal*).

bee stings
See *insect stings*.

behavioural problems in children
Behavioural problems range from mild and short-lived periods of unacceptable behaviour, which are common in most children, to more severe problems such as conduct disorders and refusal to go to school. Behavioural problems may occasionally occur in any child; specialist management is called for when the problems become frequent and disrupt school and/or family life. Some behavioural problems can occur whatever the family or home situation of the child. In some cases, however, stressful external events, such as moving home or parental divorce, may produce periods of problem behaviour.

Behavioural problems that are common in young children include sleeping problems, such as waking repeatedly in the night. In toddlers, *breath-holding attacks*, *tantrums*, separation anxiety, and *head-banging* are problems best dealt with by a consistent and controlled approach. Problems with *toilet-training*

BEHAVIOURAL PROBLEMS BY AGE

- **Babies up to 18 months**
  Sleeping and feeding difficulties, colic, crying

- **Toddlers and children 1–4 years**
  Head-banging, tantrums, biting, breath-holding attacks, separation anxiety, poor social interaction, difficulty in changing from one activity to another, toilet training problems

- **Early childhood 4–8 years**
  Nail-biting, thumb-sucking, aggression, clinginess, anxiety about illness and death, nightmare, enuresis

- **Middle childhood/adolescence 9–18 years**
  Lying, stealing, smoking, truancy, disobedience, aggression, low achievement in school, drug or alcohol use, running away, sexual promiscuity

B

are usually avoided if the training is delayed until the child is physically and emotionally ready.

In children between the ages of four and eight years, minor behavioural problems, such as *thumb-sucking* and nail-biting, clinginess, bedwetting (see *enuresis, nocturnal*), and disruption during the night due to *nightmares*, are so common as to be almost normal. Such problems are best dealt with by using a positive approach that concentrates on rewarding good behaviour. In most cases, the child grows out of the problem, but medical help may be needed.

behaviourism

An American school of *psychology* founded by John Broadus Watson early in the 20th century. He argued that, because behaviour, rather than experience, was all that could be observed in others, it should constitute the sole basis of psychology.

behaviour therapy

A collection of techniques, based on psychological theory, that are used to change abnormal behaviour or to treat anxiety. Behaviour therapy is based on two main ideas: that repeated exposure to a feared experience under safe conditions will render it less threatening, and that desirable behaviour can be encouraged by using a system of rewards, often self-administered. Although still occasionally used, behaviour therapy has largely been superseded by *cognitive-behavioural therapy* (CBT). This is based on the idea that psychological problems result from erroneous or negative ways of thinking (cognitions) and can therefore be helped by amending those faulty cognitions.

TYPES

Specific behaviour therapy techniques include exposure therapy (also known as desensitization), flooding, response prevention, and modelling.

Exposure therapy A technique that is commonly used to treat phobic disorders, such as *agoraphobia* (a fear of open spaces and/or public places), animal phobias, and fear of flying. It consists of exposing the patient to the cause of the anxiety in stages: for example, the therapist may accompany an agoraphobic patient on a short journey. At the same time, the patient is taught to cope with anxiety symptoms by using relaxation techniques. The intensity of the exposure is increased, until eventually, he or she is able to deal with the full situation.

Flooding In flooding, the patient is confronted directly and for a lengthy period with the anxiety-provoking stimulus. He or she is supported by the therapist until the fear is reduced. This technique can be emotionally traumatic and is now used less commonly.

Response prevention The patient is prevented from carrying out an obsessional task. For example, someone with a handwashing compulsion is prevented from carrying out the washing rituals. This technique is used in combination with other methods.

Modelling In this approach, the therapist acts as a model for the patient, performing the anxiety-provoking activity first, and encouraging the patient to copy.

behaviour, types A and B

Behaviours characteristic of two personality types described in the early 1970s, when studies were performed to examine the behaviour patterns of people with coronary artery disease.

It was proposed that a particular behaviour pattern (called Type A) was associated with increased vulnerability to stress-related illnesses, such as *hypertension* (high blood pressure). Type A personalities are said to feel constantly under pressure to perform many tasks at the same time, and to be competitive and self-critical. They are also impatient and easily irritated by others. In contrast to this, people with Type B personalities are said to be calmer and more relaxed.

Behçet's syndrome

A rare, multisystem disorder with recurrent *mouth ulcers* and *genital ulcers* and inflammation of the eyes, skin, joints, blood vessels, brain, and intestines.

The cause of Behçet's syndrome is unknown, but the disorder is strongly associated with HLA-B51, a genetically determined *histocompatability antigen*. It affects twice as many men as women. Treatment of Behçet's syndrome is often difficult and may involve *corticosteroid drugs* and *immunosuppressant drugs*. The condition often becomes long term.

belching

The noisy return of air from the stomach through the mouth. Swallowing air is usually an unconscious habit, which may result from eating or drinking too much and/or too quickly. Occasionally, belching may help to alleviate discomfort caused by indigestion.

belladonna

An extract of the deadly nightshade plant that has, since ancient times, been used medicinally. Belladonna contains *alkaloids* (substances containing nitrogen), such as *atropine*, that are used as *antispasmodic drugs* to treat gastrointestinal disturbances. (See also *anticholinergic drugs*.)

Bell's palsy

The most common form of *facial palsy* (facial muscle weakness).

Bence–Jones protein

An abnormal protein found in the urine of people with *multiple myeloma*, which is a cancer affecting one type of cell in the bone marrow.

bendrofluazide

The former name for the diuretic drug *bendroflumethiazide*.

bendroflumethiazide

A thiazide *diuretic drug* that is used to treat *hypertension* (high blood pressure) and *heart failure*.

bends

The nonmedical term for *decompression sickness*. The term is used especially to refer to the severe bone and joint pains that are a common symptom in divers who rise to the surface too rapidly.

benign

A term used to describe a disease that is relatively harmless. When used to refer to tumours, benign means noncancerous tumours that do not invade or destroy local tissues and do not spread to other sites within the body.

benign prostatic hyperplasia (BPH)

A medical term for noncancerous enlargement of the prostate gland (see *prostate, enlarged*).

Bennett's fracture

A fracture of the base of the thumb, which is often accompanied by partial dislocation of the joint.

benzalkonium chloride

A preservative that is widely used in eye-drops and products such as cosmetics and mouth washes.

benzocaine

A local anaesthetic (see *anaesthesia, local*) of low potency and toxicity that is commonly used as an ingredient in over-the-counter preparations for relieving the pain of conditions such as *mouth ulcers* and *sore throat*.

benzodiazepine drugs

COMMON DRUGS

SLEEPING DRUGS • Flurazepam • Loprazolam • Lormetazepam • Nitrazepam • Temazepam
SEDATIVES • Alprazolam • Chlordiazepoxide • Diazepam • Lorazepam • Oxazepam

A group of sedative drugs given for short periods either as *sleeping drugs* for *insomnia* or to control the symptoms of *anxiety* (see *tranquillizer drugs*). Common benzodiazepine drugs include diazepam, which is used as a tranquillizer, and nitrazepam, which is used to relieve insomnia. Benzodiazepine drugs may also be used in the management of alcohol withdrawal and in the short-term control of an epileptic seizure. The drugs are also sometimes abused for their sedative effects.

HOW THEY WORK

Benzodiazepine drugs promote sleep and relieve anxiety by interfering with chemical activity in the brain and nervous system. This reduces the communication between nerve cells and depresses brain activity.

POSSIBLE ADVERSE EFFECTS

Adverse effects of benzodiazepines include excessive daytime drowsiness, dizziness, and forgetfulness. Unsteadiness and slowed reactions may also occur. In addition, the drugs may cause paradoxical effects, such as excitement or aggression, in some people. If taken with alcohol, benzodiazepines may increase the alcohol's effect to a dangerous extent.

Tolerance to benzodiazepines can develop after as little as three days, and there is a high risk of users becoming physically and psychologically dependent on the drugs, even after only a few weeks' use. For these reasons, most doctors are reluctant to prescribe the drugs unless they are absolutely necessary, and then usually only for a maximum period of four weeks.

When benzodiazepine treatment is stopped suddenly, withdrawal symptoms may occur. These may include anxiety, restlessness, confusion, and nightmares. People who have been taking benzodiazepines in the long term need to have the drugs gradually withdrawn over the course of several months in order to prevent the occurrence of withdrawal symptoms.

benzoyl peroxide

An *antiseptic* agent used in a variety of topical preparations for the treatment of *acne* and fungal skin infections (see *fungal infections*). In acne, benzoyl peroxide also works by removing the surface layer of skin, thereby unblocking sebaceous glands.

benzylpenicillin

A type of *penicillin drug* that is given by injection.

bereavement

The emotional reaction following the death of a loved one. The expression of grief is individual to each person, but there are recognized stages of bereavement, each of which is characterized by a particular attitude.

STAGES OF BEREAVEMENT

In the first stage of bereavement, which may last from three days to three months, there is often a feeling of numbness and an unwillingness to recognize the death. These emotions are defence mechanisms against admitting, and therefore accepting, the loss and the associated pain. Often, the reality of the death does not penetrate completely at this time, and many people continue to behave as though the dead person were still alive. Hallucinations, in which the deceased person is seen or sensed, are a common experience among the recently bereaved. This sensation can be quite comforting for some people, but others may find it disturbing.

Once the numbness wears off, the person may be overwhelmed by feelings of anxiety, anger, and despair that can develop into a depressive illness (see *depression*). Gastrointestinal disturbances, insomnia, malaise, agitation, and tearfulness are also common.

Gradually, but usually within two years, the bereaved person adjusts to the loss and begins to look more towards the future. This process can involve periods of pain and despair, alternating with periods of enthusiasm and interest.

SUPPORT AND COUNSELLING

Family and friends can often provide the support a bereaved person needs. Outside help is sometimes required and may be given by a social worker, health visitor, member of the clergy, or self-help group. For some people, when depression, apathy, and lethargy impede their chances of recovery, specialized *counselling* or *psychotherapy* is necessary. (See also *stillbirth*.)

beriberi

A nutritional disorder resulting from a lack of *thiamine* (vitamin B_1) in the diet. Thiamine, found in wholemeal cereals, meat, green vegetables, potatoes, and nuts, is essential for the metabolism of carbohydrates. Without it, the brain, the nerves, and the muscles (including the heart muscle) are not able to function properly. In developed countries, the illness is seen only in people who are starving or those who have an extremely restricted diet, such as alcoholics.

SYMPTOMS AND SIGNS

There are two forms of the illness: "dry" and "wet" beriberi. In dry beriberi, thiamine deficiency mainly affects the nerves and skeletal muscles. The symptoms include numbness, a burning sensation in the legs, and muscle wasting. In severe cases, the affected person becomes virtually paralysed, emaciated, and bedridden.

In wet beriberi, the main problem is *heart failure* (reduced ability of the heart to pump blood around the body). This in turn causes *oedema* (swelling caused by fluid accumulation) in the legs and sometimes also in the trunk and face. Other symptoms of wet beriberi include poor appetite, rapid pulse, and breathlessness. Without treatment, heart failure worsens and can lead to death.

TREATMENT

Beriberi is treated with thiamine, given either orally or by injection, which usually brings about a complete cure. A permanent improvement in diet is also required to prevent recurrence.

Bernard–Soulier syndrome

A *genetic disorder* in which platelets (the *blood cells* responsible for initiating blood clotting) do not function properly. The syndrome is characterized by abnormal bleeding in the skin and internal organs.

berry aneurysm

An abnormal swelling that occurs at the junction of *arteries* supplying the brain. Berry aneurysms are usually due to a congenital (present at birth) weakness in the artery wall. They may occasionally rupture, which results in a *subarachnoid haemorrhage*. (See also *aneurysm*; *intracranial aneurysm*.)

berylliosis

An occupational disease caused by the inhalation of dust or fumes containing the metallic element beryllium. Short exposure to high concentrations of beryllium may lead to an episode of severe *pneumonitis* (lung inflammation). Exposure over a number of years to lower concentrations may lead to permanent lung and liver damage.

Treatment with *corticosteroid drugs* can reduce damage to the lungs. In most cases, the introduction of safe working practices prevents exposure to dangerous levels of beryllium.

Best's disease

A *genetic disorder* in which the macula (part of the light-sensitive retina at the back of the eye) is abnormal. The disorder is congenital (present from birth) and results in progressive loss of vision.

beta-blocker drugs

COMMON DRUGS

CARDIOSELECTIVE •Atenolol •Betaxolol •Bisoprolol •Celiprolol •Metoprolol
NONCARDIOSELECTIVE •Acebutolol •Carvedilol •Labetolol •Nadolol •Oxprenolol •Pindolol •Propranolol •Sotalol •Timolol

A group of drugs, also known as beta-adrenergic blocking agents, prescribed principally to treat heart and circulatory disorders such as *angina pectoris* (pain in the chest due to an insufficient supply of blood to the heart muscle) and cardiac *arrhythmias* (abnormal heartbeat). They may also be used to treat *hypertension* (high blood pressure), but are not usually recommended as first-line treatment. The drugs block the effects of the *sympathetic nervous system*, which releases *adrenaline* (epinephrine) and *noradrenaline* (norepinephrine) at nerve endings known as beta receptors.

There are two types of beta receptor: beta$_1$ and beta$_2$. Beta$_1$ receptors are present mainly in the heart and beta$_2$ are found in the lungs, blood vessels, and elsewhere in the body. Certain beta-blockers (such as atenolol, bisoprolol and metoprolol) are termed cardioselective and, because they act mostly on beta$_1$ receptors, are used principally to treat heart disease such as angina, hypertension, and cardiac *arrhythmia*. These drugs are sometimes given after a *myocardial infarction* (heart attack) to reduce the likelihood of further damage to the heart muscle.

Other types of beta-blocker, such as oxprenolol, propranolol, and timolol, may be given to prevent *migraine* attacks by acting on blood vessels in the head. They are also used to reduce the physical symptoms of *anxiety* and to control the

HOW **BETA-BLOCKERS** WORK

Beta-blockers block specific sites on body tissues where neurotransmitters (chemicals released from nerve endings) bind. These sites are called beta receptors, and there are two types: beta$_1$ receptors, found in heart tissue, and beta$_2$ receptors, found in the lungs, blood vessels, and other tissues. At these receptors, two chemicals, adrenaline (epinephrine) and noradrenaline (norepinephrine), are released from nerve endings in the sympathetic nervous system, the part of the involuntary nervous system that enables the body to deal with stress, anxiety, and exercise. These neurotransmitters bind to beta receptors to increase the force and speed of the heartbeat, to dilate the airways to increase air flow to the lungs, and to dilate blood vessels.

Cardioselective beta-blockers bind predominantly to beta$_1$ receptors; noncardioselective beta-blockers bind to both types. Beta-blockers slow the heart rate and reduce the force of contraction of heart muscle. These effects can be used to slow a fast heart rate and regulate abnormal rhythms.

Beta-blockers prevent attacks of angina pectoris by reducing the work performed by the heart muscle and therefore the heart's oxygen requirement. High blood pressure is reduced because the rate and force at which the heart pumps blood into the circulation is lowered.

The effect of blocking beta receptors on muscles elsewhere in the body is to reduce the muscle tremor of anxiety and an overactive thyroid gland. Beta-blockers may help to reduce the frequency of migraine attacks by preventing the dilation of blood vessels surrounding the brain, which is what causes the headache. In glaucoma they lower pressure in the eye by reducing fluid production in the eyeball.

Normal
Adrenaline (epinephrine) and noradrenaline (norepinephrine) can be released either from the adrenal gland or from sympathetic nerve endings. They bind to beta$_1$ and beta$_2$ receptors in tissues around the body.

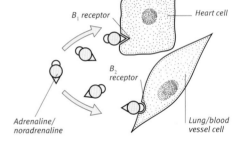

Cardioselective beta-blockers
Cardioselective beta-blockers occupy predominantly B$_1$ receptors, preventing adrenaline (epinephrine) and noradrenaline (norepinephrine) from binding to them. This reduces the stimulating action of adrenaline and noradrenaline on heart tissue. Cardioselective beta-blockers do not block B$_2$ receptors, thereby allowing adrenaline (epinephrine)/ noradrenaline (norepinephrine) to act on other tissues around the body.

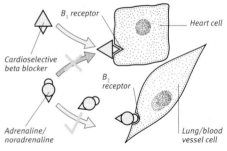

Noncardioselective beta-blockers
Noncardioselective beta-blockers occupy both B$_1$ and B$_2$ receptors, reducing the stimulating action of adrenaline (epinephrine) and noradrenaline (norepinephrine) on tissues around the body.

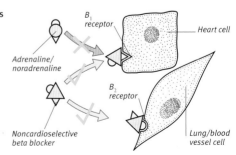

symptoms of *thyrotoxicosis* (an overactive thyroid gland). Beta-blockers such as timolol are sometimes given in the form of eye-drops to treat *glaucoma*; they work by lowering fluid pressure in the eyeball. (See also the illustrated box.)

POSSIBLE ADVERSE EFFECTS
Beta-blocker drugs may precipitate *asthma*, which can be dangerous, and they are therefore not usually prescribed for anybody who has, or has had, asthma. The drugs may worsen the symptoms of *bronchitis* and some other lung diseases, may reduce an individual's capacity for strenuous exercise, and may also reduce the flow of blood to the limbs, causing cold hands and feet. In addition, sleep disturbance and depression can be side effects of beta-blockers. Anyone taking beta-blockers should not suddenly stop; a severe recurrence of previous symptoms and a significant rise in blood pressure may result.

betahistine

A drug that is used in the treatment of the inner-ear disorder *Ménière's disease*. Betahistine reduces the frequency and severity of the characteristic attacks of nausea and vertigo.

beta interferon

A type of *interferon* (a protein produced naturally by body cells) sometimes used in the treatment of *multiple sclerosis*.

beta-lactam antibiotics

A group of *antibiotic drugs* that includes the penicillins and the cephalosporins. Beta-lactam antibiotics work by altering chemical activity in bacteria, thereby killing them.

beta-lactamase

An enzyme, also known as *lactamase*, that inactivates antibiotic drugs such as penicillins. Bacteria that produce this enzyme are therefore resistant to treatment with these kinds of antibiotics.

betamethasone

A *corticosteroid drug* used in the treatment of inflammation. Betamethasone is applied to the skin as a cream to treat contact *dermatitis* and *eczema*. The drug is also prescribed as nasal spray to treat allergic *rhinitis* (hay fever) and is taken by mouth to treat some cases of *asthma* and *arthritis*.

Adverse effects of betamethasone are unlikely with short-term use. However, prolonged topical use of the drug can cause thinning of the skin and may aggravate any infection that has developed. Taken orally over a prolonged period or in high doses, betamethasone can cause adverse effects typical of other corticosteroid drugs.

betel nut

The seed of the tropical palm ARECA CATECHU, which, when chewed, acts as a stimulant and digestive. Chewing betel nuts is associated with an increased risk of *mouth cancer*.

Betnovate

A brand name for the corticosteroid drug *betamethasone*, which is used in topical preparations.

bezafibrate

A *lipid-lowering drug* used to reduce blood cholesterol levels.

bezoar

A ball of food and mucus, vegetable fibre, hair, or other indigestible material in the stomach. Trichobezoars, which are composed of hair, may form in the stomachs of children or emotionally disturbed adults who nibble at, or pull out and swallow, their hair.

Symptoms include loss of appetite, constipation, nausea and vomiting, and abdominal pain. If trichobezoars pass into the intestines, they may cause a blockage (see *intestine, obstruction of*). Bezoars can be removed by *endoscopy* or conventional surgery.

bi-

A prefix meaning two or twice, as in bilateral (two-sided).

bicarbonate of soda

See *sodium bicarbonate*.

biceps muscle

The name given to any muscle that originates as two separate parts, which then fuse. The term biceps muscle is commonly used to refer to the biceps brachii muscle of the upper arm, which bends the arm at the elbow and rotates the forearm. Another example is the biceps femoris muscle, located at the back of the thigh, which bends the leg at the knee and extends the thigh.

bicornuate uterus

An abnormally shaped uterus that divides into two halves in its upper part. Bicornuate literally means "having two horns".

bicuspid

A term meaning to have two cusps (curved, pointed structures). Bicuspid describes certain *heart valves* and is used as an alternative name for a premolar tooth (see *teeth*).

bifocal

A spectacle lens with two different focal lengths. Glasses with bifocal lenses make corrections both for close and distant vision. (See also *myopia*; *hypermetropia*.)

biguanides

Oral hypoglycaemic drugs (see *hypoglycaemics, oral*) used in the treatment of type 2 *diabetes mellitus*. Metformin, which is the only available type of biguanide drug, reduces the production of glucose in the liver and also increases the uptake of glucose by the body's cells. (See also *antidiabetic drugs*.)

bilateral

A term that means affecting both sides of the body, or affecting both organs if they are paired (for example, both ears in bilateral deafness).

bile

A greenish-brown alkaline liquid that is secreted by the *liver*. Bile carries away

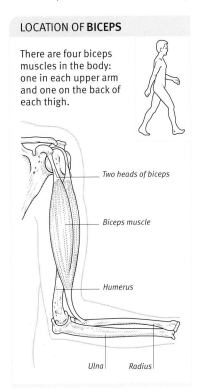

LOCATION OF BICEPS

There are four biceps muscles in the body: one in each upper arm and one on the back of each thigh.

Two heads of biceps

Biceps muscle

Humerus

Ulna   Radius

waste products formed in the liver and also helps to break down fats in the small intestine for digestion.

The waste products in bile include the pigments *bilirubin* and biliverdin, which give bile its greenish-brown colour; bile salts, which aid in the breakdown and absorption of fats; and *cholesterol*. Bile passes out of the liver through the *bile ducts* and is then concentrated and stored in the gallbladder. After a meal, bile is expelled and enters the duodenum (the first section of the small intestine) via the common bile duct. Most of the bile salts are later reabsorbed into the bloodstream to be recycled by the liver into bile. Bile pigments are excreted in the faeces. (See also *biliary system*; *colestyramine*.)

bile duct

Any of the ducts through which *bile* is carried from the *liver* to the gallbladder and then on to the duodenum (the first section of the small intestine).

The bile duct system forms a network of tubular canals. Canaliculi (small canals) surround the liver cells and collect the bile. The canaliculi join together to form ducts of increasing size. The ducts emerge from the liver as the two hepatic ducts, which join within or just outside the liver to form the common hepatic duct. The cystic duct branches off to the gallbladder; from this point the common hepatic duct becomes the common bile duct and leads into the duodenum. (See also *biliary system*.)

bile duct cancer

See *cholangiocarcinoma*.

bile duct obstruction

A blockage or constriction of a bile duct (see *biliary system*). Obstruction of a bile duct results in the accumulation of bile in the liver (*cholestasis*) and *jaundice* (yellowing of the skin and the whites of the eyes) due to a buildup of *bilirubin* (bile pigment) in the blood. Prolonged obstruction of the bile duct can lead to secondary *biliary cirrhosis*, which is a serious form of liver disease.

CAUSES

The most common cause of bile duct obstruction is *gallstones*. Other causes include a tumour affecting the pancreas (see *pancreas, cancer of*) and cancer that has spread from elsewhere in the body. *Cholangiocarcinoma* (cancer of the bile ducts) is a rare cause of a blockage. Bile duct obstruction is known to be a rare

side effect of certain drugs. It may also be caused by *cholangitis* (inflammation of the bile ducts), trauma (such as injury during surgery), and, rarely, by *flukes* or worms.

SYMPTOMS

Bile duct obstruction causes "obstructive" jaundice, which is characterized by pale-coloured faeces, dark urine, and a yellow skin colour. There may also be itching. Other symptoms of bile duct obstruction depend on the cause of the blockage; for example, there may be abdominal pain (with gallstones) or weight loss (with cancer).

TREATMENT

Treatment depends on the cause. It may involve *ERCP* (a minimally invasive procedure used for diagnosis and treatment that involves the use of X-rays and a viewing tube), *lithotripsy* (shock-wave treatment), drug therapy, or conventional surgery.

bilharzia

Another name for the tropical parasitic disease *schistosomiasis*.

biliary atresia

A rare *congenital* disorder in which some or all of the *bile ducts* fail to develop or develop abnormally. As a result, *bile* is unable to drain from the liver (see *cholestasis*). Unless the atresia can be treated, secondary *biliary cirrhosis* (a serious liver disorder) will develop and may prove fatal. Symptoms include *jaundice*, usually beginning a week after birth, and the passing of dark urine and pale faeces. Treatment is by surgery to bypass the bile ducts. If this fails, or if the jaundice recurs, a *liver transplant* is required.

biliary cirrhosis

An uncommon form of liver *cirrhosis* that results from problems with the bile ducts. There are two types of biliary cirrhosis. One is an *autoimmune disorder* and is known as primary biliary cirrhosis. Secondary biliary cirrhosis occurs as a result of a longstanding blockage. In both types of the condition, liver function is impaired due to *cholestasis* (accumulation of bile in the liver).

Primary biliary cirrhosis principally affects middle-aged women and seems to be linked with a malfunction of the *immune system*. In this disorder, the bile ducts within the liver become inflamed and are destroyed. Symptoms include itching, *jaundice* (a yellowish discolora-

tion of the skin and the whites of the eyes), an enlarged liver, and sometimes abdominal pain, fatty diarrhoea, and *xanthomatosis* (deposits of fatty material under the skin). *Osteoporosis* may also develop. Symptoms of liver cirrhosis and *liver failure* may occur after a few years. Drugs can be used to minimize complications and to relieve symptoms such as itching, but a *liver transplant* is the only cure.

Secondary biliary cirrhosis results from prolonged *bile duct obstruction* or *biliary atresia* (abnormal bile ducts). Symptoms and signs include abdominal pain and tenderness, liver enlargement, fevers and chills, and sometimes blood abnormalities. Treatment is the same as for bile duct obstruction.

biliary colic

A severe pain in the upper right quadrant of the abdomen that is usually caused by the gallbladder's attempts to expel *gallstones* or by the movement of a stone in the *bile ducts*. The pain may be felt in the right shoulder (see *referred pain*) or may penetrate to the centre of the back. Episodes of biliary colic often last for several hours and may recur, particularly after meals.

Injections of an *analgesic drug* and *antispasmodic drug* may be given to relieve the colic. The presence of gallstones can be confirmed by tests such as *cholecystography*, *ultrasound scanning*, or *ERCP* (a minimally invasive procedure involving the use of X-rays and a viewing tube that may be used for diagnosis and treatment).

biliary system

The organs and ducts in which *bile* is formed, concentrated, and carried from the *liver* to the duodenum (the first part of the small intestine). Bile is secreted by liver cells and collected by a network of *bile ducts* that carry the bile out of the liver via the hepatic duct. The cystic duct branches off the hepatic duct and leads to the gallbladder, where the bile is concentrated and stored. Beyond this junction, the hepatic duct becomes the common bile duct, which opens into the duodenum at a controlled orifice known as the ampulla of Vater. The presence of fat in the duodenum following a meal prompts the secretion of a hormone that opens the ampulla of Vater. This causes contraction of the gallbladder, which squeezes stored bile into the duodenum.

The main disorders affecting the biliary system are *gallstones*, congenital *biliary atresia* and *bile duct obstruction*. (See also *gallbladder, disorders of*.)

biliousness

A condition in which bile is brought up to the mouth from the stomach. Biliousness is also used as a nonmedical term for nausea and vomiting.

bilirubin

The main pigment in *bile*. Bilirubin is produced by the breakdown of *haemo-globin*, the pigment in red blood cells. Very high levels of bilirubin cause the yellow pigmentation of *jaundice*. Products formed from the breakdown of bilirubin make faeces brown.

Billings' method

A technique (also known as the mucus inspection method) in which a woman notes changes in the characteristics of mucus produced by her cervix. The technique is employed to predict ovulation for the purposes of *contraception* or *family planning*.

Billroth's operation

A type of partial *gastrectomy* in which the lower part of the stomach is surgically removed. Previously used in the treatment of *peptic ulcers*, the operation is now rarely performed due to the introduction of effective drug treatment for peptic ulcers.

Binet test

The first *intelligence test* that attempted to measure higher mental functions rather than more primitive abilities. The Binet test was devised in 1905.

FUNCTION OF THE **BILIARY SYSTEM**

The biliary system consists of the bile ducts leading from the liver and gallbladder, the gallbladder itself, and associated structures. The system drains waste products from the liver into the duodenum and aids the process of fat digestion through controlled release of fat-emulsifying agents (contained in bile).

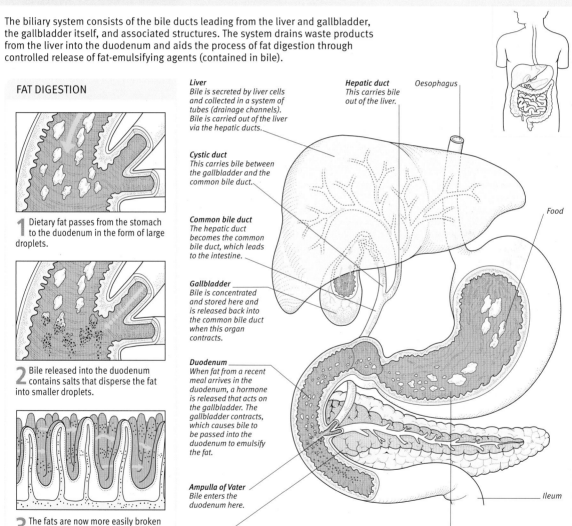

FAT DIGESTION

1 Dietary fat passes from the stomach to the duodenum in the form of large droplets.

2 Bile released into the duodenum contains salts that disperse the fat into smaller droplets.

3 The fats are now more easily broken down by lipase, an enzyme made by the pancreas, and absorbed through the intestinal lining.

Liver
Bile is secreted by liver cells and collected in a system of tubes (drainage channels). Bile is carried out of the liver via the hepatic ducts.

Cystic duct
This carries bile between the gallbladder and the common bile duct.

Common bile duct
The hepatic duct becomes the common bile duct, which leads to the intestine.

Gallbladder
Bile is concentrated and stored here and is released back into the common bile duct when this organ contracts.

Duodenum
When fat from a recent meal arrives in the duodenum, a hormone is released that acts on the gallbladder. The gallbladder contracts, which causes bile to be passed into the duodenum to emulsify the fat.

Ampulla of Vater
Bile enters the duodenum here.

Pancreas
In response to the presence of fat in the duodenum, the pancreas produces hormones that stimulate contraction of the gallbladder and cause the ampulla of Vater to open so that bile flows into the duodenum.

Hepatic duct
This carries bile out of the liver.

Oesophagus

Food

Ileum

Stomach
Fat and other products of digestion pass from the stomach to the duodenum.

binge–purge syndrome

An alternative term for the eating disorder *bulimia*.

bio-

A prefix describing a relationship to life, as in biology, the science of life.

bioavailability

The proportion of a drug that reaches the target organs and tissues, usually expressed as a percentage of the dose administered. Intravenous administration of a drug results in 100 per cent bioavailability because the drug is injected directly into the bloodstream. Drugs taken orally have a much lower bioavailability. Preparations that have equal bioavailabilities are described as bioequivalent. (See also *drug*.)

biochemistry

A science that studies the chemistry of living organisms, including human beings. The human body is made up of millions of cells and the chemical processes involved in providing these cells with energy, eliminating their wastes, repairing damage, promoting cell growth, and causing cell division are all studied by biochemists.

Life is maintained by a huge number of chemical reactions that occur inside cells. These reactions link together in a complex way and together make up the *metabolism* of the body. The reactions that produce energy and break down food and body structures are termed catabolism; those that build up body structures and store food are termed anabolism. Overall regulation of these chemical processes is a principal function of *hormones,* which are secreted into the bloodstream by the *endocrine glands*; regulation of individual reactions is carried out by *enzymes* (substances that promote biochemical reactions).

Certain vital chemical processes take place in every cell in the body. Other, more specific chemical processes are confined to specialized cells that make up the tissues of particular organs. For example, liver cells store and chemically modify the digestion products of food.

A constant interchange of substances occurs between the cell fluids and the blood and urine, and much information can be obtained about chemical changes inside cells by regularly measuring amounts of the various minerals, gases, enzymes, hormones, and proteins in the different body fluids. Such biochemical tests may be used to make or confirm a diagnosis, as well as to screen for a particular disease and monitor its progress. The most commonly used biochemical tests are performed on *blood*; such tests include *liver function tests* and *kidney function tests*. Biochemical tests can also be performed on urine (see *urinalysis*) as well as on all other body fluids.

biofeedback training

A technique in which a person uses information about a normally unconscious body function, such as blood pressure, to gain conscious control over that function. This training may help to treat stress-related conditions, including certain types of *hypertension* (high blood pressure), *anxiety*, and *migraine*.

HOW IT IS DONE

The doctor connects the patient to a recording instrument that can measure one of the unconscious body activities, such as blood pressure, heart rate, muscle tension, the quantity of sweat on the skin, brain waves, or stomach acidity. The patient receives information (feedback) on the changing levels of these activities from changes in the instrument's signals, for example a flashing light or sound changing tone.

After some experience with the technique, the person starts to become aware of how he or she is feeling whenever there is a change of signal. By using *relaxation techniques*, the person learns to change the signals by conscious control of the function. Once acquired, control can be exercised without the instrument.

biological clock

A popular term for the inherent timing mechanism that supposedly controls physiological processes and cycles in living organisms. (See also *biorhythms*.)

biology

The scientific study of all living organisms, including animals, plants, and microorganisms. It involves the study of the structure and functions of organisms, their relationships with other organisms, and their interactions with the environment.

biomechanical engineering

A discipline that applies engineering methods and principles to the body to explain how it functions and to treat disorders. Applications include the design of artificial joints and heart valves, pacemakers, and kidney dialysis machines.

biopsy

A diagnostic test involving the removal of small amounts of tissue or cells from the body for microscopic examination. A biopsy is an accurate method of diagnosing many illnesses, including cancer. Microscopic examination of tissue (see *histology*) or of cells (see *cytology*) usually gives a correct diagnosis.

HOW IT IS DONE

There are several types of biopsy. In excisional biopsy, the whole abnormal area is removed for study. Incisional biopsy involves cutting away a small sample of skin or muscle for analysis. In a needle biopsy, a needle is inserted through the skin and into the organ or tumour to be investigated. Aspiration biopsy uses a needle and syringe to remove cells from a lump (see box). Guided biopsy uses *ultrasound scanning* or *CT scanning* to locate the area of tissue to be biopsied and follow the progress of the needle. In endoscopic biopsy, an *endoscope* (viewing tube) is passed into the organ to be investigated and an attachment is used to take a sample from the lining of accessible hollow structures such as the lungs, stomach, and bladder. In an open biopsy, a surgeon opens a body cavity to reveal a diseased organ or tumour and removes a sample. Prompt analysis, in some cases by *frozen section* (in which the tissue is frozen and thinly sliced), can enable the surgeon to decide whether to remove the entire diseased area immediately.

OBTAINING RESULTS

Biopsy samples are analysed by *staining*; dyes are used to show up structures or identify constituents such as *antibodies* or *enzymes*. Tissue may be tested with specific antibodies in the investigation of infection and inflammation. In some cases, a tissue *culture* (cultivation of tissue cells in a growing medium) may be required. (See also *endometrial biopsy*; *excision*; *kidney biopsy*; *liver biopsy*.)

biorhythms

Physiological functions that vary in a rhythmic way (for example, the menstrual cycle, which repeats approximately every 28 days in fertile women).

Most biorhythms are based on a daily, or circadian (24-hour), cycle. Our bodies are governed by an internal clock, which is itself regulated by *hormones* (chemicals released by *endocrine glands*). Periods of sleepiness and wakefulness may be affected by the level of *melatonin* secreted by the pineal gland

ASPIRATION **BIOPSY**

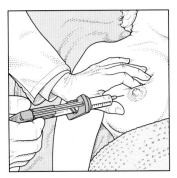

1 A fine needle attached to a syringe is inserted into the lump, and fluid or cells are sucked out to be examined under a microscope. The syringe can be held in a device that withdraws the plunger. Usually no anaesthetic is necessary, but local anaesthetic may be sometimes be used.

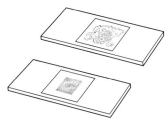

2 Before examination any fluid may be spun at high speed in a centrifuge and a small amount placed on a slide.

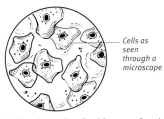

Cells as seen through a microscope

3 The cells are then fixed (preserved) and finally stained for viewing. The cytologist examines individual cells for abnormalities, paying particular attention to the size, shape, and structure of the nucleus.

in the brain. Release of melatonin is stimulated by darkness and suppressed by light. Cortisol, a hormone secreted by the adrenal glands, also reflects sleeping and waking states, being low in the evening and high in the morning.

When the normal regular division between night and day is distorted by travelling quickly to another time zone, the internal clock is disrupted and the result is *jet-lag*.

biotechnology

The use of living organisms such as *bacteria* in industry and science (for example, in drug production).

bioterrorism

The use of disease-causing organisms (such as *anthrax* and *smallpox*) as an act of violence and intimidation.

biotin

A vitamin of the B complex (see *vitamin B complex*) that is essential for the breakdown of fats.

biphosphonate drugs

See *bisphosphonate drugs*.

bipolar disorder

An illness, also known as manic-depressive illness, characterized by swings in mood between the opposite extremes of severe *depression* and overexcitability (*mania*). Initially, the mood disturbance may consist of depression or mania but eventually it alternates between the two. In a severe form that is sometimes referred to as manic-depressive psychosis, there may also be grandiose ideas or negative delusions

CAUSES

Abnormalities in brain biochemistry or in the structure and/or function of certain nerve pathways in the brain may be the underlyting cause of bipolar disorder. An inherited tendency may also be a causative factor.

TREATMENT AND OUTLOOK

Bipolar disorder is almost always treated with drugs, often in combination with other therapies. *Antidepressant drugs* are used to treat depression; *ECT* (electroconvulsive therapy) may also be used if depression is severe. *Antipsychotic drugs* are given to control manic symptoms. *Lithium* or *carbamazepine* are used to prevent relapses. In severe cases, bipolar disorder often needs hospital treatment. *Group therapy*, *family therapy*, and individual *psychotherapy* may be useful in treatment. *Cognitive-behavioural therapy* may also be helpful.

With treatment, most patients improve or remain stable. Even those with severe illness may be restored to near-normal health with lithium.

bird-fancier's lung

Also known as pigeon-fancier's lung, a form of allergic *alveolitis* (inflammation of the lungs) caused by inhalation of dust from bird droppings.

bird flu

See *avian influenza*.

birth

See *childbirth*.

birth canal

The passage from the cervix (neck of the womb) to the vaginal opening through which the baby passes during *childbirth*.

birth control

Limitation of the number of children born, either to an individual or within a population. (See also *contraception; family planning*.)

birth defects

Abnormalities that are obvious at birth or detectable early in infancy. Also called congenital defects, they encompass minor abnormalities, such as *birthmarks*, and serious disorders such as *spina bifida* (failure of the spinal column to close properly). Birth defects may occur as the result of a variety of factors, but in many cases no obvious cause can be found.

CHROMOSOME DEFECTS

Some children are born with more or fewer than the normal 23 pairs of *chromosomes* (threadlike structures in the cell nuclei that carry genetic information). *Down's syndrome*, a condition in which there is an extra copy of one of the chromosomes, is one of the most common *chromosomal abnormalities*.

GENETIC OR HEREDITARY DEFECTS

These may be inherited from one or both parents (see *gene*; *genetic disorders*). Genetic defects obvious at birth include *albinism* (lack of normal pigmentation in the skin, hair, and eyes) and *achondroplasia* (abnormally short stature).

DRUGS AND OTHER HARMFUL AGENTS

Certain drugs and chemicals (known as *teratogens*) can damage the fetus if the mother takes or is exposed to them during early pregnancy. Teratogenic drugs include *thalidomide* (now rarely prescribed) and *isotretinoin*, which is used in the treatment of severe *acne*. Alcohol can affect the development of the brain and face (see *fetal alcohol syndrome*).

IRRADIATION

Irradiation of the embryo at an early stage of development, for example, if a woman is X-rayed before she is aware of her pregnancy, can cause abnormalities.

INFECTIONS

If a woman contracts certain infections during pregnancy, there is a chance that they may cause birth defects. For example,

B

rubella (German measles) in early pregnancy can cause fetal abnormalities, including deafness, cataract (clouding of the lens of the eye), and heart disease. *Toxoplasmosis* (infection with a parasite found in cats' faeces), can also be passed on to the fetus, causing damage to the eyes, liver, and other organs.

OTHER COMMON DEFECTS

Abnormalities in the embryo's development can damage the brain and spinal cord, causing defects such as spina bifida and *hydrocephalus* (a buildup of fluid in the brain). In congenital heart disorders (see *heart disease, congenital*), there is a structural abnormality in the heart that may interfere with normal blood flow. *Cleft lip and palate* result from a failure of the two sides of the fetal face and palate to join completely.

DETECTION

Ultrasound scanning and blood tests during pregnancy can identify women at high risk of having a baby with a birth defect. Further tests such as *chorionic villus sampling*, *amniocentesis*, or *fetoscopy* may then be carried out.

PREVENTION

Some birth defects can be prevented, or the risks minimized; for example, by rubella immunization before pregnancy, folic acid supplements before and in early pregnancy, and by avoiding teratogens during pregnancy.

birthing chair

A specially designed chair to support a woman during *childbirth*. In the opinion of many doctors, sitting, as opposed to lying down, can help to shorten labour.

birth injury

Damage sustained by a baby during *childbirth*. Minor injuries, such as bruising and swelling of the scalp during a vaginal delivery (see *cephalhaematoma*) are common. More serious injury can occur, particularly if the baby is large and has difficulty passing through the birth canal. A *breech delivery* may result in injury to nerves in the baby's shoulder, causing temporary paralysis in the arm. The face may be paralysed temporarily if the facial nerve is traumatized by forceps during delivery. Fractured bones are another hazard of difficult deliveries, but the bones usually heal easily. (See also *birth defects*; *brain damage*.)

birthmark

An area of discoloured skin that is present at birth, or appears very soon afterwards. Birthmarks include *moles*, freckles, and other types of melanocytic *naevi* (a variety of flat, brown to blue-grey skin patches), strawberry marks (bright red, usually protuberant areas), and port-wine stains (purple-red, flat, often large areas). The latter two are types of *haemangioma* (malformation of blood vessels). Strawberry marks often become larger in the first year, but most disappear after the age of nine. Port-wine stains seldom fade, but some can be reduced by *laser treatment* during adulthood.

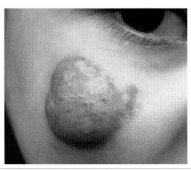

Birthmark
Strawberry marks, a common type of birthmark caused by malformation of blood vessels, are usually bright red, protuberant, and spongy.

birthpool

A pool of warm water in which a woman can sit to help relieve pain during labour (see *childbirth*).

birth, premature

See *prematurity*.

birth, preterm

See *preterm birth*.

birth rate

A measurement of the number of births in a particular year in relation to the size of the population.

birthweight

A baby's weight at birth, which usually ranges from 2.5 to 4.5 kg and in the UK averages about 3.5 kg. Birthweight depends on a number of factors, including the size and ethnic origin of the parents. Baby boys weigh, on average, slightly more than baby girls. Babies who weigh less than 2.5 kg at birth are considered to be of low birthweight. Causes include *prematurity* and undernourishment in the uterus. Abnormally high birthweight may be due to unrecognized or poorly controlled *diabetes mellitus* in the mother.

bisacodyl

A type of stimulant *laxative drug* that works by stimulating the intestinal wall into contracting, increasing the speed at which faecal matter passes through.

bisexuality

Sexual interest in members of both sexes that may or may not involve sexual activity.

bismuth

A metal, salts of which are used in tablets to treat *peptic ulcer* and in creams and suppositories to treat *haemorrhoids* (piles). Bismuth preparations taken by mouth may colour the faeces black. The tongue may darken and, occasionally, nausea and vomiting may occur.

bisphosphonate drugs

Drugs used in the prevention or treatment of *osteoporosis*. They are also used to slow bone metabolism (for example, in *Paget's disease*) and to reduce the high calcium levels in the blood associated with destruction of bone by secondary cancer growths.

bite

See *occlusion*.

bites, animal

Any injury inflicted by the mouthparts of an animal, which may range from the puncture wounds of bloodsucking insects to the massive injuries caused by shark or crocodile attacks. Teeth, especially those of carnivores, can inflict widespread mechanical injury. Severe injuries and lacerations to major blood vessels can lead to heavy blood loss and physiological *shock*. Serious infection may occur as a result of bacteria in the animal's mouth being transferred in the bite, and *tetanus* is a particular hazard. In countries where *rabies* is present, any mammal may potentially harbour the rabies virus and transmit it via a bite.

TREATMENT

Medical advice should be sought for all but minor injuries, and in all cases if there is a risk of rabies. The treatment usually includes cleaning and examination of the wound. The wound will usually be left open and dressed, rather than stitched, as closing it can encourage the multiplication of bacteria. Preventive *antibiotic drug* treatment and an anti-tetanus injection may also be given. If there is any possibility that the animal might be infected with rabies, antirabies vaccine is given; people who have not been previously immunized against rabies are also given *immunoglobulin*. (See also *bites, human*; *insect bites*; *snake bites*; *spider bites*; *venomous bites and stings*.)

bites, human

Wounds that are caused by one person biting another. Human bites rarely result in serious tissue damage or blood loss; but infection from any microorganisms in the mouth is likely, particularly if the bite is deep. For example, there is a risk of *tetanus* infection, and transmission of *hepatitis B*, *hepatitis C*, *herpes simplex*, and *HIV*.

Bitot's spots

Grey, foamy patches that appear on the *conjunctiva* (the mucous membrane covering the front of the eye). Bitot's spots, which are made up of keratinized (horny) cells, are associated with *vitamin A* deficiency.

black death

The medieval name for bubonic *plague*, which in past epidemics killed 50 per cent of its victims. One feature of the disease is bleeding under the skin, causing bluish-black bruises, hence the name.

black eye

A dark discoloration of the skin around the eye, usually following an injury. The discoloration is due to blood collecting under the skin (see *bruise*). Because the skin around the eye is loose and thin, bruising is darker than on other parts of the body. A cold compress held over the eye can help to relieve the discomfort.

blackhead

Also called a comedo, a semi-solid, black-capped plug of keratin and sebum that blocks the outlet of a sebaceous (oil-forming) gland in the skin. Blackheads occur most commonly on the face, chest, shoulders, and back.

They are associated with increased sebaceous gland activity and are one of the features of most types of *acne*.

blackout

A common term for loss of consciousness (see *fainting*).

black teeth

See *discoloured teeth*.

blackwater fever

An occasional, life-threatening complication of falciparum *malaria* (the most dangerous form of malaria). Symptoms include loss of consciousness, fever, vomiting, and very dark urine (due to pigment from destroyed *red blood cells* being filtered into the urine).

bladder

The hollow, muscular organ situated in the lower abdomen that acts as a reservoir for *urine*. The bladder lies within,

---

ANATOMY OF THE **BLADDER**

The bladder is a hollow organ that holds urine. It is situated behind the pubic bone and is protected by the pelvis. The ureters carry urine to the bladder from the kidneys. When the sphincter at the lowest part of the bladder is relaxed, urine is passed into the urethra and out of the body.

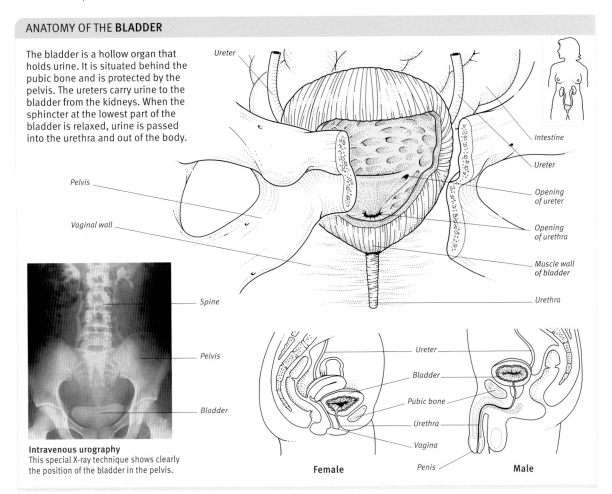

Intravenous urography
This special X-ray technique shows clearly the position of the bladder in the pelvis.

and is protected by, the *pelvis*. The average adult bladder can hold about 0.5 litres of urine before the need to pass urine is felt.

The bladder walls consist of muscle and an inner lining. Two tubes called *ureters* carry urine to the bladder from the kidneys. At the lowest point of the bladder is the opening into the *urethra* (outflow tube), known as the bladder neck. This is normally kept closed by a ring of muscle (the urethral sphincter).

FUNCTION

The bladder's function is to collect and store urine until it can be expelled from the body. Full control over bladder function takes several years to develop. In infants, emptying of the bladder is an entirely automatic, or *reflex*, reaction. When the bladder fills with urine and is stretched beyond a certain point, nerve signals are sent to the spinal cord. Signals from the spinal cord then cause the urethral sphincter to relax and the principal bladder muscle to contract, thereby expelling urine via the urethra.

Children develop complete bladder control at varying ages. Most are dry at night by the age of five years, but some take longer (see *enuresis, nocturnal*).

Defective bladder function, leading to problems such as incontinence (see *incontinence, urinary*) and *urinary retention*, can have a variety of causes. (See also *bladder disorders* box.)

bladder cancer

See *bladder tumours*.

bladder outflow obstruction

See *prostate, enlarged*; *urinary retention*.

bladder tumours

Growths originating in the inner lining of the bladder. *Papillomas* (small wart-like growths) often recur and eventually become cancerous. Other, more malignant, growths may extend not only into the bladder cavity, but also through the bladder wall to involve nearby organs, such as the colon, rectum, prostate gland, or uterus. Bladder cancer is more common in smokers and workers in the dye and rubber industries.

SYMPTOMS

Haematuria (blood in the urine) is the main symptom of bladder cancer. A tumour may obstruct the point at which a ureter enters the bladder, causing back pressure and pain in the kidney region, or the urethral exit, causing difficulty in passing, or retaining, urine.

DIAGNOSIS AND TREATMENT

Bladder tumours are diagnosed with urine tests to check for cancer cells, *cystoscopy* (passage of a viewing tube up the urethra into the bladder) and biopsy (tissue sampling for microscopic analysis) of the abnormal area.

If they are small, the tumours can be treated by heat or removed surgically during cystoscopy; in such cases, chemotherapeutic drugs may also be inserted into the bladder. Tumours tend to recur within the bladder, so regular follow-up cystoscopy and urine testing is usually

---

DISORDERS OF THE **BLADDER**

The most important causes of bladder problems are infection, tumours, calculi (stones), and impairment of the bladder's nerve supply.

Infection

Bacterial infection of the bladder, which causes inflammation of the bladder wall (see *cystitis*), is particularly common in women. The short female urethra makes it relatively easy for bacteria to enter from outside the body. In men, infection is usually associated with obstruction of urine flow from the bladder by, for example an enlarged prostate gland (see *prostate, enlarged*) or bladder tumours.

Tumours

Bladder tumours may be cancerous or noncancerous and are more common in men than in women. They are usually painless in the early stages, the first symptoms being blood in the urine (see *haematuria*) or *urinary retention*, in which the bladder cannot be emptied. All bladder tumours need careful follow-up because, left untreated, noncancerous bladder tumours may become cancerous.

Calculi

Bladder stones (see *calculus, urinary tract*) are mostly caused by the crystallization of substances, such as calcium, in the urine. They mainly affect men and usually result from a longstanding urinary tract infection and/or incomplete emptying of the bladder.

Nerve impairment

Damage to the nerves controlling the bladder can prevent normal bladder function and lead either to incontinence (see *incontinence, urinary*) or to urinary

retention. The most common cause is spinal cord injury or tumours. Bladder control can be affected by degeneration of nerves in conditions such as *diabetes mellitus*, *multiple sclerosis*, or *dementia*.

Other disorders

An unstable or *irritable bladder* is a common condition, particularly in women, in whom the bladder wall is especially sensitive to being stretched. Weakness of the muscles at the bladder neck, causing *stress incontinence*, is also common in women, particularly after childbirth. Tension or anxiety can cause frequent urination.

In children, delayed bladder control (see *enuresis, nocturnal*) is most often due to delayed maturation of the nervous system. Injury to the bladder is rare but may occur if the pelvis is fractured when the bladder is full.

INVESTIGATION

Various methods are used to investigate bladder disorders. Urinary tract infection is diagnosed by tests on a sample of urine. The bladder can be viewed directly by *cystoscopy* (insertion of a viewing tube). *Ultrasound scanning* is often performed, particularly if stones are suspected. X-ray procedures include voiding *cystourethrography*, which normally shows only the bladder and urethra, and intravenous *urography*, which shows the whole urinary tract except the urethra. *Urodynamics*, which may involve X-rays, are studies carried out to investigate bladder control problems. *Cystometry* measures bladder capacity in relation to pressure.

---

necessary. Bladder tumours that have spread through the bladder wall may be treated by *radiotherapy* or by the removal of part or all of the bladder.

Blalock shunt

A surgical procedure in which a connection is made between one of the two subclavian arteries (which normally deliver oxygen-rich blood to the neck and arms) and one of the pulmonary arteries (which carry blood from the right side of the heart to the lungs for oxygenation). The shunt may be used as a temporary treatment for congenital heart disorders, such as *tetralogy of Fallot*, in which oxygen-depleted blood is diverted back to the heart before it reaches the lungs. The shunt redirects the oxygen-depleted blood to the lungs. The improved blood oxygen levels allow the child to survive and grow until corrective surgery is possible.

bland diet

An easily digested diet that is free from possible irritants to the digestive tract, such as spicy foods and raw vegetable fibre. A bland diet is often advised following abdominal surgery or for people with gastrointestinal disorders.

blast cell

An immature *cell* that later develops into a specialized cell. For example, *white blood cells* begin as blast cells in the bone marrow and eventually form different types of mature white blood cells that are then released into the bloodstream. The presence of certain blast cells may indicate illness. For example, blast cells are found in the blood in acute leukaemia (see *leukaemia, acute*). (See also *stem cell*.)

blast injury

Tissue damage due to the effects of blast waves generated by an explosion. The eardrums and digestive tract are particularly at risk; the air within the ear and hollow parts of the gut transmits the waves in all directions, often resulting in severe damage.

blastocyst

A cell cluster that develops from a fertilized *ovum* and grows into an *embryo* (see *fertilization*).

blastomycosis

A type of *fungal infection* that can affect the lungs and other internal organs.

bleaching, dental

A cosmetic procedure for lightening certain types of *discoloured teeth*, including nonvital "dead" teeth. It involves painting oxidizing agents on to the surface of the teeth. Laser or ultraviolet light may also be shone on to the painted teeth to speed up the lightening process. Repeat treatments are usually necessary to achieve significant tooth lightening.

bleb

Another term for a *blister*.

bleeding

Loss of blood from the *circulatory system*, which may be caused by damage to the blood vessels or by a *bleeding disorder*. Bleeding may be visible (external) or concealed (internal). Rapid loss of more than 10 per cent of the blood volume can cause symptoms of *shock*, with fainting, pallor, and sweating.

The speed with which blood flows from a cut depends on the type of vessel damaged: blood usually oozes from a capillary, flows from a vein, and spurts from an artery. If an injury does not break open the skin, the blood collects around the damaged blood vessels just beneath the skin and forms a *bruise*.

Any lost blood that mixes with other body fluids such as sputum (phlegm) or urine will usually be noticed quite readily; bleeding from the lining of the digestive tract may make vomit or faeces appear darker than usual. Internal bleeding may not be discovered until severe *anaemia* develops.

bleeding disorders

A group of conditions characterized by bleeding in the absence of injury or by abnormally prolonged and excessive bleeding following injury. Bleeding disorders are the result of defects in the mechanisms by which bleeding is normally stopped: the coagulation of blood, the plugging of damaged blood vessels by platelets (the smallest type of blood cell), and the constriction of blood vessels (see *blood clotting*).

Defects in the coagulation system tend to cause deep bleeding into the gastrointestinal tract, muscles, and joint cavities. Defects of the platelets or blood vessels usually cause superficial bleeding into the skin, the gums, or the lining of the intestine or the urinary tract.

COAGULATION DEFECTS

These disorders are usually due to a deficiency of or abnormality in the *enzymes* (coagulation factors) that are involved in blood clotting. Clot formation is very slow and the clots are weak and do not seal blood vessels securely. Coagulation defects may be *congenital* (present at birth) or may be acquired later in life.

Congenital The main congenital coagulation defects are *haemophilia*, *Christmas disease*, and *von Willebrand's disease*. In all of these, one coagulation factor is either absent from the blood or present only in small amounts. Haemophilia and Christmas disease are similar disorders, resulting from deficiencies of two different coagulation factors: factor VIII and factor IX respectively. Inheritance of these disorders is sex-linked (see *genetic disorders*) and normally only males are affected. Von Willebrand's disease is an inherited disorder in which there is a platelet and a factor VIII defect; it affects both sexes about equally.

Individuals with one of these disorders may suffer from bruising, internal bleeding, abnormally heavy menstrual periods, and excessive bleeding from wounds. In severe cases, there may be recurrent bleeding into joints, such as the knee.

Acquired Acquired defects of blood coagulation factors may develop at any age due to severe liver disease, digestive system disorders that prevent the absorption of *vitamin K* (which is needed to make certain coagulation factors), or the use of *anticoagulant drugs*.

Disseminated intravascular coagulation (DIC) is an acquired disorder that is complex and serious. It may be the result of an underlying infection or of a cancerous tumour. In this condition, platelets accumulate and clots develop within small blood vessels; coagulation factors are used up faster than they are able to be replaced, and severe bleeding may result.

Tests and treatment Coagulation disorders are investigated by *blood-clotting tests*. If such a disorder is severe, it is treated by replacing the missing factor. Factors are extracted from fresh blood or from fresh frozen plasma, or genetically engineered factors may be used. Paradoxically, anticoagulants are sometimes used to suppress excess clotting activity in DIC, which results in a reduction in bleeding.

PLATELET DEFECTS

Bleeding may occur if there are too few platelets in the blood, a condition called *thrombocytopenia*. The main feature of this disorder is surface bleeding into the skin and gums, and there are multiple small bruises.

Occasionally, the platelets are present in normal numbers but function abnormally, causing bleeding. Platelet defects may be inherited, they may be associated with the use of certain drugs (including *aspirin*), or arise as a complication of certain bone marrow disorders such as *leukaemia*. Platelets can be destroyed by *autoimmune disorders* that may have been triggered by an infection or by drug treatment.

Platelet defects are investigated by blood tests. Bleeding due to a lack of platelets may be treated with intravenous platelet transfusions. In some cases, oral *corticosteroid drugs* are prescribed.

BLOOD VESSEL DEFECTS

In rare cases, abnormal bleeding is the result of a blood-vessel defect or *scurvy* (a disorder that is caused by a deficiency of *vitamin C*). Elderly people and patients on long-term courses of *corticosteroid drugs* may suffer mild abnormal bruising due to loss of skin support to the smallest blood vessels. Treatment is rarely required in these cases.

bleeding gums

See *gingivitis*.

bleeding, occult

Bleeding that is not obvious to the naked eye (such as that which occurs within the intestine) and that may be detected only by tests. (See also *occult blood, faecal*).

bleeding time

An assessment of the functioning of platelets (the tiny cell fragments within the blood that play a vital role in *blood clotting*) by measuring the speed at which they form plugs to stem bleeding from damaged blood vessels. Two small cuts are made in the forearm and the time taken for the bleeding from these cuts to stop is recorded.

blepharitis

Inflammation of the eyelids, with redness, irritation, and scaly skin at the lid margins. Blepharitis may cause burning and discomfort in the eyes and flakes or crusts on the lashes. The condition is common, tends to recur, and is sometimes associated with dandruff of the scalp or *eczema*. Severe blepharitis may lead to *corneal ulcers*. In many cases, treatment of associated dandruff with an antifungal shampoo will result in improvement of the blepharitis.

blepharoplasty

A cosmetic operation to remove drooping, wrinkled skin from the upper and/or lower eyelids. Blepharoplasty is usually performed under local anaesthetic (see *anaesthesia, local*).

blepharospasm

Prolonged, involuntary contraction of one of the muscles controlling the eyelids, causing them to close. It may be

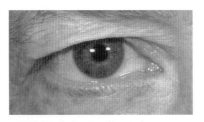

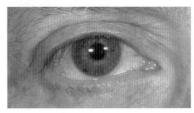

Appearance before (top) and after (bottom)
Blepharoplasty involves the removal of a crescent-shaped section of skin and underlying fat from each eyelid.

due to *photophobia* (abnormal sensitivity of the eyes to light), to damage to the *cornea* (the transparent dome that forms the front part of the eyeball), or to *dystonia* (abnormal muscle rigidity), for which *botulinum toxin* (a muscle relaxant) treatment is highly effective.

blind loop syndrome

A condition in which a redundant area or dead end (blind loop) in the small intestine becomes colonized with bacteria. The bacteria break down bile salts, which are necessary for the absorption of fat and certain vitamins. This results in poor absorption of fats and abnormal faeces. Blind loop syndrome may result from surgery or a *stricture* (narrowing) in the intestine as a result of a disorder such as *Crohn's disease*. It is characterized by *steatorrhoea* (pale yellow, foul-smelling, fatty, bulky faeces that are difficult to flush away), tiredness, and weight loss. *Antibiotic drug* treatment is usually effective, but the condition may recur if the underlying abnormality cannot be corrected.

blindness

Inability to see. Definitions of blindness and partial sight vary. In the UK, blindness is defined as a corrected *visual acuity* of 3/60 or less, or a *visual field* of no more than 20 degrees, in the better eye.

CAUSES

Loss of vision may result from injury to, or disease or degeneration of, the eyeball; the optic nerve or the nerve pathways that connect the eye to the brain; or the brain itself.

Eyeball Normal vision depends on an uninterrupted passage of light from the front of the eye to the light-sensitive retina at the back. Anything that prevents light from reaching the retina can cause blindness.

Various disorders can lead to the clouding of the cornea at the front of the eye. These disorders include *Sjögren's syndrome* (in which the eyes become excessively dry), *vitamin A* deficiency, chemical damage, infections, and injury. *Corneal ulcers*, which most commonly develop after severe infections, can cause blindness due to scarring of the cornea. *Uveitis* (inflammation of the iris, ciliary body, or choroid) can also cause loss of vision.

Cataract (cloudiness of the lens) is another common cause of blindness. It is usually the result of the lens becoming less transparent in old age, but is occasionally present from birth or develops in childhood.

Diabetes mellitus, *hypertension* (high blood pressure), or injury can all cause bleeding into the cavity of the eyeball and a subsequent loss of vision. Bleeding into the fluid in front of the lens (see *hyphaema*) or behind the lens (see *vitreous haemorrhage*) can also result in loss of vision.

Disorders of the retina that may result in blindness include age-related *macular degeneration* (degeneration of the central area of the retina, which occurs in old age); *retinopathy* due to diabetes or to hypertension; *retinal artery occlusion* or *retinal vein occlusion* (blockage of the blood flow to and from the retina); *retinal detachment*; certain types of tumour, such as *retinoblastoma* and malignant melanoma affecting the eye (see *melanoma, malignant*); and *retinal haemorrhage* (bleeding into the retina), caused by diabetes, hypertension, vascular disease, or injury.

In *glaucoma*, excessive fluid pressure within the eyeball causes degeneration of nerve fibres at the front end of the optic nerve.

Nerve pathways The light energy that is received by the retina is transformed into nerve impulses that travel along the optic nerve and nerve pathways into the brain. Loss of vision may result if the conduction of these nerve impulses is impaired.

Reasons for damage to nerve pathways include pressure caused by a tumour in the orbit (the bony cavity that contains the eyeball); a reduced blood supply to the optic nerve, which may be caused by diabetes mellitus, hypertension, a tumour, injury, or *temporal arteritis* (inflammation of arteries in the scalp); *optic neuritis* (inflammation of the optic nerve that may occur in *multiple sclerosis*); the toxic (poisonous) effects of certain chemicals; and certain nutritional deficiencies.

Brain Nerve impulses from the retina eventually arrive in a region of the *cerebrum* (the main mass of the brain) called the visual cortex. Blindness can result if there is pressure on the visual cortex from a *brain tumour* or a *brain haemorrhage*, or if the blood supply to the visual cortex has been reduced following a *stroke*.

DIAGNOSIS AND TREATMENT

It is frequently possible to detect the cause of blindness by direct examination of the eye, using such techniques as *ophthalmoscopy*, *slit-lamp examination*, and *tonometry*. The conduction of nerve impulses can be measured by means of *evoked responses*.

Treatment of blindness depends on the underlying cause. If the loss of vision cannot be corrected, the patient may then be registered as legally blind or partially sighted, and will become eligible for certain benefits and services. (See also *eye*; *vision, loss of*.)

blind spot

The small, oval-shaped area on the retina of the eye where the optic nerve leaves the eyeball. The area is not sensitive to light because it has no light

LOCATION OF **BLIND SPOT**

The blind spot is a minute area on the retina that lacks light receptors and is therefore not light-sensitive.

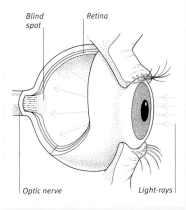

Blind spot | Retina

Optic nerve | Light-rays

receptors (nerve endings responsive to light). The blind spot can also be used to describe the part of the *visual field* in which objects cannot be detected.

blister

A collection of fluid beneath the outer layer of the skin that forms a raised area. The fluid is serum that has leaked from blood vessels in underlying skin layers after minor damage; it provides protection for the damaged tissue.

Common causes of blisters are *burns* and friction. Blisters may also occur in some skin diseases, including *eczema*, *epidermolysis bullosa*, *impetigo*, *erythema multiforme*, *pemphigus*, *pemphigoid*, and *dermatitis herpetiformis*, and in some types of *porphyria*. Small blisters develop in *chickenpox*, *herpes zoster* (shingles), and *herpes simplex*. Blisters are generally best left intact; large or unexplained blisters need medical attention.

bloating

Distension of the abdomen, commonly due to wind in the stomach or intestine (see *abdominal swelling*).

blocked nose

See *nasal congestion*; *nasal obstruction*.

blocking

The inability to express true feelings or thoughts, usually due to emotional or mental conflict. In Freudian-based *psychotherapy*, blocking is thought to result from the repression of painful emotions in early life. A very specific form of thought blocking occurs in *schizophrenia*: trains of thought are persistently interrupted involuntarily to be replaced by unrelated new ones.

blood

The red fluid that circulates in the body's veins, arteries, and capillaries. Blood is pumped by the heart via the arteries to the lungs and all other tissues and is then returned to the heart in veins (see *circulatory system*). Blood is the body's transport system and also plays an important role in the defence against infection. An average adult has about 5 litres of blood.

Almost half the blood's volume consists of *blood cells*, including red blood cells (erythrocytes), which carry oxygen to the tissues; white blood cells (leukocytes), which defend the body against infection; and platelets (thrombocytes), which are involved in *blood clotting*. The

rest of the blood volume is made up of plasma, a watery, straw-coloured fluid containing proteins, sugars, fats, salts, and minerals.

Nutrients are transported in the bloodstream to the tissues after absorption from the intestinal tract or after release from storage depots such as the liver. Waste products, including *urea* and *bilirubin*, are carried in the plasma to the kidneys and liver respectively.

Plasma proteins include fibrinogen, which is involved in blood clotting; *immunoglobulins* (also called antibodies) and *complement*, which are part of the *immune system*; and *albumin*. Hormones are also transported in the blood to their target organs.

blood–brain barrier

A system of tight, impermeable junctions between the cells that form the walls of the capillaries (tiny blood vessels) within the *central nervous system*. The blood–brain barrier has a protective function; it allows only certain substances and drugs in the bloodstream to gain access to the central nervous system, especially to the brain.

blood cells

Cells, also called blood corpuscles, that are present in blood for most or part of their lifespan. They include red blood cells (which make up about 45 per cent of the volume of normal blood), white blood cells, and platelets. All blood cells are made in the bone marrow by a series of divisions from a single type of cell called a *stem cell*.

RED BLOOD CELLS

These cells are also known as RBCs, red blood corpuscles, or erythrocytes. They transport oxygen from the lungs to the tissues (see *respiration*).

Formation Red blood cells are formed from stem cells in the bone marrow by a process called erythropoiesis, which takes about five days. Their formation requires an adequate supply of nutrients, including iron, amino acids, and the vitamins B_{12} and folic acid. The rate at which RBCs are formed is influenced by a hormone called erythropoietin, which is produced by the kidneys.

Immature red blood cells that have just been released into the bloodstream from the bone marrow are called reticulocytes; within two to four days, these develop into mature cells.

Structure and function In 1 cubic mm of blood there are approximately 5 million

CONSTITUENTS OF **BLOOD**

Blood is pumped around the body in veins and arteries, transporting oxygen from the lungs to the tissues and carbon dioxide from the tissues to the lungs. Blood also carries nutrients such as sugars, fats, and proteins that have been absorbed from the intestine and hormones produced by a variety of glands. Waste products that are released from cells are carried in the blood to be broken down in the liver or excreted from the kidneys.

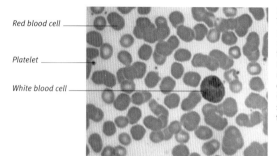

Red blood cell

Platelet

White blood cell

Normal blood smear
This is the appearance of normal blood under a microscope. The dominant feature is the abundance of red blood cells, which make up almost half of the volume of blood. One white blood cell (a lymphocyte) can be clearly seen; the platelets are the tiny dark particles.

White blood cells
These cells protect the body against infection and fight it when it occurs. They are bigger than red blood cells but fewer in number. Each of the three main types (granulocytes, monocytes, and lymphocytes) plays a different role in dealing with infection.

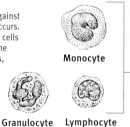

Monocyte

Granulocyte   **Lymphocyte**

Plasma

Plasma
The fluid part of the blood that consists mostly of water. It carries substances such as proteins, fats, glucose, and salts.

Red blood cells

Red blood cells
These disc-shaped cells are formed in the bone marrow and carry oxygen from the lungs to the rest of the body. They have a large surface area and a flexible shape.

Platelets
The smallest type of blood cell produced in the bone marrow. They play an important role in blood clotting.

Platelets

Layer containing white blood cells and platelets

Red blood cells

---

red blood cells, each of which is disc-shaped, about 0.0075 mm in diameter, and thicker around the edge than at the centre. This shape gives each cell a relatively large surface area, which helps it absorb and release oxygen molecules, and allows it to distort as it squeezes through narrow blood vessels. The surface structure of red blood cells varies slightly among individuals, and this provides the basis for classifying blood into groups (see *blood groups*).

RBCs are packed with large quantities of *haemoglobin*, a pigmented protein that contains iron. Haemoglobin binds (combines chemically) with oxygen to form oxyhaemoglobin, which carries oxygen to body tissues. Oxyhaemoglobin is responsible for the bright red coloration of oxygenated blood, which flows mainly through the arteries. Most venous blood is darker because it contains the unbound (deoxygenated) form of haemoglobin.

Every RBC also contains *enzymes* (substances that promote biochemical reactions), minerals, and sugars that provide energy for the cell's *metabolism* (chemical processes) and maintain its shape, structure, and elasticity.

Aging and destruction The normal lifespan of RBCs in the circulation is about 120 days. As they age, their internal chemical machinery wears out, they lose elasticity, and they become trapped in small blood vessels in the spleen and other organs; they are then destroyed by a type of white blood cell called a macrophage. Most of the components of haemoglobin molecules are reused, but some are broken down to form the waste product *bilirubin*.

Disorders Abnormalities can occur in the rate at which RBCs are produced or destroyed; in their numbers; and in their shape, size, and haemoglobin content, all of which may cause forms of *anaemia* and *polycythaemia* (see *blood disorders box*).

WHITE BLOOD CELLS

These are also called WBCs, white blood corpuscles, or leukocytes. They help to protect the body against infection and fight infection when it occurs. White blood cells are bigger than red blood cells (up to 0.015 mm in diameter) but are far less numerous (about 7,500 per cubic mm of blood). They generally spend a shorter part of their lifespan than red blood cells in the blood itself. The three main types of WBC are granulocytes (also called polymorphonuclear leukocytes), monocytes, and *lymphocytes*.

Granulocytes Granulocytes are further classified as neutrophils, eosinophils, or basophils, each type having a specific role. The most important are neutrophils, which isolate and destroy invading bacteria. Neutrophils remain in the blood for only about six to nine hours before moving through blood-vessel walls into tissues. Eosinophils play a part in allergic reactions and increase in numbers in response to certain parasitic infections. Basophils are involved in inflammatory and allergic reactions.

Monocytes These cells also play an important role in the *immune system*.

DISORDERS OF THE **BLOOD**

Abnormalities can occur in any of the components of blood: in red blood cells, white blood cells, platelets, and the numerous constituents of plasma.

There are various types of *anaemia* (a reduced level of the oxygen-carrying pigment haemoglobin in the blood), which is by far the most common blood disorder. Some abnormalities of the blood are inherited; others may be the result of various diseases, such as cancer, or be caused by poisoning by infective organisms, toxins, or drugs.

Genetic disorders

Some blood disorders are inherited (genetic) and are present from birth (congenital). Such disorders include *sickle cell anaemia* and *thalassaemia*, in which the red blood cells are abnormally fragile, and *haemophilia*, in which there is a deficiency of one of the blood clotting factors.

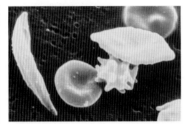

Sickle-cell anaemia
This electron micrograph shows a red blood cell deformed by sickle-cell anaemia (left). On the right is another red cell that has started to sickle.

Nutritional disorders

Heavy or persistent blood loss, most commonly as a result of menstruation, may mean that iron (an essential component of the red cell pigment haemoglobin) is lost faster than it can be replaced in the diet (see *anaemia, iron-deficiency*). Deficiencies of the vitamins B_{12} or folic acid interfere with the production of red blood cells in bone marrow and give rise to abnormally large, deformed red blood cells (see *blood; anaemia, megaloblastic*).

Cancer

There are various types of bone marrow cancer, all of which affect the blood. *Leukaemia* causes an overgrowth of abnormal white blood cells and destroys healthy bone marrow. In *polycythaemia*, too many red blood cells are produced. Another bone marrow cancer, *multiple myeloma*, can cause an excess of certain proteins in the blood plasma. Secondary deposits that have spread from cancers elsewhere in the body may also involve the bone marrow.

Clotting disorders

Defects in the blood platelets and in blood clotting mechanisms may lead to *bleeding disorders*, such as haemophilia and *disseminated intravascular coagulation (DIC)*. Liver disease may cause deficiencies of some clotting factors. Unwanted clot formation (see *thrombosis*) may have any of a variety of causes, such as a mutation

in the gene that controls production of a clotting factor (see *factor V*, for example) or use of oral contraceptives. People with *Hughes' syndrome* are also at increased risk of thrombosis.

Other disorders

Blood poisoning may be caused by the multiplication of bacteria in the blood (see *septicaemia*) or by toxins released by bacteria (see *toxaemia*). Poisoning can also be caused by toxins such as carbon monoxide and lead.

Some drugs can cause blood abnormalities. For example, thiazide *diuretic drugs* may depress production of white blood cells and/or platelets; *methotrexate* may interfere with red cell production; and too high a dose of *anticoagulant drugs* can cause abnormal bleeding.

Albumin, which is an important protein in blood plasma, may become deficient as a result of either liver or kidney disease.

INVESTIGATION

Blood disorders are investigated principally by various blood tests, such as *blood count*, *blood film*, and *blood-clotting tests*. Levels of vitamins and minerals, such as iron, may also be measured. In some cases, a bone marrow *biopsy* may also be required.

They circulate in the bloodstream for about one to three days.
Lymphocytes Lymphocytes are usually formed in the lymph nodes, rather than in the bone marrow. They play an important role in the immune system, roving throughout the body between the bloodstream, the lymph nodes, and the channels between lymph nodes. Lymphocyte cells may survive for anywhere between three months and ten years.

There are two principal types of lymphocyte: T-lymphocytes (also known as T-cells) and B-lymphocytes (also called B-cells). T-lymphocytes are responsible for delayed hypersensitivity reactions (see *allergy*) and are also involved in protection against cancer. T-lymphocytes manufacture chemicals (called lymphokines) that affect the functioning of

other cells. T-lymphocytes can be classified according to their surface marker proteins. For example, T-lymphocytes with CD4 surface marker proteins are particularly important in monitoring HIV infection. In addition, T-lymphocytes moderate the activity of B-lymphocytes, which form the antibodies that can act to prevent a second attack of certain infectious diseases.
Disorders The *leukaemias* are *blood disorders* in which there is uncontrolled overproduction of white blood cells in the bone marrow. Other disorders arise when white blood cells are not produced in sufficient numbers.

PLATELETS

Platelets, which are also called thrombocytes, are the smallest type of blood cell (0.002 mm to 0.003 mm in diameter).

There are about 300,000 of them per cubic mm of blood. Like other blood cells, they originate in the bone marrow. Platelets survive in the blood for about nine days.
Function Platelets circulate in the blood in an inactive state until brought into action by certain circumstances, when they begin to stick to blood-vessel walls and to each other. These activities play an important part in *blood clotting*, which helps wounds to heal. However, the accumulation of platelets can, occasionally, lead to the formation of clots in blood vessels (see *thrombosis*).

BLOOD CELLS IN DIAGNOSIS

The numbers, shapes, and appearance of the various types of blood cell are of great value in the diagnosis of disease (see *blood count*; *blood film*).

HOW **BLOOD** CLOTS

Clotting describes the solidification of blood anywhere in the body. Clotting occurs almost immediately at the site of a cut and helps to limit blood loss by sealing damaged blood vessels. However, if abnormal clotting occurs in major blood vessels, a heart attack, stroke, or other disorder may occur. The clotting process has two main parts – platelet activation and the formation of fibrin filaments.

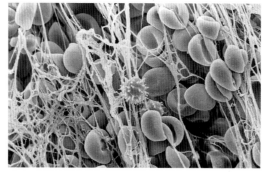

Red blood cells enmeshed in fibrin filaments
Fibrin is formed by a chemical change from a soluble protein, fibrinogen, which is present in the blood. The fibrin molecules aggregate to form long filaments, which enmesh blood cells (see left) to form a solid clot. The conversion of fibrinogen to fibrin is the last step of the "coagulation cascade", a series of reactions in the blood that are triggered by injury to the tissues and activation of platelets.

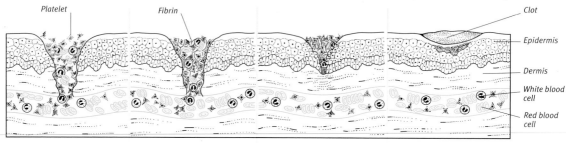

Platelet *Fibrin* *Clot* *Epidermis* *Dermis* *White blood cell* *Red blood cell*

1 Platelets are activated by coming into contact with damaged blood vessel walls, where they become sticky and then clump at the site of injury and adhere to the damaged blood-vessel wall.

2 Chemicals released by the platelets and damaged tissues stimulate coagulation factors within the blood to form filaments of fibrin at the site of injury.

3 The fibrin filaments enmesh the platelets along with red and white blood cells.

4 Once the cut blood vessel is plugged by the mass of fibrin, platelets, and red and white blood cells, the fibrin filaments contract to form a solid clot.

blood clot

See *thrombus*.

blood clotting

The process of blood solidification. Blood clotting is important in stemming bleeding from damaged blood vessels. However, blood clots can also form inside major blood vessels, leading to a *myocardial infarction* (heart attack) or to a *stroke* (see *thrombosis*).

CLOTTING MECHANISM

When a blood vessel is damaged, it constricts immediately to reduce blood flow to the area. The damage sets off a series of chemical reactions, leading to the formation of a clot to seal the injury. First, platelets around the injury site are activated, becoming sticky and adhering to the blood-vessel wall. The activated platelets then release chemicals that, in turn, activate coagulation factors. These factors, together with *vitamin K*, act on fibrinogen, a substance found in blood, converting it to fibrin. Strands of fibrin form a kind of meshwork, which traps red blood cells to form a clot.

ANTICLOTTING MECHANISMS

There are several anticlotting mechanisms that prevent the formation of unwanted blood clots. These mechanisms include prostacyclin (a *prostaglandin*), which prevents platelet aggregation (the first stage of blood clotting), and plasmin, which breaks down fibrin (see *fibrinolysis*). Blood flow washes away active coagulation factors; and the liver deactivates excess coagulation factors.

CLOTTING DEFECTS

Defects in blood clotting may result in *bleeding disorders*. Excessive clotting, or thrombosis, may be due to an inherited increase or defect in a coagulation factor (see *factor V*); the use of oral contraceptives; a decrease in the level of enzymes that inhibit coagulation; or sluggish blood flow through a particular area. Treatment is usually with *anticoagulant drugs* such as heparin or warfarin.

blood-clotting tests

Laboratory tests used to screen for and diagnose *bleeding disorders*. Such disorders usually result from deficiencies or abnormalities of blood coagulation factors or of platelets (see *blood clotting*). The tests are also used to monitor treatment with *anticoagulant drugs*; excessive doses of these drugs could cause bleeding. (See also *international normalized ratio*.)

blood count

A test, also called full blood count, that measures the *haemoglobin* concentration and the numbers of red blood cells, white blood cells, and platelets in 1 cubic mm of blood. The proportion of various white blood cells is measured and the size and shape of the red and white cells is also noted.

A blood count is the most commonly performed blood test and is important for diagnosing *anaemia* or confirming the presence of an infection to which cells in the blood have responded. It is also used to diagnose disorders such as *leukaemia* and *thrombocytopenia* (abnormally low platelet levels).

About 1 to 2 ml of blood is required for a blood count, which is usually performed by an automatic analyser.

blood culture

A laboratory test performed on a sample of *blood* to determine the presence of microorganisms such as bacteria. (See also *culture*.)

blood donation

The process of giving blood for use in *blood transfusion*. Blood donors give up to 500 ml of blood (about one-tenth of total blood volume), usually about twice a year. Donated blood is routinely tested for a range of infectious agents, such as *hepatitis B* and *hepatitis C*, and antibodies to *HIV*. After being classified into *blood groups*, the blood is stored in a blood bank, either whole or separated into its components (see *blood products*).

Apheresis is a specific type of blood donation in which only a particular component of blood (such as plasma, platelets, or white blood cells) is withdrawn from the donor.

blood film

A test that involves smearing a drop of blood on to a glass slide for examination under a microscope. The blood film is stained with dyes to make the blood cells show up clearly.

The test allows the shape and appearance of blood cells to be checked for any abnormality, for example the sickle-shaped red blood cells characteristic of *sickle cell anaemia*. The relative proportions of the different types of white blood cells can also be counted. This examination, known as a differential white cell count, may be helpful in diagnosing infection or *leukaemia*. Blood films are also used in diagnosing infections in which the parasites can be seen inside the red blood cells; an example of such an infection is *malaria*.

Blood film tests are usually carried out together with a full *blood count*.

blood gases

Measurement of the concentrations of oxygen and carbon dioxide in the blood. The acidity–alkalinity (pH) and bicarbonate levels are also measured. The test is carried out on a sample of blood that has been taken from an artery, usually at the wrist or the groin. It is useful in diagnosing and monitoring *respiratory failure*. Bicarbonate and acidity reflect the *acid–base balance* of the body, which may be disturbed in conditions such as diabetic ketoacidosis, aspirin poisoning, *hyperventilation* (overbreathing), or repeated vomiting.

Blood oxygen can also be monitored continuously without the need to take blood samples by using an *oximeter*.

blood glucose

The level of *glucose* in the blood. Abnormally high blood glucose (sometimes called blood sugar) levels may be an indication of *diabetes mellitus*. (See also *hyperglycaemia*; *hypoglycaemia*.)

blood glucose monitoring

A method of analysing a person's blood *glucose* (sugar) levels that requires only a drop of blood taken from a pinprick on the fingertip. The blood is applied to a test strip, which has an area impregnated with a chemical that reacts with the glucose in the blood sample. The glucose level is shown either by a visible colour change on the strip or by placing the strip in a digital meter. People with *diabetes mellitus* must perform regular blood glucose monitoring tests to monitor their blood glucose control. (See also *hyperglycaemia*; *hypoglycaemia*.)

blood groups

Systems of classifying blood according to the different *antigens* (marker proteins) on the surface of *red blood cells* (RBCs) and the *antibodies* in the blood plasma. The antigens affect the ability of the RBCs to provoke an *immune response*. The two principal blood grouping systems used are the ABO system and the rhesus system.

ABO GROUPS

In this system, the presence or absence of two types of antigen (A and B) on the

surface of the red blood cells determines a person's blood group. People with the A antigen (blood group A) have anti-B antibodies; people with the B antigen (blood group B) have anti-A antibodies; those with both antigens (blood group AB) have neither type of antibody; and those with neither antigen (blood group O) have both types of antibody.

RHESUS FACTORS

The rhesus system involves several antigens, the most important of which is called factor D. People with this factor are Rh-positive; those without it are Rh-negative. The importance of the Rh group relates mainly to pregnancy in Rh-negative women because, if the baby is Rh-positive, the mother may form antibodies against the baby's blood (see *rhesus incompatibility*).

USES

Blood group typing is essential for safe *blood transfusion*. The ABO and rhesus groups are used to categorize blood stored in blood banks, so that donor blood that is compatible with that of the patient can be selected before transfusion takes place.

Because a person's blood group is inherited, identification of blood group may be used in paternity testing. Genetic analysis allows identification of the blood of a person with virtual certainty (see *genetic fingerprinting*).

blood level

The concentration of a given substance in the blood plasma or serum that may be measured by *blood tests*.

blood loss

See *bleeding*.

blood poisoning

A common name for *septicaemia* with *toxaemia*, a life-threatening illness that is caused by multiplication of bacteria and formation of toxins in the bloodstream. Septicaemia may occur as a complication of an infection in an organ or tissue. In some infective conditions, *septic shock* may be caused by toxins that are released by bacteria. Treatment for blood poisoning is with *antibiotic drugs* and intensive therapy for shock. (See also *bacteraemia*.)

blood pressure

The pressure exerted by the flow of blood through the main arteries. The pressure at two different phases is measured. Systolic, the higher pressure, is

---

BLOOD GROUP COMPATIBILITY

Compatibilty depends on whether blood is being donated or received. For example, people with AB blood can donate only to other AB people but can receive blood from any group.

		Donor blood group			
		A	B	AB	O
Recipient blood group	A	○	●	●	○
	B	●	○	●	○
	AB	○	○	○	○
	O	●	●	●	○

Key	○ Compatible	● Incompatible

Blood pressure measurement is a routine part of a physical examination. A sphygmomanometer measures blood pressure as systolic, when the heart contracts, and diastolic, when it relaxes. An inflatable cuff attached to the sphygmomanometer is wrapped around the upper arm and inflated then deflated while a doctor listens to the blood flow through an artery using a stethoscope.

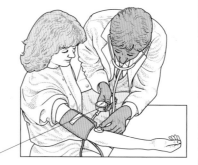

Sphygmomanometer

created by the contraction of the ventricles of the *heart*. Diastolic, the lower pressure, is recorded during relaxation of the ventricles between heartbeats; it reflects the resistance of all the small arteries in the body and the load against which the heart must work. The pressure wave that is transmitted along the arteries with each heartbeat is easily felt as the *pulse*.

Blood pressure is measured using a *sphygmomanometer* and is expressed as millimetres of mercury (mmHg). Blood pressure varies with age, between individuals, and at different times in the same individual. A healthy young adult usually has a blood pressure reading, at rest, of about 120/80 (120 mmHg systolic and 80 mmHg diastolic pressure). A sustained level of high blood pressure is called *hypertension*; abnormally low pressure is termed *hypotension*.

blood products

Donated blood (see *blood donation*) that is separated into its components: red cells, white cells, platelets, and plasma. Each blood product has a specific lifespan and use in *blood transfusion*. Leukodepleted red cells (blood with the plasma removed) are used to treat individuals with acute bleeding or some forms of chronic *anaemia* and babies with *haemolytic disease of the newborn*. Washed red cells (with white blood cells and/or plasma proteins removed) are used when a person requires repeated transfusions since there is less risk of an *allergy* to any of the blood components developing.

Platelets may be given through transfusions for people with blood-clotting disorders. Patients who have life-threatening infections may be treated with granulocytes, a type of white blood cell.

Fresh frozen plasma is used to correct many types of *bleeding disorder* because plasma contains all the clotting factors. Plasma substitutes may be used to treat *shock* due to severe blood loss, until sufficient compatible whole blood becomes available. Purified albumin preparations are used for people who have *nephrotic syndrome* and chronic liver disease.

Concentrates of blood clotting factors VIII and IX are used in the treatment of the conditions *haemophilia* and *Christmas disease*. *Immunoglobulins* (also called antibodies), which are extracted from blood plasma, can be given by injection (see *immunoglobulin injection*) to protect those people who are unable to produce their own antibodies or have already been exposed to an infectious agent. Immunoglobulins may also be given to provide short-term protection against *hepatitis A*. Immunoglobulins are given in large doses to treat certain *autoimmune disorders*.

blood smear

See *blood film*.

blood spot screening tests

A series of tests carried out in the first week of birth on a small sample of a baby's blood to check for several rare but potentially serious disorders. The blood sample is obtained by pricking the baby's heel and collecting the blood on a special card. The card is then tested for various disorders, including *phenylketonuria* (an inherited metabolic disorder), congenital *hypothyroidism* (underactivity of the thyroid gland), *sickle cell anaemia* (an inherited disorder of red blood cells), and, in some areas, *cystic fibrosis* (an inherited disorder that can affect the lungs and digestive system) and *MCADD* (an inherited metabolic disorder).

blood sugar

See *blood glucose*.

blood test, haematological

Analysis of a sample of blood to provide information about its cells and proteins and the chemicals, gases, antigens, and antibodies it contains. Haematological blood tests are used to check respiratory function, the immune system, metabolism, hormonal balance, and the health of the major organs. The tests look at the numbers, appearance, shape, and size of blood cells and assess the function of clotting factors in the blood.

TYPES

Important haematological blood tests are *blood count* and *blood group* tests if a blood transfusion is needed. Biochemical tests measure chemicals in the blood (see *acid–base balance*; *kidney function tests*; and *liver function tests*). Microbiological tests (see *immunoassay*) look for microorganisms that are in the blood, such as occurs in septicaemia. Immunological tests also look for antibodies in the blood, which may confirm immunity to an infection.

blood transfusion

The infusion of large volumes of blood or of *blood products* directly into the bloodstream to remedy severe blood loss or to correct chronic *anaemia*. In an exchange blood transfusion, nearly all of the recipient's blood is replaced by donor blood.

HOW IT IS DONE

Before a transfusion, a sample of the recipient's blood is taken to identify his or her *blood group*, which is then matched with suitable donor blood. The donor blood is transfused into an arm vein through a plastic cannula (a tube with a smooth tip). Usually, each unit (about 500 ml) of blood is given over one to four hours; in an emergency, 500 ml may be given within a couple of minutes. The blood pressure, body temperature, and pulse of the patient are monitored during the procedure.

COMPLICATIONS

If mismatched blood is accidentally introduced into the circulation, antibodies in the recipient's blood may cause the donor cells to burst, leading to *shock* or *kidney failure*. Less severe reactions can produce fever, chills, or a rash. Reactions can also occur as the result of an allergy to a particular component of the transfused blood. The risk of infection is extremely small. All blood used for transfusion is carefully screened for a number of infectious agents, including *HIV* (the *AIDS* virus) and *hepatitis B* and *hepatitis C*.

In elderly or in severely anaemic patients, a blood transfusion can overload the circulation, which may lead to heart failure. In patients with chronic anaemia who need regular transfusions over the course of many years, excess iron may accumulate in the body (a condition called haemosiderosis) and damage organs such as the heart, liver, and pancreas. Treatment with the drug *desferrioxamine* to remove excess iron may be needed in this case.

blood transfusion, autologous

The use of a person's own blood, which had been donated at an earlier time, for *blood transfusion*. An autologous transfusion eliminates the slight but serious risk of contracting an infectious illness from contaminated blood. Another advantage is that there is no risk of a reaction occurring as a result of incompatibility between the donor and recipient blood.

blood transfusion, incompatible

A *blood transfusion* in which the recipient's blood and the donor's blood are mismatched. As a result, *antibodies* that are present in the recipient's circulation lead to destruction of the transfused *red blood cells*. This can have serious consequences, including *kidney failure* and occasionally even death. Careful crossmatching of blood in the laboratory make incompatible transfusions rare.

blood vessels

A general term for arteries, veins, and capillaries (see *circulatory system*).

blue baby

An infant with a cyanotic (bluish) complexion, especially visible on the lips and tongue, caused by a relative lack of oxygen in the blood. This is usually due to a structural defect of the heart or the major arteries leaving the heart. Such defects may need to be corrected surgically (see *heart disease, congenital*).

blue naevus

A type of *naevus* (skin blemish) with a dark blue or black coloration and a clearly defined border. Blue naevi are made up of a collection of pigment-producing cells called *melanocytes* and are not cancerous.

blurred vision

Indistinct, or fuzzy, visual images. Blurred vision, which should not be confused with *double vision* (diplopia), can occur in one eye or both, for episodes of varying lengths of time, and can develop gradually or suddenly. The usual cause of longstanding blurred vision is a refractive error such as *astigmatism* (unequal curvature of the front of the eye), *hypermetropia* (longsightedness), or *myopia* (shortsightedness), all of which can be corrected by glasses or contact lenses. After the age of 40, *presbyopia* (reduced ability to focus on near objects) becomes more common.

Vision may also be blurred or impaired as a result of damage, disease, or abnormalities of parts of the eye or its connections to the brain. Blurred vision as a result of disease is most commonly caused by *cataract* or *retinopathy*.

blushing

Brief reddening of the face, and sometimes the neck, caused by widening of the blood vessels close to the skin's surface. Blushing is often an involuntary reaction to embarrassment. In some women, blushing is a feature of the *hot flushes* that occur during the *menopause*. Flushing of the face also occurs in association with *carcinoid syndrome*.

B-lymphocyte

A type of *white blood cell*, also referred to as a B-cell. B-lymphocytes play a vital part in the *immune system*, the body's natural defence mechanism, by producing *antibodies* (special proteins) to find and destroy harmful microorganisms.

BMI

The abbreviation for *body mass index*.

BMR

The abbreviation for *basal metabolic rate*.

body contour surgery

Surgery to remove excess fat, skin, or both, from the body, especially from the abdomen, thighs, and buttocks. One of the most commonly performed operations is abdominal wall reduction (abdominoplasty). To miminize scarring, a less invasive procedure, such as suction lipectomy (liposuction), may be performed. In this operation, a hollow tube inserted through a small skin incision is used to break up large areas of fat. The fat is then sucked out through the instrument.

All body contour surgery carries a risk of complications, including wound infection. Minor irregularities and some dimpling of the skin commonly occur following liposuction.

body dysmorphic disorder

A psychiatric disorder in which a person suffers intense anxiety about an imagined defect in part of his or her body.

body image

A person's perception of the different parts of his or her own body.

body mass index (BMI)

A value used as an indicator of whether a person is a healthy weight, underweight, or overweight. Although BMI indicates the degree of fatness, it is not a direct measure of body fat.

A person's BMI is calculated by dividing his or her weight (in kilograms) by his or her height (in metres) squared (i.e. the height multiplied by itself). A BMI of 18.4 or less is classed as underweight; 18.5–24.9 is classed as a healthy weight; 25–29.9 is classed as overweight; 30-39.9 is classed as obese; and a BMI over 40 is classed as very obese. These are general figures that apply to most healthy adults under the age of 60. They are not applicable to children or people over 60; people with chronic health problems; women who are pregnant or breast-feeding; or athletes, weight-trainers, or similar groups of people with a high proportion of muscle.

body odour

The smell caused by the action of *bacteria* on sweat. It is most noticeable in the armpits and around the genital area, where the *apocrine glands* contain proteins and fatty materials favourable to bacterial growth.

body temperature

See *temperature*.

boil

An inflamed, pus-filled area of skin, usually an infected hair follicle. A more severe and extensive form of boil involving several hair follicles is known as a *carbuncle*. The usual cause of a boil is infection with the bacterium STAPHYLO-COCCUS AUREUS. Recurrent boils may occur in people with known or unrecognized *diabetes mellitus* or in those with other conditions in which general resistance to infection is impaired.

Treatment sometimes involves *antibiotic drugs*. However, a boil that is opened surgically to release the pus usually heals rapidly without the need for drug treatment.

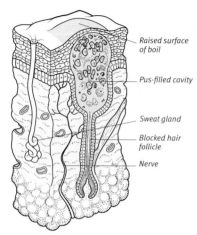

Cross-section of a boil
Following bacterial infection of the hair follicle, there is a buildup of pus, and a raised tender lump appears on the surface of the skin.

bolus

A soft mass of chewed food that is produced by the action of the tongue, the teeth, and the saliva to facilitate swallowing of the food. The term bolus is also used to describe a single dose of a drug that is rapidly injected into a vein.

bonding

The reciprocal process by which a strong tie, both psychological and emotional, is established between a parent and a newborn child. The process of

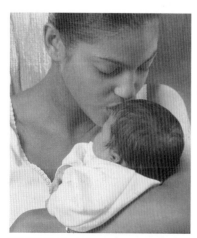

The bonding process
By the maintenance of close physical contact, bonding gradually becomes established.

bonding may be delayed if a baby is premature or ill and has to be separated from his or her parents immediately after birth (for example, by being placed in an incubator).

bonding, dental

Techniques that use plastic resins and acrylic or porcelain veneers and inlays to repair, restore, or cosmetically improve the *teeth*. Dental bonding may sometimes be used as an alternative to crowning (see *crown, dental*) and can also be used to protect the teeth.

bone

The structural material of the *skeleton* that provides a rigid framework for the muscles and protects certain organs of the body. In combination with the joints and the muscles, the bones form the locomotor system.

STRUCTURE

Bone consists of several layers. The surface has a thin covering known as the periosteum, a membrane that contains a network of blood vessels and nerves. Beneath the periosteum is an inner shell of hard (also called compact or cortical) bone composed of columns of bone cells (osteoclasts and osteoblasts). Each column has a central hollow (haversian canal) that is important for the nutrition, growth, and repair of the bone. The direction of the haversian canals corresponds with the mechanical forces acting on the bone.

Inside the hard shell, bone has a central meshlike structure (which is known as spongy, cancellous, or trabecular bone). The cavity in the centre of certain bones, and the spaces in spongy bone, contain *bone marrow*, in which the red blood cells, platelets, and most of the white blood cells are formed.

GROWTH

Bone is continuously reabsorbed by osteoclasts and replaced by osteoblasts. The osteoblasts encourage deposition of calcium phosphate on the protein framework of the bone; the osteoclasts remove it. The actions of these cells are controlled by growth hormone, secreted by the pituitary gland, the sex hormones oestrogen and testosterone, the adrenal hormones, the thyroid hormone thyrocalcitonin, and parathyroid hormone. These hormones also work to maintain the level of calcium in the blood.

Most bones begin to develop in the embryo during the fifth or sixth week of pregnancy, at which time they take the form of *cartilage*. This cartilage begins to be replaced by hard bone, in a process known as *ossification*, at around the seventh or eighth week of pregnancy; this process is not complete until early adult life. At birth, many bones consist mainly of cartilage, which ossifies later in life. The *epiphyses* (the growing ends of the long bones) are separated from the bone shaft (*diaphysis*) by the epiphyseal plate. Some bones in the body, such as certain skull bones, do not develop from cartilage, and these are known as membranous bones.

bone abscess

A localized collection of pus in a bone (see *osteomyelitis*).

bone age

A measure of skeletal maturity used to assess physical development in children. *X-rays*, which show how much bones have grown in a particular body area, are used to determine bone age. (See also *age*.)

bone cancer

Malignant growth in bone. Bone cancer may originate in the bone itself (primary bone cancer) or, more commonly, may occur as a result of cancer spreading from elsewhere in the body (secondary, or metastatic, bone cancer).

PRIMARY BONE CANCER

Cancers that originate in the bone are rare; the type of primary bone cancer that occurs most often is *osteosarcoma*. Other types include *chondrosarcoma* and *fibrosarcoma*. Cancers can also start in the bone marrow, but these are not usually considered to be bone cancers (see *multiple myeloma* and *leukaemia*). The treatment of primary bone cancer will depend on the extent to which the disease has spread. If it remains confined to bone, it may be possible to remove the cancer and fill the defect with a *bone graft*. In other cases, amputation may be recommended. *Radiotherapy* or *chemotherapy*, or both, may also be needed.

SECONDARY BONE CANCERS

The cancers that spread most readily to form secondary bone cancer are those of the breast, lung, prostate, thyroid, and kidney. These bone metastases occur commonly in the spine, pelvis, ribs, and skull. Pain is usually the main symptom. Affected bones are abnormally fragile and may fracture easily. Bone cancer that affects the spine may cause collapse or crushing of vertebrae, damaging the

STRUCTURE OF **BONE**

Bone consists of several layers: a thin, membranous surface and an inner, dense shell surrounding spongy material in which the bone marrow lies.

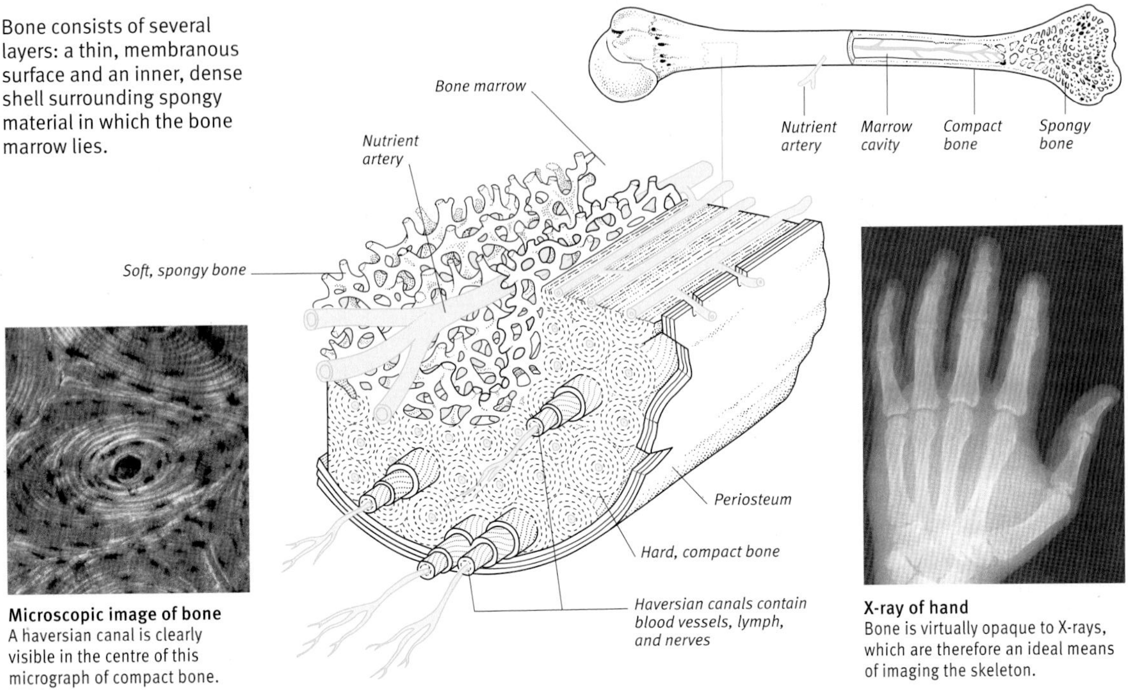

Bone marrow

Nutrient artery

Soft, spongy bone

Nutrient artery

Marrow cavity

Compact bone

Spongy bone

Periosteum

Hard, compact bone

Haversian canals contain blood vessels, lymph, and nerves

Microscopic image of bone
A haversian canal is clearly visible in the centre of this micrograph of compact bone.

X-ray of hand
Bone is virtually opaque to X-rays, which are therefore an ideal means of imaging the skeleton.

spinal cord and causing weakness or paralysis of one or more limbs.

Secondary bone cancers from the breast and prostate gland may respond to treatment with *hormone antagonists*. Other treatments that may be used include radiotherapy, chemotherapy, and surgery.

bone conduction

A method of transmitting sound that is tested during investigation into the cause of impaired *hearing*.

A vibrating tuning fork is held next to the ear. The base of the fork is then placed against the bone behind the ear. If the deafness is the result of an outer- or middle-ear problem (conductive deafness), the sound will be heard better when the tuning fork is held behind the ear. The bone transmits sound directly to the inner ear, bypassing the outer and middle ear. (See also *deafness*; *hearing tests*.)

bone cyst

An abnormal cavity in a bone. Bone cysts typically develop at one end of a long bone and may be discovered only by chance after a fracture at the site of the cyst. Minor surgery to scrape out the

cyst and fill the cavity with bone chips usually cures the condition; many small cysts do not actually require treatment.

bone density

The compactness of *bone* in relation to its volume. A decrease in bone density is a normal part of aging, but excessive loss of bone density (see *osteoporosis*) can lead to *fractures*. An increase in bone density (see *osteosclerosis*) occurs in some disorders, such as *osteopetrosis* and *Paget's disease*. Bone density is measured by a *DEXA scan*, a type of *densitometry* that uses low-dose X-rays.

bone graft

A surgical operation in which small pieces of bone are taken from one part of the body in order to repair or replace abnormal or missing bone elsewhere. The bone graft eventually dies, but it acts as a scaffold upon which strong new bone grows.

Bone is most commonly taken from the iliac crests (upper parts of the hip bones). They contain a large amount of inner, spongy bone, which is very useful for getting grafts to "take". Other common sources are the ribs (for curved bone) and the ulna in the forearm.

bone imaging

Techniques that show the structure or function of bones. *X-rays* are commonly used for diagnosing fractures and injuries. More detailed information is provided by *tomography*, *CT scanning*, or *MRI*, which can show tumours, infections, and the effects of diseased bone on surrounding tissues. *Radionuclide scanning* detects areas in the skeleton where there is high bone-cell activity. This type of scanning is used mainly to determine if cancer has spread to the bones. A *DEXA scan* is used to evaluate bone density.

bone marrow

The soft fatty tissue found in bone cavities; it may be red or yellow. Red bone marrow is present in all bones at birth and is the factory for most *blood cells*. During the teens, red bone marrow is gradually replaced in some bones by less active yellow marrow. In adults, red marrow is confined principally to the spine, sternum, (breastbone), pelvis (hip bones), ribs, scapulae (shoulderblades), clavicles (collarbones), and skull bones.

Stem cells within the red marrow are stimulated to form blood cells by the hormone erythropoietin. Yellow marrow is composed mainly of connective

DISORDERS OF **BONE**

Bone is affected by the same types of disorders as other body tissues, but its hard, rigid structure makes for extra complications. If a bone receives a direct blow or suffers from repeated stress, it may *fracture*. If it becomes infected (due to *osteomyelitis* or a *bone abscess*, for example), the resulting inflammation may interfere with the blood supply, leading to death of part of the bone.

Genetic disorders

Several inherited conditions may affect bone growth; these include *achondro–plasia* and *osteogenesis imperfecta*. Such disorders often result in short stature.

Nutritional disorders

Lack of calcium and vitamin D in the diet may result in *rickets* in children and *osteomalacia* in adults; in both conditions the bones become soft and lose their shape.

Hormonal disorders

If the pituitary gland produces excess growth hormone before puberty, this results in excessive growth of the bones tissue and fat. If the body needs to increase its rate of blood formation, some of the yellow marrow will be replaced by red. Sometimes marrow fails to produce sufficient numbers of normal blood cells, as occurs in aplastic anaemia (see *anaemia, aplastic*) or when marrow has been displaced by tumour cells. In other cases, marrow may over-produce certain blood cells, as occurs in *polycythaemia* and *leukaemia*.

and other organs, leading to *gigantism*. Excess parathyroid hormone may lead to *bone cysts*. Osteoporosis (loss of bone density) is common in women following the menopause, when oestrogen levels fall.

Tumours

Several different types of cancerous and noncancerous growth can arise from bone (see *bone cancer* and *bone tumour*). In addition, the bones are a common site for secondary tumours (metastases) that have spread from cancerous tumours elsewhere in the body.

Other disorders

Paget's disease involves thickening of some areas of the bones, while other areas become spongy.

INVESTIGATION

Bone disorders are investigated using imaging techniques such as *X-rays*, *CT scanning*, *radionuclide scanning*, and *densitometry*; by *biopsy*; and *blood tests*.

bone marrow biopsy

A procedure to obtain a sample of cells from the bone marrow (an aspiration biopsy) or a small core of bone with marrow inside (a trephine biopsy). The sample is usually taken, under local *anaesthesia*, from the sternum (breast-bone) or iliac crests (upper part of the hip bones). Microscopic examination gives information on the development of the blood components and on the presence of cells foreign to the marrow. It is useful in the diagnosis of many blood disorders, including *leukaemia* and *anaemia*. It can also show whether bone marrow has been invaded by *lymphoma* or cells from other tumours.

bone marrow transplant

The technique of using normal red *bone marrow* to replace cancerous, defective, or diseased bone marrow in a patient. In allogeneic bone marrow transplantation (BMT), healthy marrow is taken from a donor with a very similar tissue-type to the recipient's (often a brother or sister). In autologous BMT, the patient's own healthy bone marrow is harvested while his or her disease is in remission and is reinfused at a later time. Generally, BMT is used only in the treatment of serious, potentially life-threatening blood and immune system disorders, including aplastic anaemia (see *anaemia, aplastic*), *sickle cell anaemia*, and *leukaemia*.

The term "bone marrow transplant" is often used interchangeably with "stem cell transplant". Strictly, a bone marrow transplant uses cells only from bone marrow whereas a stem cell transplant may use cells from bone marrow, blood, or stored umbilical cord blood.

HOW IT IS DONE

Before transplantation, all of the recipient's bone marrow is destroyed with *cytotoxic drugs* or radiation to prevent rejection of the donated cells and to kill any cancer cells present. The donor bone marrow is transfused into the circulation from where cells find their way to the bone marrow cavities and start to grow.

In autologous BMT, the patient's bone marrow is stored by *cryopreservation* (freezing). Before being frozen, the marrow is usually treated to eliminate any undetected cancerous cells. If the patient's disease recurs, the stored bone marrow can then be reinfused.

COMPLICATIONS

The major risks with BMT are infection during the recovery period and rejection (known as *graft-versus-host disease*, or GVHD). *Immunosuppressant drugs* are used to prevent and treat rejection. The risk of GVHD may be reduced by removing the T-cells (see *T-lymphocyte*) from the marrow using monoclonal antibodies before it is reinfused. GVHD does not occur with autologous BMT.

bone metastases

Cancerous *tumours* in bone, also known as secondary bone cancers, that have spread from a cancer in another part of the body (see *bone cancer*). The bones of the ribs, pelvis, skull, and spine are particularly affected.

bone pain

An unpleasant sensation (see *pain*) felt in a part of the skeleton (see *musculo-skeletal pain*). Bone pain is frequently described as constant and gnawing, and it may disturb sleep. There are many possible causes of bone pain, including trauma of the bone (see *fracture*), infection (see *osteomyelitis*), disorders of the bone itself (such as *Paget's disease*), and *bone tumours*. (See also *osteoid osteoma*; *osteomalacia*; *sickle cell anaemia*.)

bone resorption

Loss of *bone* tissue. Bone resorption and the laying down of new bone tissue are continuous processes. With increasing age, resorption exceeds new bone formation, and the bone tissue gradually becomes thinner. However, in certain disorders (for example, *osteoporosis*), resorption takes place more rapidly and to a greater extent, causing weakening of bone and increased risk of *fractures*.

bone tumour

A bone swelling that may be cancerous (see *bone cancer*) or noncancerous. The most common type of noncancerous bone tumour is an *osteochondroma*. Other types of bone tumour are *osteoma*

PERFORMING A **BONE MARROW TRANSPLANT**

Normal bone marrow is used to replace malignant or defective marrow. In the allogeneic procedure, healthy marrow is taken from a donor. In the autologous procedure, the patient's own healthy marrow is used.

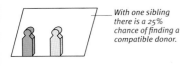

With one sibling there is a 25% chance of finding a compatible donor.

With three siblings there are three opportunities for a 25% chance of finding a donor.

Finding a donor
The more siblings one has, the greater the chance of finding a donor. With three or more siblings, the chances are good.

1 Before transplantation, all the recipient's bone marrow is destroyed by treatment with drugs or radiation. Destroying the marrow kills any cancer cells.

2 Using general anaesthesia, bone marrow is aspirated from the donor's iliac crests and/or sternum. Up to one litre is removed. The transplanted marrow grows quickly to occupy the bone spaces.

3 After aspiration, the bone marrow is transfused intravenously into the patient. The bone marrow cells find their way through the circulation into the patient's marrow cavities, where they start to grow.

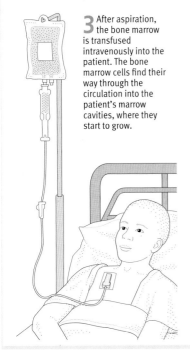

SITES OF **BONE MARROW**

Red or yellow in colour, bone marrow is a soft, fatty tissue found in the cavities of bones. In newborn babies, red bone marrow is present in all bones; during the teen years, most is replaced by yellow marrow. The marrow used for transplants is red.

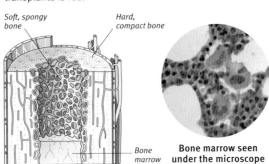

Soft, spongy bone

Hard, compact bone

Bone marrow

Bone marrow seen under the microscope

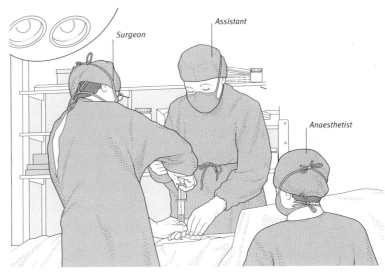

Surgeon

Assistant

Anaesthetist

DONOR ASPIRATION

With the donor lying face down, a hollow aspiration needle, which has a stylet (a thin, sharp lance) within it, is introduced into the bone (iliac crests)

The stylet is then removed. Bone marrow is sucked out through the cortex into a syringe connected to the needle.

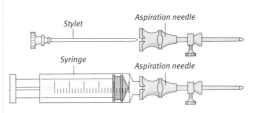

Stylet

Aspiration needle

Syringe

Aspiration needle

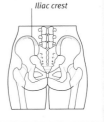

Iliac crest

B

and chondroma (see *chondromatosis*). Treatment is needed only if the tumour becomes large or causes symptoms by pressing on other structures. In such cases, it can be removed by surgery. Osteoclastoma (also called a giant cell tumour), which usually occurs in the arm or leg of a young adult, is tender and painful and has to be removed.

booster

A follow-up dose of *vaccine*, given to reinforce or prolong immunity after an initial course of *immunization*.

borborygmi

The medical name for *bowel sounds* that are audible without a stethoscope.

borderline personality disorder

A personality disorder that falls between neurotic and psychotic levels. Mood changes are often rapid and inappropriate. Angry outbursts are common, as are impulsive, self-damaging acts such as gambling or suicide attempts.

Bordetella pertussis

A species of *bacteria* that may infect the human respiratory tract and is responsible for causing *whooping cough*.

Bornholm disease

One of various names for epidemic *pleurodynia*, an infectious viral disease that causes severe chest pains and fever.

Borrelia

A genus of spiral-shaped *bacteria* transmitted through tick bites (see *ticks and disease*). BORRELIA species cause *relapsing fever* (which is characterized by recurrent bouts of fever) and *Lyme disease*.

bottle-feeding

Infant feeding using a milk preparation usually based on modified cow's milk. This formula milk contains similar proportions of protein, fat, lactose (milk sugar), and minerals to those in human milk, but it lacks the protective antibodies that are present in breast milk. Vitamins are added.

In some cases, medical problems in the mother or child may make *breast-feeding* impossible or undesirable, in which case bottle-feeding is recommended. However, bottle-fed babies are at higher risk of gastrointestinal infections than breast-fed babies and may be more likely to develop allergic disorders. (See also *feeding, infant*.)

Botox

A brand name for *botulinum toxin*.

botulinum toxin

A potentially lethal toxin produced by the bacterium CLOSTRIDIUM BOTULINUM. The toxin causes *botulism*, a rare but serious form of *food poisoning*. Medically, botulinum toxin is used in tiny doses as a *muscle-relaxant drug* to control muscle spasms in disorders such as *blepharospasm* (spasm of the eyelids), *facial spasm*, and spasmodic *torticollis* (spasm of the neck muscles). It is also sometimes used to treat severe *hyperhidrosis* (excessive sweating). Cosmetically, botulinum toxin is used to temporarily reduce wrinkles.

botulism

A rare but serious form of poisoning caused by eating improperly canned or preserved food contaminated with a toxin produced by the bacterium CLOSTRIDIUM BOTULINUM. The toxin causes progressive muscular paralysis as well as other disturbances of the central and peripheral nervous systems. CLOSTRIDIUM BOTULINUM produces spores that resist boiling, salting, smoking, and some forms of pickling. The spores multiply only in the absence of air and thrive in canned or poorly preserved food. Ingestion of even minute amounts of the toxin can lead to severe poisoning.

SYMPTOMS
The symptoms of botulism first occur within 8 to 36 hours of ingesting contaminated food. They include difficulty in swallowing and speaking; nausea and vomiting; and double vision. Prompt treatment is vital. In infants, the toxin can form in the body after the ingestion of foods contaminated with the bacterium, such as honey. (See also *food poisoning*.)

Bouchard's node

A bony swelling that forms on the middle finger joint in a person with *osteoarthritis*. (See also *Heberden's node*.)

bougie

A rod-shaped instrument used for insertion into tubular organs, such as the urethra, during investigations or treatment. It may also be used to stretch a narrowed area.

bovine spongiform encephalopathy (BSE)

Commonly known as "mad cow disease", a neurological disorder in cattle that can be transmitted to humans through the consumption of infected meat, causing *Creutzfeldt–Jakob disease*. (See also *encephalopathy*.)

bowel

A common name for the large and/or small *intestines*.

bowel disorders

Any disorder that affects the *intestine*. Common bowel disorders are *inflammatory bowel disease* and *irritable bowel syndrome (IBS)*. (See also *intestine* disorders box; *intestine, cancer of*; *intestine, obstruction of*; *intestine, tumours of*.)

bowel movements, abnormal

See *faeces, abnormal*.

bowel sounds

Sounds made by the passage of air and fluid through the *intestine*. Absent or abnormal bowel sounds may indicate a disorder. Those that are audible without a stethoscope are known as borborygmi and are a normal part of the digestive process, but they may be exaggerated by anxiety and some intestinal disorders.

Bowen's disease

A rare skin disorder that is characterized by the formation of a flat patch of red, scaly skin, most commonly on the face or the hands. Bowen's disease may become cancerous.

Treatment includes surgical removal of the diseased skin, or its destruction by freezing, *cauterization*, laser treatment, or topical chemotherapy.

bowleg

An outward curving of bones in the legs that results in wide separation of the knees when the feet are together. Bowlegs are common in very young children, and they are a normal part of development. In most cases, the curve straightens as the child grows. If the bowing is severe, is on one side only, or persists beyond the age of three, a doctor should be consulted. Surgery may be needed. Rarely, leg deformity is a result of bone disease, particularly *rickets* (a vitamin D deficiency) in children.

Bowman's capsule

A cup-shaped membrane within the kidney's *nephron* containing a *glomerulus* (a cluster of tiny blood vessels called capillaries). Here, blood is filtered into the kidney tubule.

BP

The abbreviation for *blood pressure*.

brace, dental

See *orthodontic appliances*.

brace, orthopaedic

An appliance worn to support part of the body or hold it in a fixed position. A brace may be used to correct or halt the development of a deformity, to aid mobility, or to relieve pain. (See also *caliper splint*; *splint*.)

brachial artery

The *artery* that runs down the inner side of the upper arm, between the armpit and the elbow.

brachialgia

Pain or stiffness in the arm that is often accompanied by pain, tingling and/or numbness of the hands or fingers, and weak hand grip. It may be a symptom of underlying disorders such as *frozen shoulder* or nerve compression from *cervical osteoarthritis*.

brachial plexus

A group of large nerve trunks formed from nerve roots of the lower part of the cervical spine (in the neck) and upper part of the thoracic spine (in the chest). These nerve trunks divide into the musculocutaneous, axillary, median, ulnar, and radial nerves, which control muscles in and receive sensation from the arm and the hand. Injuries to the brachial plexus can cause loss of movement and sensation in the arm.

In severe injuries, there may be damage to both the upper and the lower nerve roots of the brachial plexus, producing complete paralysis of the arm. The paralysis may be temporary if the nerve fibres are not torn. It may be possible to repair nerve roots that have been torn by nerve grafting, which is a *microsurgery* procedure, but if a nerve root has become separated from the spinal cord, surgical repair will not be successful. Apart from injuries, the brachial plexus may be compressed by the presence of a *cervical rib* (extra rib).

brachytherapy

A form of *radiotherapy* in which radioactive material is placed in or near the area or tissue being treated (often a tumour). *Interstitial radiotherapy* and intracavitary radiotherapy (see *intracavitary therapy*) are types of brachytherapy.

bradycardia

An abnormally slow heart rate. Most people have a heart rate of between 60 and 100 beats per minute. Many athletes and healthy people who exercise regularly and vigorously have slower rates. In others, bradycardia may indicate an underlying disorder such as *hypothyroidism* or *heart block*. Bradycardia may also occur as a result of taking *beta-blocker drugs*. Profound or sudden bradycardia may cause a drop in blood pressure that results in fainting (see *vasovagal attack*).

bradykinin

A *polypeptide* (protein molecule) that forms naturally in the blood as part of the inflammatory process. Bradykinin is a powerful vasodilator (it causes the widening of blood vessels). Bradykinin also allows fluid to leak from the blood vessels; stimulates pain receptors; and causes contraction of the smooth muscle in internal organs such as the lungs or intestines.

Braille

A system of embossed dots, now accepted for all written languages, that enables blind people to read and write. The system is based on six raised dots, which can be combined in different ways to form symbols.

There are two types of Braille. In grade I, each symbol represents an individual letter or punctuation mark. In grade II, which is the more widely used, symbols represent common letter combinations or words.

brain

The major organ of the *nervous system*, located in the *cranium* (skull). The brain receives, sorts, and interprets sensations from the nerves that extend from the *central nervous system* (brain and spinal cord) to the rest of the body; it initiates and coordinates nerve signals involved in activities such as speech, movement, thought, and emotion.

An adult brain weighs about 1.4 kg and has three main structures: the *brainstem*; the *cerebellum*; and the largest part, the *cerebrum*, which consists of left and right hemispheres.

CEREBRUM

Each hemisphere in the cerebrum has an outer layer called the cortex, consisting of grey matter, which is rich in nerve-cell bodies and is the main region in the brain for conscious thought, sensation, and movement. Beneath the cortex are tracts of nerve fibres called white matter, and, deeper within the hemispheres, are the *basal ganglia* (paired nerve cell clusters). The surface of each of the hemispheres is divided by fissures (sulci) and folds (gyri) into distinct lobes (occipital, frontal, parietal, and temporal lobes), named after the skull bones that overlie them. A thick band of nerve fibres called the corpus callosum connects the hemispheres.

The cerebrum encloses a central group of structures including the *thalami* and the *hypothalamus*, which has close connections with the *pituitary gland*. Encircling the thalami is a complex of nerve centres called the *limbic system*. These structures act as links between parts of the cerebrum and the brainstem lying beneath the thalami.

BRAINSTEM AND CEREBELLUM

The brainstem is concerned mainly with the control of vital functions such as breathing and blood pressure. The cerebellum at the back of the brain controls balance, posture, and muscular coordination. Both of these regions operate at a subconscious level.

MENINGES AND CEREBROSPINAL FLUID

The brain and spinal cord are encased in three layers of membranes known as *meninges*. *Cerebrospinal fluid* circulates between these membrane layers and within the four main brain cavities, which are known as *ventricles*. This fluid helps to nourish and cushion the brain.

BLOOD SUPPLY

The brain as a whole has an extensive blood supply. Blood comes from a circle of arteries fed by the internal *carotid arteries* (which run up each side of the front of the neck to enter the base of the skull) and from two vertebral arteries that run parallel to the spinal cord. The brain receives about 20 per cent of the blood from the heart's output.

brain abscess

A collection of pus, surrounded by inflamed tissues, within the brain or on its surface. The most common sites are the frontal and temporal lobes of the *cerebrum* in the forebrain.

Brain abscesses may occur after a head injury, but most cases result from the spread of infection from elsewhere in the body, such as the middle ear or the sinuses. Another cause of a brain abscess is an infection following a pene-trating brain injury. Multiple brain abscesses may occur

STRUCTURE OF THE **BRAIN**

The brain has three main parts: the brainstem (an extension of the spinal cord), the cerebellum, and the cerebrum, much of which consists of the two large cerebral hemispheres. Each hemisphere consists of an outer layer, or cortex, which is rich in nerve cells and called grey matter, and inner areas rich in nerve fibres, called white matter. The surface of each hemisphere is thrown into folds called gyri, separated by fissures called sulci. The two hemispheres are linked by a thick band of nerve fibres, the corpus callosum. Deep within the forebrain are various central structures, which include the thalamus, hypothalamus, basal ganglia, and pituitary gland.

The brain has the consistency of jelly and, in adults, weighs about 1.4 kg. It is protected by membranous coverings (known as meninges) within the skull.

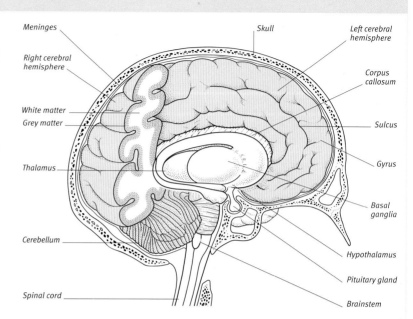

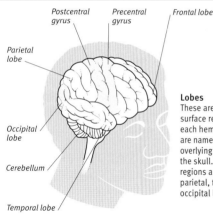

Lobes
These are broad surface regions of each hemisphere that are named after the overlying bones of the skull. The four main regions are the frontal, parietal, temporal, and occipital lobes.

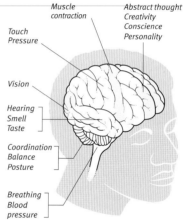

Special areas
Some areas of the brain are associated with specific functions – for example, the occipital lobe with vision and the cerebellum with balance and coordination. Touch and pressure sensation is perceived within the postcentral gyrus. Muscle movements are controlled from the precentral gyrus; speech is controlled from an area in the frontal lobe of the dominant hemisphere.

IMAGING THE BRAIN

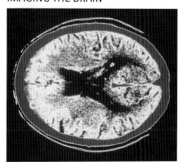

CT scanning
CT scans produce images as "slices" through the head. The scan above shows bleeding into the brain tissue (a cerebral haemorrhage).

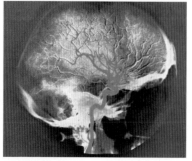

Angiography
This technique makes blood vessels clearly visible. The angiogram above shows the carotid artery and its branches.

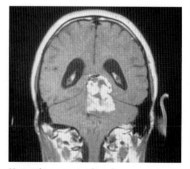

Magnetic resonance imaging
MRI produces three-dimensional or cross-sectional images. This MRI shows a tumour (the white area to the right of centre) in the cerebellum.

as a result of blood-borne infection, most commonly in patients with a heart-valve infection (see *endocarditis*).

Symptoms of a brain abscess include headache, drowsiness, vomiting, visual disturbances, fever, and seizures. There may also be other symptoms, such as speech disturbances, that are due to local pressure. Treatment is with *antibiotic drugs* and surgery. A *craniotomy* may be needed to open and drain the abscess. Untreated, brain abscesses can cause permanent damage and can be fatal. Despite treatment, scarring can cause *epilepsy* in some cases.

brain contusion

Bruising of the brain accompanied by loss of consciousness, which occurs as the result of an injury. (See also *brain damage*; *concussion*.)

brain damage

Degeneration or death of nerve cells and tracts within the brain that may be localized to a particular area of the brain or may be diffuse.

DIFFUSE DAMAGE

One of the most common causes of diffuse brain damage is prolonged cerebral *hypoxia* (an insufficient supply of oxygen to the brain), which may occur in a baby during a difficult birth. Other causes of diffuse damage to the brain tissue include *cardiac arrest* (cessation of the heartbeat), *respiratory arrest* (cessation of breathing), drowning, certain types of poisoning, and *status epilepticus* (prolonged seizures).

Diffuse brain damage may also occur gradually as a result of exposure to environmental pollutants, such as lead or mercury compounds (see *Minamata disease*), or if nerve-cell poisons build up in the brain, as occurs in untreated *phenylketonuria*. Other possible causes of diffuse brain damage include brain infections such as *encephalitis*.

LOCALIZED DAMAGE

Localized brain damage may occur as the result of a *head injury*, *stroke* (damage to part of the brain caused by an interruption to its blood supply), *brain tumour*, or *brain abscess*.

At birth, a raised blood level of the bile pigment bilirubin (see *haemolytic disease of the newborn*) can cause local damage to the *basal ganglia* (nerve clusters deep within the brain). This leads to a condition called *kernicterus*. Brain damage that occurs before, during, or after birth may result in *cerebral palsy*.

OUTCOME

Diffuse damage to the brain may result in *learning difficulties* and severe physical disability. Localized brain damage may cause specific deficits in brain function, such as disturbances of movement or speech (see *speech disorders*). Nerve cells and tracts in the brain and spinal cord cannot repair themselves once they have been damaged, but some return of function may be possible with training, as patients learn to use other parts of the brain. (See also *Structure of the brain* box.)

brain death

The irreversible cessation of all functions of the brain, including those of the brainstem. (See also *death*.)

brain failure

See *brain syndrome*, *organic*.

brain haemorrhage

Bleeding within or around the brain caused either by injury or by the spontaneous rupture of a blood vessel. There are four types of brain haemorrhage:

DISORDERS OF THE **BRAIN**

Defects and disorders of the brain have numerous causes, including infection, injury, *brain tumour*, or a lack of blood or oxygen (see *hypoxia*). Brain cells destroyed by injury or disease cannot be replaced, so any resulting loss in function can be difficult to reverse.

Because the brain is encased within the skull, any space-occupying tumour, *brain abscess*, or *haematoma* (large blood clot) creates raised pressure, which can impair the function of the whole brain.

Brain disorders that are localized in a small region may affect a specific function, such as speech (see *aphasia*). However, more often, damage is more diffuse and the symptoms can be varied and numerous.

The brain may also be damaged by a blow to the head (see *head injury*).

Congenital defects

Some brain disorders are congenital (present from birth) due to genetic or chromosomal disorders, as in *Down's syndrome*. Structural defects during fetal development include *hydrocephalus* (water on the brain) and *anencephaly* (congenital absence of the brain).

Impaired blood and oxygen supply

Brain cells can survive only a few minutes without oxygen. A reduced supply may occur at birth, causing *cerebral palsy*. Later in life, choking or arrest of breathing and heartbeat can cause hypoxia (oxygen lack).

From middle age onwards, *cerebrovascular disease*, which impairs the blood supply to one or more regions of the brain, is the most important cause of brain disorders. If an artery within the brain becomes blocked or ruptures, leading to haemorrhage, the result is a *stroke*.

Infection

Encephalitis (infection within the brain) may be due to a virus. *Meningitis* (infection of the membranes surrounding the brain) is generally due to bacterial infection.

Creutzfeldt–Jakob disease is a rare, fatal brain disease associated with an infective agent called a prion, which, in some cases, has been linked with *bovine spongiform encephalopathy* (BSE), a disease in cattle.

Degenerative disorders

Multiple sclerosis is a progressive disease of the brain and spinal cord. Degenerative brain diseases include *Alzheimer's disease* and *Parkinson's disease*.

Other disorders

Emotional or behavioural disorders are often called psychiatric illnesses, but the distinction between these and neurological disorders is unclear. In many illnesses, such as *depression* and *schizophrenia*, there may be an underlying disturbance of brain chemistry.

INVESTIGATION

Procedures used to investigate brain disorders and function include tests of reflexes and of mental and physical abilities. Electrical activity may be measured with an *EEG*. Physical abnormalities can be found using *brain imaging* techniques such as *angiography*, *CT scanning*, or *MRI*.

subdural, extradural, subarachnoid, and intracerebral (see the illustrated box). Extradural and subdural haemorrhages are usually caused by a blow to the head (see head injury). Subarachnoid and intracerebral haemorrhages tend to occur spontaneously due to rupture of aneurysms or small blood vessels in the brain.

brain imaging

Techniques that can provide pictures of the brain. Brain imaging techniques are used to detect injury or disease of the brain and include X-rays, angiography, CT scanning, MRI (magnetic resonance imaging), PET (positron emission tomography) scanning, and SPECT (single photon emission CT).

INVESTIGATION OF BRAIN STRUCTURE

CT scanning gives images of the brain substance; it provides clear pictures of the ventricles (fluid-filled cavities) and can reveal tumours, blood clots, strokes, aneurysms, and abscesses.

MRI (magnetic resonance imaging) produces very detailed images of the brain's structure. This technique is also used to detect patches of abnormal brain tissue, as seen in multiple sclerosis.

Angiography involves the injection of a contrast medium that shows up the blood vessels in the brain on X-ray. It is used to investigate aneurysms and other circulatory disorders.

INVESTIGATION OF BRAIN FUNCTION

PET and SPECT scanning are specialized forms of radionuclide scanning that use small amounts of radioactive material to provide information about brain function as well as structure. They enable blood flow and metabolic activity in the brain to be measured.

Functional magnetic resonance imaging (fMRI) can be used to determine which parts of the brain are activated by different sensations or activities, such as sight or movement of the fingers. This technique is used to assess how the brain is working.

Ultrasound scanning, through the fontanelles (holes where the skull bones have yet to fuse), can detect bleeding in the brain only in premature or very young babies; ultrasound waves cannot penetrate the bones of a mature skull.

brainstem

A stalk of nerve tissue that forms the lowest part of the brain and links with the spinal cord. The brainstem acts partly as a highway for messages travelling between other parts of the brain

SITES OF **BRAIN HAEMORRHAGE**

Haemorrhages within the skull fall into four main types – extradural, subdural, subarachnoid, and intracerebral – according to the site of the bleeding in relation to the brain and its protective coverings (the meninges). The causes and effects of the bleeding and the outlook for the patient vary depending on which type the haemorrhage falls into.

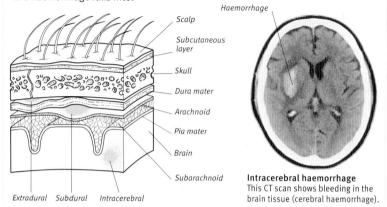

Scalp
Subcutaneous layer
Skull
Dura mater
Arachnoid
Pia mater
Brain
Subarachnoid
Haemorrhage

Extradural   Subdural   Intracerebral

Intracerebral haemorrhage
This CT scan shows bleeding in the brain tissue (cerebral haemorrhage).

and spinal cord. It also connects with 10 of the 12 pairs of cranial nerves (which emerge directly from the underside of the brain) and controls basic functions such as breathing, vomiting, and eye reflexes. Brainstem activities are below the level of consciousness, and they operate mainly on an automatic basis.

STRUCTURE

The brainstem is composed of three main parts: the midbrain, pons, and medulla. Attached to the back of the brainstem is a separate part of the brain, the cerebellum, which is concerned with balance and coordinated movement. Running longitudinally through the middle of the brainstem is a canal; this widens in the pons and medulla to form the fourth ventricle (cavity) of the brain, which contains the circulating cerebrospinal fluid.

Midbrain The midbrain is the smallest section of the brainstem. This part contains the nuclei (nerve-cell centres) of the third and fourth cranial nerves, which control eye movements and the size and reactions of the pupil. It also contains cell groups, such as the substantia nigra, involved in smooth coordination of limb movements.

Pons The pons contains thick bundles of nerve fibres that connect with the cerebellum. It also houses the nuclei for the fifth to eighth cranial nerves, and relays sensory information from the ear, face, and teeth, as well as the signals that

move the jaw, adjust facial expressions, and produce some eye movements.

Medulla The medulla resembles a thick extension of the spinal cord. It contains the nuclei of the ninth to 12th cranial nerves. by which it receives and relays taste sensations from the tongue and

LOCATION OF THE **BRAINSTEM**

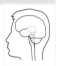

The brainstem is a 7.5 cm-long stalk of nerve cells and fibres that joins the upper spinal cord to the rest of the brain.

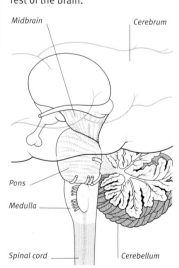

Midbrain
Cerebrum
Pons
Medulla
Spinal cord
Cerebellum

relays signals to muscles involved in speech and in tongue and neck movements. The medulla also contains the "vital centres" (groups of nerve cells that regulate the heartbeat, breathing, blood pressure, and digestion (information on which is relayed via the 10th cranial nerve (see *vagus nerve*).

Reticular formation Throughout the brainstem are numerous nerve-cell groups known collectively as the reticular formation. This network alerts the higher brain centres to sensory stimuli that may require a conscious response. Our sleep/wake cycle is controlled by the reticular formation.

DISORDERS

The brainstem is susceptible to the same disorders that afflict the rest of the central nervous system (see *brain, disorders of*). Damage to the medulla's vital centres is rapidly fatal; damage to the reticular formation may cause *coma*. Damage to specific cranial nerve nuclei can sometimes lead to specific effects. For example, damage to the seventh cranial nerve (the facial nerve) leads to *facial palsy*. Degeneration of the substantia nigra in the midbrain is thought to be a cause of *Parkinson's disease*.

brain syndrome, organic

Disorder of consciousness, intellect, or mental functioning that is of organic (physical), as opposed to psychiatric, origin. Possible causes include degenerative diseases, most notably *Alzheimer's disease*; infections; certain drugs; or the effects of injury, *stroke*, or tumour.

SYMPTOMS

Symptoms of acute organic brain syndrome range from mild confusion to stupor or *coma*. They may also include disorientation, memory loss, hallucinations, and delusions (see *delirium*). In the chronic form, there is a progressive decline in intellect, memory, and behaviour (see *dementia*). Treatment is more likely to be successful with the acute form. In chronic cases, irreversible brain damage may already have occurred. (See also *psychosis*.)

brain tumour

An abnormal growth in or on the brain. Although they are not always cancerous, all brain tumours are serious due to the buildup of pressure they cause within the brain and the compression of adjoining brain areas, both of which may occur as the tumour grows and expands. Expansion of a brain tumour

within the rigid skull may also result in damage to the normal tissue that surrounds the tumour.

TYPES

Brain tumours may be primary growths arising directly from tissues within the skull or metastases (secondary growths) that have spread via the bloodstream from cancerous tumours elsewhere in the body, particularly from those in the lung or breast.

The cause of primary brain tumours is not known. About 60 per cent are *gliomas* (which are frequently cancerous), and arise from the brain tissue. Other primary tumours include *meningiomas*, which arise from the meningeal membranes covering the brain; *acoustic neuromas*, which arise from the acoustic nerve; and *pituitary tumours*, which arise from the tissue of the pituitary gland. Most of these tumours are noncancerous, but their relatively large size can cause local tissue damage.

Some types of primary brain tumour affect mainly children. These include two types of glioma called *medulloblastoma* and cerebellar *astrocytoma*. Primary brain tumours virtually never spread (metastasize) outside the central nervous system.

Secondary growths (metastases) are always cancerous and may be found in more than one organ.

SYMPTOMS

Compression of brain tissue or nerve tracts near the tumour may cause muscle weakness, loss of vision, or other sensory disturbances, speech difficulties, and epileptic seizures.

The presence of a growing tumour can increase pressure in the skull, causing severe, persistent headache, visual disturbances, vomiting, dizziness, impaired mental functioning, abnormal behaviour, personality changes, and seizures. *Hydrocephalus* (excess fluid in the brain) may occur if the tumour obstructs the circulation of cerebrospinal fluid.

DIAGNOSIS AND TREATMENT

Many different *brain imaging* techniques may be used to locate the site of a brain tumour and to establish its size and the extent of its spread.

In some cases, complete removal of a brain tumour may be possible using guidance from MRI scanning during surgery. In such cases, the patient may be cured. However, many tumours are inaccessible or too extensive for removal. In cases where a tumour cannot be completely removed, as much as possible will be cut away to relieve pressure.

For primary and secondary tumours, *radiotherapy* or *anticancer drugs* may also be given. *Corticosteroid drugs* and diuretic drugs are often prescribed temporarily to reduce the size of a tumour and any associated swelling of brain tissues, and reduce intracranial pressure (*ICP*).

bran

The fibrous outer covering of grain that cannot be digested. The fibre is used as a bulk-forming *laxative* to prevent constipation (see *fibre, dietary*).

branchial disorders

Disorders due to abnormal development, in an embryo, of the branchial arches (paired segmented ridges of tissue in each side of the throat). Such disorders include branchial cyst and branchial *fistula*.

A branchial cyst is a soft swelling, containing fluid that may be either clear or puslike, that appears on the side of the neck in early adulthood. Treatment of a branchial cyst is usually with surgical removal.

A branchial fistula occurs between the back of the throat and the external surface of the neck, where it appears as a small hole, usually noted at birth. A hole in the neck that does not extend to the back of the throat is a branchial cleft sinus. A branchial fistula or cleft sinus may discharge mucus or pus and may be removed surgically.

brash, water

See *waterbrash*.

Braxton Hicks' contractions

Short, relatively painless contractions of the uterus during pregnancy. They may be felt in late pregnancy and are sometimes mistaken for labour pains.

BRCA1 and BRCA2

Two *genes* associated with many cases of inherited *breast cancer* and ovarian cancer (see *ovary, cancer of*). Normally, these genes suppress tumour formation but when certain mutations (changes) are present in them, tumour suppression is impaired, which results in an increased cancer risk.

breakbone fever

A tropical viral illness, which is also called *dengue*, that is spread by mosquitoes. The symptoms include high fever and severe joint and muscle pain.

breakthrough bleeding

Bleeding or staining ("spotting") from the vagina between menstrual periods in women taking an oral contraceptive. The bleeding is most common during the first few months of taking the pill and is caused by incomplete suppression of the monthly buildup of the *endometrium* (lining of the uterus). (See also *vaginal bleeding*.)

breast

Either of the two mammary glands, which, in women, provide milk to nourish a baby and are secondary *sexual characteristics*. The male breast is an immature version of the female breast.

DEVELOPMENT AND STRUCTURE

At puberty, a girl's breasts begin to develop: the areola (circular area of pigmented skin around the nipple) swells and the nipple enlarges. This is followed by an increase in glandular tissue and fat.

The adult female breast consists of between 15 and 20 lobes of milk-secreting glands embedded in fatty tissue. The ducts of these glands have their outlet in the nipple. The areolar skin contains sweat glands, sebaceous glands, and hair follicles. Bands of fine ligaments determine the breast's height and shape.

The size, shape, and general appearance of a woman's breasts may vary throughout the menstrual cycle, during pregnancy and lactation, and following the menopause.

BREAST FUNCTION

During pregnancy, the hormones *oestrogen* and *progesterone*, secreted by the ovaries and placenta, cause the milk-producing glands in the breasts to develop and become active. These two hormones also cause the nipples to enlarge.

Just before and immediately after childbirth, the glands in the breast produce a watery fluid known as *colostrum*. The production of this fluid is replaced by milk production a few days later. Milk production and release are stimulated by the hormone *prolactin*.

breast abscess

A collection of pus in the mammary gland, usually in a woman who is lactating (producing milk). Breast abscesses develop if acute *mastitis* (infection of the breast tissue) is not treated promptly and occur most commonly during the month after a woman's first delivery.

The initial symptoms of a breast abscess are the same as those of acute mastitis. The abscess develops in one area, which becomes very firm, red, and extremely painful. Treatment involves *antibiotic drugs* and repeated *aspiration* (withdrawal by suction) of the pus using a needle and syringe. In rare cases, surgical drainage may be needed.

breast awareness

A woman's familiarity with the appearance and feel of her breasts, which allows her to recognize both normal and abnormal changes. Doctors recommend that women develop breast awareness in order to improve the chance of detecting *breast cancer* at an early stage. (Women over 50 should also have regular *mammography*.)

Breast awareness has replaced the more formal technique of breast self-examination because there is no evidence that the routine self-examination technique is any more effective at detecting potentially serious changes than the more relaxed breast awareness. Therefore it is now recommended that women simply become familiar with the look and feel of their breasts at different times in a way that suits them.

NORMAL BREASTS

Every woman's breasts are unique so what is normal for one woman may not be for another. Also, a woman's breasts vary in appearance and feel depending on her age and the stage of her menstrual cycle (if premenopausal). The important thing is for a woman to become familar with what is normal for her personally.

However, there are general differences at different times of life. Before the menopause, the breasts tend to feel different at different times during the menstrual cycle. In the days preceding a period, the milk-producing glands become active and the breasts may feel lumpy and tender. After the menopause, the milk-producing glands are no longer active and the breasts tend to be less firm, softer, and not lumpy. After a hysterectomy, the breasts usually show the usual monthly changes until the time at which menopause would have occurred.

CHANGES TO BE AWARE OF

There are many possible causes for changes in the breasts, and most are not serious. However, they need to be

THE FEMALE **BREAST**

The breast is made up of lobes of glands set in fatty tissue, the ducts of which have their outlet at the nipple. The areola contains sweat glands, sebaceous glands, and hair follicles.

Fat
Skin
Areola
Nipple
Milk duct
Lobules
Fatty tissue
Pectoral muscle

A mammogram
An X-ray of a healthy breast. The dense white areas are fibrous tissues that support the fat nodules.

DISORDERS OF THE **BREAST**

Disorders of the breast are mostly minor and respond to treatment. Problems are most commonly caused by infection, hormonal changes, and tumours.

Infection

Mastitis (bacterial infection of breast tissue) often occurs with breast-feeding, usually due to a blocked milk duct. Untreated, it may lead to a *breast abscess*.

Hormonal changes

Breast pain and tenderness is common just before menstruation or when a woman is taking hormones. Before menstruation, breasts may increase in size and become lumpy. Such lumps shrink when menstruation is over. Hormonal disorders may, rarely, cause *galactorrhoea* (abnormal production of milk). In men, *gynaecomastia* (abnormal breast development) may occur as a result of hormonal disturbance or treatment with certain drugs.

Tumours

The majority of *breast lumps* are non-cancerous tumours, such as *cysts* (fluid-filled sacs) and *fibroadenomas* (thickened areas of milk-producing tissue). More rarely, *breast cancer* may occur.

INVESTIGATION

Disorders of the breast may be discovered during *breast awareness* or physical examination by a doctor. Special investigations for the breast include *biopsy* (removal of a small sample of tissue for analysis) and *mammography*.

checked by a doctor without delay because there is a small chance that they could be an early sign of breast cancer.

The changes to look out for are any lumps or thickened areas of tissue in one breast or armpit that are different from the corresponding part of the other breast or armpit; any alterations in the shape or outline of the breasts, particularly changes that occur when the arms are moved or the breasts are lifted; any dimpling or puckering of the skin of the breasts; any pain or discomfort in one breast that is different from usual; any rash on or around the nipple, or any bleeding or moist areas on the nipple that do not heal readily; any change in nipple position; and any discharge from the nipple (unless you are breast-feeding and it is a milky discharge).

breastbone

The common name for the *sternum*, the front part of the *thorax* (chest).

breast cancer

A cancerous tumour of the breast. Breast cancer is the most common type of cancer in women. One woman in every 11 who lives to old age will develop breast cancer at some point in her life. Breast cancer can also rarely develop in men. The advancement of techniques for early diagnosis and treatment of breast cancer has improved overall survival rates.

CAUSES

Current theories regarding the causes of breast cancer are focused on hormonal and genetic influences. However, the principal risk factor is age, with a woman's chance of developing the disease doubling every ten years of her life.

The incidence of breast cancer is higher than average in women whose menstrual periods began at an early age and in those whose *menopause* was late in commencing. The risk is also higher in women who did not have children, women who had their first child late in life, and women who did not breast-feed long-term. Women whose mothers or sisters had breast cancer are also at increased risk. Diet may also play a part; breast cancer is more common in countries in which the typical diet contains a lot of fat. Obesity and moderate to heavy alcohol intake also increase the risk. *Hormone replacement therapy (HRT)* may slightly increase the chance of developing breast cancer; the risk increases with the length of time HRT has been taken.

Breast cancer in women under the age of 50 may be linked to genetic factors and several genes have been identified, notably *BRCA1 and BRCA2*, mutations (changes), which are thought to account for about 10 per cent of all breast cancers. Women with one or more relatives who have developed the disease in their 30s or 40s may wish to seek specialist genetic advice.

SYMPTOMS AND SIGNS

The first sign of breast cancer is often a painless lump. However, it is important to note that nine out of ten breast lumps are not cancerous. Other symptoms of breast cancer may include a dark discharge from the nipple, retraction (indentation) of the nipple, and an area of dimpled, creased skin over the lump. In the majority of cases, only one breast is affected.

An abnormality may sometimes be detected during a routine *mammography*, which is offered every three years to all women between the ages of 50 and 70.

INVESTIGATION AND TREATMENT

If a lump is detected in the breast, an imaging procedure, such as mammography or *ultrasound scanning*, will be carried out. Cells will then be collected from the lump by fine-needle *aspiration*, a type of *biopsy* in which a hollow needle attached to a syringe is inserted into the breast and a small sample of cells is sucked out for analysis.

A small cancerous tumour that is not thought to have spread outside the breast is removed surgically, along with a surrounding margin of normal tissue. *Lymph nodes* in the armpit are usually removed at the same time. Larger cancers may require *mastectomy* (surgical removal of the whole breast). Surgery can be combined with or followed by *mammoplasty* (breast reconstruction) to help reduce the psychosexual impact of the disease.

Any further treatment depends on the size of the tumour; whether or not there is evidence of spread to the lymph nodes; and the sensitivity of the tumour cells to hormones, which is assessed in the laboratory using a technique known as oestrogen receptor testing. The woman's age and whether or not she has gone through the menopause are also significant factors in determining appropriate treatment.

After surgery, most women have a course of *radiotherapy* to any remaining breast tissue and to the armpit, and/or *chemotherapy* (treatment with *anticancer drugs*). *Tamoxifen*, an oral anti-oestrogen drug, is commonly prescribed following surgery for breast cancer to reduce the risk of recurrence. Drugs such as *trastuzumab* may be used to treat certain types of early-stage cancer and some cases of advanced cancer.

Women who are approaching the menopause may be offered treatment to bring on an early menopause if the tumour is oestrogen-sensitive.

Secondary tumours in other parts of the body, which may be present at the time of the initial diagnosis or may develop years after apparently successful treatment, are treated with anticancer drugs and hormones.

OUTLOOK
A complete cure or years of good health can usually be expected after treatment for early breast cancer. Regular check-ups are required to detect recurrence or the development of a new cancer in the other breast. Mammograms should be performed periodically for this reason. If the cancer recurs, it can be controlled, sometimes for years, by drugs and/or radiotherapy. (See also *breast awareness*.)

breast cyst

A fluid-filled lump that forms within the milk-producing tissue of the breast. Breast cysts most commonly affect women in their 30s and 40s, especially in the years leading up to the *menopause*. A lump can be diagnosed as a cyst by *ultrasound scanning*, a *mammography*, or by withdrawing fluid from it with a syringe and needle (see *aspiration*), which usually results in the lump disappearing. About half of all women with a breast cyst will develop future cysts. Any new breast lump should be seen by a doctor to confirm the diagnosis.

breast enlargement surgery

A type of *mammoplasty*.

breast-feeding

The natural method of infant feeding during the period between birth and weaning. Human milk contains the ideal balance of nutrients for a baby and provides valuable *antibodies* (proteins made by the immune system) against infections. For the first few days after childbirth, the breasts produce a watery fluid known as *colostrum*. Milk flow is stimulated by the baby's sucking and is usually established in about three to four days.

Breast-feeding problems may occur as a result of engorged breasts and cracked nipples or if the baby has problems sucking; a breast-feeding advisor may be able to help with these difficulties. Breast-feeding can sometimes cause infection of the breast tissue (see *mastitis*) that leads to a *breast abscess*. In such cases, treatment with *antibiotic drugs* may mean that it is possible to continue breast-feeding.

breast implant

An artificial structure surgically introduced into the breast to increase its size (see *mammoplasty*).

breast lump

Any mass, swelling, or cyst that can be felt in the breast tissue. At least 90 per cent of lumps are noncancerous; the rest are cancerous (see *breast cancer*).

Many women have generally lumpy breasts, with the lumps more obvious before a period. Once known as *fibrocystic disease* or *fibroadenosis*, this is now considered to be a variation of normal. Lumpy breasts do not increase the risk of breast cancer, but any new or distinct lump should be medically assessed. In a young woman, a single lump is likely to be a noncancerous *fibroadenoma*. This growth is usually round, firm, and rubbery, causes no pain, and can be moved about beneath the skin. In an older woman, a lump is more likely to be a noncancerous, fluid-filled *breast cyst*.

Breast awareness may help to detect any changes. Treatment depends on the cause and type of lump. Cysts can be drained in a simple outpatient procedure. Other lumps may need to be removed surgically.

breast pump

A device that is used to draw milk from overfull breasts during lactation (see *breast-feeding*). A breast pump may also be used to express milk for future use or to feed a baby who is unable to suckle.

breast reconstruction

See *mammoplasty*.

breast reduction

See *mammoplasty*.

breast self-examination

See *breast awareness*.

breast tenderness

Soreness or tenderness of the breasts, frequently accompanied by a feeling of fullness. Breast tenderness is extremely common. In most women it is cyclical, varying in severity in response to the hormonal changes of the menstrual cycle. The breasts are usually most tender before a period (see *premenstrual syndrome*). The condition tends to affect both breasts and may be aggravated by stress or caffeine. Breast tenderness may also be noncyclical, caused by muscle strain or *mastitis*. During lactation, it may be due to engorgement of the breasts with milk. Rarely, tenderness may be due to a *breast cyst* or to *breast cancer*. Examination by a doctor will exclude any underlying problems.

Women with large breasts are more likely to suffer from both cyclical and noncyclical breast tenderness.

Cyclical tenderness may be relieved by reduced caffeine intake, relaxation exercises for stress, a well-fitting bra, or weight loss to reduce breast size. If these measures do not work, hormonal treatment may be recommended.

breath-holding attacks

Periods during which a toddler holds his or her breath, usually as an expression of pain, frustration, or anger. The child usually becomes red or even blue in the face after a few seconds, and may faint. Breathing quickly resumes as a natural reflex, ending the attack. Breath-holding does not cause damage and is usually outgrown.

breathing

The process by which air passes into and out of the lungs to allow the blood to take up *oxygen* and dispose of *carbon dioxide*. Breathing is controlled by the respiratory centre in the *brainstem*. On inhalation, the diaphragm contracts and flattens. The intercostal muscles (the muscles between the ribs) contract and pull the ribcage up and out. The resulting increase in volume in the chest cavity causes the lungs to expand, and the reduced pressure draws air into the lungs. On exhalation, the chest muscles and diaphragm relax, causing the ribcage to sink and the lungs to contract, squeezing air out.

In normal, quiet breathing, less than a tenth of the air in the lungs passes out to be replaced by the same amount of fresh air (the tidal volume). This new air mixes with the stale air (the residual volume) already held in the lungs. The normal breathing rate for an adult at rest is 13 to 17 breaths per minute. (See also *respiration*.)

breathing difficulty

Laboured or distressed breathing that includes a change in the rate and depth of breathing or a feeling of breathlessness. Some degree of breathlessness is normal after exercise, particularly in unfit or overweight people. Breathlessness at rest is always abnormal and is usually due to disorders that affect the airways (see *asthma*), lungs (see *pulmonary disease, chronic obstructive*), or cardiovascular system (see *heart failure*). Severe anxiety can result in breathlessness, even when the lungs are normal (see *hyperventilation*). Damage to the breathing centre in the brainstem due to a *stroke* or *head injury* can affect breathing. This may also happen as a side effect of certain drugs. *Ventilator* assistance is sometimes needed.

At high altitudes the amount of oxygen in the air is reduced. Consequently, the lungs have to work harder in order to provide the body with sufficient oxygen (see *mountain sickness*) and a degree of breathlessness is therefore normal, although it should gradually diminish as the body becomes acclimatized to the lower oxygen concentration.

Breathlessness may occur in severe anaemia because abnormal or low levels of the oxygen-carrying pigment *haemoglobin* means that the lungs need to work harder to supply the body with oxygen. Breathing difficulty that intensifies on exertion may be caused by reduced circulation of blood through the lungs. This may be due to *heart failure* (reduced pumping efficiency of the heart), *pulmonary embolism* (blockage of blood vessels in the lungs by clots), or *pulmonary hypertension* (increased pressure in the arteries in the lungs).

Breathing difficulty due to air-flow obstruction may be caused by chronic *bronchitis*, asthma, an allergic reaction, or *lung cancer*. Breathing difficulty may also be due to inefficient transfer of oxygen from the lungs into the bloodstream. Temporary damage to the lung tissue may be due to *pneumonia, pneumothorax* (collapsed lung), *pulmonary oedema* (fluid in the lung), or *pleural effusion* (fluid around the lung). Permanent lung damage may be due to *emphysema*, a condition in which the small air sacs in the lungs are destroyed.

Chest pain (for example, due to a broken rib) that is made worse by chest or lung movement can make normal breathing difficult and painful, as can *pleurisy* (inflammation of the membrane that lines the lungs and chest cavity). Pleurisy is associated with pain in the lower chest and often in the shoulder tip on the affected side.

Abnormalities of the skeletal structure of the thorax (chest), such as severe *scoliosis* or *kyphosis*, may cause difficulty in breathing by impairing the normal movements of the ribcage.

BREATHING

In an adult, inhalation and exhalation occur between 13 and 17 times a minute at rest and up to 80 times a minute during vigorous exertion. A normal, resting inhalation takes in about 400 ml of air; a deep breath, up to 4 litres.

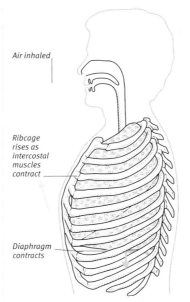

Air inhaled

Ribcage rises as intercostal muscles contract

Diaphragm contracts

Inhalation
Air is drawn into the lungs as the intercostal muscles (between the ribs) contract, causing the ribcage to rise, and the diaphragm contracts and flattens.

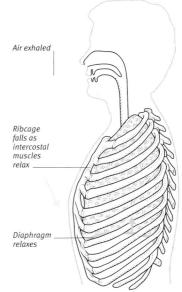

Air exhaled

Ribcage falls as intercostal muscles relax

Diaphragm relaxes

Exhalation
Air is expelled from the lungs as the intercostal muscles relax, causing the ribcage to fall, and the diaphragm relaxes and resumes its domed shape.

breathing exercises

Techniques for learning to control the rate and depth of breathing. They aim to teach people to inhale through the nose, while expanding the chest, and then to exhale fully through the mouth, while contracting the abdominal muscles. The exercises are used after chest surgery and for people with chronic obstructive pulmonary disease (see *pulmonary disease, chronic obstructive*), who often tend to have difficulty breathing effectively. Breathing exercises can also help people with *anxiety disorders* and may also help to relieve the symptoms of *asthma*.

In *yoga*, deep, rhythmic breathing is used to achieve a state of relaxation. During *childbirth*, breathing exercises can relax the mother and may also help to control the contractions of the uterus and reduce pain. (See also *physiotherapy*.)

breathing stoppage

The cessation of *breathing* (see *apnoea*). Breathing may be stopped by an *airway obstruction*, by damage to the brainstem (for example, following a *stroke*), by *Cheyne–Stokes respiration*, and, in children, by *breath-holding attacks*. (See also *choking*.)

breathlessness

A feeling of laboured breathing. Breathlessness is a normal response to exercise or exertion (and may occur with even mild exertion in unacclimatized people at high altitude), but may also be caused by some underlying disorders (see *breathing difficulty*).

breath test

A procedure used to check for infection of the digestive tract by HELICOBACTER PYLORI, the bacterium associated with *peptic ulcers*. The test involves drinking a substance that can be broken down by the bacterium. The breakdown process produces a chemical that passes into the bloodstream and is then breathed out. A machine detects the substance's presence in the breath, confirming infection with the bacterium.

breech delivery

A birth in which the fetus presents buttocks first. Many fetuses lie in a breech position before week 32 of pregnancy, but most of them turn by week 36. The three per cent that do not turn may be in one of three types of breech presentation: in a complete breech, the fetus is curled up; in a frank breech, the fetus's legs are extended and the feet are close to the face; in a footling breech, one or both feet are positioned over the cervix. In many twin pregnancies, one twin is in a breech position.

A mother whose fetus is in a breech presentation may be offered a procedure to turn the fetus around after week 36 of pregnancy, because this usually makes birth easier. For some breech deliveries, a *caesarean section* may be recommended.

bridge, dental

False teeth attached to natural teeth on either side of a gap left by one or more missing teeth (see the illustrated box). Adhesive bridges, which are attached to, but do not damage, the teeth on either side of the gap are now available in certain situations. (See also *denture*.)

Bright's disease

An alternative name for the kidney disorder *glomerulonephritis*.

Briquet's syndrome

An alternative name for *somatization disorder*, a psychiatric illness.

brittle bones

Bones with an increased tendency to fracture. They are a feature of *osteoporosis* and may occur in people who are taking *corticosteroid drugs*, are immobile, or have certain hormonal disorders. In *osteomalacia*, the bones are soft and tend both to become deformed and to fracture. The inherited disorder *osteogenesis imperfecta* is a rare cause of brittle bones and frequent fractures and is usually detected in infancy.

brittle diabetes

A former term for type 1 (insulin-dependent) *diabetes mellitus* in which it is difficult to maintain blood sugar levels within an acceptable range.

Broca's area

An area of the frontal lobe (usually the left lobe in right-handed people) of the cerebral cortex (the outer layer of the *brain*) that is responsible for speech origination. Damage to Broca's area may result in *aphasia* (a complete loss of previously acquired language skills).

Brodmann areas

Areas of the cerebral cortex (outer layer of the *brain*), that are numbered one to 47. Each area contains nerve cells that correspond to specific functions, such as sight, hearing, and movement.

broken leg

See *femur, fracture of*; *fibula*; *tibia*.

broken nose

Fracture of the nasal bones or dislocation of the cartilage that forms the bridge of the nose (see *nose, broken*).

broken tooth

See *fracture, dental*.

broken veins

A term that is commonly used to refer to *telangiectasia*, a condition in which the small blood vessels under the surface of the skin enlarge and give the impression of being "broken". The skin on the nose and cheeks is most commonly affected and may also have a reddened appearance.

bromocriptine

A drug used to suppress production of *prolactin* (a hormone) to treat conditions such as noncancerous pituitary tumours (see *prolactinomas*; *acromegaly*). Bromocriptine may also be used to suppress milk production after childbirth and to treat *Parkinson's disease*. Side effects include nausea and vomiting; high doses may cause drowsiness and confusion.

bronchial asthma

See *asthma*.

bronchiectasis

A lung disorder in which one or more bronchi (air passages leading from the trachea) are abnormally widened and distorted, with damaged linings. Bronchiectasis commonly develops during childhood and was once associated with infections such as *measles* and *pertussis* (whooping cough). The condition may also be a complication of *cystic fibrosis*. Bronchiectasis results in pockets of long-term infection within the airways and the continuous production of large volumes of green or yellow sputum (phlegm). Extensive bronchiectasis may cause shortness of breath.

Symptoms are usually controlled with *antibiotic drugs* and *postural drainage*, a

---

FITTING A **BRIDGE**

The most common type of bridge consists of one or more false teeth attached to a crown on each side of a gap. The natural teeth are shaped to receive the crowns, which are then cemented into place.

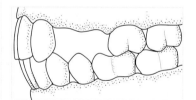

1 Two complete teeth are missing. A bridge of two false teeth and two crowns can be attached.

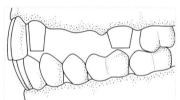

2 The two healthy teeth are shaped so that they can receive the crowns on either side of the gap.

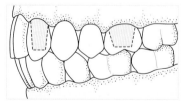

3 The bridge, which is mounted on a cast-metal subframe (not shown), is cemented on to the healthy teeth on either side of the gap.

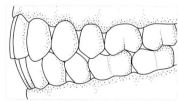

4 The finished bridge is in position, showing the new porcelain teeth; the metal base to which they are cemented is concealed.

technique that clears secretions from the lungs. If the condition is confined to one area of lung, surgical removal of the damaged area may be recommended.

bronchiole

One of many small airways of the *lungs*. Bronchioles branch from larger airways (bronchi) and subdivide into progressively smaller tubes before reaching the alveoli (see *alveolus, pulmonary*), where gases are exchanged.

bronchiolitis

An acute viral infection of the lungs, mainly affecting babies and young children, in which the bronchioles (the airways branching off the bronchi) become inflamed. A common cause is the respiratory syncytial virus (RSV).

Symptoms include rapid breathing, a cough, and fever. In mild cases no treatment may be necessary, although humidifying the air may enable the infant to breathe more easily. Sometimes a *bronchodilator drug* may be prescribed to widen the airways and help breathing. In severe cases, hospital admission may be necessary so that *oxygen therapy* can be given. If treatment is prompt, the infant usually recovers within a few days.

bronchitis

Inflammation of the bronchi, the large air passages to the lungs. It results in a cough that may produce considerable quantities of sputum (phlegm) and may be acute or chronic. Both types are more common in smokers and in areas with high atmospheric pollution. (See also *bronchitis, acute*; *bronchitis, chronic*.)

bronchitis, acute

A form of *bronchitis*, usually due to a viral infection, that develops suddenly but often clears up within a few days. Bacterial infection of the airways may be a complication. Smokers, babies, the elderly, and people with lung disease are particularly susceptible. Symptoms include wheezing, shortness of breath, and a cough producing yellow or green sputum. There may also be pain behind the sternum (breastbone) and fever.

Symptoms may be relieved by drinking plenty of fluids and inhaling steam or using a humidifier. Most cases clear up without further treatment, although secondary bacterial infection may require antibiotic drugs. Acute bronchitis may be serious in people who already have lung damage.

bronchitis, chronic

Smoking-induced inflammation of the airways associated with *emphysema*, in which the air sacs in the lungs are destroyed. The combination of chronic bronchitis and emphysema is known as chronic obstructive pulmonary disease (see *pulmonary disease, chronic obstructive*). Symptoms include a productive cough and progressive breathlessness.

bronchoconstrictor

A substance that causes narrowing of the airways. Bronchoconstrictors, such as *histamine*, are released during an allergic reaction (see *allergy*) and may provoke an *asthma* attack. The effect can be reversed by a *bronchodilator drug*.

bronchodilator drugs

COMMON DRUGS

SYMPATHOMIMETICS • Bambuterol • Eformoterol • Ephedrine • Epinephrine • Fenoterol • Salbutamol • Salmeterol • Terbutaline

ANTICHOLINERGICS • Ipratropium bromide • Tiotropium

XANTHINES • Aminophylline • Theophylline

Drugs that widen the bronchioles (small airways in the lungs) to improve air flow and breathing. They are especially used to treat *asthma* and chronic obstructive pulmonary disease (see *pulmonary disease, chronic obstructive*), in which the lungs are inflamed and damaged.

TYPES

There are three main types of bronchodilator drug. Sympathomimetics (such as *salbutamol*) are used primarily for the rapid relief of *breathing difficulty*. Anticholinergics (such as ipratropium) and xanthines (such as *aminophylline*) are more frequently used for the long-term prevention of attacks of breathing difficulty. Bronchodilators can be given by *inhaler*, in tablet form, or, in severe cases, by *nebulizer* or injection.

SIDE EFFECTS

The main side effects of sympathomimetic bronchodilators are palpitations and trembling. Anticholinergics may cause dry mouth, blurred vision, and, rarely, difficulty in passing urine. Xanthines may cause headaches, nausea, and palpitations.

bronchography

An *X-ray* procedure used for examining the bronchi, which are the two main air passages of the lungs. Once used to diagnose *bronchiectasis* (widening and distortion of the bronchi), this method has now been largely replaced by other imaging techniques, especially *CT scanning*, and by *bronchoscopy*.

bronchopneumonia

The most common form of *pneumonia*. In bronchopneumonia, inflammation is spread throughout the lungs in small patches around the airways; in lobar pneumonia, it is confined to one lobe.

bronchoscopy

Examination of the bronchi, the main airways of the lungs (see *bronchus*), by means of an *endoscope* (viewing tube) known as a bronchoscope. Bronchoscopes may be rigid or flexible.

WHY IT IS DONE

Bronchoscopy is performed to inspect the bronchi for abnormalities, such as *lung cancer* and *tuberculosis*; to collect samples of mucus; to obtain cells; and to take *biopsy* samples from the airways or lungs. A bronchoscope with special attachments is used to carry out treatments such as removing inhaled foreign bodies, destroying abnormal growths, and sealing off damaged blood vessels. (See also *Bronchoscopy* box, overleaf.)

bronchospasm

Temporary narrowing of the bronchi (the air passages to the lungs). Bronchospasm is caused by contraction of the muscles in the walls of the bronchi, by inflammation of the lining of the bronchi, or by a combination of both. Contraction may be triggered by the release of substances during an allergic reaction (see *allergy*). When the airways are narrowed, the air is reduced, causing wheezing or coughing.

Asthma is the most common cause of bronchospasm. Other possible causes include respiratory infection, chronic obstructive pulmonary disease (see *pulmonary disease, chronic obstructive*), in which the lungs are inflamed and damaged, *anaphylactic shock* (a potentially life-threatening hypersensitivity reaction), or allergic reaction to chemicals.

bronchus

A large air passage in a lung. Each lung has one main bronchus, originating at the end of the trachea (windpipe). This main bronchus divides into smaller branches known as segmental bronchi, which further divide into *bronchioles*.

bronchus, cancer of

See *lung cancer*.

HOW **BRONCHODILATORS** WORK

When bronchioles become narrow following contraction of the muscle layer and swelling of the mucous lining, the passage of air is impeded. Bronchodilator drugs relax the muscles surrounding bronchioles by acting on the nerve signals that govern muscle activity.

Sympathomimetic and anticholinergic drugs interfere with nerve signals passed to the muscles through the autonomic nervous system. Sympathomimetics enhance the action of neurotransmitters that encourage muscle relaxation. Anticholinergics block the neurotransmitters that trigger muscle contraction. Xanthine drugs relax muscle in the bronchioles by a direct effect on the muscle fibres; however, their precise action is not fully understood.

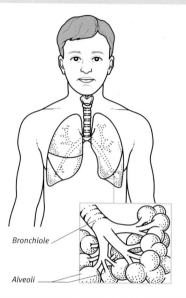

Bronchiole

Alveoli

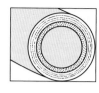

Normal bronchioles
The muscle surrounding the bronchioles is relaxed, leaving the airway open.

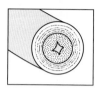

During an asthma attack
The muscle contracts and the lining swells, narrowing the airway.

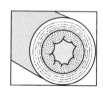

After drug treatment
The muscles relax, opening the airway, but the mucous lining remains swollen.

BRONCHOSCOPY

There are two kinds of bronchoscope. The rigid type is a hollow tube that is passed into the bronchi via the mouth and requires a general anaesthetic. The flexible, fibre-optic bronchoscope (a narrower tube formed from light-transmitting fibres) can be inserted through either the mouth or nose. It is used after giving only a mild sedative and/or local anaesthetic and it reaches further into the lungs. Both types of bronchoscope can be fitted with forceps for taking tissue samples and the instrument also has attachments for performing laser therapy and cryosurgery. (See also *endoscopy*.)

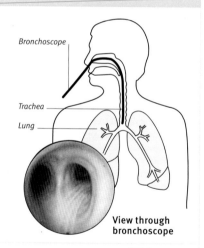

Bronchoscope

Trachea

Lung

View through bronchoscope

BRONCHOSCOPE

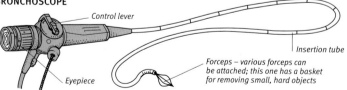

Control lever

Insertion tube

Forceps – various forceps can be attached; this one has a basket for removing small, hard objects

Eyepiece

bronze diabetes

An outdated term for *haemochromatosis*, a rare genetic disorder in which excess *iron* is deposited in tissues; this may lead to bronze skin coloration and the development of *diabetes mellitus*.

brown fat

A special type of fat found in infants and some animals. Located mainly between and around the shoulderblades, brown fat provides energy and helps infants to maintain a constant body temperature.

Brown–Sequard syndrome

A combination of symptoms associated with damage to a part of the *spinal cord*. There is loss of pain and temperature sensation on the opposite side of the body below the damage, and weakness and stiffness of muscles below the damage on the same side of the body.

brow presentation

A rare form of *malpresentation* in which the head of the fetus is bent slightly backwards and its brow lies against the mother's cervix. Vaginal delivery is not possible if this presentation persists throughout labour, and a *caesarean section* is then required.

brucellosis

A rare bacterial infection, caused by various strains of BRUCELLA, which may be transmitted to humans from affected cattle, goats, and pigs. The infection may also be transmitted in unpasteurized dairy products.

Brucellosis causes high fever, sweating, poor appetite, joint aches, headache, backache, weakness, and depression. Rarely, severe untreated cases lead to *pneumonia* or *meningitis* (inflammation of the membranes surrounding the brain and spinal cord). In long-term brucellosis, bouts of the illness recur over months or years, and the depression can be severe. The disease is treated with *antibiotic drugs*.

bruise

A discoloured area under the skin caused by leakage of blood from damaged capillaries (tiny blood vessels). The blood initially appears blue or black; as the *haemoglobin* (the red pigment in blood) breaks down, the bruise turns a yellowish colour.

A bruise that does not fade after about week, that appears for no apparent reason, or that is severe after only minor injury, may indicate a *bleeding disorder*. (See also *black eye*; *purpura*.)

bruits

The sounds that are made in the heart, arteries, or veins when the blood circulation becomes turbulent or when it flows abnormally fast. This may happen when blood vessels widen (as in an *aneurysm*), when they become narrowed by disease (as in *arteriosclerosis*), or when heart valves are narrowed or damaged (as in *endocarditis*). Bruits can be heard by a doctor through a *stethoscope*. (See also *carotid bruit*.)

bruxism

Rhythmic grinding or clenching of the teeth that usually occurs during sleep. The main causes are emotional stress and minor discomfort when the teeth are brought together. Continued bruxism may wear away the teeth.

BSE

The abbreviation for *bovine spongiform encephalopathy*.

bubo

An inflamed and swollen *lymph node*, usually in the groin or armpit. Buboes usually occur as the result of a bacterial infection such as *plague* or a *sexually transmitted infection*.

bubonic plague

The most common form of *plague*, characterized by the development of a *bubo* (a swollen lymph node) in the groin or armpit.

buccal

A term that refers to the cheek or mouth. Buccal preparations of some drugs are available. Placed between the cheek and gum, they dissolve and are absorbed directly into the blood circulation.

buck teeth

Prominent upper incisors (front teeth) that protrude from the mouth. Orthodontic treatment of buck teeth involves repositioning the teeth with a removable brace (see *brace, dental*) or a fixed *orthodontic appliance*.

Budd–Chiari syndrome

A rare disorder in which the veins draining blood from the liver become blocked or narrowed. Blood accumulates in the liver, which swells. *Liver failure* and *portal hypertension* (raised pressure in the vein carrying blood to the liver) result.

Treatment is aimed at removing the cause of the obstruction to the draining of blood from the liver; this may be a blood clot, pressure on the veins from a liver tumour, or a congenital (present from birth) abnormality of the veins. In most cases, treatment has only a limited effect and, unless a *liver transplant* can be carried out, the disease is generally fatal within two years.

budesonide

A *corticosteroid drug* used in the prevention of bronchial *asthma* attacks. Budesonide is administered using an *inhaler*. Adverse effects, which include hoarseness, throat irritation and, rarely, fungal infections, can be reduced by rinsing the mouth after administration of the drug.

Buerger's disease

A rare disorder, also known as thromboangiitis obliterans, in which the nerves, arteries, and veins in the legs, and sometimes the arms, become severely inflamed. The blood supply to the toes and fingers becomes cut off, eventually causing *gangrene* (tissue death). Buerger's disease is most common in men under the age of 45 who smoke heavily.

buffalo hump

A lump of fat under the skin on the back of the neck. A buffalo hump may develop following long-term treatment with high doses of *corticosteroid drugs* or as a result of *Cushing's syndrome*.

building-related illnesses

Another term for the group of symptoms known as *sick building syndrome*.

bulbar palsy

Weakness of the muscles involved in talking and swallowing, causing slurred speech, hoarseness, difficulty in swallowing, and choking on food and drink. Bulbar palsy may be caused by damage to the muscles' nerve supply, as in *motor neuron disease*, or disease of the muscles themselves, as in *muscular dystrophy*.

bulimia

A psychiatric illness that is characterized by bouts of overeating, usually followed by self-induced vomiting or excessive use of *laxatives*. Most people suffering from bulimia are girls or women between the ages of 15 and 30. In some cases, the symptoms coexist with those of *anorexia nervosa*.

Repeated vomiting can lead to dehydration and loss of potassium, which may cause weakness and cramps, and also causes tooth damage due to the gastric acid in vomit. Treatment of bulimia includes supervision and regulation of the person's eating habits, *psychotherapy* (such as *cognitive-behavioural therapy*), and, in some cases, antidepressant drugs (*see selective serotonin reuptake inhibitors*).

bulk-forming agent

A type of *antidiarrhoeal drug* that absorbs water, thereby making stools less liquid. Bulk-forming agents are also used as *laxatives*, stimulating bowel movement by softening the faeces and increasing their bulk.

bulla

A large air- or fluid-filled bubble that is usually found in the lungs or skin. Lung bullae in young adults are usually *congenital* (present from birth). In later life, lung bullae develop in patients with *emphysema*, a disorder in which the air sacs in the lungs are gradually destroyed. Skin bullae are large, fluid-filled *blisters* with a variety of causes, including the bullous disease *pemphigus*.

bull-neck

Swelling of the neck caused by severely swollen *lymph glands*, often related to infections in the tonsils and throat. (See also *diphtheria*.)

bullous pemphigoid

An alternative term for *pemphigoid*, a skin disease in which large, tense blisters develop.

bumetanide

A powerful, short-acting loop *diuretic drug* used to treat *oedema* (accumulation of fluid in tissues) resulting from *heart failure*, *nephrotic syndrome* (damage to the kidney's filtering units), or *cirrhosis*. It may be given by injection for the emergency treatment of *pulmonary oedema* (accumulation of fluid in the lungs). Side effects may include rash and muscle pain.

bundle

Also known as a fascicle, a cluster of nerve or muscle fibres.

bundle branch block

See *heart block*.

bunion

A thickened pad of tissue or a fluid-filled bursa (sac) overlying a deformed big-toe joint. The underlying cause is an abnormal outward projection of the big toe called a *hallux valgus*. Small bunions can usually be remedied by wearing well-fitting shoes and a special toe pad to straighten the big toe. Large bunions may require surgery to realign the joint and relieve the pressure.

buphthalmos

A large, prominent eyeball in an infant due to congenital *glaucoma* (increased pressure inside the eyeball). The condition is usually treated with surgery to reduce the pressure; otherwise, the child's sight is progressively damaged.

HOW **BUNIONS** FORM

A bunion results from the rubbing of a shoe against an abnormal outward projection of the joint at the base of the big toe (a hallux valgus), leading to irritation and inflammation. The joint abnormality is often due to wearing narrow, pointed shoes with high heels, although it can also result from an inherited weakness in the joint.

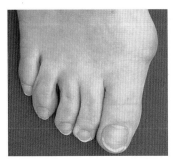

Bunion
Valgus deformity of the joint between the first metatarsal bone and the adjoining phalanx.

---

bupivacaine

A long-acting local anaesthetic (see *anaesthesia, local*) often used as a *nerve block* during *childbirth* and in *epidural anaesthesia* and *spinal anaesthesia*. Side effects are uncommon, but high doses may cause blood pressure to fall.

bupropion

Another name for *amfebutamone*, a drug used, togther with self-help measures, as an aid to stopping smoking.

Burkitt's lymphoma

A cancer of lymph tissues (see *lymphatic system*) characterized by the development of tumours within the jaw and/or the abdomen. Associated with infection with the *Epstein–Barr virus*, Burkitt's lymphoma almost exclusively affects children living in the low-lying, moist, tropical regions of Africa and New Guinea. *Anticancer drugs* or *radiotherapy* give a partial or complete cure in approximately 80 per cent of cases. (See also *lymphoma*.)

burns

Tissue damage caused by contact with heat, electricity, chemicals, or radiation. Burns are classified, according to the severity of skin damage, as first-, second-, or third-degree (or superficial, partial thickness, or full thickness).

FIRST-DEGREE BURNS

A first-degree burn causes reddening of the skin and affects only the epidermis, (topmost layer of skin). These types of burns usually heal quickly, but the damaged skin may peel away after a day or two. *Sunburn* is a common example of a first-degree burn.

SECOND-DEGREE BURNS

A second-degree burn extends into, and damages, the dermis (deep layer of skin), sometimes causing the formation of blisters. Because some of the dermis is left to recover, these types of burns usually heal without leaving scars, unless they are very deep.

THIRD-DEGREE BURNS

A third-degree burn destroys the full skin thickness and may extend to the muscle layer beneath the skin. The affected area will look white or charred; if the burn is very deep, muscles and bones may be exposed. Even if very localized, third-degree burns will need specialist treatment and possibly skin grafts to prevent scarring.

ELECTRICAL BURNS

Electrical burns can cause extensive tissue damage with minimal external skin damage. The electric current may cause heart damage.

EFFECTS AND COMPLICATIONS

Extensive first-degree burns (such as sunburn) cause pain, restlessness, fever, and headache, but are not life-threatening. A second- or third-degree burn that affects more than ten per cent of the body surface causes *shock*, with lowered blood pressure and a rapid pulse, due to massive fluid loss from the burned area. Shock may be fatal if this fluid is not replaced intravenously.

When the skin is burned it can no longer protect the body from contamination by airborne bacteria. The infection of extensive burns may cause fatal complications if effective treatment with *antibiotic drugs* is not available.

Victims who have inhaled smoke may develop inflammation of the lungs and may need specialist care for burns of the eyes and respiratory passages.

TREATMENT

A burn is covered with a non-stick dressing to keep the area moist. *Analgesic drugs* are given if necessary and antibiotics are prescribed if there is any infection. For extensive second-degree burns, which may be slow to heal or carry a high risk of infection, a topical antibacterial agent, such as silver sulfadiazine, is used. Third-degree burns always require *skin grafts*, which are used early to minimize scarring. Extensive burns may require *plastic surgery*.

burping

Another term for *belching*.

burr hole

A hole made in the skull by a special drill with a rounded tip (burr). The hole relieves pressure on the brain that often results from bleeding inside the skull, usually due to a *head injury*. Burr holes may be part of a *craniotomy* (in which a section of skull is removed for access to the brain) and may be life-saving.

bursa

A fluid-filled sac that acts as a cushion at a pressure point, often where a tendon or muscle crosses bone or other muscles. The important bursae are found around the knee, elbow, and shoulder joints.

bursitis

Inflammation of a *bursa* (a fluid-filled sac) causing pain and swelling. Bursitis may result from pressure, friction, or injury to the membrane surrounding a

BURNS

Superficial burns cause the skin to redden and peel but, unless extensive, need no treatment. Burns that blister usually heal well but can be fatal if they affect a large area of the body. Burns that extend beyond the skin layers may damage fat, nerves, and muscle; and healing is slow because they are likely to require skin grafting.

The skin

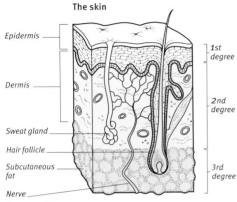

Epidermis

Dermis

Sweat gland

Hair follicle

Subcutaneous fat

Nerve

1st degree

2nd degree

3rd degree

Degrees of burns
Burns are divided into three categories. First-degree (superficial) burns affect the epidermis and the skin may peel; second-degree (partial thickness) burns extend into the dermis and cause blisters; third-degree (full thickness) burns destroy the whole of the skin's thickness.

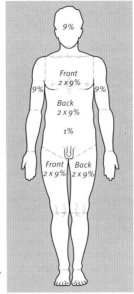

9%

Front
2 x 9%

9%   9%

Back
2 x 9%

1%

Front   Back
2 x 9%   2 x 9%

Skin surface area
For assessment of burns, the body is divided into roughly nine per cent areas. This varies slightly In young children because the head is larger in relation to the body.

---

joint, or to infection. Prepatellar bursitis (also known as housemaid's knee), for example, is the result of prolonged kneeling on a hard surface. Treatment is by avoiding further pressure and by taking *nonsteroidal anti-inflammatory drugs*. *Antibiotic drugs* may be necessary if the bursa is infected.

buserelin

A synthetic form of the hormone *gonadorelin* that is used to treat *endometriosis* (a disease of the lining of

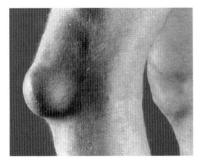

Prepatellar bursitis
This condition, which is caused by inflammation of a bursa, produces a fluid-filled swelling in front of the kneecap.

the uterus), infertility, and cancer of the prostate gland.

butterfly rash

Also called a butterfly patch, a red, blotchy, butterfly-shaped skin eruption that appears on the cheeks and across the bridge of the nose in some people with the *autoimmune disease* (one in which the immune system attacks the body's own tissues) systemic *lupus erythematosus*. (See also *rash*.)

buzzer and pad system

A device used to treat bedwetting (see *enuresis, nocturnal*). A pad that detects moisture is placed in the bed and is attached to a buzzer that sounds when the pad becomes wet with urine. The person is woken up as soon as he or she starts to pass urine and gradually learns to wake up before starting to pass urine.

bypass operations

Surgical procedures that are used to bypass blockages or narrowing. The term "bypass" usually refers to operations on arteries, although blockages in

the digestive system can also be treated with bypass operations.

The most common type of bypass operation is *coronary artery bypass*, which is used to treat *coronary artery disease*, (a condition in which the arteries have become blocked or narrowed by *atherosclerosis*). Obstructions can be bypassed by using sections of healthy artery or vein from elsewhere in the body or using tubing made from a synthetic material such as dacron.

Intestinal bypass operations are most often performed to treat cancer patients in whom the tumour is too extensive to be removed surgically. The blocked area is bypassed by joining together the sections of bowel above and below the blockage.

byssinosis

A lung disease caused by the dust that is produced during the processing of flax, cotton, hemp, or sisal.

Byssinosis causes a feeling of tightness in the chest and shortness of breath that may become chronic (of long duration) if exposure to the causative agent continues.

Bronchodilator drugs and other drugs used to treat asthma can relieve the symptoms of byssinosis. Good ventilation and the use of safety equipment, such as breathing masks, reduce the risk of developing the disease.

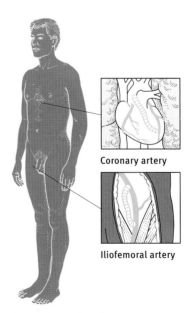

Coronary artery

Iliofemoral artery

Common bypass locations
The coronary artery and the iliofemoral vessels are the most common locations for bypasses.

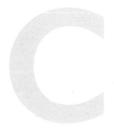

cachexia

A condition of severe weight loss and decline in health caused by a serious underlying disease, such as cancer or tuberculosis, or by starvation.

cadaver

A dead human body used as a source of transplant organs or for anatomical study and dissection.

cadmium poisoning

The toxic effects of cadmium, a tinlike metal. Poisoning as a result of inhalation of cadmium fumes is an industrial hazard, the effects of which depend on the duration and severity of exposure. Eating vegetables grown in cadmium-rich soil, or the consumption of food or drink stored in cadmium-lined containers, can also cause poisoning.

Short-term exposure to cadmium may lead to *pneumonitis* (inflammation of the lungs). Exposure over a long period can lead to urinary tract *calculi* (stones), *kidney failure*, or *emphysema* (a form of permanent lung damage).

caecum

The first section of the large intestine, joining the *ileum* (the end of the small intestine) to the ascending *colon*. The *appendix* projects from the caecum. (See also *digestive system*.)

caesarean section

An operation to deliver a baby from the mother's uterus through a horizontal or, less commonly, a vertical incision in the abdomen. A caesarean section is performed if vaginal delivery would be difficult or dangerous for the mother or the baby, for example, if there is *fetal distress*, *placenta praevia*, or *pre-eclampsia*.

A caesarean section may be performed using either an *epidural anaesthesia* or general anaesthesia (see *anaesthesia, general*). The procedure for performing a caesarean section is shown in the illustrated box (see opposite page).

After the operation, the mother is given *analgesic drugs* (painkillers) as required. If there are no complications, she and the baby can usually leave hospital about four to five days after the operation.

café au lait spots

Coffee-coloured patches on the skin that may occur on any part of the body. Café au lait spots are usually oval in shape and may measure several centimetres across. Generally, the presence of a few of these spots is not significant. However, larger numbers of them may be a sign of *neurofibromatosis*, a hereditary disorder of the sheaths that surround nerve fibres.

caffeine

A *stimulant drug* that is found in coffee, tea, cocoa, and cola drinks. Caffeine reduces fatigue, improves concentration, makes the heart pump blood faster, and has a diuretic effect.

CAFFEINE LEVELS

The strength and preparation method determine exact amounts of caffeine present (in mg per cup).

Drink	Caffeine	
Tea, weak	50mg	
Tea, strong	80mg	
Coffee, weak	80mg	
Coffee, strong		200mg
Cocoa	10–17mg	
Cola	43–75mg	

Large quantities of caffeine may produce side effects such as agitation and tremors. A regular high intake may lead to increased *tolerance*, so that people need to increase their caffeine intake to obtain the equivalent stimulant effect. In people who consume large amounts of caffeine, withdrawal symptoms (see *withdrawal syndrome*), such as headaches and tiredness, may occur after a few hours without caffeine.

Caffeine may be used in some drug preparations, particularly in combination with *analgesic drugs* (painkillers) and with *ergotamine* in preventive treatments for migraine.

caisson disease

An alternative term for *decompression sickness*. It usually occurs when a person surfaces too quickly after a deep dive.

calamine

A preparation of zinc oxide and iron oxide that is applied to the skin as an ointment, lotion, or dusting powder to relieve irritation and itching. Calamine has a protective, cooling, and drying effect on the skin.

calcaneal bursitis

Inflammation of the bursa (fluid-filled pad) that cushions the *calcaneus* (heel bone) and prevents friction at the back of the heel (see *bursitis*). The condition causes pain and swelling but usually clears up with rest and the use of *anti-inflammatory drugs*.

calcaneus

The heel bone. The calcaneus is one of the tarsal (ankle) bones and is the largest bone in the *foot*. The *Achilles tendon* runs between the back of the calcaneus and the calf muscles; the tendon controls upward and downward movements of the foot.

DISORDERS

The calcaneus may be fractured by a fall from a height on to the heel. Minor fractures do not usually cause problems and can be treated by placing the affected foot and leg in a *cast*. A more serious fracture, with compression of the bone, may cause permanent damage to the joints involved in turning the foot in and out, leading to pain and stiffness that are aggravated by walking.

The point at which the Achilles tendon joins the calcaneus may become strained by excessive or prolonged stress from the pull of the tendon (in some *running injuries*, for example). In children, this area may be inflamed and painful (see *osteochondrosis*) because the bone is still growing.

LOCATION OF THE CALCANEUS

The calcaneus is the largest of the tarsal bones. It projects backwards beyond the leg bones.

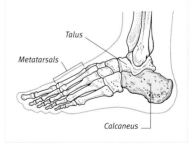

PROCEDURE FOR A **CAESAREAN SECTION**

A caesarean section allows delivery of a baby through a horizontal or vertical cut in the abdominal and uterine walls. The mother is given epidural anaesthesia, so that she remains conscious during the procedure, or general anaesthesia.

HOW IT IS DONE

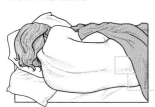

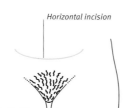

Vertebra

Spinal cord

Epidural space

Skin   Catheter

1 First, epidural anaesthesia is carried out to temporarily numb the abdomen by deadening the nerves leading to it. A needle is introduced into the epidural space and a catheter is threaded through it. A local anaesthetic is injected down the catheter. A catheter is also inserted into the bladder to empty it.

Horizontal incision

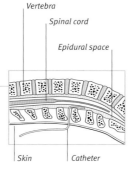

2 The abdomen is then opened, usually through a horizontal incision made just above the pubic bone. This type of cut heals most effectively. The resulting scar is hardly noticeable and comes below the "bikini line".

WHY IT IS DONE

A caesarean can be elective (planned) in cases of breech presentation; placenta praevia (where the placenta is lying close to or across the cervix); the mother's ill health; or, most commonly, if there were problems in previous caesareans that still exist (such as the mother having a small pelvis). Elective caesarean is sometimes requested by the parents for social reasons.

An emergency caesarean is needed in cases of *fetal distress* (lack of oxygen); unsuccessful induction of labour; or bleeding (such as in placental abruption (premature separation) or placenta praevia).

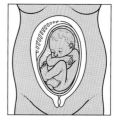

Breech presentation

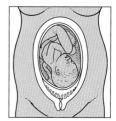

Placenta praevia

3 The amniotic fluid is drained off by suction. The baby is delivered through an incision in the lower part of the uterus. The umbilical cord is cut and the afterbirth removed. The incisions in the uterus and abdomen are then sewn up. The mother is given an injection of ergometrine and oxytocin to make the uterus contract and stop any bleeding.

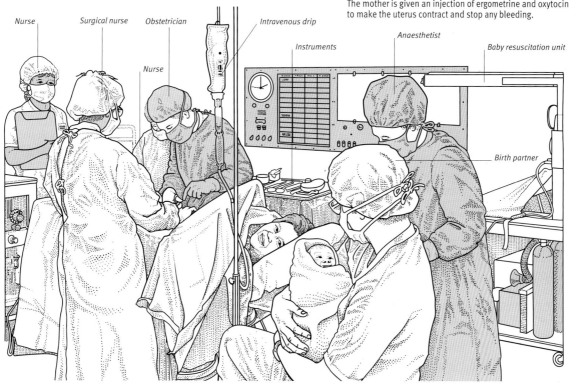

Nurse   Surgical nurse   Obstetrician   Intravenous drip   Anaesthetist   Baby resuscitation unit

Nurse   Instruments

Birth partner

C

The tendons of the sole of the foot are fixed under the calcaneus, and the associated muscles are important in supporting the arches of the foot. Inflammation around these tendons (as occurs in plantar *fasciitis*) causes pain and tenderness under the heel when standing or walking. A calcaneal spur (a bony protrusion) occurs in some people with plantar fasciitis and also, occasionally, in those with healthy feet.

calciferol

A former name for vitamin D₂. This vitamin is now more commonly known as ergocalciferol (see *vitamin D*).

calcification

The deposition of *calcium* salts in body tissues. Calcification is part of the normal processes of bone and teeth formation and the healing of fractures. It also occurs in injured muscles, in arteries affected by *atherosclerosis*, and when blood calcium levels are raised by disorders of the *parathyroid glands*.

calcification, dental

The deposition of *calcium* salts in developing teeth. Primary teeth (see *eruption of teeth*) begin to calcify in a fetus at between three and six months gestation. Calcification of permanent teeth (other than the wisdom teeth) begins between birth and four years.

Certain tooth conditions can cause abnormal calcification. In amelogenesis imperfecta, an enamel disorder (see *hypoplasia, enamel*), teeth have a thin, grooved covering due to incomplete calcification. Another cause is absorption of high levels of fluoride (see *fluorosis*) and drugs, such as *tetracycline*, that are taken in pregnancy.

calcinosis

The abnormal deposition of *calcium* salts in the skin, muscles, or *connective tissues*, forming *nodules*. Calcinosis occurs in connective tissue disorders such as *scleroderma*. (See also *calcification*.)

calcipotriol

A derivative of *vitamin D* that is used in topical treatments for the skin condition *psoriasis*.

calcitonin

A *hormone* produced by the *thyroid gland* that helps to control blood *calcium* levels by slowing the rate at which calcium is lost from the bones.

WHY IT IS USED

A synthetic form of calcitonin used in the treatment of *Paget's disease*, in which the bones grow abnormally and become deformed, causing pain and an increased risk of fracture. Injections of calcitonin can generally halt abnormal bone formation in about a week and can relieve pain within a few months.

Calcitonin is also used in the treatment of *osteoporosis* (thinning of the bones) and *hypercalcaemia* (abnormally high levels of calcium in the blood), which may be caused by overactivity of the *parathyroid glands* or by *bone cancer*. It helps to relieve the nausea and vomiting that result from hypercalcaemia by rapidly reducing the blood level of calcium.

SIDE EFFECTS

Calcitonin causes minimal side effects. Gastrointestinal reactions, such as nausea, vomiting, and diarrhoea, usually diminish with continued use.

calcium

The body's most abundant mineral, calcium is essential for cell function, muscle contraction, the transmission of nerve impulses from nerve endings to muscle fibres, and for *blood clotting*. Calcium phosphate is the hard, basic constituent of teeth and bones. Dietary sources of calcium include dairy products, eggs, and green, leafy vegetables.

CONTROL OF CALCIUM LEVELS

Vitamin D and certain hormones help to control the overall amount of calcium in the body. They act by regulating the amount of calcium that is absorbed from food and the amount filtered out from the blood by the kidneys and excreted in the urine.

The levels of calcium in the blood are controlled by the actions of two hormones: parathyroid hormone, which is produced by the *parathyroid glands*, and *calcitonin*, which is produced by the thyroid gland. When the level of calcium in the blood falls to a low level, the parathyroid glands release more parathyroid hormone, which raises the blood calcium level by helping to release calcium from the enormous reservoir in the bones. When the blood calcium level rises significantly, the thyroid gland releases more calcitonin. This hormone counteracts the effects of parathyroid hormone, thereby lowering the level of calcium in the blood.

DISORDERS OF CALCIUM METABOLISM

Abnormally high levels of calcium in the blood (*hypercalcaemia*) or abnormally low levels (*hypocalcaemia*) may seriously disrupt cell function, particularly in muscles and nerves. (See also *mineral supplements*.)

calcium carbonate

A *calcium* salt used in some *antacid drugs*, which can be taken for the treatment of indigestion.

calcium channel blockers

COMMON DRUGS

- Amlodipine • Diltiazem • Felodipine
- Isradipine • Lacidipine • Lercanidipine
- Nicardipine • Nifedipine • Verapamil

Drugs used in the treatment of *angina pectoris* (chest pain due to impaired blood supply to the heart muscle), *hypertension* (high blood pressure), and certain types of cardiac *arrhythmia* (irregular heartbeat).

HOW THEY WORK

Calcium channel blockers work by interfering with the movement of *calcium* across the membranes of muscle cells in blood vessels and in the heart muscle itself. This action decreases the work of the heart in pumping blood, reduces the pressure of blood flow through the body, and improves blood circulation through the heart muscle.

The drugs also slow the passage of nerve impulses through the heart's internal conduction system, which helps to correct certain types of arrhythmia.

SIDE EFFECTS

The side effects of calcium channel blockers are mainly related to their action of increasing the blood flow through tissues. These effects include headaches, swollen ankles, flushing, and dizziness. Adverse effects tend to diminish with continued treatment.

calculus

A hard deposit in the body. Calculus may form on the surface of the teeth (see *calculus, dental*). Alternatively, it may be a small, hard, crystalline mass that forms in a body cavity from certain substances in fluids such as bile, urine, or saliva. Such calculi (also called stones) can occur in the gallbladder and bile ducts (see *gallstones*), kidneys, ureters, bladder (see *calculus, urinary tract*), or in the salivary ducts.

Although some calculi do not cause any symptoms, some can cause severe pain, in which case they may need to be dissolved, shattered, or surgically removed from the body cavity.

C

calculus, dental

A hard, crustlike deposit, also called tartar, found on the crowns and roots of the teeth. Calculus forms when mineral salts in saliva are deposited in existing *plaque*, a coating of mucus and debris that forms on the teeth.

TYPES
There are two types of dental calculus. Supragingival calculus is a yellowish or white deposit that forms above the gum margin, on the crowns of teeth in areas close to the openings of *salivary gland* ducts. Subgingival calculus forms below the gum margin, is more evenly distributed around all the teeth, and is brown or black.

Both types of calculus are hard and are therefore difficult to remove; the subgingival variety may be more difficult to remove because of its location and degree of calcification.

EFFECTS AND TREATMENT
The toxins present in calculus can lead to gum inflammation (see *gingivitis*), which may progress to destruction of the supporting tissues (see *periodontitis*). Calculus should be removed on a regular basis by professional *scaling*. Careful attention to *oral hygiene* may reduce the recurrence of dental calculus.

calculus, urinary tract

A stone in the kidneys, ureters, or bladder that is formed from crystallized substances in the urine.

TYPES AND CAUSES
Kidney and ureteral stones Most stones that form in the kidneys and ureters are composed of calcium oxalate or other salts crystallized from the urine. These stones may be associated with a diet that is rich in oxalates (which are found, for example, in leafy vegetables and tea); high levels of *calcium* in the blood due to *hyperparathyroidism* (overactivity of the parathyroid glands); or chronic dehydration.

Other types of kidney or ureteral stone are associated with *gout* and certain cancers. Stones that develop in these locations due to chronic *urinary tract infection* are termed "infective". Kidney stones that fill the entire network of urine-collecting ducts at the top of the ureter are called staghorn calculi, due to their shape.

Bladder stones In developing countries, bladder stones usually occur as a result of dietary deficiencies. In developed countries, they are usually caused by an obstruction to urine flow from the

bladder and/or a longstanding urinary tract infection. The composition of the stones is related to the acidity or alkalinity of the urine.

SYMPTOMS
The most common symptom of a stone in the kidney or ureter is *renal colic*, a severe pain in the back, under the ribs, that often spreads into the groin. This pain may be accompanied by nausea and vomiting. There may also be *haematuria* (blood in the urine). A bladder stone usually causes difficulty and pain on passing urine.

DIAGNOSIS AND TREATMENT
Investigation of a suspected calculus usually starts with microscopic examination of the urine, which may reveal red blood cells and the presence of crystals. The degree of acidity or alkalinity of the urine may reflect the type of stone involved. The site of a stone

can usually be confirmed by a plain X-ray, although *ultrasound scanning* or *CT scanning* may also be used.

Renal colic is treated with bed rest and an *analgesic drug* (painkiller). With an adequate fluid intake, small stones are usually passed in the urine without causing problems. The first line of treatment for larger stones in the urinary tract is often ESWL (extracorporeal shock-wave *lithotripsy*, a procedure that uses ultrasonic waves or shock waves to disintegrate the stones. Alternatively, *cystoscopy* can be used to crush and remove stones in the bladder and lower ureter. In some cases, surgery may be needed to remove the stones.

calendar method

A method of *contraception*, also called the rhythm method, based on abstaining from sexual intercourse around the

---

URINARY TRACT **CALCULI**

Calculi form in the urinary tract when certain substances in the urine become overly concentrated. The substances form crystals, which grow into stones. Some stones may be associated with recurrent episodes of *urinary tract infection*. Symptoms vary according to the site of the stone. Small stones may be passed in the urine and cause no symptoms. Some stones, however, may lodge in a ureter, causing *renal colic* (a sudden, severe pain in the small of the back that moves towards the groin) and haematuria (blood in the urine). In the bladder, stones may settle over the outlet, which can cause difficulty in passing urine, a poor flow rate, and dribbling. Any obstruction to urine flow may result in rapid kidney damage and acute, severe infection (*pyelonephritis*).

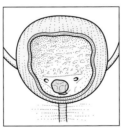
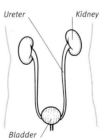
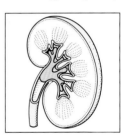

Ureter Kidney

Bladder

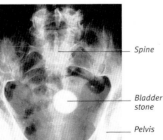

Spine

Bladder stone

Pelvis

X-ray of a bladder stone
A large bladder stone, such as the one that can be clearly seen in this X-ray, can make the passing of urine both difficult and painful.

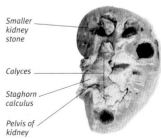

Smaller kidney stone

Calyces

Staghorn calculus

Pelvis of kidney

Staghorn calculus
Here, a staghorn calculus has filled the entire pelvis and calyces of the kidney, producing a cast of them. A smaller stone has formed in the medulla (central area).

time of *ovulation* (the release of an egg from a woman's ovary). This time is calculated on the basis of the length of her previous menstrual cycles. The calendar method is unreliable because a woman's menstrual cycle may vary. There are now more scientific and effective contraceptive methods of this type (see *contraception, natural methods*).

calf muscles

The muscles extending from the back of the knee to the heel. The gastrocnemius muscle starts behind the knee and forms the bulky part of the calf; beneath it lies the soleus muscle which starts at the back of the *tibia* (shin). These two muscles join to form the *Achilles tendon*, which connects them to the heel. Contraction of the calf muscles pulls the heel up and is important in walking, running, and jumping.

LOCATION OF **CALF MUSCLES**

The gastrocnemius muscle and the soleus muscle at the back of the leg join to form the Achilles tendon.

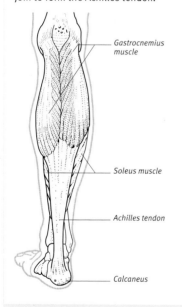

- Gastrocnemius muscle
- Soleus muscle
- Achilles tendon
- Calcaneus

calf pain

Various disorders may be responsible for pain in the calf. Common causes include *cramp*, muscle strain, and *sciatica* (inflammation of the sciatic nerve). More rarely, pain in the calf muscles may be due to blood clots in leg veins (see *thrombosis, deep vein*). This disorder is a particular risk if a person has been

immobile for a long time – for example, after surgery or during a long journey by air. Another possible problem is *claudication* (cramping pain often due to narrowing of the arteries). In this last condition, pain is often caused by walking and relieved by rest.

caliper splint

An *orthopaedic* device that corrects or controls a deformed leg or supports a leg weakened by a muscular disorder, allowing an affected person to stand and walk. For example, a person who has lost the ability to flex the foot upward and, as a result, drags the toes on the ground with each step can be fitted with a splint that keeps the foot permanently at right angles to the leg, thereby allowing walking.

A caliper splint consists of one or two vertical metal rods attached to leather or metal rings that are worn around the affected limb. A splint extending just below the knee is sufficient to control the position of the ankle. Longer splints may be jointed to allow movement of the knee.

callosity

See *callus, skin*.

callus, bony

A diffuse growth of new, soft bone that forms as part of the healing process in a *fracture*. As healing continues, the callus is replaced by harder bone, and the original shape of the bone is restored.

callus, skin

An area of thickened skin, usually on the hands or feet, caused by regular or prolonged pressure or friction. A *corn* is a callus on a toe. If corns are painful, the thickened skin can be pared away by a chiropodist using a scalpel.

caloric test

A method of finding out whether the *labyrinth* in the inner ear is diseased. A caloric test may be performed as part of investigations into *vertigo* (dizziness) and hearing loss.

The outer-ear canal is briefly flooded with water of different temperatures, above and below normal body temperature. This flooding sets up convection currents in the semicircular canals in the inner ear. If the labyrinth is normal, *nystagmus* (rapid reflex flickering of the eyes) occurs for a predictable period. If the labyrinth is diseased, this response

is either absent or reduced. The presence and duration of nystagmus may be observed directly or recorded electrically using *electronystagmography*.

calorie

A unit of energy. One calorie is the amount of energy that is needed to raise the temperature of 1 gram of water by 1°C. The term "calorie" is also used in medicine and *dietetics* to mean "kilocalorie", which is a larger unit of energy equal to 1,000 calories.

Normally, when a person's calorie intake matches the amount of energy expended, body weight remains constant. If intake exceeds expenditure, weight is usually gained; if expenditure exceeds intake, weight is usually lost. In general, fats contain more calories than proteins or carbohydrates.

Energy can also be measured in joules: 1 calorie equals 4.2 joules. (See also *calorimetry*; *diet and disease*.)

calorie requirements

See *energy requirements*.

calorimetry

The measurement of the *calorie* (energy) value of foods or the energy expenditure of a person. In direct calorimetry, a small measure of food is burned up inside a sealed container, which is immersed in water. The resultant rise in water temperature is used to calculate the calorie value.

Energy production in humans can be measured by oxygen uptake. Every litre of oxygen taken into the body produces 4.8 kilocalories of energy. The level of energy production is calculated by comparing the percentage of oxygen in air that is inhaled and exhaled.

Calpol

A brand name for paediatric preparations containing *paracetamol*, an *analgesic* and antipyretic (fever-reducing) drug.

camouflaging preparations

Creams or powders that are applied to the skin to conceal skin disfigurements, such as *birthmarks* and scars.

Campbell de Morgan's spot

A small (1–3 mm), bright red, domed spot, also known as a cherry angioma, that appears on the trunk or limbs. A Campbell de Morgan's spot is a type of *haemangioma* (a noncancerous blemish). The spots are harmless. They are caused by weakening of the walls of capillaries in the dermis (the inner layer of the skin). Campbell de Morgan's spots are common in adults, especially elderly people.

Campylobacter

A group of bacteria that are among the most common causes of gastrointestinal disorders. Campylobacter bacteria are harboured by animals and can be passed on to humans through contaminated food, especially in poultry, causing *food poisoning*. These bacteria also cause a form of *colitis*, an inflammatory disease of the colon.

canal

A narrow tubular passage or channel in the body, such as the *ear* canal, which leads from the outer to the middle ear, or the alimentary canal, which is part of the *digestive system*.

cancer

Any of a group of diseases that are characterized by abnormal and unrestrained growth of cells in body organs or tissues. Cancerous tumours can form in any tissue in the body but they most commonly develop in major organs, such as in the lungs, breasts, intestines, skin, stomach, or pancreas. Cancerous tumours can also develop in the nasal sinuses, the testes or ovaries, or the lips or tongue. Cancers may also develop in the tissues of the bone marrow that form blood cells (see *leukaemia*) and in the lymphatic system, the muscles, or the bones.

Cancers differ from benign (noncancerous) *neoplasms* (growths) in that they spread and infiltrate surrounding normal tissue. The tumours can cause blockages in hollow organs, such as within the digestive tract. They can also destroy nerves and erode bone. Cancer cells may also spread through the blood vessels or lymphatic system to other organs to form secondary tumours, known as metastases (see *metastasis*).

CAUSES

Tumour-forming cells develop when the *oncogenes* (genes controlling cell growth and multiplication) in a cell or cells undergo a series of changes. A small group of abnormal cells develop that divide more rapidly than normal, lack differentiation (they no longer perform their specialized task), and may escape the normal control of hormones and nerves.

Possible causes of cancer include environmental factors (such as sunlight and pollutants), alcohol consumption, dietary factors, and, most particularly, smoking, which is responsible for more cancers than any other agent. All of these factors may provoke critical changes within body cells in people who are already susceptible to developing cancer. Susceptibility to certain cancers may be inherited.

SYMPTOMS

Cancer symptoms depend on the site of the growth, the tissue of origin, and the extent of the tumour. They may be a direct feature of the growth (for example, lumps or skin changes) or may result from disruption of the function of a vital organ or blockage of a part of the body by the tumour. Unexplained weight loss is a feature of many different types of cancer.

DIAGNOSIS

Screening tests (see *cancer screening*) are increasingly being used to detect early signs of certain types of cancer in people who are thought to be at risk. Early detection of cancer optimizes the chance of a cure; for this reason, screening for breast cancer, cancer of the cervix, and intestinal cancer has reduced

mortality from these tumours. Diagnosis of cancer after symptoms have appeared is based on a physical examination, and confirmed by *biopsy* (removal of a sample of abnormal tissue for microscopic analysis) and imaging tests.

There are four main types of procedure used to detect cancer: cytology (cell) tests, imaging techniques, chemical tests, and direct inspection.

TREATMENT AND OUTLOOK

Many cancers are now curable, usually by combinations of surgery, *radiotherapy*, and *anticancer drugs*. For details of a specific type of cancer, refer to the article on that organ (for example, see *lung cancer*; *stomach cancer*).

cancerphobia

An intense fear of developing cancer, out of proportion to the actual risk, that significantly affects the life of the sufferer. An individual who has cancerphobia may become convinced that symptoms such as headaches, skin problems, constipation, or difficulty in swallowing, are signs of cancer. Patterns of behaviour that are typical of *obsessive–compulsive disorder* (for example, prolonged washing rituals) may be adopted in an attempt to reduce the

TREATMENT OF **CANCER**

The treatment of many cancers is still primarily surgical. Excision of an early tumour will often give a complete cure. There may be small, undetectable metastases (secondary tumours) at the time of operation, so surgery is commonly combined with radiotherapy and anticancer drugs. The aim of these treatments is to suppress or arrest the rate of cell division in any tumour cells left after surgery. Anticancer drugs often have unpleasant side effects because it is sometimes difficult to direct specific drugs to their target, and normal cells and tissues may be disrupted along with the tumour cells.

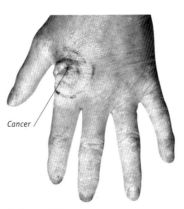

Cancer

Before radiotherapy
The photograph shows a skin cancer on the back of the hand before treatment.

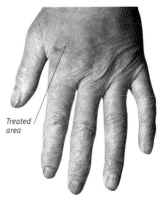

Treated area

After radiotherapy
This was the appearance a few weeks later, after a course of radiotherapy.

C

TESTS USED TO DETECT **CANCER**

Cytology tests	These tests reveal the presence of abnormal cells. One example is the *cervical smear test*, an investigation in which cells are brushed from the cervix (neck of the uterus) and examined microscopically to detect	potential or early cancer of the cervix. Another example is urine cytology, used to detect bladder cancer. Cells can also be removed from solid lumps; this procedure is often carried out on breast lumps.
Imaging techniques	Imaging tests can sometimes reveal changes in the appearance of tissue that are suggestive of cancer. One such test is a low-dose X-ray used in *mammography* to detect early breast cancer. Another is *ultrasound scanning*; for example, pelvic	ultrasound scans can detect cancer of the ovary. *CT scanning* and *MRI* provide detailed images of internal anatomy and are particularly useful for showing inaccessible areas, such as the brain and the back of the abdominal cavity.
Chemical tests	Tests on blood, urine, or faeces can show the presence of substances suggestive of cancer. For example, microscopic amounts of blood in the	faeces may be due to cancer of the colon; high blood levels of prostate specific antigen (PSA) are sometimes due to prostate cancer.
Viewing techniques	Viewing tests involve looking inside a hollow organ using an *endoscope* (a viewing tube). They are usually performed only when cancer is already suspected. Examples	include *colonoscopy*, *gastroscopy*, *cystoscopy*, and *laparoscopy* (viewing of the colon, stomach, bladder, and abdominal cavity, respectively).

risk of cancer. *Psychotherapy*, including *behaviour therapy*, may be of benefit. (See also *phobia*.)

cancer screening

Tests that are carried out to detect cancer before symptoms have developed. Cancer screening is used particularly for groups of people who are thought to be susceptible because of their age, occupation, lifestyle, or genetic predisposition. Early detection often increases the chance of a cure. Tests for cancers of the cervix (see *cervical smear test*), breast (see *mammography*), bladder, and colon have proved effective in reducing mortality from these conditions.

cancrum

The medical term for canker or ulceration. It mainly refers to the mouth and lips, when the condition is known as cancrum oris. (See also *noma*.)

candidiasis

Infection by the fungus CANDIDA ALBICANS, also known as thrush or moniliasis. Candidiasis affects areas of mucous membrane in the body, most commonly the vagina and the inside of the mouth. In infants, candidiasis can occur in conjunction with *nappy rash*.

CAUSES

The fungus is normally present in the mouth and the vagina, but in some situations it may multiply excessively. Candidiasis may occur if *antibiotic drugs* destroy the harmless bacteria that control the growth of the fungus, or if the body's resistance to infection is lowered. Certain disorders, for example *diabetes mellitus*, and the hormonal changes that occur during pregnancy or with *oral contraceptives* may also encourage growth of the fungus.

Candidiasis can be contracted by having sexual intercourse with an infected partner. The infection is far more common in women than in men.

SYMPTOMS

Symptoms of vaginal infection include a thick, white discharge, genital irritation, and discomfort on passing urine. Less commonly, the penis is infected, usually causing *balanitis* (inflammation of the head of the penis). Oral candidiasis produces sore, creamy-yellow, raised patches inside the mouth.

Candidiasis may spread from the genitals or mouth to other moist areas of the body. It may also affect the gastrointestinal tract, especially in people with impaired immune systems, such as those taking *immunosuppressant drugs* or who have HIV (the virus that leads to *AIDS*).

DIAGNOSIS AND TREATMENT

Candidiasis is diagnosed by examination of a sample taken from the white discharge or from patches.

The condition is treated topically with *antifungal drugs* such as clotrimazole or with oral antifungals. The drugs are given in the form of creams, vaginal pessaries, or throat lozenges. Treatment of candidiasis is usually successful, but the condition may recur.

Canesten cream

A brand name for the *antifungal drug* clotrimazole, used to treat fungal infections of the skin and genitals (for example, *candidiasis*).

canine tooth

See *teeth*.

cannabis

A preparation that is derived from the hemp plant CANNABIS SATIVA and usually used to produce euphoria and hallucinations (see *marijuana*).

cannula

A smooth, blunt-ended tube that is inserted into a blood vessel, lymphatic vessel, or body cavity, in order to introduce or withdraw fluids.

Cannulas are used for *blood transfusions* and *intravenous infusions* and for draining *pleural effusions* (fluid around the lungs). If necessary, a cannula may be left in place for several days if continuous testing of, or introduction of, fluids is required.

canthus

The anatomical term for the corner of the *eye* (the angle at which the upper and lower eyelids meet).

capacity, iron-binding

A measure of the level of transferrin, a protein that acts in addition to *haemoglobin* (the oxygen-carrying pigment in the blood) to bind and transport iron in the blood. Measuring iron-binding capacity may help to establish the cause of *anaemia* (a reduced level of haemoglobin in the blood).

Transferrin is formed mainly in the *liver*. The amount produced is determined by the amount of iron that is stored in the body. When iron stores are low, as occurs in iron-deficiency anaemia (see *anaemia, iron-deficiency*), more transferrin is produced to enable the blood to carry as much iron as possible. The level of transferrin and the iron-binding capacity of the blood are thereby raised, although the level of iron in the body is low.

C

capacity, vital

The maximum volume of air, usually around 4.5 litres, that can be expelled from the lungs following maximum inhalation. Vital capacity is measured as part of lung function tests (see *pulmonary function tests*).

cap, cervical

A flexible contraceptive device that is placed directly over the *cervix* to prevent sperm from entering it (see *contraception, barrier methods of*).

cap, duodenal

See *duodenal cap*.

Capgras' syndrome

The delusion (false belief) that a relative or friend has been replaced by an identical impostor. Capgras' syndrome, also known as the "illusion of doubles", is seen most frequently in patients with paranoid *schizophrenia* but can also occur in some organic brain disorders (see *brain syndrome, organic*) and *affective disorders*.

capillary

Any of the vessels that carry blood between the smallest arteries, or arterioles, and the smallest veins, or venules (see *circulatory system*). Capillaries form a fine network throughout the body's organs and tissues. Their thin walls are permeable; as a result, they allow blood and cells to exchange constituents such as oxygen, glucose, carbon dioxide, and water (see *respiration*).

Capillaries open and close to blood flow according to the requirements of different organs for oxygen and nutrients. For example, when a person is running, most of the capillaries in the leg muscles are open, but at rest many are closed. The opening and closing of skin capillaries helps to regulate *temperature*. The blood flow through each capillary is controlled by a tiny circle of muscle at its entrance.

DISORDERS

A direct blow to an area of the body may rupture the capillary walls, causing bleeding under the skin, which in turn results in swelling and bruising.

Capillaries become more fragile in elderly people, in people taking high doses of *corticosteroid drugs*, and in those suffering from *scurvy* (vitamin C deficiency). All such people have a tendency to develop *purpura* (small areas of bleeding under the skin which often appear as reddish-purple patches).

capillary haemangioma

See *haemangioma*.

Caplan's syndrome

A combination of *rheumatoid arthritis* and *pneumoconiosis* (a lung disorder that is caused by inhalation of certain mineral dusts). In Caplan's syndrome, large areas of fibrous (scar) tissue form in the lungs, often causing severe shortness of breath.

capping, dental

See *crown, dental*.

capsule

An anatomical structure enclosing an organ or body part. For example, the liver, kidneys, joints, and eye lenses are all enclosed in capsules.

The term "capsule" is also used to describe a soluble, elongated shell, usually made of gelatine, which contains a drug to be taken by mouth. The coating of some capsules prevents potentially irritant drugs from being released into the stomach, or allows drugs to be released slowly to enable them to be taken less frequently.

capsulitis

Inflammation of a *capsule*, a structure that encloses an organ or joint. One example of capsulitis is *frozen shoulder*.

STRUCTURE OF **CAPILLARIES**

These minute blood vessels have thin, permeable walls, which allow the transfer of oxygen, glucose, and water from blood to tissues.

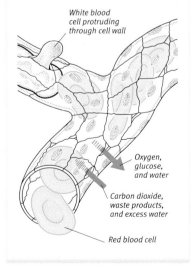

White blood cell protruding through cell wall

Oxygen, glucose, and water

Carbon dioxide, waste products, and excess water

Red blood cell

captopril

An *ACE inhibitor drug*. These drugs are used in the treatment of *hypertension* (high blood pressure), *heart failure*, and diabetic *nephropathy* (kidney damage).

caput

The Latin word for "head". The term is commonly used of the caput succedaneum: a soft, temporary swelling in the scalp of newborn babies, which is caused by pressure during labour. The word "caput" was once also used to refer to the face, skull, and associated organs; to the origin of a muscle; or to any enlarged extremity, such as the caput femoris, the head of the femur (thigh bone).

carbamazepine

An *anticonvulsant drug* that is chemically related to the *tricyclic antidepressants*. Taken orally or as suppositories, carbamazepine reduces the frequency of seizures that are caused by abnormal nerve signals in the brain and is used mainly in the long-term treatment of *epilepsy*. The drug is also prescribed to relieve the severe pain of *trigeminal neuralgia* and as a mood-stabilizing drug in the treatment of psychiatric disorders such as *bipolar disorder*.

To prevent side effects (which may include dizziness, drowsiness, nausea, and blurred vision), carbamazepine is usually started at a low dose and is gradually increased.

carbaryl

An insecticide that is prescribed to treat head *lice* and *crab lice*. Carbaryl is applied topically, either as a water-based liquid or as an alcohol-based lotion. However, the drug must not come into contact with the eyes or with areas of broken skin. The lotion is considered unsuitable for small children and people with asthma because they may be affected by the alcoholic fumes.

carbimazole

A drug used to treat *hyperthyroidism* (overactivity of the thyroid gland). Because carbimazole is slow to take effect, and its full benefits may not be felt for several weeks, *beta-blockers* may be given to relieve symptoms in the interim.

Long-term treatment with carbimazole may reduce the production of blood cells by the bone marrow, and regular blood counts are therefore required. Side effects may include headaches, dizziness, joint pain, and nausea.

C

carbocisteine

A type of *mucolytic drug* that is used to thin sputum, making it easier to cough up. Carbocisteine may be helpful in chronic obstructive pulmonary disease (see *pulmonary disease, chronic obstructive*) and *cystic fibrosis*.

carbohydrates

A group of compounds that are composed of carbon, hydrogen, and oxygen that provide the body with its main source of energy. They include sugars (simple carbohydrates) and starches (complex carbohydrates).

TYPES AND SOURCES

Carbohydrates are found in many foods, the principal ones being fruits, vegetables, cereals, and pulses, and fall into two main groups: available carbohydrates and unavailable carbohydrates.

The main available carbohydrates are starches and sugars, which are metabolized into glucose for the body's use. Unavailable carbohydrates, such as cellulose, cannot be broken down by digestive *enzymes* and make up the bulk of dietary fibre (see *fibre, dietary*).

CARBOHYDRATE METABOLISM

The different types of carbohydrates are processed by the body in different ways. Monosaccharides (also known as simple sugars), which include glucose, galactose, and fructose, can all be absorbed unchanged from the intestine into the bloodstream. The disaccharides (also known as double sugars), which include sucrose, maltose, and lactose, need to be broken down into simple sugars before they can be absorbed. Starches also have to be broken down into simple sugars

---

TYPES OF **CARBOHYDRATE**

Monosaccharides are the simplest, consisting of a single saccharide molecule. Disaccharides consist of two linked saccharide molecules. Polysaccharides consist of a long chain of many saccharide molecules. Starch is an important carbohydrate and a major constituent in the diet.

- **Monosaccharides**
  glucose, galactose, fructose

- **Disaccharides**
  sucrose, lactose, maltose

- **Polysaccharides**
  starches, cellulose

---

before they can be absorbed. The breakdown process is carried out by enzymes (chemical catalysts) in the digestive tract.

The simple sugars (mainly glucose) are then absorbed through the intestinal wall and into the bloodstream for distribution throughout the body. Some glucose is burned up immediately (see *metabolism*) in order to generate energy for cells that need a constant supply, such as brain cells and red blood cells. Galactose and fructose are converted to glucose in the liver to be used by body cells. Surplus glucose is transported to the liver, muscles, and fat cells where it is converted into *glycogen* and fat for storage.

When blood glucose levels are high, glucose storage is stimulated by *insulin*, a hormone that is secreted by the *pancreas*. When blood glucose levels become low, insulin secretion diminishes and *glucagon*, another hormone produced by the pancreas, stimulates the conversion of stored glycogen to glucose for release into the bloodstream. Fat cannot be converted to glucose, although it can be used as a fuel to conserve glucose.

In the disorder *diabetes mellitus*, carbohydrate metabolism is disturbed by a deficiency of insulin or resistance of body cells to its effects.

carbolic acid

See *phenol*.

carbon

A nonmetallic element that is present in all the fundamental molecules of living organisms, such as *proteins*, *fats*, and *carbohydrates*, and well as in some inorganic molecules, such as *carbon dioxide*, *carbon monoxide*, and *sodium bicarbonate*. Pure carbon is the major constituent of diamond, coal, charcoal, and graphite.

carbon dioxide (CO_2)

A colourless, odourless gas. Carbon dioxide consists of one carbon atom linked to two oxygen atoms and has the chemical formula CO_2. The gas is present in small amounts in the air and is an important by-product of *metabolism* in cells. It is produced by the breakdown of substances such as carbohydrates and fats to produce energy. It is then carried in the bloodstream to the lungs, where it is exhaled.

Carbon dioxide helps to control the rate of respiration: when a person exer-

---

CARBOHYDRATE METABOLISM

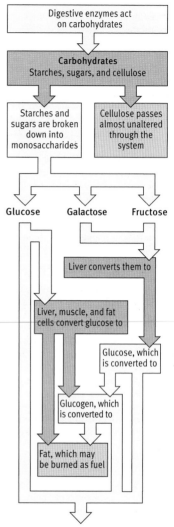

Glucose is absorbed into the bloodstream for distribution throughout the body or is used directly by body cells.

---

cises, CO_2 levels in the blood rise, causing the person to breathe more rapidly in order to expel carbon dioxide and to take in more *oxygen*.

Carbon dioxide that is compressed and cooled to -75°C becomes solid *dry ice*, which is used in *cryosurgery* (destruction of diseased tissues by freezing).

carbon monoxide (CO)

A colourless, odourless, poisonous gas. Carbon monoxide consists of one carbon atom linked to one oxygen atom and has the chemical formula CO. It is produced by inefficient combustion of organic substances (such as coal, gas, and oil) and is present in vehicle exhaust fumes and tobacco smoke.

POISONING

Carbon monoxide is toxic because it binds with *haemoglobin* (the oxygen-carrying molecule in red blood cells), which prevents the blood from carrying oxygen to the body tissues. As a result, the tissues are deprived of oxygen, and asphyxiation occurs. The initial symptoms of acute high-level carbon monoxide poisoning include dizziness, headache, nausea, and faintness. Continued inhalation of the gas may lead to loss of consciousness, permanent brain damage, and even death. Low-level exposure to carbon monoxide over a period of time may cause fatigue, nausea, diarrhoea, abdominal pain, and general malaise.

carbon tetrachloride (CCl4)

A colourless, poisonous, volatile chemical with a characteristic odour. Carbon tetrachloride consists of one carbon atom linked to four chlorine atoms and has the chemical formula CCl_4. Formerly used in domestic dry-cleaning fluids, its use is now restricted to industry.

Carbon tetrachloride is an extremely dangerous chemical, and it can cause dizziness, confusion, and liver and kidney damage if a significant amount of the chemical is inhaled or swallowed.

carbuncle

A cluster of interconnected *boils* (painful, pus-filled, inflamed hair roots). Carbuncles are usually caused by infection with the bacterium STAPHYLOCOCCUS AUREUS. The back of the neck and the buttocks are the most common sites. The swellings mainly affect people with reduced immunity, particularly those with *diabetes mellitus*.

Treatment is usually with an *antibiotic drug*. In addition, the application of hot *compresses* may encourage the pus-filled heads of the boils to burst, which relieves pain. Occasionally, incision and drainage (together with removal of the core of the carbuncle) may be necessary if a carbuncle is persistent, and drainage and healing have not occurred spontaneously.

carcinogen

Any agent that is capable of causing *cancer*, such as tobacco smoke, high-energy *radiation*, or asbestos fibres.

CHEMICAL CARCINOGENS

Chemicals form the largest group of carcinogens. Major types include polycyclic aromatic hydrocarbons (PAHs), which occur in tobacco smoke, pitch, tar fumes, and soot. Exposure to PAHs may lead to cancer of the respiratory system or skin. In addition, certain aromatic amines used in the chemical and rubber industries may cause bladder cancer after prolonged exposure.

PHYSICAL CARCINOGENS

The best-known physical carcinogen is high-energy radiation, such as nuclear radiation and *X-rays*. Radiation may also come from *ultraviolet light*, for example in sunlight. Another known physical carcinogen is asbestos (see *asbestos-related diseases*).

Exposure to radiation may cause cancerous changes in cells, especially in cells that divide quickly; for example changes in the precursors of white blood cells in the bone marrow causes *leukaemia*. The level of risk depends on the dosage and duration of exposure to the carcinogen. Over many years, exposure to ultraviolet radiation in sunlight can cause skin cancer.

BIOLOGICAL CARCINOGENS

Only a few biological agents are known to cause cancer in humans. SCHISTOSOMA HAEMATOBIUM, one of the blood flukes responsible for the tropical disease *schistosomiasis*, can cause cancer of the bladder; and ASPERGILLUS FLAVUS, a fungus that produces the poison *aflatoxin* in stored peanuts and grain, is believed to cause liver cancer.

Viruses that are associated with cancer include some strains of the human papillomavirus, which are linked to cervical cancer; the hepatitis B and C viruses, which are linked to liver cancer; and some types of herpes virus, which are associated with *Kaposi's sarcoma* and *Burkitt's lymphoma* (the latter is specifically associated with the herpes virus known as the *Epstein-Barr virus*).

AVOIDANCE OF CARCINOGENS

In industry, known carcinogens may be banned. Alternatively, as in the nuclear industry and hospital X-ray departments, they may be allowed if their use is considered essential, if exposure is strictly limited, and if regular medical screening is provided for workers using them.

Outside industry, people are exposed to very few known, unavoidable, high-risk carcinogens. Any substance that could possibly be carcinogenic, such as a food additive, a cosmetic, or a chemical

for use in drugs, must be screened by an official body (such as the Medicines and Healthcare products Regulatory Agency – MHRA – which assesses drugs in the UK) before it can be manufactured.

carcinogenesis

The development of a *cancer* caused by the action of *carcinogens* (factors that cause cancer) on normal cells. Carcinogens are believed to alter the *DNA* in cells, particularly in *oncogenes* (genes that control the growth and division of cells). An altered cell divides abnormally fast, passing on the genetic changes to its offspring cells. Thus, a group of cells is established that is not affected by the body's normal restraints on growth.

carcinoid syndrome

A rare condition caused by an intestinal or lung tumour, called a carcinoid, which secretes excessive amounts of the hormone *serotonin* and often also other chemicals, such as *bradykinin*. Carcinoid syndrome is characterized by bouts of facial flushing, diarrhoea, and wheezing, but symptoms usually occur only if the tumour has spread to the liver or has arisen in a lung.

Carcinoid tumours in the intestine, lung, and, more rarely, the liver are sometimes removed surgically, but, in most cases, surgery is unlikely to be of benefit. In these circumstances, symptoms may be relieved by drugs such as *octreotide*, which often inhibits the growth of the tumour.

carcinoid tumour

A type of hormone-secreting cancerous tumour. Carcinoids most often occur in the small intestine or rectum but occasionally also develop in the lungs. (See also *carcinoid syndrome*.)

carcinoma

Any cancerous tumour (see *cancer*) that arises from cells in the covering surface layer or lining membrane of an organ. A carcinoma is distinguished from a *sarcoma*, which is a cancer arising in bone, muscle, or connective tissue. The most common cancers of the lungs, breast, stomach, skin, cervix, colon, and rectum are carcinomas.

carcinoma in situ

The earliest, usually curable, stage of a cancer. In this stage, the disease has not yet spread from the surface layer of cells in an organ or other tissue.

C

carcinomatosis

The presence of cancerous tissue in different sites of the body due to the spread of *cancer* cells from a primary (original) cancerous tumour.

SYMPTOMS

The symptoms of carcinomatosis may include weight loss, lack of energy, and various other problems depending on the sites of the metastases (secondary tumours). For example, metastases in the lungs may cause coughing and breathlessness; those that develop in the liver may cause jaundice.

DIAGNOSIS AND TREATMENT

A diagnosis of carcinomatosis may be confirmed by *X-rays* or by *radionuclide scanning* of the bones and lungs, by biochemical tests, or in the course of an operation. *Anticancer drugs* or *radiotherapy* may be given to destroy the metastases. The condition will not be improved by removing the primary tumour unless the tumour is producing a hormone that directly stimulates the growth of metastases.

cardiac aneurysm

Ballooning of an area of a ventricle (lower chamber) of the heart, usually as a result of damage following a *myocardial infarction* (heart attack). (See also *ventricular aneurysm*.)

cardiac arrest

A halt in the pumping action of the heart. Cardiac arrest occurs when the heart's rhythmic muscular contractions stop, and usually results from abnormal electrical activity. It causes sudden collapse, loss of consciousness, and the absence of pulse and breathing.

CAUSES

The most common cause of cardiac arrest is a *myocardial infarction* (heart attack). Other possible causes include *respiratory arrest*, *electrical injury*, loss of blood, *hypothermia*, drug overdose, and *anaphylactic shock* (an extremely severe type of allergic reaction).

DIAGNOSIS AND TREATMENT

The survival of the patient depends on prompt restoration of the heartbeat and the oxygen supply to the brain. *Cardiopulmonary resuscitation* may be used to maintain the circulation until the heartbeat resumes.

A diagnosis of cardiac arrest can only be confirmed by monitoring the electrical activity of the heart using *ECG*. This helps medical personnel distinguish between ventricular fibrillation (the rapid, uncoordinated contraction of individual heart muscle fibres) and asystole (the complete absence of heart muscle activity), which are the two abnormalities of heart rhythm that can lead to cardiac arrest.

Ventricular fibrillation may be corrected by *defibrillation* (application of an electric shock to the heart). Asystole is more difficult to reverse but may respond to injection of *adrenaline* (epinephrine) or an electrical *pacemaker*.

OUTLOOK

In general, recovery after ventricular fibrillation is more likely than after a cardiac arrest triggered by asystole.

cardiac arrhythmia

See *arrhythmia, cardiac*.

cardiac asthma

Difficulty in breathing that is similar to asthma but is the result of *pulmonary oedema* (fluid on the lungs); the oedema, in turn, is due to *heart failure* (the inability of the heart to cope with its workload). Attacks of cardiac asthma usually occur at night. The disorder is not related to bronchial *asthma* and requires different treatment.

cardiac catheter

See *catheterization, cardiac*.

cardiac cycle

The sequence of events, lasting for less than a second, that make up each beat of the *heart*. A heartbeat has three phases: diastole, atrial systole, and ventricular systole. In diastole, the heart relaxes. During atrial systole, the *atria* (upper chambers of the heart) contract, and in ventricular systole, the *ventricles* (the heart's lower chambers) contract. The *sinoatrial node* (the heart's natural pacemaker) regulates the timing of the phases by sending electrical impulses to the atria and the ventricles.

cardiac dysrhythmia

See *dysrhythmia, cardiac*.

cardiac massage

Rhythmic compression of the heart. Cardiac massage is performed when the heart has stopped beating, in order to maintain blood circulation, especially to vital organs such as the brain. It involves repeatedly squeezing the heart to force blood out of it and into the circulatory system, then releasing the pressure on the heart so that it fills with blood again. Cardiac massage is continued until the heart resumes beating or the person is declared dead.

There are two main types: *external cardiac massage*, which involves pressing on the chest to squeeze the heart, and *internal cardiac massage*, when the exposed heart is massaged by hand. (See also *cardiopulmonary resuscitation*.)

cardiac muscle

See *muscle*.

cardiac neurosis

Excessive anxiety about the condition of the heart. Cardiac neurosis usually follows a *myocardial infarction* (heart attack) or heart surgery, but sometimes occurs when the person has had no previous heart trouble.

A person who has cardiac neurosis experiences symptoms that are typical of heart disease, such as breathlessness and chest pain, and may be reluctant to exercise or work for fear of having a heart attack. Medical investigation reveals no physical problem, however.

Psychotherapy (such as *cognitive-behavioural therapy*) may help an affected person to overcome the anxiety and resume a normal, active life.

cardiac oedema

An abnormal buildup of fluid in body tissues that is caused by *heart failure* (inability of the heart to cope with its workload). (See also *oedema*.)

cardiac output

The volume of blood pumped by the heart each minute. Cardiac output is a measure used to assess how efficiently the heart is working. At rest, a healthy adult's heart pumps between 2.5 and 4.5 litres of blood per minute. During exercise, this figure may rise to as much as 30 litres per minute. A low output during exercise may indicate damage to the heart muscle or major blood loss.

cardiac stress test

Also know as an exercise *ECG*, one of a group of tests used to assess the function of the *heart* in people who experience chest pain, breathlessness, or palpitations during exercise. The test establishes whether the patient has *coronary artery disease* (in which the blood supply to the heart muscle is impaired).

An ECG machine records the patterns of the heart's electrical activity while the heart is stressed. This is usually achieved by the patient exercising on a treadmill or stationary bicycle. Specific changes in the electrical pattern as exercise levels increase indicate *angina pectoris* (chest pain due to impaired blood supply to the heart muscle).

Cardiac stress testing may also be used in conjunction with *radionuclide scanning* or *angiography* in order to identify damaged areas of heart muscle.

cardiology

The study of the function of the *heart* and the investigation, diagnosis, and medical treatment of disorders of the heart and blood vessels, such as *atherosclerosis* (fat deposits on the artery walls) and *hypertension* (high blood pressure).

Some disorders reduce the pumping efficiency of the heart. They include arrhythmias (abnormalities in the rate or rhythm of the heartbeat; see *arrhythmia, cardiac*), *coronary artery disease* (in which the blood supply to the heart muscle is impaired), *cardiomyopathy* (in which the heart muscle itself is abnormal), and *heart valve* disorders.

Some babies are born with structural defects of the heart and/or the major blood vessels that emerge from it (see *heart disease, congenital*). Diseases of the lungs and blood vessels can also have adverse effects on heart function.

Many people with heart problems are treated by their general practitioners, but some may be referred to a cardiologist (a heart specialist). Investigations may include *echocardiography* (imaging the heart using ultrasound), *MRI* (magnetic resonance imaging), *radionuclide scanning*, and *ECG* (electrocardiography, which measures the electrical activity of the heart). If coronary artery disease is suspected, a *cardiac stress test* may be done and the cardiologist may perform coronary *angiography* (taking X-ray images of blood vessels) and possibly also widen any blocked blood vessels (see *angioplasty, balloon*). A cardiologist may refer a patient to a cardiovascular surgeon if surgical treatment is required.

cardiomegaly

Enlargement of the *heart*. This condition may take the form of *hypertrophy* (thickening) of the heart muscle or of dilation (increase in volume) of one or more of the heart chambers.

CAUSES

Hypertrophy of the heart muscle occurs in conditions in which the heart has to work harder than normal to pump blood. These disorders include *hypertension* (high blood pressure), which causes the wall of the left ventricle to thicken; *pulmonary hypertension* (raised blood pressure in the lungs), in which the wall of the right ventricle thickens; thyroid disease; severe *anaemia*; and a type of *cardiomyopathy* (disease of the heart muscle) in which the walls of one or both ventricles may become thickened.

Dilation of a heart chamber may be due to heart valve incompetence (failure of a valve to close properly after a contraction). In *aortic insufficiency*, failure of the aortic valve to close completely allows blood to flow back from the aorta into the left ventricle after each contraction, eventually enlarging the chamber.

SYMPTOMS

Symptoms of cardiomegaly may not occur until the heart has enlarged to the point where it cannot cope with additional stress (for example, as a result of exercise or infection). The heart's reduced pumping efficiency leads to *heart failure*, with symptoms of breathlessness and ankle swelling.

DIAGNOSIS AND TREATMENT

Cardiomegaly is diagnosed by a physical examination, *chest X-ray*, and *ECG* (measurement of the electrical activity of the heart). Treatment is directed at the underlying cause.

cardiomyopathy

Any disease of the heart muscle that weakens the force of cardiac contractions, thereby reducing the efficiency of blood circulation. Cardiomyopathies may be the result of infectious, metabolic, nutritional, toxic, autoimmune, or degenerative disorders. However, in many cases, the cause is unknown.

TYPES

There are three principal forms of the condition: hypertrophic, dilated, and restrictive cardiomyopathy.

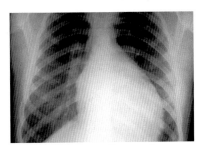

Chest X-ray showing cardiomyopathy
The heart has become greatly enlarged as a result of the heart-muscle abnormality.

In hypertrophic cardiomyopathy, the heart muscle is abnormally thickened. This condition is usually inherited.

In dilated cardiomyopathy, which is often of unknown cause, *metabolism* (chemical activity) of the heart muscle cells is abnormal and the heart's walls tend to balloon out under pressure.

Restrictive cardiomyopathy is a condition in which the heart walls are unusually inflexible, so that the heart cannot fill sufficiently with blood. It is often caused by scarring of the endocardium (the inner lining of the heart) or by *amyloidosis* (infiltration of the muscle with a starchlike substance).

SYMPTOMS AND SIGNS

Symptoms of cardiomyopathy include fatigue, palpitations, and chest pain. Palpitations may be due to an abnormal heart rhythm such as *atrial fibrillation* (rapid, uncoordinated contractions of the upper chambers of the heart).

The condition may lead to *heart failure*, in which the pumping action of the heart becomes less efficient. Symptoms of heart failure include breathing difficulty and *oedema* (abnormal fluid accumulation in body tissues).

DIAGNOSIS

A *chest X-ray* may show enlargement of the heart, and *echocardiography* (an ultrasound technique for imaging the structure and movement of the heart) may show thickened heart muscle. A *biopsy* (small tissue sample removed for microscopic analysis) of heart muscle may reveal muscle cell abnormalities.

TREATMENT

Symptoms of cardiomyopathy may be treated with *diuretic drugs* to control heart failure and *antiarrhythmic drugs* to correct the abnormal heart rhythm. In many cases, heart muscle function deteriorates, and the only remaining option is a *heart transplant*.

cardiopulmonary bypass

The procedure by which the circulation of blood around the body is maintained while the heart is stopped during heart surgery. A *heart–lung machine* is used to maintain the supply of oxygenated blood to the body tissues.

cardiopulmonary resuscitation

The administration of life-saving measures to a person who has suffered a *cardiac arrest* (in which the heart stops pumping blood). A person in cardiac arrest shows no sign of breathing and has no detectable pulse or heartbeat.

C

Brain damage is likely if the brain is starved of blood, and therefore oxygen, for more than three to four minutes.

First, five rescue breaths (see *rescue breathing*) are given, followed by 30 chest compressions applied to the lower breastbone (see *external cardiac massage*). Then two rescue breaths are given followed by 30 compressions, and this cycle of two breaths then 30 compressions is continued until medical help arrives or the casualty recovers. Even if the casualty does recover, he or she should still go to hospital.

cardiotocography

See *fetal heart monitoring*.

cardiovascular

A term that means "pertaining to the heart and blood vessels".

cardiovascular disorders

Disorders of the heart (see *heart* disorders box), blood vessels, and blood circulation (see *arteries, disorders of*; *veins, disorders of*).

cardiovascular surgery

The branch of surgery that is concerned with the heart and blood vessels. Cardiovascular surgery can be divided into two main areas.

One area, sometimes called cardiothoracic surgery, includes operations to prevent or repair damage to the heart itself and to the major blood vessels within the chest cavity. Cardiothoracic surgery is used, for example, to help treat damage due to congenital heart disease (see *heart disease, congenital*) or a *myocardial infarction* (heart attack).

The second area, which is known as vascular surgery, is concerned with the treatment of blood vessels elsewhere in the body, such as in the legs. (See also *coronary artery bypass*; *heart transplant*; *heart valve surgery*.)

cardioversion

The restoration of normal heart rhythm, usually by applying an electric shock to the chest. Cardioversion is also sometimes known as *defibrillation*.

carditis

A general term for inflammation of any part of the heart or its linings. There are three types. *Myocarditis* (inflammation of the heart muscle) is usually caused by a viral infection. *Endocarditis* (inflammation of the internal lining of the heart) is usually due to a bacterial infection. *Pericarditis* (inflammation of the outer covering of the heart) is usually the result of a viral or bacterial infection but may be associated with a *myocardial infarction* (heart attack) or an autoimmune disorder, such as systemic *lupus erythematosus*.

caries, dental

The gradual erosion of enamel (the hard covering of a tooth) and dentine (the softer substance that lies beneath the enamel). This condition is more commonly known as tooth decay.

CAUSES

The main cause of dental caries is *plaque*, a sticky substance consisting of food deposits, saliva by-products, dead cells from the lining of the mouth, and bacteria that collects on the surface of teeth. The breakdown of food deposits by bacteria creates acid that eats into the enamel to form cavities. Left unchecked, decay spreads to the dentine, and as the cavity enlarges, bacteria may invade and destroy the pulp tissue at the core of the tooth.

SYMPTOMS

Initial decay usually occurs on the grinding surfaces of the back teeth and on areas around the gum line. In the early stages, dental caries does not usually cause any symptoms. Advanced decay causes toothache (see *pulpitis*), however, which may be aggravated by eating very sweet, hot, or cold food. Sometimes advanced decay can also cause halitosis (bad breath).

TREATMENT

Treatment consists of drilling away the area of decay and filling the cavity (see *filling, dental*). In advanced decay, it may be necessary to remove the infected pulp and replace it with a filling (see *root-canal treatment*) or to extract the tooth (see *extraction, dental*).

PREVENTION

The risk of dental caries occurring can be reduced by cutting down on sugar consumption, practising good *oral hygiene*, and visiting the dentist regularly for check-ups. Water *fluoridation* and the use of fluoride toothpaste also helps to prevent caries.

CAUSES OF **CARIES** (TOOTH DECAY)

The primary cause of tooth decay is dental *plaque*, a sticky substance that forms on the teeth. Plaque consists of food remains, saliva by-products, and the bacteria that live in the mouth. The bacteria feed mainly on the fermentable carbohydrates (simple sugars and starches) in food, and, in breaking them down, create an acid that gradually destroys enamel, forming a cavity. If the process is not checked, the dentine is eroded next, enlarging the cavity and enabling the bacteria to invade the pulp at the centre of the tooth.

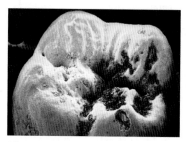

Micrograph of dental caries
The surface enamel of this decaying molar tooth is being broken down.

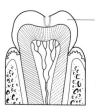

Enamel

1 Acid produced in the breakdown of food gradually destroys enamel, forming a cavity.

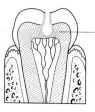

Dentine

2 Unchecked, decay spreads to the dentine.

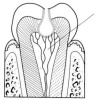

Pulp cavity

3 The cavity continues to enlarge, enabling the bacteria to invade exposed pulp at the tooth's centre.

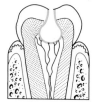

4 If untreated, the infected pulp will die and the tooth will be destroyed.

C

carotenaemia

A harmless condition in which blood levels of *carotene*, an orange pigment in certain vegetables, are very high as a result of excessive intake of these foods. Carotenaemia may cause temporary yellowing of the skin, especially on the palms and soles. Unlike *jaundice*, carotenaemia does not cause yellowing of the whites of the eyes.

carotene

A yellow or orange pigment found in carrots, tomatoes, and leafy green vegetables. The most important form of carotene is beta-carotene, an *antioxidant*. Beta-carotene is converted in the intestines into retinol (see *vitamin A*), which is essential for vision and healthy skin. Excessive intake of foods containing carotene may cause *carotenaemia* (temporary yellowing of the skin).

carotid artery

Any of the main arteries of the neck and head. There are two common carotid arteries (left and right), each of which divides into two main branches (internal and external).

The left carotid artery arises from the *aorta* and runs up the neck on the left side of the *trachea* (windpipe). The right carotid artery arises from the subclavian artery (which branches off the aorta) and follows a similar route on the right side of the neck. Just above the level of the *larynx* (voicebox), each carotid artery divides to form an external carotid artery and an internal carotid artery.

The external arteries have multiple branches that supply most of the tissues in the face, scalp, mouth, and jaws. The internal arteries enter the skull to supply the brain and eyes. At the base of the brain, branches of the two internal carotids and the basilar artery join to form a ring of blood vessels called the circle of Willis. Narrowing of these vessels may be associated with *transient ischaemic attack (TIA)*; obstruction of them causes a *stroke*.

The carotid arteries have two specialized sensory regions in the neck: the carotid sinus, which monitors blood pressure, and the carotid body, which monitors the oxygen content of the blood and helps to regulate breathing. The carotid artery is one of the points at which the *pulse* can be measured. (See also *carotid bruit*; *carotid doppler scanning*; *carotid sinus syndrome*.)

LOCATION OF **CAROTID ARTERY**

The common carotid artery runs up each side of the neck and divides to form internal and external branches.

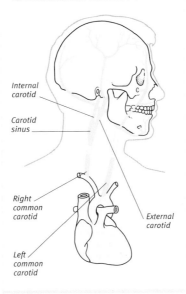

Internal carotid

Carotid sinus

Right common carotid

Left common carotid

External carotid

carotid bruit

An abnormal noise in a *carotid artery* (one of the major arteries supplying the neck and head), which is due to turbulent blood flow. A doctor can hear the noise with a stethoscope placed on the side of a person's neck, over the artery. A carotid bruit indicates narrowing (stenosis) of the artery, usually due to fatty deposits on the blood vessel lining (see *atherosclerosis*).

carotid doppler scanning

A method for assessing blood flow through the *carotid arteries* (the major arteries supplying the neck and head) by the use of *ultrasound scanning*. Carotid doppler scanning is used to investigate certain disorders, such as carotid artery stenosis (narrowing of the artery), *transient ischaemic attacks*, and *stroke*, that may be the result of narrowing of the common carotid arteries and their branches.

An ultrasound transducer is moved over each side of the neck in the area of the carotid arteries. The transducer emits ultrasound waves, which are reflected off the moving blood cells and blood-vessel walls to produce an image on a screen. This image reveals any narrowing of the arteries or turbulence in blood flow.

carotid sinus syndrome

A condition mainly affecting elderly people, in which the carotid sinus, a structure within the common *carotid artery* of the neck that regulates blood pressure, is overly sensitive.

The carotid sinus is a pocket in the artery at the point where the vessel divides to form two branches. It contains sensors that continually monitor blood pressure. When the blood pressure is raised, the sinus sends messages to the brain, which signals blood vessels to widen and the heart rate to slow, thus lowering the pressure.

In carotid sinus syndrome, the sinus reacts too readily: simply turning the neck suddenly or coughing can trigger the sensors. As a result, the brain slows the heart rate and lowers blood pressure excessively, causing the affected person to faint. This problem may be avoided by the insertion of a *pacemaker*, which will help to maintain a normal heart rate, overriding any inappropriate messages from the carotid sinus.

carpal tunnel syndrome

Numbness, tingling, and pain in the thumb, index finger, and middle fingers. Carpal tunnel syndrome is caused by compression of the *median nerve* at the wrist. The carpal tunnel, through which the nerve passes, is a narrow gap formed by the carpal bones of the wrist and a ligament that lies over them. The condition may affect one or both of the hands and is sometimes accompanied by weakness in the thumb. Symptoms may be worse at night.

CAUSES

Carpal tunnel syndrome is common among people who use computer keyboards, who make constant, repetitive hand movements. The condition also occurs without obvious cause in middle-aged women. In addition, it is quite common in pregnancy; in women who have begun using *oral contraceptives*; in those who suffer from *premenstrual syndrome*; and in men and women who suffer from *rheumatoid arthritis*, *myxoedema* (thickening and coarsening of the skin and other body tissues), and *acromegaly* (a condition in which there is abnormal enlargement of the skull, jaw, hands, feet, and internal organs).

TREATMENT

Treatment depends on the underlying cause. It may include wrist splints, *nonsteroidal anti-inflammatory drugs*, or *diuretic drugs*. Persistent symptoms may

C

be treated by the injection of a *cortico-steroid drug* under the ligament. Alternatively, the ligament may be cut surgically in order to relieve pressure on the nerve.

carpopedal spasm

Involuntary contraction of muscles in the hands and feet. Carpopedal spasm is due to low levels of calcium in the blood. This problem, in turn, may be caused by *hyperventilation* (abnormally rapid breathing) or by disorders such as *hypoparathyroidism*.

carpus

The eight bones of the *wrist*.

carrier

A person who is able to pass on an infectious or inherited disease without actually suffering from it themselves.

car sickness

See *motion sickness*.

cartilage

A type of *connective tissue* (a material that holds body structures together) made up of varying amounts of the gel-like substance *collagen*. Cartilage is not as hard as *bone*, but it nevertheless forms an important structural component of various parts of the skeletal

---

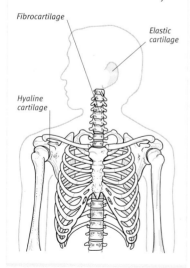

TYPES OF **CARTILAGE**

The three main types of cartilage have different amounts of collagen, vary in toughness and elasticity, and exist at different sites in the body.

Fibrocartilage

Elastic cartilage

Hyaline cartilage

---

system, including the *joints*. Much of the fetal skeleton is formed entirely of cartilage. During childhood, the cartilage is gradually converted to bone by a process known as *ossification*.

TYPES

There are three main types of cartilage: hyaline cartilage, fibrocartilage, and elastic cartilage. Each type is composed of a different proportion of collagen and has a particular function.

Hyaline cartilage is a tough, smooth tissue that lines the surfaces of joints, such as the knee, providing an almost frictionless layer over the bony parts of the joint. If the lining becomes worn (as occurs in *osteoarthritis*) or damaged, the movement of that joint may be painful or severely restricted.

Fibrocartilage contains a large proportion of collagen and is solid and strong. This type of cartilage makes up the discs that are situated between the bones of the spine (see *disc, intervertebral*). It also forms the shock-absorbing pads of tissue within joints.

Elastic cartilage is soft and rubbery. It is found in structures such as the outer ear and the *epiglottis*.

caruncle

A general term for a small, fleshy swelling. Caruncles can be normal, such as the red, raised tissue in the inner corner of the eye. Some are abnormal, appearing as polyp-like growths; this type may be found, for example, at the opening of the urethra (the tube by which urine leaves the bladder).

Casal's necklace

A red rash forming a clearly defined ring around the neck. It is a symptom of *pellagra*, a disorder caused by lack of the B vitamin niacin in the diet.

caseous abscess

An *abscess* (collection of pus) containing matter that resembles curds or cottage cheese. Caseous abscesses are most commonly due to *tuberculosis*.

cast

A rigid casing applied to a limb or other part of the body to hold a broken bone or dislocated joint in position as it heals. Most casts are made of bandages impregnated with polyurethane resin or *plaster of Paris*, which are applied while wet and harden as they dry. Casts are removed using an electric saw that cuts through the cast but does not damage the skin.

castor oil

A colourless or yellow-tinged oil that is obtained from the leaves of the castor oil plant, RICINUS COMMUNIS. Zinc and castor oil are combined in a soothing ointment to treat conditions such as *nappy rash*. Castor oil was once used as a laxative but is no longer recommended for this purpose.

castration

The surgical removal of the testes (see *orchidectomy*). The term "castration" is sometimes also used to refer to removal of the ovaries (see *oophorectomy*).

Castration is performed when the testes or ovaries are diseased. It may also be carried out in order to reduce the level of *testosterone* (a male sex hormone produced in the testes) or of *oestrogen* (a female sex hormone produced in the ovaries) in people who have certain types of *cancer* that are stimulated by these hormones.

Orchidectomy and oophorectomy are performed less frequently since the introduction of *gonadorelin* analogues, which are drugs that also act to reduce the amount of testosterone and oestrogen produced by the body.

catabolism

Any chemical process in which complex substances are broken down in the body cells into simpler substances, releasing energy into the cells; for example, the breakdown of intracellular fat to provide energy. The opposite process of building up complex substances from simpler ones (building proteins from amino acids, for example) is called *anabolism*. (See also *biochemistry*; *metabolism*.)

catalepsy

A physical state in which the muscles of the face, body, and limbs stay in a semirigid, statuelike position for minutes, hours, or even days. Catalepsy sometimes occurs in people who have *schizophrenia* or *epilepsy* but may also be due to brain disease or certain drugs.

catalyst

A substance, such as an *enzyme*, that increases the rate of a chemical reaction without being permanently changed itself by that reaction.

cataplexy

A sudden loss of muscle tone, causing an involuntary collapse without loss of consciousness. Triggered by intense emotion, particularly laughter, it occurs almost exclusively in sufferers of sleep disorders such as *narcolepsy*.

cataract

Loss of transparency of the *lens* of the *eye*, due to changes in its protein fibres. At an advanced stage, the front part of the lens becomes densely opaque, but the cataract never causes total blindness. A densely opalescent lens still transmits light, but the clarity and detail of the image is lost. Cataract usually occurs in both eyes, but in most cases one eye is more seriously affected than the other.

CAUSES
Almost everyone over 65 has some degree of cataract; the condition might be considered part of the normal aging process. Regular exposure to *ultraviolet light* increases the risk.

Other causes of cataract include an injury to the eye, particularly if a foreign body enters the lens. Cataract is also common in people with *diabetes mellitus* and may develop at an earlier age if blood sugar levels are not well controlled. Long-term use of *corticosteroid drugs* may contribute to cataract.

Congenital cataract may be due to an infection of the mother in early pregnancy, especially with *rubella* (German measles), or to the toxic effects of certain drugs in pregnancy. It may also be associated with *Down's syndrome* or the rare genetic disorder *galactosaemia*.

SYMPTOMS
Cataract is entirely painless and causes only visual symptoms. The onset of symptoms is almost imperceptible, although night driving may be affected in the early stages and bright lights may appear to be surrounded by haloes. There is slow, progressive loss of visual acuity (increasing blurring of vision). The person may become shortsighted and notice disturbances in colour perception.

TREATMENT
When vision has become significantly impaired, *cataract surgery* is performed to remove the lens and replace it with an implant. Provided the eye is otherwise healthy, cataract surgery generally gives excellent results.

cataract surgery

Removal of the *lens* from the eye. Cataract surgery is done to restore sight in people whose vision is impaired by a *cataract*. The lens is usually replaced with a plastic implant during the operation. Alternatively, for young people

and those with other eye disorders, a contact lens or spectacle lens fitted after the operation may be preferable.

catarrh

Oversecretion of mucus by inflamed *mucous membranes* (see *rhinitis*), sinuses (see *sinusitis*) or air passages.

catatonia

A state in which a person becomes mute or adopts a bizarre, rigid pose. The eyes usually remain open and the person may seem awake, but they make no voluntary movements. The state is seen in a rare form of *schizophrenia* and some types of brain disease.

PROCEDURE FOR **CATARACT SURGERY**

In a normal, healthy lens there is no interference with the passage of light rays. Even when peripheral opacities develop, vision is not limited until the central zone is affected. Dense nuclear opacities, however, such as that shown on the right, cause deteriorating vision. The affected lens cannot be restored to its former transparency, hence the need for surgical replacement.

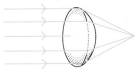
Dense nuclear cataract

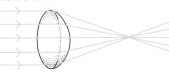
Normal lens

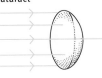
Peripheral cataract

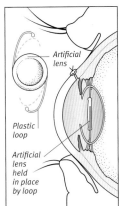
Appearance of cataract
In preparation for surgery, measurements are taken of the cornea and the eye's length to calculate the power of the lens implant that will be needed to restore vision fully. The surgery itself is straightforward and is usually carried out under local anaesthesia. Instruments of remarkable delicacy and precision are used for the procedure, which is usually performed with the help of an operating microscope.

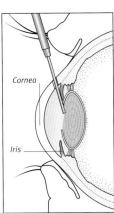
Cornea

Iris

1 An ultrasound probe is inserted into the lens capsule through a small incision in the cornea. The incision is made using a diamond tipped instrument.

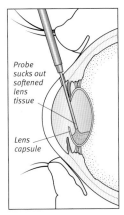
Probe sucks out softened lens tissue

Lens capsule

2 The ultrasound probe softens the lens by emitting sound waves. It then sucks out the softened lens tissue. Only the front part of the lens capsule is removed.

Artificial lens

Plastic loop

Artificial lens held in place by loop

3 An artificial lens is placed inside the lens capsule. The incision in the cornea is left to heal naturally, or it may be closed with a few surgical stitches.

catharsis

A word that means purification or cleansing. The term "catharsis" is used in medicine to refer to the process of cleaning out the bowels. In addition, the term was used by Sigmund Freud in *psychoanalytic theory* to describe the expression of previously repressed feelings and memories. Freud believed that the revival of "forgotten" memories and the expression of the emotions associated with them could bring relief from anxiety, tension, and a variety of other psychological symptoms.

cathartic

A term that means "having the power to purify or cleanse". A cathartic drug stimulates movement of the bowels (see *laxative drugs*).

catheter

A flexible tube that is inserted into the body to drain or introduce fluids or to carry out other functions. Catheters are commonly used to drain urine from the bladder (see *catheterization, urinary*). Other procedures using catheters may be performed in order to investigate the condition of the heart (see *catheterization, cardiac*), to widen obstructed blood vessels, or to control bleeding. (See also *balloon catheter*.)

catheterization, cardiac

A procedure in which a fine, sterile *catheter* (flexible tube) is introduced into the heart through a vein or artery in the arm or leg. Cardiac catheterization may be used to diagnose and treat congenital heart disease (see *heart disease, congenital*), *coronary artery disease*, and some disorders of the heart valves.

Cardiac catheterization may be used diagnostically to measure pressure in the chambers of the heart; to take samples of blood or tissue for laboratory analysis; or to introduce radiopaque dye (a substance opaque to X-rays) into the arteries in order to make the heart cavities visible on X-ray (see *angiography*). Cardiac catheterization may be used therapeutically to widen narrowed coronary arteries (see *angioplasty, balloon*) or to widen narrowed heart valves (see *valvuloplasty*).

The procedure causes little discomfort and is performed under local anaesthesia (see *anaesthesia, local*). A small incision is made in an artery or vein near the skin surface, and the catheter is introduced into the vessel. The tube is passed along the blood vessels and into the heart.

catheterization, urinary

The insertion of a sterile *catheter* (a flexible tube) into the *bladder* in order to drain urine from the body.

WHY IT IS DONE

Urinary catheterization is carried out when a person is unable to empty the bladder normally or is incontinent (see *incontinence, urinary*). The procedure is also performed during certain operations in which a full bladder might block the surgeon's view of surrounding organs; in bladder function tests such as *cystometry* and *cystourethrography*; and to monitor urine production in critically ill patients.

HOW IT IS DONE

There are two principal techniques: urethral catheterization (described in the illustrated box below), and suprapubic catheterization.

Suprapubic catheterization is used if it is not possible to pass a catheter up the urethra (for example, if the urethra is abnormally narrow). This form of catheterization involves the insertion of a catheter into the bladder directly through the abdominal wall, and this is carried out under local anaesthesia (see *anaesthesia, local*).

cation

An *ion* of positive charge. An example of a cation is the sodium ion in saline solution. (See also *electrolyte*.)

cation exchange resin

A type of drug used to remove excess *potassium* that has accumulated in the body because of *renal failure*.

CAT scanning

An abbreviation for computerized axial tomographic scanning, which is commonly known as *CT scanning*.

cat-scratch fever

An uncommon disease that develops in people (mostly children) who have suffered a scratch or bite from a cat. The fever is due to infection with a bacterium called BARTONELLA HENSELAE.

URETHRAL **CATHETERIZATION** OF THE BLADDER

A urinary catheter is usually passed into the bladder through the urethra. First, the doctor or nurse cleans the opening of the urethra with antiseptic solution to avoid introducing infection into the urinary tract. He or she then applies a local anaesthetic gel to the urethra. The procedure usually takes about 10 minutes.

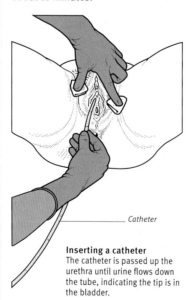

Catheter

Inserting a catheter
The catheter is passed up the urethra until urine flows down the tube, indicating the tip is in the bladder.

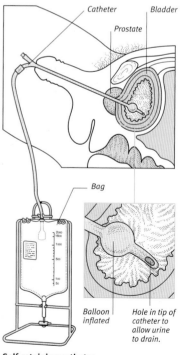

Catheter   Bladder
Prostate
Bag
Balloon inflated   Hole in tip of catheter to allow urine to drain.

Self-retaining catheter
If the catheter is to remain in the bladder, a self-retaining type is used. This catheter has a balloon at its tip that can be inflated and filled with sterile water.

SYMPTOMS

The main symptom, appearing three to ten days after the bite or scratch, is a swollen *lymph node* near the affected area. The node may become painful and tender, and an infected blister may develop at the site of the injury. A fever, rash, and headache may occur.

DIAGNOSIS AND TREATMENT

Diagnosis of cat-scratch fever is confirmed by *biopsy* (removal of a small sample of tissue for microscopic analysis) of the swollen lymph node and by a skin test. *Analgesic drugs* (painkillers) may be used to relieve the fever and headache. In most cases, the illness clears up completely within two months.

cats, diseases from

Cats carry various parasites and infectious organisms that can be spread to humans. Some of these are specific to cats; others may also affect dogs.

SPECIFIC DISEASES

The most serious disease that can be contracted from an infected cat is *rabies*. Anyone who is bitten by a cat (or any other animal) in a country where rabies is present should seek medical advice without delay.

Cat-scratch fever is an uncommon illness that is caused by infection with the bacterium BARTONELLA HENSELAE following a scratch or bite from a cat.

Cats commonly carry the *protozoan* (single-celled parasite) TOXOPLASMA GONDII, which causes the disease *toxoplasmosis*. Infection with the parasite, which is usually from contact with a cat's faeces, is not generally serious, but it can have severe effects in pregnant women. Infections in early pregnancy can lead to *miscarriage* or severe malformation of the fetus. Later in pregnancy, infections can result in nervous system disorders in the fetus and may even lead to blindness in early childhood.

Cat faeces may also carry eggs of the cat roundworm, a possible cause of *toxocariasis*. Rarely, a larva from an ingested roundworm egg migrates to and lodges in an eye, causing deterioration of vision or blindness. Children who have been playing in sand or soil that has been contaminated by cat faeces are at risk of coming into contact with the worm eggs.

Other cat-related disorders in humans include *tinea* (fungal infections of the skin, hair, or nails), particularly ringworm, (ringlike fungal patches, often on the scalp), bites from cat fleas, and allergic reactions to dander (scales from animal skin, hair, or feathers) that may cause *asthma* or *urticaria* (nettle rash).

PREVENTION

Diseases from cats can be avoided by good hygiene, such as hand-washing, particularly after touching a cat. All pets should have regular worming and flea treatment and veterinary care if ill.

cauda equina

A "spray" of nerve roots resembling a horse's tail that descends from the lower *spinal cord* and occupies the lower third of the spinal canal.

caudal

This word is used to refer to the lower end of the *spine*. The word "caudal" means "of the tail".

caudal block

A type of *nerve block* in which a local anaesthetic is injected into the lower part of the spinal canal (the central space within the spine). Caudal block may be used to anaesthetize the buttocks and genitals as part of *obstetric* and gynaecological procedures.

cauliflower ear

Painful, swollen distortion of the pinna (ear flap) resulting from blows or friction that have caused bleeding in the soft *cartilage* of the ear.

Immediate treatment following an injury involves the use of ice-packs to reduce the swelling. In severe cases, a doctor may drain blood from the ear and apply a pressure bandage.

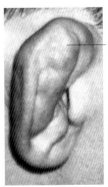

Affected area

Example of cauliflower ear
Following injury to the ear, there has been bleeding into the soft cartilage. The ear flap has been deformed, with loss of the normal folds of skin.

causalgia

A persistent, burning pain, usually in an arm or leg. Causalgia most often occurs as a result of injury to a nerve by a deep cut, limb *fracture*, or gunshot wound. The skin overlying the painful area may be red and tender, or blue, cold, and clammy. The condition may be aggravated by light sensations, such as touch, or by emotional factors.

In some cases, treatment with *antidepressant drugs* or *anticonvulsant drugs* is effective. A few people benefit from *sympathectomy*, in which nerves supplying the affected area are severed.

caustic

Describes substances that have a burning or corrosive action on body tissues or a burning taste. An example is caustic soda, the common name for sodium hydroxide. Caustic agents such as silver nitrate are used to destroy warts.

cauterization

The application of a heated instrument to destroy tissues, stop bleeding, or promote healing. Cauterization may be used to treat conditions such as *haemorrhoids* (piles) and *cervical ectopy*. It has been largely replaced by *electrocoagulation* (use of high-frequency electric current and, increasingly, laser to seal blood vessels).

Caverject preparations

A brand name for preparations of *alprostadil*, a *prostaglandin drug* used to treat *erectile dysfunction*.

cavernous sinus thrombosis

Blockage of a venous *sinus* (a channel for venous blood located deep inside the skull behind an eye socket) by a *thrombus* (an abnormal blood clot). Cavernous sinus thrombosis is usually a complication of a bacterial infection in an area drained by the veins entering the sinus. At first, only the veins behind one eye are affected, but within a few days the thrombosis may spread to the sinus behind the other eye.

CAUSES

Among the infections that can lead to cavernous sinus thrombosis are *cellulitis* (a severe skin infection) of the face, infections of the mouth, eye, or middle ear, *sinusitis* (infection of the air spaces of the facial skull), and *septicaemia* (infection in the bloodstream).

SYMPTOMS

Symptoms of cavernous sinus thrombosis include severe headache, high fever, pain and loss of sensation in and above the affected eye due to the pressure on the fifth cranial nerve, and *proptosis* (protrusion of the eyeball) due to swelling around and behind the eye. In some cases, vision may become blurred

C

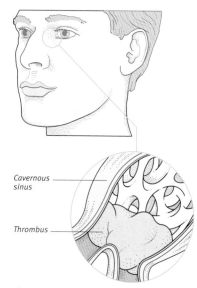

Cavernous sinus

Thrombus

Thrombus in cavernous sinus
The clot obstructs blood flow in the cavernous sinus, causing pressure behind the eye socket.

and eye movements may be paralysed due to pressure on the *optic nerve* and other cranial nerves.

TREATMENT
Treatment with *antibiotic drugs* and *anticoagulant drugs* can save vision. Left untreated, blindness will result, and the infection may eventually prove fatal.

cavity, abdominal
See *abdomen*.

cavity, dental
A hole in a tooth, commonly caused by dental caries (see *caries, dental*).

cavity, oral
See *mouth*.

cavity, pelvic
The area of the body that lies below the abdomen. Framed by the pelvic bones and lower spine, it contains the lower digestive and urinary organs, nearly all of the reproductive organs in females, and part of the reproductive system in males.

cavity, pleural
The space between the two layers of the *pleura* (membrane) that lines the chest wall and the outside of the lungs.

CD4 count
A blood test used to monitor *HIV infection* and *AIDS* that involves counting the number of CD4 *lymphocytes* (white blood cells that fight infection) in a blood sample. CD4 lymphocytes are destroyed by HIV, and reduced levels of them indicate the progression of HIV. A CD4 count can also be used to monitor the effectiveness of treatment.

cefaclor
A common antibiotic that belongs to the group of *cephalosporin drugs*.

cefadroxil
A *cephalosporin drug*, which is used to treat bacterial infections.

cefalexin
A *cephalosporin drug*, which is used to treat bacterial infections.

cefotaxime
A *cephalosporin drug*, which is used to treat bacterial infections.

cefuroxime
A *cephalosporin drug*, which is used to treat bacterial infections.

celecoxib
A COX-2 inhibitor drug (a type of *nonsteroidal anti-inflammatory drug*) used to relieve the pain and inflammation of *rheumatoid arthritis* and *osteoarthritis*. Side effects include nausea and diarrhoea. Abdominal discomfort may also occur, but can be minimized by taking the drug with food. COX-2 inhibitors are associated with an increased risk of heart disease and stroke and are not generally recommended for people who have had, or are at risk of having, a heart attack or stroke.

cell
The basic structural unit of all living organisms. The human body comprises billions of cells, which are structurally and functionally integrated to perform the complex tasks necessary for life. In spite of variations in their size and function, most of the body's cells have a similar form.

CELL MEMBRANE
Each cell is a microscopic bag containing liquid cytoplasm. It is surrounded by a membrane that regulates the passage of useful substances (such as oxygen and nutrients) into the cell and of waste materials (such as carbon dioxide) and manufactured substances (such as hormones) out of the cell. Some cells, such as those lining the small intestine, have microvilli, projections that increase the cells' surface area to facilitate absorption.

NUCLEUS
All cells, except red blood cells, have a *nucleus*. The nucleus controls all major cell activities by regulating the amount and types of *proteins* made in the cell. Inside the nucleus are *chromosomes*, which are made of the nucleic acid *DNA*. This acid contains the instructions for *protein synthesis*, which are carried into the cytoplasm by a type of *RNA* (another nucleic acid) and are decoded in particles called ribosomes. The nucleus also contains a spherical structure called the nucleolus, which plays a role in the production of ribosomes.

ORGANELLES
In the cytoplasm there are various tiny structures called organelles, each with a particular role. Energy is generated by *mitochondria* breaking down sugars and fatty acids. Substances that would damage the cell if they came into contact with the cytoplasm are contained in particles called lysosomes and peroxisomes. A system of membranes in the cytoplasm, called the endoplasmic reticulum, transports materials through the cell. Flattened sacs called the Golgi complex receive and process proteins from the endoplasmic reticulum.

Enzymes and hormones are secreted by vesicles (small saclike structures) at the cell surface. Some waste products and other materials are transported and stored in vacuoles (spaces created by the cytoplasm). The cytoplasm has a network of fine tubes (microtubules) and filaments (microfilaments) known as the cytoskeleton, which gives the cell a definite shape.

cell death
See *apoptosis*.

cell division
The processes by which cells multiply. *Mitosis* is the most common form, giving rise to daughter cells identical to the parent cells. *Meiosis* produces egg (see *ovum*) and *sperm* cells that differ from their parent cells in that they have only half the normal number of *chromosomes*.

cellular immunity
The part of the body's *immune system* that attacks and destroys harmful cells directly rather than by using *antibodies* (proteins that combat infection).

Lymphocytes (a type of white blood cell) mount a response against infectious organisms and other abnormal cells, such as cancer cells. There are two

CELL TYPES

Despite their fundamental similarities in structure, the cells of the body are differentiated so that they can perform a variety of specific tasks, such as carrying oxygen (red blood cells), destroying invading microorganisms (white blood cells), and making hormones (secretory cells in glands). Some cells (nerve cells, for instance) cannot be replaced once they have been destroyed, while other cells (those that form toe- and fingernails, for instance) regrow and continue to function even after a person's death. There are four main types of cells, which are grouped according to their primary functions.

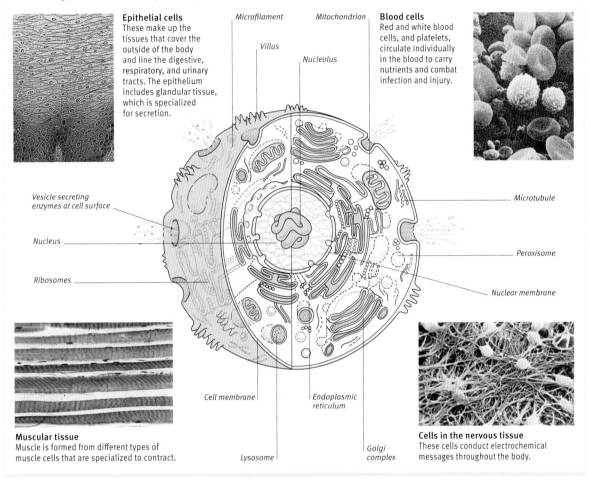

Epithelial cells
These make up the tissues that cover the outside of the body and line the digestive, respiratory, and urinary tracts. The epithelium includes glandular tissue, which is specialized for secretion.

Microfilament

Villus

Mitochondrion

Nucleolus

Blood cells
Red and white blood cells, and platelets, circulate individually in the blood to carry nutrients and combat infection and injury.

Vesicle secreting enzymes at cell surface

Nucleus

Ribosomes

Microtubule

Peroxisome

Nuclear membrane

Cell membrane

Endoplasmic reticulum

Lysosome

Golgi complex

Muscular tissue
Muscle is formed from different types of muscle cells that are specialized to contract.

Cells in the nervous tissue
These cells conduct electrochemical messages throughout the body.

principal types of lymphocytes: T-lymphocytes, which provide cellular immunity, and B-lymphocytes, which produce antibodies. T-lymphocytes recognize specific antigens (substances that the body identifies as foreign), including cancer cells and cells infected by viruses. One group of T-lymphocytes, known as killer T-cells, attach themselves to the abnormal cells and release toxic proteins that destroy them. (See also *humoral immunity*.)

cellulite

The popular term for the subcutaneous fat that gives the skin a dimpled, or orange-peel, appearance, especially on the thighs and buttocks. Cellulite usually affects women rather than men. The cause is not known, although genetic and/or hormonal factors may be involved.

cellulitis

A bacterial infection of the skin and the tissues beneath it, which usually affects the lower legs but can occur anywhere on the body. Cellulitis is most commonly caused by streptococci bacteria, which enter the skin via a wound.

The symptoms include fever and chills; and the affected area is hot, red and swollen. Cellulitis is more severe in people with reduced immunity, such as those who have an *immunodeficiency disorder*. Untreated cellulitis at the site of a wound may progress to *bacteraemia* (bacterial infection of the blood) and *septicaemia* (blood poisoning). Facial infections may spread to the eye socket.

Treatment is with *antibiotic drugs* such as benzylpenicillin and flucloxacillin, or *erythromycin*. (See also *erysipelas*.)

cellulose

A *carbohydrate* consisting of chains of glucose (a simple sugar). Cellulose is the main constituent of plant cell walls. Because it cannot be digested, cellulose is an important source of dietary fibre (see *fibre, dietary*).

C

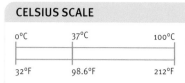

0°C	37°C	100°C
32°F	98.6°F	212°F

Celsius scale

A temperature scale in which the melting point of ice is defined as zero degrees (0°C) and the boiling point of water is 100 degrees (100°C). On this scale, the normal body temperature in humans is 37°C. The scale is named after the Swedish astronomer Anders Celsius (1701–1744). "Centigrade" is an obsolete name for the same scale.

To convert a Celsius temperature to Fahrenheit, multiply the figure by 1.8, then add 32. To convert Fahrenheit to Celsius, subtract 32, then multiply by 0.56. (See also *Fahrenheit scale*.)

cementum

Bonelike tissue surrounding the root of a tooth (see *teeth*).

centigrade scale

The obsolete name for the *Celsius scale*.

centrally acting antihypertensive drugs

A type of *antihypertensive drug* used in the treatment of *hypertension* (high blood pressure). Centrally acting antihypertensives, such as *clonidine* and *methyldopa*, act on the mechanism in the brain that controls blood-vessel size.

central nervous system

The anatomical term for the *brain* and *spinal cord*, often abbreviated to CNS. The central nervous system is made up of neurons (nerve cells) and supporting tissue, and works in tandem with the *peripheral nervous system* (PNS), which carries signals between the CNS and the rest of the body.

The CNS receives sensory information from organs such as the eyes and ears, and from sensory receptors in the body. It analyses this information, then initiates an appropriate motor response in the body, such as contracting a muscle. (See also *nervous system*.)

central venous pressure

The pressure within the right *atrium*, the chamber of the heart that receives oxygen-depleted blood from the body. Central venous pressure is measured by means of a fine tube, attached to a monitor, that is passed through a vein close to the heart and into the right atrium. By monitoring the pressure, doctors can estimate the volume of blood circulating around the body. This action may be of value following severe haemorrhage and in cases where the blood pressure is too low to deliver an adequate blood supply to organs and tissues (see *shock*).

centrifuge

This is a machine that separates the different components of a body fluid for analysis. When a fluid such as blood is spun at high speed around a central axis, groups of particles of varying density, such as red and white blood cells, are separated by centrifugal force and can be analysed independently.

cephalexin

An alternative spelling of cefalexin, a common *cephalosporin drug*.

cephalhaematoma

An extensive, soft swelling on the scalp of a newborn baby. Cephalhaematoma is caused by bleeding into the space between the skull and its fibrous covering (the periosteum or pericranium) due to pressure exerted on the baby's head during delivery. The swelling is neither painful nor serious and it gradually subsides, although this process may take several weeks.

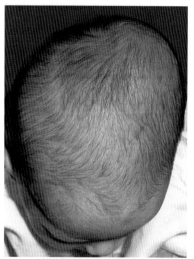

Cephalhaematoma
This baby was born with a cephalhaematoma on one side of the scalp at the back of the head. The condition is not serious and the swelling gradually subsides over a period of a few weeks.

cephalic

Relating to the head, as in cephalic presentation, the head-first position of a baby in the birth canal.

cephalopelvic disproportion

A complication of childbirth (see *childbirth, complications of*) in which the mother's pelvis is too narrow in proportion to the size of the baby's head.

cephalosporin drugs

COMMON DRUGS
- Cefaclor • Cefadroxil • Cefalexin • Cefotaxime
- Cefpodoxime • Ceftazidime • Cefuroxime

A large group of *antibiotic drugs*, derived from the fungus CEPHALOSPORIUM ACREMONIUM, which are effective against a wide range of infections. Cephalosporins are used to treat ear, throat, and respiratory tract infections and conditions, such as *urinary tract infections* and *gonorrhoea*, in which the causative bacteria are resistant to other types of antibiotic.

HOW THEY WORK
Cephalosporin drugs interfere with the development of bacterial cell walls and inhibit the production of protein in the bacterial cells. As a result, the bacteria die. Some types of bacteria, however, produce an enzyme (a protein that acts as a catalyst) called beta-lactamase that can inactivate some of the older cephalosporin drugs. Newer cephalosporins are not affected by this enzyme.

SIDE EFFECTS
Occasionally, cephalosporin drugs may cause allergic reactions, such as rash, itching, and fever. Rarely, *anaphylactic shock* (a very severe allergic reaction) occurs. Other side effects include diarrhoea, *colitis* (inflammation of the colon), and *blood disorders*.

cerebellar ataxia

Jerky, staggering gait and other uncoordinated movements caused by disease of, or damage to, the *cerebellum*. Other features may include *dysarthria* (slurred speech), hand tremor, and *nystagmus* (abnormal jerky eye movements).

Causes include *stroke*, *multiple sclerosis*, *brain tumour*, damage as a result of *alcohol dependence*, and an inherited disorder of the cerebellum.

cerebellar syndrome

A collection of symptoms, due to certain types of brain disorder, that include tremor, speech disturbance, and abnormal eye movements (*nystagmus*) and gait.

cerebellum

A region of the brain at the back of the skull, behind the *brainstem*. The cerebellum is concerned primarily with the maintenance of posture and balance and the coordination of movement.

STRUCTURE

The cerebellum is linked to the *brainstem* by thick nerve tracts. It consists of two hemispheres. From the inner side of each hemisphere arise three nerve fibre stalks, which link with different parts of the brainstem and carry signals between the cerebellum and the rest of the brain. Nerve fibres from the stalks fan out towards the deep folds of the *cortex* (outer part) of each cerebellar hemisphere, which consists of layers of what is often referred to as *grey matter* (interconnected nerve cells).

FUNCTION

Information about the body's posture and the state of contraction or relaxation in its muscles is conveyed from muscle tendons and the labyrinth in the inner ear via the brainstem to the cerebellum. Working with the *basal ganglia* (nerve cell clusters deep within the brain), the cerebellum uses this data to fine tune messages sent to muscles from the motor cortex in the *cerebrum* (the main mass of the brain).

LOCATION OF **CEREBELLUM**

The cerebellum is situated behind the brainstem and is connected to it by a collection of nerve tracts.

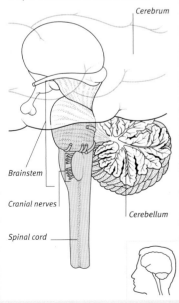

Cerebrum

Brainstem

Cranial nerves

Cerebellum

Spinal cord

DISORDERS

Disease or damage to the cerebellum may result in *cerebral ataxia*, which is characterized by jerky, staggering gait, slurred speech, and other uncoordinated movements of the body. *Alcohol intoxication* impairs cerebellar function and may produce similar symptoms.

cerebral haemorrhage

Bleeding that occurs within the brain due to a ruptured blood vessel (see *intracerebral haemorrhage*; *stroke*).

cerebral malaria

A potentially fatal complication of *malaria* that affects the brain and causes loss of consciousness.

cerebral oedema

An abnormal accumulation of fluid in the *brain*. The resulting compression of brain tissues may cause symptoms such as headache and visual disturbances. There are various causes for cerebral oedema, including injury, *anoxia* (lack of oxygen), and poisoning.

cerebral palsy

A disorder of posture and movement that results from damage to the developing brain before, during, or just after birth, or in early childhood. Cerebral palsy is nonprogressive. It varies in severity from slight clumsiness of hand movement and gait to complete immobility.

CAUSES

In most cases, damage occurs before or at birth, sometimes as a result of cerebral *hypoxia* (an inadequate supply of oxygen to the brain). More rarely, the cause is a maternal infection that spreads to the baby in the uterus.

In rare cases, cerebral palsy is caused by *kernicterus*, which results from an excess of bile pigment in babies with *haemolytic disease of the newborn*. Possible causes after birth include *encephalitis* (inflammation of the brain tissue), *meningitis* (inflammation of the protective membranes covering the brain), *head injury*, or *intracerebral haemorrhage* (bleeding within the brain).

SYMPTOMS

Cerebral palsy may not be recognized until well into the baby's first year. Initially, the infant may have hypotonic (floppy) muscles, be difficult to feed, and show delay in sitting up without support. An affected child may go on to develop *spastic paralysis* (abnormal muscle stiffness), *athetosis* (involuntary writhing movements), or *ataxia* (loss of coordination and balance). Other nervous system disorders, such as hearing defects or epileptic seizures, may be present. About 70 per cent of children have mental impairment, but the rest are of normal or high intelligence.

DIAGNOSIS AND TREATMENT

If the condition is suspected from the symptoms and from neurological and developmental assessments, imaging tests such as *CT scanning* and *MRI* may be performed to identify brain damage.

Although there is no cure for cerebral palsy, much can be done to help and a team of professionals working with the family can maximize the child's ability to function. *Physiotherapy* can help a child to develop muscular control and maintain balance. *Speech therapy* may improve speech and communication. Drugs such as *muscle relaxants* can be used to control spasms and *botulinum toxin* injected into muscles makes them less stiff and increases joint mobility.

cerebral thrombosis

The formation of a *thrombus* (blood clot) in an artery in the brain. The clot may block the artery, cutting off blood, nutrients, and oxygen to the region of brain tissue supplied by the artery. This problem may result in a *stroke*.

cerebrospinal fluid

A clear, watery fluid that circulates between the ventricles (cavities) within the *brain*, the central canal in the *spinal cord*, and the space between the brain and spinal cord and their protective coverings, the *meninges*. Cerebrospinal fluid functions as a shock-absorber, helping to prevent or reduce damage to the brain and spinal cord after a blow to the head or back. It contains glucose, proteins, salts, and white blood cells.

Examination of the fluid, samples of which are usually obtained by *lumbar puncture*, is used in the diagnosis of many conditions affecting the brain and spinal cord, including *meningitis* and *subarachnoid haemorrhage*.

Accumulation of cerebrospinal fluid within the skull during the development of the fetus, or in infancy, may cause the skull to become enlarged (a condition known as *hydrocephalus*).

cerebrovascular accident

Any sudden rupture or blockage of a blood vessel in the brain. The problem causes serious bleeding and/or local obstruction to blood circulation, and leads to a *stroke* (damage to part of the brain due to interrupted blood supply).

Blockage may be due to *thrombosis* (clot formation) or to *embolism* (a clot fragment, or an air bubble carried in the circulation). Rupture of vessels may result in different patterns of bleeding: *intracerebral haemorrhage* (bleeding in the brain) or *subarachnoid haemorrhage* (bleeding around the brain).

cerebrovascular disease

Any disease affecting an artery supplying blood to areas inside the brain. Such diseases include *atherosclerosis* (narrowing of the arteries) and defects in arterial walls that cause *aneurysm* (a balloon-like swelling in an artery).

The disease may eventually cause a *cerebrovascular accident*, which commonly results in a *stroke*. Extensive narrowing of blood vessels throughout the brain can be a cause of *dementia*.

cerebrum

The largest and most developed part of the *brain*, and the site of most conscious and intelligent activities.

STRUCTURE

The main components of the cerebrum are two large hemispheres that grow out from the upper part of the *brainstem* (an extension of the spinal cord). The surface of the cerebrum is made up of a series of folds called gyri, which are separated by fissures called sulci, with a deep longitudinal fissure separating the two hemispheres.

The four main surface regions of each hemisphere – the frontal, parietal, temporal, and occipital lobes – are named after the bones that are overlying them. Each hemisphere has a central cavity, called a *ventricle*, that is filled with *cerebrospinal fluid*. This cavity is surrounded by an inner layer, consisting of clusters of nerve cells called the *basal ganglia*. There is a middle layer of *white matter* composed mainly of nerve fibres, which carry information between particular areas of the *cortex* and between the cortex, central brain, and *brainstem*. The outer surface layer of each hemisphere is the cerebral cortex, which is also known as the *grey matter*, where much of the sensory information from organs such as the eyes and the ears is processed. A thick band of fibres called the corpus callosum carries nerve signals between the two cerebral hemispheres.

STRUCTURE OF THE **CEREBRUM**

The cerebrum dwarfs the rest of the brain. Much of its surface is hidden within the folds, as shown by the vertical cross-section below.

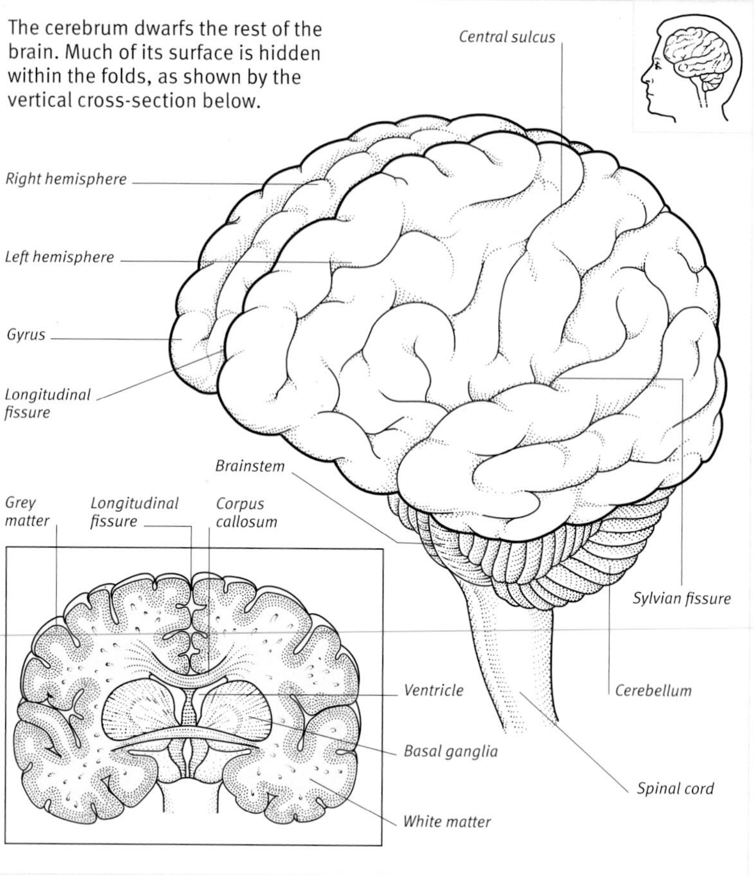

Right hemisphere

Left hemisphere

Gyrus

Longitudinal fissure

Central sulcus

Brainstem

Sylvian fissure

Cerebellum

Spinal cord

Grey matter

Longitudinal fissure

Corpus callosum

Ventricle

Basal ganglia

White matter

FUNCTION

Specific sensory processing takes place in separate regions. For example, visual perception is located in a part of the occipital lobe called the visual cortex.

The cortex also contains motor areas concerned with initiating signals for movements of the skeletal muscles. Linked to the sensory and motor areas of the cortex are association areas. These regions integrate information from various senses and also perform functions such as comprehension and recognition, memory storage and recall, thought, and decision-making.

Some cortical functions are localized to one dominant hemisphere (the left in almost all right-handed and many left-handed people). Two clearly defined areas in the dominant hemisphere are Wernicke's area, which is responsible for the comprehension of spoken and written language, and Broca's area, which is concerned with language expression.

DISORDERS

Damage to particular areas of the cerebrum may cause specific syndromes. For example, damage to the frontal lobe may cause mental apathy, whereas a parietal lobe injury may result in geographical disorientation. Disease of the temporal lobe may cause *amnesia* (memory loss), and visual defects may result from occipital lobe damage.

Quite often, however, cerebral disease causes nonspecific symptoms such as convulsions and headaches.

cerumen

The medical term for *earwax*.

Cerumol

A brand-named preparation used for the removal of *earwax*.

cervical

This term can mean either relating to the neck or relating to the *cervix* (the neck of the uterus).

C

cervical cancer

See *cervix, cancer of.*

cervical dysplasia

The former term for *cervical intraepithelial neoplasia* (CIN).

cervical ectopy

Formerly known as cervical erosion, a condition affecting the *cervix* (the neck of the uterus) in which a layer of mucus-forming cells that are more characteristic of the inner lining of the cervix appear on its outside surface. There is no loss of tissue or ulceration of the cervix. The tissue may, however, be more fragile, and tend to bleed and secrete more mucus, than normal.

CAUSES

Cervical ectopy may be present from birth. Other possible causes include pregnancy and long-term use of *oral contraceptives.*

SYMPTOMS

Most women with cervical ectopy have few or no symptoms. Some, however, experience vaginal bleeding at unexpected times and may have a vaginal discharge. The cervix has a fragile, reddened area on the surface.

DIAGNOSIS AND TREATMENT

The condition is often detected during a routine *cervical smear test.* Only women with symptoms need treatment. Affected tissue may be destroyed using *cauterization* (application of a heated instrument), *cryosurgery* (freezing), *diathermy* (heat), or *laser treatment.*

cervical erosion

The former term for *cervical ectopy.*

cervical incompetence

Abnormal weakness of the *cervix* (the neck of the uterus) that can result in recurrent *miscarriages.* Normally, the cervix remains closed until the onset of labour. An incompetent cervix may gradually widen under the weight of the fetus from about the 12th week of pregnancy onwards, or may suddenly open during the second trimester.

DIAGNOSIS AND TREATMENT

The condition is detected by a *pelvic examination* or by *ultrasound scanning.* Treatment is with a suture (stitch) applied like a purse string around the cervix at about the 12th week of pregnancy. The suture is left in position until the pregnancy is at or near full term and is then cut to allow the mother to deliver the baby normally.

cervical intraepithelial neoplasia

Also known as CIN (and formerly called cervical dysplasia), abnormalities in the cells of the cervix (the neck of the uterus). CIN is not itself cancer but some cases may develop into cancer.

TYPES

There are three grades of CIN: mild (CIN1), moderate (CIN2), and severe (CIN3), based on the severity of the changes in cervical cells. In mild CIN, abnormal cells may return to a normal state without treatment. Severe CIN, left untreated, may progress to cervical cancer (see *cervix, cancer of*).

CAUSES

The cause of CIN is not known but risk factors include smoking, having unprotected sex at an early age or with many partners, and exposure to *human papillomavirus.*

DIAGNOSIS AND TREATMENT

CIN is diagnosed by examining cervical cells obtained from a *cervical smear test.* Further tests, such as *colposcopy* and *biopsy*, may be performed to determine the extent to which abnormal cells have penetrated into the cervix. The treatment depends on the severity of the condition. Mild CIN may not require treatment because the cells may return to normal, although regular monitoring is necessary. Persistent mild CIN and moderate or severe CIN are treated by destroying or removing the abnormal tissue, either by a method known as LLETZ (large loop excision of the transformation zone), which involves using a heated wire loop, passed through the vagina, to remove the abnormal tissue, or by *cone biopsy.*

cervical mucus method

A form of contraception based on identifying days on which to abstain from sexual intercourse and thereby avoid pregnancy. This technique involves monitoring the changes in the mucus secreted by a woman's *cervix.* (See *contraception, natural methods of.*)

cervical osteoarthritis

A degenerative disorder, also called cervical spondylosis, that affects the joints between the cervical *vertebrae* (the bones in the neck). Cervical osteoarthritis mainly occurs in middle-aged and elderly people, but occasionally the degeneration begins earlier due to an injury, such as a whiplash neck injury sustained in a road traffic accident.

TREATING **CERVICAL INTRAEPITHELIAL NEOPLASIA (CIN)**

Some cases of CIN may need treatment to destroy or remove the area of abnormal tissue (the transformation zone). The main methods of treatment are LLETZ (large loop excision of the transformation zone) and cone biopsy. All treatments are carried out through the vagina and it is usual to have slight bleeding or a discharge for a few days afterwards.

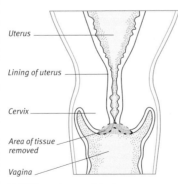

Uterus

Lining of uterus

Cervix

Area of tissue removed

Vagina

LLETZ (large loop excision)
This is used mainly when the abnormal tissue is localized around the opening of the cervix. It uses a heated wire loop to remove the abnormal tissue, and is usually done under local anaesthesia.

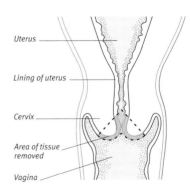

Uterus

Lining of uterus

Cervix

Area of tissue removed

Vagina

Cone biopsy
This method is used when the abnormal tissue extends in towards the uterus. In the procedure, which is done under either local or general anaesthesia, a larger cone-shaped area of the cervix is removed.

SYMPTOMS

The main symptoms of cervical osteoarthritis are neck pain and stiffness. Pressure on the nerves between affected vertebrae may cause pain in the arms and shoulders, numbness tingling and weakness in the hands. Symptoms tend to flare up from time to time with periods of mild discomfort between.

Other symptoms, such as dizziness, unsteadiness, and double vision when turning the head, may also occur as a result of pressure on blood vessels running through the vertebrae to the brain. Rarely, pressure on the spinal cord can cause weakness or paralysis in the legs and loss of bladder control.

DIAGNOSIS AND TREATMENT

X-rays and other imaging procedures, such as *CT scanning* or *MRI* (magnetic resonance imaging), are used to diagnose cervical osteoarthritis.

Treatment of severe neck pain and stiffness may include *heat treatment*, supporting the neck in a collar (usually only as a short-term measure), and *analgesic drugs* (painkillers). *Physiotherapy* may improve neck posture and movement and is useful when the pain has eased. Pressure on the spinal cord may be relieved by surgery (see *decompression, spinal canal*).

cervical rib

A *congenital* abnormality, which is of unknown cause, in which the lowest of the seven cervical *vertebrae* (neck bones) has overdeveloped to form an extra *rib* that lies parallel to and above the first normal rib. The abnormality can vary

LOCATION OF **CERVICAL RIB**

The overdeveloped seventh cervical vertebra forms a rib parallel to a normal one.

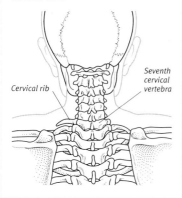

Cervical rib

Seventh cervical vertebra

CERVICAL SMEAR

Cervical smear tests are carried out routinely every three years for women aged 25 to 49 then every five years for women aged 50 to 64. The procedure is risk-free, although it may be slightly uncomfortable, and the actual collection of the cells from the cervix takes only a few seconds.

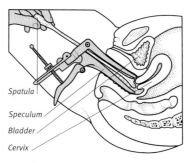

Spatula

Speculum

Bladder

Cervix

Procedure for cervical smear
The woman lies on her back with her legs bent and relaxed so that they fall open at the knees. The vagina is held open with a speculum. Cells are collected with a spatula or a special brush and either smeared on to a glass slide or put in a special liquid for later microscopic examination.

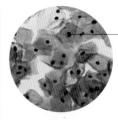

Normal cell nucleus

Normal cells as seen under the microscope

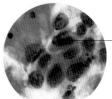

Large dark-stained nucleus of abnormal cell

Abnormal cells as seen under the microscope

from a small, bony swelling to a fully developed rib and it may occur on only one or on both sides.

SYMPTOMS

In many cases, there are no symptoms. If the rib presses on the lower *brachial plexus* (the group of nerves passing from the spinal cord into the arm), however, there may be pain, numbness, and pins-and-needles affecting both the forearm and hand.

DIAGNOSIS AND TREATMENT

An *X-ray* will show the presence of a cervical rib, but other possible causes of pain and tingling in the hand or arm (such as *carpal tunnel syndrome* or a *disc prolapse*) still need to be excluded.

Exercises to strengthen the shoulder muscles and improve posture may bring relief. Severe or persistent symptoms may require surgery to remove the rib.

cervical smear test

A test used to detect *cervical intraepithelial neoplasia* (abnormal changes in the cells of the *cervix*) that could develop into cancer (see *cervix, cancer of*). A cervical smear test can also detect some infections of the cervix, such as *human papillomavirus*, some types of which cause genital warts (see *warts, genital*).

A cervical smear test is routinely carried out every three years for women aged 25 to 49, and then every five years for women aged 50 to 64.

HOW IT IS DONE

The vagina is held open with a speculum and a spatula or fine brush is passed through the vagina to the cervix. A small sample of cells is taken from the surface of the cervix using the spatula or brush. The cell sample is then put on to a glass slide for examination under a microscope or placed in a special liquid (a method known as liquid-based cytology) and sent for later microscopic examination.

If the cells appear normal when examined under a microscope, nothing further needs to be done. If the cells show abnormalities, further smears or other tests, such as *colposcopy* or *biopsy*, may be required.

cervical spondylosis

An alternative name for the neck disorder *cervical osteoarthritis*.

cervicitis

Inflammation of the *cervix* (the neck of the uterus). The condition is usually due to a sexually transmitted infection, such as *gonorrhoea*, *chlamydial infections*, genital herpes (see *herpes, genital*), or genital warts (see *warts, genital*). However, cervical infection may also result from injury to the cervix during childbirth or surgery.

SYMPTOMS

Cervicitis often does not produce symptoms, although there may be a vaginal

ANATOMY OF THE **CERVIX**

The cervix contains a central canal for the passage of sperm and menstrual blood and for childbirth. The canal and outer surface of the cervix are lined with two types of cells: mucus-secreting glandular cells and protective squamous cells.

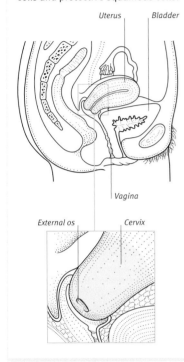

Uterus   Bladder

Vagina

External os   Cervix

discharge, irregular vaginal bleeding, burning pain when passing urine, and lower abdominal pain.

COMPLICATIONS
If it is left untreated, cervicitis can spread to cause *endometritis* (inflammation of the lining of the uterus), *salpingitis* (inflammation of the fallopian tubes), or *pelvic inflammatory disease*.

If a pregnant woman has cervicitis, her baby may be infected during delivery, resulting in *neonatal ophthalmia* (eye infection) or, less commonly, *pneumonia* due to chlamydial infection.

DIAGNOSIS AND TREATMENT
The condition is diagnosed by means of internal examination and by taking swabs of the vaginal discharge, which are then analysed in order to verify the identity of the organism that is responsible for the condition.

Treatment of cervictis is with *antibiotic drugs* or *antiviral drugs*. However, if symptoms persist, the area may be cauterized

by *electrocoagulation* (application of an electric current), *cryotherapy*, (freezing), or *laser treatment*.

cervix

A small, cylindrical organ, several centimetres in length and less than 2.5 cm in diameter, comprising the lower part and neck of the *uterus* (womb). The cervix separates the body and cavity of the uterus from the *vagina*. The fibrous, smooth muscle tissue of the cervix creates a form of sphincter (circular muscle), which can stretch open in *pregnancy* and *childbirth*.

FUNCTION
The cervical canal runs through the cervix. It allows the passage of blood during *menstruation* and of *sperm* from the vagina into the uterus following sexual intercourse, and forms part of the birth canal during childbirth. After puberty, mucus is secreted by the glandular cells in the canal to assist the entry of sperm into the upper cervix. In addition, the mucus protects the sperm and provides them with energy.

During pregnancy, the internal muscle fibres enlarge, thereby lengthening the cervix and acting as a barrier for the retention of the fetus. Towards the end of pregnancy, the cervix begins to shorten in readiness for labour and delivery. During labour the cervical canal widens up to 10 cm to allow the baby to pass from the uterus. Soon after childbirth, the muscles in the cervix contract and the canal returns to its original size.

DISORDERS
The cervix may be injured, or may develop infections or other disorders (see disorders of the cervix box, below). Such

conditions are usually investigated by means of a *pelvic examination*, a *cervical smear test*, or swabs taken from the cervix. In cases of suspected cancer or a precancerous condition, a *colposcopy* (inspection of the cervix with a viewing instrument) may be performed.

cervix, cancer of

One of the most common forms of cancer affecting women worldwide. Cancer of the *cervix* has well-defined precancerous stages in which abnormal changes occur in cells on the surface of the cervix (see *cervical intraepithelial neoplasia*). These types of changes can be detected by a *cervical smear test*. In many cases, this detection allows early treatment leading to a complete cure. If left untreated, however, cancer of the cervix may spread to the organs in the *pelvis*.

TYPES
There are two main types of cervical cancer: the squamous type and a much rarer form called adenocarcinoma.

The squamous type of cervical cancer is associated with some types of *human papillomavirus* (HPV), which may be acquired during sexual intercourse. The other factors that predispose a woman to developing this type of cancer are smoking, starting to have sex at an early age, having many sexual partners, and having a depressed immune system.

The second type of cervical cancer, adenocarcinoma, sometimes occurs in women who have never had sexual intercourse. Its causes are unknown.

SYMPTOMS
In many cases, cancer of the cervix is detected before symptoms develop. If the

DISORDERS OF THE **CERVIX**

The *cervix* (neck of the uterus) may be susceptible to injuries, infections, tumours, and other conditions.

Injury
Minor injury to the cervix may occur during childbirth, particularly if labour is prolonged. Persistent damage to muscle fibres as a result of injury may lead to *cervical incompetence*.

Infection
The most common cervical infections are sexually transmitted infections, such as *gonorrhoea*, *chlamydial infections*, and *trichomoniasis*. Viral infections of the

cervix include those due to the *human papillomavirus* and the herpes simplex virus (see *warts, genital*; *herpes, genital*).

Tumours
Polyps are noncancerous growths that occur on the cervix. Cancerous growths (see *cervix, cancer of*) are preceded by changes in the surface cells (*cervical intraepithelial neoplasia*), which can be detected by a *cervical smear test*.

Other disorders
Cervical ectopy is a condition in which mucus-secreting cells form on the outside of the cervix.

condition is advanced, there may be vaginal bleeding or a bloodstained discharge at unexpected times, such as between periods, after sexual intercourse, or after the menopause. There may be pain if the cancer has spread into the deeper parts of the cervix and then out into the pelvic tissues.

DIAGNOSIS AND TREATMENT
Following an abnormal smear test result, *colposcopy* (inspection of the cervix with a viewing instrument) or a *cone biopsy* may be carried out to diagnose the condition.

Early cancer may be treated with surgery to remove or destroy the abnormal tissue. In more advanced cases affecting the pelvic organs, *radiotherapy* and *chemotherapy* may be given. In certain cases, radical surgery in which the bladder, vagina, cervix, uterus, and rectum are removed may be recommended.

A vaccine against human papillomavirus is available to protect against strains of the virus associated with cervical cancer. In the UK this vaccine will be routinely offered to all girls aged 12 to 13.

cestodes

The scientific name for tapeworms, a group of long, flat, multisegmented parasites (see *tapeworm infestation*).

cetirizine

An *antihistamine drug* that is used to relieve the symptoms of certain conditions such as allergic *rhinitis* (hay fever) and *urticaria* (nettle rash).

cetrimide

An *antiseptic* that is used in many preparations for cleansing the skin.

Chagas' disease

An infectious parasitic disease found only in parts of South and Central America. Chagas' disease is spread by insects commonly called cone-nosed or assassin bugs. The *parasites* live in the bloodstream and can affect the heart, intestines, and nervous system.

Symptoms include swelling of the *lymph nodes* and fever. Long-term complications include damage to the heart. The drug nifurtimox kills the parasites but has unpleasant side effects.

chalazion

A round, painless swelling in the upper or lower eyelid caused by obstruction of one of the *meibomian glands*, which lubricate the edges of the eyelids.

Chalazions are sometimes called meibomian cysts. They can occur at any age and may be more common in people suffering from the skin conditions *acne*, *rosacea*, or seborrhoeic *dermatitis*.

If the cyst becomes infected, the eyelid becomes more swollen, red, and painful. A large swelling putting pressure on the *cornea* at the front of the eye can cause blurring of vision. About one-third of chalazions disappear without treatment, but large cysts may need to be removed surgically.

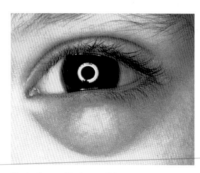

Chalazion on the lower lid
Small chalazions often disappear spontaneously. Larger ones may need to be removed surgically.

challenge, food

See *exclusion diet*.

chancre, hard

An *ulcer*, usually on the genitals, that develops during the first stage of *syphilis* (a sexually transmitted infection).

chancroid

A sexually transmitted infection, found mainly in the tropics, that is characterized by enlargement of the lymph nodes in the groin and painful genital *ulcers*. Chancroid is caused by the bacterium HAEMOPHILUS DUCREYI. Prompt treatment of the condition with *antibiotic drugs* is usually effective.

chapped skin

Sore, cracked, rough skin, usually on the hands and face (particularly the lips), caused by dryness. Chapping is caused by the lack, or removal, of the natural oils that keep skin supple. It tends to occur in cold weather or after repeated washing or wetting.

Chapping can be prevented by wearing protective gloves or applying *barrier creams* before immersing the hands in water, then drying the skin well. Areas of chapped skin can be treated with hand or face cream.

charcoal

A form of carbon that is used in medicine mainly as an adsorbent agent (a substance that binds to toxins) in the emergency treatment of some types of poisoning and drug overdose.

Charcot–Marie–Tooth disease

An inherited muscle-wasting disease of the legs (see *peroneal muscular atrophy*).

Charcot's joint

A joint damaged by repeated injuries that go unnoticed due to loss of sensation in the area (see *neuropathic joint*).

check-up

See *examination, physical*.

cheilitis

Inflammation, cracking, and dryness of the lips. There are several possible causes of cheilitis, including ill-fitting dentures, a local infection, an allergy to cosmetics, excessive sunbathing, or deficiency of riboflavin (vitamin B_2). Treatment is given for the underlying cause; in the meantime, a soothing skin cream can help to relieve the soreness.

chelating agents

Chemicals to treat metal poisoning, which act by combining with metals such as lead, arsenic, and mercury to form less toxic substances. *Penicillamine* is a commonly used chelating agent.

chemical formula

See *formula, chemical*.

chemical pathology

See *pathology, chemical*.

chemosis

Swelling of the *conjunctiva* (the membrane covering the eye and lining the eyelid). Chemosis is most commonly associated with allergic and infective *conjunctivitis*. Treatment may include the use of eyedrops containing an *antihistamine drug* or *antibiotic drug*.

chemotherapy

The term usually used to refer to treatment with *anticancer drugs*. The word "chemotherapy" may also describe the use of *antibiotic drugs* to treat infectious diseases, particularly tuberculosis.

Chemotherapy for cancer works by destroying cancer cells or preventing them from multiplying. The drugs also affect healthy tissues, however, so the treatment is often given in short courses, with drug-free periods in between to allow normal cells to recover. Normal tissues often affected include bone marrow (causing anaemia), the mouth, the intestinal lining, the hair follicles, and the ovaries and testes; sometimes causing severe side effects.

chenodeoxycholic acid

A constituent of *bile* that is necessary for the absorption of fat from the diet and also for the excretion of *cholesterol*.

cherry angioma

An alternative name for a *Campbell de Morgan's spot* (a small, bright red, non-cancerous spot on the trunk or limbs).

cherry-red spot

A red spot that can be seen on the *retina* of infants who have the inherited metabolic disorder *Tay–Sachs disease*.

cherubism

An inherited disease, also known as familial fibrous dysplasia of the jaw. Cherubism is so called because it produces swelling at either side of the jaw, giving the face a cherubic appearance.

chest

The upper part of the trunk. The chest, also known as the *thorax*, extends from the base of the neck down to the *diaphragm muscle*.

chest compression

Another name for *external cardiac massage*. Chest compressions are carried out as part of the life-saving technique *cardiopulmonary resuscitation*.

chest pain

Pain in the chest often has no serious cause, but in some cases it may be a symptom of an underlying disorder requiring urgent treatment. The pain may be in the chest wall (in the skin, the underlying muscles, or the ribs) or in an organ within the chest.

CAUSES

Common causes of pain in the chest wall are a strained muscle or an injury, such as a broken rib. A sharp pain that travels from the back of the chest around to the front may be due to pressure on a nerve root where it leaves the spine; nerve compression may result from disorders such as *osteoarthritis* of the *vertebrae*. Pain in the side of the chest may be caused by *pleurodynia*

(inflammation of the muscles between the ribs and of the diaphragm muscle, associated with a viral infection). The viral infection *herpes zoster* (shingles) may cause severe pain along the course of a nerve in the chest wall. In *Tietze's syndrome*, inflammation at the junctions of the rib *cartilages* causes pain on the front of the chest wall.

A common cause of pain within the chest is *gastro-oesophageal reflux disease* (regurgitation of acid from the stomach into the *oesophagus*); this problem may cause heartburn, a pain behind the sternum (breastbone). More serious causes include disorders involving the lungs, such as *pleurisy* (inflammation of the membranes surrounding the lungs and lining the inside of the chest wall). Pleurisy may be due to *pneumonia* (inflammation of the lungs due to infection) or, rarely, *pulmonary embolism* (a blood clot that has lodged in an artery in the lung). Cancerous lung tumours (see *lung cancer*; *mesothelioma*) may also cause pain as they enlarge in size and press on the *pleura* and the ribs.

Pain in the centre of the chest may be due to a heart disorder. The common disorder *angina pectoris* produces pain that may spread from the chest to the

throat, jaw, or arms. It is caused by an inadequate blood supply to the heart, commonly due to *coronary artery disease*. *Myocardial infarction* (heart attack) causes a similar pain to angina but is usually more severe and is not relieved by rest. Acute *pericarditis* (inflammation of the membrane covering the heart) produces severe pain that may be relieved slightly when the person leans forwards. *Mitral valve prolapse* may cause sharp pain, usually on the left side of the chest.

Chest pain may also be a result of *anxiety* and emotional stress (see *hyperventilation*; *panic attack*).

TREATMENT

The treatment of chest pain depends on the underlying cause. For example, *antibiotic drugs* may be given for chest pain due to pneumonia, and surgery is needed to treat some lung tumours or some cases of coronary artery disease.

chest thrust

A first-aid technique to unblock the airway of a baby who is *choking*.

chest X-ray

A medical test, usually to examine the heart or lungs. Chest X-rays are used to confirm diagnoses of heart disorders,

---

DIAGNOSING **CHEST PAIN**

To make an accurate diagnosis of the underlying cause, it is important for the patient to describe the location, quality (e.g. burning, pressing, or sharp), severity, and duration of the pain, any factors that relieve it or make it worse, and any other symptoms, such

as breathing difficulty. In addition, the doctor will do a physical examination, including listening to chest sounds with a stethoscope and feeling for areas of tenderness in the chest wall. He or she may also arrange for other diagnostic procedures to be carried out.

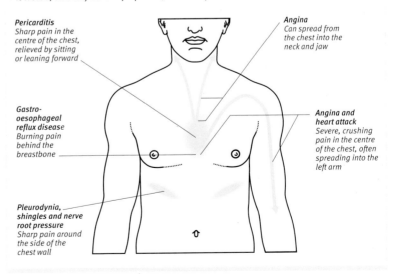

Pericarditis
Sharp pain in the centre of the chest, relieved by sitting or leaning forward

Gastro-oesophageal reflux disease
Burning pain behind the breastbone

Pleurodynia, shingles and nerve root pressure
Sharp pain around the side of the chest wall

Angina
Can spread from the chest into the neck and jaw

Angina and heart attack
Severe, crushing pain in the centre of the chest, often spreading into the left arm

such as enlargement of a heart chamber, or lung diseases, such as tuberculosis or lung cancer. They may also be used to examine the ribs after an injury. The procedure is simple, quick, and painless. (See also *X-rays*.)

Cheyne–Stokes respiration

An abnormal pattern of breathing in which the rate and depth of respiration vary rhythmically. Cheyne–Stokes respiration is characterized by repeated cycles, each lasting a few minutes, of deep, rapid breathing that becomes slower and shallower and then stops for between 10 and 20 seconds.

The pattern of Cheyne–Stokes respiration may be due to a malfunction in the part of the brain that controls breathing (as occurs in some cases of *stroke* and *head injury*). It may be due to *heart failure* or occur in healthy people at high altitude, especially during sleep.

chickenpox

A common, mild infectious disease, also called varicella, most often occurring in children. Symptoms are a rash and slight fever. In adults, chickenpox is uncommon but usually more severe. An attack gives lifelong immunity, but the causative virus remains dormant in nerves and may reappear later in life to cause *herpes zoster* (shingles).

CAUSE AND SYMPTOMS

Chickenpox is caused by the varicella zoster virus, which is spread in airborne droplets. A widespread rash develops 10 to 21 days after infection and consists of clusters of small, red, itchy spots that become fluid-filled blisters within a few hours. After several days, the blisters dry out to form scabs.

Scratching the blisters can lead to secondary infection and scarring. In adults, or in anyone whose immune system is suppressed by drug treatment or illness, serious complications involving the lungs can occur.

People with chickenpox are highly contagious from about two days before the rash appears to about a week afterwards. Nonimmune pregnant women should be particularly careful to avoid children with chickenpox or anyone with shingles, because the disease may be serious in pregnancy and newborn babies could suffer a severe attack.

TREATMENT AND PREVENTION

In most cases, no specific treatment is needed. *Paracetamol* helps to reduce fever, and *calamine* lotion may be used to relieve itching. Anyone at high risk who has been exposed to the virus may be given treatment with *immunoglobulin*, which may prevent the condition from developing. In severe cases of chickenpox, in both children and adults, *aciclovir* (an antiviral drug) is given.

A vaccine against chickenpox is available but is not part of the routine childhood immunizations in the UK. However, it may be given to certain groups of adults or children at risk of contracting or passing on the disease.

chigoe

A painful, itchy swelling, about the size of a pea, caused by a sand flea that lives in sandy soil in Africa and tropical America. When stepped on, the flea penetrates the skin of the feet and lays eggs. Chigoe fleas should be removed with a sterile needle, and the wounds treated with an antiseptic.

chilblain

An itchy, purple-red swelling, usually on a toe or a finger. Chilblains are caused by excessive constriction (narrowing) of small blood vessels below the surface of the skin in cold weather. They are most common in young children and elderly people, and women are more susceptible to them. They generally heal without treatment.

child abuse

Maltreatment of children. Child abuse includes physical injury, *sexual abuse*, emotional mistreatment, and/or neglect; it occurs at all levels of society.

Child abuse can cause severe physical and psychological damage in the victims. In addition, being deprived or ill-treated in childhood may predispose some affected people to repeat the pattern of abuse with their own children.

childbed fever

See *puerperal fever*.

childbirth

The event during which a baby leaves the mother's *uterus* (womb) and enters the outside world. The process of childbirth, known as labour, normally takes place between 38 and 42 weeks of pregnancy, as timed from the mother's last menstrual period.

For most women who receive a high standard of medical care during pregnancy (see *antenatal care*) and delivery, childbirth presents no serious problems.

The development of specialized equipment and the availability of *blood transfusions* and *antibiotic drugs* have made childbirth much safer for both mother and baby. In developing countries, however, the number of women who die from childbirth remains high (see *maternal mortality*).

ONSET OF LABOUR

It is often difficult to determine precisely when labour has started. During the last three months of pregnancy, the uterus begins to contract in preparation for the birth. Such contractions, called *Braxton Hicks' contractions* may be mistaken for the onset of labour. However, when the contractions become progressively more painful and when they occur more regularly and with shorter intervals between each contraction, labour has probably started.

At the onset of labour, the *cervix* (the neck of the uterus) becomes thinned and softened and then begins to dilate with each contraction. During this time, there may be a "show", which is when the mucous plug that blocks the cervical canal during pregnancy is expelled as a bloody discharge. "Breaking of the waters", which is the rupture of the *amniotic sac* (the fluid-filled membranous bag that protects the fetus in the uterus), may occur either as a slow trickle of fluid from the vagina or as a sudden gush.

STAGES OF LABOUR

Childbirth occurs in three stages (see the illustrated box opposite for details).

The first stage of childbirth covers the period lasting from the onset of labour to the point when the woman's cervix is fully dilated, which is when the opening has widened to about 10 cm in diameter. The duration of this stage varies from woman to woman and from birth to birth.

The second stage of labour lasts from full dilation of the cervix until the delivery of the baby. In this stage, the mother feels the urge to push with each strong contraction. As the baby's head descends into the mother's *vagina*, the baby rotates to face the mother's back. Once the baby's head is delivered, the rest of the body follows with the next contractions. After delivery, the umbilical cord, which connects the baby to the *placenta*, is clamped and cut.

In the third stage of labour, the delivery of the placenta (the afterbirth) takes place. This event happens within about ten minutes of the baby's birth.

STAGES OF **CHILDBIRTH**

At the onset of labour, painful and regular uterine contractions begin and the cervix (the neck of the womb) starts to dilate (widen). The mother is usually examined vaginally every two to four hours to assess the extent of dilation. The duration of the first stage of labour depends on several factors, but primarily on whether the baby is the mother's first or a subsequent child. *Fetal heart monitoring* is often carried out, and the frequency, strength, and duration of the mother's contractions are recorded. During the second stage of labour, the contractions become stronger and the woman feels the urge to push; however, she is advised to push only during a contraction. Once the baby is delivered, he or she is usually laid on the mother's abdomen, but may first be warmed, dried, and checked by a midwife or doctor.

THE FIRST STAGE

With the first contractions, the normally thick, tough cervix becomes thinned and softened and is gradually pulled up until it becomes effaced (merged with the walls of the uterus). The cervix then begins to dilate (stretch open) with each contraction. It is fully dilated when the opening is about 10 cm in diameter. This stage of labour can take 12 hours or more for first babies, but only a few hours for subsequent babies.

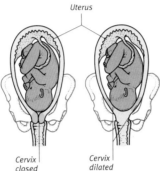

Uterus

Cervix closed

Cervix dilated

THE SECOND STAGE

As the baby's head descends, it reaches the pelvic floor muscles, which cause the head to rotate until eventually the baby's chin is pointing down towards the mother's rectum. As the baby is pushed further down the birth canal, the mother's anus and perineum (the area between the vulva and anus) begin to bulge out, and soon the baby's head can be seen at the opening of the vagina. As the head emerges, the perineal tissues are stretched very thin; sometimes it is necessary to perform an episiotomy (cutting of the tissues under local anaesthetic) to prevent them from tearing. As soon as the baby's head emerges, it turns, usually aided by the midwife, so it is once more in line with the body. With the next few contractions, one shoulder is delivered at a time; then the rest of the baby slides out. After delivery, the cord is clamped and cut.

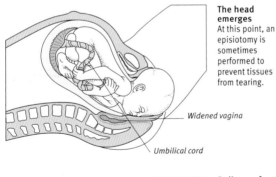

The head emerges
At this point, an episiotomy is sometimes performed to prevent tissues from tearing.

Widened vagina

Umbilical cord

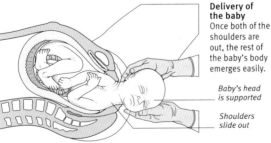

Delivery of the baby
Once both of the shoulders are out, the rest of the baby's body emerges easily.

Baby's head is supported

Shoulders slide out

ELECTRONIC FETAL MONITORING

This may be performed if the fetus is at risk, or as a routine check. The fetal heart rate and the mother's uterine contractions are recorded.

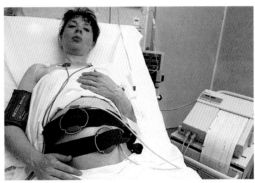

Fetal monitoring devices
In the procedure shown above, the baby's heartbeat is detected by a metal plate strapped to the lower belt. A plate beneath the upper belt detects the contractions. An alternative method is to attach an electrode to the baby's head; the electrode is linked to the monitor by a wire passed through the mother's vagina.

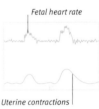

Fetal heart rate

Uterine contractions

THE THIRD STAGE

Three to 10 minutes after the birth, the placenta (afterbirth) separates from the uterine wall and is removed by gentle traction on the cord. Drugs such as ergometrine or oxytocin may be used to aid its expulsion and to reduce bleeding. Rarely, the placenta may have to be manually removed, under general or epidural anaesthetic, by an obstetrician. Any tears or incisions are cleaned and stitched. This may be done while the mother holds her baby.

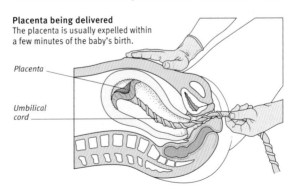

Placenta being delivered
The placenta is usually expelled within a few minutes of the baby's birth.

Placenta

Umbilical cord

PAIN RELIEF IN LABOUR AND DELIVERY

Method	Why given	Possible effects on baby
Narcotic analgesics	Routine pain relief during labour	Baby may be less responsive at birth, and may have respiratory problems, but these effects are reversible
Epidural	Routine pain relief during labour, delivery of twins, breech delivery, and caesarean section	Effects are uncommon unless mother's blood pressure falls
Nitrous oxide	Pain relief during labour and delivery; used for short periods only	None
Pudendal block	Forceps delivery	None
Local anaesthetic into perineum	Forceps delivery or episiotomy	None
General anaesthesia	Caesarean section	Baby may show reduced responsiveness at birth

PAIN RELIEF
Pain relief is available during normal labour and delivery. There are various forms, including opioid *analgesic drugs*, *epidural anaesthesia*, and *pudendal block*. (See also *childbirth, complications of*; *childbirth, natural*.)

childbirth, complications of
Problems that occur during *labour* and delivery. Complications may affect the mother, the baby, or both. Some are potentially life-threatening, especially to the baby if they impair the baby's oxygen supply (see *fetal distress*).

MATERNAL PROBLEMS
If contractions begin, or if the membranes rupture, before the 37th week of pregnancy, premature labour may occur, with the delivery of a small, immature baby (see *prematurity*).

Premature rupture of the *amniotic sac* (the fluid-filled, membranous bag that protects the fetus in the uterus) can lead to infection in the *uterus*, requiring prompt delivery of the baby and treatment with *antibiotic drugs*.

Slow progress in the first stage of a normal labour may be due to inadequate contractions of the uterus. It is usually treated with intravenous infusions of synthetic *oxytocin*. If the mother cannot push strongly enough, or if the contractions are ineffective in the second stage of labour, the baby may be delivered by *forceps delivery*, *vacuum extraction*, or *caesarean section*.

Rarely, *eclampsia* (convulsions associated with raised blood pressure) may develop during labour. This disorder requires treatment with *anticonvulsant drugs* and oxygen, and a caesarean section will be necessary.

Bleeding before labour (*antepartum haemorrhage*) or during labour may be caused by premature, partial separation of the *placenta* from the wall of the uterus. Less commonly, it may result from a condition called *placenta praevia*, in which the placenta lies over the opening of the *cervix*. Blood loss after the delivery (*postpartum haemorrhage*) is usually due to failure of the uterus to contract after delivery, or to retention of part of the placenta.

FETAL PROBLEMS
If the baby lies in the breech position (see *breech delivery*), or in any other *malpresentation* (not lying in the normal head-down position in the uterus), caesarean section may be necessary.

Multiple pregnancies (see *pregnancy, multiple*) carry an increased risk of problems during delivery due to the difficulty of predicting the position of the second or subsequent babies. It is also more likely that babies in multiple pregnancies will be born prematurely.

FETAL–MATERNAL PROBLEMS
If the mother's pelvis is too small in proportion to the head of her baby (a condition known as cephalopelvic disproportion), the baby may have to be delivered by caesarean section.

childbirth, natural
The use of relaxation and other techniques to help cope with pain and minimize the use of drugs and medical intervention during *childbirth*.

child development
The acquisition of physical, mental, and social skills in children. Although there is wide variation in individual rates of progress, most children develop certain skills within predictable age ranges (see the illustrated boxes opposite and on p.166 for the typical age ranges at which key skills develop).

FACTORS AFFECTING DEVELOPMENT
The capability for acquiring new skills is dependent upon the maturity of the child's nervous system. Individual rates of maturity are determined genetically and modified by environmental factors in the *uterus* and after birth. For example, premature children miss out on a portion of the growing time in the uterus; therefore, the time that they take to progress should be calculated from the full-term pregnancy date, not the actual date of birth.

Sight and hearing are both crucial to a child's general developmental progress; any defect in these areas will affect the child's ability to watch, listen, learn, and imitate. Intelligence also affects the speed of development.

Speaking to and playing with children is essential for their language development and to help them practise new physical skills. Introducing children to other children also provides them with a great deal of stimulation and helps develop social skills.

DEVELOPMENTAL MILESTONES
Development is assessed in early childhood by looking at the child's abilities in four major areas: physical skills; hearing and language; vision and fine movement; and social behaviour and play. Children acquire particular skills at widely recognized stages known as developmental milestones.

All children acquire skills in much the same order (for example, a child will not learn to stand before learning to sit); however, the rate at which these skills are acquired varies enormously from child to child. A child may develop more rapidly in one area than in another. A more detailed assessment is required only if a child's progress is significantly slower than average or if a parent is concerned for other reasons (see *developmental delay*).

child guidance

A form of care provided by a multidisciplinary diagnosis and advice team, which helps children suffering from emotional or behavioural problems (see *behavioural problems in children*). Indications of such problems include poor performance at school, disruptive or withdrawn behaviour, breaking the law, and *drug abuse*.

Child guidance professionals include the specialists such as psychiatric social workers, psychiatrists, and psychologists. These people often work closely together in hospital paediatric departments, in schools, or in child-guidance clinics.

Various methods of assessment and therapy may be employed, depending on the age of the child and the problem involved. For young children, *play therapy* may be used to help with diagnosis. Older children may be offered *counselling*, *psychotherapy*, or *group therapy*. *Family therapy* may be of benefit in cases where there are relationship difficulties between child and one or both parents.

chill

A shivering attack accompanied by chattering teeth, pale skin, goose pimples, and feeling cold. Chill frequently precedes a fever. Repeated or severe shivering suggests serious illness.

Chinese medicine

Traditional Chinese medicine is based on the theory that a universal life-force, called chi, manifests itself in the body as two complementary qualities called *yin and yang*. According to this belief, vigorous yang and restraining yin must be in balance, and the chi must flow evenly for good health.

Treatments for illness aim to restore the balance between yin and yang and normalize the flow of chi in the body. They include Chinese *herbal medicine*, physical techniques such as *acupressure* and *acupuncture*, and *t'ai chi*.

chiropody

The examination, diagnosis, treatment, and prevention of diseases and disorders of the foot and its related structures, including the toes, toenails, skin of the feet, and the ankles. A practitioner of chiropody is called a chiropodist.

CHILD DEVELOPMENT: 0–18 MONTHS

Locomotion

By 6 months
Babies can lift up their heads and chests and roll from front to back and back to front. They can sit up with support, bounce up and down, and bear weight on their legs if supported.

9 months
Babies try to crawl, sit without support, and pull themselves up to standing or sitting positions. They can step purposefully on alternate feet if they are supported.

1 year
Children can crawl on hands and knees and walk around furniture (holding on). They may be able to walk alone or with one hand held.

18 months
Children can walk well with feet closer together. They can stoop to pick up objects, run with care, walk upstairs with one hand held, and crawl backwards downstairs.

Vision and fine movement

By 6 months
Babies look intently at everything and everybody. They follow moving objects with their eyes and reach for objects with one or both hands. Objects are transferred from hand to hand and brought to the mouth.

9 months
Babies are visually very alert. Their grasp involves mostly the index and middle fingers. They can manipulate objects with both hands, but have difficulty voluntarily releasing grasped objects.

1 year
Children can grasp small objects well and release grasped objects easily. Both hands are used equally. They can hold a block in each hand and bang the blocks together.

18 months
Children can build a tower of three blocks (when shown), enjoy turning pages of a book, can grip a crayon, scribble, and make dots. They may use one hand more than the other.

Hearing, understanding, and speech

By 6 months
Babies turn their heads to locate sources of sound and have begun to understand the tone of their mother's voice. They enjoy making vowel sounds and tuneful noises. They laugh and squeal.

9 months
Babies listen to sounds and understand "no" and other words. They babble in long strings (making sounds such as ba-ba, da-da, ma-ma) and start using sound to attract attention. (Deaf babies' utterances are monotonous and do not develop in complexity.)

1 year
Children turn when they hear their own name spoken. They have some understanding of how other people feel; they know what most household objects are used for; they may babble meaningfully to themselves; and they may say two or three words.

18 months
Children comprehend short communications spoken directly to them but do not understand the difference between statements, commands, and questions. Vocabulary may contain six to 20 words.

Social behaviour and play

By 6 months
Babies enjoy looking at their images in mirrors and playing peekaboo games. They can grasp objects and can also shake, bang, and otherwise manipulate them. They will not, however, look for objects that are shown and then hidden. They are shy with strangers.

9 months
Babies look for objects that are shown and then hidden, thus showing the beginnings of memory. They imitate hand clapping, wave bye-bye, and show great determination in getting objects. They continue to be shy with strangers.

1 year
Children spend less time putting objects in their mouths and more time releasing objects by throwing them, dropping them, putting them in boxes. They play pat-a-cake and like to be around a familiar adult to whom they demonstrate affection.

18 months
Children actively explore their homes. They enjoy moving things into and out of boxes and looking at picture books. They use spoons and cups and can take off their shoes and socks. They are also determined, impetuous, selfish, and cannot be reasoned with. They alternate between clinging to a familiar adult and struggling to break free.

CHILD DEVELOPMENT: 2–5 YEARS

Locomotion

2 years	3 years	4 years	5 years
Children can climb furniture and walk up and down stairs (using two feet to each step).	Children can climb with agility, throw and kick balls, ride tricycles, and run around corners.	Children walk up and down stairs with one foot on each step, and can stand, walk, and run on tiptoe.	Children can stand and hop on one foot, and are skilful in rolling, sliding, and swinging.

Vision and fine movement

2 years	3 years	4 years	5 years
Children can build towers of six or seven blocks, can unscrew a lid, and show a definite right- or left-handedness.	Children hold crayons with an adult grasp and can undo buttons, but may need help buttoning them up. Their handedness is clearly established.	Children hold a pencil with a mature grasp, can copy simple letters (i.e. O,T, H or V), and can build a tower of more than 10 blocks.	Children can match 10 or 12 colours, can copy many more letters, and can draw the full body of a person with a recognizable head and facial features.

Hearing, understanding, and speech

2 years	3 years	4 years	5 years
Children begin to listen to general conversation. They obey simple instructions and can use 50 or more words meaningfully. They constantly talk to themselves and can put two or more words together to communicate.	Children listen to conversation and enjoy nursery stories. They understand the difference between statements, commands, and questions. They have large vocabularies and speak clearly in sentences; there may be some errors.	Children can repeat softly spoken words at a distance of 1 m. They speak fluently and with correct grammar, and can provide their full names, ages, and addresses. They tell long stories, confusing fact and fantasy.	Children enjoy reciting rhymes, telling stories, and having books read to them.

Social behaviour and play

2 years	3 years	4 years	5 years
Children ask the names of everything and enjoy participating in nursery rhymes and songs. They ask for food and drink and indicate toilet needs. They begin to play with toys more imaginatively, though they may not like to share them. They are constantly demanding and will throw tantrums if their desires are thwarted.	Children constantly ask questions. They can dress and undress and eat with a fork and spoon. They are dry and clean during the day and sometimes at night. Three-year-olds can play with toys imaginatively and will share with others. They can be reasoned with and have fewer tantrums. They are also more affectionate to younger siblings.	Children continue asking questions constantly. They are more independent and skilful in dressing, undressing, eating, and washing. They need to play with other children and can share with others. They can understand past, present, and future.	Children ask the meaning of abstract words. They like to build complex structures out of bricks or other objects. They continue in imaginative and dramatic play. They enjoy companionship and understand the need for rules and fair play. They have an understanding of time and are generally sensible, restrained, and independent.

chiropractic

A system of treatment for a range of disorders, that is based on manipulation of the spine. The main principle of chiropractic is the theory that disease stems from the misalignment of bones.

chlamydial infections

A group of infectious diseases caused by chlamydiae, a group of bacteria that can multiply only by invading the cells of another life-form.

TYPES

Two main species of chlamydiae cause disease in humans. They can be treated with *antibiotic drugs*.

The first species, CHLAMYDIA TRACHOMATIS, is responsible for some sexually transmitted infections, including about half of all cases of *nongonococcal urethritis* in men and *pelvic inflammatory disease* in women. It can also cause the tropical eye disease *trachoma*.

A second species, CHLAMYDIA PSITTACI, is responsible for *psittacosis*. This is a rare form of pneumonia that is transmitted to humans from birds.

Chlamydia is also responsible for a type of pneumonia (see *Chlamydia pneumoniae*).

Chlamydia pneumoniae

An infectious organism that can cause a mild form of *pneumonia*, which occurs particularly in young adults.

Chlamydia psittaci

An organism that mainly affects birds but can occasionally spread to people who are in contact with pigeons, parrots, parakeets, or poultry. It causes a type of pneumonia called *psittacosis*.

Chlamydia trachomatis

An organism that belongs to the chlamydiae group and has several strains. In men, it is a major cause of the sexually transmitted infection *nongonococcal urethritis*, which may cause a discharge from the penis. In women, the infection usually causes no symptoms, but can lead to *pelvic inflammatory disease*, which is a major cause of *infertility*, *ectopic pregnancy*, and *miscarriage*. A baby born to a woman with chlamydial infection may acquire an acute eye disorder called neonatal *ophthalmia*.

In some parts of Africa and Asia, certain strains of CHLAMYDIA TRACHOMATIS cause *trachoma*, a serious eye disease that is the most common cause of blindness worldwide.

chloasma

A skin condition, also called melasma, in which blotches of pale brown pigmentation appear on the face, notably on the forehead, nose, and cheeks. The condition is aggravated by sunlight. Chloasma sometimes develops during pregnancy. More rarely, it is associated with the menopause or the use of *oral contraceptives*. The areas of abnormal pigmentation usually fade in time, but the condition may recur.

chloral hydrate

A type of *sleeping drug*.

chlorambucil

An *anticancer drug* that is used in the treatment of some types of cancer, such as *Hodgkin's disease*.

chloramphenicol

An *antibiotic drug* commonly used as drops to treat superficial eye infections. Chloramphenicol is also used to treat life-threatening infections of unknown cause. Rarely, tablets or injections are associated with aplastic *anaemia*.

chlorate poisoning

The toxic effects of chemicals called chlorates, which are present in some defoliant weedkillers.

Symptoms of chlorate poisoning include ulceration of the mouth, abdominal pain, and diarrhoea. Chlorates can also cause kidney and liver damage, corrosion of the intestines, and *methaemoglobinaemia* (a harmful chemical change in the blood pigment *haemoglobin*). Even small doses of chlorates can be fatal, and immediate medical help is therefore essential if chlorate poisoning is suspected.

chlordiazepoxide

A *benzodiazepine drug* mainly used in the treatment of *anxiety*.

chlorhexidine

A type of disinfectant mainly used to cleanse the skin before surgery or before taking a blood sample.

chlorine

A poisonous, yellowish-green gas with powerful bleaching and disinfectant properties. If inhaled in even very small amounts, chlorine gas is highly irritating to the lungs; inhalation of large amounts is rapidly fatal.

chloroform

A colourless liquid producing a vapour that was formerly used as a general anaesthetic (see *anaesthesia, general*). However, chloroform is associated with liver damage and heart problems and safer drugs are now used instead.

chloroquine

A drug used mainly in the prevention and treatment of *malaria*. It is also a *disease-modifying antirheumatic drug* used to treat systemic *lupus erythematosus* and *rheumatoid arthritis*.

Possible side effects of chloroquine include nausea, headache, diarrhoea, rashes, and abdominal pain. Long-term use may damage the retina of the eye.

chlorphenamine

An *antihistamine drug* that is used to treat a number of allergic conditions such as allergic *rhinitis* (hay fever), allergic *conjunctivitis*, *angioedema* (allergic facial swelling) and *urticaria* (nettle rash). Chlorphenamine is also a component of some *cold remedies*.

chlorpheniramine

An alternative name for *chlorphenamine*.

chlorpromazine

A widely prescribed *antipsychotic drug* used to relieve symptoms of major psychotic illnesses such as *schizophrenia* and *mania*. The drug reduces delusional and hallucinatory experiences and may have an effect on irritability and overactivity. It is also used as an *antiemetic drug* to treat nausea and vomiting, especially when these problems are the result of treatment with other drugs, radiotherapy, or anaesthesia.

Chlorpromazine may cause *photosensitivity* (increased sensitivity of the skin to sunlight) and, in some cases, *parkinsonism* (a movement disorder), slow reactions, and blurred vision.

chlorpropamide

A drug that is used to treat *diabetes mellitus* (see *hypoglycaemics, oral*).

choanal atresia

A *congenital* abnormality of the *nose* in which one or both of the nasal cavities are not fully developed.

chocolate cyst

A brown swelling in an *ovary*. Chocolate cysts may develop in *endometriosis*, a condition in which endometrial tissue (which forms the lining of the uterus) is found in sites outside the uterus. The colour is the result of clotted blood within the cysts.

choking

Partial or complete inability to breathe due to obstruction of the airways. If the airway is completely blocked, total suffocation will occur if the obstruction is not cleared promptly.

In mild choking (partial obstruction of the airway), breathing is still possible and coughing usually clears the obstruction. If choking is severe (complete or almost complete blockage of the airway), breathing is not possible and first aid may be life-saving.

For adults and children, make the victim bend forward and give five sharp blows between the shoulderblades. If this does not clear the obstruction, give five abdominal thrusts (also known as the Heimlich manoeuvre): place your fist in the middle of the upper abdomen, just below the ribcage, grasp your fist with the other hand, and pull sharply inwards and upwards five times. If these do not clear the obstruction, repeat the cycle of five back blows and five abdominal thrusts until the airway obstruction clears.

For babies, lay the victim face-down along one arm with the head lower than the body. Support the head and shoulders with one hand and give five sharp blows to the upper part of the back with the other hand. If this does not clear the obstruction, turn the baby face-up along the other arm, put two fingers on the lower half of the breastbone, and give five sharp downward thrusts at the rate of one every three seconds. If this fails, repeat the cycle of five back blows and five chest thrusts until the obstruction clears.

If the obstruction cannot be cleared by first-aid techniques, a doctor may need to perform an emergency *tracheostomy* (making an opening in the windpipe).

cholangiocarcinoma

A cancerous growth in one of the *bile ducts*. Cholangiocarcinoma causes *jaundice* and weight loss.

cholangiography

An imaging procedure involving the use of a *contrast medium* (a substance that is opaque to *X-rays*) to make the *bile ducts* visible on X-rays. It is used to diagnose biliary stones (which are similar to *gallstones*, but they develop in the bile ducts instead of the gallbladder) and narrowing or tumours of the bile ducts. *ERCP* (endoscopic retrograde cholangiopancreatography) is one of the main methods of cholangiography. *Ultrasound scanning* and *MRI* can also be used to locate biliary stones.

C

cholangitis

Inflammation of any of the bile ducts, such as the common bile duct, which leads from the liver and gallbladder to the small intestine (see *biliary system*). There are two forms of the condition: acute ascending cholangitis and sclerosing cholangitis.

ACUTE ASCENDING CHOLANGITIS

This form of cholangitis is usually due to bacterial infection of the duct and its bile. The infection, in turn, generally results from blockage of the duct – for example, by a gallstone (see *bile duct obstruction*). The infection spreads up the duct and may affect the liver. The main symptoms of acute ascending cholangitis are recurrent bouts of *jaundice*, abdominal pain, chills, and fever.

Mild attacks are treated with *antibiotic drugs* and fluids. Severe attacks may be accompanied by life-threatening *septicaemia* (blood poisoning) and *kidney failure*. In these cases, the infected material may be drained from the bile duct during surgery or *endoscopy* (a procedure in which instruments are passed through a viewing tube).

SCLEROSING CHOLANGITIS

In this rare condition, all the bile ducts within and outside the liver become narrowed. This causes *cholestasis* (stagnation of the bile in the liver), chronic jaundice, and itchiness of the skin, and the liver is progressively damaged.

The drug *colestyramine* may relieve itching. The only other treatment available is a *liver transplant*.

chole-

A prefix that means "relating to the *bile* or the *biliary system*", as in cholecystitis (inflammation of the gallbladder).

cholecalciferol

An alternative name for *colecalciferol*, also called vitamin D₃ (see *vitamin D*).

cholecystectomy

Surgical removal of the *gallbladder*. Cholecystectomy is usually performed to deal with the presence of troublesome *gallstones*. It is also used in cases of acute *cholecystitis* (inflammation of the gallbladder) and as an emergency treatment for rupture of the gallbladder or *empyema* (accumulation of pus).

Cholecystectomy may be carried out by conventional surgery or, more commonly, by *minimally invasive surgery* using a *laparoscope* (a viewing tube through which instruments can be passed).

cholecystitis

Acute or chronic painful inflammation of the *gallbladder*. Acute cholecystitis is usually caused by a *gallstone* obstructing the outlet from the gallbladder. The bile trapped inside the gallbaldder becomes more concentrated and irritates the gallbladder walls. Bacterial infection of the bile may result.

The main symptom of acute cholecystitis is severe, constant pain in the right side of the abdomen under the

CHOLECYSTECTOMY

Surgical removal of the gallbladder (cholecystectomy) is most often carried out when the gallbladder contains gallstones. The procedure is usually performed by minimally invasive ("keyhole") surgery using a laparoscope (as shown here), although conventional surgery may still sometimes be used. Both methods are performed under general anaesthesia. Laparoscopic surgery takes longer than conventional surgery but requires only small incisions, enabling most patients to make a full recovery more quickly.

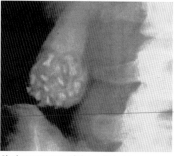

Cholecystogram of the gallbladder
Gallstones, which become more prevalent with age, are revealed by a cholecystogram (X-ray image of the gallbladder).

Sites of incision
- Liver
- Stomach
- Gallbladder

Suction instrument

Instrument

Instrument

Laparoscope

Gallbladder

Liver

Procedure for cholecystectomy
The abdominal cavity is inflated with gas to provide a clear view, then a laparoscope fitted with a video camera is introduced through a small incision. Further instruments are passed through other incisions. While watching the monitor, the surgeon removes the gallbladder, ensuring that there is no leakage from the bile duct or blood vessels.

ribs. The pain is accompanied by fever and, occasionally, *jaundice* (yellowing of the skin and whites of the eyes).

Repeated mild attacks of acute cholecystitis can lead to a chronic form of the condition, in which the gallbladder shrinks, its walls thicken, and it ceases to store bile. Symptoms include indigestion, pains in the upper abdomen, nausea, and belching; they may be aggravated by eating fatty foods.

TREATMENT AND COMPLICATIONS
Treatment of cholecystitis usually involves the use of *analgesic drugs*, *antibiotic drugs*, and an intravenous infusion of nutrients and fluids. In some affected people, complications develop. These may include *peritonitis* (inflammation of the lining of the abdominal cavity), if the gallbladder bursts, and *empyema* (an accumulation of pus). Both of these complications require urgent surgical treatment. *Cholecystectomy* (removal of the gallbladder) is the usual treatment for chronic cholecystitis.

cholecystography

An X-ray procedure in which a *contrast medium* (a substance that is opaque to X-rays) is used for viewing of the *gallbladder* and common *bile duct*. The technique of cholecystography is usually used for the detection of *gallstones* but has largely been replaced by *ultrasound scanning* of the gallbladder.

cholecystokinin

A *hormone* that is produced in the *duodenum* (the first section of the small intestine) in response to the ingestion of fats and certain other food substances. Cholecystokinin stimulates the *gallbladder* to release bile into the duodenum, and triggers the secretion of digestive enzymes from the *pancreas*, thus aiding the breakdown of foods to release nutrients. Cholecystokinin is also found in the brain, where it has a function as a *neurotransmitter*.

choledochal cyst

A widening of the common bile duct, which carries the digestive juice bile from the liver and gallbladder to the *duodenum*. The disorder is congenital (present at birth), but symptoms may not develop until early adulthood; they consist of abdominal pain and jaundice (yellow coloration of the skin and eyes due to the accumulation of bilirubin, a bile pigment). Surgery is needed to correct the abnormality.

cholelithiasis
See *gallstones*.

cholera

An infection of the small intestine by the bacterium VIBRIO CHOLERAE. The disease causes profuse watery diarrhoea, which can lead to dehydration and death in severe untreated cases.

CAUSE AND INCIDENCE
Infection is acquired by ingesting contaminated food or water. Outbreaks of the disease occur regularly in northeast India, but worldwide cholera is controlled by sanitation.

SYMPTOMS
Cholera starts suddenly, between one and five days after infection, with diarrhoea that is often accompanied by vomiting. More than 500 ml of fluid may be lost each hour and, if this fluid is not replaced, severe dehydration and then death may occur within hours. The fluid loss is caused by the action of a toxin produced by the cholera bacterium that greatly increases the passage of fluid from the bloodstream into the large and small intestines.

TREATMENT
Treatment of cholera is by *oral rehydration therapy* and, in severe cases, by *intravenous infusion* of rehydration fluids. *Antibiotic drugs* help eradicate the infection and can shorten the period of diarrhoea. After adequate rehydration, affected people usually make a full recovery from the infection.

PREVENTION
Cholera is controlled worldwide by the improvement of sanitation, and in particular by ensuring that sewage is not permitted to contaminate water supplies used for drinking. Travellers planning to visit cholera-infected areas are advised to consume only water that has been boiled, or bottled drinks from reliable sources. An oral cholera vaccine is available for travellers to endemic or epidemic areas.

cholestasis

Stagnation of *bile* in the small *bile ducts* within the liver, leading to *jaundice* and liver disease. The obstruction to the flow of bile may be intrahepatic (within the liver) or extrahepatic (in the bile ducts outside the liver).

CAUSES
Intrahepatic cholestasis may develop as a result of viral hepatitis (see *hepatitis, viral*) or as an adverse effect of various drugs. The flow of bile will improve

gradually as the inflammation from hepatitis subsides or when a causative drug is discontinued.

The bile ducts outside the liver can become blocked by abnormalities such as gallstones or tumours (see *bile duct obstruction*). Rarely, the ducts are absent from birth (see *biliary atresia*).

TREATMENT
Bile duct obstruction and biliary atresia are often treated surgically to ensure or restore the free passage of bile from the liver to the duodenum.

cholestatic jaundice

Jaundice (yellow discoloration of the skin) that occurs as a result of *cholestasis* (obstruction in the flow of bile to the intestine).

cholesteatoma

A rare but serious condition in which skin cells proliferate and grow inwards from the ear canal into the middle ear. Cholesteatoma usually occurs as a result of long-standing *otitis media* (a middle-ear infection) together with a defect in the eardrum (see *eardrum, perforated*). If left untreated, it may grow and damage the small bones in the middle ear and surrounding structures.

Cholesteatoma needs to be removed surgically through the eardrum or by *mastoidectomy* (removal of the mastoid bone, which is located behind the ear, together with the cholesteatoma).

cholesterol

A fat-like substance that is an important constituent of body cells and also is involved in the formation of *hormones* and bile salts. Cholesterol is made by the liver from various foods, especially those containing saturated fats (see *fats and oils*), although a small amount is absorbed directly from cholesterol-rich foods such as eggs and shellfish.

Both cholesterol and fats (triglycerides) are transported in the blood as lipoproteins. These are particles with a core made of varying proportions of cholesterol and triglycerides, and an outer layer made of proteins.

CHOLESTEROL-RELATED DISEASES
High blood cholesterol levels increase the risk of *atherosclerosis* (accumulation of fatty deposits on the lining of the arteries) and with it the risk of *coronary artery disease* or of *stroke* (damage to part of the brain due to interruption of its blood supply). In general, cholesterol transported in the bloodstream as low-

C

density lipoproteins (LDLs) or as very low-density lipoproteins (VLDLs) – so-called "bad" cholesterol – is a risk factor for these conditions, while cholesterol in the form of high-density lipoproteins (HDLs) – "good" cholesterol – seems to protect against arterial disease.

Levels of cholesterol in the blood are influenced by diet, weight, genetic factors, and metabolic diseases such as *diabetes mellitus*. Cholesterol levels can be measured by blood tests. They are measured in millimoles per litre (mmol/L). The optimum level is less than 5.0. However, about two in three adults in the UK have levels above 5.0.

A higher than optimum level of blood cholesterol may require dietary modification (including reducing saturated fat intake and eating more oily fish) and exercise. Sometimes, however, medication (such as *simvastatin*) may be necessary to reduce the cholesterol level and lower the risk of arterial disease.

cholesterolosis

Abnormal deposits of *cholesterol* in the lining of the gallbladder that may be associated with the development of *gallstones*. Cholesterolosis is also sometimes known as strawberry gallbladder because of the appearance of an affected gallbladder.

cholestyramine

An alternative spelling for the lipid-lowering drug *colestyramine*.

cholic acid

One of the acids contained in *bile*.

cholinergic crisis

A condition that affects people with *myasthenia gravis* who are undergoing treatment with *cholinesterase inhibitors*. The problem is caused by an overdose of cholinesterase inhibitors. During a cholinergic crisis, the muscle weakness that is associated with myasthenia gravis worsens dramatically, and needs emergency medical treatment.

cholinesterase inhibitors

COMMON DRUGS
• Neostigmine • Pyridostigmine

A group of drugs, also known as anticholinesterases, that are used to relieve muscle weakness that results from myasthenia gravis. In this disease, abnormal activity of the immune system causes the destruction of receptors on muscle cells that bind with acetylcholine, a neurotransmitter that makes the muscles contract. Cholinesterase inhibitors block the action of acetylcholinesterase, the enzyme that normally breaks down acetylcholine, allowing the neurotransmitter more time to act. The drugs are also used to reverse the effects of muscle-relaxant drugs given with general anaesthesia.

chondritis

Inflammation of *cartilage* (connective tissue composed of the gel-like substance collagen). It is usually caused by pressure, stress, or injury.

Costochondritis is inflammation of the cartilage between the ribs and the sternum (breastbone). This condition causes tenderness over the sternum and pain if pressure is exerted on the ribs at the front of the chest. Chondritis may also affect the cartilage lining the hip and knee joints; this inflammation may eventually lead to *osteoarthritis*.

chondro-

A prefix denoting a relationship to *cartilage*, as in chondrocyte, a cell that produces cartilage.

chondrocalcinosis

The presence of calcium pyrophosphate in joint cartilage. The condition, which occurs in *pseudogout* (a form of arthritis), causes pain and swelling.

chondroma

A noncancerous tumour composed of *cartilage*, affecting the bones. Chondromas most often occur in the hands and feet (see *chondromatosis*).

chondromalacia patellae

A painful knee disorder, one cause of anterior knee pain, in which the *cartilage* (connective tissue composed of the gel-like substance collagen) behind the patella (kneecap) is damaged. Adolescents are most commonly affected.
CAUSE
Chondromalacia patellae may result from knee injuries or sporting activities in which the knee is bent for long periods. This action may weaken the inner part of the quadriceps muscle (which is at the front of the thigh), causing the patella to tilt when the knee is straightened and rub against the lower end of the *femur* (thigh bone). The rubbing causes the cartilage that covers both bones to roughen, causing pain and tenderness.

TREATMENT
Treatment of chondromalacia patellae is with *analgesic drugs* (painkillers) and exercises to strengthen the thigh muscles. Rarely, surgery is needed.

chondromatosis

A condition in which multiple noncancerous tumours, called *chondromas*, arise in the bones, most commonly in the bones of the hands and feet. The tumour cells consist of *cartilage* (connective tissue composed of the gel-like substance collagen). Chondromatosis usually causes no symptoms.

chondrosarcoma

A cancerous growth of *cartilage* (connective tissue composed of the gel-like substance collagen). Chondrosarcoma occurs within or on the surface of large bones, such as the femur (thigh bone), causing pain and swelling.

The condition usually appears in middle age. The tumour may develop slowly from a noncancerous tumour (see *chondroma; dyschondroplasia*) or may grow rapidly from an area of previously normal bone. If a limb is affected, *amputation* of the *bone* above the tumour usually results in a permanent cure. Treatment of sites such as the pelvis or ribs is more difficult.

chordae tendineae

Stringlike strands of fibre that attach the flaps of the mitral and tricuspid *heart valves* to the walls of the ventricles (lower heart chambers). The chordae tendineae, which are popularly known as the heartstrings, prevent the valves from turning inside out.

chordee

Abnormal curvature of the penis, usually downwards. Chordee most often occurs in males with *hypospadias*, a birth defect in which the opening of the urethra lies on the underside of the penis instead of at the tip. It is usually corrected by surgery, between the ages of one and three years.

chorea

A condition that is characterized by irregular, rapid, jerky movements, usually affecting the face, limbs, and trunk. The movements are involuntary and, unlike tics, they are not predictable but occur at random. Chorea disappears during sleep. The disorder is sometimes combined with athetosis (continued writhing movements); this combined condition is known as *choreoathetosis*.

TYPES AND CAUSES

Chorea arises from disease or disturbance of structures lying deep within the brain (in particular, the paired nerve cell groups called the *basal ganglia*). The condition is a feature of *Huntington's disease* and *Sydenham's chorea*. It may also occur in pregnancy, when it is called chorea gravidarum. In addition, chorea may be a side effect of certain drugs, including *oral contraceptives*; certain drugs for psychiatric disorders; and drugs for treating *Parkinson's disease*.

TREATMENT

If the cause of chorea is an underlying disease, the condition may be treated with drugs that inhibit the nerve pathways concerned with movement. If chorea has occurred as a side effect of a drug, the drug may be withdrawn and a substitute provided.

choreoathetosis

A condition characterized by uncontrollable movements of the limbs, face, and trunk. In this disorder, the jerky, rapid movements typical of *chorea* are combined with the slower, continuous writhing movements of *athetosis*.

Choreoathetosis may occur in children with *cerebral palsy*. It may also be a side effect of certain drugs.

choriocarcinoma

A rare, cancerous *tumour* that develops from placental tissue (see *placenta*) in the uterus. Choriocarcinoma usually

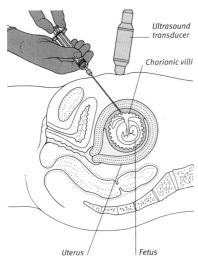

Chorionic villus sampling via the abdomen
A few chorionic villi are sucked from the placenta through a hollow needle inserted into the abdomen.

occurs as a complication of a *hydatidiform mole* (a noncancerous tumour that arises in placental tissue); however, it sometimes develops after a normal pregnancy, a miscarriage, or an abortion. Occasionally, the tumour may not appear until months or even years after the pregnancy that gave rise to it.

SYMPTOMS

There may be no early symptoms. The tumour may become apparent because of persistent bleeding from the vagina after a miscarriage or abortion, or for more than eight weeks following childbirth. If it is left untreated, the tumour destroys the walls of the uterus; and the cancer may also spread in the bloodstream to the vagina and vulva and then to the liver, lungs, brain, and bones.

DIAGNOSIS AND TREATMENT

Any woman who has been treated for a hydatidiform mole is screened regularly by *ultrasound scanning*. Blood and urine levels of human chorionic gonadotrophin (HCG), a hormone normally produced by the placenta, are also measured because high levels of this hormone in the body are associated with choreocarcinoma.

Treatment with *anticancer drugs* is usually successful. *Hysterectomy* (surgical removal of the uterus) may also be necessary. Following treatment, HCG levels are regularly monitored for between two and five years.

chorion

One of the two membranes that surround the *embryo*. The chorion lies outside the *amnion*, has small fingerlike projections called the chorionic villi, and develops into the *placenta*.

chorionic gonadotrophin

See *gonadotrophin, human chorionic*.

chorionic villi

The short, fingerlike projections that extend from the surface of the *chorion* (the membrane that surrounds a fetus). (See also *chorionic villus sampling*; *villus*.)

chorionic villus sampling (CVS)

A method of diagnosing genetic abnormalities in a *fetus*. The test involves taking a small sample of tissue from the *chorionic villi* at the edge of the *placenta* for *chromosome analysis*. The cells of the chorionic villi have the same chromosome makeup as those from the fetus, so they can be used to detect any fetal genetic abnormalities.

STRUCTURE OF **CHOROID**

The choroid lines the inside of the eyeball. It thickens around the lens to form the ciliary body. Muscles stretching between the choroid and the lens contract to adjust the shape of the lens in focusing.

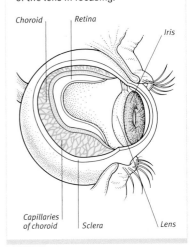

CVS is offered to women at a higher-than-normal risk of having a child with a genetic disease, such as *thalassaemia*, or a chromosomal abnormality, such as *Down's syndrome*. It is normally performed between the 10th and 13th weeks of pregnancy and can be carried out via the abdomen or vaginally, depending on the position of the placenta. CVS slightly increases the risk of a *miscarriage* occurring.

choroid

A layer of tissue at the back of the *eye*, beneath the *retina*. The choroid contains a network of blood vessels that supply nutrients and oxygen to the retina and to the surrounding tissues in the eye.

choroiditis

Inflammation of the *choroid* (the layer of tissue at the back of the eye). It may occur on its own or as part of a generalized inflammation affecting the whole eye (see *uveitis*). The condition is often the result of infections such as *toxocariasis* or *toxoplasmosis*, or, more rarely, of *sarcoidosis*, *syphilis*, or *histoplasmosis*, although it sometimes has no obvious cause. Chorioditis is painless but causes blurring of vision.

Treatment includes *corticosteroid drugs* to reduce inflammation and *antibiotic drugs* for any causative infection.

choroid plexus

A network of thin-walled blood vessels in the *eye* or *brain*. The choroid plexus of the eye supplies blood to the *retina*. In the brain, the choroid plexus lines the *ventricles* (cavities) and produces *cerebrospinal fluid*.

Christmas disease

A rare genetic bleeding disorder in which there is deficient production of one of the proteins in blood that is needed for blood coagulation (see *blood clotting*).

Christmas disease has similar features to *haemophilia*. However, the deficient proteins are different. In Christmas disease the deficiency is of a protein called factor IX, while in haemophilia the deficiency is of the protein factor VIII.

chromium

A metallic element that plays a vital role in the activities of several *enzymes* (substances that control the rate of chemical reactions) in the body. It is needed in only minute amounts (see *trace elements*). In excess, it is toxic. It causes inflammation of the skin, and, if inhaled, damages the nose. Chromium fumes may increase the risk of *lung cancer*.

chromosomal abnormalities

Variations from normal in the number or structure of *chromosomes* contained in a person's cells. In most cases, the chromosomal abnormality is present in all of the body's cells. The possible effects range from virtually none to a lethal condition, depending on the particular type of abnormality.

CAUSES

The cause of a chromosomal abnormality is generally a fault in the process of chromosome division, either during the formation of an egg or sperm, or during the first few divisions of a fertilized egg. Occasionally, a parent passes on an abnormal arrangement of his or her own chromosomes.

TYPES

Chromosomal abnormalities are classified according to whether they involve the 44 autosomes (pairs of very similar chromosomes) or the two *sex chromosomes* (X and Y). A whole extra set of chromosomes per cell is called polyploidy; this is lethal in early pregnancy.

AUTOSOMAL ABNORMALITIES

These abnormalities cause physical and mental defects of varying severity. Some types of autosomal abnormality, known

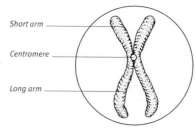

Appearance of a dividing chromosome
Just after a chromosome has copied itself, the copies are joined at a constriction (centromere) that divides them into long and short "arms".

as trisomies, involve the presence of an extra chromosome on one of the 22 pairs of autosomes. The most common trisomy is *Down's syndrome*, which is caused by the presence of three number 21 chromosomes (which is the reason Down's syndrome is also sometimes known as trisomy 21).

Sometimes, part of a chromosome is missing, as in *cri du chat syndrome*. In *translocation*, a part of a chromosome is joined to another, causing no ill effects in the person but a risk of abnormality in his or her children.

SEX CHROMOSOME ABNORMALITIES

Normally, a female has two X chromosomes and a male has an X and a Y. Abnormalities may occur if there are missing or extra sex chromosomes.

In *Turner's syndrome*, a girl is born with only a single X chromosome in her cells instead of the normal complement of two. The condition causes physical abnormalities, defective sexual development, and infertility.

In boys, one or more extra X chromosomes causes *Klinefelter's syndrome*. This condition results in defective sexual development and infertility.

The presence of an extra X chromosome in women or of an extra Y chromosome in men normally has no physical effect but increases the risk of mild learning difficulties.

DIAGNOSIS

If suspected, chromosomal abnormalities can be diagnosed by *chromosome analysis* in early pregnancy, using *amniocentesis* or *chorionic villus sampling*.

Because chromosomal abnormalities affect every one of a person's cells, no cure is possible. Many disorders caused by autosomal chromosome defects result in early death. Others, such as Down's syndrome, are compatible with survival but cause physical and mental disability. Hormonal or surgical treatment, or a combination, can help to

correct some of the developmental defects caused by Klinefelter's and Turner's syndromes.

Anyone who has a child or other family member affected by a chromosomal abnormality may wish to consider *genetic counselling* to establish the risk of his or her future children being affected by the condition.

chromosome analysis

Study of the *chromosomes* in cells to find out if a *chromosomal abnormality* is present or to establish its nature.

WHY IT IS DONE

Some pregnancies are associated with a higher-than-average risk of the baby having a chromosomal abnormality. Risk factors include an older mother, the birth of a previous child with a chromosomal defect, or a defect or *translocation* (rearrangement) in the mother's or the father's chromosomes. In many cases, there are no identifiable risk factors, and so all pregnant women are offered a preliminary blood test (see *antenatal screening*) to identify those at high risk of a fetal abnormality. If the fetus is at high risk, a sample of cells is taken for chromosome analysis. If a serious abnormality, such as *Down's syndrome*, is identified, the parents will be offered termination of the pregnancy (see *abortion, induced*) and *genetic counselling* to assess the risk of a subsequent pregnancy being affected.

Chromosome analysis is also carried out when a baby is stillborn without an obvious cause, or when a baby is born with abnormal physical characteristics that suggest a chromosomal defect, such as *Turner's syndrome*.

The analysis of the sex chromosomes may be carried out in order to establish the chromosomal sex of a child whose genitals have an ambiguous appearance (see *genitalia, ambiguous*); to confirm or to exclude the diagnosis of *chromosomal abnormalities*; or to investigate *infertility*.

HOW IT IS DONE

Fetal cells for analysis can be obtained by *amniocentesis* or *chorionic villus sampling*. Chromosome analysis in children and adults uses white blood cells taken from a blood sample.

chromosomes

Threadlike structures in the nuclei (see *nucleus*) of cells that carry inherited information in the form of genes, which govern cell activity and function. The number of genes on each chromosome varies from about 2,960 on chromosome 1 to about 230 on the Y chromosome; the total number of genes on the full set of chromsomes is about 20,000 to 25,000.

The genes of each chromosome are arranged in single file along a long double filament of *DNA*. The sequence of chemical units (known as bases) in the DNA provides the coded instructions for cellular activities. Each cell contains the chemical machinery for decoding these instructions (see *genetic code*; *nucleic acids*).

All of the body cells (except for egg or sperm cells) carry the same chromosomal material, which has been copied by a process of *cell division* from the original material in the fertilized egg. Each human cell normally contains 46 chromosomes made up of 23 pairs. Half of each pair of chromosomes comes from the mother and half from the father.

TYPES OF CHROMOSOMES
In each set of chromosomes, 22 pairs are autosomal, which are the same in both sexes, and the remaining pair are the sex chromosomes.

There are two types of sex chromosome, called X and Y. In females, the sex chromosomes are a matched pair of X chromosomes. In males, one is an X

and the other is a Y. The mother's egg contributes an X chromosome to every offspring. The father's sperm contributes the other chromosome in the pair: an X in girls or a Y in boys.

The Y chromosome is thought to provide all of the information required for the development of male sexual characteristics. In the absence of the Y chromosome, the female pattern of development takes place.

CHROMOSOME DIVISION
When a cell divides, all of its components, including the chromosomes, are duplicated into the two offspring cells. The process by which most body cells divide is called *mitosis*. Shortly before cell division, the DNA in each chromosome is copied; if viewed under a microscope, chromosomes at this stage appear as double rods joined at an area called the centromere. As cell division proceeds, the duplicated chromosomes are pulled apart, divided at the centromeres, so that each daughter cell will receive a single copy of each of the usual 46 chromosomes.

When egg or sperm cells are formed, by a process called *meiosis*, there are two important departures from the normal process of chromosome division. First, after the DNA has been

copied (before division takes place), some sections of chromosomal material are exchanged between the two members of each chromosome pair. This helps to ensure that each of a person's eggs or sperm contains a different combination of chromosomal material, and this is the reason why siblings (with the exception of identical twins) have a unique appearance. Next, the cells undergo two consecutive divisions. Therefore, the original parent cell gives rise to four separate egg or sperm cells, each of which has only 23 chromosomes, half the full complement.

DISORDERS
Defective chromosome division during the formation of eggs and sperm (or, more rarely, during the first few divisions of a fertilized egg) can lead to various *chromosomal abnormalities*. The precise nature of the abnormality can be investigated by detailed *chromosome analysis*. (See also *genetic disorders*.)

chronic
A term that is used to describe a disorder or a set of symptoms that has persisted over a long time. The term "chronic illness" implies a continuing disease process with progressive deterioration (sometimes despite treatment).

PROCEDURE FOR **CHROMOSOME ANALYSIS**

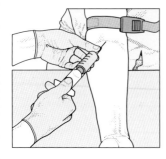

1 In antenatal testing, a collection of fetal cells is obtained by amniocentesis or by chorionic villus sampling. In a test on a baby, child, or adult, white blood cells are obtained from a sample of blood.

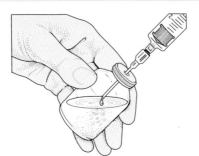

2 The cells are suspended in a medium containing substances that encourage them to divide. Chemicals are then added that stop the cells from dividing at a stage where their chromosome content is most easily visible.

3 The cells are spread on a microscope slide and stained. A selected few (in which the chromosomes are clearly visible and well separated) have their nuclei photographed or are closely examined through a high-powered microscope.

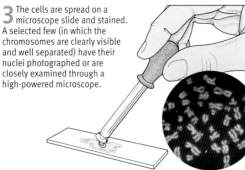

4 The chromosomes are matched up and arranged into the 22 pairs of autosomes and the sex chromosomes. A study of the complete set will reveal any abnormalities.

1 2 3   4 5
6 7 8 9 10 11 12
13 14 15   16 17 18
19 20   21 22   X Y
Male   Female

C

CHROMOSOMES: EGG AND SPERM CELLS

These differ from other body cells in that they contain only 23 chromosomes – one from each of the 22 autosome pairs plus an X chromosome (in the case of an egg) and either an X or a Y (in the case of a sperm). Because they have only half the normal complement, they are called haploid, while other cells are diploid.

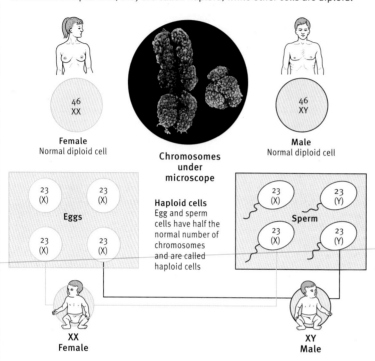

Female
Normal diploid cell
46
XX

Chromosomes under microscope

Male
Normal diploid cell
46
XY

Eggs
23 (X)   23 (X)
23 (X)   23 (X)

Haploid cells
Egg and sperm cells have half the normal number of chromosomes and are called haploid cells

Sperm
23 (X)   23 (Y)
23 (X)   23 (Y)

XX
Female

XY
Male

Chronic disorders are usually contrasted with *acute* disorders, which are of sudden onset and are short in duration.

A chronic illness produces little change in symptoms from day to day, and an affected person may be able, to carry out normal activities. The term "acute", in contrast, suggests rapid onset of severe symptoms such as high fever, intense pain, or breathlessness, with a rapid change in the person's condition from one day to the next.

A person with a chronic disease may suffer an acute exacerbation (flare-up) of symptoms. On the other hand, people who have had a *stroke* or some other acute illness may be left with permanent disabilities, but their condition is not chronic.

chronic bronchitis

See *pulmonary disease, chronic obstructive*.

chronic fatigue syndrome

Also known as myalgic encephalo-myelitis, or ME, a condition that causes extreme fatigue over a prolonged period, often several years. It is most common in women aged between 25 and 45.

CAUSES

The cause is unclear. In some cases, it develops after a viral infection or stressful event such as bereavement. In other cases, there is no preceding illness or event.

SYMPTOMS

The main symptom is persistent, over-whelming tiredness. Other symptoms vary, but commonly include impair-ment of short-term memory or concentration, sore throat, tender *lymph nodes*, muscle and joint pain, muscle fatigue, unrefreshing sleep, and head-aches. The syndrome is often associated with *depression* or *anxiety*.

DIAGNOSIS

There is no specific diagnostic test for chronic fatigue syndrome, and investi-gations of the condition are usually aimed at excluding other possible caus-es of the symptoms, such as *anaemia*. A physical examination, blood tests, and a psychological assessment may be car-ried out. If no cause for the condition can be found, diagnosis is made from the symptoms.

TREATMENT

There is no known cure but commonly tried treatments include graded exercise and *cognitive-behavioural therapy*. *Anti-depressant drugs* may also sometimes be prescribed. Chronic fatigue syndrome is a long-term disorder, but may clear up after several years.

chronic glaucoma

See *glaucoma*.

chronic heart failure

See *heart failure*.

chronic obstructive lung disease

See *pulmonary disease, chronic obstructive*.

chronic obstructive pulmonary disease

See *pulmonary disease, chronic obstructive*.

chronological age

The most common measurement of an individual's *age*.

Churg–Strauss syndrome

A condition characterized by vasculitis (inflammation in the walls of small blood vessels), which mainly affects adults in their thirties who have *asthma*. It is thought to be due to an allergy of unknown cause.

The vasculitis can cause a variety of symptoms, depending on the parts of the body that are affected. Common problems include abdominal pain, if the bowel is involved, and skin rashes. The disease may be severe or even life-threatening, although in most cases it responds well to treatment with oral *corticosteroid drugs*. The drug treatment may need to be continued, at a low dose, for some time to prevent a recur-rence of the condition.

chylomicron

A globule of fat (see *fats and oils*) that is carried into the bloodstream from the intestine following the digestion of a meal containing fat.

ciclosporin

An *immunosuppressant drug* that is used following *transplant surgery*. The drug reduces the risk of tissue rejection and the need for large doses of *corticosteroid drugs*. Ciclosporin may need to be taken indefinitely after a transplant. It is also a *disease-modifying antirheumatic drug* and is used to treat *rheumatoid arthritis* and other *autoimmune disorders*. In addition, ciclosporin may be used in the treatment of severe *eczema* and *psoriasis*.

Because ciclosporin suppresses the immune system, it increases susceptibility to infection. Swollen gums and increased hair growth are fairly common side effects. The drug may also cause kidney damage, so people taking the drug need regular monitoring of kidney function.

cilia

Hairlike, mobile filaments that exist on the surface of some epithelial cells (see *epithelium*). Cilia are found in particularly abundant amounts in the linings of the respiratory tract, where they move rhythmically to propel dust and mucus out of the airways.

ciliary body

A structure in the *eye* containing muscles that alter the shape of the *lens* to adjust focus. (See also *accommodation*.)

cimetidine

An *H₂-receptor antagonist*, which is a type of *ulcer-healing drug*. Cimetidine can be taken in tablet or liquid form, or it may be injected. The drug promotes healing of gastric and duodenal ulcers (see *peptic ulcer*) and also reduces the symptoms of *oesophagitis* (inflammation of the gullet).

Side effects include fatigue, dizziness, and skin rashes. Rarely, the drug may cause *erectile dysfunction* and *gynaecomastia* (breast enlargement in men).

CIN

The abbreviation for *cervical intraepithelial neoplasia*.

cinnarizine

An *antihistamine drug* used to control nausea and vomiting due to travel sickness, or to reduce nausea and vertigo in disorders of the inner ear such as *labyrinthitis* and *Ménière's disease*. Side effects of cinnarizine may include drowsiness, lethargy, a dry mouth, and blurred vision.

ciprofloxacin

An *antibiotic drug* used to treat infections of the respiratory, gastrointestinal, and urinary tracts. It may also be used as an initial treatment for *anthrax*.

circadian rhythms

Any pattern of physiological functions that is based on a cycle approximately 24 hours long (also called a diurnal rhythm). One example of this pattern is the daily cycle of sleeping and wakefulness. (See also *biorhythms*.)

circulation, disorders of

Conditions affecting the flow of blood around the body. (See *arteries, disorders of*; *veins, disorders of*.)

circulatory collapse

A life-threatening condition in which the circulatory system is unable to maintain an adequate blood flow to the body's organs and tissues (see *shock*). Circulatory collapse can occur when the heart stops beating (see *cardiac arrest*), or it may be due to loss of blood or problems with the blood vessels.

circulatory system

The *heart* and *blood vessels*, which together are responsible for maintaining continuous flow of blood through the body. Also known as the cardiovascular system, the circulatory system provides the tissues with a supply of oxygen and nutrients, and carries away carbon dioxide and other waste products.

STRUCTURE AND FUNCTION

The circulatory system has two main parts: the systemic circulation, which supplies blood to the whole body apart from the lungs; and the pulmonary circulation to the lungs, which supplies the blood with fresh oxygen (see *circulatory system* box, overleaf).

Oxygen-rich blood from the pulmonary circulation enters the systemic circulation via the left *ventricle* of the heart. The ventricle pumps it under high pressure into the *aorta* (the body's main artery), from where it travels through arteries and smaller arterioles to all parts of the body. Within the body tissues, the arterioles branch into networks of fine blood vessels known as capillaries. Oxygen and nutrients pass from the blood through the thin capillary walls and into the tissues; carbon dioxide and other waste products pass in the opposite direction. Deoxygenated blood is returned to the heart via venules (small veins), veins, and the *venae cavae* (the two principal veins in the body).

Within the systemic circulation, there is also a bypass (the portal circulation) that carries nutrient-rich blood from the stomach, intestine, and other digestive organs via the portal vein to the *liver*. Nutrients and other substances pass into the liver cells for processing, storage, breakdown, or re-entry into the general circulation. Blood passes out of the liver through the hepatic vein and rejoins the main systemic circulation via the inferior (lower) vena cava.

Venous blood returns to the right atrium of the heart to enter the pulmonary circulation. It is pumped from the right ventricle through the pulmonary artery to the lungs, where carbon dioxide is exchanged for oxygen. The reoxygenated blood then returns via the pulmonary veins to the heart and re-enters the systemic circulation.

On its journey from the heart to the body tissues, blood is forced along the arteries at high pressure. In contrast, blood flowing through the veins and back to the heart is at low pressure. It is kept moving by muscles in the limbs, which compress the veins and thus squeeze blood through them, and by valves in the veins that prevent the blood from flowing backwards. (See also *lymphatic system*; *respiration*.)

circumcision

Surgical removal of the foreskin of the *penis*. Circumcision may be medically required to treat *phimosis* (a tight foreskin that causes ballooning on urination), recurrent attacks of *balanitis* (infection under the foreskin due to retained secretions), or *paraphimosis* (painful compression of the shaft of the penis by a retracted foreskin). It may also be performed for religious, cosmetic, or social reasons.

circumcision, female

Removal of all or some parts of the female external genitalia: the *clitoris*, labia majora, and labia minora (see *labia*). Female circumcision is sometimes combined with narrowing of the entrance to the *vagina*.

Female circumcision is common in certain parts of Africa but has no valid medical purpose. It can cause retention of urine and injuries during sexual intercourse and childbirth.

cirrhosis

A condition of the *liver* that results from long-term damage to liver cells. In cirrhosis, bands of fibrosis (internal scarring) develop, leaving *nodules* of regenerating cells that are inadequately

C

CIRCULATORY SYSTEM

The heart and blood vessels create a continuous flow of blood around the body to provide tissues with oxygen and nutrients. The circulatory system also removes waste products. The systemic circulation deals with the supply of blood to all parts except the lungs; the pulmonary (lung) circulation reoxygenates the blood.

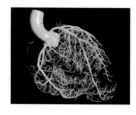

Resin cast of coronary arteries
The photograph on the left shows a resin cast of the arteries that supply oxygenated blood to all parts of the heart muscle. The larger vessels are called the coronary arteries. They branch off the root of the aorta, the largest artery in the body, which receives oxygenated blood directly from the heart.

SYSTEMIC CIRCULATION

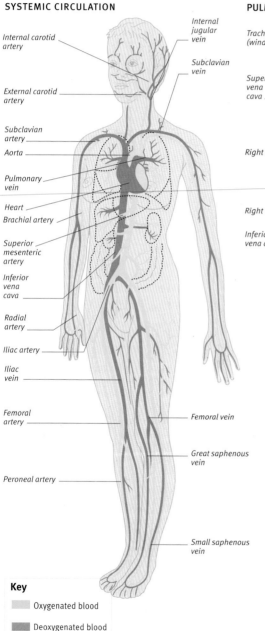

Internal carotid artery

Internal jugular vein

Subclavian vein

External carotid artery

Subclavian artery

Aorta

Pulmonary vein

Heart

Brachial artery

Superior mesenteric artery

Inferior vena cava

Radial artery

Iliac artery

Iliac vein

Femoral artery

Femoral vein

Great saphenous vein

Peroneal artery

Small saphenous vein

Key

Oxygenated blood

Deoxygenated blood

PULMONARY CIRCULATION

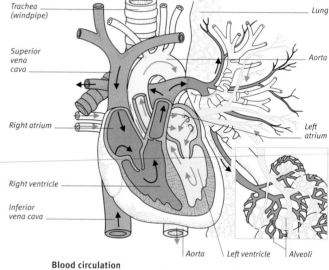

Trachea (windpipe)

Superior vena cava

Right atrium

Right ventricle

Inferior vena cava

Lung

Aorta

Left atrium

Aorta

Left ventricle

Alveoli

Blood circulation
The right side of the heart receives deoxygenated blood from the systemic ("body") circulation via the venae cavae. The heart pumps this blood to the lungs, where it is oxygenated and returns to the left side of the heart (pulmonary circulation). It is then pumped via arteries to the tissues, where the blood releases oxygen. Deoxygenated blood then returns to the heart.

CAPILLARY NETWORK

All tissues contain a network of tiny capillaries. Blood enters these vessels from the arterioles and is drained by venules.

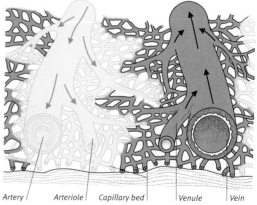

Artery | Arteriole | Capillary bed | Venule | Vein

supplied with blood. Liver function is gradually impaired; the liver no longer effectively removes toxic substances from the blood (see *liver failure*). The distortion and fibrosis also lead to *portal hypertension* (abnormally high blood pressure in the veins leading from the intestines and spleen to the liver).

CAUSES
The most common cause of cirrhosis is excessive *alcohol* consumption. Another possible cause is one of the forms of chronic *hepatitis* (inflammation of the liver). Other causes, which are rare, include disorders of the *bile ducts*; *haemochromatosis*, in which increased iron absorption occurs; *Wilson's disease* (an increase in copper absorption); *cystic fibrosis*, which causes obstruction of the bile ducts with mucus; and *heart failure*.

SYMPTOMS AND COMPLICATIONS
Cirrhosis may go unrecognized until symptoms such as mild *jaundice*, *oedema* (an accumulation of fluid in body tissues) and vomiting of blood develop. There may be enlargement of the liver and spleen. Men may experience loss of body hair and enlargement of the breasts due to an imbalance in sex hormones caused by liver failure.

Complications of cirrhosis include *ascites* (an accumulation of fluid in the abdominal cavity), *oesophageal varices* (enlarged veins within the oesophagus wall), and *hepatoma* (liver cancer). Cirrhosis may also cause toxins to build up in the brain, producing symptoms such as confusion and coma (see *hepatic encephalopathy*).

TREATMENT
Treatment is focused on slowing the rate at which liver cells are being damaged, if possible by treating the cause. Any complications will also be treated. In some cases, however, the cirrhosis progresses and a *liver transplant* may need to be considered.

cisplatin
An *anticancer drug* used to treat some cancers of the *testis* and the *ovary*.

citalopram
An *antidepressant drug* belonging to a group called selective serotonin reuptake inhibitors (SSRIs). Citalopram takes up to four weeks to reach its full effect; it gradually improves the user's mood, energy levels, and level of interest in everyday activities. Citalopram is also used to treat panic disorder. It is not usually prescribed for patients under 18.

The drug may cause gastrointestinal problems such as nausea, vomiting, or diarrhoea, but these usually diminish with continued use. In some people, citalopram may also cause drowsiness, an effect that may possibly be increased by alcohol, and therefore people taking the drug should avoid activities such as driving until they have learned how strongly citalopram affects them.

CJD
Abbreviation for *Creutzfeldt–Jakob disease*.

CK
Abbreviation for *creatine kinase*.

clamp
An instrument used during surgical procedures to compress the cut end of an organ or blood vessel temporarily.

clap
A slang term for *gonorrhoea*.

clarithromycin
An *antibiotic drug* that belongs to the macrolide group. Clarithromycin is used to treat infections of the skin and the respiratory tract.

classic migraine
A type of *migraine* attack accompanied by an aura (neurological disturbances), nausea, and vomiting.

claudication
A cramplike pain in a muscle, most often in the legs, due to inadequate blood supply. Claudication in the legs is usually caused by blockage or narrowing of arteries due to *atherosclerosis* (see *peripheral vascular disease*). In intermittent claudication, pain is felt in the calves after walking a certain distance and is relieved by rest. A rarer cause is spinal *stenosis* (narrowing of the spinal canal), causing pressure on the nerve roots that pass into either leg.

claustrophobia
An intense fear of being in enclosed spaces, such as lifts or tunnels, or of being in crowded areas. The usual treatment is *behaviour therapy* involving techniques that gradually lessen the patient's anxiety. (See also *phobia*.)

clavicle
The anatomical name for the collarbone. The two clavicles, one on each side, form joints with the top of the sternum

The two clavicles run across the front of each shoulder, joining the top of the sternum to each scapula. They help to support the arms.

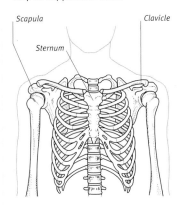

Scapula   Clavicle

Sternum

(breastbone) and the scapula (shoulderblade). The clavicles support the arms and transmit forces from the arms to the central skeleton.

Most fractures of the clavicle occur as a result of a fall on to the shoulder or on to an outstretched arm. When the clavicle is broken, the arm must be supported in a sling, and a figure-of-eight bandage must be used to keep the fractured bone ends together. Healing of a fractured clavicle typically takes about three weeks.

clavulanic acid
A substance that inhibits the action of beta-lactamase (an enzyme that is found in certain bacteria and which makes those bacteria resistant to antibiotics). Clavulanic acid itself possesses no antibacterial properties, but it is combined with the penicillin drug *amoxicillin* to produce the antibiotic drug *co-amoxiclav*. This combination is more powerful than amoxicillin alone because it inactivates bacteria such as STAPHYLOCOCCUS AUREUS, which would otherwise be resistant to amoxicillin.

claw-foot
A deformity of the foot in which the arch of the foot is exaggerated and the tips of the toes turn under.

Claw-foot may be congenital (present from birth) or it may occur as a result of damage or disruption to the nerve or blood supply to the muscles of the foot. Surgery may improve the condition.

claw-hand

A deformity in which the fingers are permanently curled. It is caused by injury to the *ulnar nerve*, which controls the muscles of the thumb and fingers. Treatment includes repairing the nerve by using splints to hold the fingers straight, or cutting a tendon in the wrist to allow the fingers to straighten.

claw-toe

A deformity of unknown cause in which the end of one or more affected toes bends downwards so that the toe curls under. A painful *corn* may form on the tip of the toe or on the top of the bent joint. Protective pads can relieve pressure from footwear. In severe cases, surgery may be required.

cleft lip and palate

A split in the upper lip and/or palate that is present at birth. Cleft lip is a vertical, usually off-centre split in the upper lip; it may be a small notch, or may extend to the nose. The gum may also be cleft, and the nose may be crooked. The term "harelip" refers only to a midline cleft lip, which is rare. Cleft palate is a gap that may extend from the back of the palate to behind the teeth and be open to the nasal cavity. The condition is often accompanied by other problems such as partial deafness and possibly other *birth defects*.

CAUSES
In many cases the cause is unknown. However, certain drugs taken during pregnancy, such as some anticonvulsants and corticosteroids, may be associated with the condition. Genetic factors may be involved in some cases.

TREATMENT
Surgery to repair a cleft lip may be undertaken in the first few days after birth or when the baby is about three months of age. Surgery improves the child's appearance; after repair, speech defects are rare. A cleft palate is usually repaired when an infant is about six to nine months old, but further surgery, *orthodontic* treatment, and *speech therapy* may be required.

cleidocranial dysplasia

Also called cleidocranial dysostosis, a rare, autosomal dominant *genetic disorder* causing malformation of the bones, particularly those in the skull and shoulders. An affected person typically has absent or underdeveloped *clavicles* (collarbones), and can move the shoul-ders forwards so that they almost touch. The sutures (fixed joints) of the *skull* bones take longer than normal to fuse together. There may also be abnormalities in the structure of the pelvis, fingers, teeth, and *vertebrae* (bones of the spinal column).

clemastine

An *antihistamine drug* that is used to relieve the symptoms of allergic conditions such as *urticaria* (nettle rash) and allergic *rhinitis* (hay fever). Because clemastine can cause drowsiness, driving and hazardous work should be avoided.

clergyman's knee

Inflammation of the *bursa* (the fluid-filled sac) that cushions the pressure point above the tibial tubercle (the bony prominence just below the knee). The condition is caused by prolonged kneeling. (See also *bursitis*.)

climacteric

See *menopause*.

clindamycin

An *antibiotic drug* that may be prescribed as a skin preparation to treat *acne* or in creams to treat bacterial vaginal infections. It may also be given as tablets or by injection to treat some bone and joint infections, as prophylaxis for *endocarditis* (infection of the membrane lining the heart), and to treat falciparum *malaria*.

Clindamycin can have serious side effects. In particular, the drug may cause a potentially life-threatening form of bowel inflammation known as antibiotic-associated colitis.

clinical diagnosis

A procedure in which a doctor determines the nature of a disorder on the basis of an individual's description of his or her symptoms and a physical examination. Unlike *pathological diagnosis*, a clinical diagnosis does not depend on the analysis of tissue specimens taken from the body.

clinical pharmacology

The branch of *pharmacology* that deals with the use of drugs in patients in hospitals and in the community.

clinical psychology

The branch of *psychology* (the scientific study of mental processes) concerned with the diagnosis and treatment of emotional and behavioural problems.

clinical trial

See *trial, clinical*.

clioquinol

An *antibacterial drug* and *antifungal drug* used as a constituent of ear drops to treat infections of the outer ear. It is also included in some skin preparations.

clip

A small device used to hold a wound closed or prevent leakage from a blood vessel. Specialized clips are used in female sterilization operations (see *sterilization, female*) to seal the fallopian tubes.

clitoridectomy

An operation to remove the *clitoris* (see *circumcision, female*).

clitoris

A small, sensitive, erectile organ that is part of the female genitalia. It is partly enclosed in the *labia* and covered by a fold of skin called the *prepuce*, or hood. The clitoris swells and becomes more sensitive during sexual stimulation.

clobazam

A type of *benzodiazepine* drug used in the treatment of *anxiety* and *epilepsy*.

clobetasone

A *corticosteroid drug*, used as a cream or an ointment to treat inflammatory skin conditions, such as *eczema*.

clomifene

A drug used to treat female *infertility* caused by failure to ovulate. Minor side effects may include hot flushes, head-

LOCATION OF **CLITORIS**

The clitoris is a part of the external genitals in females. It is located just below the pubic bone, and is partly enclosed within the labia.

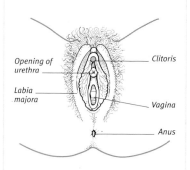

ache, nausea, breast tenderness, and blurred vision. More seriously, *ovarian cysts* occasionally develop, but they shrink when the dose is reduced. The drug may also cause multiple births.

clomipramine

A *tricyclic antidepressant drug*, which is used as a treatment for *depression*. Side effects include dry mouth, blurred vision, and constipation.

clonazepam

A *benzodiazepine drug* used mainly as an *anticonvulsant drug* to prevent and treat epileptic fits (see *epilepsy*). It also prevents *petit mal* attacks in children. Side effects include drowsiness, dizziness, fatigue, and irritability.

clone

An exact copy. In medicine, the term "clone" usually refers to duplicates of cells, genes, or organisms.

Clones of cells are all descended from one original cell. In many types of cancer, cells are thought to be derived from one abnormal cell. Clones of genes are copies of a single gene. In research, several clones of a gene can be made so the gene can be studied in detail. Clones of organisms can be produced by removing the nuclei from cells of a donor individual and transplanting them into the egg cells of another individual. The eggs mature into living plants or animals that are all identical to the donor.

clonic

Relating to the abnormal muscle contractions known as *clonus*, which are sometimes a sign of a brain or spinal cord disorder.

clonic convulsion

A form of *seizure* in which there are uncontrolled, jerking movements of the limbs and body (see *clonus*). Clonic convulsions are a feature of some types of *epilepsy*.

clonidine

An *antihypertensive drug* that controls hypertension (high blood pressure) by acting on the part of the brain that regulates the size of blood vessels. Clonidine is also used to control hot flushes in menopausal women and to treat some cases of migraine. Possible side effects of the drug include constipation, drowsiness, dry mouth, and

dizziness. Caution should be taken if high doses of the drug are suddenly stopped because this can cause a dangerous rise in blood pressure.

clonus

A series of rapid, abnormal *muscle* contractions. Clonus is a sign of damage to nerve fibres that carry impulses from the motor cortex in the *cerebrum* of the brain to a particular muscle. It may occur in the wrist, knee, ankle, or toe in response to stretching of the muscles in that area. It may also be a feature of seizures (see *clonic convulsion*).

clopidogrel

An *antiplatelet drug* used to help prevent strokes or heart attacks in people at risk of these conditions, particularly those who have previously had them. Possible side effects of the drug include indigestion, abdominal pain, and diarrhoea. With prolonged use there is also an increased risk of internal and/or external bleeding, especially in people who are also taking aspirin.

closed-angle glaucoma

An alternative term for acute *glaucoma*.

closed fracture

A type of *fracture*, also known as a simple fracture, in which the broken bone ends do not penetrate the overlying skin.

Clostridium

Any of a group of rod-shaped *bacteria*. Clostridia are found in soil and in the gastrointestinal tracts of humans and animals. They produce powerful toxins and are responsible for potentially life-threatening diseases such as *botulism*, *tetanus*, and *gangrene*.

clot

See *blood clotting*.

clotrimazole

A topical *antifungal drug* used to treat yeast infections, especially *candidiasis*, and fungal infections such as *tinea* (ringworm). Side effects are very rare, although some people may experience burning and irritation on the surface of the skin where the drug was applied.

clotting factor

A circulating protein that is activated during the *blood clotting* process. There are a number of clotting factors, which

are involved in a complex series of chemical reactions leading to the formation of a blood clot.

clotting time

The time taken for blood to coagulate, which is measured in tests by the observation of a blood sample under laboratory conditions. (See also *blood-clotting tests*.)

cloudy urine

An abnormality in the appearance of *urine*, which may be caused by a *urinary tract infection* or the presence of salts. (See also *urine, abnormal*.)

clove oil

An oil distilled from the dried flower-buds of EUGENIA CARYOPHYLLATA that is used mainly as a flavouring in pharmaceuticals. Clove oil is sometimes used as a remedy for toothache.

clozapine

A type of *antipsychotic drug* used to treat *schizophrenia* in patients who have not responded well to other forms of treatment or who have had severe side effects from more conventional drugs. Clozapine helps to control severe resistant schizophrenia, allowing the person to lead a more normal life. A person taking the drug needs to have regular blood tests because it may seriously decrease the number of *white blood cells*.

clubbing

Thickening and broadening of the fingertips and ends of the toes, which is usually accompanied by increased curving of the nails. Clubbing is associated with certain chronic lung diseases, such as *lung cancer*, *bronchiectasis*, and fibrosing *alveolitis*; with some types of heart abnormalities; and, rarely, with the inflammatory bowel diseases *Crohn's disease* and *ulcerative colitis*.

club-foot

A deformity of the foot that is present from birth (see *talipes*).

clumping

The common name for agglutination, a process in which tiny particles that the body identifies as foreign (see *antigen*), such as the proteins on the surfaces of bacteria or foreign red blood cells, stick together to form visible masses. This process is an immune system reaction caused by antibodies (proteins manu-

C

factured by the immune system; see *antibody*) called agglutinins. Particles of a particular antigen will only clump together in the presence of the specific agglutinin to that antigen.

Looking for clumping can be used as a means of determining people's blood groups. In blood typing, samples of a person's blood are mixed with antibodies against the blood types A and B to see if clumping occurs with either of these antibodies, neither, or both (see *blood groups*). In *cross-matching*, a sample of a person's blood is mixed with a sample of blood from a possible donor; if the red blood cells clump together, it shows that the two samples of blood are of incompatible types. In addition, bacteria can be identified by using samples that contain agglutinins to specific bacteria (as, for example, in the *latex fixation test*).

cluster headaches

Brief but severe headaches that recur several times a day over a period lasting from a few weeks to about two months. They tend to affect one side of the head or face, often in a characteristic pattern, and may also cause pain and watering of the eye. The cause is uncertain, but in some people they may be triggered by alcohol.

Cluster headaches may be treated with injections of *sumatriptan* (a *serotonin agonist* that is also used to treat migraine) or inhalation of pure oxygen. *Ergotamine* is also sometimes used to treat cluster headaches.

CMV

The abbreviation for *cytomegalovirus*, a type of *herpes* virus.

CNS

The abbreviation for *central nervous system* (the brain and spinal cord).

CNS stimulants

Drugs that increase mental alertness (see *stimulant drugs*).

coagulation, blood

The main mechanism by which blood clots are formed. Coagulation involves a complex series of reactions in the blood *plasma* (see *blood clotting*).

coal tar

A thick, black, sticky substance that is distilled from coal. Coal tar is a common ingredient in many ointments and medicinal shampoos that are prescribed for certain skin and scalp disorders, such as *psoriasis* and some types of *dermatitis* and *eczema*.

co-amilofruse

A combined preparation that contains the diuretic drugs *amiloride* and *furosemide* (frusemide).

co-amoxiclav

A *penicillin drug* containing a mixture of *amoxicillin* and *clavulanic acid*. It is a more powerful antibiotic than amoxicillin alone, so it is used to treat infections caused by strains of bacteria that are resistant to amoxicillin.

coarctation of the aorta

A *congenital* heart defect of unknown cause, in which there is narrowing in a section of the *aorta* that supplies blood to the lower body and legs. To compensate for this problem the heart has to work harder than normal, thereby causing *hypertension* (high blood pressure) in the upper part of the body.

SYMPTOMS

Symptoms of coarctation of the aorta usually appear in early childhood. They include headache, weakness after exercise, cold legs, and, rarely, breathing difficulty and swelling of the legs due to *heart failure*. Associated abnormalities include a heart *murmur*, weak or absent pulse in the groin, lack of synchronization between the groin and wrist pulses, and blood pressure that is higher in the arms than in the legs.

DIAGNOSIS AND TREATMENT

Diagnosis may be made by *aortography*, *MRI* (magnetic resonance imaging), and/or chest X-ray. Surgery to correct the defect is usually performed in early childhood.

Coat's disease

A disease that causes a progressive deterioration in vision. It is congenital (present at birth) but usually begins in childhood, and affects boys more than girls. The cause is unknown.

In Coat's disease, the capillaries (tiny blood vessels) supplying the retina become damaged and leak fluid (a process called exudation). As a result, the retina does not function properly. Usually, only one eye is affected. Vision may be impaired in the centre of the visual field or around the edges. In some cases, a squint develops. There is also a risk of retinal detachment.

Diagnosis involves viewing the retina through an ophthalmoscope, and by imaging the blood vessels using *fluorescein* dye. Treatment may involve sealing the capillaries by phototherapy (treatment with light rays) or cryotherapy (treatment with cold). If given early enough, it may stabilize the disease and may even improve vision. In some cases, the disease stabilizes by itself.

cobalamin

A complex molecule that contains *cobalt* and is part of *vitamin B₁₂*.

cobalt

A metallic element. Cobalt is found in foods as a constituent of *vitamin B₁₂*. A radioactive form is used in *radiotherapy*.

Cobb syndrome

A very rare disorder in which spinal cord *angiomas* (noncancerous tumours of the blood or lymph vessels) occur together with arteriovenous malformations (abnormal connections between arteries and veins) in the overlying skin. It is congenital (present from birth) but is almost never inherited.

The symptoms usually appear in childhood or adolescence; they include weakness, paralysis, loss of sensation, and loss of bowel and bladder control.

Treatment includes surgery to block the blood flow to the abnormal vessels (see *embolization*) and to relieve pressure on the spinal cord (see *decompression, spinal canal*).

co-beneldopa

A preparation containing the drugs benserazide and *levodopa*; co-beneldopa is used in the treatment of *Parkinson's disease*.

cocaine

A drug obtained from the leaves of the coca plant ERYTHROXYLON COCA. In the past, cocaine was used as a local anaesthetic (see *anaesthesia, local*) for minor surgical procedures, but it has largely been replaced by other anaesthetics due to its potential for abuse.

Cocaine affects the brain, producing euphoria and increased energy. These effects have led to its illicit use (see *drug abuse*). Regular inhalation of the drug can damage the lining of the nose and may eventually cause perforation of the septum (the tissue separating the two sides of the nose). Continued use of the drug can cause dependence (see *drug dependence*), and, if high doses are taken, may result in *psychosis*, which can cause users to become violent. Overdose of cocaine can cause seizures and *cardiac arrest*.

Crack, which is a purified form of cocaine, produces a more rapid and intense reaction; and deaths have occurred as a result of the drug's adverse effects on the heart.

cocci

Spherical *bacteria*, some of which cause infections in humans (see *staphylococcal infections*; *streptococcal infections*).

coccus

The singular of *cocci*.

coccydynia

A pain in the region of the *coccyx*. Coccydynia may result from a blow to the base of the spine in a fall, prolonged pressure due to poor posture when sitting, or the use of the lithotomy position (lying on the back with hips and knees bent) during childbirth. The pain usually eases in time. Treatment may include heat, injections of a local anaesthetic, and *manipulation*.

coccyx

A small, triangular bone, commonly called the tailbone, made up of four tiny bones fused together at the base of the *spine*. Together with a larger bone called the *sacrum*, situated just above it, the coccyx forms the back section of the *pelvis*. There is very little movement between the coccyx and sacrum, and later in life the two structures commonly become fused together.

cochlea

The spiral-shaped organ situated in the *labyrinth* of the inner ear that enables *hearing*. A structure known as the *organ of Corti*, inside the cochlea, can detect sound vibrations of different frequencies and converts them into electrical impulses. These electrical impulses are then transmitted to the brain via the *vestibulocochlear nerve*. Sound waves of different frequencies stimulate different areas inside the cochlea, enabling us to hear and differentiate between a wide variety of sounds.

cochlear implant

A device that is used to treat profoundly deaf people who are not helped by hearing aids. Unlike a hearing aid,

ANATOMY OF **COCCYX**

The coccyx consists of four fused bones at the base of the spine. With the sacrum, it forms the back of the pelvis.

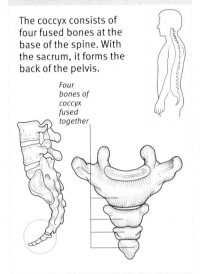

Four bones of coccyx fused together

which amplifies sounds, a cochlear implant converts sounds into electrical signals that are relayed to the cochlear nerve deep in the inner ear (see *cochlear implant box*, below).

The implant consists of tiny electrodes that are surgically implanted in the cochlea, and a receiver that is embedded in the skull just behind and above the ear. A microphone, sound processor, and transmitter are worn externally. A cochlear implant does not restore normal hearing, but it enables

patterns of sound to be detected. Combined with lip-reading, it may enable speech to be understood.

Cockayne's syndrome

An autosomal recessive *genetic disorder* that causes premature aging (see *progeria*), deterioration of the nervous system, and dwarfism (see *short stature*). Affected people also have very thin skin that is extremely sensitive to the effects of sunlight. In addition, there may be visual problems due to degeneration of the retina (see *retinitis pigmentosa*) or atrophy (wasting away) of the *optic nerve*; *deafness*; and *learning difficulties*. The age at which symptoms appear and the course of the disease vary from one individual to another.

There is no cure for the aging or the neurological symptoms, but an affected person can protect his or her skin from sun damage by avoiding exposure to ultraviolet light, or by applying a sunblock to protect areas of exposed skin when outdoors in sunlight.

co-codamol

A compound *analgesic drug* containing *paracetamol* and *codeine*.

codeine

An *opioid analgesic drug* derived from the opium poppy plant. Codeine is useful for relieving mild to moderate pain and may be combined with other analgesic drugs (such as paracetamol) in

COCHLEAR IMPLANT

Sounds picked up by the microphone are converted into electronic signals by the sound processor and relayed to the external transmitter, which sends them through the skin to the receiver. The waves then travel along the wire to the electrodes in the cochlea, where sound is normally received.

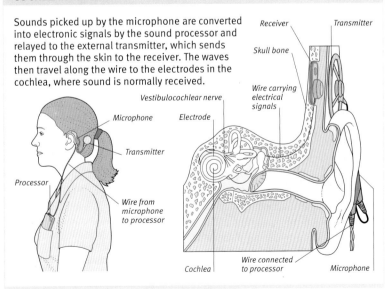

C

painkilling preparations. Codeine is also used as a *cough remedy* and as an *anti-diarrhoeal drug*.

Codeine may cause dizziness and drowsiness, especially if taken with alcohol. If used for long periods, it may cause constipation and be habit-forming.

cod-liver oil

A pale yellow oil obtained from the liver of fresh cod, which is a valuable source of *vitamin A* and *vitamin D*.

co-dydramol

A compound *analgesic drug* (painkiller) that contains *paracetamol* and dihydrocodeine.

coeliac disease

A condition, sometimes called gluten-sensitive enteropathy, that results from *hypersensitivity* to *gluten*, a protein found in wheat, rye, barley, and some other cereals. Exposure to foods containing gluten causes an abnormal immune response in which the lining of the small intestine is damaged. The condition leads to *malabsorption* and results in vitamin and mineral deficiencies.

CAUSES AND SYMPTOMS
Coeliac disease tends to run in families, and varies in severity. The disorder may first appear during infancy, or may not develop until adulthood.

In babies, symptoms usually develop within six months of the introduction of gluten into the diet. The baby may become listless and irritable, develop vomiting and diarrhoea, and become dehydrated and seriously ill. Babies and children may also fail to grow or to gain weight, and may suffer from muscle wasting, especially around the buttocks. In adults, symptoms that include tiredness, breathlessness, abdominal pain, diarrhoea, vomiting, and swelling of the legs may develop over several months. In addition, a chronic, distinctive rash called *dermatitis herpetiformis* may occur.

Damage to the intestinal lining and malabsorption cause weight loss and result in faeces that are bulky and foul-smelling. The resulting vitamin and mineral deficiencies can lead to *anaemia* and skin problems. Some affected people suffer damage to the intestinal lining but never develop symptoms.

DIAGNOSIS AND TREATMENT
Diagnosis may be made by specialized blood tests but in most cases *jejunal biopsies*, in which tissue samples from the lining of the jejunum (the central part of the small intestine) are taken for examination, are also performed.

Coeliac disease is treated by a life-long gluten-free diet, which can relieve symptoms within weeks of its introduction. Specially manufactured foods, such as gluten-free flour and pasta, are available. Without such treatment, there may be a long-term risk of cancers developing in the small intestine.

coenzyme

A nonprotein chemical, occurring naturally in the body, that plays a role in assisting the proper functioning of some types of *enzyme* (proteins that regulate chemical reactions in the body). (See also *NAD*.)

Coffin–Siris syndrome

An autosomal *genetic disorder* characterized by absence or underdevelopment of the tips of the little finger and little toe. Other features include *hirsutism* (excessive hair), *hypotonia* (lack of muscle tone) and weak joints, and *learning difficulties*.

cognition

Mental processes by which knowledge is acquired. Such cognitive processes include perception, problem-solving, and reasoning.

cognitive–behavioural therapy

A method of treating psychological disorders such as *anxiety*, *depression*, *panic disorder*, *post-traumatic stress disorder*, and *chronic fatigue syndrome*. It is based on the idea that problems arise from a person's faulty cognitions (erroneous ways of perceiving the world and oneself). In cognitive–behavioural therapy, the patient is helped to identify negative or false cognitions and then encouraged to try out new thought strategies. For example, a patient may be asked to keep a diary of his or her thoughts and feelings, in order to identify triggers for distress, and may be taught techniques for responding differently to upsetting thoughts.

cognitive dissonance

A state of mental or emotional tension caused by inconsistency and disagreement among different aspects of a person's thoughts, beliefs, values, and behaviour. (For example, a person may buy a well-made pair of shoes but find that they are actually uncomfortable.) People may try to reduce such tension by reinterpreting or rationalizing the situation. (For example, the person with the uncomfortable shoes may persuade him- or herself that the shoes will become more comfortable with wear.)

cogwheel rigidity

A term that is sometimes used for a characteristic muscle stiffness seen in people with *Parkinson's disease*. When the limbs of an affected person are passively moved, the muscles stretch in a series of small jerks.

coil

The common name for any of the various types of intrauterine contraceptive device (see *IUD*; *Mirena*).

coitus

Another term for *sexual intercourse*.

coitus interruptus

A method of contraception (see *contraception, withdrawal method of*) in which the man withdraws his penis from the woman's vagina before *ejaculation* occurs. Coitus interruptus is unreliable because sperm can be released before orgasm occurs, and it may cause *psychosexual dysfunction* in men and women.

colchicine

A drug extracted from the autumn crocus (COLCHICUM AUTUMNALE). Colchicine is used to treat acute attacks of *gout* and to reduce their frequency. Side effects include vomiting and diarrhoea.

cold abscess

An *abscess* caused by infection with the *tuberculosis* bacterium. A cold abscess does not usually produce redness and heat, hence its name.

cold, common

A common viral infection that causes inflammation of the mucous membranes lining the nose and throat.

CAUSES
There are at least 200 highly contagious viruses that are known to cause the common cold. These organisms are easily transmitted in minute airborne droplets sprayed from the coughs or sneezes of infected people. In many cases, cold viruses are also spread to the nose and throat by hand-to-hand contact with an infected person, or by handling objects that have become contaminated with the virus.

SYMPTOMS AND TREATMENT

The symptoms of a cold typically include a stuffy or runny nose, sore throat, headache, and cough. They usually intensify over 24–48 hours (unlike the symptoms of *influenza*, which tend to worsen rapidly over a few hours).

Most colds clear up by themselves within a week. Affected people can take simple measures to cope with symptoms; for example, mild *analgesic drugs* or *cold remedies* may help to relieve aches and pains, and *cough remedies* can soothe a cough. Sometimes, however, infection spreads and may cause *laryngitis*, *tracheitis*, acute *bronchitis*, *sinusitis*, or *otitis media*. In these cases, a bacterial infection may develop on top of the viral infection, and *antibiotic drugs* may be needed to treat it. (Antibiotics are ineffective against viruses, so they will not cure colds.)

cold injury

Localized tissue damage caused by chilling of part of the body. Cold injury is distinct from *hypothermia*, which refers to chilling of the whole body.

The most serious form of cold injury is *frostbite*. In this condition, an area of skin and flesh becomes frozen, hard, and white as a result of exposure to very cold, dry air. Sometimes there is restriction of the blood supply to the affected area. Another type of cold injury, *immersion foot*, occurs when the legs and feet are kept cold and damp for hours or days. The main risk of both frostbite and immersion foot is that the blood flow will be slowed to such an extent that the tissues die and, as a result, develop *gangrene*. Less serious forms of cold injury include *chilblains* and *chapped skin*.

cold remedies

Preparations used to relieve symptoms of colds (see *cold, common*). The main ingredient of cold remedies is usually a mild *analgesic drug*, such as *paracetamol* or *aspirin*, which helps to relieve aches and pains. Other common ingredients include *antihistamine drugs* and *decongestant drugs*, designed to reduce nasal congestion; *caffeine*, which acts as a mild stimulant; and *vitamin C*.

cold sore

A small skin blister, usually around the mouth, commonly caused by a strain of the *herpes simplex* virus called HSV1 (herpes simplex virus type 1).

CAUSES AND SYMPTOMS

The first attack of the virus often occurs in childhood and may be symptomless or may cause a flulike illness with painful mouth and lip ulcers, called *gingivostomatitis*. The virus then lies dormant within nerve cells, but may occasionally be reactivated and cause cold sores.

Reactivation of the virus may occur after exposure to hot sunshine or a cold wind, during a common cold or other infection, or in women around the time of their *menstrual periods*. Prolonged attacks may occur in people whose immunity to infection has been reduced due to illness or treatment with *immunosuppressant drugs*.

In many cases, an outbreak of cold sores is preceded by tingling in the lips, followed by the formation of small blisters that enlarge, causing itching and soreness. Within a few days the blisters burst and become encrusted. Most disappear within a week.

TREATMENT

The antiviral drug *aciclovir*, applied as a cream, may prevent cold sores if used at the first sign of tingling. Using sunscreen may reduce the likelihood of recurrence.

colecalciferol

An alternative name for vitamin D₃ (see *vitamin D*).

colectomy

The surgical removal of part or all of the *colon* (the major part of the large intestine, which produces faeces).

WHY IT IS DONE

Partial colectomy is usually carried out to remove damaged or distorted sections of colon. It may be performed to treat severe cases of *diverticular disease* (in which abnormal pouches form in the colon wall); to cut out a cancerous tumour (see *colon, cancer of*); or to remove a narrowed part of the intestine that is causing a blockage to the passage of faeces.

Total colectomy is performed to treat severe cases of *ulcerative colitis*, when the condition cannot be controlled by drugs. It may also be performed on individuals with familial polyposis (see *polyposis, familial*), an inherited condition in which large numbers of growths develop in the colon.

HOW IT IS DONE

In a partial colectomy, the diseased section of the colon is removed, and the ends of the severed colon are joined. A temporary *colostomy* (which allows the discharge of faeces from the large intestine through an artificial opening in the abdominal wall) may be needed until the rejoined colon has healed.

In a total colectomy, the whole of the large intestine is removed, either with or without the *rectum*. If the rectum is removed, an *ileostomy* (similar to a colostomy, but using the small intestine) may be performed.

RECOVERY

The colon usually functions normally after a partial colectomy. However, after a total colectomy the large intestine's ability to absorb water from faeces is reduced, which can result in diarrhoea, and *antidiarrhoeal drugs* may therefore be required.

colestyramine

A *lipid-lowering drug* used to treat some types of *hyperlipidaemia* (high levels of fats in the blood). Colestyramine is also used to treat diarrhoea in disorders such as *Crohn's disease*.

colic

A term that means "pertaining to the colon". The term "colic" also refers to a severe, spasmodic form of abdominal pain that occurs in waves of increasing intensity. (See also *biliary colic*; *colic, infantile*; *colic, uterine*; *renal colic*.)

colic, biliary

See *biliary colic*.

colic, infantile

Episodes of irritability and excessive crying in otherwise healthy infants. The condition is thought to be due to muscle spasms in the intestines.

A baby that suffers an attack of colic cries or screams incessantly, draws up his or her legs towards the stomach, and may become red in the face and possibly also pass wind. The baby will not respond to normal methods of comforting, such as feeding or cuddling. Colic often tends to be worse in the evenings; the symptoms may also be made worse by tiredness or stress.

Colic can be very distressing, but it is harmless. Usually, The condition first appears at the age of three to four weeks, and it clears up without treatment by about the age of 12 weeks. Carers should seek medical help, however, if additional symptoms, such as fever, develop, or if they are finding it difficult to cope with the baby.

colic, renal

See *renal colic*.

colic, uterine

Cramping abdominal pains that are usually associated with menstruation. (See also *dysmenorrhoea*.)

coliform bacteria

A group of rod-shaped *bacteria* that inhabit the intestine. Coliform bacteria include ESCHERICHIA and other genera that are sometimes associated with gastrointestinal illnesses.

colistin

One of the *polymyxin* group of *antibiotic drugs*. Colistin is used in *topical* preparations for eye and skin conditions. It may also be given orally to destroy bacteria in the large intestine, in people who are particularly susceptible to infection. In addition, colistin may be used in a *nebulizer* in order to treat lung infections. The drug is used only to treat infections that are resistant to other antibiotic drugs because it is toxic and may cause damage to kidney and nerve tissue.

colitis

Inflammation of the *colon*. Colitis causes diarrhoea, usually containing blood and mucus. Other symptoms may include abdominal pain and fever.

CAUSES

Colitis is a feature of the inflammatory bowel disorders *ulcerative colitis* and *Crohn's disease*. It may also be associated with other conditions that cause inflammation in the colon or rectum, such as *diverticular disease* or *proctitis*, or with cancer (see *colon, cancer of*). In addition, it may result from infection with various types of microorganism, such as *campylobacter* and *shigella* bacteria, viruses, or *amoebae*. One form of colitis may be provoked by *antibiotic drugs*; the drugs destroy bacteria that normally live in the intestine and allow CLOSTRIDIUM DIFFICILE, a bacterium that causes irritation, to proliferate.

DIAGNOSIS

Investigations into colitis may include examination of a sample of faeces for microorganisms or for obvious or hidden blood (see *faecal occult blood test*); *sigmoidoscopy* or *colonoscopy* (viewing of the inside of the colon); *biopsy* (tissue sampling) of the inflamed areas or ulcers; and a barium enema (see *barium X-ray examinations*).

TREATMENT

If the cause is an infection, antibiotics may be needed. Crohn's disease and ulcerative colitis are treated with *corticosteroid* and *immunosuppressant drugs*, together with a special diet. In some cases, surgery may be required.

collagen

A tough, fibrous *protein*. Collagen is the body's major structural protein, forming an important part of *tendons*, *bones*, and *connective tissue*.

collagen diseases

See *connective tissue disease*s.

collapse

A nonmedical term for a state of prostration or extreme exhaustion. It may also be used to describe a fainting fit or loss of consciousness. The medical term *circulatory collapse* refers to a life-threatening condition in which the blood no longer circulates effectively.

collarbone

The common name for the *clavicle*.

collar, orthopaedic

A soft foam or stiffened device that is worn around the neck to relieve pain or give additional support.

Colles' fracture

A break in the *radius* (one of the bones of the forearm) just above the wrist, in which the wrist and hand are displaced backwards, restricting movement and causing swelling and severe pain. The fracture is usually the result of putting out a hand to lessen the impact of a fall. It is more common in elderly people, due to weakening of the bones by aging or *osteoporosis*.

The broken bones are manipulated back into place and set in a *cast*. Healing of the bones takes up to six weeks. Hand and wrist movements usually return to normal, but there may be minor wrist deformity.

Collet–Sicard syndrome

A condition resulting from damage to the *cranial nerves* that control muscles in the tongue and throat. It is usually due to a *head injury* or to compression of the nerves by a tumour. The syndrome causes paralysis of muscles in the tongue, palate, throat, larynx (voicebox), and neck on one side. There is no cure, but the cause is treated if possible.

collodion

A syrupy mixture of *ether*, *alcohol*, and pyroxylin used in skin preparations for minor cuts and abrasions. Collodion acts by evaporating rapidly to leave a protective film over the area.

colloid

A form of fluid that is similar to a suspension (a fluid consisting of insoluble particles of a substance suspended in a liquid). Particles in a suspension are large and heavy enough to be separated from the liquid in a *centrifuge*. A colloid has smaller, lighter particles that can only be separated out of the liquid by spinning at a very high speed. In medicine, *plasma proteins* are separated from blood and sometimes used in colloid preparations to treat *shock*. The term "colloid" also refers to a material that contains protein and is found in the *thyroid gland*.

coloboma

A rare *birth defect* in which a gap exists in the tissues of the eye. The gap may be in the eyelid or in part of the eyeball, such as the *iris*, *retina*, or *choroid*. A coloboma in the iris will be visible as a black notch, or as a gap stretching from the pupil to the edge of the iris.

The condition results from incomplete development of the eyes while the baby is still an *embryo*; this problem may, in turn, be linked to certain *chromosomal abnormalities*. Coloboma may range from minor to severe. In some cases, it may cause *blurred vision* or decreased *visual acuity*.

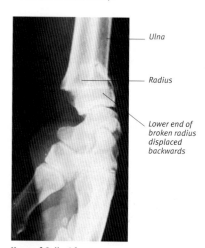

Ulna

Radius

Lower end of broken radius displaced backwards

X-ray of Colles' fracture
This X-ray clearly shows that the lower end of the broken radius has been pushed back. This gives a classic "dinner fork" appearance when the wrist is viewed from the side.

colon

The major part of the large *intestine*.

STRUCTURE

The colon is a segmented tube, about 1.3 m long and 6.5 cm wide, that forms a large loop in the abdomen. It consists of four sections: the ascending, transverse, and descending colons, and the S-shaped sigmoid colon, which connects with the rectum.

The colon consists of four layers. It has a tough outer membrane that protects it from damage. The next layer comprises muscles that contract and relax rhythmically to move the intestinal contents along (see *peristalsis*). Inside the muscular layer is a submucous coat containing blood vessels and lymph vessels (see *lymphatic system*). The innermost layer produces mucus, which helps to lubricate the passage of waste material.

FUNCTIONS

The main functions of the colon are to absorb water and mineral salts from food residue and to concentrate the remaining waste products. The material that remains after digestion enters the colon from the small intestine. As this substance passes through the colon, the water and salts contains are absorbed into blood vessels in the submucous coat. The waste material becomes increasingly concentrated and is finally expelled from the rectum as *faeces*. (See also *digestive system*; *intestine, disorders of*.)

colon, cancer of

A *malignant* tumour of the *colon* (the major part of the large intestine). Cancers of the colon or of the rectum (the lower part of the colon), which are generally referred to as colorectal cancer, are among the most common forms of cancer. They most often occur in people over the age of 60.

CAUSES

A genetic basis has been found for some types of colon cancer. Up to one in three cases are associated with a family history of colon disease. In particular, an inherited disorder called familial adenomatous *polyposis* (in which large numbers of polyps develop in the colon) greatly increases the risk. In the majority of cases, however, the precise cause is not known. Contributory factors include diet: eating a lot of meat and fatty foods and not enough fibre may increase the risk. The disease also sometimes occurs in association with *ulcerative colitis* and *Crohn's disease*.

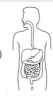

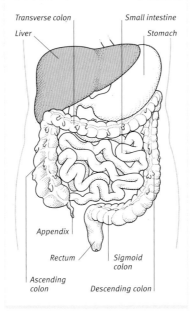

Transverse colon

Small intestine

Liver

Stomach

Appendix

Rectum

Sigmoid colon

Ascending colon

Descending colon

SYMPTOMS

The first symptoms of colon cancer include an inexplicable change in bowel movements (either constipation or diarrhoea), blood mixed in with the faeces, and pain in the lower abdomen. Sometimes, however, there are no symptoms until the tumour has grown large enough to cause an obstruction in the intestine (see *intestine, obstruction of*) or perforate it (see *perforation*).

DIAGNOSIS, TREATMENT, AND SCREENING

A preliminary diagnosis is made on the basis of the symptoms, physical examination (possibly including a *rectal examination*), and testing a sample of faeces for blood (see *faecal occult blood test*). If these indicate cancer is a possibility, further tests may be performed. These additional tests may include *sigmoidoscopy* or *colonoscopy* to view the inside of the colon, biopsy (removal of a tissue sample for analysis), barium enema (see *barium X-ray examinations*), and *CT scanning* or *MRI*.

In most cases, treatment of colon cancer is with a partial *colectomy*. In this procedure, the diseased area of colon is removed, together with a surrounding area of healthy tissue, and the cut ends of the colon are rejoined. Surgery may be combined with *radiotherapy* or *chemotherapy*. The outlook depends on how far the cancer has spread, but colon cancer that is treated in its early stages can be cured.

Regular screening using the faecal occult blood test (FOBT) and colonoscopy is offered to those at high risk of colon cancer, and a general screening programme (using FOBT) for those aged 60 to 69 is being phased in.

colon, disorders of

See *intestine, disorders of*.

colon, irritable

See *irritable bowel syndrome*.

colonization

The multiplication of foreign organisms, such as *bacteria*, in a host body. (This process is not necessarily harmful.) The term "colonization" is also used to refer to the development of *cancer* cells in an area to which they have spread that is separate from the primary tumour.

colonoscopy

The viewing of the inside of the *colon* using a flexible endoscope (fibre-optic instrument) known as a colonoscope, which is introduced through the *anus* and guided along the colon. Colonoscopy is used to investigate symptoms such as bleeding from the anus and to detect physical abnormalities such as inflammation (see *colitis*), growths (see *polyps*), and *cancer*. Instruments may be passed through the colonoscope to take *biopsy* specimens or remove polyps. (See also *endoscopy*.)

colon, spastic

See *irritable bowel syndrome*.

Colorado tick fever

A viral illness transmitted by the bites of infected ticks. It occurs in the mountain areas of the western United States, usually in early summer. Symptoms appear 3–6 days after a tick bite; they include flulike chills and fever, severe headache, nausea, and sometimes a red, raised rash. The illness usually lasts for a few days, subsides, then returns for a further few days. The virus can, however, remain in the blood for several months.

Treatment involves removal of the tick as soon as possible and taking *analgesic drugs* (painkillers) if necessary. Tick bites can be prevented by wearing clothing that covers the arms and legs and tucking trouser legs into socks. (See also *ticks and disease*.)

colorectal cancer

A general term referring to cancer of the colon (see *colon, cancer of*) and/or of the rectum (see *rectum, cancer of*).

colostomy

An operation in which part of the *colon* is brought to the surface of the skin through an incision in the abdominal wall. The exposed part is formed into a *stoma*, an artificial opening through which *faeces* are discharged into a bag attached to the skin. A colostomy may be either temporary or permanent.

A temporary colostomy may be performed at the same time as a partial *colectomy* (removal of part of the colon) to allow the remainder of the colon to heal without faeces passing through and contaminating it. The colostomy is closed when the rejoined colon has healed. A permanent colosto-my is needed if the rectum or anus has been removed (for example, to treat colon cancer) and normal defaecation is therefore impossible.

colostrum

A thick, yellowish fluid that is produced by the breasts during the first few days after childbirth, before being replaced by breast milk. Colostrum contains less fat and sugar, but more minerals and protein, than breast milk. It also has a high content of *lymphocytes* (white blood cells) and *immunoglobulins*, which help to protect the baby against infections.

colour blindness

See *colour vision deficiency*.

colour vision

The ability to see and distinguish the different parts of the colour spectrum, which consists of electromagnetic radiation (energy waves) with a range of wavelengths between about 400 and 700 nanometres (millionths of a millimetre). Different wavelengths trigger nerve signals in the *retina* (the light-sensitive layer of cells at the back of the eye); these signals pass to the brain and are interpreted as violet, indigo, blue, green, yellow, orange, and red.

RETINAL FUNCTION

As light falls on the retina, it strikes light-sensitive cells called rods and cones. The rods can detect all visible light, but only the cones can distinguish colour. There are three types of cone: red-sensitive, blue-sensitive, and green-sensitive. Each of these types of cone responds more strongly to a particular part of the light spectrum. The cones are most concentrated in a central area of the retina called the *fovea*; for this reason, colour vision is most accurate for objects that are viewed directly. Colour vision is, therefore, poor at the periphery of vision.

When light hits a cone, it causes a structural change in the pigment within the cone, which in turn causes the cone to emit an electrical signal. This signal passes to the brain via the *optic nerve*. Colour perception requires a minimum level of light; below this level, everything is perceived only by the rods and is seen as various shades of grey. (See also *colour vision deficiency*; *eye*; *perception*; *vision*.)

colour vision deficiency

Any abnormality in *colour vision* that causes a person to have difficulty in distinguishing between certain colours.

TYPES

The most common type of colour vision deficiency is the reduced ability to discriminate between red and green. Most cases of red–green colour vision deficiency are the result of defects in the light-sensitive cells in the *retina*. These defects are usually inherited, and tend to be sex-linked (see *genetic disorders*); the majority of sufferers are male, while females are unaffected, but they can pass on the disorder to their children. Occasionally, defects may be acquired as a result of diseases of the retina or the optic nerve, or they are caused by injury. There are two forms of red–green deficiency. A person with a severe green deficiency has difficulty in distinguishing between oranges, greens, browns, and pale reds. A severe red deficiency causes all shades of red to appear dull.

A much rarer colour vision deficiency exists in which blue cannot be distinguished. This condition may be inherited, or it may be due to degeneration of the retina or the optic nerve. Mono-

---

PROCEDURE FOR **COLOSTOMY**

An incision is made in the abdominal wall and part of the colon is pulled through. In a temporary colostomy, a small loop is exposed, and an opening is made in it large enough for faeces to pass through. If the rectum and anus have been removed, the cut end of the colon is brought to the skin surface. The edges of the opening or severed end are stitched to the skin at the edges of the abdominal incision to create a stoma (artificial opening) through which faeces will be expelled.

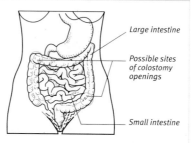

- Large intestine
- Possible sites of colostomy openings
- Small intestine

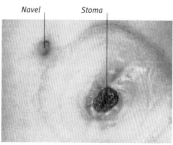

Position of the stoma
A colostomy bag is attached over the stoma to collect faeces. After a bowel movement, it is either replaced or emptied.

Navel   Stoma

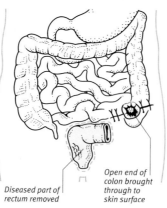

Diseased part of rectum removed

Open end of colon brought through to skin surface

Permanent colostomy

---

chromatism (the total absence of colour vision) also exists, but this deficiency is very rare.

colposcopy

Viewing of the *cervix* (the neck of the uterus) using a magnifying instrument called a colposcope. Colposcopy is carried out to detect areas of precancerous tissue (see *cervical intraepithelial neopla-*sia) or early cervical cancer (see *cervix, cancer of*). Removal of tissue samples (see *biopsy*) or treatment to remove any abnormal areas can be performed during colposcopy.

coma

A state of unconsciousness and unresponsiveness to external stimuli (for example, pinching) or internal stimuli (such as a full bladder). Coma results from disturbance or damage to areas of the *brain* involved in conscious activity or maintenance of consciousness – in particular, parts of the *cerebrum* and *brainstem*, and central regions of the brain, especially the *limbic system*.

Conditions that can produce coma include severe *head injury*; disorders such as *stroke* or *cardiac arrest*, in which

---

COLOUR VISION

Light, consisting of radiation of various wavelengths, is focused on the retina. At the back of the retina, light-sensitive rod and cone cells are stimulated to emit electrical impulses.

The impulses then travel through cells called bipolar cells to a layer called the ganglion cells, where some initial processing occurs, before passing to the brain via the optic nerve.

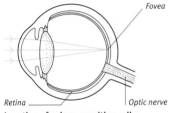

Location of colour-sensitive cells
The rods and cones are located at the back of the retina. Behind them is a darkly pigmented layer of cells, which reduces light scattering. Colour vision depends on the cones, which are concentrated in an area called the fovea.

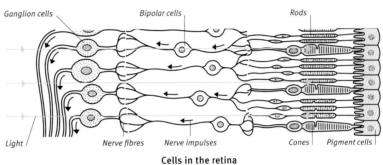

Cells in the retina

Key

– – – – Blue-sensitive cones
——— Green-sensitive cones
· · · · · Red-sensitive cones

Colour response of cones (right)
There are three classes of cone. One of these (red-sensitive) responds best to light of long wavelengths; another (blue-sensitive) to light of short wavelengths; and the third (green-sensitive) to intermediate wavelengths.

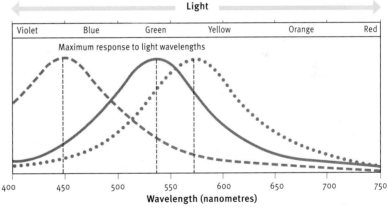

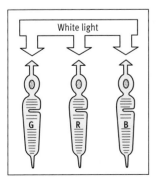

Response to white light
White light consists of a mixture of all wavelengths (colours), and it therefore stimulates all three classes of cone to signal equally. This pattern of response is interpreted as whiteness by the brain.

Key
G Green-sensitive
R Red-sensitive
B Blue-sensitive

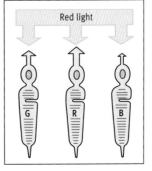

Response to red light
Light with a long wavelength (red light) produces a strong response from red-sensitive cones, a weak response from blue-sensitive cones, and an intermediate response from green-sensitive cones. This pattern of signalling is interpreted as the colour red by the brain.

part or all of the brain tissue is deprived of blood; or infectious disorders that affect the brain, such as *meningitis* and *encephalitis*. In addition, excessively high or low blood levels of certain substances may result in coma; for example, a person with *diabetes mellitus* may become comatose if his or her blood level of glucose (sugar) rises or falls to an abnormal degree.

SYMPTOMS

There are varying depths of coma. In less severe forms, the affected person may make small movements and respond to certain stimuli. In a deep coma, the person does not make any movements or respond to any stimulus. However, even people in deep comas may show some automatic responses, for example breathing unaided and blinking. If the lower brainstem is damaged, however, vital body functions are impaired, and artificial ventilation and maintenance of the circulation are necessary to keep the person alive.

OUTLOOK

If brain damage is minor and reversible, the person may make a full recovery, but deep coma due to severe trauma may result in long-term neurological problems such as muscle weakness or changes in behaviour.

A person in a deep coma (known as a *persistent vegetative state*) may be kept alive for years provided the brainstem is still functioning. Complete and irreversible loss of brainstem function leads to *brain death* (the permanent cessation of all brain functions).

combination drug

A preparation containing more than one active substance.

comedo

Another name for a *blackhead*.

commensal

A *bacterium* or other organism that normally lives in or on the body without either harming or benefiting its host.

comminuted fracture

A type of *fracture* in which the bone shatters into more than two pieces. A severe blow, such as an impact occurring in a car accident, may result in a comminuted fracture.

common cold

See *cold, common*.

communicable disease

Any disease due to a microorganism or parasite that can be transmitted from one person to another. (See also *contagious*; *infectious disease*.)

compartment syndrome

A painful *cramp* due to compression of a group of muscles within a confined space. It may occur when muscles are enlarged due to intensive sports training or to an injury such as *shin splints*. Cramps induced by exercise usually disappear when the exercise is stopped. Severe cases may require *fasciotomy* to improve blood flow and prevent development of a permanent *contracture*.

compensation

The adjustment made by an organ to make up for changes in body function or structure. An example of compensation is the increased size of one kidney when the other has been removed.

complement

A collection of *proteins* in the *plasma* (the fluid part of *blood*) that helps to destroy foreign cells and is an important part of the *immune system*.

complementary medicine

A group of therapies, often described as "alternative", that may be used to complement or act as an alternative to conventional medicine. Such treatments fall into three broad categories: touch and movement (as in *acupuncture*, *massage*, and *reflexology*); medicinal (as in *naturopathy*, *homeopathy*, and Chinese medicine); and psychological (as in *biofeedback*, *hypnotherapy*, and *meditation*).

complete heart block

See *heart block*.

complete miscarriage

The expulsion from the uterus of an embryo or a fetus together with its membranes and placenta (see *abortion*).

complex

A term used in medicine to mean a group or combination of related signs and symptoms that form a syndrome (as in *Eisenmenger complex*), or a collection of substances of similar structure or function (as in *vitamin B complex*). In psychology, a complex (for example, the *Oedipus complex*) denotes a group of unconscious ideas and memories that have emotional importance.

compliance

The degree to which patients follow medical advice.

complication

A condition resulting from a preceding disorder or from its treatment.

compos mentis

Latin for "of sound mind".

compound

A term used in chemistry to describe a substance that contains two or more chemically combined elements. In *pharmacy*, a compound is a preparation that contains a number of ingredients.

compound fracture

A type of *fracture*, also known as an open fracture, in which a broken bone breaks through the overlying skin. In this type of fracture, there is a high risk of infection.

compress

A pad of lint or linen applied, under pressure, to an area of skin. Cold compresses soaked in ice-cold water or wrapped around ice help to reduce pain, swelling, and bleeding under the skin after an injury (see *ice pack*). Hot compresses increase the circulation and help to bring *boils* to a head. A dry compress may be used to stop bleeding from a wound or may be coated with medication to help treat infection.

compression syndrome

A collection of localized neurological symptoms, such as numbness, tingling, discomfort, and muscle weakness, that is caused by pressure on a *nerve*.

compulsive behaviour

See *obsessive–compulsive disorder*.

computed tomography

Another name for *CT scanning*.

computer-aided diagnosis

The use of computer technology in certain diagnostic tests and procedures. It involves the use of probability-based computer systems to produce a list of the most likely diagnoses from a patient's symptoms and medical history. However, such technology is not currently in common use. Computers may also be programmed to interpret visual data, such as abnormal cells, and may be used to analyse samples from certain types of blood test and *cervical smear tests*. They are also used in imaging procedures such as *CT scanning* and *MRI*.

concealed haemorrhage

Internal loss of blood (see *bleeding*).

conception

The *fertilization* of a woman's *ovum* (egg) by a man's *sperm*, followed by implantation of the resulting *blastocyst* (the growing mass of fertilized cells) in the lining of the *uterus*. This process marks the beginning of *pregnancy*. (See also *contraception*; *infertility*.)

concussion

Brief *unconsciousness*, usually following a violent blow to the head. The loss of consciousness is due to a brief disturbance of the electrical activity in the brain. Common symptoms following concussion include confusion, inability to remember events that occurred just prior to the injury, dizziness, blurred vision, and vomiting.

Anyone who has been concussed, however briefly, should see a doctor as soon as possible. Persistent symptoms, or new ones such as drowsiness, difficulty in breathing, repeated vomiting, or visual disturbances, could signify brain damage or an *extradural haemorrhage*, and medical advice should be sought without delay. Repeated concussion can cause *punch-drunk* syndrome. (See also *head injury*.)

conditioning

The formation of a specific physical or behavioural response to a particular *stimulus* in the environment.

CLASSICAL CONDITIONING

In classical conditioning, a stimulus that consistently evokes a particular response is paired repeatedly with a second stimulus that would not normally produce the response. Eventually, the second stimulus begins to produce the response whether or not the first stimulus is present. This phenomenon was shown by the physiologist Ivan Pavlov. He observed that dogs salivated in anticipation of food (an unconditioned response to a stimulus). He then devised a procedure in which a bell was rung every time a dog was given food; once the procedure had been repeated several times, the dog began to salivate every time it heard the bell (a conditioned response to a stimulus) even if no food was presented.

OPERANT CONDITIONING

In operant conditioning, attempts are made to modify behaviour by rewarding or punishing a subject (animal or human) every time the subject shows a particular response to a specific stimulus. A response that is rewarded will be reinforced and will become more frequent, whereas a response that is punished will be inhibited and will become less frequent.

USE IN MEDICINE

Behavioural psychology (see *behaviour therapy*) is based on the idea that inappropriate behaviour patterns in some psychological disorders are learned through conditioning. It is thought that these patterns can be modified by the same process of conditioning.

condom

A barrier method of *contraception* in the form of a thin latex rubber or plastic sheath that is placed over a man's *penis* before sexual *intercourse*. Condoms also provide some protection against *sexually transmitted infections*.

condom, female

A barrier method of *contraception* in the form of a sheath that is inserted into a woman's *vagina* before sexual *intercourse*. Female condoms also offer some protection against *sexually transmitted infections*.

conduct disorders

Repetitive and persistent patterns of aggressive and/or antisocial behaviour, such as vandalism, substance abuse, and persistent lying, in children or adolescents. (See also *behavioural problems in children*; *adolescence*.)

conduction

The movement of particular forms of energy, such as nerve impulses and sound waves, through a system.

conductive deafness

Deafness caused by faulty *conduction* of sound from the outer to the inner *ear*. Causes include excess earwax or fluid in the middle ear (see *glue ear*).

conduit

A channel or tube that conveys fluid. Conduits may be created surgically to redirect the flow of body fluids. The most common form of artificially constructed conduit is an ileal conduit, which is created from part of the small intestine to divert urine out of the body when the bladder has had to be removed (see *cystectomy*).

condyle

A round projection on the end of a *bone* that fits into a hollow on another bone to form a joint; an example of a condyle is the elbow.

condyloma

A warty skin growth that usually occurring in moist areas of the body, for example the genitals. The most common type of condyloma is caused by the human papillomavirus (see *genital warts*). Condylomata are highly infectious flattened growths that may develop around the genitals in the secondary stage of *syphilis*.

condyloma acuminatum

See *warts, genital*.

cone

A type of light-sensitive cell located in the *retina* of the eye. Cones play a major role in *colour vision*.

cone biopsy

A surgical procedure, performed under local or general anaesthesia, in which a conical or cylindrical section of tissue from the lower part of the *cervix* (neck of the uterus) is removed. A cone biopsy is performed following an abnormal result of a *cervical smear test* if the extent of the precancerous or cancerous area (see *cervical intraepithelial neoplasia*) cannot be seen by *colposcopy* (inspection of the cervix with a viewing instrument). In some cases, a cone biopsy itself may be curative. (See also *cervix, cancer of*).

confabulation

The use of a fictional story to make up for gaps in memory. The phenomenon occurs most commonly in chronic alcoholics who suffer from *Wernicke–Korsakoff syndrome*. It may also occur in people with *head injuries*.

confidentiality

The ethical principle that a doctor does not disclose any information given in confidence by a patient, even after death of the patient.

The patient's *consent* is necessary before a doctor supplies confidential information to another party, such as an insurance company, an employer, or a

C

lawyer. Doctors must, however, disclose information about patients when required to do so by law, or when they are faced with injuries or disorders that indicate a serious crime. Doctors are also required to notify health authorities about patients with specified infectious diseases.

Treatment of young children is usually discussed with the parents, but an older child's request for confidentiality is generally respected if the doctor feels that he or she is competent enough to understand the issues involved.

confusion

An acute or chronic disorganized mental state in which thought, memory, and reasoning are impaired.

CAUSES AND SYMPTOMS

Acute confusion can arise as a symptom of *delirium*, in which brain activity is affected by fever, drugs, poisons, or injury. People with acute confusion may also have *hallucinations* and behave in a violent manner. Chronic confusion is often associated with *alcohol dependence*, the long-term use of *antianxiety drugs*, and certain physically based mental disorders. Many of the conditions that cause chronic confusion (for example, *dementia*) are progressive. Features of such conditions include absent-mindedness, poor short-term memory, and a tendency to be repetitive.

TREATMENT

If the underlying cause of confusion can be treated, there may be marked improvement. *Sedative drugs* can be of benefit in acute confusion.

congenital

A term meaning "present at birth". Congenital abnormalities (sometimes called *birth defects*) may be inherited. Alternatively, they may result from damage or infection occurring either in the *uterus* or at the time of birth.

congenital adrenal hyperplasia

See *adrenal hyperplasia, congenital*.

congenital amputation

See *amputation, congenital*.

congestion

A term that usually refers to the accumulation of excess *blood*, *tissue fluid*, or *lymph* in part of the body.

A major cause of congestion is an increased blood flow to an area due to inflammation. Another possible cause is

reduced drainage of blood from an affected area, as can occur in *heart failure*, in venous disorders such as *varicose veins*, and in *lymphatic disorders*. (See also *nasal congestion*.)

congestive heart failure

See *heart failure*.

conjoined twins

See *twins, conjoined*.

conjunctiva

The transparent membrane covering the *sclera* (white of the eye) and lining the inside of the eyelids. Cells in the conjunctiva produce a fluid that lubricates the lids and the *cornea*.

conjunctival haemorrhage

An alternative term for *subconjunctival haemorrhage* (bleeding in the white of the eye).

conjunctivitis

Inflammation of the *conjunctiva*, causing redness, discomfort, and discharge from the affected eye.

TYPES AND SYMPTOMS

There are two common types: infective conjunctivitis, caused by bacteria or viruses; and allergic conjunctivitis, an allergic response to substances such as cosmetics and pollen. Both types may have similar symptoms. In infective conjunctivitis, the discharge contains pus and may result in the eyelids being stuck together on waking in the morn-

LOCATION OF **CONJUNCTIVA**

This transparent membrane covers the sclera (white of the eye) and lines the inside of the eyelids.

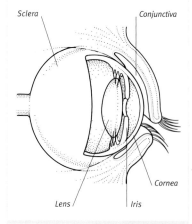

Sclera

Conjunctiva

Cornea

Lens

Iris

ings. In allergic conjunctivitis, the discharge is clear and the eyelids are often swollen and itchy.

Other, less common forms of conjunctivitis include neonatal *ophthalmia* (infective eye disease in newborns), *keratoconjunctivitis* (inflammation of the conjunctiva and cornea), and *trachoma* (a form of chlamydial infection).

TREATMENT

Bacterial infections may be treated with eyedrops or ointment containing an *antibiotic drug*. Viral conjunctivitis often disappears without the need for treatment. Allergic conjunctivitis may be treated with eyedrops that contain cromoglicate, an *antihistamine*, or a *corticosteroid drug*.

connective tissue

The material that supports, binds, or separates the various structures of the body. *Tendons* and *cartilage* are made up of connective tissue. This type of tissue also forms the matrix (basic substance) of *bone* and the nonmuscular structures of *arteries* and *veins*.

connective tissue diseases

Certain *autoimmune disorders* (disorders in which the immune system attacks the body's own tissues) that often affect blood vessels and produce secondary damage to *connective tissue*. Connective tissue diseases include *rheumatoid arthritis*, *polyarteritis nodosa*, systemic *lupus erythematosus*, *systemic sclerosis*, and *dermatomyositis*.

Conn's syndrome

A disorder caused by the secretion of excessive amounts of the hormone *aldosterone*. The overproduction of this hormone is caused by a noncancerous tumour of one of the *adrenal glands*. (See also *aldosteronism*.)

consciousness

A state of alertness in which a person is fully aware of his or her thoughts, surroundings, and intentions.

consent

Also sometimes referred to as informed consent, the legal term describing a patient's agreement to a doctor performing an operation, arranging drug treatment, or carrying out a diagnostic test. The patient's consent is also needed before a doctor supplies confidential information to another party, such as an insurance company, an employer, or a lawyer. Consent is valid only if the patient has been fully informed about the purpose of that particular procedure, the likely outcome, and any complications and side effects. In addition, valid consent can only be given by people (of any age) who are legally competent – that is, able to understand the particular medical issues involved and any advice given by a health professional. For people who are not legally competent, a relative may give or withhold consent on their behalf. (See also *confidentiality*.)

constipation

The infrequent or difficult passing of hard, dry *faeces*. Constipation may be uncomfortable but in the short term is usually harmless.

CAUSES
The most common cause of constipation is insufficient fibre in the diet (see *fibre, dietary*), because fibre assists the propulsion of waste matter through the *colon*. Other common causes include lack of regular bowel movements due to poor toilet-training in childhood or repeatedly ignoring the urge to move the bowels. Constipation in elderly people may be due to immobility or to weakness of the muscles of the abdomen and the pelvic floor.

Occasionally, constipation is a symptom of an underlying disorder. This is especially likely if it is part of a persistent change in bowel habits in someone over the age of 40, or if it is accompanied by other symptoms such as blood in the faeces, pain on moving the bowels, or weight loss. Conditions that may cause constipation include *haemorrhoids*, *anal fissure*, *irritable bowel syndrome*, and narrowing of the colon due to disorders such as *diverticular disease* or cancer (see *colon, cancer of*).

TREATMENT
Self-help measures such as establishing a regular bowel routine, increasing the amount of fibre in the diet, and drinking more fluids are usually beneficial. Prolonged use of *laxative drugs* should be avoided, because this can impair the normal functioning of the colon.

constriction

A narrowed area in the body, or the process of narrowing.

contact dermatitis, allergic

A type of *dermatitis* caused by an allergic skin reaction to a substance that is harmless for most people. Common causes include nickel and rubber. (See also *irritant dermatitis*.)

contact lenses

Thin, shell-like, transparent discs fitted over the *cornea* of the eye that are used to correct defective vision. Contact lenses are most commonly used for the correction of *myopia* (shortsightedness) and *hypermetropia* (longsightedness). In addition, noncorrective lenses are available for cosmetic use, for example to change eye colour.

TYPES
There are several types. Hard plastic lenses give good vision; they are also long-lasting and durable, inexpensive, and easy to maintain. Sometimes, however, these lenses are difficult for the wearers to tolerate and may fall out. Hard gas-permeable lenses are more comfortable because they allow oxygen to pass through to the eye, but are less durable. Soft lenses are the most comfortable because of their high water content. Disposable soft lenses are for single use only; extended-wear lenses are worn for up to a month.

Other types of contact lenses include rigid scleral lenses, which cover the whole of the front of the eye and are used to disguise disfigurement; bifocal contact lenses; and toric contact lenses, which have an uneven surface curvature and can correct *astigmatism*.

PROBLEMS
Hard plastic lenses may cause abrasion of the cornea if they are worn for too long. People who wear soft lenses sometimes develop sensitivity of the eyes and eyelids. Any type of contact lens may cause redness of the eye. The most serious complication of using contact lenses is infection of the eye, which can occasionally cause permanent damage to the cornea and affect vision; meticulous hygiene lowers the risk. (See also the illustrated box *Care and insertion of contact lenses*, overleaf.)

contact tracing

A service provided by clinics treating *sexually transmitted infections*, in which all contacts of a person diagnosed as having a sexually transmitted infection are traced and then encouraged to be examined and treated to help prevent the spread of infection. Contact tracing is also used in cases of other infections, especially *tuberculosis*, *meningitis*, and imported *tropical diseases*.

contagious

A term used to describe a disease that can be transferred from person to person by ordinary social contact. All contagious diseases, such as the common cold or chickenpox, are *infectious*. The term "contagious" does not apply to the many *infectious diseases*, such as typhoid, syphilis, or AIDS, which are spread by other means.

continuous positive airway pressure (CPAP)

A method of *ventilation* (mechanically assisted breathing) in which the air pressure inside a patient's airways is kept above atmospheric pressure.

continuous positive pressure ventilation (CPPV)

A rarely used method of *ventilation* (mechanically assisted breathing) in which positive pressure is applied to the airways to produce each inhalation.

contraception

The control of fertility to prevent *pregnancy*. Contraception can be achieved by a variety of methods. Some forms prevent *ovulation* in the woman; others stop *sperm* from meeting an *ovum* in the *fallopian tube* (preventing *fertilization*), or prevent a fertilized ovum from implanting in the *uterus*.

Some contraceptive methods involve changes in sexual activity; such methods include total or periodic abstinence from intercourse (see *contraception, natural methods of*) and *coitus interruptus*, in which sexual intercourse is stopped before ejaculation occurs. Other methods, known as barrier methods (see *contraception, barrier methods of*), involve the use of condoms to prevent sperm from coming into contact with eggs. Hormonal methods, including the use of *oral contraceptives*, implants, and injections (see *contraceptives, injectable*), prevent conception by altering the hormone balance in a woman's body. Further forms of contraception include the use of intrauterine devices (see *IUDs*); postcoital methods (see *contraception, emergency*); or sterilization of the male (see *vasectomy*) or female (see *sterilization, female*).

contraception, barrier methods of

The use of a device and/or a chemical that will physically stop *sperm* from reaching an *ovum*, thus preventing *fertilization* and pregnancy. Barrier methods

C

CARE AND INSERTION OF **CONTACT LENSES**

The care of hard contact lenses may require the use of several chemical solutions. A cleaning solution is used to remove deposits of mucus and protein from the lenses. A wetting solution is used before inserting a lens in the eye. A further solution may also be used for storage; if used, a storage solution must be washed off before a contact lens is inserted.

Soft contact lenses absorb any chemicals with which they come into contact, so the solutions used must be weaker. Disinfection with a chemical or heating system is needed to prevent contamination and eye infection. Two or three solutions may be necessary, but intermittent cleaning with a third system, such as an enzyme tablet or an oxidizing agent, may also be required.

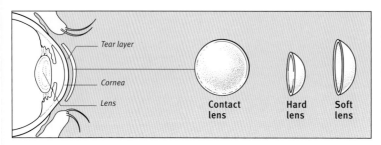

Tear layer

Cornea

Lens

Contact lens

Hard lens

Soft lens

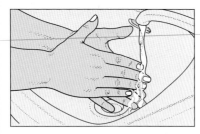

1 Before touching lenses, wash your hands thoroughly under running water and take care to rinse off all traces of soap. Remove the lens from its container; for a hard lens, you may prefer to do this with a rubber sucker. Rinse the lens thoroughly in the wetting solution. Do not use tapwater.

Inverted lens

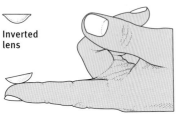

2 Place the contact lens on the tip of your index finger. If it is a soft lens, make sure that it has not turned inside out. If it has, you will see an out-turned rim.

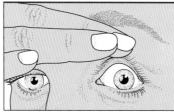

3 Keep both eyes open. Hold the upper lid of one eye open, and look straight ahead or at the lens as you bring it up to your eye.

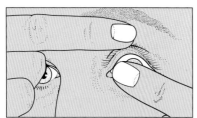

4 Place the contact lens on your eye, over the iris and pupil. Look downwards and then release the lid. If necessary, the lens may be centred by gently massaging the eyelid. The photograph on the right shows a hard lens correctly positioned.

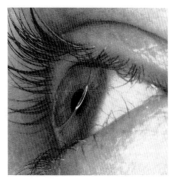

and *spermicides* (preparations that kill sperm), when used together correctly, can be highly effective in preventing conception. Barrier methods of contraception also help to prevent the sexual transmission of diseases such as *HIV*, genital herpes (see *herpes, genital*), and viral hepatitis (see *hepatitis, viral*).

The male *condom*, a latex sheath that covers the penis, is one of the most widely used barrier contraceptives. The female condom (see *condom, female*), which lines the vagina, is similar to the male condom but is larger.

Other barrier methods that are used by women include the diaphragm and the cap. The diaphragm (see *diaphragm, contraceptive*) is a hemispherical dome of thin rubber with a metal spring in the rim to hold it in place against the vaginal wall, blocking the entrance to the *cervix*. It is used with a spermicide. A cervical cap (see *cap, cervical*) is an alternative to the diaphragm.

Spermicides, in the form of aerosol foams, creams, gels, and pessaries, are placed in the vagina as close as possible to the cervix shortly before sexual intercourse. Although some condoms are precoated with spermicide, not all types of spermicide should be used with rubber barrier devices. (See also the illustrated box opposite.)

contraception, emergency

Measures to avoid *pregnancy* following unprotected *sexual intercourse*. There are two main methods: hormonal and physical. In the first, high-dose oral *progesterone* (the "morning after" pill) should be taken in a single dose, as soon as possible after unprotected sexual intercourse: preferably within 12 hours, but no later than 72 hours afterwards. In the physical method, an *IUD* is inserted by a doctor within five days of unprotected sex. Both methods are thought to work by preventing a fertilized egg from implanting in the uterus. (See also the illustrated box opposite.)

contraception, hormonal methods of

The use by women of synthetic *progestogen drugs*, often combined with synthetic *oestrogens*, to prevent conception. The combined pill (see *oral contraceptives*), the best-known form of hormonal contraception, contains both an oestrogen and a progestogen; it acts by suppressing *ovulation* (the release of an egg from an ovary). Progestogen

METHODS OF **CONTRACEPTION**

Forms of contraception include natural, barrier, hormonal, and postcoital methods. Most are for use by women. Another option is sterilization, surgery that disrupts part of the male or female reproductive system to render a person permanently infertile.

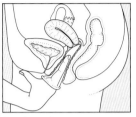

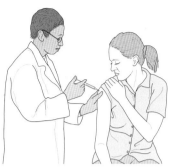

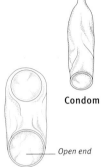

Condom

Female condom

Female condom
The female condom is placed in the vagina with the open end extending just beyond the vaginal opening.

Open end

Male condom
Condoms should be checked for holes and air squeezed from the tip to prevent bursting. They may be used with a spermicide. On withdrawal, the rim should be held to stop the condom slipping off.

Hormone injection
A progestogen is injected by a doctor or nurse into a muscle in the woman's arm or buttock. The hormone is released into her body over a period of 8 or 12 weeks, after which time the procedure is repeated.

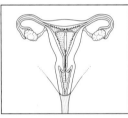

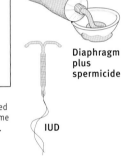

Diaphragm plus spermicide

IUD

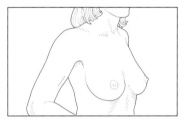

IUD in position
An IUD is a small piece of moulded plastic with strings attached. Some contain copper or a progestogen. The IUD is fitted in the uterus to stop fertilized eggs implanting.

Diaphragm in position
A diaphragm is a rubber dome held in place over the cervix by means of a coiled metal spring in its rim. It physically prevents sperm from reaching the cervix.

Hormonal implant
A flexible rod containing a progestogen hormone is inserted into the woman's arm, under the skin, where it releases progestogen into the blood.

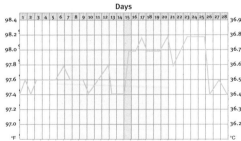

Days

	1	2	3	4	5	6	7	8	9	10	11	12	13	14	15	16	17	18	19	20	21	22	23	24	25	26	27	28	

98.4 — 36.9
98.2 — 36.8
98.0 — 36.7
97.8 — 36.6
97.6 — 36.5
97.4 — 36.4
97.2 — 36.3
97.0 — 36.2
°F — °C

Temperature method
This natural form of contraception involves charting a woman's temperature to see whether ovulation has taken place. The temperature should be taken at the same time each day, on waking. Ovulation precedes a temperature rise. A rise in temperature for three days means the end of the fertile time.

Minipill (progestogen-only pill; POP)

Pill

The pill
Contraceptive pills contain oestrogen to prevent ovulation, and/or a progestogen, which changes the cervical mucus to prevent sperm penetration, or alters the uterine lining to prevent implantation.

STERILIZATION

This procedure offers an almost completely safe and reliable form of birth control; it is usually irreversible. It does not affect sex hormones, so a man produces sperm-free semen and a woman produces normal eggs that do not reach the uterus.

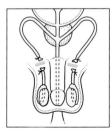

Male sterilization (vasectomy)
The vas deferens (tube from a testis to the urethra) on each side is cut so sperm cannot enter the urethra.

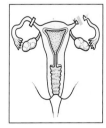

Female sterilization
A laparoscope (viewing tube) is inserted, under anaesthetic, through the abdominal wall. An instrument is passed through it to cut or seal the fallopian tubes.

C

drugs make cervical mucus thick and impenetrable to sperm. They also cause thinning of the *endometrium* (lining of the uterus), which reduces the chance of a fertilized egg implanting successfully. The progestogen *desogestrel* also inhibits ovulation, which makes it more relaible than other progestogen-only pills (POPs).Progestogens can be given as pills, as *contraceptive implants* under the skin, as patches, or by injection (see *contraceptives, injectable*), or they can be released into the uterus by some *IUDs*. (See also the illustrated box on the previous page.)

contraception, natural methods of

Methods of avoiding conception that do not involve the use of any contraceptive hormones or devices.These methods are based on attempts to pinpoint a woman's fertile period around the time of *ovulation*, so that sexual *intercourse* can be avoided at this time.

The *calendar method* is based on the assumption that ovulation takes place around 14 days before menstruation. Due to its high failure rate, it has been largely superseded by other methods.

The *temperature method* is based on the normal rise of a woman's body temperature in the second half of the menstrual cycle, after ovulation has occurred. The woman takes her temperature each day using an ovulation thermometer. Sex is considered to be safe only after there has been a rise in temperature lasting at least three days.

The *cervical mucus method* involves attempting to pinpoint the fertile period by charting the appearance and amount of cervical mucus during the menstrual cycle. Certain recognized changes in the mucus occur before and often at ovulation. The *symptothermal method* is a combination of the temperature and mucus methods. Fertility devices are also available that work by measuring hormone levels in the urine to predict fertile days. (See also the illustrated box on the previous page.)

contraception, postcoital

See *contraception, emergency*.

contraception, withdrawal method of

See *coitus interruptus*.

contraceptive

Any agent that reduces the likelihood of *conception*. (See also *contraception*.)

contraceptive implant

A hormonal method of *contraception* in which a long-acting *progestogen drug* is inserted under the skin inside the upper arm. An implant consists of a small, flexible rod that steadily releases the drug into the bloodstream. It functions continually for several years.

contraceptives, injectable

A hormonal method of *contraception* in which long-acting *progestogen drugs* are injected every two to three months. Injectable contraceptives are a very effective form of contraception, but they may cause menstrual disturbances, weight gain, headaches, and nausea, especially in the first few months.

contractions, uterine

Rhythmic, squeezing muscular spasms that occur in the walls of the *uterus* before and during *childbirth* in order to expel the baby from the uterus. Regular contractions indicate the start of *labour* and increase in strength and frequency throughout the first stage. (See also *Braxton Hicks' contractions*.)

contracture

A deformity that is caused by shrinkage of tissue in an area of skin, muscle, or a tendon and that may restrict the movement of a joint. Skin contractures commonly occur as a result of scarring following extensive burns or other injuries. Other types of contracture are caused by inflammation and shrinkage of *connective tissues*; examples of these include *Dupuytren's contracture* and *Volkmann's contracture*.

contraindication

Factors in a patient's condition that would make it unwise to pursue a certain line of treatment.

contrast enema

A *contrast medium* (a substance that is opaque to X-rays) that is introduced into the large intestine through the anus and which enables the colon and rectum to be seen in outline on an X-ray. (See also *barium X-ray examinations*.)

contrast medium

A substance that is opaque to *X-rays* and is introduced into hollow or fluid-filled parts of the body to render them visible on X-ray film. Barium is one of the most commonly used contrast media (see *barium X-ray examinations*).

controlled drug

One of a number of drugs that are subject to restricted use because of their potential for abuse. Controlled drugs include opiates such as *cocaine* and *morphine*, *amphetamine drugs*, and *barbiturate drugs*.

controlled trial

A scientific method of testing the effectiveness of new treatments or comparing different treatments.

In a typical controlled drug trial, two comparable groups of patients with the same illness are given courses of apparently identical treatment. Only one group, however, actually receives the new treatment; the second group (the control group) is given a *placebo* (a harmless substance containing no active ingredients). Alternatively, the control group may be given an established drug that is known to be effective. After a predetermined period, the two groups are assessed. If the patients on the new treatment show a greater improvement than those on the placebo (or those on an existing treatment), this result proves that the drug has a beneficial effect.

Controlled trials must be conducted "blind" (meaning that the patients do not know which treatment they are receiving). In a "double-blind" trial, neither the patients nor the doctors who assess them know who is receiving which treatment.

contusion

Bruising to the skin and underlying tissues from a "blunt" injury such as an abrasion (graze) or an impact.

convergent squint

A type of *squint* in which the abnormal eye is directed too far inwards towards the other eye.

conversion disorder

A psychological disorder, formerly called hysteria, in which repressed emotions appear to be unconsciously converted into physical symptoms such as blindness, loss of speech, or paralysis. Conversion disorder is generally treated by *psychotherapy*.

convulsion

See *seizure*.

convulsion, febrile

Twitching or jerking of the limbs with loss of consciousness that occurs in a child after a rapid rise in body temperature. Febrile convulsions are common and usually affect children between the ages of six months and five years.

CAUSES

The convulsions are due to immaturity of the temperature-lowering mechanism in the brain; the mechanism allows the child's body temperature to rise too rapidly in response to infections such as *measles* or *influenza*.

TREATMENT AND PREVENTION

Treatment includes making sure the child cannot injure him- or herself during the seizure by placing padding (such as pillows or towels) around the child; however, do not try to hold the child down. Loosen any clothing around the child's neck, and remove anything from the child's mouth that may interfere with breathing (such as food or vomit) but do not put anything into the child's mouth. Stay with the child during the seizure and when it has stopped, place him or her in the *recovery position*, which will keep the airway open and prevent inhalation of vomit. You should also seek immediate medical help. Seizures can often be prevented in susceptible children by giving *paracetamol* or *ibuprofen* at the first signs of fever.

OUTLOOK

Most children who have one or more febrile convulsions suffer no long-term effects. However, there is a very small risk of developing *epilepsy*, which is increased in children who have a pre-existing abnormality of the brain or nervous system, or children with a family history of epilepsy.

Cooley's anaemia

See *thalassaemia*.

COPD

The abbreviation for chronic obstructive pulmonary disease (see *pulmonary disease, chronic obstructive*).

copper

A metallic element that is an essential part of several *enzymes* (substances that regulate chemical reactions in the body). Copper is required by the body in only minute amounts (see *trace elements*). An excess in the body may occur as a result of the rare inherited disorder *Wilson's disease*.

cordotomy

A surgical procedure in which certain bundles of nerve fibres within the *spinal cord* are severed. Cordotomy is carried out to relieve persistent, severe pain that has not responded to other treatment. It is most frequently performed to treat pain in the lower trunk and legs, especially in people who have cancer.

cord, spermatic

See *spermatic cord*.

cord, testicular

See *spermatic cord*.

cord, umbilical

See *umbilical cord*.

cord, vocal

See *vocal cords*.

corn

A small area of thickened skin on a toe or other part of the foot. A corn is caused by the pressure of a tight-fitting shoe. The dead skin cells form a hard plug that extends down into the skin tissues. Pressure on this plug can cause pain. If a corn is painful, a spongy ring or corn pad can be placed over it to relieve the pressure. If the corn persists, the area of thickened skin can be removed by a chiropodist.

cornea

The transparent, thin-walled surface that forms the front of the eyeball. The cornea has two main functions. It helps to focus light rays on to the *retina* at the back of the eye, and protects the front of the eye from debris and injury.

The cornea is joined at its circumference to the *sclera* (white of the eye); the black *pupil* and the coloured *iris* are visible beneath it. There are three main

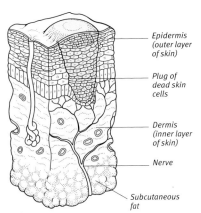

Cross-section of a corn
A plug of dead skin cells extends through the epidermis into the dermis, which has a nerve supply. Pressure on the plug can cause pain.

layers. The outermost layer (the epithelium) protects the eye and absorbs oxygen and nutrients from tears. The central layer (the stroma) is by far the thickest and gives the cornea its form. The inner layer (the endothelium) expels excess fluid from the cornea, thus keeping the tissues transparent.

For the cornea to stay healthy, it must be kept moist and clean. It is kept moist by a film of *tears*, which are produced by the *lacrimal gland* and by the mucus- and fluid-secreting cells in the eyelids and *conjunctiva*. Further protection is provided by the eyelids, which blink or close to keep out debris. In addition, the cornea is very sensitive, and immediately registers the presence of any injury or foreign body.

corneal abrasion

A scratch or defect in the *epithelium* (outer layer) of the *cornea* caused by a small, sharp particle in the eye (see *eye, foreign body in*) or by an injury. Corneal abrasions usually heal quickly but may cause severe pain and *photophobia*.

Treatment of a corneal abrasion includes covering the eye with a patch and *analgesics* to relieve pain. If the ciliary muscles go into spasm, eyedrops containing cycloplegic drugs may be used to paralyse the ciliary muscle. *Antibiotic* eyedrops are usually given to prevent bacterial infection (which can lead to a *corneal ulcer*).

corneal graft

The surgical transplantation of donor corneal tissue to replace a damaged *cornea*. In most grafts, tissue is taken from a human *donor* after death. The success rate of corneal grafts is generally high, because the cornea has no blood vessels; this reduces access for white blood cells, which could otherwise cause *rejection* of the donor tissue.

corneal transplant

See *corneal graft*.

corneal ulcer

A break, erosion, or open sore in the *cornea*. It usually affects the outer layer of the cornea, but in some cases may penetrate down to the middle layer.

Corneal ulcers are commonly caused by a *corneal abrasion*. They may also be due to chemical damage, or infection with *bacteria*, *fungi*, or *viruses* (particularly *herpes virus*). Eye conditions such as *keratoconjunctivitis sicca* and eyelid

LOCATION OF **CORNEA**

The cornea is a transparent, thin-walled dome forming the front of the eyeball, over the iris. It consists of five layers of differing thickness.

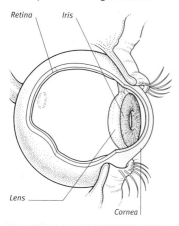

Retina
Iris
Lens
Cornea

deformities such as *entropion* or *ectropion* increase the risk of a corneal ulcer.

Ulcers are revealed by introducing *fluorescein* dye into the eye. Infections and predisposing eye conditions are treated according to their cause. A superficial, noninfectious ulcer usually heals quickly; if it fails to do so, it may be treated with a "bandage" contact lens or with *tarsorrhaphy* (temporary sealing of the eyelids).

coronary

Any structure that encircles another like a crown. The term is usually used to refer to the *coronary arteries*, which surround the heart and supply it with blood It is also sometimes used as a nonmedical term for a heart attack (see *myocardial infarction*).

coronary artery

Either of the two main *arteries* that supply the heart tissues with oxygen-rich blood. These vessels, known as the left and right main coronary arteries, arise directly from the *aorta* (the main artery in the body). The term "coronary artery" is also applied to any of the arteries that branch off from the main coronary arteries, such as the left circumflex artery and the left anterior descending artery. Blockage of a coronary artery as a result of *atherosclerosis* (an accumulation of fatty deposits in the artery) can lead to *myocardial infarction*. (See also *coronary artery disease*.)

coronary artery bypass

A major heart operation that is carried out in order to bypass *coronary arteries* that have become narrowed or blocked (usually as a result of *atherosclerosis*). The procedure involves using healthy blood vessels (such as a mammary artery from the chest or a vein from the leg) to improve blood flow to the heart muscle. A coronary artery bypass is performed if symptoms of coronary artery disease have not been relieved by drugs, or if balloon *angioplasty* (a surgical procedure used to widen blocked arteries) and insertion of a *stent* (rigid tube) is inappropriate or has failed.

Before surgery, sites of blockage are identified using an imaging procedure called *angiography*. Usually, a *heart–lung machine* is needed to maintain the circulation during the operation, although sometimes *minimally invasive surgery* may be used to bypass the artery, thereby avoiding the need to stop the heart.

The long-term outlook is good following a coronary artery bypass. However, the grafted vessels may also eventually become blocked by atherosclerosis. (See also *Coronary artery bypass* box, opposite.)

DISORDERS OF THE **CORNEA**

Various injuries or conditions can affect the sensitive cornea.

Injury

A *corneal abrasion* (scratch) can become infected and progress to a *corneal ulcer*. Penetrating corneal injuries can cause scarring, which may lead to impairment of vision. Chemical injuries can result from contact with a corrosive substance such as an acid or alkali.

In *actinic keratopathy*, the outer layer of the cornea is damaged by ultraviolet light. In exposure keratopathy, damage occurs as a result of reduced protection from the tear film and blink reflex.

Infection

The cornea can be infected by viruses, bacteria, or fungi. Some infections can cause ulceration, the *herpes simplex* virus being especially dangerous.

Inflammation

True inflammation of the cornea (called *keratitis*) is uncommon because the cornea contains no blood vessels.

coronary artery disease

Narrowing of the coronary arteries, which supply blood to the heart, leading to damage or malfunction of the heart. The most common heart disorders due to coronary artery disease are *angina pectoris* (chest pain due to insufficient oxygen reaching the heart) and *myocardial infarction* (heart attack).

CAUSES

The usual cause is *atherosclerosis*, in which fatty plaques develop on artery linings. An affected vessel can become totally blocked if a blood clot forms or lodges in the narrowed area.

Atherosclerosis has many interrelated causes, including smoking, a high-fat diet, lack of exercise, being overweight, and raised blood cholesterol levels. Other risk factors include a genetic predisposition and diseases such as *diabetes mellitus* and *hypertension*.

SYMPTOMS

In its early stages, coronary artery disease often produces no symptoms. The first sign is frequently the chest pain of angina, or an actual heart attack.

Coronary artery disease may also cause arrhythmias (abnormalities in the heartbeat); in severe cases, arrhythmia

Congenital defects

Rare congenital defects include microcornea (a cornea that is smaller than normal) or megalocornea (one that is bigger than normal) and *buphthalmos*, or "ox-eye", in which the entire eyeball is distended as a result of *glaucoma* (raised fluid pressure in the eyeball).

Degeneration

Degenerative conditions of the cornea include calcium deposition, thinning, and spontaneous ulceration. Such conditions occur mainly in elderly people, and are more common in previously damaged eyes.

Other disorders

Other disorders include: *keratomalacia*, which may result from vitamin A deficiency; *keratoconjunctivitis sicca* (dry eye); corneal dystrophies, such as *keratoconus*, in which the cornea becomes thinner and cone-shaped; and oedema, in which fluid builds up inside the cornea and impairs vision.

CORONARY ARTERY BYPASS

This procedure is now the most common and successful major heart operation in the Western world. Each year some 20,000 people in the UK undergo the operation, which can relieve them from dependence on drug treatment for heart disease and restore them to active life.

Site of incision

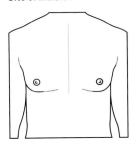

HOW IT IS DONE

Coronary artery bypass is a major procedure, requiring two surgeons and lasting up to five hours.

1 The first surgeon makes an incision down the centre of the patient's chest. The heart is then exposed by opening the pericardium.

2 Simultaneously, several incisions are made in the leg, and a length of vein removed.

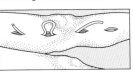

3 The heart is stopped and a heart-lung bypass machine takes over the task of pumping oxygenated blood through the body.

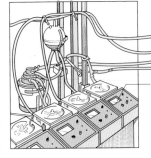

Heart-lung machine

4 The section of the vein taken from the leg is then sewn to the aorta and to a point below the blockage. If several arteries are blocked, they can be bypassed by using other sections from the same leg vein, or an arterial graft may be taken from the chest.

5 The heart-lung machine is disconnected and the patient's heart is restarted by giving it an electric shock.

WHY IT IS DONE

Narrowed coronary arteries cannot supply the heart muscle with sufficient blood, and, as a result, it becomes starved of oxygen. This may cause angina (chest pain) or damage to the heart tissue. By joining lengths of blood vessel (from a vein in the leg, as shown here, or the mammary artery in the chest) to the aorta and to a point below the blockages, the obstructed sections of coronary artery can be bypassed.

Before the operation

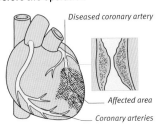

Diseased coronary artery

Affected area

Coronary arteries

After the operation

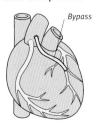

Bypass

First surgeon prepares heart for bypass

Anaesthetist

Second surgeon removes vein from leg

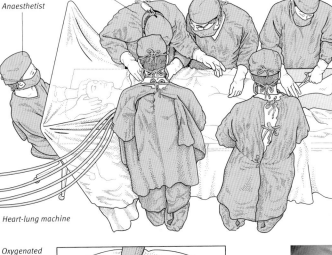

Oxygenated blood from heart-lung machine

Superior vena cava (tied off)

Deoxygenated blood to heart-lung machine

Inferior vena cava (tied off)

Pericardium

Aorta

Bypass

Wire suture

Coronary arteries

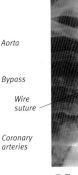

6 Finally, the breastbone is wired together, and the pericardium and chest are sewn up.

C

C

can cause *cardiac arrest* (in which the heart stops beating). In elderly people, it may lead to *heart failure*, in which the heart gradually becomes less and less efficient at pumping blood.

TREATMENT

Treatment of coronary artery disease is with drugs such as glyceryl trinitrate and other *nitrate drugs*, *beta-blockers*, *calcium channel blockers*, *potassium channel activators*, and *vasodilator drugs*. *Aspirin* to thin the blood and *statins* to lower the blood cholesterol level may be advised. Lifestyle changes, such as stopping smoking, eating a low-fat diet, and losing any excess weight, are also of vital importance.

If drug treatment fails to relieve the symptoms or if there is extensive narrowing of the coronary arteries, blood flow may be improved by balloon *angioplasty* and insertion of a *stent* or by *coronary artery bypass* surgery.

coronary care unit

A specialist ward for the care of acutely ill patients who may have suffered a *myocardial infarction* (heart attack) or another serious cardiovascular disorder.

coronary heart disease

An alternative name for *coronary artery disease*.

coronary thrombosis

A condition in which a *thrombus* (blood clot) narrows or blocks one of the *coronary arteries*, thereby preventing sufficient oxygen from reaching a section of the heart muscle. In most cases, the thrombus forms in a blood vessel that has already been narrowed by *atherosclerosis*. Sudden blockage of a coronary artery will cause a *myocardial infarction* (heart attack).

coroner

A public officer appointed to inquire into a cause of death when it is unknown or when unnatural causes are suspected.

cor pulmonale

Enlargement of, and strain upon, the right side of the *heart* that is caused by one of several chronic lung diseases. Damage to the lungs leads to *pulmonary hypertension* (abnormally high blood pressure in the arteries that supply the lungs). The resulting back pressure of blood puts strain on the heart, and may eventually cause right-sided *heart failure* with *oedema*.

corpus callosum

The band of nerve fibres that forms a connection between the two hemispheres of the *brain*.

corpus cavernosum

One of two cylindrical bodies of erectile tissue that is found in both the *clitoris* and the *penis*. The spongy structure of the corpus cavernosum allows the tissue to become rigid when it becomes filled with blood.

corpuscle

Any minute body or cell, particularly red and white blood cells or certain types of *nerve* ending.

corpus luteum

A small tissue mass in the *ovary* that develops from a ruptured egg *follicle* after *ovulation* (the release of an egg). The corpus luteum secretes the female sex hormone *progesterone*, which causes the endometrium (lining of the uterus) to thicken in preparation for implantation of a fertilized egg. If fertilization does not occur, the corpus luteum shrinks and dies.

corrosive oesophagitis

A type of *oesophagitis* that is caused by swallowing caustic chemicals.

corset

A device that is worn around the trunk to treat spinal injuries or deformities.

cortex

The outer layer of certain organs, such as the brain or kidneys.

corticosteroid drugs

COMMON DRUGS

- Beclometasone • Betamethasone
- Cortisone • Dexamethasone
- Fludrocortisone • Hydrocortisone
- Prednisolone • Triamcinolone

A group of drugs that are chemically similar to *corticosteroid hormones*, which are produced by the *adrenal glands*.

WHY THEY ARE USED

Corticosteroid drugs are used as hormone replacement therapy in *Addison's disease* and when the *adrenal glands* or *pituitary gland* have been destroyed by disease or have been removed. The drugs are also used to treat inflammatory intestinal disorders, such as *ulcerative colitis* and *Crohn's disease*, and as an urgent treatment for the inflammation in the artery supplying the retina that occurs in *temporal arteritis*.

Other uses of corticosteroid drugs include the treatment of *autoimmune diseases* such as systemic *lupus ery-*

HOW **CORTICOSTEROIDS** WORK

When given as hormone replacement therapy (such as in Addison's disease), corticosteroids supplement or replace natural hormones. Large doses have an anti-inflammatory effect (right) because they reduce the body's production of prostaglandin (natural chemicals that cause inflammation in damaged tissues such as an arthritic joint). They also suppress the immune system by reducing release and activity of white blood cells.

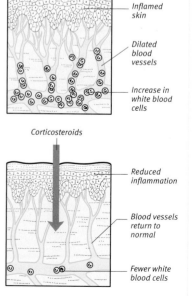

Inflamed skin

Dilated blood vessels

Increase in white blood cells

Corticosteroids

Reduced inflammation

Blood vessels return to normal

Fewer white blood cells

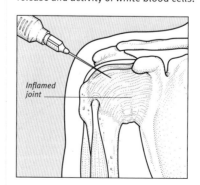

Inflamed joint

thematosus and *rheumatoid arthritis*, and the treatment of *asthma*, *eczema*, and *allergic rhinitis*. Corticosteroid drugs are also used to prevent organ rejection following *transplant surgery* and in the treatment of some types of cancer, such as *lymphoma* or *leukaemia*. In addition, injections of corticosteroids may be administered to relieve pain in disorders such as *tennis elbow* and *arthritis*.

POSSIBLE ADVERSE EFFECTS

Side effects are uncommon when corticosteroid drugs are used in the form of cream or taken by inhaler. However, tablets taken in high doses for long periods may cause *diabetes mellitus*, *hypertension*, *osteoporosis*, *oedema*, *peptic ulcer*, *Cushing's syndrome*, inhibited growth in children, and, in rare cases, *cataract* or *psychosis*. High doses of the drugs also impair the *immune system*, increasing the risk of serious infections such as *septicaemia* and *tuberculosis*; and *chickenpox* can be life-threatening in people taking corticosteroids.

Long-term treatment suppresses production of corticosteroid hormones by the adrenal glands, and sudden withdrawal may lead to *adrenal failure*, which can be life-threatening. For this reason, anyone who is taking or has recently been taking corticosteroids should carry a steroid treatment card and inform a doctor before undergoing any other form of medical treatment.

corticosteroid hormone

Any of a variety of hormones that is produced by the cortex of the *adrenal glands*. There are two main groups of corticosteroid hormone: *glucocorticoids* (such as *hydrocortisone*, cortisone, and corticosterone) and *mineralocorticoids* (such as *aldosterone*). (See also *corticosteroid drugs*; *steroid hormones*.)

corticotropin

An alternative name for *ACTH* (adrenocorticotrophic hormone).

Corti, organ of

See *organ of Corti*.

cortisol

An alternative name for *hydrocortisone*, a corticosteroid hormone that is produced by the *adrenal glands*.

cortisone

A *corticosteroid hormone* that is produced synthetically. Cortisone is sometimes used as a replacement hormone in the

treatment of *Addison's disease*. Side effects of the hormone include *peptic ulcer* and bleeding in the stomach.

Corynebacterium

A genus of gram-positive (see *Gram's stain*), rod-shaped bacteria. Corynebacteria cause disease, including *diphtheria* in humans and various types of infection in domestic animals and birds.

coryza

A term for the nasal symptoms of the common cold (see *cold, common*).

cosmesis

A term used for any procedures that are carried out to improve a person's appearance or to correct a disfiguring physical defect, such as *cosmetic surgery*, *cosmetic dentistry*, or the use of make-up to cover physical flaws.

cosmetic dentistry

Procedures to improve the appearance of the *teeth* or prevent further damage to the teeth and/or *gums*. Cosmetic dentistry procedures include fitting an *orthodontic appliance* to correct teeth that are out of alignment or an incorrect bite (see *malocclusion*); fitting a *crown* or *veneer*; *bonding* to treat chipped or stained teeth; *bleaching* of discoloured teeth; and replacing amalgam fillings with tooth-coloured ones.

cosmetic surgery

Any operation that is performed to improve appearance rather than to cure or treat disease. Cosmetic surgery techniques include the removal of skin blemishes or *dermabrasion*; *rhinoplasty* to alter the shape or size of the nose; *face-lifts*; *mammoplasty* to reduce or enlarge the breasts; *body contour surgery* to remove excess body fat and tissue; *hair transplants*; *blepharoplasty* to remove excess skin on the eyelids; and mentoplasty to alter the size or shape of the chin.

As with any surgical procedure, all forms of cosmetic surgery carry the risk of side effects from the anaesthetic, and of complications arising from the operation itself.

costal

A term meaning "relating to the *ribs*", as in the costal cartilages, which connect the ribs to the breastbone.

TYPES OF **COSMETIC SURGERY**

There is a range of cosmetic surgery procedures for various parts of the body. The sites of some of the more commonly performed operations are shown below. The procedures vary in the permanency of their results and in the likelihood of achieving a satisfactory appearance.

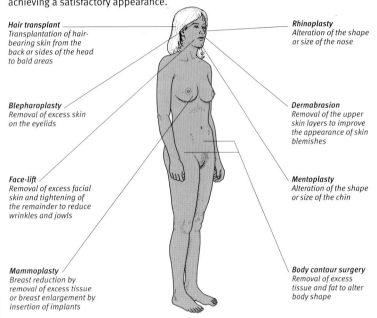

Hair transplant
Transplantation of hair-bearing skin from the back or sides of the head to bald areas

Blepharoplasty
Removal of excess skin on the eyelids

Face-lift
Removal of excess facial skin and tightening of the remainder to reduce wrinkles and jowls

Mammoplasty
Breast reduction by removal of excess tissue or breast enlargement by insertion of implants

Rhinoplasty
Alteration of the shape or size of the nose

Dermabrasion
Removal of the upper skin layers to improve the appearance of skin blemishes

Mentoplasty
Alteration of the shape or size of the chin

Body contour surgery
Removal of excess tissue and fat to alter body shape

C

costalgia

Pain that occurs around the chest as a result of damage to a *rib* or to one of the *intercostal nerves* beneath the ribs. Damage to an intercostal nerve most commonly results from an attack of the viral infection *herpes zoster* (shingles). The pain is difficult to treat and has a tendency to persist.

Costen's syndrome

A term that is sometimes used to describe facial pain due to *temporomandibular joint* disorders.

costosternal

A combined term sometimes used to describe the junction of the *ribs* and the *sternum* (breastbone).

cot death

See *sudden infant death syndrome*.

co-trimoxazole

An *antibacterial drug* that is a combination of trimethoprim and sulfamethoxazole. Because of rare but potentially serious side effects, co-trimoxazole is now used to treat certain infections only in circumstances in which they cannot be treated with other drugs. Its main use is in the treatment of *pneumocystis pneumonia, toxoplasmosis, and nocardiosis*.

cough

A *reflex* action that helps to clear the airways of sputum, a foreign body, or any other irritant or blockage. A cough is described as "productive" when it brings up mucus or sputum and "unproductive" or "dry" when it does not.

CAUSES

Many coughs are due to irritation of the airways by dust, smoke (see *cough, smoker's*), or a viral infection of the upper respiratory tract (see *cold, common; laryngitis; pharyngitis; tracheitis*). Coughing is also a feature of *bronchitis, asthma, pneumonia,* and *lung cancer*.

TREATMENT

Over-the-counter *cough remedies* are available, but, in general, they just ease symptoms. More specific treatment is directed at the underlying disorder.

coughing up blood

A symptom, known medically as haemoptysis, caused by the rupture of a blood vessel in the airway, lung, nose, or throat. The coughed-up blood may appear as bright-red or rusty-brown streaks, clots in the sputum, a pinkish froth, or, more rarely, blood alone. In all cases, medical assessment is needed.

CAUSES

Many disorders can cause haemoptysis. The most common are infections, such as *pneumonia* or *bronchitis*; and congestion and rupture of blood vessels in the lungs due to *heart failure*, *mitral stenosis*, or *pulmonary embolism*. A cancerous tumour can also produce haemoptysis by eroding the wall of a blood vessel.

DIAGNOSIS AND TREATMENT

Investigations into coughing up blood include *chest X-ray*, blood tests, and sometimes *bronchoscopy* or *CT scanning*. In some cases, no underlying cause is found. Treatment depends on the cause. but stopping smoking is essential in all cases.

cough remedies

Over-the-counter medications used for treating a *cough*. There are various preparations, but the effectiveness of most is unproven. *Expectorant* cough remedies are purported to encourage expulsion of sputum. Cough suppressants, which control the coughing reflex, include some *antihistamine drugs* and *codeine*. They may be helpful in controlling coughing at night that prevents sleep; however, they cause drowsiness and may cause constipation as well.

cough, smoker's

A recurrent cough due to *smoking*. The cough is usually triggered by accumulation of thick sputum in the airways as a result of inflammation caused by tobacco smoke. Giving up smoking will usually stop the cough, but it may take time. In general, the longer a person has been smoking, the longer it takes for the cough to clear. Smokers with a persistent cough should seek medical advice, particularly if the cough changes, because smoking is associated with *lung cancer*.

counselling

Advice and psychological support from health professionals to help people deal with personal difficulties. It is used to address problems at work, school, or in the family; give advice on medical, sexual, and marital problems; help deal with addictions; and give support during life crises. Types of counselling include *genetic counselling*, trauma counselling, and *sex therapy*. In most cases counselling is a one-to-one activity, but it may also be carried out in small groups. (See also *child guidance; family therapy; marriage guidance; psychotherapy*.)

Cowden's disease

An autosomal dominant *genetic disorder*, also called multiple hamartoma syndrome, in which noncancerous growths develop in tissues, including the skin, mouth, and intestines. Skin growths may include flat-topped, flesh-coloured lesions on the face. Multiple polyps may grow in the intestines.

People with the disease are also at increased risk of developing certain cancers, particularly thyroid cancer, colorectal cancer, and, in women, breast and ovarian cancer. There is no specific treatment for the condition.

cowpox

An infection caused by the vaccinia virus, which usually affects cows. This virus was used in the past to confer immunity against *smallpox*.

coxa vara

A deformity of the *hip* in which the angle between the neck and head of the *femur* (thigh bone) and the shaft of the femur is reduced, resulting in shortening of the leg, pain and stiffness in the hip, and a limp. The most common cause is a fracture to the neck of the femur or, during adolescence, injury to the developing part of the head of the femur. Coxa vara can also occur if the bone tissue in the neck of the femur is soft, a condition that may be *congenital* or the result of a bone disorder such as *rickets* or *Paget's disease*. Treatment may include surgery (see *osteotomy*).

COX-2 inhibitor drugs

A group of *nonsteroidal anti-inflammatory drugs* (NSAIDs) used mainly to relieve the pain and inflammation of *rheumatoid arthritis* and *osteoarthritis*. Examples of COX-2 inhibitors include *celecoxib*, etoricoxib, and lumiracoxib. COX-2 inhibitors cause less stomach irritation as a side effect than do other NSAIDs, although they may still cause abdominal discomfort, which can be minimized by taken the drugs with food.

COX-2 inhibitors are associated with an increased risk of heart disease and strokes and are therefore not generally recommended for people who have had a heart attack or stroke or who are at risk of these conditions.

coxsackievirus

One of a group of *viruses* responsible for a broad range of diseases. There are two main types of coxsackievirus: A and

B. The best known of the type A infections is *hand, foot, and mouth disease*, a common childhood disorder characterized by blistering of skin around the mouth, hands, and feet. Type B viruses can cause serious illnesses such as *meningitis*, *pericarditis*, and *pneumonia*.

CPAP

The abbreviation for *continuous positive airway pressure*.

CPPV

The abbreviation for *continuous positive pressure ventilation*.

crab lice

See *pubic lice*.

crack

A popular term for a highly potent, fast-acting form of *cocaine*.

cracked heel

See *heel, cracked*.

cradle cap

A skin condition, common in babies and most prevalent between the age of three and nine months, in which thick, yellow scales occur in patches over the scalp. Cradle cap, a form of *seborrhoeic dermatitis*, may also occur on the face, neck, behind the ears, and in the nappy area. It is not clear why cradle cap occurs, but it is not due to poor hygiene.

Cradle cap is harmless as long as the skin does not become infected. It can be treated by daily use of a simple shampoo. Alternatively, warm olive oil may be rubbed into the baby's scalp and left on overnight to loosen and soften the scales, which can be washed off the following day. A mild ointment that contains an *antifungal drug* and a *corticosteroid drug* may be prescribed if the skin becomes inflamed.

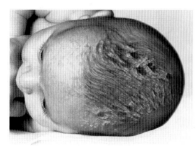

Appearance of cradle cap
Thick, yellow, scaly patches occur on the scalp of babies, most commonly between the age of 3 and 9 months. It is not clear why cradle cap occurs.

cramp

A painful spasm in a muscle that is caused by excessive and prolonged contraction of the muscle fibres. The affected muscle may feel hard and tender to the touch.

Cramps often occur as a result of increased muscular activity, which causes a buildup of *lactic acid* and other chemicals in the muscles, and leads to small areas of muscle-fibre damage. Repetitive movements, such as writing (see *cramp, writer's*) or sitting or lying in an awkward position may also result in cramps. In addition, cramps may follow profuse sweating because loss of sodium salts disrupts muscle cell activity.

Massaging or stretching the muscles involved may bring relief. A drug containing *quinine* may be given for recurrent night cramps. Recurrent, sudden pain in a muscle not associated with hardness of the muscle may be caused by *peripheral vascular disease*.

cramp, writer's

Painful spasm in the hand muscles following repetitive movements, which makes writing or typing impossible.

Crandall's syndrome

A rare *congenital* disorder that runs in families and is characterized by twisted, brittle hairs, sensorineural *deafness*, and *hypogonadism* (underdevelopment of the *ovaries* or *testes*). The condition is associated with deficiencies of *luteinizing hormone* and *growth hormone*.

cranial nerves

Twelve pairs of *nerves* that emerge from the underside of the *brain*. Each of the cranial nerves has a number as well as a name; the numbers are used to indicate the sequence in which the nerves emerge from the brain. (see the illustrated box overleaf.)

Certain cranial nerves primarily carry sensory information from the ears, nose, and eyes to the brain. These nerves are the *vestibulocochlear nerve* (hearing and balance), *olfactory nerve* (smell), and *optic nerve* (vision). Other cranial nerves carry motor impulses that move the muscles in the head and neck. They are the *oculomotor nerve*, the *trochlear nerve*, and the *abducent nerve* (producing eye movements); the *spinal accessory nerve* (producing head and shoulder movements); and *hypoglossal nerve* (producing tongue movements).

Some cranial nerves have both sensory and motor functions. They are the *facial nerve* (facial expressions, taste, and the secretion of saliva and tears), the *trigeminal nerve* (facial sensation and jaw movements), and the *glossopharyngeal nerve* (taste and swallowing). The *vagus nerve* has branches to all the main digestive organs, as well as to the heart and the lungs. It is a major component of the *parasympathetic nervous system*, which is concerned with maintaining automatic body functions such as breathing, the heartbeat, and digestion.

craniopharyngioma

A rare, non-hormone-secreting tumour of the *pituitary gland*. Symptoms of a craniopharyngioma may include headaches, vomiting, and defective vision. If the tumour develops in childhood, the child's growth may be stunted and sexual development may not occur.

Craniopharyngiomas are usually surgically removed. If left untreated, they may cause permanent brain damage.

craniosynostosis

The premature closure of one or more of the joints (sutures) between the *skull* bones in infants. If all of the joints are involved, the growing *brain* may be compressed and there is a risk of brain damage due to the increased pressure inside the skull. If the abnormality is localized, the head may be deformed. Craniosynostosis may occur before birth and may be associated with other *birth defects*. It may also occur in an otherwise healthy baby, or in a baby with a disorder such as *rickets*.

If the brain has been compressed, an operation may be performed to separate the fused skull bones.

craniotomy

Temporary removal of a section of the skull to enable surgery on the *brain*. It may be carried out to take a sample of tissue for analysis, remove a *tumour*, or drain an *abscess* or blood clot. (See also the illustrated box, p.203.)

cranium

The part of the *skull* around the *brain*.

C-reactive protein

A protein produced by the body in response to inflammation. The blood level of this protein is measured to screen for and evaluate the treatment of inflammatory conditions.

CRANIAL NERVES

All but two of the cranial nerve pairs connect with nuclei in the brainstem. The olfactory and optic nerves, in contrast, link directly with parts of the cerebrum. The nerves emerge through openings in the cranium (skull); many then divide into branches. Certain cranial nerves are principally concerned with transmitting sensory information from organs such as the ears, nose, and eyes to the brain.

Others carry motor impulses that move the tongue, eyes, and facial (and other) muscles, or stimulate glands such as the salivary glands. A few nerves have both sensory and motor functions. The 10th, or *vagus nerve*, is one of the most important parts of the *parasympathetic nervous system*, and has branches to the main digestive organs, the heart, and the lungs.

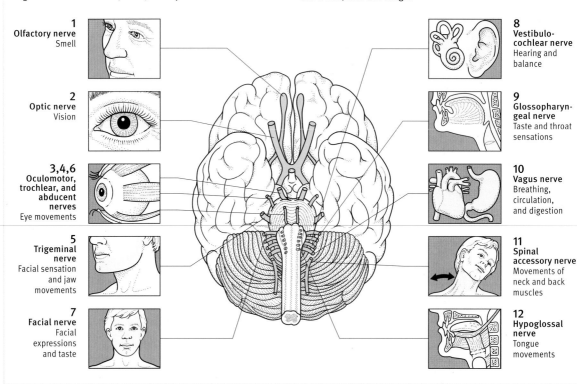

1
Olfactory nerve
Smell

2
Optic nerve
Vision

3,4,6
Oculomotor, trochlear, and abducent nerves
Eye movements

5
Trigeminal nerve
Facial sensation and jaw movements

7
Facial nerve
Facial expressions and taste

8
Vestibulo-cochlear nerve
Hearing and balance

9
Glossopharyn-geal nerve
Taste and throat sensations

10
Vagus nerve
Breathing, circulation, and digestion

11
Spinal accessory nerve
Movements of neck and back muscles

12
Hypoglossal nerve
Tongue movements

cream

A thick, semi-solid preparation with moisturizing properties, used to apply medications to the skin.

creatine kinase

An *enzyme* (a protein that alters the rate of a chemical reaction in the body) found in muscle. After damage to muscle cells, including those of the heart, creatine kinase leaks into the blood. Increased levels of the enzyme can be detected by special tests (see *muscle enzymes*). Different types of creatine kinase exist in different types of muscle. If blood tests show a raised level of the form found in heart muscle, it may indicate that a *myocardial infarction* (heart attack) has occurred. Raised levels of the form found in skeletal muscles may indicate a range of disorders, from muscle injury to diseases such as *muscular dystrophy*.

creatinine

A waste product from chemical proc-esses in the muscles. The kidneys filter it from the blood for excretion in *urine*.

creatinine clearance

A type of *kidney function test* in which the level of *creatinine* in the blood and the urine is measured. The blood level is measured, then the urine is collected and tested over 24 hours to measure the level of creatinine being excreted. The two levels are compared; if there is a high level of creatinine in the blood but a low level in the urine, it shows that the kidneys are not effectively clearing creatinine from the body.

crepitation

A crackling sound in the lungs (heard through a *stethoscope*) due to a build-up of fluid. (See also *auscultation*.)

crepitus

A grating sound or sensation caused by rough surfaces inside the body rubbing together. Crepitus may be felt or heard when the ends of a broken bone rub against each other, or when *cartilage* on the surfaces of a joint has worn away due to *osteoarthritis*. Faint crepitus may be heard in the lung as a result of abnormalities such as inflammation in *pneumonia*.

The term also describes the crackling sound made when an air pocket under the skin (see *emphysema, surgical*), or an area of gas *gangrene*, is pressed.

cretinism

A *congenital* condition in infants that is characterized by stunted growth, failure of normal development, *learning difficulties*, and coarse facial features. Cretinism occurs when the *thyroid gland* produces insufficient amounts, or fails to produce any at all, of the thyroid hormone *thyroxine* at birth. However, newborn babies are routinely screened for thyroid hormones (see *blood spot screening tests*) so that the condition can be recognized at an early stage and replacement therapy with thyroxine can be given. (See also *hypothyroidism*.)

Creutzfeldt–Jakob disease

A rare, progressive degenerative disease of the *brain*. Creutzfeldt–Jakob disease (CJD) is thought to be caused by accumulation in the brain of a *prion* (an abnormal type of infectious protein). A similar agent causes scrapie in sheep and *bovine spongiform encephalopathy* (BSE) in cattle.

TYPES
One form of CJD largely affects middle-aged or elderly people, and appears to have no obvious cause. A second form occurs in younger people. and this form is associated with contamination during brain surgery or transplants from infected people, or with treatment using infected human growth hormone or *gonadotrophins*.

A third form, new variant (nv) CJD, was first identified in 1995 and affects people in their teens and 20s. It is thought to be acquired by eating beef infected with BSE. This form causes pathological changes in the brain that are similar to the changes found in cattle suffering from BSE. Another variant of the disease is hereditary.

SYMPTOMS
Symptoms are broadly similar for all forms of the disease. Slowly progressive *dementia* (deterioration in brain function) and *myoclonus* (sudden muscular contractions) occur; coordination diminishes; the intellect and personality deteriorate; and blindness may develop. As the disease progresses, speech is lost and the body becomes rigid.

OUTLOOK
There is no treatment for Creutzfeldt–Jakob disease, and death usually occurs within two to three years.

cri du chat syndrome

A rare *congenital* condition that causes severe *learning difficulties*, abnormal facial appearance, low birth weight, and short stature. It is characterized by a cat-like cry in infancy. Cri du chat syndrome is caused by a *chromosomal abnormality*. There is no treatment. (See also *genetic counselling*.)

Crigler–Najjar syndrome

A rare *genetic disorder* in which there is an absence or lack of the liver enzyme that breaks down *bilirubin* (the yellowish pigment in the digestive juice *bile*) for excretion. The condition appears in early childhood.

Children with Crigler–Najjar syndrome have jaundice (yellowing of the skin and whites of the eyes, due to a buildup of bilirubin in the blood). In some children, the liver enzyme is completely absent, and the condition is fatal by about two years of age. Some other children may just have insufficient amounts of the enzyme, and may live into adulthood. A *liver transplant* may be the only effective treatment for Crigler–Najjar syndrome.

crisis

A term for a turning point in the course of a disease (either the onset of recovery or deterioration). The word is also used to describe a distressing and difficult episode in life.

crisis intervention

The provision of immediate advice or help, by agencies such as mental health and social services departments, to people who have acute psychiatric or sociomedical problems.

critical

A term used to mean "seriously ill" or to describe a crucial state of illness from which a patient may not recover.

Crohn's disease

A chronic inflammatory disease that can affect any part of the gastrointestinal tract from the mouth to the anus. Crohn's disease can occur at any age, but people in their mid-20s are most likely to be affected. it is more common in women than men.

PROCEDURE FOR **CRANIOTOMY**

Before the operation, all or part of the patient's scalp is shaved. After a general anaesthetic has been given, layers of skin, muscle, and membrane are cut away from the skull at the planned operation site and the bone is cut with a saw (see below). The "lid" of bone is then either folded back on a "hinge" of muscle or removed completely. The dura (the outermost of the three membranes that surround the brain) is then opened to reveal the inner membranes and the brain.

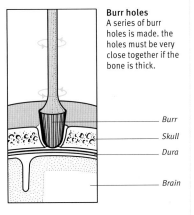

Burr holes
A series of burr holes is made. the holes must be very close together if the bone is thick.

Burr
Skull
Dura
Brain

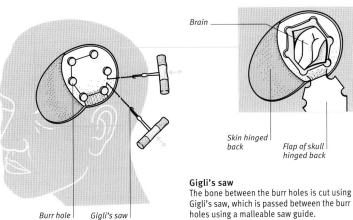

Burr hole | Gigli's saw

Brain

Skin hinged back | Flap of skull hinged back

Gigli's saw
The bone between the burr holes is cut using Gigli's saw, which is passed between the burr holes using a malleable saw guide.

C

The most common site of inflammation is the terminal ileum (the end of the small intestine where it joins the large intestine). The wall of the intestine becomes extremely thick due to continued chronic inflammation, and deep, penetrating ulcers may form. The disease tends to be patchy; areas of the intestine that lie between the diseased parts may appear to be normal, but are usually mildly affected.

CAUSES

The cause is unknown, but genetic and environmental factors seem to be involved. It is possible that the disease is caused by an abnormal immune response to an *antigen* (foreign protein). Smoking increases the risk, and worsens the condition once developed.

The risk of developing Crohn's disease is higher in people who have a close relative with the disorder.

SYMPTOMS

In young people, the ileum is usually involved. The disease causes spasms of abdominal pain, diarrhoea and chronic sickness, loss of appetite, anaemia, and weight loss. The ability of the small intestine to absorb nutrients from food is reduced. In elderly people, it is more common for the disease to affect the rectum and cause rectal bleeding.

Crohn's disease can also affect the colon (the major part of the large intestine), causing bloody diarrhoea. In rare cases, it also affects the mouth, oesophagus, stomach, and duodenum (the upper part of the small intestine).

Complications may affect the intestines or may develop elsewhere in the body. The thickening of the intestinal wall may narrow the inside of the intestine so much that an obstruction occurs (see *intestine, obstruction of*).

About three in ten affected people develop a fistula (abnormal passageway). Internal fistulas may develop between loops of intestine. External fistulas, from the intestine to the skin of the abdomen or around the anus, may cause leakage of faeces (see *faecal fistula*).

Abscesses (pus-filled pockets of infection) form in about one in five people. Many abscesses occur around the anus, but some occur within the abdomen.

Complications in other parts of the body may include inflammation of various parts of the eye, severe arthritis affecting various joints of the body, *ankylosing spondylitis* (an inflammation of the spine), skin disorders, liver disease, and *gallstones*.

DIAGNOSIS

A physical examination may reveal tender abdominal swellings that indicate thickening of the intestinal walls. *Sigmoidoscopy* (examination of the lower, or sigmoid, colon and the rectum with a viewing instrument) may confirm the diagnosis. X-rays using barium follow-through or barium enemas (see *barium X-ray examinations*) will show thickened loops of intestine with deep fissures.

It may be difficult to differentiate between Crohn's disease when it is affecting the colon and *ulcerative colitis*, an inflammatory bowel disease limited to the large intestine. However, *colonoscopy* (examination of the colon using a flexible viewing instrument) and *biopsy* (the removal of a sample of tissue for microscopic examination) can confirm the diagnosis. *CT scanning*, *MRI* (magnetic resonance imaging), and ultrasound scanning may also be used to detect complications such as abscesses.

TREATMENT

The aim of treatment is to bring about long-term remission of the disease. It may involve high doses of *corticosteroid drugs* or *mesalazine* and related drugs; *immunosuppressant drugs*; or monoclonal antibody treatment with *infliximab*; in some cases, a combination of these drugs may be used. *Antibiotic drugs* may also be given to combat infection. In severe cases, *enteral feeding* (in which easily digestible food is given through a tube directly into the intestines) may be necessary. Once the disease is in remission, normal feeding can be resumed and the dose of corticosteroids can be reduced.

Surgical treatment to remove damaged sections of the intestine is avoided whenever possible because the disease may recur in other parts of the intestine. However, many people with the condition do need surgery at some stage to treat problems such as perforation or blockage of the intestine.

OUTLOOK

Some people in whom the disease is localized remain in normal health indefinitely and seem to be cured.

cromoglicate

See *sodium cromoglicate*.

crossbite

A type of *malocclusion* (an abnormal relationship between the upper and lower teeth) in which some or all of the lower front teeth overlap the upper front teeth. A molar crossbite, in which the upper and lower back teeth overlap, can also occur.

cross-eye

A type of *strabismus* (squint) in which one of the eyes turns inwards relative to the other, or in which both eyes turn inwards towards each other.

cross-matching

A procedure to determine compatibility between the blood of a person who requires a *blood transfusion* and that of a *donor*. Red blood cells from one person are combined with *serum* (the clear fluid that separates from blood when it clots) from the other. Clumping of red blood cells indicates the presence of *antibodies*, showing that the blood is not compatible.

croup

A common disorder in infants and young children, in which narrowing and inflammation of the airways causes hoarseness, stridor (a grunting noise during breathing), and a barking cough.

Croup may be caused by a viral or bacterial infection affecting the *larynx*, epiglottis (see *epiglottitis*), or *trachea*. Most cases are due to a viral infection and are generally mild. Other causes include *diphtheria*, *Haemophilus influenzae b* (Hib), *allergy*, spasm due to insufficient *calcium* levels in the blood, and inhalation of a *foreign body*.

Humidifying the air can help to ease breathing. In more severe cases, hospital treatment may be required so that *corticosteroid drugs* administered through a *nebulizer* and oxygen can be given. If the infection is bacterial, it is treated with *antibiotic drugs*.

Crouzon's syndrome

An autosomal dominant *genetic disorder* that causes facial deformities. Affected people have eyes that protrude (see *exophthalmos*) and are spaced widely apart; a *squint*; an abnormally tall skull; a large, beaked nose; and an underdeveloped upper jaw, which makes the lower jaw look as if it is protruding.

crowding, dental

See *overcrowding, dental*.

crown

The name for the top of the head. The word is also used of the visible part of a tooth. (See also *crown, dental*; *crowning*.)

C

crown, dental

An artificial replacement for the crown of a decayed, discoloured, or broken *tooth*. A crown made from porcelain is usually used on front teeth, but back teeth need the greater strength of a crown made from gold or porcelain fused to metal.

A crown may be fitted by filing the tooth to form a peg and cementing the crown over the top of it. For a badly decayed or weakened tooth, it may be necessary to remove the natural crown, perform *root-canal treatment*, then fit the artificial crown on to a post that is cemented in the root canal. For details on how crowns are fitted, see the illustrated box below.

crown–heel length

A routine measurement of the length of a newborn baby, taken from the *crown* of the head to the heels.

crowning

The popular name given to the phase in the second stage of labour (see *childbirth*) when the baby's head first appears at the mother's vaginal opening.

cruciate ligament

One of the two *ligaments* in the knee that pass over each other to form a cross. The ligaments form connections between the *femur* and *tibia* inside the knee joint and prevent overbending and overstraightening at the knee.

crush syndrome

Damage to a large amount of *muscle* (usually as a result of a serious accident), which causes *kidney failure*. The damaged muscles release proteins into the bloodstream, temporarily impairing kidney function. As a result, some substances normally excreted in the urine build up to toxic levels in the blood. If left untreated, crush syndrome may be fatal, but *dialysis* allows the kidneys time to recover.

crutch palsy

Weakness or *paralysis* of muscles in the wrist, fingers, and thumb in people who walk with a crutch under the armpit. Crutch palsy is due to pressure on the *nerves* supplying these muscles. It does not occur if elbow crutches are used.

crying in infants

A normal response in babies to needs or discomforts, such as hunger or thirst. Most healthy babies stop crying when their needs are attended to. In a few cases, persistent crying may be due to a physical cause such as intolerance of cow's milk or an illness (such as an ear or throat infection, or a viral fever).

cryo-

A prefix meaning "ice cold". It is used of medical procedures that involve the use of freezing or low temperatures.

cryopreservation

The preservation of living cells or tissue samples by freezing. The technique is used to store human eggs for *in vitro fertilization*, sperm for *artificial insemination*, or *plasma* and blood obtained from people with rare blood groups.

cryosurgery

The use of temperatures below freezing to destroy tissue, or the use of cold during surgical procedures to produce *adhesion* between an instrument and an area of body tissue.

Cryosurgery causes only minimal scarring. It is used to treat cancerous tumours in sites where heavy scarring can block vital openings, such as in the *cervix*, the liver, and the intestines. It may be used in eye operations, for example in treating *retinal detachment*. It is also used for removing *warts*, *skin tags*, some *birthmarks*, and some skin cancers, and to treat *haemorrhoids*.

cryotherapy

The use of cold or freezing temperatures or substances in treatment. (See also *cryosurgery*.)

HOW **CROWNS** ARE FITTED

The tooth is filed down to form a peg over which the replacement is fitted. An impression of the peg and the natural tooth is taken and a replica is made. Using this replica as a model, the artificial crown is constructed.

Cast full crown

Porcelain fused to metal crown

Porcelain jacket crown

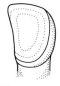

Three-quarter crown

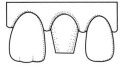

1 A cracked or broken tooth, or one that has been heavily filled, can be replaced by a crown.

2 The damaged area of the tooth is removed and the remaining part is shaped to receive the crown.

3 The artificial crown, a hollow shell, is fitted over the shaped tooth and then cemented in place.

POST CROWNS

If the natural tooth is badly decayed or has been weakened, its crown is removed and a post crown is fitted.

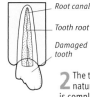

Root canal
Tooth root
Damaged tooth

1 This tooth is so decayed that a retaining peg cannot be fashioned.

2 The tooth's natural crown is completely removed.

Root canal filled
Tooth trimmed

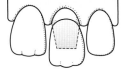

Gold post in root canal

Crown

3 A gold post is cemented into the root canal and the crown is then cemented over the post.

cryptococcosis

A rare infectious disorder caused by inhaling the fungus CRYPTOCOCCUS NEOFORMANS, which is found especially in soil contaminated with pigeon faeces. The most serious form that the infection can take is *meningitis*. Another form of infection causes growths in the lungs, resulting in chest pain and a cough, or on the skin, causing a rash of ulcers. Most cases of cryptococcosis occur in people with reduced immunity, such as those with *AIDS*.

Cryptococcal meningitis is diagnosed from a sample of spinal fluid. A combination of the antifungal drugs *amphotericin B* and flucytosine is usually prescribed to treat the infection. Most cases in which only the lungs are infected need no treatment.

cryptophthalmus

A *birth defect* in which the opening between the upper and lower eyelids is absent. (See also *Fraser's syndrome*.)

cryptorchidism

A developmental disorder of male infants in which the testes fail to descend normally into the scrotum (see *testis, undescended*).

cryptosporidiosis

A type of diarrhoeal infection caused by *protozoa*, which may be spread from person to person or be transmitted from domestic animals to people. The disease causes watery diarrhoea and sometimes fever and abdominal pain. It is most common in children but also occurs in people with AIDS.

In most cases, *rehydration therapy* is the only treatment needed. In people whose *immune system* is suppressed, however, the infection may be much more severe. Such people may need to be admitted to hospital for treatment with intravenous fluids and *antidiarrhoeal drugs*.

CSF

The abbreviation for *cerebrospinal fluid*.

CS spray

A noxious powder, also known as CS gas or tear gas, that is used in aerosol form as a means of riot control. CS spray causes severe irritation of the eyes, airways, and skin, and sometimes nausea and vomiting. Its effects are short-lived, usually lasting for only a few minutes.

CT scanning

A diagnostic technique in which the combined use of a computer and a machine emitting *X-rays* produces cross-sectional images of the body tissues.

A CT (computed tomography) scanner is a machine that is shaped like a doughnut that rotates around the patient's body. The machine contains one or more X-ray sources and, on the opposite side, some X-ray detectors. Unlike a conventional X-ray image, which shows only a few levels of tissue density, the X-ray detector can register hundreds of levels of density. It sends

PERFORMING A CT SCAN

CT scanning combines the use of a computer and X-rays emitted by a rotating machine to produce cross-sectional images. Before the scan is carried out, a contrast medium may be injected to make blood vessels, organs, or abnormalities show up more clearly; for scans of the intestines, a drink of contrast medium may be given to highlight loops of intestine.

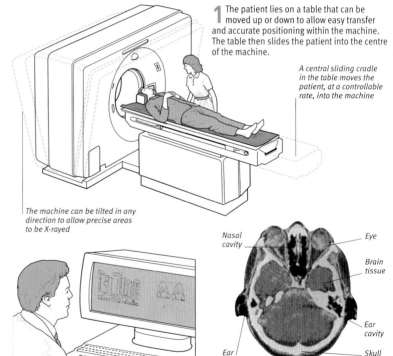

1 The patient lies on a table that can be moved up or down to allow easy transfer and accurate positioning within the machine. The table then slides the patient into the centre of the machine.

A central sliding cradle in the table moves the patient, at a controllable rate, into the machine

The machine can be tilted in any direction to allow precise areas to be X-rayed

Nasal cavity

Eye

Brain tissue

Ear cavity

Ear

Skull

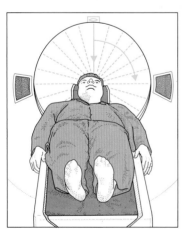

2 The scanner rotates around the patient. As it does so, it sends a large number of X-ray beams, each of low dosage and lasting only a fraction of a second, through the patient's body at different angles.

3 Detectors in the scanner record the amount of X-rays absorbed by different tissues. This information is sent to a computer, which converts it into an image (such as the section through the head, above) for a radiologist to interpret.

this information to a computer, which processes the data and shows the results as an image on a monitor. CT images usually show the body as "slices", in which the different tissues can be seen in detail. In some machines, this information can be used to produce a three-dimensional reconstruction of the area scanned.

CT scanning has revolutionized the diagnosis and treatment of *tumours*, *abscesses*, and haemorrhages in the brain, as well as *head injuries* and *strokes*. The procedure is also used to locate and show tumours, to investigate a wide range of diseases, and to aid needle *biopsy* in organs of the trunk.

Newer types of CT scanners use a spiral technique: the scanner rotates around the body as the patient is moved slowly forwards on a bed, causing the X-ray beams to follow a spiral course. Images can be made of hollow organs such as the colon (a procedure known as "virtual colonoscopy"). For some procedures, injected or swallowed contrast media (chemicals that are opaque to X-rays) may be used to make certain tissues more easily visible.

The images produced during CT scanning can be stored digitally or on conventional X-ray film. (For details of the procedure, see *Performing a CT scan* box, opposite.)

cuff

A body structure that consists of muscle and tendon fibres and encircles a *joint*. (See also *rotator cuff*.)

culture

A growth of bacteria or other microorganisms, cells, or tissues cultivated artificially in the laboratory.

Microorganisms are collected from the site of an infection and cultured in order to produce adequate amounts so that tests to identify them can be performed. Cells from a fetus may be cultured to diagnose disorders prenatally. Healthy cells may be cultured for the study of chromosomes (see *chromosome analysis*). Some types of tissue, such as skin, may be cultured to produce larger amounts that can be used for grafting (see *skin graft*) to repair areas of tissue that have been lost or damaged – by burns, for example. Other tissues are cultivated to provide a medium in which viruses can be grown and identified in the laboratory; viruses will only multiply within living cells.

cupping

An ancient procedure in which the practitioner draws blood to the skin surface by applying a heated vessel to the skin. It produces an inflammatory response thought to relieve *bronchitis*, *asthma*, and musculoskeletal pains.

curare

An extract from the bark and juices of various trees that is used by South American Indians as an arrow poison. Curare kills by producing muscle *paralysis*. Synthetic compounds that are related to curare are sometimes used to produce paralysis during surgery.

cure

The process of restoration to normal health after an illness. The word "cure" usually means the disappearance of a disease rather than simply a halt in its progress. A treatment that ends an illness may also be called a cure.

curettage

The use of a surgical instrument called a *curette* to scrape abnormal tissue, or samples for analysis, from the lining of a body cavity or from the skin. (See also *D and C*.)

curettage, dental

The scraping of a cavity or other dental surface with a *curette* (a narrow, spoon-shaped instrument). Dental curettage is one method that is used to remove the lining of periodontal pockets and diseased tissue from root surfaces in *periodontitis*. This enables the healthy underlying tissue to reattach itself to the root surface.

curette

A spoon-shaped surgical instrument used for scraping away material or tissue from an organ, cavity, or surface.

Curling's ulcer

A type of *stress ulcer* that occurs specifically in people who have suffered extensive skin burns.

Cushing's syndrome

A hormonal disorder caused by an abnormally high level of *corticosteroid hormones* in the blood. Cushing's syndrome is characterized by a reddened, moon-shaped face, wasting of the limbs, thickening of the trunk, and a humped upper back. Other symptoms include *acne*; stretch marks on the skin; bruising; *osteoporosis* (loss of bone density); susceptibility to infection and *peptic ulcers*; and, in women, increased hairiness. Mental changes frequently also occur, causing *depression*, *insomnia*, *paranoia*, or *euphoria*. *Oedema*, *hypertension*, and *diabetes mellitus* may develop. In children, growth may be suppressed.

The excess of hormones is most commonly due to prolonged treatment with *corticosteroid drugs*. Such cases of Cushing's syndrome are usually mild. In other cases, high hormone levels are due to overactivity of the *adrenal glands* because of an *adrenal tumour*, or due to a *pituitary tumour* affecting production of *ACTH* (adrenocortocotrophic hormone), which in turn stimulates the adrenal glands.

Cushing's syndrome that occurs as a result of treatment with corticosteroid drugs usually disappears when the dose of the drug is gradually reduced. In cases of Cushing's syndrome that are caused by an adrenal gland tumour, the tumour will be removed surgically. If the cause of the disease is a pituitary tumour, the tumour may be removed surgically or it may be shrunk by irradiation and drug treatment. In both of these cases, surgery is followed by *hormone replacement therapy*.

cushion

Any soft body structure resembling a pad or cushion, such as a *bursa*.

cusp

A tapering point, such as on a tooth. The term also refers to the flaps of the *heart valves*.

cusp, dental

One of the protrusions found on the grinding surface of a *tooth*.

cutaneous

Relating to the skin.

cutaneous anthrax

See *anthrax*.

cutaneous horn

See *horn, cutaneous*.

cutdown

Creation of a small skin incision in order to gain access to a *vein*, to take blood or to give intravenous fluid. This procedure is sometimes needed when a vein cannot be identified through the skin, in conditions such as *shock*.

cuticle

The outermost layer of skin. The term commonly refers to the thin flap of skin at the base of a nail, and also to the outer layer of a hair shaft.

CVA

The abbreviation for *cerebrovascular accident*.

CVP

The abbreviation for *central venous pressure* (the pressure in the right atrium of the heart).

CVS

The abbreviation for *chorionic villus sampling*, and for *cardiovascular system*.

cyanide

Any of a group of salts of hydrocyanic acid. Most of these substances are extremely poisonous, and their inhalation or ingestion can rapidly lead to breathlessness and *paralysis*, followed by unconsciousness and death. Certain cyanides are eye irritants and are used in tear gases.

cyanocobalamin

An alternative name for *vitamin B₁₂*.

cyanosis

A bluish coloration of the skin or mucous membranes caused by an abnormally high level of deoxygenated *haemoglobin* in the blood. Cyanosis confined to the hands and feet is not serious; it is usually due to slow blood flow, often as a result of exposure to cold. A blue tinge to the lips and tongue, however, could be caused by a serious heart or lung disorder such as chronic obstructive *pulmonary disease* or *heart failure*.

cyclopenthiazide

A *thiazide diuretic* drug that is used to reduce *oedema* associated with *heart failure* and kidney disorders, and to treat *hypertension* (high blood pressure). Side effects of this drug include lethargy, loss of appetite, leg cramps, dizziness, rash, and *erectile dysfunction*.

cyclophosphamide

An *anticancer drug* used in the treatment of *Hodgkin's disease* and *leukaemia*. It is also used as a *disease-modifying anti-rheumatic drug* to treat *rheumatoid arthritis* and as an *immunosuppressant drug* to treat systemic *lupus erythematosus*.

cycloplegia

Paralysis of the ciliary muscle of the eye, which makes *accommodation* difficult. In some circumstances, cycloplegia may be induced by cycloplegic drugs to facilitate eye examinations.

cyclosporin

An alternative spelling for *ciclosporin*.

cyclothymia

A personality characteristic typified by marked changes of mood from cheerful, energetic, and sociable to gloomy, listless, and withdrawn. Mood swings may last for days or months and may follow a regular pattern.

Cymalon

A brand name for an over-the-counter preparation containing sodium bicarbonate, sodium carbonate, citric acid, and sodium citrate. This preparation is commonly used to relieve the symptoms of *cystitis*.

cyproterone acetate

A drug that blocks the action of *androgen hormones*. It is used to treat prostate cancer (see *prostate, cancer of*) and occasionally to reduce male sex drive. It is also used combined with ethinylestradiol as a treatment for severe *acne* in women. Side effects include weight gain and an increased risk of blood clots.

cyst

An abnormal but usually harmless lump or swelling filled with fluid or semi-solid material. Cysts occur in body organs or tissues. There are various types, including *sebaceous cysts*, *dermoid cysts*, *ovarian cysts*, *breast cysts*, *Baker's cysts*, and cysts that form around parasites in diseases such as hydatid disease or amoebiasis. Cysts may need to be removed surgically if they disrupt the function of body tissues.

cyst-/cysto-

Relating to the *bladder*, as in *cystitis* (inflammation of the bladder).

cystectomy

The surgical removal of part or all of the *bladder*. The procedure is used for treating bladder cancer (see *bladder tumours*). Radical cystectomy (in which all of the bladder is removed) is followed by the construction of an alternative channel for *urine*, usually ending in a *stoma* in the lower abdomen

(see *urinary diversion*). In men, the *prostate gland* and *seminal vesicles* are also removed, usually resulting in *impotence*. In women, the *uterus*, *ovaries*, and *fallopian tubes* are removed. After radical cystectomy, the patient has to wear an external pouch to collect urine.

cysticercosis

An infection, which is rare in developed countries, caused by the larvae of the pork *tapeworm*. The disease is characterized by the presence of *cysts* in the muscles and brain, which are formed by the worms during their larval stage.

cystic fibrosis

A serious and potentially fatal *genetic disorder*, characterized by a tendency to develop chronic lung infections combined with an inability to absorb fats and other nutrients from food. The main characteristic feature of cystic fibrosis (CF) is the secretion of sticky, viscous mucus in the nose, throat, airways, and intestines.

CAUSES
CF is caused by an inherited defect in a *gene*. The defect is recessive, which means that one faulty gene must be inherited from each parent before any abnormality appears. People with only one defective gene have no symptoms but are carriers and can pass the gene on to their children. About 1 in 25 people carry the defective gene, and about 1 in 2,500 babies is born with CF.

The defective gene causes a biochemical abnormality in which the faulty movement of ions across cell membranes affects mucus formation. As a result, the mucus-forming glands in several organs do not function properly. Most seriously, the glands in the lining of the bronchial tubes produce thick mucus, which predisposes the person to chronic lung infections. Another serious malfunction is poor or absent secretion of pancreatic enzymes, which are involved in the breakdown and absorption of fats in the intestine. The sweat glands are also affected and excrete excessive amounts of salt.

SYMPTOMS AND COMPLICATIONS
The course and severity of CF vary. Typically, a child passes unformed, pale, oily, foul-smelling *faeces* and may fail to thrive. Often, growth is stunted and the child has recurrent respiratory infections. Without prompt treatment, *pneumonia*, *bronchitis*, and *bronchiectasis* may develop, causing lung damage.

Most males and some females are infertile. Excessive salt loss from sweating may lead to *heatstroke* and collapse.

DIAGNOSIS AND TREATMENT

A prenatal diagnosis can be made by genetic analysis of samples from *chorionic villus sampling* or *amniocentesis*. Newborn babies can be screened for the disease using the *blood spot screening test*. If the tests indicate that a baby may have CF, a sweat test to look for high levels of salt in the sweat may be offered.

If CF is confirmed, doctors will discuss available treatments. Prompt treatment with intensive *physiotherapy*, *bronchodilator drugs*, and *antibiotics* helps to reduce the severity and frequency of lung infections; and lung function may be improved by dornase alfa, a genetically engineered version of a human enzyme, administered by *nebulizer*. *Pancreatin* and a protein- and calorie-rich diet are given to bring about weight gain and encourage more normal faeces. Supervision of the treatment is best carried out from a special centre staffed by paediatricians, nurses, and physiotherapists with particular knowledge of the disease.

OUTLOOK

The highly specialized treatment now available for people with CF maximizes their chances of a reasonable quality of life. About 9 in 10 children survive into their teens; many live well into their 40s. Progressive respiratory failure is the usual cause of death, but in some cases a heart–lung transplant may be considered.

HOW **CYSTECTOMY** IS DONE

Radical cystectomy is a major procedure performed under general anaesthesia. An incision is made in abdomen, and the ureters are cut and tied. The bladder and other lower abdominal organs are removed. The stoma is then formed from part of the small intestine. After the operation, the patient is given intravenous infusions of fluids, salt, and glucose until the intestines are functioning normally again.

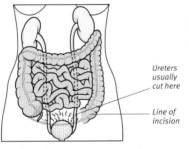

Ureters usually cut here

Line of incision

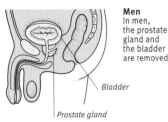

Men
In men, the prostate gland and the bladder are removed

Bladder

Prostate gland

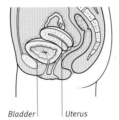

Women
In women, the uterus, fallopian tubes, ovaries, and part of the vagina (as well as the bladder) are removed

Bladder | Uterus

Large intestine

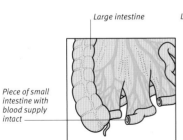

Piece of small intestine with blood supply intact

Formation of the stoma
A short section of small intestine, with its blood vessels, is detached from the remainder of the intestines. The two ureters are joined to this loop of intestine. One end of the loop is then sealed, and the other inserted through the abdominal wall to form the stoma.

Large intestine | Kidney | Ureter

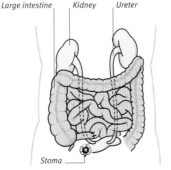

Stoma

Urine expulsion
Urine produced by the kidneys is channelled via the ureters and intestinal loop to the stoma, where it leaves the body.

---

cystinosis

A rare *genetic disorder* in which the *amino acid* cystine accumulates in cells throughout the body.

The juvenile form of cystinosis becomes apparent in the first year of life, at which time cystine deposits damage the eyes, resulting in impaired vision. The deposits also lead to potentially fatal *kidney failure*.

In the adult form, which is less severe, the main symptoms are eye problems, including extreme sensitivity to light (see *photophobia*). The kidneys are much less likely to be affected in adults than in children.

cystinuria

An inherited disorder (see *metabolism, inborn errors of*) in which the kidneys are unable effectively to process certain *amino acids* (the chemical compounds that make up proteins). Cystinuria is inherited in an autosomal recessive manner (see *genetic disorders*) and occurs in around one in 1,000 births.

Under normal circumstances, blood is filtered as it passes through the *kidneys*; a wide range of substances is removed, then useful compounds, such as amino acids, are reabsorbed. In cystinuria, this process does not work effectively. As a result, high levels of four amino acids, particularly cystine, occur in the urine. This excess cystine can result in the development of a rare form of kidney stones (see *renal calculi*) in both adults and children.

Cystinuria is usually detected in people who have symptoms of kidney stones, or in those who have passed stones that, on analysis, are found to contain cystine. The diagnosis can be confirmed by urine tests that measure the levels of amino acids. Treatment involves drinking large amounts of fluids regularly in order to dilute the urine and reduce the concentration of cystine. If the levels of cystine remain high, the drug *penicillamine* may be required to help prevent the formation of new stones.

cystitis

Inflammation of the lining of the *bladder* that is usually the result of a bacterial infection.

CAUSES

Cystitis is more common in women than in men because the *urethra* is short, so it is relatively easier for the bacteria that cause the disorder to pass into the bladder. A bladder *calculus* (stone), a *bladder tumour*, or a *urethral stricture* can obstruct urine flow and increase the risk of infection. In men, cystitis is rare; it usually occurs when an obstruction, such as an enlarged prostate gland (see *prostate, enlarged*), compresses the urethra. Cystitis in children is often associated with a structural abnormality of the *ureters*, which allows *reflux* (backward flow) of urine towards the kidneys.

The use of catheters (see *catheterization, urinary*) also carries the risk of infection. People with *diabetes mellitus* are especially susceptible to urinary tract infections because they have higher-than-normal levels of glucose in their urine which encourages growth of bacteria.

SYMPTOMS

The main symptoms are a frequent urge to pass *urine* and a burning pain on urinating. The urine may be foul-smelling or may contain blood. There may also be fever and chills, and lower abdominal discomfort. However, in children there are frequently no symptoms relating to the urinary tract, and they may have only generalized symptoms, such as fever and vomiting.

TREATMENT

Symptoms of mild cystitis may be relieved by drinking plenty of fluids, which helps to flush out the bladder. Any bacterial infection is treated with *antibiotic drugs* in order to prevent bacteria from spreading upwards to the kidneys and causing *pyelonephritis* (infection of the kidneys).

cystocele

A swelling in the front of the *vagina* that forms where the *bladder* pushes against weakened tissues in the vaginal wall. A cystocele may be associated with a prolapsed uterus (see *uterus, prolapse of*). Occasionally, a cystocele may pull the urethra out of position, causing *stress incontinence* or incomplete emptying of the bladder, which may in turn lead to infection of the retained urine (see *cystitis*).

Pelvic floor exercises may help to relieve symptoms. Surgery may be performed to lift and tighten the tissues at the front of the vagina.

cystometry

A procedure that is used to assess the function of the *bladder* and also to investigate urinary *incontinence* or poor bladder emptying; it is also used to detect abnormalities of the nerves that

supply the bladder. In this procedure, a catheter is inserted into the bladder, then the internal pressure is measured as the bladder is filled and then emptied. (See *urodynamics*.)

cystoscopy

The examination of the *urethra* and *bladder* using a cystoscope inserted up the urethra. A cystoscope is a viewing instrument, which can be rigid or flexible, sometimes with a camera at the tip (see *endoscopy*).

Cystoscopy is used to inspect the bladder for calculi (stones), bladder tumours, sites of bleeding and infection, and, in children, to investigate vesicoureteric reflux. Cystoscopy is also used to take urine samples from the ureters so that doctors can look for infection or tumour cells. Radiopaque dye may be injected into the ureters by means of the cystoscope during the X-ray procedure of retrograde pyelography (see *urography*).

Certain treatments can also be performed through the cystoscope. These include the removal of bladder tumours or calculi and the insertion of *stents* (narrow tubes) into a ureter to relieve an obstruction.

cystostomy

The surgical creation of a hole in the *bladder*. Cystostomy is usually carried out to drain *urine* in cases where the

introduction of a *catheter* (flexible tube) would be either inadvisable or simply impossible.

cystourethrography, voiding

An *X-ray* procedure that is used for studying the *bladder* during the passing of urine. Voiding cystourethrography is most commonly used in young children to detect abnormal *reflux* of urine (backflow of urine up the ureters) as the bladder empties. (See *urodynamics*.)

-cyte

A suffix denoting a *cell*. For example, a leukocyte is a white blood cell; an *erythrocyte* is a red blood cell.

cyto-

A prefix that means "related to a *cell*", as in cytology, the study of cells.

cytokine

A protein that is released by cells in response to the presence of harmful organisms such as *viruses*. Cytokines (such as *interferons*) bind to other cells, thereby activating the immune response (see *immune system*).

cytokine inhibitors

A group of drugs that are used to treat some cases of active *rheumatoid arthritis*, severe active *Crohn's disease*, moderate to severe *ulcerative colitis*, and severe active psoriatic arthritis. Examples of

PROCEDURE FOR **CYSTOSCOPY**

Cystoscopy involves passing a viewing instrument (cystoscope) up the urethra and into the bladder under local or general anaesthesia. There is no risk of damage to the genital organs or urinary tract, although the patient may feel some discomfort when passing urine for the first few days afterwards.

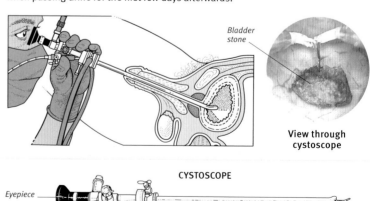

Bladder stone

View through cystoscope

CYSTOSCOPE

Eyepiece

Sheath

Forceps

CYTOLOGY METHODS

Cells for examination are obtained in several ways, depending on the part of the body being investigated. Cells from body surfaces may be collected by scraping or swabs; those from internal structures may be obtained by biopsy or aspiration.

Improvements in collection techniques have made it possible to take cells from previously inaccessible sites. If a cytologist can make a diagnosis from cells removed in these ways, the patient may be spared an exploratory operation.

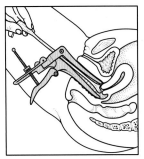

Cells from the cervix
The vagina is held open with a speculum. Cells are scraped from the surface of the cervix with a spatula (above) or a special brush.

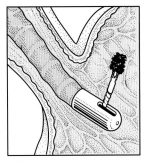

Cells from the respiratory tract or oesophagus
These cells are usually obtained by using an endoscope fitted with a small brush or suction tube.

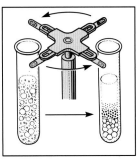

Cells from body fluids
These cells are obtained either by passing the fluid through a filter or centrifugation (spinning the fluid rapidly to separate out the cells).

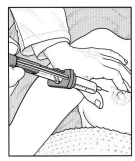

Aspiration biopsy
In this procedure, a very fine needle is passed into a suspected tumour and a biopsy sample of cells is withdrawn.

cytokine inhibitors include infliximab, etanercept, and adalimumab. Because of the serious side effects of these drugs, they are given only under specialist supervision and then only when other treatments are unsuitable or have proved to be unsuccessful.

cytology

The study of cells. The main use of cytology is to detect abnormal cells; it is widely used to screen for cancer (as in the *cervical smear test*) or to confirm a diagnosis of cancer, and is increasingly used in antenatal screening to detect certain fetal abnormalities. Examination of cells from body fluids helps doctors to determine the cause of conditions such as *pleural effusion* (fluid in the pleural cavity around the lungs) and *ascites* (abnormal accumulation of fluid in the abdominal cavity); for example the tests can identify whether cancer or infection is present.

Cells are collected by procedures such as scraping or fine-needle aspiration *biopsy*. For antenatal tests, cells from the fluid that surrounds and cushions the fetus in the uterus are obtained by means of *amniocentesis* or *chorionic villus sampling*.

cytomegalovirus

One of the most common of the *herpes* viruses. Cytomegalovirus (CMV) infection causes infected cells to appear enlarged. The virus may produce an illness that is similar to glandular fever (see *mononucleosis, infectious*), but usually there are no symptoms. Individuals with impaired immunity are more seriously infected. CMV in a pregnant woman can cause birth defects and brain damage in the baby.

cytopathology

The microscopic study of *cells* in health and disease. (See also *cytology*.)

cytopenia

A general term for a deficiency of any of the various types of blood cells. Specific types of cytopenia include *neutropenia* (deficiency of neutrophils, a type of white blood cell) and thrombocytopenia (deficiency of platelets).

cytoplasm

The jellylike substance that contains the internal structures of a *cell*. Cytoplasm is 90 per cent water, but it also also contains enzymes, amino acids, and other chemicals that are required for cell function.

cytotoxic drugs

A group of *anticancer drug*s that kill or damage abnormal *cells*. Cytotoxic drugs may also damage or kill healthy cells, especially those that multiply rapidly, such as the cells in hair follicles or those in the intestinal lining.

cytotoxic T-cell

Also known as a killer T-cell or a CD8 lymphocyte, a type of white *blood cell* that plays an important role in the immune system. Cytotoxic T-cells destroy abnormal or cancerous cells and cells that are infected with viruses. Cytotoxic T-cells also play a role in rejection of tissue and organ transplants.

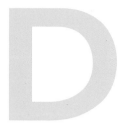

D

dacryocystitis

Inflammation of the tear sac, usually resulting from the blockage of the tear duct. The condition sometimes occurs in infants if the tear duct has not developed normally. In adults, it may follow inflammation in the nose or an injury. The cause is often unknown.

Symptoms include pain, redness, and swelling between the inner corner of the eyelids and the nose. Infection may occur and cause a discharge.

The obstruction may be cleared by flushing the tear duct with saline. *Antibiotic* eye-drops or ointment are given for infection. In infants, massaging the tear sac may clear a blockage. Surgery to drain the tear sac (dacryocystorhinostomy) is occasionally necessary.

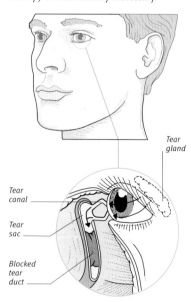

Mechanism of dacryocystitis
Inflammation of the tear sac may occur when the duct through which tears drain away from the tear sac becomes blocked.

dactylitis

Inflammation of the fingers or toes. Dactylitis sometimes occurs in people who have the inherited blood disorder *sickle cell anaemia*. Less commonly, the condition can be associated with *tuberculosis* or *syphilis* infection.

Daktacort

A brand name for a cream containing a combination of synthetic *hydrocortisone* (a corticosteroid drug) and *miconazole* (an antifungal drug). Daktacort is used to treat inflamed skin conditions, such as *eczema* and *dermatitis*, where a fungal infection is also suspected.

Daktarin

A brand name for *miconazole*, an antifungal drug used in the treatment of *athlete's foot* and other common fungal skin infections. Daktarin gel is used to treat oral thrush (see *candidiasis*).

Dalacin

A brand name for *clindamycin*, an antibiotic that may be applied to the skin to treat severe *acne* or as a vaginal cream in the treatment of bacterial vaginal infections. Due to its toxic side effects, Dalacin is given as tablets or by injection only for serious infections.

danazol

A drug used for treating *endometriosis* (a condition in which fragments of the uterine lining occur elsewhere in the pelvic cavity), severe pain and tenderness in noncancerous breast disease, and *menorrhagia* (heavy periods).

Danazol suppresses the release of *gonadotrophin hormones* (pituitary hormones that stimulate activity in the ovaries), which in turn reduces the production of the hormone oestrogen. This action usually prevents ovulation and causes irregularity or absence of menstrual periods.

Possible adverse effects include nausea, rash, and weight gain. Pregnancy should be avoided while taking danazol.

D and C

An abbreviation for dilatation and curettage, a gynaecological procedure in which the cervix (neck of the *uterus*) is dilated, then the *endometrium* (lining of the uterus) is scraped away and a sample is removed for analysis. D and C was once used to diagnose disorders of the uterus, but has largely been replaced by hysteroscopy, an endoscopic technique for viewing the uterus lining or taking a *biopsy* (tissue sample) from the lining. Endometrial biopsies can also be taken using a small vacuum suction device.

dander

Minute scales shed from an animal's skin, hair, or feathers. Dander from humans and pets floats in the air or settles on surfaces, making up a large proportion of household dust. Some people are allergic to animal dander and develop the symptoms of allergic *rhinitis* (hay fever) or of *asthma* if they inhale the scales.

dandruff

A harmless condition in which dead skin is shed from the scalp, often as white flakes. The usual cause is seborrhoeic *dermatitis*. Frequent use of antidandruff shampoo usually controls dandruff.

danthron

See *dantron*.

dantrolene

A *muscle-relaxant drug* used to relieve muscle spasm caused by *spinal injury*, *stroke*, or neurological disorders such as *cerebral palsy*. The drug does not cure the underlying disorder but often improves mobility. Dantrolene is also used in the treatment of malignant *hyperthermia* (a sudden, severe rise in body temperature brought on by general anaesthesia).

dantron

A stimulant *laxative drug* used to treat constipation in the terminally ill. Constipation is common in these patients as a side effect of treatment with opioid *analgesic drugs* (painkillers). Dantron may colour the urine red.

dapsone

An *antibacterial drug* used to treat *Hansen's disease* (leprosy), *dermatitis herpetiformis*, and *pneumocystis pneumonia*. The drug may cause nausea, vomiting, and, rarely, damage to the liver, red blood cells, and nerves.

Darier's disease

A rare, progressive skin disorder, also known as keratosis follicularis, that is inherited as an autosomal dominant genetic trait (see *genetic disorders*). The disease is characterized by the development of a number of greasy, pigmented *papules* (raised spots) on the scalp, the face and neck, behind the ears, and along the middle of the back.

daydreaming

The conjuring up of pleasant or exciting images or situations in one's mind during waking hours.

day surgery

Surgical treatment carried out in a hospital or clinic without an overnight stay. The proportion of all operations performed on a day-surgery basis has risen substantially in recent years. Modern anaesthetics and surgical techniques, in particular *minimally invasive surgery*, allow a swifter recovery than in the past, so that patients can often return home within a few hours of surgery.

DDAVP

A brand name for *desmopressin*, which is a synthetic form of *ADH* (antidiuretic hormone).

DDT

The abbreviation for the insecticide dichlorodiphenyltrichloroethane. DDT was once widely used in the fight against diseases transmitted by insects. However, some insects have developed resistance to the toxic effects of DDT, and this resistance can be passed on to their offspring. (See also *pesticides*.)

deafness

Complete or partial loss of hearing in one or both ears. There are two types of deafness: conductive deafness, caused by faulty propagation of sound from the outer to the inner ear; and sensorineural deafness, in which there is a failure in the transmission of sounds to the brain.

CAUSES

The most common cause of conductive deafness in adults is *earwax. Otosclerosis*, a condition in which the stapes (a small bone in the middle ear) loses its normal mobility, is a less common cause. In children, conductive deafness is usually due to *otitis media* (middle-ear infection) or *glue ear* (accumulation of sticky fluid in the middle ear). In rare cases, deafness results from a ruptured eardrum (see *eardrum, perforated*).

Sensorineural deafness may be present from birth. This type of deafness may result from a *birth injury* or damage resulting from maternal infection with *rubella* in early pregnancy. Damage to the inner ear may also occur soon after birth as the result of severe neonatal *jaundice*.

In later life, sensorineural deafness can be due to damage to the cochlea and/or labyrinth of the inner ear. It may result from prolonged exposure to loud noise, or be caused by *Ménière's disease*, certain drugs, or some viral infections. The cochlea and labyrinth also degenerate naturally with old age, resulting in *presbyacusis*.

Sensorineural deafness due to damage to the acoustic nerve may be the result of an *acoustic neuroma* (a noncancerous tumour that develops on the nerve).

SYMPTOMS AND SIGNS

A baby who is congenitally deaf fails to respond to sounds, and, although crying is often normal, he or she does not babble or make the usual baby noises that lead to speech. In an adult who has started to become deaf, sounds heard are not only quieter than before, but may be distorted and less clear.

Deafness may be accompanied by *tinnitus* (noises in the ear) and *vertigo* (dizziness and loss of balance). Sometimes deafness can lead to confusion and sometimes to *depression*.

DIAGNOSIS

All newborn babies are given a *hearing test* in the first few weeks of life to detect congenital deafness. For older children and adults, examination of the ear with an *otoscope* (a viewing instrument with a light attached) can show if the outer-ear canal is blocked by wax, or if the eardrum is inflamed, perforated, or has fluid behind it. After a physical examination, hearing tests may be performed; these tests can determine whether deafness is conductive or sensorineural.

TREATMENT

The treatment depends on the exact cause of the deafness. Removal of excess earwax remedies conductive deafness in many cases. Otosclerosis is generally treated by an operation known as *stapedectomy*, in which the stapes is replaced with an artificial substitute. Glue ear may also be treated by surgery (see *myringotomy*) and by the insertion of a *grommet* (a small tube that allows fluid to drain away from the middle ear).

Many children who are born deaf can learn to communicate effectively, often by using sign language. *Cochlear implants* (electrodes implanted in the inner ear that can receive sound signals) may help profoundly deaf adults and children, but they are not suitable for everyone. People who have sensorineural deafness usually need *hearing-aids* to increase the volume of sound reaching the inner ear. *Lip-reading* is invaluable for people who have difficulty hearing, whatever the type and severity of their deafness. Various other aids, such as an amplifier for the earpiece of a telephone, are available to help deaf people perform everyday tasks. (See also *ear*; *hearing*.)

DEAFNESS

Some possible causes of deafness
The part of the ear affected in each case is shown. Some of the problems (e.g. earwax, which affects the outer ear, and glue ear, which affects the middle ear) cause conductive deafness; others (e.g. drug toxicity and Ménière's disease, which affect the inner ear) cause sensorineural deafness.

D

death

Permanent cessation of all vital functions. The classic indicators of death are the permanent cessation of heart and lung function, and, in almost all cases, these remain the criteria by which death is certified. *Brain death* is the irreversible cessation of all functions of the entire brain, including the *brainstem* (the part of the brain that controls involuntary actions such as breathing).

The diagnosis of death under normal circumstances, when the individual is not on a *ventilator*, is based on the absence of breathing, absence of heartbeat, and on the pupils being fixed wide open and unresponsive to light.

When an individual has been placed on a ventilator machine, the criteria for diagnosing brain death are based on clear evidence of irreversible damage to the brain; persistent deep *coma*; no attempts at breathing when the patient is taken off the ventilator; and complete lack of brainstem function. (See also *death, sudden*; *mortality*.)

death rate

See *mortality*.

death rattle

A noisy form of breathing resulting from the retention of *sputum* (mucous material) in the airways of a dying person who is no longer able to swallow it or cough it up. Although unpleasant for the person's companions, it does not appear to cause distress to him or her.

death, sudden

Unexpected death in a person who previously seemed to be healthy. The most common cause of sudden death in adults is *cardiac arrest* (cessation of the heartbeat). *Cardiomyopathy* (disease of the heart muscle) may cause sudden death at any age, and its presence may have been unsuspected. Sudden death may also occur as a result of *stroke* or in people with unsuspected *myocarditis* (inflammation of the heart muscle) or *pneumonia*. Less common causes of a sudden death include *anaphylactic shock* (a severe allergic reaction), a severe attack of *asthma*, and *suicide*.

In infants, death without warning is termed *sudden infant death syndrome* (SIDS), or cot death.

The sudden death of a person of any age must be reported to the coroner, who decides whether there should be an *autopsy* (postmortem examination).

death, sudden infant

The sudden, unexpected death of an infant that cannot be explained. See *sudden infant death syndrome (SIDS)*.

debility

Generalized weakness and lack of energy. It may be due to a physical disorder (such as *anaemia*) or to a psychological disorder (such as *depression*).

debridement

Surgical removal of foreign material and/or dead, damaged, or infected tissue from a wound or burn in order to expose healthy tissue. Such treatment promotes the healthy healing of badly damaged skin, muscle, and other tissues in the body.

decalcification, dental

The dissolving of minerals in a tooth. Dental decalcification is the first stage of tooth decay. It is caused by bacteria in *plaque* acting on the refined carbohydrates (mainly sugars) in food to produce acid, which, after prolonged or repeated exposure, causes changes to occur on the surface of the tooth. If the decalcification penetrates the enamel layer, it spreads into the dentine and permits bacteria to enter the inner pulp. (See also *caries, dental*.)

decay, dental

See *caries, dental*.

decerebrate

The state of being without a functioning *cerebrum*, the main controlling part of the brain. This situation occurs if the *brainstem* is severed, which effectively isolates the cerebrum.

decidua

The lining of the *uterus* (womb) during the course of pregnancy. The surface layers of the decidua are shed from the body during *childbirth*.

deciduous teeth

See *primary teeth*.

decompensation

The loss of an organ's ability to meet the requirements of the body. The term "decompensation" is usually used to describe lessening function in an organ that has been progressively damaged by disease. For example, if the heart decompensates, it becomes unable to maintain an adequate circulation.

The word can also be used with regard to mental illness, as in *depression*, when an individual may lose his or her usual compensation mechanisms (strategies by which a person makes up for real or imagined deficiencies) and suddenly deteriorates.

decomposition

The gradual breakdown of organic matter (such as food or dead tissue) into other chemical compounds by way of bacterial and/or fungal action, heat, or other processes.

decompression sickness

A hazard of divers and of others who work in or breathe compressed air or other mixtures of gases. Decompression sickness is also called "the bends". It results from gas bubbles forming in the tissues and impeding the flow of blood.

CAUSE

At depth, divers accumulate inert gas in their tissues from the high-pressure gas mixture they breathe (see *scuba-diving medicine*). Problems can usually be avoided by allowing the excess gas in their tissues to escape slowly into the lungs during controlled slow ascent or release of pressure. If the ascent is too rapid and the pressure falls too quickly, gas can no longer be held within the tissues and is released as bubbles.

SYMPTOMS

Bubbles of gas may block blood vessels, causing symptoms such as skin itching

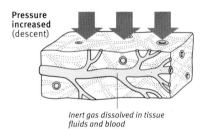

Inert gas dissolved in tissue fluids and blood

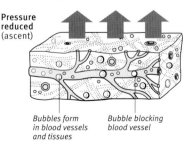

Bubbles form in blood vessels and tissues   *Bubble blocking blood vessel*

How decompression sickness occurs
On ascent, pressure is reduced rapidly and the gas may form bubbles that may, in turn, cause symptoms. Divers avoid this by ascending slowly.

and mottling and severe pain in and around the larger joints. Symptoms of nervous system impairment (such as leg weakness or visual disturbances) are particularly serious, as is a painful, tight feeling across the chest.

TREATMENT

Divers with decompression sickness are immediately placed inside a recompression chamber. Pressure in the chamber is raised, causing the bubbles within the tissues to redissolve. Subsequently, the pressure in the chamber is slowly reduced, allowing the excess gas to escape safely via the lungs.

OUTLOOK

If treated promptly by recompression, most divers with the "bends" make a full recovery. In serious, untreated cases, however, there may be long-term complications such as partial paralysis. Repeated episodes may lead to degenerative disorders of the bones or joints.

decompression, spinal canal

Surgery to relieve pressure on the spinal cord or a nerve root emerging from it (see *microdiscectomy*). Pressure may have various causes, including a *disc prolapse* ("slipped" disc); a tumour or abscess of the spinal cord; or a tumour, abscess, or fracture of the ver-

tebrae. Any of these conditions can cause weakness or paralysis of the limbs and loss of bladder control.

To treat major disc prolapses and tumours, a *laminectomy* (removal of the bony arches of one or more vertebrae) to expose the affected part of the cord or nerve roots may be performed.

Recovery after treatment depends on the severity and duration of the pressure, the success of the surgery in relieving the pressure, and whether any damage is sustained by the nerves during the operation.

decongestant drugs

Drugs that are used to relieve *nasal congestion*, commonly in people with upper *respiratory tract infections*. They work by narrowing blood vessels in the membranes lining the nose. This action reduces swelling, inflammation, and the amount of mucus produced buy the nasal lining. Common drugs include ephedrine, xylometazoline, and phenylephrine. Small amounts of these drugs are present in many over-the-counter cold remedies.

Taken by mouth, decongestant drugs may cause tremor and palpitations. Adverse effects are unlikely with nose drops, but if taken for several days they

become ineffective and symptoms may then recur or worsen despite continued treatment. Decongestants may not be suitable for people who have certain medical conditions and they must be avoided by people taking MAOIs (*monoamine oxidase inhibitors*, a group of *antidepressant drugs*).

decubitus

The position of reclining or lying down, as in a decubitus ulcer (see *bedsore*).

decubitus ulcer

See *bedsore*.

decussation

A point at which two or more structures in the body cross over each other to the opposite side. An example is the point at which nerve fibres intercross in the *central nervous system*.

deep vein thrombosis

See *thrombosis, deep vein*.

DEET

The commonly used abbreviation for diethyltoluamide, the active ingredient in many insect repellents. It can be applied to the skin and clothing and helps prevent bites from many types in insects, including the mosquitoes that transmit *malaria*, *dengue*, and *West Nile virus*. Deet is not generally recommended for use on children.

defaecation

The expulsion of waste material as *faeces* from the body through the anus.

defence mechanisms

Techniques used by the mind to lessen unpleasant or unwelcome emotions, impulses, experiences, or events, and to avoid external or internal conflict.

TYPES

The principal defence mechanism is repression, which is the suppression of unacceptable thoughts. Other types of defence mechanism include displacement, rationalization, projection, reaction formation, and isolation.

In displacement, dangerous thoughts or feelings are redirected at a harmless object; for example, someone who is angry at another person may kick the furniture instead of hitting that person. Rationalization involves reinterpreting thoughts or actions in a more acceptable way; for example, a person may criticize someone else but claim "It's for

D

THE ACTION OF DECONGESTANTS

Decongestants work by narrowing blood vessels in the membranes that line the nose. This action reduces swelling, inflammation, and the amount of mucus produced by the nasal lining.

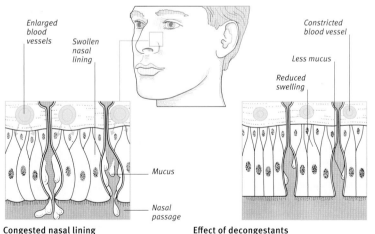

Congested nasal lining
When blood vessels enlarge in response to infection or irritation, increased amounts of fluid pass into the lining, which swells and produces more mucus.

Effect of decongestants
Chemicals stimulate constriction of the blood vessels in the nasal lining, which reduces swelling, mucus production, and nasal congestion.

your own good". In projection, a person attributes his or her own faults to someone else, for example by thinking "that person hates me" when in fact he or she hates that person. In reaction formation, an unacceptable feeling is hidden by actions that suggest the opposite; for example, someone may disguise hatred for another person by showing great concern for that person. In the mechanism of isolation, unpleasant memories (for example, of being assaulted) are retained but the feelings that go with them are hidden, so that a person may recall such an event apparently without emotion.

defibrillation

Also known as cardioversion, the administration of one or more brief electric shocks to the heart, usually via two metal plates, or paddles, placed on the chest over the heart. It is performed to return the heart's rhythm to normal in some types of *arrhythmia* (irregular or rapid heartbeat), such as *atrial fibrillation* or *ventricular fibrillation*.

Defibrillation can be carried out as an emergency procedure to treat ventricular fibrillation, which is a cause of *cardiac arrest* and most commonly occurs after a heart attack (see *myocardial infarction*). It can also be used as a planned treatment, in which case it is performed under a brief general *anaesthesia*. Breathing may be maintained by artificial means for the duration of the procedure.

deficiency anaemia

A type of anaemia. See *anaemia, iron-deficiency*; *pernicious anaemia*.

defluoridation

The removal of excess fluoride from drinking water to prevent *fluorosis* (mottling of tooth enamel) in consumers. (See also *fluoridation*; *fluoride*.)

defoliant poisoning

The toxic effects of plant poisons that cause leaves to drop off. Defoliants are poisonous if swallowed. Examples of defoliants include sodium *chlorate*, potassium chlorate, phenoxy herbicides, *paraquat, dioxin*, and hexachlorobenzene.

deformity

Any malformation or distortion of part of the body. Deformities may be congenital (present from birth), or they may be acquired as a result of injury, disorder, or disuse.

Most congenital deformities are relatively rare. Among the more common are club-foot (*talipes*) and *cleft lip and palate*. Injuries that can cause deformity include burns, torn muscles, and broken bones. Disorders that may cause deformity include certain nerve problems, some deficiencies, such as *rickets*, and *Paget's disease* of the bone. Disuse of a part of the body can lead to deformity through stiffening and *contracture* of unused muscles or tendons.

Many deformities can be corrected by orthopaedic techniques, *plastic surgery*, or specific exercises.

degeneration

Physical and/or chemical changes in cells, tissues, or organs that reduce their efficiency. Degeneration is a feature of aging and may also be due to disease processes. Other known causes include injury, reduced blood supply, poisoning (by alcohol, for example), or a diet deficient in a specific vitamin. (See also *degenerative disorders*.)

degenerative disorders

A term covering a wide range of conditions in which there is progressive impairment in the structure and function of a body system, organ, or tissue. The number of specialized cells or structures in the organ affected is usually reduced, and cells are replaced by *connective tissue* or scar tissue.

Degenerative nervous system disorders include *Alzheimer's disease, motor neuron disease, Huntington's disease*, and *Parkinson's disease*. Degenerative disorders of the eye include Leber's *optic atrophy* and senile *macular degeneration*. Degenerative disorders of the joints include *osteoarthritis*. Muscle degeneration occurs in *muscular dystrophies*.

Some degree of hardening of the arteries seems to be a feature of normal aging. However, in certain people degenerative changes in the muscle coat of the arteries are unusually severe, and calcium deposits may be seen on *X-rays* (as in Monckeberg's sclerosis, which is a type of *arteriosclerosis*).

In most cases, little can be done to slow the progress of the disease, but it is often possible to relieve symptoms with drug treatment.

Degos syndrome

A rare disorder that affects the linings of small and medium-sized arteries throughout the body, particularly in the skin, intestine, and nervous system, causing the vessels to become blocked. The cause is unknown.

The disease typically produces multiple small skin lesions that initially appear as red, raised spots and then form depressed, white scars. Lesions may then form in arteries supplying other parts of the body, such as the intestine and the nervous system. This development may cause severe or even life-threatening problems, such as *stroke* from lesions that have formed in the brain and perforation of the intestine by lesions that penetrate through the intestinal wall (see *peritonitis*).

dehiscence

The splitting open of a partly healed wound. The term is most commonly used to refer to the splitting open of a surgical incision that has been closed with sutures or clips.

dehydration

A condition in which a person's *water* content is at a dangerously low. level Water accounts for about 60 per cent of a man's body weight and about 50 per cent of a woman's. The total content of water (plus mineral salts and other substances dissolved in the body fluids) must be kept within fairly narrow limits to enable the healthy functioning of cells and tissues.

CAUSES

Dehydration occurs due to inadequate intake of fluids or excessive fluid loss. The latter may occur as a result of severe or prolonged vomiting or diarrhoea, or in people who have poorly controlled *diabetes mellitus, diabetes insipidus*, and certain types of *kidney failure*. Children are particularly susceptible to dehydration due to diarrhoea.

SYMPTOMS

The symptoms of severe dehydration are extreme thirst; dry lips and tongue; an increase in heart rate and breathing rate; dizziness; confusion; lethargy; and eventual *coma*. The skin looks dry and loses its elasticity. Any urine passed is small in quantity and dark-coloured. If there is also salt depletion (for example, due to heavy sweating), there may be headaches, cramps, and pallor.

TREATMENT

It is important to drink plenty of fluids. In cases of persistent vomiting and diarrhoea, *rehydration therapy* is required; salt and glucose rehydration mixtures are available from chemists.

In severe cases of dehydration, fluids may be given intravenously; the water/salt balance is carefully monitored by blood tests and adjusted as necessary.

déjà vu

French for "already seen". A sense of having already experienced an event that is happening at the moment. Frequent occurrence may sometimes be a symptom of *temporal lobe epilepsy.*

delayed allergy

A type of *hypersensitivity* reaction that, unlike most forms of *allergy*, does not develop immediately on exposure to a particular *allergen.*

Delayed allergies, also called type IV hypersensitivity reactions, may result from bacterial, viral, fungal, or protozoal infections or from *vaccination* with a live virus vaccine. Examples of such delayed allergic reactions include *contact dermatitis* and the body's response to infection in *tuberculosis.*

delayed dentition

The late *eruption of teeth.* The term "delayed dentition" may refer to the eruption of the first deciduous teeth (see *primary teeth*) after the end of the 13th month of life or to the eruption of the first *permanent teeth* after the seventh year of life. Delayed dentition is a feature of various conditions that result in generally restricted growth (see *short stature*), such as *hypothyroidism.*

delayed puberty

Onset of *puberty* (sexual maturation) after the age of 14. In most cases, the child is simply developing at a slower rate than normal, a tendency that often runs in families, but in some cases there may be an underlying disorder.

One possible underlying cause of delayed puberty is underproduction of sex hormones. Rarely, the condition results from a problem with the *hypothalamus* or the *pituitary gland*, which are responsible for secreting sex hormones; a genetic abnormality affecting sexual development, such as *Klinefelter's syndrome* in boys or *Turner's syndrome* in girls; or a long-term illness, such as *Crohn's disease.* Certain lifestyle factors, such as excessive exercise or an inadequate diet, may also delay puberty.

Treatment depends on the underlying cause. If delayed puberty runs in the child's family, no action may be needed. In some cases, however, conditions causing delayed puberty may also lead to *infertility*, so the child may need further investigations in the future if he or she wishes to have children.

delayed shock

A common term for severe mental or physical reactions that may occur some time after a traumatic event (see *post-traumatic stress disorder*; *shock*; *stress.*)

delinquency

Criminal behaviour in a young person who is below the official age at which he or she can be prosecuted. The term is often extended to include behaviour such as *drug abuse*, playing truant, or running away from home. Delinquency is probably a result of a combination of social, psychological, and biological factors. *Child guidance* or *family therapy* may be recommended. Persistent offenders may be sent to special schools, taken into care, or made wards of court.

delirium

A state of acute mental confusion, commonly brought on by physical illness. Symptoms vary according to personality, environment, and the severity of illness. They may include failure to understand events or remember what has been happening, restlessness, mood swings, hallucinations, and panic. Fever and disturbances of body chemistry are often contributory factors.

Children and older people are most susceptible to delirium, particularly as a result of infection, following surgery, or when there is a pre-existing brain disturbance (such as *dementia* in an elderly person). Drugs, poisons, and alcohol are common precipitants.

delirium tremens

A state of confusion accompanied by trembling and vivid hallucinations. It usually arises in chronic alcoholics after withdrawal or abstinence from alcohol. Early symptoms include restlessness, agitation, trembling, and sleeplessness. The person may then develop a rapid heartbeat, fever, and dilation of the pupils. Sweating, confusion, hallucinations, and convulsions may also occur.

Hospital admission for treatment is usually necessary. Treatment consists of rest, rehydration, and sedation. Vitamin injections, particularly of thiamine (see *vitamin B complex*), may be given, because some symptoms are linked to thiamine deficiency.

delivery

The expulsion or extraction of a baby from the mother's uterus. In most cases, the baby lies lengthwise in the uterus with its head facing downwards; it is delivered head first through the vaginal opening by a combination of uterine contractions and the mother's pushing (see *childbirth*).

If the baby is lying in an abnormal position (see *breech delivery*; *malpresentation*), if uterine contractions are weak, or if the baby's head is large in relation to the size of the mother's pelvis (known as *cephalopelvic disproportion*), a *forceps delivery* or *vacuum extraction* may be required. If a vaginal delivery is impossible or dangerous to the mother or the baby, a *caesarean section* is necessary.

deltoid

The triangular muscle of the shoulder region that forms the rounded flesh of the outer part of the upper arm, and passes up and over the shoulder joint. The wide end of the muscle is attached to the scapula (shoulderblade) and the clavicle (collarbone). The muscle fibres meet to form the apex of the triangle, which is attached to the humerus (the upper-arm bone) at a position about halfway down its length.

The central, strongest part of the deltoid muscle raises the arm sideways. The front and back parts of the muscle are used to twist the arm.

LOCATION OF THE **DELTOID**

The deltoid muscle of the shoulder region forms the rounded, outer part of the upper arm and is attached to the scapula and clavicle.

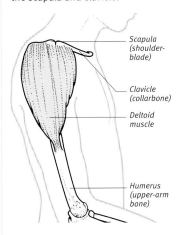

Scapula (shoulderblade)

Clavicle (collarbone)

Deltoid muscle

Humerus (upper-arm bone)

delusion

A fixed, irrational idea not shared by others and not responding to reasoned argument. The central idea in a paranoid delusion involves persecution or jealousy; for instance, a person may falsely believe that he or she is being poisoned or that a partner is persistently unfaithful (see *paranoia*).

Persistent delusions are an indication of serious mental illness, particularly *schizophrenia* and *manic–depressive illness*. (See also *hallucination*; *illusion*.)

demand pacemaker

A permanent artificial cardiac *pacemaker* (a device that sends electrical impulses to the *heart* to maintain a regular *heartbeat*) that discharges impulses only when the *heart rate* is abnormal. Such a pacemaker may be set to function only if the heart rate slows, or alternatively to override an abnormally rapid rate. (See also *fixed-rate pacemaker*.)

demasculinization

The loss, in a male, of normal male secondary sexual characteristics (see *sexual characteristics, secondary*). This includes reduced facial hair growth, along with testicular *atrophy* (wasting away of the testes) and shrinkage of the *prostate* gland. Demasculinization may occur in a range of conditions in which the testes are damaged or diseased. It may also result from disorders such as *cirrhosis* and *kidney failure*, which interfere with the processing in the body of the female sex hormone *oestrogen*. (See also *feminization*; *intersex*; *masculinization*; *sex determination*.)

dementia

A condition characterized by a generalized deterioration in brain function. Dementia most commonly affects the elderly; about 1 in 20 people over the age of 65, and up to 1 in 5 people over the age of 80, have the disorder.

CAUSES AND TYPES

Dementia is usually caused by damage to brain tissue. It is most commonly due to *Alzheimer's disease*, which causes changes in the structure and chemistry of the brain. The second most common form is *multi-infarct dementia*. In this condition, narrowed or blocked arteries in the brain deprive the tissue of blood and oxygen; repeated small *strokes* (episodes of tissue damage due to a lack of blood) occur, causing deterioration that develops gradually and in stages. Other,

rare forms of dementia include Lewy body dementia (in which small, spherical structures called Lewy bodies appear in the brain tissue); *AIDS*-related dementia; and deterioration that occurs as a result of progressive brain disorders such as *Parkinson's disease*.

In a small proportion of cases (mainly in people younger than 65), dementia is due to a treatable cause such as a head injury, a *brain tumour*, *encephalitis*, *alcohol dependence*, a vitamin or hormone deficiency, or a side effect of certain medications.

SYMPTOMS

The main symptoms of dementia are progressive memory loss, disorientation, and confusion. The affected person may not remember recent events, he or she may become easily lost in a familiar neighbourhood, and may be confused over days and dates. These symptoms may gradually come on and they may be hardly noticeable at first; in addition, the person may cover up any problems by *confabulation* (making up explanations in order to fill the gaps in his or her memory).

Sudden outbursts or embarrassing behaviour may be the first obvious signs of dementia. Unpleasant personality traits may be magnified; families of those affected may have to endure accusations, unreasonable demands, or even assault. *Paranoia*, *depression*, and *delusions* may occur as the disease progresses. Irritability or anxiety gives way to indifference towards all feelings and events. Personal care and hygiene are neglected, and speech becomes incoherent. Eventually, affected people may need total nursing care.

TREATMENT

The rare cases of dementia due to a treatable underlying cause may be significantly improved or even cured by appropriate treatment of the cause. However, most types of dementia do not fall into this category and treatment is based on the management of symptoms. In such cases, the affected person should be kept clean and well-nourished, in comfortable surroundings, and with good nursing care. These measures can help to ease distress for both the patient and his or her family. In some cases, encouraging the affected person to stay as mentally active as possible may be helpful.

For some people with mild to moderate Alzheimer's disease, drug treatment with *acetylcholinesterase inhibitors* such

as donepezil may improve behavioural symptoms and may also slow the deterioration in mental function. Regardless of treatment, however, Alzheimer's disease is progressive.

dementia praecox

An outdated term that was formerly used to describe severe *schizophrenia*, especially that affecting adolescents or young adults.

demineralization

Excessive loss of the *minerals* calcium and phosphate from bone. Generalized demineralization can occur as a result of immobility following an illness or injury, or may be due to a bone disease such as *osteomalacia*. Patchy demineralization can be a result of bone metastases (cancerous tumours that have spread from elsewhere in the body); this condition causes areas of bone to weaken, increasing the risk of *fractures*.

De Morgan's spots

See *Campbell de Morgan's spots*.

De Morsier's syndrome

Also called septo-optic dysplasia, a rare disorder that results from the abnormal development of the *optic disc* in the eye, the *pituitary gland*, and parts of the brain. De Morsier's syndrome causes eye problems, including blindness in one or both eyes, abnormal eye movements such as *nystagmus*, *squint*, and dilation of the pupils (rather than the normal contraction) in response to light. Other symptoms of the syndrome include *seizures*, *hypotonia* (poor muscle tone), and hormonal problems, commonly a deficiency in growth hormone leading to short stature.

Treatment aims to relieve symptoms such as hormonal deficiencies, and to provide *rehabilitation* for affected people who have impaired vision.

demyelination

Breakdown of the fatty sheaths that surround and electrically insulate nerve fibres. The sheaths provide nutrients to the nerve fibres and are vital to the passage of electrical impulses along them. Demyelination "short-circuits" the functioning of the nerve, which causes loss of sensation, coordination, and power in specific areas of the body. The affected nerves may be within the *central nervous system* (CNS), comprising the brain and the spinal cord, or may be

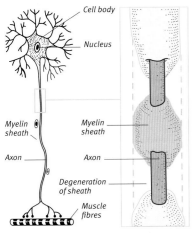

Mechanism of demyelination
The fatty myelin sheaths that surround and insulate nerve fibres break down, causing the affected nerves to "short-circuit".

part of the *peripheral nervous system*, which links the CNS to sense receptors, muscles, glands, and other organs throughout the body.

Patches of demyelination are visible on *MRI* (magnetic resonance imaging) scans of the brain in people who have *multiple sclerosis*, a disease with symptoms that include blurred vision, muscle weakness, and loss of coordination. The cause of the demyelination in multiple sclerosis is not known. In many cases of the disease, episodes of demyelination alternate with periods in which there is partial or complete recovery of nerve function.

In the rare disorder *encephalomyelitis*, there is inflammation of nerve cells in the CNS and sometimes also areas of demyelination along the nerves.

dendritic ulcer

A type of *corneal ulcer* (affecting the transparent dome that forms the front of the eyeball) with threadlike extensions that branch out from the centre. Dendritic ulcers are commonly due to infection with *herpes simplex* virus.

denervation

The loss of the *nerve* supply to an area of skin, a muscle, an organ, or another body part. Nerves may be damaged by injury or by disease, or as a result of surgery. A denervated area loses all sensation, and its functioning may be impaired; for example, muscles may become paralysed. In some cases, the affected nerves may regrow, but often the damage is permanent.

dengue

A tropical disease caused by a virus spread by the mosquito *AEDES AEGYPTI*. The symptoms include fever, headache, rash, and joint and muscle pains, which often subside after about three days. There is no specific treatment for dengue. Preventive measures consist of protecting against mosquito bites (see *insect bites*), including the use of insect repellents such as *DEET*.

densitometry

An imaging technique that uses low-dose *X-rays* to measure bone density. It is used to diagnose and assess the severity of *osteoporosis* (wasting away of bone tissue), especially in the spine and the femur (thigh bone), and to assess its response to treatment.

During the procedure, X-rays are passed through the body. A computer assesses the amount of X-rays absorbed by the body and uses this information to calculate the bone density.

density

The "compactness" of a substance, defined as its mass per unit volume. In radiology, the term relates to the amount of radiation absorbed by a structure being X-rayed. Bone absorbs radiation well and appears white on X-ray film. A lung, which contains mostly air, absorbs little radiation and is dark on the film. The same is true for images obtained by *CT scanning* and *MRI*. (See also *specific gravity*.)

dental emergencies

Injuries or disorders of the teeth and gums that require immediate treatment because of severe pain and/or because delay could lead to poor healing or to complications. A tooth that has become dislodged by injury can often be reimplanted (see *reimplantation, dental*) into the gum successfully if this is done without delay. A partly dislodged tooth should be manipulated back into the socket in the gum immediately.

SCOPE OF **DENTAL EXAMINATION**

A dental examination includes an assessment of the condition of the teeth, of the gums, of the mouth, and of the bone that supports the teeth.

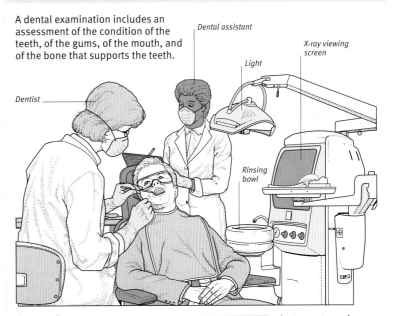

Constructing a dental record
During the dental examination, the dentist checks for the presence or absence of individual teeth. Any abnormalities and all fillings are recorded (by the dentist's assistant).

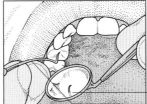

Instruments used
The dentist uses a mirror to see the backs of the teeth and into the back of the mouth; a metal instrument is used to probe for dental cavities or chipped teeth.

Mirror
Probe

D

TYPES OF DENTAL X-RAY

There are three types of X-ray. Each of the different types is useful for revealing particular dental problems.

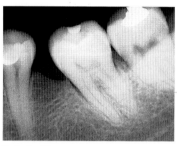

Periapical X-rays
These X-rays give detailed pictures of whole teeth and the surrounding gums and bone. They show unerupted or impacted teeth, root fractures, abscesses, cysts, tumours, and the characteristic bone patterns of some skeletal diseases. The film, in a protective casing, is placed in the patient's mouth and is held in position behind the teeth to be X-rayed.

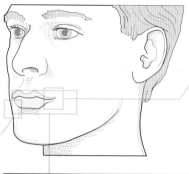

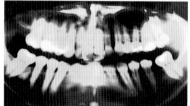

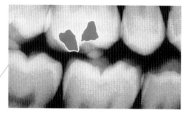

Bite-wing X-rays
These X-rays show the crowns of the teeth. They are useful for detecting areas of decay between teeth and changes in bone that are caused by periodontal (gum) disease. The film is in a holder with a central tab on to which the patient bites.

Panoramic X-rays
These X-rays show all the teeth and surrounding structures on one large film. They are invaluable for finding unerupted or impacted teeth, cysts, jaw fractures, or tumours. Pictures are recorded continuously on to film as the camera swings around from one side of the jaw to the other.

Other dental emergencies include a broken tooth (see *fracture, dental*); severe *toothache*, which may be due to an abscess (see *abscess, dental*); Vincent's disease (see *gingivitis, acute ulcerative*), which causes ulceration, and bleeding of the gums; and eruption of wisdom teeth that cut into the tongue.

dental examination

An examination of the mouth, gums, and teeth by a dentist as a routine check or during the assessment of a suspected problem.

Routine examinations are recommended so that tooth decay (see *caries, dental*), gum disease (see *gingivitis*), or *mouth cancer* can be detected and treated at an early stage, before they cause serious damage. During the examination, the dentist uses a metal instrument to probe for dental cavities, chipped teeth, or fillings. (See the box on p.219.) *Dental X-rays* are sometimes carried out to detect problems, for example with the jaw, that may not be visible. The dentist also checks the bite (how well the upper and the lower teeth come together). Regular examinations in children enable a dentist to monitor the replacement of primary teeth by permanent, or secondary, teeth. Referral for *orthodontic* treatment may be made.

dental extraction

See *extraction, dental*.

dental floss

A fine thread or tape, usually made of nylon, that is used to remove plaque (see *plaque, dental*) and food particles from hard-to-reach areas between the teeth and around the line of the gums (see *flossing*). Floss may be waxed or unwaxed, and some types contain fluoride. Flossing should be carried out regularly, in addition to toothbrushing.

dental impaction

See *impaction, dental*.

dental X-ray

An image of the teeth and jaws that provides information for the detection, diagnosis, and treatment of conditions that can threaten oral and general health. The part to be imaged is placed between a tube emitting *X-rays* and a photographic film. Because X-rays are unable to pass easily through hard tissue, a shadow of the teeth and bone is seen on the film. There are three types of dental X-ray : periapical X-ray, bite-wing X-ray, and panoramic X-ray.

Periapical X-rays are taken using X-ray film held behind the teeth. They give detailed images of whole teeth and the surrounding tissues. They can show unerupted or impacted teeth, root fractures, abscesses, cysts, and tumours, and can help diagnose some skeletal diseases. Bite-wing X-rays show the crowns of

the teeth and can detect areas of decay and changes in bone due to *periodontal disease*. Panoramic X-rays show all the teeth and the surrounding structures on one large film. They can show unerupted or impacted teeth, as well as cysts, jaw fractures, or tumours.

The amount of radiation received from dental X-rays is extremely small; however, routine dental X-rays should be avoided during pregnancy.

dentifrice

A paste, powder, or gel used with a toothbrush to clean the teeth. Dentifrice usually contains a mild abrasive, along with detergents, colourings and flavourings, binding and moistening agents, and thickening agents. It also usually has *fluoride* added and, sometimes, desensitizing agents and antibacterials.

dentigerous cyst

A fluid-filled *cyst* (lump or swelling) surrounding the crown of an unerupted tooth (see *eruption of teeth*). This type of cyst may produce swelling or resorption (loss of substance) of the adjacent tooth roots. Treatment is by extraction of the affected tooth and by surgical removal of the cyst.

dentine

The hard tissue that surrounds the pulp of a tooth (see *teeth*).

dentistry

The science or profession concerned with the teeth and their supporting structures. Most dentists work in general dental practice; others practise a specialized branch of dentistry.

Dentists in general practice undertake all aspects of dental care. They may refer patients to a consultant in one of the specialized branches of dentistry, such as *orthodontics* (correction of the alignment of teeth), *prosthetics* (fitting of bridgework and dentures), *endodontics* (treatment of diseases of the tooth pulp), and *periodontics* (treatment of disorders affecting the tissues supporting the teeth).

Dental hygienists carry out scaling (removal of hard deposits on the teeth) and demonstrate methods to keep the teeth and gums healthy.

dentition

The arrangement, number, and type of teeth in the mouth. In young children, primary dentition comprises 20 teeth (incisors, canines, and molars). These teeth are replaced between the ages of 6 and 13 years by the secondary (permanent) dentition. Secondary dentition comprises 32 teeth (incisors, canines, premolars, and molars). Often, the third molars (wisdom teeth) do not erupt until the age of 18–25, or even older in some cases; sometimes, they fail to erupt at all. (See also *eruption of teeth*.)

denture

An appliance that replaces missing natural teeth. A denture consists of a metal and/or acrylic (hard plastic) base that is mounted with acrylic teeth. The artificial teeth are matched to the person's original teeth. Denture baseplates, which are created from impressions taken from the upper and lower gums, fit the mouth accurately.

deodorant

A substance that removes unpleasant odours, especially body odours.

deossification

The loss or removal of *bone* tissue, as in *osteoporosis*. (See also *ossification*.)

deoxygenation

In *respiration*, the release of *oxygen* from red *blood cells* to supply other tissues.

deoxyribonucleic acid

See *DNA*; *nucleic acids*.

dependence

Psychological or physical reliance on persons or drugs. An infant is dependent on its parents, but, as he or she grows, this dependence normally wanes. Some adults never become fully independent (see *dependent personality*).

Alcohol and drugs may induce physical or emotional dependence in users; a person who has a dependency may develop physical symptoms, such as sweating or abdominal pains, or become distressed if deprived of the drug. (See also *alcohol dependence*; *drug dependence*.)

dependent oedema

A form of *oedema* (the accumulation of fluid in body tissues) that mainly affects the lower parts of the body. It may be a feature of congestive *heart failure*. Oedema affecting the ankles may have various possible causes, such as immobility, *varicose veins*, and *pregnancy*.

dependent personality

A *personality disorder* characterized by an inability to function without significant guidance from others, feelings of helplessness when alone or when close relationships end, and a fear of separation. Other features of a dependent personality include difficulty in making decisions, low self-esteem, and hypersensitivity to criticism.

Dependent personality disorder is of unknown cause and normally first manifests itself in early adulthood. There is no specific treatment for the condition, but *psychotherapy* may gradually help sufferers to make their own choices. Medication, for example with *antianxiety drugs* or *antidepressant drugs*, may be effective in relieving associated symptoms in some cases.

depersonalization

A state of feeling unreal, in which an individual has a sense of detachment from self and surroundings. Depersonalization is frequently accompanied by *derealization*, in which the world is experienced as unreal. It is rarely serious and usually comes on suddenly and may last for moments or for hours. Depersonalization most often occurs in people who have *anxiety disorders*. Other causes include certain drugs and *temporal lobe epilepsy*.

depilatory

A chemical hair remover, such as barium sulphide, supplied as a cream and applied for cosmetic reasons or to treat *hirsutism* (excessive hairiness in women).

Depixol

A brand name for flupentixol, an *antipsychotic drug* used in the treatment of *schizophrenia* and other related illnesses. The drug may be given either orally or by injection. Possible adverse effects include an increased risk of *parkinsonism* (a set of neuromuscular symptoms including tremors, muscle rigidity, and slow movements).

Depo-provera

A brand name for *medroxyprogesterone*, a long-acting *progestogen drug* that is given by *depot injection* as a contraceptive. It is similar to *progesterone hormone*, a natural female sex hormone.

TYPES OF **DENTURES**

Partial dentures
Partial dentures are used when only some of the teeth are missing. They fill unsightly gaps, make chewing easier, maintain clear speech, and keep the remaining teeth in the correct position. Teeth on either side of a gap may tip (making cleaning more difficult) or drift (placing unnatural stress on the tissues of the mouth). Partial dentures are held in place by metal clasps that grip adjacent teeth or by clasps combined with metal rests (extensions of the denture plate that rest on the surface of the tooth).

Full dentures
Full dentures are needed when there are no teeth left in the mouth. They stay in place by resting on the gum ridges and, in the case of upper dentures, by suction. Fitting is sometimes delayed after extraction of teeth to allow the gums to shrink and change shape as they heal.

Immediate dentures
Immediate dentures are fitted immediately after extraction of teeth. They protect the gum and control bleeding from extraction sites. Since a toothless period is avoided, they are particularly useful for replacing front teeth. However, they can be expensive and require follow-up visits so that they continue to fit comfortably. They may also need replacing within a short time.

D

depot injection

An intramuscular injection of a drug that gives a slow, steady release of its active chemicals into the bloodstream. Release of the drug is slowed by the inclusion of substances such as oil or wax, and can be made to last for hours, days, or weeks.

A depot injection can be useful for patients who may not take their medication correctly. It also prevents the necessity of giving a series of injections over a short period. Drugs that may be given by depot injection include hormonal contraceptives (see *contraception, hormonal methods of*), *corticosteroid drugs*, and *antipsychotic drugs*. Side effects may arise due to the uneven release of the drug into the bloodstream.

depressed skull fracture

A fracture in which a part of a skull bone is pushed inwards towards the *brain* (see *skull, fracture of*). A depressed skull fracture usually results from a high-energy blow to a small surface area of the skull.

depression

Feelings of sadness, hopelessness, and a loss of interest in life, combined with a sense of reduced emotional well-being. Most people experience these feelings from time to time, usually as a normal response to an upsetting event; for example, it is natural to feel depressed when a close relative dies. When a person's behaviour and physical state are also affected, however, this is an indication that the symptom is part of a depressive illness.

Depression that occurs without any apparent cause, deepens, and persists may occur as part of a variety of psychiatric illnesses. Some people who suffer from depression are eventually diagnosed as having *bipolar disorder*, a condition characterized by episodes of depression alternating with mania (periods of overly excitable mood and uncontrolled behaviour).

SYMPTOMS

Symptoms vary with the severity of the condition. In a person suffering from mild depression, the main symptoms are anxiety and a variable mood; the person may also have fits of crying that occur for no apparent reason. More severe depression may cause loss of appetite, difficulty in sleeping, tiredness, loss of interest in social activities, and impaired concentration; movement and thinking may also become slower. Alternatively, the opposite occurs, and the person may become extremely anxious. People who are severely depressed may have thoughts of committing *suicide* and feelings of worthlessness. *Hallucinations* or *delusions* may occur in extreme cases.

CAUSES

Often, there is no single obvious cause, and a combination of factors may be involved. Depression may be triggered by physical illnesses (such as a viral infection), by hormonal disorders (such as *hypothyroidism*), or by the hormonal changes that occur following childbirth (see *postnatal depression*). Certain drugs, such as *oral contraceptives*, may contribute to the condition. Inheritance may play a part in bipolar disorder. Some people become depressed in the winter (see *seasonal affective disorder syndrome*), probably in response to the long hours of darkness.

Aside from these causes, there are social and psychological factors that may play a role. Depression may also be related to the number of disturbing changes or events in a person's life.

INCIDENCE

Depression is the most common serious psychiatric illness. The World Health Organization ranks it fourth in the ten leading causes of disease worldwide. One person in six is estimated to suffer some degree of depression in their lifetime, and one person in 20 develops clinical depressive illness.

Depression is particularly common in people over 50, and appears to be more common in women; twice as many women as men seek help for the condition. This difference may result from the fact that women are more prepared to seek help for their symptoms, while men may be more likely to express their discontent in the form of problems such as alcohol abuse and violence.

TREATMENT

There are three main forms of treatment for depression, depending on the type and severity of the illness.

Treatment usually includes a form of *psychotherapy*, given either individually or in a group. This form of treatment is most useful for people whose personality and life experiences are the main causes of their illness. Types of therapy range from *counselling* to help deal with practical problems to more structured approaches such as *cognitive–behavioural therapy* or *psychoanalysis*.

Antidepressant drugs may be very effective, with up to seven in ten affected people responding well to the first drug that is offered. Antidepressants are not addictive. Many drugs, however, do not start to take effect until about two weeks into treatment, and all types need to be continued after the symptoms of depression have cleared.

ECT (electroconvulsive therapy) is not often used in the UK, but it is still considered to be an effective treatment for people suffering from severe depression for whom other treatments have been ineffective. ECT may be life-saving, but it can cause mild, temporary memory impairment.

OUTLOOK

Depression often recurs; up to three-quarters of people who have needed hospital treatment for depression will have another episode within ten years. However, long-term antidepressant medication and psychological therapies can greatly reduce the risk of recurrence.

Despite the effectiveness of drug treatment, suicide remains a serious risk; nearly half of all deaths in people with recurrent depression are due to suicide. This risk can, however, be substantially reduced by maintenance treatment with antidepressive drugs.

De Quervain's disease

An inflammatory condition that affects one of the *tendons* of the muscles that are used to move the *thumb*. In de Quervain's disease, the sheath (covering) of this tendon becomes so inflamed and thickened that the tendon can no longer move through the sheath smoothly, and thumb movements are painful. The inflammation is often caused by overuse of the thumb.

Treatment is with rest, *nonsteroidal anti-inflammatory drugs* (NSAIDs), and *corticosteroid drug* injections into the affected tendon sheath, which may be helpful in relieving the inflammation, but in severe cases surgery is needed to loosen the sheath.

De Quervain's thyroiditis

A form of *thyroiditis* (inflammation of the thyroid gland) that is uncommon and is caused by a viral infection; the condition often follows a viral infection of the nose and throat.

The thyroid gland, which is situated in the front of the neck, may become painful and swollen; this swelling is sometimes accompanied by fever. There is a temporary rise in thyroid hormone levels (*hyperthyroidism*) lasting for a few weeks, as damage to the thyroid gland causes it to release its hormone stores. This is followed by insufficient levels (*hypothyroidism*) when the stores then become depleted.

Aspirin is used to treat the inflammation, with a short course of the corticosteroid drug *prednisolone* given in more severe cases. During the initial pase of hyperthyroidism, *beta-blocker drugs* may be given to control symptoms. Thyroid function usually returns to normal once the illness has been treated.

Dercum's disease

Also called adiposis dolorosa, a disorder characterized by accumulation of localized, symmetrical fat deposits under the skin, mainly on the forearms and thighs. The swellings are uncomfortable or painful. Other symptoms include muscle weakness and headaches. The disease may cause death from heart failure. Dercum's disease mainly affects middle-aged women and is thought to be an autosomal dominant *genetic disorder*.

derealization

Feeling that the world has become unreal. It usually occurs together with *depersonalization* and may be caused by fatigue, *hallucinogenic drugs*, or disordered brain function.

dermabrasion

Removal of the surface layer of the skin by high-speed sanding to improve the appearance of scars, such as from *acne*, or to remove tattoos.

dermatitis

Inflammation of the skin, sometimes due to an *allergy*. Dermatitis is the same as *eczema*, and the terms can be used interchangeably. The following are types of dermatitis.

SEBORRHOEIC DERMATITIS

This condition is a red, scaly, itchy rash that develops on the face (particularly the nose and eyebrows), scalp, chest, and back. It often develops during times of stress and is probably caused by an excessive growth of yeast on the skin. *Corticosteroid drugs* and drugs that kill microorganisms may help.

CONTACT DERMATITIS

Contact dermatitis results from a reaction to some substance that comes in contact with the skin. Common causes are detergents, nickel, certain plants,

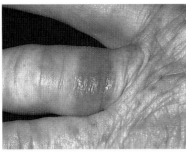

Contact dermatitis
An allergic reaction to the metal (often nickel) in a ring has produced a red, inflamed area of skin around the finger.

and cosmetics. It may be treated with topical corticosteroids. A patch test (see *skin tests*) may be performed in order to identify the cause.

PHOTODERMATITIS

This form of dermatitis occurs in people whose skin is abnormally sensitive to light. A cluster of spots or blisters occurs on any part of the body exposed to the sun (see *photosensitivity*).

dermatitis artefacta

Any self-induced damage to the skin. It may range from scratches to extensive mutilation that produces severe ulcers or other lesions. When given a medical examination, the affected person may vigorously deny having any part in causing the problem. Psychiatric assessment and treatment is required to control the behaviour. (See also *factitious disorder*.)

dermatitis herpetiformis

A chronic skin disease in which clusters of tiny, red, intensely itchy blisters occur in a symmetrical pattern, most commonly on the back, elbows, knees, buttocks, and scalp. It usually develops in adult life and is believed to be related to *coeliac disease*, a condition in which the lining of the small intestine reacts to gluten, a constituent of many cereals.

dermatology

The branch of medicine that is concerned with the *skin*, *hair*, and *nails*, and their disorders.

dermatome

An area of skin that is supplied with nerve fibres by a single spinal nerve from the cervical, thoracic, lumbar, or sacral regions of the spinal cord.

The entire body surface is an interlocking pattern of dermatomes, which is similar from one person to another.

Abnormal sensation in a dermatome signifies damage to a particular nerve root, commonly due to a *disc prolapse* ("slipped" disc).

dermatome, surgical

A surgical instrument for cutting varying thicknesses of skin for use in skin grafting procedures.

dermatomyositis

A rare *autoimmune disorder* in which the muscles and skin become inflamed. In most cases the cause is unknown, but in some instances the disease is linked to an underlying *cancer*.

Dermatomyositis causes a skin rash that may first appear on the bridge of the nose and cheeks, followed by a purple discoloration on the eyelids and sometimes a red rash over the knees, knuckles, and elbows. Muscles become weak, stiff, and painful, particularly those in the shoulders and pelvis; affected people may find that they cannot raise their hands above their head, or cannot raise themselves from a squatting position. Calcium may be deposited in the muscles, particularly in affected children.

The diagnosis is made by medical examinations, *blood tests*, and *biopsy* of muscle tissue. Treatment is with *corticosteroids* and/or *immunosuppressant drugs* and *physiotherapy*. In about half of all cases, full recovery occurs after a few years. The remainder have persistent muscle weakness. In some cases, the disease eventually affects the lungs and other organs and may be fatal.

dermatophyte infections

A group of common fungal infections affecting the skin, hair, and nails, also called *tinea* or, popularly, ringworm.

dermis

The inner layer of the *skin*.

dermographism

Abnormal sensitivity of the skin to mechanical irritation, to the extent that firm stroking leads to the appearance of itchy weals. The condition is a form of *urticaria* (nettle rash). It is most common in fair-skinned people who have a tendency to allergic conditions.

dermoid cyst

A noncancerous tumour with a cell structure similar to that of skin. The growth contains hairs, sweat glands,

D

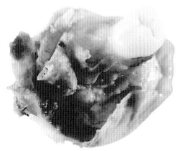

Dermoid cyst of the ovary
Dermoid cysts commonly occur in the ovaries. They can contain fragments of cartilage, bone, and, in this case, a whole tooth.

and sebaceous glands. Dermoid cysts may also contain fragments of cartilage, bone, and even teeth. The cysts can occur in various parts of the body, but they are most commonly found in the ovaries and on the skin around the head or neck, causing small, painless swellings. Dermoid cysts only rarely become cancerous.

Usually, surgical removal of the cysts is recommended. (See also *teratoma*.)

dermoid tumour

See *dermoid cyst*.

Dermovate

A brand name for clobetasol, a topical *corticosteroid drug* that is applied to the skin. Dermovate is only prescribed for severe skin disorders that have not responded to treatment with another, weaker topical corticosteroid.

De Sanctis–Cacchione syndrome

A hereditary condition that is transmitted as an autosomal recessive trait (see *genetic disorders*). De Sanctis–Cacchione syndrome is characterized by *xeroderma pigmentosum* (extreme sensitivity of the skin to sunlight), impaired intellectual development, growth retardation (see *short stature*), and underdevelopment of the gonads (the *testes* or *ovaries*).

desensitization

A technique that is used in *behaviour therapy* for the treatment of *phobias*. The patient is gradually exposed to the feared object or situation while using *relaxation techniques* to control his or her feelings. The exposure is carried out repeatedly over several weeks or months, until the person no longer feels afraid when confronted with the object or situation.

desensitization, allergy

See *hyposensitization*.

desferrioxamine

A drug used to rid the body tissues of excess *iron* that accumulates as a result of repeated blood transfusions in certain types of *anaemia*, such as aplastic anaemia and *thalassaemia*. It is also used to treat iron poisoning, and may be used to treat excess *aluminium* in people on *dialysis*.

The drug is administered by intravenous injection or by subcutaneous infusion. It may be given with *vitamin C* to boost excretion of the iron. Side effects may include gastrointestinal disturbances, dizziness, and skin reactions.

designer drugs

A group of illegally produced chemicals that mimic the effects of specific drugs of abuse. Made in illicit laboratories, they are cheap to produce and undercut the street prices of drugs. Designer drugs can cause *drug dependence* and *drug poisoning*.

TYPES
There are three major types: drugs that are derived from opioid *analgesic* drugs (painkillers) such as fentanyl; drugs that are similar to *amphetamines*, such as ecstasy; and variants of *phencyclidine* (PCP), a hallucinogenic drug.

RISKS
These highly potent drugs are not tested for adverse effects or for the strength of the tablets or capsules, making their use hazardous. For example, some derivatives of fentanyl are 20–2,000 times as powerful as morphine. Amphetamine derivatives can cause brain damage at doses only slightly higher than those required for a stimulant effect. Many designer drugs contain impurities that can cause permanent damage.

WARNING
Designer drugs carry a high risk of drug dependence, with severe *withdrawal reactions*, and of drug poisoning, causing effects such as brain damage.

desmoid tumour

A growth, usually in the abdominal wall. The tumour feels hard and it occurs most frequently in women who have had children, possibly due to stretching of abdominal muscles during pregnancy. They may also arise at the sites of old surgical incisions. Removal of the tumour is the usual treatment, but recurrence is common.

desmopressin

A synthetic form of *ADH* (antidiuretic hormone, also known as vasopressin) that is used to treat *diabetes insipidus* and bed-wetting (see *enuresis*). It is also used in the treatment of some cases of the bleeding disorders *haemophilia* and *von Willebrand's disease*.

desogestrel

A *progestogen drug* used either alone or with *ethinylestradiol* as an ingredient of some *oral contraceptives*. Progestogens make cervical mucus thick and impenetrable by sperm and cause thickening of the uterine lining, which reduces the chance of a fertilized egg implanting successfully; desogestrel also inhibits ovulation. Possible side effects of the drug include weight changes and fluid retention. There may, in addition, be nausea, vomiting, headache, depression, and breast tenderness.

desquamation

The process by which the surface of the *epidermis* (the outer layer of the skin) is shed in the form of scales or small sheets. This process is a feature of seborrhoeic dermatitis (see *dermatitis*) and *ichthyosis* (an inherited scaling condition of the skin). Desquamation of the skin may occur after illnesses involving fever, particularly *scarlet fever*.

detached retina

See *retinal detachment*.

detergent poisoning

The toxic effects that can result from swallowing cleaning agents that are present in shampoos, laundry powders, and household cleaning liquids. These effects include vomiting, diarrhoea, and swelling of the abdomen.

detoxify

To remove the toxicity (the poisonous property) from a substance or to neutralize the substance's toxic effects. Detoxification is one of the functions carried out by the *liver*.

The term "detoxification" is used to describe treatment for alcohol dependence and also a short-term diet in which toxins such as *caffeine* and *alcohol* are excluded and foods high in fats and sugar are avoided. "Detox" diets are usually based on fruits, vegetables, starches such as brown rice, and drinking plenty of water. People who follow these diets may feel refreshed afterwards, although there is no scientific evidence that the diets eliminate toxins faster than normal. Detox diets should be used only for a few days, and preferably with guidance from a doctor or dietician. They are not recommended for children or adolescents, people with *diabetes mellitus* or *eating disorders*, or those who have any other medical condition.

detrusor instability

Inappropriate contraction of the detrusor muscle in the wall of the *bladder* that causes an uncontrollable release of urine even when the bladder is not sufficiently full to trigger urination. It may have various causes, including bladder inflammation, obstruction of the bladder outlet (for example, by a stone or, in men, by an enlarged *prostate gland*), or damage to the nerves supplying the bladder. (See also *incontinence, urinary*.)

development

The process of growth and change by which an individual matures physically, mentally, emotionally, and socially. It takes place in major phases: during the first two months of pregnancy (see *embryo*), and, to a lesser extent, during the rest of pregnancy (see *fetus*); during the first five years of life (see *child development*); and then again during *puberty* and *adolescence*.

developmental delay

A term used if a baby or young child has not acquired new skills within the expected time range. Normally, new abilities and patterns of behaviour appear at given ages, and existing behaviour patterns change and sometimes disappear (see *child development*). Delays vary in severity, and may affect the development of one or more of the following: hand–eye coordination, walking, listening, language, speech, or social interaction.

GENERALIZED DELAY

A child who is late in most aspects of development usually has a generalized problem. This may be due to a severe visual or hearing impairment, limited intellectual abilities (see *learning difficulties*), or damage to the brain before, during, or after birth. For further information on possible causes of generalized delay, see the table above.

SPECIFIC FORMS OF DELAY

Delay in movement and walking often has no serious cause. In some cases, however, there are specific causes; these can include *muscular dystrophy* and *spina*

CAUSES OF DEVELOPMENTAL DELAY

- Physical or emotional deprivation (child abuse). Lack of affection, stimulation, or teaching.

- Severe visual impairment. Vision is vital for normal development in all areas. Children learn to recognize objects before learning their names, they learn about sounds by seeing which objects make which sounds, and they become motivated to crawl and walk by the desire to explore their surroundings (see *vision, disorders of*; *blindness*).

- Severe hearing impairment (see *deafness*).

- Learning difficulties.

- Damage to the brain before, during, or after birth, or in infancy. The results of damage depend on which parts of the brain are damaged and on severity (see *brain damage*; *cerebral palsy*).

- Severe, prolonged disease of any organ or body system (such as bone, heart, kidney, muscle), and nutritional disorders.

---

bifida. Delay in developing manipulative skills (the ability to pick up and use objects with the hands) is often due to lack of adequate stimulation.

Delayed speech development may have various causes. The most important is *deafness*, which may cause the child to be unresponsive to sound. *Autism* is a rare cause; in this condition, hearing is normal but the child may be unresponsive to the human voice. Another possible cause is generalized difficulty with muscle control, which may affect speech production; this may occur in children who have cerebral palsy. Damage to, or structural defects of, the speech muscles, the larynx (voicebox), or the mouth may also cause speech difficulties, as may any disorder that affects the speech area of the brain (see *aphasia*; *dysarthria*; *dysphonia*; *speech disorders*).

Children vary greatly in the age at which they gain bladder and bowel control. Usually, bowel control is acquired first. Delay in bladder control is much more common than delay in bowel control. Such delays have many possible causes (see *enuresis*; *encopresis*; *soiling*).

ASSESSMENT

Delays may first be noticed by parents; if this is the case, a health visitor or doc-

---

tor should be consulted promptly. Delays may also be detected during routine developmental checks with a health visitor, family doctor, or paediatrician. These checks are performed at various ages, but usually at birth, six weeks, six to eight months, 18 to 24 months, and five years.

A child who shows signs of developmental delay should undergo a full assessment. This will usually include a physical examination, along with *hearing tests*, *vision tests*, and a thorough developmental assessment. The child may need to undergo further investigations, such as blood tests, to check for any genetic abnormality, or referral to a specialist such as a neurologist, speech therapist, or physiotherapist.

TREATMENT

The treatment depends on the severity and probable cause of the delay. It may include a course of *speech therapy* or *family therapy*, or provision of physical aids such as *glasses* or a *hearing aid*. Parents are often of prime importance in providing help for their child. In some cases, however, the child may also benefit from being admitted to a school or special unit that provides education for children with specific difficulties.

developmental dysplasia of the hip (DDH)

Previously known as congenital hip dislocation, a disorder present at birth in which the head of the *femur* (thighbone) fails to fit properly into the cup-like socket in the *pelvis* to form a normal joint. One or both of the hips may be affected.

CAUSE AND INCIDENCE

The cause of DDH is not known. The condition is more common in girls, especially in babies born by *breech delivery* or following pregnancies in which there was an abnormally small amount of amniotic fluid surrounding the fetus.

DIAGNOSIS AND TREATMENT

DDH is usually dicovered during one of the developmental checks after birth or in early infancy. If so, an *ultrasound scan* is done to confirm the diagnosis. If the dislocation is detected in early infancy, *splints* are applied to the thigh to manoeuvre the ball of the joint into the socket and keep it in position. These splints are worn for about three months and usually correct the problem. Progress may be monitored by *ultrasound scanning* and *X-rays*. Corrective surgery may also be required.

D

D

OUTLOOK

If treatment is delayed, there may be lifelong problems with walking. Without treatment, the dislocation often leads to shortening of the leg, limping, and early *osteoarthritis* in the joint.

deviated nasal septum

See *nasal septum*.

deviation, sexual

An abnormal form of sexual behaviour, most common in men, in which sexual intercourse between adults is not the final aim. Forms of sexual deviation include *exhibitionism*, *fetishism*, *paedophilia*, and *transvestism*.

Devic's disease

A rare condition, sometimes called neuromyelitis optica, in which there is *demyelination* of the fibres in the optic nerves and the spinal cord. The condition begins with inflammation of the optic nerves (see *optic neuritis*), leading to loss of vision. There are also attacks of numbness, muscle weakness, and loss of coordination in the parts of the trunk and limbs below the diseased area of the spine. In addition, the spinal cord damage may lead to disruption of urinary and bowel control and impairment of sexual function.

dexamethasone

A *corticosteroid drug* used as eye drops in the treatment of *iritis* (inflammation of the iris), and as eardrops in the treatment of *otitis externa* (outer ear infection).

Dexamethasone is given in tablet form or by injection to treat severe *asthma* and other inflammatory disorders, and to reduce inflammation of the brain due to *head injury*, *stroke*, or a *brain tumour*. It may also be injected into an inflamed joint to relieve the symptoms of *osteoarthritis*.

Dexamethasone eye drops may cause irritation of the eyes. Prolonged use or high doses of dexamethasone tablets may cause the adverse effects common to the corticosteroid group of drugs.

dexamfetamine

A central nervous system stimulant (see *amphetamine drugs*; *stimulant drugs*) sometimes used to treat *narcolepsy* (a sleep disorder). It is also used in children with *attention deficit hyperactivity disorder* who have not responded to treatment with methylphenidate. Because of its stimulant properties, dexamfeta-

mine has become a drug of abuse. Excessive use leads to *anxiety* and *drug psychosis*. With prolonged use, physical tolerance develops: the drug's stimulant effects lessen and a higher dose must then be taken to produce the same effect. *Drug dependence* (a physical or psychological need for the drug) also develops after repeated use.

DEXA scan

Dual-energy X-ray absorptiometry, a technique that measures bone density by passing beams of low-dose radiation through bone. DEXA scans are used to assess the severity of the bone disorder *osteoporosis*. (See also *densitometry*.)

dextran

A polysaccharide (a type of *carbohydrate*) consisting of branched chains of glucose units. Dextrans that are formed by the action of bacteria on sucrose in the mouth produce *plaque* (a rough, sticky coating on the teeth), which is a major cause of tooth decay (see *caries, dental*).

Commercially manufactured preparations of synthetic dextran solution may be used in surgery or in emergency treatment for *shock*, to increase the volume of the *plasma* (the fluid part of the blood) in the circulation. Dextrans used for this purpose are known as plasma expanders.

dextrocardia

A rare condition, which is present from birth, in which the heart is situated in, and points towards, the right-hand side of the chest instead of the left. The heart may also be malformed. Sometimes, the position of the abdominal organs is also reversed, so that the liver is on the left-hand side and the stomach is on the right. The cause of dextrocardia is not known.

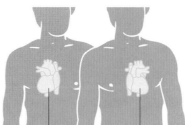

Abnormal position   Normal position

Heart positions
In dextrocardia, the heart is situated in, and points towards, the right-hand side of the chest instead of the left-hand side.

No treatment is necessary unless the heart is malformed, in which case surgical correction may be performed.

dextromethorphan

A cough suppressant that is available over the counter as an ingredient in many *cough remedies*.

dextrose

Another name for *glucose*.

diabetes, bronze

Another name for *haemochromatosis*, a rare genetic disease in which excessive amounts of iron are deposited in tissues. Bronze diabetes causes a bronze skin coloration, and sufferers often develop *diabetes mellitus*.

diabetes insipidus

A rare condition that is characterized by excessive thirst and the passing of large quantities of dilute urine. A person with diabetes insipidus may pass between five and 20 litres of urine every 24 hours, provided that this output is matched by a sufficient intake of water. If the lost water is not replaced, dehydration may occur, leading to confusion, stupor, and coma.

Diabetes insipidus usually results from a failure of the *pituitary gland* to secrete *ADH* (antidiuretic hormone), which normally regulates the amount of water excreted in the urine. This failure may be due to a disease of the pituitary gland, or may temporarily follow brain surgery. A rare form of the disease, called nephrogenic diabetes insipidus, is due to failure of the kidneys to respond to ADH.

Diagnosis mainly involves blood and urine tests. A doctor may measure output of urine over 24 hours. He or she may also measure urine output when fluid has been withheld for several hours; an affected person will continue to pass a large volume of urine. The person's response to synthetic ADH may also be tested; if the urine output remains high even after the person has taken ADH, this indicates the nephrogenic form of the disease.

Treatment of ADH-related diabetes insipidus is with desmopressin (synthetic ADH). Treatment of nephrogenic diabetes insipidus is by a low-sodium diet and thiazide *diuretic drugs*.

diabetes mellitus

A disorder that develops when the cells of the body do not receive enough *insulin*. This hormone is produced by

LIVING WITH **DIABETES MELLITUS**

As the level of glucose in the blood rises, the volume of urine required to carry it out of the body is increased, causing not only a frequent need to urinate but also constant thirst. The high levels of sugar in the blood and urine impair the body's ability to fight infection, leading to urinary tract infections (such as *cystitis* and *pyelonephritis*), vaginal yeast infections (*candidiasis*), and recurrent skin infections.

Because the body's cells are starved of glucose, the sufferer feels weak and fatigued (see right). The cells are able to obtain some energy from the breakdown of stored fat, resulting in weight loss. The chemical processes involved in this breakdown of fat are, however, defective, especially in insulin-dependent diabetics. They lead to the production of acids and substances known as ketones, which can cause coma and sometimes death.

Other possible symptoms of undiagnosed diabetes include blurred vision, boils, increased appetite, and tingling and numbness in the hands and the feet.

Symptoms will develop in every untreated person who has insulin-dependent (Type 1) diabetes, but will appear in only one-third of those who have the non-insulin-dependent form (Type 2). There are many people with Type 2 diabetes who are unaware of it. The disease is often diagnosed only after complications of the diabetes have been detected.

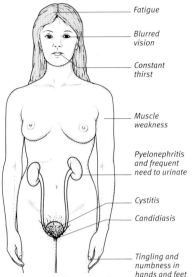

Fatigue

Blurred vision

Constant thirst

Muscle weakness

Pyelonephritis and frequent need to urinate

Cystitis

Candidiasis

Tingling and numbness in hands and feet

Symptoms of untreated diabetes mellitus

SELF-MONITORING OF BLOOD GLUCOSE LEVELS

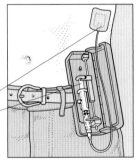

Testing of blood glucose
A spring-loaded pricking device is used to obtain blood from the fingertip. A drop of blood is spread on to a chemically impregnated strip. The strip is inserted into a digital glucose meter, which analyses the blood and gives an almost instant reading of the glucose level.

DEVICES FOR INJECTING INSULIN

Insulin can be injected using a disposable syringe and needle or a pen with refill cartridges (below), or it may be infused continuously from a portable pump (right).

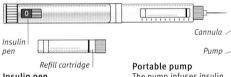

Insulin pen

Refill cartridge

Insulin pen
This device is useful if multiple daily injections are needed.

Cannula

Pump

Portable pump
The pump infuses insulin by way of a cannula inserted through the skin.

---

the *pancreas*; it normally enables body cells to take in glucose from the blood to generate energy, and enables the *liver* and fat cells to take in glucose for storage. A lack of insulin in the cells may occur because the *pancreas* produces too little, or none at all; alternatively, it may occur because the tissues are resistant to the hormone's effects.

TYPES, CAUSES, AND INCIDENCE

There are two main types of diabetes mellitus, both of which tend to run in families. Type 1 (insulin-dependent) diabetes usually develops suddenly in childhood or adolescence. This type of diabetes is an *autoimmune disorder* in which the immune system destroys insulin-secreting cells in the pancreas

and insulin production ceases. Affected people may be genetically predisposed to developing the condition; the disease process may be triggered by viral infection. People with Type 1 diabetes must have insulin or they may fall into a coma and die.

Type 2 (non-insulin-dependent) diabetes tends to develop gradually. It mainly develops in people over the age of 40, although it is becoming more common in younger people. In this type, insulin is still produced but there is not enough to meet the body's needs because the tissues become relatively resistant to its effects. Obesity and inheritance are possible contributory factors; many people who develop Type

2 diabetes are overweight, and affected people often have close relatives with the condition.

Diabetes can sometimes develop during pregnancy, a condition known as gestational diabetes (see *diabetic pregnancy*). In such cases, it usually disappears after childbirth, although women who have had gestational diabetes are at increased risk of developing Type 2 diabetes later in life.

Diabetes mellitus affects more than 120 million people worldwide. Type 2 diabetes is by far the more common form of the disease. More than two million people in the UK have been diagnosed with this type and an estimated three-quarters of a million have

D

the condition but do not know it. Type 2 diabetes is three to four times more common in black people, and about seven times more common in Asians. It also becomes more common with increasing age.

SYMPTOMS

Lack of insulin causes high levels of glucose to remain in the blood. This, in turn, results in a high level of glucose in the urine. This condition, termed *glycosuria*, causes the passage of large quantities of urine, excessive thirst, and *urinary tract infections*. Lack of glucose in the cells causes weight loss, hunger, and fatigue, and leads to chemical imbalances. For further information on the symptoms, see the illustrated box on the previous page.

In Type 1 diabetes, symptoms such as thirst, weight loss, and excessive urination usually develop rapidly over a few weeks. If it is not promptly diagnosed and treated at this stage, it may lead to *diabetic ketoacidosis*, which is a potentially fatal condition.

Type 2 diabetes may be present for months or years while causing few noticeable symptoms. It may only be diagnosed when a complication (see below), such as poor vision, is detected during a medical check-up.

COMPLICATIONS

Some complications of diabetes mellitus result from damage to capillaries (tiny blood vessels) throughout the body. These conditions include *retinopathy* (damage to the retina, which is the light-sensitive part of the eye) and *diabetic nephropathy* (kidney damage). Damage to the blood vessels supplying nerves causes *diabetic neuropathy* (damage to nerve fibres); this may first appear in the fingers and toes, then spread up the limbs. The loss of sensation, and poor circulation, may result in *ulcers* on the feet and legs. Other problems include dizziness on standing and, in men, *erectile dysfunction*.

People with diabetes have a greater risk of developing *atherosclerosis* (accumulation of fatty deposits on the lining of the arteries), *hypertension* (high blood pressure), other *cardiovascular disorders*, and *diabetic cataract* (opacity in the lens of the eye).

DIAGNOSIS AND TREATMENT

If diabetes mellitus is suspected, a urine sample will be taken and tested for the presence of glucose. The diagnosis is confirmed by a blood test to detect abnormally high levels of glucose in the

blood. If the results of this test are unclear, a glucose tolerance test may be done. The person is asked to fast for several hours, and then is given glucose; the blood and the urine are tested at 30-minute intervals to show how efficiently the body is utilizing the glucose. Tests may also be carried out to detect and assess damage to organs such as the eyes, kidneys, and heart.

Treatment aims to keep blood glucose levels as normal as possible. Dietary control is an essential element. The ideal diet for a person with diabetes resembles the sort of healthy eating plan recommended for everyone (see *diabetic diet*). If the person is overweight, and particularly if he or she has Type 2 diabetes, weight loss can be achieved by a reduced-calorie diet. Also, regular exercise and treatment with *antidiabetic drugs* may be required.

In addition to general treatment, all people with Type 1 diabetes need to take insulin regularly. Injections are usually self-administered two, three, or four times a day. The insulin doses need to be matched to activity levels and food intake. If the glucose/insulin balance is not maintained, *hyperglycaemia* (too much glucose in the blood) or *hypoglycaemia* (too little glucose in the blood) may develop. Careful monitoring of blood glucose levels is also an essential part of self-treatment. Pancreas transplants have been tried as a possible cure for the condition, as has treatment involving transplantation of islet cells (the clusters of insulin-producing cells in the pancreas). However, such treatments are still experimental.

Treatment of type 2 diabetes usually consists of dietary measures, weight reduction, exercise, and antidiabetic drugs, often *hypoglycaemic* drugs such as sulphonylureas. Some people eventually need insulin injections.

In general, careful control of blood glucose levels reduces the risk of complications or, if such problems have already developed, slows their progression. People with diabetes should have regular medical check-ups in order that any complications can be detected as early as possible. Additional tests, such as measurement of *glycosylated haemoglobin* (also known as the HbA1C test, which shows blood glucose levels over the previous three months) and urine tests to detect *proteinuria*, can improve medical control and aid early detection of problems.

OUTLOOK

With modern treatment and efficient self-monitoring, people with diabetes mellitus can usually live a normal life; however, the disease is irreversible and life expectancy is reduced.

diabetic arthropathy

Joint damage associated with *diabetes mellitus*. It results from the loss of protective pain sensation that can occur when peripheral nerves are damaged (see *diabetic neuropathy*). The condition often affects the joints in the legs; the ankle is particularly vulnerable.

Affected joints (called neuropathic joints or Charcot's joints) tend to be swollen and deformed but painless. Treatment includes fitting a special cast to reduce swelling in the limb, and the use of supportive footwear.

diabetic cataract

An opacity in the lens of the eye (see *cataract*) due to *diabetes mellitus*. The slow-growing opacities that often appear in old age (senile cataracts) tend to develop 10–15 years earlier than usual in people who have diabetes. Occasionally, young people with poorly controlled diabetes develop juvenile cataracts, which are diffuse opacities that develop rapidly. Treatment for diabetic cataract is the same as for other forms of cataract.

diabetic coma

A life-threatening state of unconsciousness and unresponsiveness, due either to *diabetic ketoacidosis* or to *hypoglycaemia*. The latter condition may be induced either by excessive doses of *oral hypoglycaemic* drugs or inadequate food intake.

diabetic diet

A nutritional regime designed to prevent complications of *diabetes mellitus* by controlling the timing and amount of *energy* intake, thereby minimizing the occurrence of *hyperglycaemia* (high blood glucose levels) or *hypoglycaemia* (low blood glucose levels).

People with diabetes should follow the same kind of healthy diet that is recommended for people in general (see *nutrition*). The diet should be rich in complex carbohydrates (such as bread and pasta), which should make up about 50 per cent of total energy intake (see *calorie*); protein should make up 10-15 per cent of energy intake; and fat should make up less than 30 per cent of energy intake. In addition, the energy intake needs to be controlled in order to maintain a healthy body weight. People who take insulin need to coordinate their meals with the times for their insulin injections.

diabetic ketoacidosis

A severe, acute complication of Type 1 *diabetes mellitus*, a condition in which the *pancreas* produces too little *insulin*. If levels of insulin are too low, the *liver* generates more glucose, but the tissues are unable to take up the glucose properly and have to break down fats to obtain energy, causing the production of acidic chemicals called ketone bodies. Diabetic ketoacidosis may be the first sign that a person has insulin-dependent diabetes, or it may develop in a person known to have the condition who has taken insufficient insulin.

The features of diabetic ketoacidosis include nausea; vomiting; deep, rapid breathing; breath that smells of acetone (like nail polish remover); and confusion. The condition can progress to severe *dehydration* and *coma*.

Treatment involves giving insulin to correct the deficiency and fluids containing salts to relieve dehydration.

diabetic maculopathy

See *maculopathy, diabetic*.

diabetic nephropathy

Kidney damage resulting from longstanding or poorly controlled *diabetes mellitus*. The disorder includes damage to capillaries (tiny blood vessels) in the kidneys and hardening of the tissues. As a result, the kidneys become less able to filter the blood efficiently. Protein may escape into the urine, depleting the body's supplies (see *nephrotic syndrome*). In severe cases, chronic *kidney failure* may develop. Many affected people have *hypertension* (high blood pressure), which may also damage blood vessels.

People with diabetes should have regular check-ups so any kidney problems can be treated as soon as possible. Checks may include urine tests for protein, as well as *kidney function tests*.

diabetic neuropathy

Any of various types of *neuropathy* (disease of or damage to the nerves) that result from longstanding or poorly controlled *diabetes mellitus*.

The most common type of diabetic neuropathy is called peripheral sensory neuropathy. In the early stages of this disorder, intermittent pain and tingling are felt in the extremities, particularly in the feet. The pain gradually worsens until, finally, pain sensation is lost to an area. People with sensory neuropathy in the feet can develop cuts, scrapes, or blisters that they may not notice. If left untreated, serious complications may result from such injuries. Daily observation of the feet is critical.

Another form of diabetic neuropathy is damage to motor nerves (which initiate movements). This problem causes weakened muscles. The foot is particularly susceptible, and may undergo a change of appearance as a result. A further form, diabetic amyotrophy, causes painful wasting of the thigh muscles.

Autonomic neuropathies affect the nerves that regulate involuntary vital functions. Symptoms and signs include postural *hypotension* (low blood pressure on standing); diarrhoea at night; inability to empty the bladder completely, which may lead to urinary tract infection; and *erectile dysfunction*. Cranial neuropathies affect nerves that supply the head and face; damage to nerves supplying the eye muscles causes impaired vision and eye pain.

diabetic pregnancy

Pregnancy associated with *diabetes mellitus*. The term "diabetic pregnancy" may refer to a pregnancy in a woman with pre-existing diabetes, or to diabetes that develops during pregnancy; in the latter case, the condition is known as gestational diabetes.

Women with established diabetes can have a normal pregnancy provided that the diabetes is well controlled. Careful control of blood glucose levels must begin well before conception. Poor control may affect the baby's growth, and increase the risk of fetal malformations and complications during pregnancy.

In gestational diabetes, the mother does not produce enough insulin to keep blood glucose levels normal. The condition is usually detected in the second half of pregnancy, when urine tests reveal the presence of glucose. Treatment is the same as for women who

STEPS IN **DIAGNOSING** A CONDITION

A doctor may go through several steps to ascertain the cause of a person's problem. The medical history, physical examination, and tests may prove vital clues. A doctor usually makes at least a provisional diagnosis before beginning any treatment because treatment can mask symptoms, making the doctor's task of establishing an exact diagnosis more difficult.

Taking the medical history
Perhaps the most important part of the diagnostic procedure is the patient's own account of his or her illness – the medical history. "Listen to the patients, they are telling you their diagnosis" is the traditional teaching given to medical students. Many doctors believe that the medical history provides the strongest basis for ascertaining a diagnosis. The added information derived from the physical examination may be small, but, at times, critical.

Conducting a physical examination
After the medical history has been obtained, the doctor has in mind a short list of probable diagnoses. A physical examination helps shorten the list. The doctor is then left with a differential diagnosis. A differential diagnosis is a group of possible diseases that could account for patterns of symptoms and signs (i.e. physical findings, such as enlargements of lymph nodes or tenderness in a specific region of the abdomen).

Ordering special tests
Next, based on his or her provisional diagnosis, the doctor may order a series of laboratory tests on the blood (and sometimes the urine) and may also arrange for diagnostic imaging of suspect organs by techniques such as ultrasound scanning, X-rays, CT scanning, MRI, or radionuclide scanning. The results of these tests either confirm the doctor's provisional diagnosis or narrow the possibilities so the doctor may be confident in making the correct diagnosis.

Using a computer
Doctors today also use computer systems and algorithms to help reach a diagnosis. Both approaches rely on analysis of large numbers of patient records to quantity probabilities and to devise an orderly series of questions – a decision tree. The main purposes of computer assistance is to remind the doctor of the full range of possible diagnoses for a particular set of symptoms, thereby making it less likely that any possibility will be overlooked. It remains the task of the doctor to integrate the facts and decide upon a diagnosis.

D

PROCEDURE FOR **DIALYSIS**

There are two methods of removing wastes from the blood and excess fluid from the body when the kidneys have failed. The first, haemodialysis, may also be used as emergency treatment in some cases of poisoning or drug overdose. It makes use of an artificial kidney (or "kidney machine") and can be carried out at home. Peritoneal dialysis needs an abdominal incision, which is performed in hospital but may also be done at home.

HOW HAEMODIALYSIS IS DONE

1 Access to the bloodstream for dialysis is obtained by a shunt (in the short term or in an emergency) or an arteriovenous fistula, in which an artery is joined surgically to a vein.

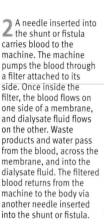

Vein | Shunt

Shunt sewn into blood vessel

Artery

2 A needle inserted into the shunt or fistula carries blood to the machine. The machine pumps the blood through a filter attached to its side. Once inside the filter, the blood flows on one side of a membrane, and dialysate fluid flows on the other. Waste products and water pass from the blood, across the membrane, and into the dialysate fluid. The filtered blood returns from the machine to the body via another needle inserted into the shunt or fistula.

WHY IT IS DONE

In people with damaged kidneys, the process of maintaining the balance of electrolytes and water, and of excreting waste products, may fail, causing harmful, even life-threatening, effects. Dialysis can take over the function of the kidneys until they start working normally again. Or dialysis can function for the kidneys for the rest of a seriously affected person's life if a kidney transplant is not performed.

Diseased kidney
The kidney on the right was removed from a person with adult polycystic kidney disease, one of many disorders that may damage kidney function to the extent that dialysis is needed.

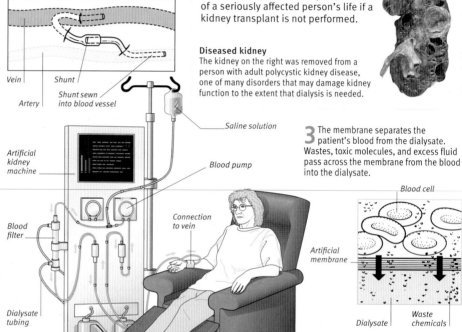

Saline solution

Artificial kidney machine

Blood pump

Connection to vein

Blood filter

Dialysate tubing

3 The membrane separates the patient's blood from the dialysate. Wastes, toxic molecules, and excess fluid pass across the membrane from the blood into the dialysate.

Blood cell

Artificial membrane

Dialysate | Waste chemicals

4 The dialysate is discarded and the purified blood returned to the patient. Each session lasts from two to six hours.

HOW PERITONEAL DIALYSIS IS DONE

1 A small abdominal incision is made, and a catheter is inserted into the peritoneal cavity. A bag of dialysate is attached to the catheter; the fluid passes into the cavity, where it is left for several hours. Used fluid is then drained out of the abdomen.

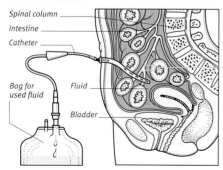

Spinal column
Intestine
Catheter

Bag for used fluid | Fluid

Bladder

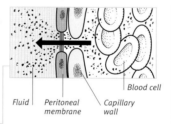

Blood cell

Fluid | Peritoneal membrane | Capillary wall

2 Waste products, and excess water from the blood vessels lining the peritoneal cavity, seep through the peritoneal membrane into the cavity and mix with the dialysate. The fluid is allowed to drain out (by the release of a clamp) through the catheter and into the empty dialysate bag.

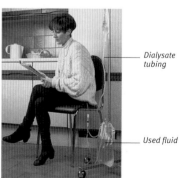

Dialysate tubing

Used fluid

3 The bag is discarded and replaced with a bag containing fresh dialysate. The procedure, which takes about an hour, can be performed during the day or overnight.

have pre-existing diabetes mellitus. Gestational diabetes disappears after the birth, but it is associated with an increased risk of the woman developing Type 2 diabetes in later life.

diabetic retinopathy

See *retinopathy*.

diagnosis

The process of identifying or finding out the nature of a disorder. The doctor listens to a patient's account of his or her illness, and may carry out a physical examination. If further information is needed, tests or imaging procedures may be ordered after a provisional diagnosis has been formed (see *Steps in diagnosing a condition* box, p.229).

diagnostic ultrasound

The use of high-frequency sound waves to form images of internal organs and so help doctors to make diagnoses (see *ultrasound scanning*). Certain forms of ultrasound scanning are used to form moving images, such as images of the flow of blood through the heart (see *Doppler echocardiography*).

dialysis

A filtering technique used to remove waste products from the blood and excess fluid from the body as a treatment for *kidney failure*.

WHY IT IS DONE

Each day, the kidneys normally filter about 1,500 litres of blood. They help to maintain the fluid and *electrolyte* balance of the body. Important minerals and nutrients, such as potassium, sodium, calcium, amino acids, glucose, and water are reabsorbed into the blood. *Urea*, excess minerals, toxins, and drugs are excreted in the urine.

Dialysis is used to perform this function in people whose kidneys have been damaged due to acute or chronic kidney failure. Without dialysis, wastes accumulate in the blood and the electrolyte levels become unbalanced; this may be life-threatening. In chronic kidney failure, patients may need to have dialysis several times a week for the rest of their lives or until they can be given a *kidney transplant*. In acute kidney failure, dialysis is carried out more intensively until the kidneys are working normally.

HOW IT IS DONE

There are two methods: haemodialysis and peritoneal dialysis. In both procedures, excess water and wastes in the blood pass across a membrane into a solution called a dialysate, which is then discarded.

Haemodialysis filters out wastes by passing blood through an artificial kidney machine. The process needs to be performed three or four times a week, and each session lasts two to six hours. In peritoneal dialysis, the abdominal cavity is filled with dialysate, which is changed regularly, and the *peritoneum* (the membrane lining the abdominal cavity) acts as a natural filter. The procedure is often carried out overnight or continuously during the day and night.

RISKS

Both types of dialysis carry the risk of upsetting body chemistry and fluid balance, which can cause complications. In addition, peritoneal dialysis carries a risk of infection in the peritoneum. Life expectancy is reduced for people on lifelong dialysis because it does not replace natural kidney function perfectly; a *kidney transplant* is therefore a better long-term option.

diamorphine

A synthetic, opioid *analgesic* similar to *morphine*; diamorphine is another name for *heroin*. It is used to relieve severe pain and to relieve distress in acute *heart failure*. Diamorphine carries the risk of dependence (see *drug dependence*). It may cause nausea, vomiting, and constipation. (See also *heroin abuse*.)

diaphragmatic hernia

The protrusion of an abdominal structure through the *diaphragm muscle* into the thorax (chest cavity). The most common form of this problem is a *hiatus hernia*, in which part of the stomach protrudes through the space in the diaphragm that is normally occupied by the *oesophagus*.

diaphragm, contraceptive

A female barrier method of contraception in the form of a hemispherical dome of thin rubber with a metal spring in the rim. The diaphragm is inserted into the vagina and positioned over the cervix. (See also *contraception, barrier methods*.)

diaphragm muscle

The dome-shaped sheet of muscle that separates the chest from the abdomen. The diaphragm is attached to the spine,

---

ANATOMY OF THE **DIAPHRAGM**

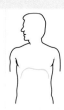

The diaphragm is attached to the spine, the lower pairs of ribs, and the lower end of the sternum (breastbone). Its muscle fibres converge on the central tendon, which is a thick, flat plate of dense fibres. There are openings in the diaphragm for the oesophagus, the phrenic nerve (which controls diaphragm movements and hence breathing), and the aorta and vena cava (the body's main blood vessels).

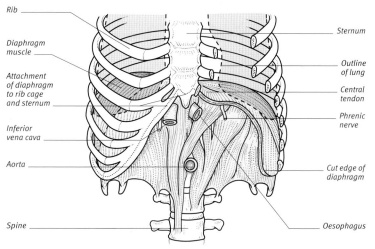

ribs, and sternum (breastbone). It has openings for the oesophagus and major nerves and blood vessels.

The diaphragm plays an important role in breathing. During inhalation, its muscle fibres contract, causing it to move downwards and drawing air into the lungs. During exhalation, the diaphragm muscle relaxes and it moves upwards, causing air to leave the lungs. (See also *breathing*.)

diaphysis

The shaft, or central portion, of a long bone, such as the *femur* (thigh-bone). During bone formation, the *epiphysis* (end of the long bone) develops independently from the diaphysis, as they are initially separated by a mass of cartilage known as the epiphyseal plate. The diaphysis and epiphysis eventually fuse to form a complete bone.

diarrhoea

An increase in the fluidity, frequency, or volume of bowel movements, as compared to the usual pattern for a particular individual. Diarrhoea may be acute or chronic. The condition can be very serious in infants and in elderly people because of the risk of severe, potentially fatal, *dehydration*.

CAUSES
Acute diarrhoea is usually a result of consuming food or water contaminated with certain bacteria or viruses (see *food poisoning*). Infective *gastroenteritis* also causes diarrhoea and may be acquired as a result of droplet infection. Other causes of acute diarrhoea include anxiety and, less commonly, *amoebiasis*, *shigellosis*, *typhoid fever* and *paratyphoid fever*, drug toxicity, *food allergy*, and *food intolerance*.

Chronic diarrhoea generally takes the form of repeated attacks of acute diarrhoea. Such a pattern may be the result of an intestinal disorder such as *Crohn's disease*, *ulcerative colitis*, cancer of the colon (see *colon, cancer of*), or *irritable bowel syndrome*. Diarrhoea that recurs, persists for more than a week, or is accompanied by blood requires medical investigation.

TREATMENT
The water and electrolytes (salts) lost during a severe attack of diarrhoea need to be replaced to prevent dehydration. Ready-prepared powders of electrolyte mixtures can be bought from chemists (see *rehydration therapy*). *Antidiarrhoeal drugs*, such as *diphenoxylate* and *lopera-*

mide may help if the diarrhoea is disabling. They should not, however, be used to treat attacks of diarrhoea in children.

diastole

The period in the heartbeat cycle when the heart muscle is at rest; it alternates with *systole*, the period of muscular contraction. (See also *cardiac cycle*).

diastolic pressure

The lowest level of *blood pressure* measured in the main arteries. Diastolic pressure is the pressure between heartbeats, when the *ventricles* (the lower chambers of the heart) are relaxed and filling with blood. Systolic pressure, the highest level of blood pressure in the main arteries, occurs when the ventricles of the heart contract.

The normal range of blood pressure varies with age and between individuals, but a young adult usually has a diastolic pressure of about 80 mmHg (mm of mercury) and a systolic pressure of about 120 mmHg. A persistently high diastolic pressure occurs in most cases of *hypertension*.

diathermy

The production of heat in a part of the body using high-frequency electric currents or microwaves. Diathermy can be used to increase blood flow and to reduce some types of deep-seated pain, for example in rheumatic or arthritic conditions. Diathermy can also be used to destroy tumours and diseased areas of tissue without causing bleeding. A diathermy knife is used by surgeons to coagulate bleeding vessels or to separate tissues without causing them to bleed (see *electrocoagulation*).

diathermy, short-wave

See *short-wave diathermy*.

diathesis

A predisposition towards certain disorders. For example, a bleeding diathesis is present when a *bleeding disorder* (such as haemophilia) makes a person susceptible to prolonged bleeding after an injury. A diathesis may be inherited or it may be acquired as a result of an illness or an injury.

diazepam

One of the *benzodiazepine drugs*, used mainly for the short-term treatment (usually a maximum of four weeks) of

severe *anxiety* and *insomnia*. Diazepam is also prescribed as a *muscle-relaxant drug*, as an *anticonvulsant drug* in the emergency treatment of *epilepsy*, and to treat alcohol withdrawal symptoms in people who are dependent on alcohol. It may also be administered intravenously in order to produce sedation in people undergoing certain medical procedures, such as *endoscopy*.

Diazepam may cause drowsiness, dizziness, and confusion; therefore, driving and hazardous work should be avoided while taking the drug. Alcohol increases the sedative effects of the drug and should not be consumed while diazepam is being used.

Like other benzodiazepines, diazepam can be habit-forming if it is taken regularly, and its effects diminish with prolonged use. People who have been taking diazepam regularly for more than two weeks should never stop their treatment suddenly; instead, they should gradually decrease the dose of the drug, under medical supervision, in order to avoid withdrawal symptoms (such as anxiety, sweating, or, rarely, after large doses, *seizures*).

DIC

See *disseminated intravascular coagulation*.

diclofenac

A *nonsteroidal anti-inflammatory drug* (NSAID) that is used to relieve pain and stiffness in *arthritis* and to hasten recovery following injury to muscles or ligaments. Possible adverse effects of the drug include nausea, abdominal pain, and peptic ulcer.

Didronel

A brand name for disodium etidronate (see *etidronate, disodium*), which is a *bisphosphonate drug*. Didronel is used to treat bone disorders such as *Paget's disease* and *osteoporosis*.

diet

See *nutrition*.

diet and disease

A variety of diseases are linked with diet. Diseases due to a deficiency of *nutrients* are a major problem in poor countries. In children, starvation or malnutrition may result in *marasmus* or *kwashiorkor*, while vitamin deficiencies may cause *rickets* or *keratomalacia* (a condition that causes blindness). Vitamin deficiencies may lead to *beriberi*, *pellagra*, or *scurvy*.

GOOD DIETARY HABITS

- Eat fresh rather than preserved, packaged, or convenience foods.

- Eat at least five portions of fruit and vegetables every day. When raw or only lightly cooked, they retain a higher nutritional value.

- Eat wholegrain products, including wholemeal bread.

- Cut down consumption of red meat; instead, eat fish, poultry, and pulses.

- Keep the fat content of your diet low and use polyunsaturated fats and vegetable oils rather than saturated fats.

- Cut down on sugar and salt in all foods.

- When choosing filling foods, eat potatoes in their skins, pasta, or rice.

In affluent countries, diseases due to deficiency are rare, occurring only in certain groups of people (such as alcoholics). Instead, many disorders are due at least partly to overconsumption of food. Overeating causes weight gain and, in severe cases, *obesity*. The latter condition places a person at increased risk of disorders such as *diabetes mellitus*, *stroke*, *coronary artery disease*, and *osteoarthritis*. Diets causing weight gain tend to be high in fats and sugar, but may be low in valuable components such as fibre and vitamins.

FATS
A diet that is high in fats, particularly saturated fats (see *fats and oils*), may contribute to *atherosclerosis* (narrowing of the arteries due to accumulation of fatty deposits on the arterial walls); this, in turn, may lead to cardiovascular diseases such as coronary artery disease, stroke, and peripheral vascular disease. A high-fat diet has also been linked with cancer of the bowel (see *colon, cancer of*) and *breast cancer*.

ALCOHOL
Overconsumption of *alcohol* can lead to *alcohol-related disorders*. In the digestive system, it may cause *cirrhosis* of the liver, *pancreatitis*, and oesophageal cancer (see *oesophagus, cancer of*); people who are dependent on alcohol also often become malnourished. Drinking too much alcohol may cause cardiovascular problems such as *hypertension* (high blood pressure) and *heart failure*; neurological disorders such as *Wernicke–Korsakoff syndrome*; and psychological or behavioural problems such as *depression* or violence.

SALT
A high salt intake may predispose a person to hypertension.

FIBRE
Fibre, found in fruit, vegetables, and grains, provides bulk, which helps the passage of food through the intestine and also aids absorption of nutrients (see *fibre, dietary*). Lack of fibre is thought to be a factor in digestive disorders such as *diverticular disease* (in which abnormal pouches form in the colon), chronic *constipation*, and *haemorrhoids*.

VITAMINS
Many people's diets contain too few natural vitamins; to remedy this problem, it is better to eat vitamin-rich foods than to take vitamin supplements. Women who are planning a pregnancy should take the recommended dose of *folic acid* supplement before conceiving and then during the first 12 weeks of pregnancy in order to reduce the risk of *neural tube defects* in the baby.

FOOD ALLERGIES
Many illnesses are commonly ascribed to *food allergy*, but it is only rarely that a definite link is proved. Nut allergies, which may cause the life-threatening reaction *anaphylaxis*, and *coeliac disease* (a reaction to the protein gluten, which is found in wheat and other cereals) are examples of genuine food allergies. (See also *nutritional disorders*.)

dietary amenorrhoea
A form of *amenorrhoea* (cessation of menstruation) caused by major weight loss, although not necessarily by a lack of food. In some cases, the weight loss is deliberate and severe (see *anorexia nervosa*). Absence of menstrual periods occurs because the loss of body fat disrupts the levels of the female sex hormone *oestrogen*.

dietary fibre
See *fibre, dietary*.

dietetics
The application of nutritional science to maintain or restore health. Dietetics involves not only a knowledge of the composition of foods, the effects of cooking and processing various foods, and dietary requirements, but also of psychological aspects of diet, such as eating habits (see *nutrition*).

diethylstilbestrol
A synthetic form of the female sex hormone *oestrogen*. It is occasionally used to treat *breast cancer* (in postmenopausal women only), and very occasionally to treat prostate cancer (see *prostate, cancer of*). Adverse effects include nausea, *oedema* (fluid retention) and breast enlargement (*gynaecomastia*) in men.

differential diagnosis
One of two or more different disorders that could be the cause of a patient's symptoms. If certain symptoms, such as abdominal pain, might be caused by various disorders, a doctor will carry out further tests, observe the patient's response to particular treatments, or monitor the course of the disease in order to arrive at the true diagnosis.

differentiation
The process by which the cells of the early *embryo*, which are almost identical and have not yet taken on any particular function, gradually diversify to form the distinct tissues and organs of the more developed embryo.

The word "differentiation" is also used in the assessment of cancer; it means the degree to which the microscopic appearance of cancerous tissue resembles normal tissue.

diffusion
The spread of a substance (by movement of its molecules) in a fluid from an area of high concentration to one of lower concentration, thus producing a uniform concentration throughout.

diflunisal
A *nonsteroidal anti-inflammatory drug* (NSAID) used to relieve joint pain and stiffness in types of *arthritis*. The drug is also given for back pain, sprains, and strains. Side effects include nausea, diarrhoea, and a rash.

DiGeorge syndrome
An *immunodeficiency disorder* that results in a failure of the *immune system's* cells to fight infection. The disorder is hereditary and congenital (present at birth). In DiGeorge syndrome, the *thymus* gland is absent or fails to develop normally. The thymus is a key part of the immune system, so its absence may allow persistent, serious infections to develop. Children with DiGeorge syndrome are susceptible to *opportunistic infections*, such as *candidiasis* (thrush),

D

THE DIGESTIVE PROCESS

Digestion starts when food enters the mouth. It continues as the food is propelled through the digestive tract by waves of muscular contractions (peristalsis). The digestive process also involves various organs (the salivary glands, liver, gallbladder, and pancreas), which produce enzymes and acids that help to break down the food.

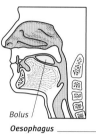

Bolus   *Bolus*

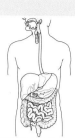

Swallowing
In the mouth, food is cut and ground by the teeth and mixed with saliva, which softens it and breaks down certain carbohydrates. After swallowing, the food mass (bolus) enters the oesophagus.

ACTION OF DIGESTIVE AGENTS

Agent or enzyme (where produced)	Digestive action
Amylase (mouth and pancreas)	Converts starch (a carbohydrate) to maltose
Sucrase, maltase, and lactase (pancreas and small intestine)	Break down vegetable and milk sugars into glucose, fructose, and galactose
Hydrochloric acid (stomach), **Pepsin** (stomach), **Trypsin** (pancreas), **Peptidase** (small intestine)	Assist in the breakdown of proteins into polypeptides, peptides, and amino acids
Lipase (pancreas) **Bile salts and acids** (liver – stored in the gallbladder)	Break down fats into glycerol and fatty acids

TIME SCALE

The approximate period food spends in each part of the digestive system is shown below.

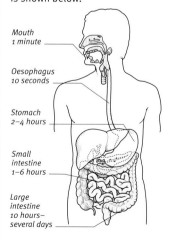

Mouth
1 minute

Oesophagus
10 seconds

Stomach
2–4 hours

Small intestine
1–6 hours

Large intestine
10 hours– several days

Oesophagus
Food is carried down the oesophagus by peristaltic action and enters the stomach.

Stomach
Food is broken down further by churning and by the action of hydrochloric acid and digestive enzymes secreted by the stomach lining. Food remains in the stomach until it is reduced to a semi-liquid consistency (chyme), when it passes into the duodenum.

Gallbladder

Bile duct

Pancreas

Duodenum
This is the first part of the small intestine. As food travels through the duodenum, it is broken down further by digestive enzymes from the liver, the gallbladder, and the pancreas.

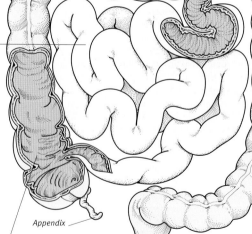

Small intestine
Additional enzymes secreted by glands in the lining of the small intestine complete the digestive process. Nutrients are absorbed through the intestinal lining into the network of blood vessels and lymph vessels that supply the intestine. Undigested matter passes into the large intestine (the colon).

Appendix

Colon
Water from undigested matter is absorbed through the lining of the colon. The residue passes into the rectum.

Rectum
Undigested matter enters this final part of the large intestine and is expelled.

Anus

and there may be evidence of failure to thrive (restricted growth). In addition, heart abnormalities and *hypocalcaemia* (abnormally low levels of calcium in the blood) may occur.

Transplants of thymus tissue, or *bone marrow transplants*, may be successful in treating the immunodeficiency.

digestion

The process by which food is broken down into smaller components that can be transported and used by the body. (See also *digestive system*).

digestive system

The group of organs responsible for *digestion*. The digestive system consists of the digestive tract (also known as the alimentary tract or canal) and various associated organs.

STRUCTURE

The *mouth*, *pharynx* (throat), *oesophagus* (gullet), *stomach*, *intestines*, and *anus* make up the digestive tract. The intestines consist of the small intestine (comprising the *duodenum*, *jejunum*, and *ileum*) and the large intestine (comprising the *caecum*, *colon*, and *rectum*). Associated organs, such as the *salivary glands*, the *liver*, and *pancreas*, secrete digestive juices that help break down food as it goes through the tract.

FUNCTION

Food and the products of digestion are moved from the throat to the rectum by *peristalsis* (waves of muscular contractions of the intestinal wall).

Food is broken down into simpler substances before being absorbed into the bloodstream. Physical breakdown is performed by the teeth, which cut and chew, and the stomach, which churns the food. Chemical breakdown of food is performed by the action of *enzymes* (biological catalysts), acids, and salts. *Carbohydrates* are broken down into simple sugars. *Proteins* are broken down into *polypeptides*, *peptides*, and *amino acids*. *Fats* are broken down into *glycerol*, glycerides, and *fatty acids*.

In the mouth, saliva lubricates food and contains enzymes that begin to break down carbohydrates. The tongue moulds food into balls (called boli) for easy swallowing. The food then passes into the pharynx, from where it is pushed into the oesophagus and is then squeezed down into the stomach. Once in the stomach, the food is mixed with hydrochloric acid and pepsin. These substances, produced by the stomach

lining, help to break down proteins. When the food has been converted to a semi-liquid consistency, it passes into the duodenum, where bile salts and acids (produced by the liver) help to break down the fats it contains. Digestive juices released by the pancreas into the duodenum contain enzymes that further break down food.

Breakdown concludes in the small intestine, carried out by enzymes that are produced by glands in the intestinal lining. Nutrients are absorbed in the small intestine through tiny projections from the intestinal wall, called villi. The food residue enters the large intestine, where much of the water it contains is absorbed by the lining of the colon. Undigested matter is expelled via the rectum and anus as *faeces*.

digit

A division, such as a *finger* or *toe*, that is located at the end of a limb.

digitalis drugs

A group of drugs extracted from plants belonging to the foxglove family. They are used to treat heart conditions such as *heart failure* and arrhythmias (see *arrhythmia, cardiac*), most commonly *atrial fibrillation* (irregular, rapid beating of the upper heart chambers). The drugs most frequently used are *digitoxin* and *digoxin*.

digital subtraction angiography

See *angiography*.

digitoxin

A long-acting *digitalis drug* that is used to treat *heart failure* and certain types of *arrhythmia* (irregular heartbeat).

digoxin

The most widely used of the *digitalis drugs*. Digoxin is used in the treatment of *heart failure* and certain types of *arrhythmia* (irregular heartbeat), such as *atrial fibrillation*. Blood tests are sometimes needed to ensure the correct digoxin dose, especially in patients with kidney disease. An excessive dose may cause headache, loss of appetite, nausea and vomiting, and visual disturbances. Digoxin occasionally disrupts the normal heartbeat, causing *heart block*.

Di Guglielmo's disease

A form of acute myeloblastic leukaemia (see *leukaemia, acute*) characterized by excessive numbers of red blood cells in the bone marrow and bloodstream.

dihydrocodeine

A type of opioid *analgesic drug* (pain-killer). Side effects of dihydrocodeine include nausea and vomiting.

dilatation

A condition in which a body cavity, passage, or opening is enlarged or stretched due to normal physiological processes (such as *childbirth*) or because of the effects of disease.

The term "dilatation" also refers to medical procedures for achieving such enlargement, as in dilatation and curettage (see *D and C*).

dilatation and curettage

See *D and C*.

dilation

A term that is sometimes used as an alternative to *dilatation*.

dilator

An instrument used for stretching and enlarging a narrowed body cavity, passage, or opening, for example to enable an investigative procedure or surgery.

diltiazem

A *calcium channel blocker* drug that is used in the treatment of *hypertension* (high blood pressure) and *angina pectoris* (chest pain due to impaired blood supply to the heart muscle). Side effects of diltiazem may include headaches, loss of appetite, nausea, constipation, and swollen ankles.

dimeticone

A silicone-based substance, also known as simeticone, that is used in *barrier creams* and as an antifoaming agent in *antacid* preparations.

dioptre

A unit of the power of *refraction* (the "strength") of a lens; the greater the power, the stronger the lens. Lenses that cause parallel light rays to converge have a positive dioptric number and are used to correct longsightedness (see *hypermetropia*). Those that cause light rays to diverge have a negative dioptric number and are used to correct shortsightedness (see *myopia*).

dioxin

The name of a highly toxic group of chemicals. Dioxins are contaminants of some defoliant weedkillers (see *defoliant poisoning*; *Agent Orange*).

D

diphenoxylate

An *antidiarrhoeal drug* that is chemically related to the opioid *analgesic drugs* (painkillers). Diphenoxylate lessens the contractions of the muscles in the walls of the intestines, thereby reducing the frequency of bowel movements.

diphtheria

A bacterial infection that causes a sore throat, fever, and sometimes serious or even fatal complications. Diphtheria is caused by the bacillus CORYNEBACTERIUM DIPHTHERIAE. The disease is now rare in developed countries as a result of mass *immunization*.

SYMPTOMS

The infection may begin in the throat or in the skin. In the throat, multiplication of bacteria causes the formation of a membrane that may cover the tonsils and spread up over the palate or down to the larynx (voicebox) and the trachea (windpipe), causing *breathing difficulty* and a husky voice. Other symptoms include enlarged *lymph nodes* in the neck, an increased heart rate, and mild fever. If infection is confined to the skin, the bacteria may produce a yellowish lesion covered by a hard membrane.

Life-threatening symptoms occur only in people who are not immune to the disease. They are caused by a toxin that is released by the bacteria and affects the heart and nervous system. Occasionally, a victim collapses and dies within a day of developing throat symptoms. More often, the victim is recovering from diphtheria when *heart failure* or paralysis of the throat or limbs develops. These complications can occur up to seven weeks after the onset of infection in the throat.

TREATMENT

Diphtheria is treated with antibiotics; in addition, an antitoxin is given to neutralize the bacterial toxin. If severe breathing difficulties develop, a *tracheostomy* (insertion of a breathing tube into the windpipe) may also be necessary.

PREVENTION

In the UK, children are given immunity against diphtheria in a single combined vaccine. At the age of 2, 3, and 4 months, the vaccine is combined with vaccine against tetanus, pertussis (whooping cough), polio, and HAEMOPHILUS INFLUENZAE type b, or Hib (DTaP/IPV/Hib); at 3 years 4 months to 5 years, it is combined with vaccine against tetanus, pertussis, and polio (DTaP/IPV or dTaP/IPV); and at 13 to 18 years, it is combined with tetanus and polio vaccine (Td/IPV).

diplegia

Paralysis affecting both sides of the body (both legs and, to a lesser extent, both arms). (See also *spastic diplegia*.)

diplopia

The medical term that is used to describe *double vision*.

dipsomania

A form of *alcohol dependence* in which periods of excessive drinking and craving for drink alternate with periods of relative sobriety.

dipyridamole

A drug that reduces the stickiness of platelets in the *blood* and thereby helps to prevent the formation of abnormal blood clots within arteries. Dipyridamole may be used with *aspirin* or *warfarin* to prevent the formation of blood clots following *stroke* or *transient ischaemic attack* or in people who have artificial heart valves.

Possible adverse effects may include headache, flushing, and dizziness.

disability

A loss or impairment of normal functioning or activity as the result of a physical or mental impediment. (See also *handicap*; *rehabilitation*.)

disaccharide

A *carbohydrate* comprising two linked *monosaccharide* units. Lactose, maltose, and sucrose are all disaccharides.

discectomy

A procedure in which part or all of a damaged intervertebral disc (see *disc, intervertebral*) is surgically removed. Discectomy relieves the symptoms of *disc prolapse* (in which an intervertebral disc ruptures and part of its pulpy core protrudes) by relieving the pressure that the protruding tissue places on nerves or nerve roots.

discharge

A visible emission of fluid from an orifice or a break in the skin (such as a wound or burst boil). A discharge may be a normal occurrence, as in some types of *vaginal discharge*, but it could also be due to an infection or to inflammation, as occurs, for example, in *rhinitis* (inflammation of the lining of the nasal passages), *urethritis* (infection of the urethra), or *proctitis* (infection of the rectum).

disciformis, keratitis

A form of *keratitis* (inflammation of the cornea at the front of the eye) in which a disc-like opacity forms in the corneal tissue, usually as an *immune response* to a viral infection.

disc, intervertebral

One of the flat, circular, platelike structures containing *cartilage* that line the joints between adjacent *vertebrae* (bones) in the *spine*. Each intervertebral disc is composed of a fibrous outer layer and a soft, gelatinous core. The discs act as shock absorbers to cushion the vertebrae during movements of the spine. With increasing age, intervertebral discs become less supple and more susceptible to damage from injury; one of the most common problems is *disc prolapse* ("slipped" disc).

disclosing agents

Dyes that make the *plaque* deposits on teeth more visible so that they can be seen and removed.

discoid lupus erythematosus

A form of the chronic autoimmune disorder *lupus erythematosus* that is confined to the skin. It causes a red, itchy, scaly rash to appear, particularly on the face and scalp, behind the ears, and on any parts of the body that are exposed to sunlight. The disorder most commonly occurs in women between the ages of 25 and 45, and tends to run in families. Over a period of several years, discoid lupus erythematosus may subside and recur repeatedly with different degrees of severity. Diagnosis is by a skin *biopsy*, and treatment is with topical corticosteroid drugs or drugs such as hydroxychloroquine.

discoloured teeth

Teeth vary in colour from individual to individual and, in general, secondary teeth are darker in colour than primary teeth. In addition, teeth often get darker with age. The term discoloured teeth, however, refers to teeth that are abnormally coloured or stained.

EXTRINSIC STAINS

Extrinsic stains (those found on the tooth's surface) are common. They are usually easily removed by polishing and can be prevented by regular tooth cleaning. Smoking tobacco produces a brownish-black deposit on the teeth. Pigment-producing bacteria can leave a visible, usually green, line along the teeth, especially in children. Some dyes in foodstuffs can cause yellowing; dark brown spots may be due to areas of thinned enamel stained by foods. Some bacteria produce an orange-red stain. Stains may also follow the use of drugs containing metallic salts.

INTRINSIC STAINS

Intrinsic stains (within the tooth's substance) are permanent, but they can be reduced by *bleaching*. Causes include the death of the pulp inside the tooth or the removal of the pulp during *root-canal treatment*. The antibiotic drug *tetracycline* can be absorbed by developing teeth, and may cause yellowing of the teeth if given to children.

Mottling of the tooth enamel occurs if excessive amounts of fluoride are consumed during development of the enamel (see *fluorosis*). *Hepatitis* (liver disease) during infancy may lead to dis-coloration of the primary teeth. The teeth of children with *congenital* malformation of the *bile ducts* may be similarly affected.

TREATMENT

Many stains can be covered or diminished with whitening toothpastes or with cosmetic dental procedures such as *bonding* and bleaching.

disc, optic

See *optic disc*.

disc prolapse

A common disorder of the *spine*, in which one of the pads between the vertebrae (see *disc, intervertebral*) ruptures and part of its pulpy core protrudes. Commonly known as a slipped disc, it causes painful and at times disabling pressure on a nerve root or, less commonly, on the spinal cord. The lower back is most commonly affected, but disc prolapse can affect any of the vertebrae, including those in the neck.

CAUSES

A prolapsed disc may sometimes be caused by a sudden strenuous action but it usually develops gradually, due to degeneration of the discs with age.

SYMPTOMS

Symptoms depend on the location of the affected disc. If the sciatic nerve root is compressed, it causes *sciatica*, which may be accompanied by numbness and tingling, and, eventually, by weakness in the muscles of the leg. A prolapsed disc in the neck causes neck pain and stiffness and weakness in the arm and hand.

DIAGNOSIS AND TREATMENT

Diagnosis is usually made from the symptoms, although a *CT scan* or *MRI* scan of the spine may sometimes be done to confirm the diagnosis.

PHYSICAL AIDS FOR THE **DISABLED**

A variety of specially designed or adapted articles are available to help disabled people carry out everyday activities. Such aids include prostheses, supports, and mobility aids to improve disabled people's general functioning, as well as items designed to help them perform specific tasks more easily.

Devices that help vision, hearing, and movement improve the ability of disabled people to cope with all aspects of daily life. Such devices include walking frames, glasses, hearing-aids, artificial limbs, corsets, and wheelchairs. For people with very severe conditions, ventilators, home dialysis, and artificial feeding devices are used to sustain life.

There are various household aids available that can help people to cook, feed themselves, wash, dress, use the toilet, and get in and out of beds and chairs. Specially designed furniture and other devices can help disabled parents to care for their children. Sexual aids can facilitate an active sex life.

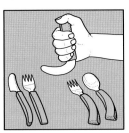

Tap turner
A device that helps with gripping and turning taps.

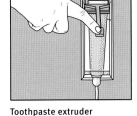

Tongs
Extending tongs to pick up dropped items. The tongs close up to fit in a pocket or handbag.

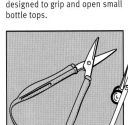

Bottle opener
A small hand-held device designed to grip and open small bottle tops.

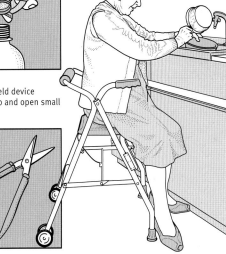

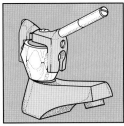

Cutlery
A range of knives, forks, and spoons with thick, moulded handles for easy manipulation.

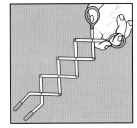

Toothpaste extruder
A wall-mounted device that dispenses toothpaste with minimal finger pressure.

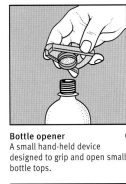

Scissors
Self-opening scissors with easy-grip handles.

"A" frame
A lightweight walking frame that doubles as a seat and can be folded flat.

D

SYMPTOMS AND TREATMENT OF **DISC PROLAPSE**

A prolapsed disc in the lower back causes low back pain and, if a sciatic nerve root is compressed, *sciatica* (pain running down the back of the leg from the buttock to the ankle), sometimes accompanied by numbness and tingling. Low back pain and sciatica are usually aggravated by coughing, sneezing, bending, and sitting for long periods. Prolonged pressure on the sciatic nerve can lead to weakness in the muscles of the leg.

A prolapsed disc in the neck causes neck pain and stiffness. If the disc compresses the root of a nerve that supplies the arm, there will be tingling and weakness in that arm and hand.

In rare cases, pressure is exerted on the spinal cord itself, sometimes leading to paralysis of the legs and loss of bladder or bowel control.

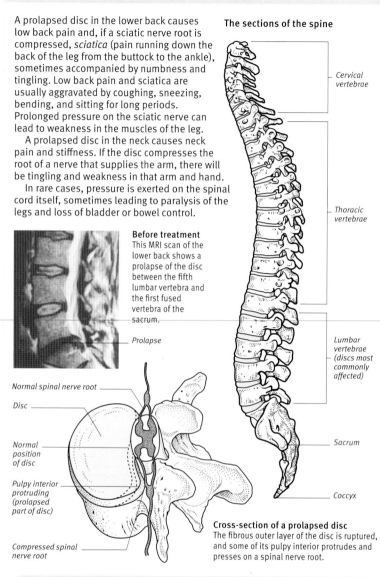

The sections of the spine

Cervical vertebrae

Thoracic vertebrae

Lumbar vertebrae (discs most commonly affected)

Sacrum

Coccyx

Before treatment
This MRI scan of the lower back shows a prolapse of the disc between the fifth lumbar vertebra and the first fused vertebra of the sacrum.

Prolapse

Normal spinal nerve root

Disc

Normal position of disc

Pulpy interior protruding (prolapsed part of disc)

Compressed spinal nerve root

Cross-section of a prolapsed disc
The fibrous outer layer of the disc is ruptured, and some of its pulpy interior protrudes and presses on a spinal nerve root.

TREATMENT

Disc prolapse often responds to analgesics, and special exercises (see *physiotherapy*) are helpful. Patients are usually advised to be as mobile as possible. For resting or sleep, they should lie flat on a supportive mattress, with the head supported and the shoulders, hips, and ankles aligned to ease pressure on the spine. If these measures fail and nerve root compression is causing muscle weakness, an operation may relieve the pressure (see *discectomy*; *decompression, spinal canal*).

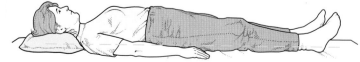

In most cases, the symptoms improve on their own within about six weeks, as the swelling around the protruding disc tissue subsides. During this period, *analgesic drugs* such as *paracetamol* can help relieve pain. Patients are usually advised to keep as mobile as possible, and physiotherapy may be helpful. However, if the pain is severe, a short period of bed rest may be advised. In very severe cases, surgical techniques, such as decompression of the spinal canal (see *decompression, spinal canal*) or removal of the protruding material and repair of the disc (see *discectomy*) may be necessary.

disc, slipped

See *disc prolapse*.

disease

Illness or abnormal functioning of a body part or parts due to a specific cause, such as an infection, and identifiable by certain *symptoms* and *signs*.

disease-modifying antirheumatic drugs

A diverse collection of antirheumatic drugs, known as DMARDs, that are used to relieve the symptoms and slow the progression of *rheumatoid arthritis* and psoriatic arthritis (a form of arthritis that sometimes occurs as a complication of *psoriasis*). DMARDs are not effective in treating osteoarthritis. Examples of DMARDs include *auranofin*, *azathioprine*, *chloroquine*, *ciclosporin*, *cyclophosphamide*, *gold*, hydroxychloroquine, *methotrexate*, *penicillamine*, *sodium aurothiomalate*, and *sulfasalazine*.

DMARDs not only improve the symptoms and signs of inflammatory joint disease, but they also slow the course of the illness. (In contrast, *nonsteroidal antiinflammatory drugs* relieve symptoms but do not alter the progress of the disease.) DMARDs work by modifying the body's immune response and directly suppressing the disease process.

In general, DMARDs may need to be used for several months before the full effects are felt. Many specialists therefore recommend starting therapy early to prevent or delay the progression of joint damage. Treatment with a combination of DMARDs may be more effective than a single drug, and may enable lower doses of each drug to be used, reducing the risk of adverse effects.

Possible side effects depend on the drug taken. They include diarrhoea, rash, *anaemia* (a reduced blood level of haemoglobin), *leukopenia* (a low white blood cell count), and increased susceptibility to infection. Regular *blood tests* and urine tests (see *urinalysis*) are needed during treatment to monitor the effects of DMARDs on the bone marrow, kidneys, and liver.

disinfectants

Substances that kill microorganisms and thus prevent infection. The term is usually applied to strong chemicals that are used to decontaminate objects.

dislocation, joint

Complete displacement of the two bones in a joint so that they are no longer in contact, usually as a result of injury. (Displacement that leaves the bones in partial contact is called *subluxation*.) It is usually accompanied by tearing of the joint ligaments and damage to the membrane encasing the joint.

SYMPTOMS AND COMPLICATIONS

Dislocation restricts or prevents the movement of the joint; it is usually very painful. The affected joint looks misshapen and swells. Injuries that are severe enough to cause dislocation often also cause *fractures*. In some cases, dislocation is followed by complications such as *paralysis*.

TREATMENT

The joint may be X-rayed to confirm dislocation and check for fracture. The bones are then manipulated back into their proper position, or an operation is performed to reset them. The bones are then immobilized in a *splint* or *cast* to allow healing to take place.

disodium etidronate

See *etidronate disodium*.

disopyramide

An *antiarrhythmic drug* that is used to treat an abnormally rapid heartbeat, as may occur after a *myocardial infarction* (heart attack). It reduces the force of heart muscle contraction. As a result, it may aggravate pre-existing *heart failure*. Other possible side effects include dry mouth and constipation.

disorder

Any abnormality of physical or mental function.

disorientation

Confusion as to time, place, or personal identity. Speech and behaviour tend to be muddled, and the affected person often cannot answer questions about time, date, present location, name, or address. Disorientation is usually due to a *head injury*, *intoxication*, or a chronic brain disorder, such as *dementia*. It may occasionally be due to *somatization disorder* (a psychological illness). (See also *confusion*; *delirium*.)

dispense

To prepare and distribute medicines to a patient according a doctor's *prescription*.

displacement

The transference of feelings from one object or person to another. Displacement is usually performed consciously to obtain emotional relief in a manner that will not cause harm to oneself or to another person. Some psychotherapists believe that displacement is an unconscious *defence mechanism*.

dissecting aneurysm

An *aneurysm* (ballooning of an artery) that usually affects the first part of the *aorta*. It is caused by a tear in the inner layer of the arterial wall, which results in the inner layer peeling away from the outer layer. This results in blood collecting in the space between the inner and outer layers.

A dissecting aneurysm may rupture or may compress the blood vessels leaving the aorta, producing *infarction* (localized tissue death due to lack of blood supply) in the organs supplied by them. The patient will suffer from severe chest pain that often spreads to the back or the abdomen. Surgical repair may help relieve the symptoms.

dissection

Cutting of body tissues during surgery or for the purpose of anatomical study.

disseminated intravascular coagulation (DIC)

A type of *bleeding disorder* in which abnormal clotting of blood leads to a depletion of coagulation factors in the blood; the consequence may be severe and spontaneous bleeding.

disseminated lupus erythematosis

An alternative name for systemic *lupus erythematosus*.

disseminated tuberculosis

A state in which the infectious disease *tuberculosis* has spread from the site of the original infection to affect several other parts of the body, either via the *lymphatic system* or in the bloodstream (see *miliary tuberculosis*).

dissociative disorders

A group of psychological conditions in which a particular mental function becomes cut off from the rest of the mind. Examples of dissociative disorders include hysterical amnesia (see *hysteria*), *fugue*, *multiple personality disorder*, and *depersonalization*. (See also *conversion disorder*.)

dissociative reaction

A psychological *defence mechanism* in which a person views unpleasant ideas or events, such as being assaulted, in a n unusually detached way in order to protect himself or herself from overwhelming feelings such as fear. In more severe cases, certain mental processes are split off from the rest of a person's mental activity and may function independently (see *dissociative disorders*).

dissonance

A term that is used in social psychology to describe a state that arises when an individual has minimal awareness of any discord, disagreement, or conflict within himself or herself. (See also *cognitive dissonance*.)

distal

A term describing a part of the body that is further away from another part with respect to a central point of reference, such as the trunk. For example, the fingers are distal to the arm. The opposite of distal is *proximal*.

disulfiram

A drug that acts as a deterrent to drinking *alcohol*. It is prescribed for people who request help in overcoming *alcohol dependence*. Treatment with the drug is usually combined with a counselling programme.

Disulfiram causes a buildup of acetaldehyde in the body when alcohol is ingested, even in the small amounts that may be present in some foods, medicines, and toiletries such as mouthwashes. This causes flushing, headache, nausea, thirst, dizziness, faintness, and palpitations. Symptoms may start within 10 minutes of drinking alcohol and can last for several hours. Occasionally, large amounts of alcohol taken during treatment can cause unconsciousness.

dithranol

A drug that is used in the treatment of the skin condition *psoriasis*. Dithranol is prescribed as an ointment, paste, or cream and works by slowing the rate at which skin cells multiply. This effect can be boosted by ultraviolet light treatment (see *phototherapy*). Dithranol can cause skin inflammation.

diuretic drugs

Drugs that help to remove excess water from the body by increasing the amount that is lost as *urine*. Diuretic drugs are used in the treatment of a variety of disorders, including *hypertension* (high blood pressure), *heart failure*, the eye condition *glaucoma*, *nephrotic syndrome* (a kidney disorder), and *cirrhosis* of the liver.

TYPES

There are various types of diuretic drug, which differ markedly in their speed and mode of action. Thiazide diuretics cause a moderate increase in urine production. Loop diuretic drugs are fast-acting, powerful drugs that are often used as an emergency treatment for heart failure. Potassium-sparing diuretics are used along with thiazide and loop diuretics, both of which may cause the body to lose too much potassium. Carbonic anhydrase inhibitors block the action of the enzyme carbonic anhydrase, which affects the amount of bicarbonate ions in the blood; these drugs increase urine output moderately but are effective only for short periods of time. Osmotic diuretics are used to maintain urine output following serious injury or major surgery.

POSSIBLE ADVERSE EFFECTS

Diuretics may cause chemical imbalances in the blood. The most common is hypokalaemia (low blood levels of potassium). This is usually treated with potassium supplements or potassium-sparing diuretic drugs. A diet rich in potassium may also be helpful. Some diuretics raise the blood level of uric acid, which increases the risk of *gout*. Certain diuretic drugs increase the blood glucose level, which may precipitate or worsen *diabetes mellitus*.

diurnal rhythms

A biological pattern that is based on a daily cycle; also called *circadian rhythms*. (See also *biorhythms*.)

diverticula

Small sacs or pouches that protrude externally from the wall of a hollow organ (such as the colon). They are thought to be caused by pressure forcing the lining of the organ though areas of weakness in the wall. Their presence in the walls of the intestines is characteristic of *diverticular disease*.

diverticular disease

The presence of small protruding sacs or pouches called diverticula in the intestinal wall, and the symptoms or complications caused by them. The term *diverticulosis* signifies the presence of diverticula in the intestine. *Diverticulitis* is a complication produced by inflammation in one or more diverticula.

diverticulitis

Inflammation of *diverticula* (abnormal pouches) in the wall of the intestine, particularly in the *colon*. Diverticulitis is a form of *diverticular disease* and a complication of *diverticulosis*.

SYMPTOMS AND COMPLICATIONS

The symptoms include fever, abdominal pain, vomiting, and rigidity of the abdomen. Intestinal haemorrhage may cause bleeding from the rectum.

Diverticula may perforate, or abscesses may form in the tissue around the colon, leading to *peritonitis* (inflammation of the lining of the abdomen). Other complications include intestinal bleeding, narrowing in the intestine, or a *fistula* (an abnormal channel between one part of the intestine and another).

TREATMENT

Diverticulitis usually subsides with bed rest and *antibiotics*. In severe cases, a liquid diet or *intravenous infusion* may be required. Surgery may be needed, in which the diseased section of the intestine is removed and the remaining sections are then joined back together. Some patients are given a temporary *colostomy* (an operation in which part of the colon is attached to the abdominal wall to form an opening for the discharge of faeces).

diverticulosis

A form of *diverticular disease* in which *diverticula* (abnormal pouches) exist in the wall of the intestine, particularly in

---

HOW **DIURETICS** WORK

The normal filtration process of the kidneys (which takes place in the tubules) removes water, salts (mainly potassium and sodium), and waste products from the bloodstream. Most of the salts and water are returned to the bloodstream, but certain amounts are expelled from the body together with the waste products in the urine.

Diuretics interfere with this normal kidney action. Osmotic, loop, and thiazide diuretics reduce the amount of sodium and water taken back into the blood, thus increasing the volume of urine. Modifying filtration in this way reduces the blood's water content. Less water in the blood causes excess water in the tissues to be expelled in urine.

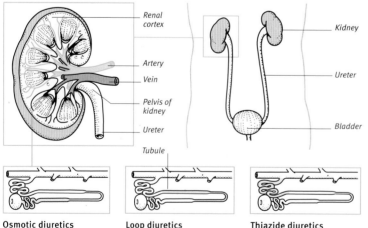

Renal cortex
Artery
Vein
Pelvis of kidney
Ureter
Tubule

Kidney
Ureter
Bladder

Osmotic diuretics
These act on the first part of the tubules to reduce the reabsorption of water into the bloodstream.

Loop diuretics
These drugs take effect on the middle part of the tubules and block sodium and chloride reabsorption.

Thiazide diuretics
This group acts on the last part of the tubules to reduce the reabsorption of sodium into the bloodstream.

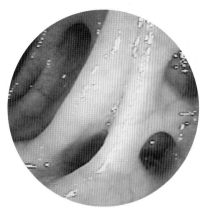

Diverticulosis of the colon
Diverticula (pouches) are clearly visible in this endoscopic view of the wall of the colon. The condition is thought to be due to a low-fibre diet.

the *colon*. Complications of diverticulosis may include intestinal bleeding and *diverticulitis*. The cause is believed to be a lack of fibre in the diet (see *fibre, dietary*). Diverticulosis is very rare in developing countries, where high-fibre foods make up much of the diet.

SYMPTOMS
Symptoms occur in only a minority of people with diverticulosis. They usually result from spasm or cramp of the intestinal muscle near diverticula. Many patients have symptoms similar to those of *irritable bowel syndrome*, including abdominal pain, a bloated sensation, and changes in bowel habits. In severe cases of diverticulosis, intestinal haemorrhage can lead to bleeding from the rectum.

DIAGNOSIS AND TREATMENT
Diagnosis is made by a barium enema (see *barium X-ray examinations*) or *endoscopy* (direct inspection using a viewing tube) of the intestine. In people with cramps, a high-fibre diet, fibre supplements, and *antispasmodic drugs* may relieve the symptoms. A high-fibre diet also reduces the incidence of complications. Whe adding fibre to the diet, it is important to increase fluid intake. Bleeding from diverticula usually subsides without treatment, but surgery is an option.

diving medicine
See *scuba-diving medicine*; *decompression sickness*.

Dixarit
A brand name for *clonidine*, an *antihypertensive drug* that is also used in the treatment of *migraine* and, in menopausal women, *hot flushes*.

dizziness
A sensation of unsteadiness and lightheadedness. Dizziness may be a mild, brief symptom that occurs by itself, or it may be part of a more severe, prolonged attack of *vertigo* (a condition typified by a spinning sensation) with nausea, vomiting, sweating, or fainting.

CAUSES
Most attacks are harmless and are due to a fall in the pressure of blood to the brain. This can occur when getting up quickly from a sitting or lying position (called *postural hypotension*). Similar symptoms may result from a *transient ischaemic attack*, in which there is a temporary, partial blockage in the arteries that supply the brain.

Other possible causes include tiredness, stress, fever, *anaemia*, *heart block* (impairment of electrical activity in the heart muscle), *hypoglycaemia* (low blood sugar levels), and *subdural haemorrhage* (bleeding between the outer two membranes that cover the brain).

Dizziness as part of vertigo is usually due to a disorder of the inner ear, the *acoustic nerve*, or the *brainstem*. The principal disorders of the inner ear that can cause dizziness and vertigo are *labyrinthitis* and *Ménière's disease*. Disorders of the acoustic nerve, such as *acoustic neuroma*, are rare causes of dizziness and vertigo. Brainstem disorders that can cause dizziness and vertigo include a type of *migraine*, *brain tumours*, and *vertebrobasilar insufficiency*.

TREATMENT
Brief episodes of mild dizziness usually clear up after taking a few deep breaths or after resting for a short time.

Severe, prolonged, or recurrent dizziness should be investigated by a doctor. Treatment depends on the underlying cause. For example, certain cases of dizziness and vertigo due to a disorder of the inner ear are treated with *antiemetic drugs* or *antihistamine drugs*.

dizygotic twins
Nonidentical *twins*, also called fraternal twins. Dizygotic twins are the result of the simultaneous *fertilization* of two egg cells (*ovum*). They each have a *placenta* of their own and may be of different sexes. (See also *monozygotic twins*.)

DLE
Discoid lupus erythematosus.

DMARDs
See *disease-modifying antirheumatic drugs*.

DMSA scan
A type of *kidney imaging* technique (see *radionuclide scanning*).

DNA
The abbreviation for deoxyribonucleic acid. DNA is the principal molecule carrying genetic information in almost all organisms; the exceptions are certain viruses that use *RNA*.

DNA is found in the *chromosomes* of cells; its double-helix structure allows the chromosomes to be copied exactly during the process of cell division. A special form of DNA exists in mitochondria, the tiny energy-producing structures within cells (see *mitochondrial DNA*). Sections of DNA can also be created artificially (see *recombinant DNA*) during genetic engineering. (See also *meiosis*; *mitosis*; *nucleic acids*.)

DNA fingerprinting
See *genetic fingerprinting*.

dobutamine
A drug that is used in the treatment of *heart failure* and *shock*, and sometimes after *cardiac arrest* (a halt in the pumping action of the heart). The drug is given by intravenous drip.

Dobutamine stimulates nerve cells in the heart to increase the heart rate and raise the blood pressure. For this reason, the drug may be used in a *cardiac stress test* to investigate potential *coronary artery disease* in cases where the patient is unable to exercise on a treadmill (see *exercise ECG*).

doctor
A qualified medical practitioner who is licensed to practise by the appropriate medical authority in his or her country, such as the General Medical Council in the UK. Suitably qualified dentists are also entitled to use the title "doctor".

dogs, diseases from
Infectious or parasitic diseases acquired from contact with dogs. They may be caused by viruses, bacteria, fungi, protozoa, worms, insects, or mites living in or on a dog. Many parasites that live on dogs can be transferred to humans, for example through stroking a dog's fur.

The most serious disease from dogs is *rabies*. The UK is free of rabies, but travellers to countries in which rabies exists should treat any dog bite with suspicion. Dog bites can cause serious bleeding and shock and may become infected.

D

Toxocariasis and *hydatid disease* are potentially serious diseases caused by the ingestion of worm eggs from dogs. In the tropics, walking barefoot on soil that is contaminated with dog faeces can lead to dog *hookworm infestation*.

Bites from dog *fleas* are an occasional nuisance. *Ticks* and *mites* from dogs, including a canine version of the *scabies* mite, are other common problems. The fungi that cause *tinea* infections in dogs can be caught by humans.

Some people become allergic to animal *dander* (tiny scales from fur or skin). They may, for example, suffer from attacks of *asthma* or *urticaria* (nettle rash) when a dog is in the house. (See also *zoonoses*.)

dominant

A term used in *genetics* to describe a *gene* that shows its effects when it is present in either a single or double dose in the genotype. Many characteristics are determined by a single pair of genes, one of each pair being inherited from each parent. A dominant gene of a pair has an effect whether there are one or two copies, unlike a recessive gene, which only has an effect when there are two copies.

A dominant gene overrides an equivalent recessive gene. For example, the gene for brown eyes is dominant, so if a child inherits a gene for brown eyes from one parent and a gene for blue eyes from the other, the child will have brown eyes.

Some genetic disorders are determined by a dominant gene, or example, *Marfan syndrome* and *Huntington's disease*. In such cases, a child will have the disease if he or she inherits the gene from one or both parents.

dominant characteristic

An inherited characteristic (external or internal physical feature) that appears in offspring even if they have inherited the *gene* for it from only one of their parents. See *dominant*.

dominant trait

An inherited *trait* (a characteristic or condition) that appears when just a single copy of the *gene* for that trait is present, as opposed to a *recessive* trait, which only appears when two copies of the appropriate gene are present. *Dominant* genes mask the presence of recessive genes, and dominant traits can be inherited from one parent alone.

domperidone

An *antiemetic drug* used to relieve nausea and vomiting associated with some gastrointestinal disorders or during treatment with certain drugs or *radiotherapy*. Adverse effects may include breast enlargement and secretion of milk from the breast.

donepezil

An *acetylcholinesterase inhibitor* that is used to treat mild to moderate *dementia* due to *Alzheimer's disease*.

donor

A person who provides blood for *transfusion*; body tissues or organs for *transplantation*; or eggs or semen for *artificial insemination*. The organs that are most frequently donated are kidneys, corneas, heart, lungs, liver, and pancreas. Certain organs can be donated during a person's lifetime; some are only used following *brain death*.

All donors should be free of cancer, serious infection (such as hepatitis B), and should not carry *HIV*. Organs for transplantation must be removed within a few hours of brain death, and before or immediately after the heartbeat has stopped. In some kidney transplants, the kidney is provided by a living donor, usually a relative whose tissues match well on the basis of *tissue-typing*. Tests are performed to ensure that both kidneys are healthy before one is removed.

Suitable related donors may also provide bone marrow for transplantation and sometimes skin for grafting. (See also *blood donation*; *bone marrow transplant*; *organ donation*; *transplant surgery*.)

Doose syndrome

A rare, inherited form of *epilepsy*. The condition is typified by muscular jerking, especially symmetrical jerking of the arms and shoulders and, in severe cases, twitching of the facial muscles. In addition, the affected person may fall to the ground and briefly lose consciousness. Doose syndrome can be treated with *anticonvulsant drugs*.

dopa

An amino acid that the body uses to form *dopamine*, an important neurotransmitter. Dopa is also formed as an intermediate stage when the body makes *epinephrine*, *norepinephrine*, and *melanin*. *Levodopa*, a form of dopa, is used to correct dopamine deficiency in people who have *Parkinson's disease*.

dopa-decarboxylase inhibitors

Drugs used in the treatment of the movement disorder *Parkinson's disease*. The two principal dopa-decarboxylase inhibitors, co-beneldopa and co-careldopa, are a combination of *levodopa* and benserazide and levodopa and carbidopa, respectively. These drugs stop levodopa from being activated except within the brain, which reduces the incidence of common side effects such as nausea and vomiting.

dopamine

A *neurotransmitter* (chemical released from nerve endings) found in the brain and around some blood vessels. It helps to control body movements: a deficiency of dopamine in the *basal ganglia* (groups of nerve cells deep in the brain) causes *Parkinson's disease*.

Synthetic dopamine is injected as an emergency treatment for shock caused by a *myocardial infarction* (heart attack) or *septicaemia* (blood infection) and as a treatment for severe *heart failure*.

Doppler echocardiography

An investigation in which blood flow through the *heart* is assessed by the use of *ultrasound* (high-frequency sound waves). An ultrasound transducer is moved over the chest in the area of the heart. The waves emitted by the transducer are reflected by blood, forming echoes that are recorded to give a picture of blood flow. This allows the direction and speed of the blood flow to be measured.

Doppler echocardiography can be used to investigate the presence of some conditions of the heart and circulation, including abnormalities of the heart valves (see *valvular heart disease*). The procedure is painless and takes between 15 and 30 minutes to perform.

Doppler effect

A change in the frequency with which waves (such as sound waves) from a source reach an observer when the source is in rapid motion with respect to the observer. Approaching sounds seem higher in pitch (frequency) than sounds that are moving away. This is due to the fact that the wavelengths of sounds from an approaching source are progressively foreshortened, whereas those from a receding source are stretched.

The Doppler effect is used in various medical *ultrasound scanning* techniques (see *Doppler ultrasonography*).

Doppler ultrasonography

A type of *ultrasound scanning* in which shifts in the frequency of ultrasonic waves are used to measure the velocity of moving structures. An emitter sends out pulses of ultrasound (inaudible, high-frequency sound) of a specific frequency. When the pulses bounce off a moving object (for example, blood flowing through a blood vessel), the frequency of the echoes is changed from that of the emitted sound. A sensor is able to detect the frequency changes and converts the data into useful information (about how fast blood is flowing, for example).

Doppler ultrasonography is widely used to detect narrowing of arteries in the neck due to *atherosclerosis* (accumulation of fatty deposits on the artery walls) and to detect blood clots in veins (as occurs in *deep vein thrombosis*). In addition, Doppler ultrasound techniques are used to monitor the fetal heartbeat, to detect air bubbles during *dialysis* and in *heart–lung machines*, and to measure blood pressure. (See also *Doppler echocardiography*.)

Dorfman–Chanarin syndrome

A very rare, autosomal recessive *genetic disorder* affecting fat metabolism (see *lipidosis*). The disease is *congenital* (present from birth). It is characterized by *ichthyosis* (thickened, scaly skin); *myopathy* (degeneration of muscle), and sometimes also defects in vision and in hearing. Blood tests show abnormal white *blood cells* containing vacuoles (tiny spaces) filled with fat.

dorsal

Relating to the back, located on or near the back, or describing the uppermost part of a body structure when a person is lying face-down. For example, dorsalgia describes pain in the back, and the dorsal part of the hand is the back of the hand. In human anatomy, the term dorsal means the same as posterior. The opposite of dorsal is *ventral* (meaning anterior or front).

dose

A term used to refer to the amount of a drug to be taken at a particular time, or to the amount of radiation to which an individual is exposed, during a session of *radiotherapy* for example. Drug dose may be expressed in terms of the weight of the active substance, the volume of liquid to be taken, or its effects on body tissues. The amount of radiation that is absorbed by body tissues during a session of radiotherapy is expressed in units called millisieverts (see *radiation units*).

dosulepin

A tricyclic *antidepressant drug* used in the treatment of *depression*. The drug has a sedative action and is particularly useful in cases of depression accompanied by *anxiety* or *insomnia*. Possible adverse effects include blurred vision, dizziness, flushing, and rash.

dothiepin

The former name for *dosulepin*.

double-blind

A type of *controlled trial* that tests the effectiveness of a particular treatment or compares the benefits of different treatments. In double-blind trials, neither the patients undergoing the treatments nor the doctors who are assessing them know which of the patients are receiving which treatment. This eliminates any expectations about which treatment will be most effective.

double contrast enema

A type of radiological investigation (see *radiology*) of the *intestine* (the main part of the digestive tract). A *contrast medium* (a substance opaque to *X-rays*) is introduced into the passage or cavity to be examined. The area is then distended (widened) by the introduction of air. A thin coating of the contrast medium is left on the walls of the intestine. As a result, the area to be examined is shown in outline on X-ray images. (See also *barium X-ray examinations*.)

double vision

Also known as diplopia, double vision is a condition in which a person sees two visual images of a single object instead of only one image. The two images are separate, but each of them is quite clearly focused.

CAUSES

It is usually a symptom of a squint, especially of paralytic squint, in which paralysis of one or more of the eye muscles impairs eye movement. Other causes include a tumour in the eyelid or a tumour or blood clot behind the eye. Double vision can also occur in *exophthalmos*, a condition in which the eyeballs protrude as the result of an underlying hormonal disorder.

TREATMENT

Double vision needs immediate investigation. The treatment depends on the underlying cause.

douche

The introduction of water and/or a cleansing agent into the vagina using a bag and tubing with a nozzle. Douching is unnecessary for hygiene and is ineffective as a method of *contraception*. It may cause infection or spread existing infection into the uterus or fallopian tubes.

Down's syndrome

A *chromosomal abnormality* that results in a variable degree of *learning difficulty* and a characteristic physical appearance in affected individuals. It is the most common chromosomal abnormality.

CAUSES

People with Down's syndrome have an extra *chromosome* (47 instead of the normal 46). They have three copies of chromosome number 21 instead of two; for this reason, the disorder is also called trisomy 21. In most cases, it is the result of a sperm or egg being formed with an extra chromosome 21, due to the failure of the chromosome 21 pair to part and enter separate cells during *meiosis*. If one of these abnormal egg or sperm cells takes part in fertilization, the baby will also have the extra chromosome. This type of abnormality is more likely if the mother is over 35.

A less common cause is a chromosomal abnormality called a *translocation*, in which part of one parent's own

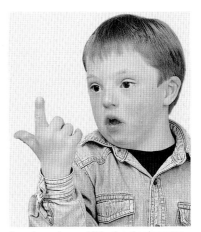

Down's syndrome child using sign language
There is a greater than normal risk of congenital deafness in Down's babies. Typical features of the condition include upward-sloping eyes that are covered at the corners, small facial features, and a large tongue that tends to stick out.

D

chromosome number 21 has joined with another chromosome. The parent is unaffected but has a high risk of having Down's children.

SYMPTOMS

Typical physical features of a person with Down's syndrome include small face and features; upward-sloping eyes with folds of skin that cover their inner corners; large tongue; flattened back to the head; short, broad hands, with a single horizontal crease on the palm (see *simian crease*); and short stature. *Learning difficulties* are very common, and range from mild to severe; however, affected people often have cheerful, friendly personalities.

People with Down's syndrome have a greater than normal risk for certain disorders. One possible problem is a heart defect at birth (see *heart disease, congenital*), which affects up to two in five babies. Others include intestinal *atresia* (a narrowing in the intestines), *hypothyroidism* (underactivity of the thryoid gland), and congenital *deafness*. Acute *leukaemia* is more common than in other children. Down's syndrome children are also more susceptible to upper respiratory tract and ear infections. Affected adults over the age of 40 have a higher than normal risk of developing *Alzheimer's disease*.

DIAGNOSIS

Screening tests in pregnancy include special blood tests and a *nuchal translucency scan* (also known as NT, a form of *ultrasound scan*). The results of these tests are combined to work out the risk of having a baby with Down's syndrome. If the results indicate that a fetus is likely to have the syndrome, *chorionic villus sampling* or *amniocentesis* are offered. In some cases, however, Down's syndrome is only recognized once the baby has been born. The diagnosis is confirmed by chromosome analysis of cells from the baby.

OUTLOOK

There is no cure for Down's syndrome and people with the condition have a lower than normal life expectancy, although some individuals survive into old age. Down's syndrome children can make the most of their capacities with appropriate environmental and educational stimulation and support. Some children learn skills such as reading and writing, and some adults may be able to work; however, most affected people cannot live independently and need long-term care.

doxazosin

An *antihypertensive drug* taken to reduce high blood pressure (see *hypertension*). Possible side effects include dizziness, headache, and nausea.

doxorubicin

An *anticancer drug* given by injection, often with other anticancer drugs. It is used in the treatment of a variety of cancers, including *lung cancer*.

doxycycline

A *tetracycline drug* used in the treatment of chronic *prostatitis*, *pelvic inflammatory disease*, *acne*, and chest infection in chronic *bronchitis*. It is also used to prevent and treat *malaria*. Taking the drug with food reduces possible side effects.

drainage angle

The gap between the outer edge of the *iris* (the coloured ring of muscle in the eye) and the *cornea* (the transparent covering of the eyeball). This structure, and the network of tissue behind it (the trabecular network), allows excess *aqueous humour* to drain from the front chamber of the eye. Blockage of the drainage angle causes acute *glaucoma*.

drain, surgical

An appliance that is inserted into a body cavity or a wound in order to release air or permit drainage of fluid. Drains range from simple soft rubber tubes that pass from a body cavity into a dressing to wide-bore tubes that connect to a collection bag or bottle. Suction drains are thin tubes containing many small holes to help collect fluid or air, which is then drawn into a vacuum bottle.

dream analysis

The interpretation of a person's dreams as part of *psychoanalysis* or *psychotherapy*. First developed by Sigmund Freud, it is based on the idea that repressed feelings and thoughts are revealed, in a disguised way, in dreams.

dreaming

Mental activity that takes place during *sleep*. Dreaming is thought to occur only during periods of REM (rapid eye movement) sleep, which last for about 20 minutes and occur four to five times a night. Compared to other phases, the REM phase of sleep is active. Blood flow and brain temperature increase, and there are sudden changes in heart rate and blood pressure.

Dreams usually closely mirror the day's preoccupations. Dreaming can be seen as a process in which the mental impressions, feelings, and ideas are sorted out. People roused during REM sleep report especially vivid dreams.

dressings

Protective coverings for *wounds* that are used to absorb blood or other body secretions, prevent contamination, or retain moisture. Pressure dressings are applied to stem bleeding or to reduce swelling at the site of injury.

Dressler's syndrome

An uncommon disorder, also known as postinfarction syndrome, that may occur following a *myocardial infarction* (heart attack) or heart surgery. Dressler's

TYPES OF **DRAINS**

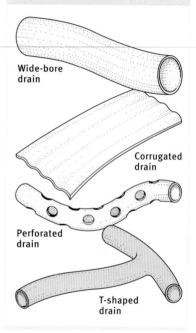

Wide-bore drain

Corrugated drain

Perforated drain

T-shaped drain

syndrome is characterized by fever, chest pain, *pericarditis* (inflammation of the membrane lining the heart), and *pleurisy* (inflammation of the membrane around the lungs). Treatment is with *aspirin* or, in severe cases, with *corticosteroid drugs*.

dribbling

Involuntary leakage of urine from the bladder (see *incontinence, urinary*) or of saliva from the mouth (drooling). Dribbling of saliva is normal in infants.

In adults, it may be due to poorly fitting dentures; alternatively, it may be the result of facial paralysis, dementia, or another disorder of the nervous system, most commonly *Parkinson's disease*. Dribbling of saliva may also be caused by an obstruction in the mouth that interferes with swallowing.

drip

See *intravenous infusion*.

drip, postnasal

See *postnasal drip*.

driving, health and

Safe driving depends in part on the health of the vehicle's driver. Any state or medical disorder that affects a driver's physical condition, or impairs mental faculties such as judgment, alertness, or speed of reaction, increases the risk of injury to the driver and also to other road users and pedestrians.

One of the most obvious hazards is being under the influence of *alcohol*. There are strict laws regarding the maximum blood alcohol level allowed, because alcohol is known to impair judgment and to slow reaction times. Illicit drugs (see *drug abuse*) have a similarly harmful effect. Some prescribed *drugs* can also affect ability to drive; for example, some antihistamines (used to treat disorders such as hay fever) can cause drowsiness. The combination of drugs and alcohol is more potent than either used alone. Other states that can be hazardous include *fatigue* and any type of *stress* reaction such as anger and *anxiety*. Driving when tired is one of the most common causes of road accidents.

Various health problems or conditions may affect a person's fitness to drive, an obvious example being impaired vision. Other examples include having had a *stroke*, having had a *pacemaker* fitted, certain physical disabilities, and some chronic conditions, such as *epilepsy* and *diabetes mellitus*. People whose fitness to drive is impaired may still be allowed to drive (possibly subject to certain restrictions) but must disclose their condition to their vehicle licensing authority and insurance company.

Regardless of the medical condition, a person must contact the vehicle licensing authority if there is any doubt or cause for concern about his or her fitness to drive.

drooping eyelid

See *ptosis*.

drop attack

A brief disturbance that affects the nervous system, causing a person to fall to the ground without warning. Unlike in *fainting*, the person may not lose consciousness, but injuries can occur from the fall. Elderly women make up the group most commonly affected.

CAUSES

The causes are not fully understood, but they may be a form of *transient ischaemic attack* (TIA) in which there is a fall in blood flow to nerve centres in the *brainstem*. Elderly men may have a drop attack while passing urine or while standing, possibly due to low blood pressure or to an abrupt alteration in heart rhythm. Akinetic seizures (a rare form of *epilepsy*) are also sometimes described as drop attacks; the sufferer falls to the ground but does not have muscular spasms.

TREATMENT

There is no treatment for drop attacks in elderly people. Akinetic seizures usually respond to *anticonvulsant drugs*.

drop, foot

See *foot-drop*.

dropped beat

A type of cardiac arrhythmia (see *arrhythmia, cardiac*) characterized by the absence of a single ventricular contraction. The next heartbeat often comes slightly early, and is more forceful than usual; this beat is often the one that is noticed, rather than the dropped one. Dropped beat is very common and may be caused by alcohol, caffeine, and some medications. Single, infrequent dropped beats are very unlikely to be due to heart disease.

dropsy

An outmoded term for generalized *oedema* (fluid accumulation in body tissues).

drowning

Death caused by suffocation and *hypoxia* (a lack of oxygen) associated with immersion in a fluid. Most often, the person inhales liquid into the lungs; but sometimes no liquid enters the lungs, a condition called dry drowning (see *drowning, dry*). People who are resuscitated after prolonged immersion are said to be victims of "near drowning". (See also *Types of drowning*, p.246.)

MECHANISM OF DROWNING

Initially, automatic contraction of a muscle at the entrance to the windpipe, a mechanism known as the laryngeal reflex, prevents water from entering the lungs; instead, the water enters the oesophagus and stomach. However, the laryngeal reflex impairs breathing and can quickly lead to hypoxia and to loss of consciousness. If the person is buoyant at this point and floats face-up, his or her chances of survival are reasonable because the laryngeal reflex begins to relax and normal breathing may then resume.

FIRST AID AND TREATMENT

An ambulance should be called and the person's condition assessed. If he or she is not breathing and/or the pulse is absent, resuscitative measures should be started (see *cardiopulmonary resuscitation; rescue breathing*) and continued until medical help arrives.

Victims can sometimes be resuscitated despite a long period immersed in very cold water (which reduces the body's oxygen needs). In all cases of successful resuscitation, the person should be sent to hospital, because life-threatening symptoms may develop some hours after rescue if water has passed from the lungs into the blood.

drowning, dry

A form of *drowning* in which no fluid enters into the lungs. Some fatal drowning cases are "dry". Victims of dry drowning have a particularly strong laryngeal reflex, which diverts water into the stomach instead of the lungs, but at the same time impairs breathing. As with cases of "wet" drowning, death occurs by suffocation.

drowsiness

A state of consciousness between full wakefulness and *sleep* or *unconsciousness*. Drowsiness is medically significant if a person fails to awaken after being shaken, pinched, and shouted at, or wakes but relapses into drowsiness.

Abnormal drowsiness must be treated as a medical emergency. It may be the result of a *head injury*, high fever, *meningitis* (inflammation of the membranes surrounding the brain and spinal cord), *uraemia* (excess urea in the blood due to *kidney failure*), or *liver failure*. Alcohol or drugs may also produce this effect. In a person with *diabetes mellitus*, drowsiness may be a result of *hypoglycaemia* (low blood sugar levels) or of *hyperglycaemia* (high blood sugar levels).

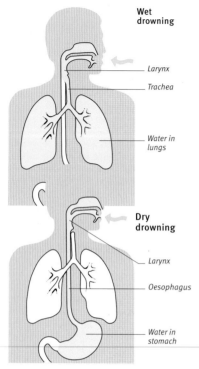

Wet drowning

Larynx

Trachea

Water in lungs

Dry drowning

Larynx

Oesophagus

Water in stomach

Types of drowning
In four-fifths of deaths due to drowning, the victim has inhaled liquid into his or her lungs. In the other fifth, no liquid is present in the lungs; this condition is called dry drowning. In both cases, death is by suffocation.

drug

A chemical substance that alters the function of one or more body organs or the process of a disease. Drugs include prescribed medicines, over-the-counter remedies, and various substances (such as alcohol, tobacco, and drugs of abuse) that are used for nonmedical purposes.

CLASSIFICATION AND LICENSING

Drugs normally have a chemical name, an officially approved generic name (see *generic drug*), and often a brand name. Most drugs for medical use are either licensed for prescription by a doctor only or can be bought over the counter at a chemist's or supermarket. However, for some drugs, low-strength preparations are available over the counter but higher strengths are available only on prescription. Some non-prescription drugs, such as paracetamol, can be bought only in limited quantities over the counter.

Most drugs are artificially produced to ensure a pure preparation with a predictable potency (strength). Some drugs are genetically engineered. A drug is classified according to its chemical make-up, or the disorder it treats, or

according to its specific effect on the body. All new drugs are tested for their efficiency and safety. In the UK, drugs are licensed by the Medicines and Healthcare products Regulatory Agency (MHRA). A licence may be withdrawn if toxic effects are reported or if the drug causes serious illness.

USES

Drugs can be used to relieve physical or mental symptoms, to replace a natural substance that is deficient, or to stop the excessive production of a *hormone* or other chemical by the body. Some drugs are given to destroy foreign organisms, such as bacteria or fungi. Others, which are known as *vaccines*, are given to stimulate the body's *immune system* to form *antibodies*.

METHODS OF ADMINISTRATION

Drugs are given by mouth or injection, or are applied directly or indirectly to the affected site via transdermal, nasal, and other direct routes (for example, to the lungs through an inhaler). Drugs that are injected take effect more rapidly than those taken by mouth because they enter the bloodstream directly. There are different routes for injection. The fastest is intravenous; intramuscular is also fast because muscles have a good blood supply; subcutaneous injection is the slowest but is easier for self-administration.

ELIMINATION

Unabsorbed drugs are broken down in the liver. Those taken orally are excreted in faeces; those that have entered the bloodstream are eliminated in urine.

ADVERSE EFFECTS

Most drugs can produce adverse effects. These effects may wear off as the body adapts to the drug. Adverse effects are more likely if there is a change in the absorption, breakdown, or elimination of a drug (caused, for example, by liver disease). Unexpected reactions sometimes occur due to a genetic disorder, an allergic reaction, or the formation of antibodies that damage body tissues. Some drugs interact with food, alcohol, or other drugs.

Many drugs can cross the placenta; some affect the growth and development of the fetus if taken by a pregnant woman. Most drugs can pass into the breast milk of a nursing mother, and some have adverse effects on the baby.

drug abuse

Use of a drug for a purpose other than that for which it is normally prescribed or recommended. Commonly abused

drugs include *stimulant drugs*, such as *cocaine* and *amphetamine drugs*; central nervous system depressants, such as *alcohol* and *barbiturate drugs*; *hallucinogenic drugs*, such as *LSD*; and narcotics (see *opioid drugs*), such as *heroin*. Some drugs are abused in order to improve performance in sports (see *sports, drugs and*; *steroids, anabolic*).

Problems resulting from drug abuse may arise from the adverse effects of the drug, accidents that occur during intoxication, or from the habit-forming potential of many drugs, which may lead to *drug dependence*.

drug addiction

Physical or psychological dependence on a drug (see *drug dependence*).

drug dependence

The compulsion to continue taking a drug, either to prevent the ill effects that occur when it is not taken, or to produce the desired effects of taking it.

TYPES

Drug dependence can be psychological or physical, or more commonly both. A person is psychologically dependent if he or she experiences craving or distress when the drug is withdrawn. In physical drug dependence, the body has adapted to the drug, causing the symptoms and signs of *withdrawal syndrome* when the drug is stopped. These symptoms are relieved if the drug is taken again.

CAUSE

Dependence develops as a result of regular or excessive drug use, and it develops most frequently with drugs that alter mood or behaviour.

SYMPTOMS AND SIGNS

Drug dependence may cause physical problems, for example lung and heart disease from smoking and liver disease from excessive *alcohol* consumption. Mental problems, such as anxiety and depression, are common during drug withdrawal. Dependence may also be linked with drug tolerance, in which increasing doses of the substance are needed to produce the same effect.

COMPLICATIONS

Complications such as *hepatitis* or *AIDS* are a particular risk for people who abuse drugs by injection. Death may occur from taking a contaminated drug or from an accidental overdose.

TREATMENT AND OUTLOOK

Controlled withdrawal programmes are available in special centres and hospitals, which usually offer gradual, supervised reductions in dose. Alternative, less harmful drugs may be given, as well as treatment for any withdrawal symptoms that may develop. Social service agencies and support groups may provide follow-up care. However, the success of treatment depends to a large extent on the motivation of the affected person. Problems often recur if people return to the circumstances that originally gave rise to the drug abuse.

drug eruption

An adverse, allergic reaction (see *allergy*) that is provoked by the ingestion or topical application of a particular *drug*. A drug eruption is usually manifested as a *rash* on the surface of the skin.

drug-induced disease

Any disorder resulting from the use of a *drug*. Examples include drug-induced *lupus erythematosus*, haemolytic anaemia (see *anaemia, haemolytic*), and *parkinsonism*. Factors that may increase the risk of drug-induced disease are age, sex, individual sensitivity, underlying disease (especially of the kidneys or liver), and the combination of drugs a patient is taking. Adverse effects associated with the use of medications may lead to hospitalization, disability, or even death. (See also *side effect*.)

drug interaction

The effect of a *drug* when it is taken in combination with other drugs or with substances such as alcohol.

drug overdose

See *drug poisoning*.

drug poisoning

The harmful effects on the body that occur as a result of an excessive dose of a particular drug.

INCIDENCE AND CAUSES

Accidental poisoning most commonly occurs in young children. Child-resistant drug containers have helped to reduce this risk. In adults, drug poisoning usually occurs in elderly or confused people who are unsure about their treatment and dosage requirements. Accidental poisoning may also occur in *drug abuse*. Deliberate self-poisoning may be a cry for help (see *suicide*; *suicide, attempted*).

Drugs that are most commonly taken in overdose include *benzodiazepine drugs*, *antidepressant drugs*, and over-the-counter drugs such as *paracetamol*.

TREATMENT

Anyone who has taken a drug overdose, and any child who has swallowed tablets belonging to someone else, needs immediate medical attention. It is important to identify the drugs that have been taken.

Treatment in hospital may involve washing out the stomach by passing water through a tube introduced into the mouth (see *lavage, gastric*). *Charcoal* may be given by mouth to reduce the absorption of the drug from the intestine into the bloodstream. To eliminate the drug, urine production may be increased by an *intravenous infusion*. Antidotes are available only for a few specific drugs. Such antidotes include *naloxone* (for *morphine*) and acetylcysteine (for paracetamol).

COMPLICATIONS

Drug poisoning may cause drowsiness, breathing difficulty, irregular heartbeat, and, rarely, cardiac arrest, fits, and kidney and liver damage. *Antiarrhythmic drugs* can be given to treat heartbeat irregularity. Fits are treated with *anticonvulsant drugs*. Blood tests to monitor liver function and careful monitoring of urine output are carried out if the drug is known to damage the liver or kidneys.

drug psychosis

A mental condition in which a person loses contact with reality during or following use of certain drugs (see *drug abuse*). Drug psychosis may be produced by drugs such as *amphetamines*, *cocaine*, *LSD* (lysergic acid diethylamide) and *cannabis*. The condition may also be caused by prescribed drugs, particularly by high doses of *corticosteroid drugs*.

Other possible effects associated with drug psychosis include abnormal behaviour, *hallucinations*, *delusions*, and extreme emotion, such as excitement or a dazed, unresponsive state. Treatment involves withdrawal from the drug and the use of *antipsychotic drugs* to relieve symptoms.

drunkenness

See *alcohol intoxication*.

drusen

Abnormal yellowish deposits that build up in the *retina* (the light-sensitive layer at the back of the eye), which can lead to a disturbance of central vision. Drusen may be a sign of age-related *macular degeneration*.

dry drowning

See *drowning, dry*.

dry eye

See *keratoconjunctivitis sicca*.

dry gangrene

A type of *gangrene*.

dry ice

Frozen *carbon dioxide*. Carbon dioxide changes from a gas to a solid when cooled, without passing through a liquid phase. Dry ice may be applied to the skin in *cryosurgery*, a freezing technique that is used, for example, to treat *warts*.

dry mouth

See *mouth, dry*.

dry socket

Infection at the site of a recent tooth extraction, causing pain, bad breath, and an unpleasant taste in the mouth. Dry

D

COMMON METHODS OF **DRUG ADMINISTRATION**

How taken	Action
By mouth	Drugs are digested and absorbed from the intestine in the same way as nutrients. How quickly the tablet or liquid works depends on how rapidly it is absorbed. This, in turn, depends on such factors as the drug's composition, how quickly the drug dissolves and the effect of digestive juices on it. Some drugs are inactivated as soon as they reach the liver and never enter the circulation.
By injection	Drugs given by injection have a very rapid effect and are given if digestive juices would destroy a drug.
Topical	These drugs have a local effect on the parts of the body that are exposed to them as well as a systemic (generalized) effect if some of the drug is absorbed into the bloodstream from the site of application.

D

socket occurs when a blood clot fails to form in the tooth socket after a difficult extraction, such as removal of a wisdom tooth (see *impaction, dental*). The clot itself may become infected, or infection may already have been present before extraction. The inflamed socket appears dry, and exposed bone is often visible.

The socket is irrigated to remove debris and may then be coated with an anti-inflammatory paste. The infection usually clears up within a few days.

DSM-IV

The fourth edition of the "Diagnostic and Statistical Manual of Mental Disorders", published by the American Psychiatric Association in 1994. An updated "Text Revision" version (DSM-IV-TR) was published in 2000. It classifies psychiatric illnesses and is widely accepted in other countries.

DTaP/IPV/Hib

A combined vaccine that provides immunity against *diphtheria*, *tetanus*, *pertussis* (whooping cough), *poliomyelitis*, and *Hib* (HAEMOPHILUS INFLUENZAE type B, a bacterium that can cause *meningitis* and *epiglottitis*). In this vaccine (and in the *DTaP/IPV or dTaP/IPV* vaccines), the polio and pertussis parts have been altered to minimize the risk of adverse effects.

HOW IT IS DONE

The injection is given in three doses to infants at two, three, and four months of age, so that they are protected as soon as possible. The childhood immunization schedule also includes a preschool booster (see *DTaP/IPV or dTaP/IPV*), and further diphtheria, tetanus, and polio boosters before leaving school. (See *Typical childhood immunization schedule*, p.414.)

PROTECTION

The vaccine provides a very high level of immunity to diphtheria, tetanus, pertussis, polio, and Hib infections.

POSSIBLE ADVERSE EFFECTS

DTaP/IPV/Hib is less likely to cause reactions than the older vaccines. Any side effects are usually mild and tend to occur within 12–24 hours of immunization. They include a slightly raised temperature, irritability and fretfulness, and a small lump, redness, and swelling at the injection site. Severe side effects are very rare.

Medical advice should be sought if a child has had a severe reaction to a previous dose of the vaccine or if a child has an acute illness when an immunization is due to be given.

DTaP/IPV or dTaP/IPV

Versions of a combined vaccine that provides immunity against *diphtheria*, *tetanus*, *pertussis* (whooping cough), and *poliomyelitis*. The DTaP/IPV version contains high-strength diphtheria vaccine; the dTaP/IPV version contains low-strength diphtheria vaccine. The combined vaccine is given as a booster to children aged between three years four months and five years old as part of the routine childhood immunization programme. (See *Typical childhood immunization schedule*, p.414.)

dual personality

See *multiple personality*.

Dubin–Johnson syndrome

An inherited disorder that is caused by an autosomal recessive genetic trait (see *genetic disorders*). Dubin–Johnson syndrome is characterized by longstanding, mild *jaundice* (yellowing of the skin and the whites of the eyes), which may not become apparent until puberty or adulthood. There is an abnormality in the transportation of *bilirubin* (the main pigment found in bile) from the *liver* to the *biliary system*, which causes the bilirubin to accumulate in the liver.

No specific treatment is available. Affected people are advised to avoid drinking alcohol, and to avoid taking a range of medications that are processed by the liver, for example *oral contraceptives*. *Genetic counselling* may be offered to prospective parents who have a family history of Dubin–Johnson syndrome.

Duchenne's dystrophy

The most common and severe form of *muscular dystrophy*.

duct

A tube or a tube-like passage leading from a gland to allow the flow of fluids, such as the tear ducts.

ductal carcinoma

Any *carcinoma* (a cancerous tumour arising from cells in an organ's surface layer or its lining membrane) of a duct (a tube or tube-like passage leading from a *gland*).

Examples of ducts that are most frequently affected by carcinomas are the pancreatic duct (see *pancreas*) and the milk ducts in the female *breast*. Ductal carcinomas of the breast that have not yet spread into the breast tissue can usually be cured by surgery.

LOCATION OF THE **DUODENUM**

The duodenum is about 25 cm long and shaped like a C; it forms a loop around the head of the pancreas.

Gallbladder

Duodenum

Pylorus

Duodenal cap

Stomach

Ampulla of Vater

Pancreas

Duke's classification

A *staging* system for *carcinomas* (cancerous tumours arising from cells in an organ's surface layer or lining membrane) in the lower gastrointestinal tract. Carcinomas of the *colon* (the main part of the large intestine) or *rectum* (the muscular tube that connects the large intestine to the anus) are classified according to this system.

dumbness

See *mutism*.

dumping syndrome

Symptoms that include sweating, fainting, and palpitations due to the rapid passage of food from the stomach into the intestine. Dumping syndrome (also known as rapid gastric emptying) is uncommon but mainly affects people who have had a *gastrectomy* (surgical removal of the stomach).

Symptoms may occur within about 30 minutes of eating (early dumping) or after 90–120 minutes (late dumping). Some very anxious people may experience the symptoms of dumping even though their stomach is intact.

CAUSES

Gastric surgery interferes with the normal mechanism for emptying food from the stomach (see *digestion*). If a meal containing a high level of carbohydrates is "dumped" too quickly from the stomach, the upper intestine may swell. This, together with excessive amounts of certain hormones released into the bloodstream, causes the symptoms of early dumping. As sugars are absorbed from the intestine, they rapidly increase the blood glucose level, causing excess *insulin* hormone release. This may, in turn, later lower the blood glucose level below normal, causing the symptoms of late dumping.

PREVENTION

A person who has had a gastrectomy can prevent symptoms by eating frequent, small, dry meals that contain no refined carbohydrates. Symptoms may also be prevented by resting for an hour or so after a meal.

duodenal cap

The upper area of the first part of the *duodenum*; this is revealed in a *barium X-ray examination*.

duodenal ulcer

A raw area in the wall of the *duodenum* (the first part of the small intestine) due to erosion of its inner surface lining. Duodenal and gastric (stomach) ulcers are types of *peptic ulcer*, and have similar causes, symptoms, and treatment.

duodenitis

Inflammation of the *duodenum* (the first part of the small intestine), producing vague gastrointestinal symptoms. It is diagnosed by oesophagogastroduodenoscopy (see *gastroscopy*): examination of the walls of the upper digestive tract with a flexible viewing instrument. The treatment for duodenitis is similar to that for a duodenal ulcer (see *peptic ulcer*).

duodenum

The first part of the small intestine. The duodenum begins at the duodenal cap, just beyond the pylorus (the muscular valve at the lower end of the stomach). It extends to the ligament of Treitz, which marks the boundary with the second part of the small intestine (the jejunum). (See *Location of the duodenum*, opposite page.)

The duodenum is about 25 cm long and C-shaped; it forms a loop around the head of the *pancreas*. Ducts from the pancreas, *liver*, and *gallbladder* feed into it through a small opening. Digestive enzymes in the pancreatic secretions and chemicals in the bile are released into the duodenum through this opening.

duplex kidney

Two fused kidneys on one side of the body. Another structural abnormality of the kidney is duplex renal pelvis, in which a single kidney has two renal pelvises (urine-collecting chambers). A third possibility is duplex ureter, in which there are two ureters leading from one kidney. The ureters may open into the bladder, or, in females, one may open into the vagina. These malformations arise during formation in the *embryo*. Surgical correction may be necessary to prevent complications such as infections.

duplex uterus

Duplication of part or all of the *uterus*. There may be two uteri joined to one vagina, or two uteri with two vaginas.

A more common condition is *septate uterus*, in which a band of tissue (septum) divides the uterine cavity into two spaces instead of one.

Dupuytren's contracture

A disorder of the hand in which one or more fingers become fixed in a bent position. In about half of the cases, both hands are affected. In most cases there is no apparent cause, but the disease may be, in part, inherited. Men over the age of 40 are most often affected.

The tissues just under the skin in the fingers or palm become thickened and shortened, which causes difficulty in straightening the fingers. Surgery can correct deformity of the fingers, but in some cases the condition recurs.

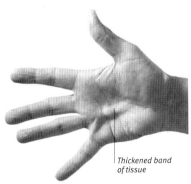

Thickened band of tissue

Dupuytren's contracture
A band of tissue in the hand thickens and contracts, gradually pulling the fingers into a permanently bent position.

dura mater

The outer of the three membranes (*meninges*) covering the brain.

Duroziez's disease

A congenital (present at birth) form of *mitral stenosis* (a narrowing of the opening of the mitral valve, which is situated on the left side of the *heart*).

dust diseases

Lung disorders caused by dust particles inhaled and absorbed into the lung tissues. There, they may cause *fibrosis* (formation of scar tissue) and progressive lung damage. The main symptoms are a cough and breathing difficulty. It may take at least 10 years of exposure to dusts containing coal, silica, talc, or asbestos before serious lung damage develops (see *pneumoconiosis*). Hypersensitivity to moulds on hay or grain may lead to allergic *alveolitis*.

Preventive measures, such as the installation of dust extraction machinery, have reduced the incidence of dust diseases, and replacements have been found for especially hazardous substances such as asbestos.

DVT

Deep vein thrombosis (see *thrombosis, deep vein*).

dwarfism

See *short stature*.

dydrogesterone

A drug that is derived from the female sex hormone *progesterone*. It is used to treat *premenstrual syndrome* and certain menstrual problems (see *menstruation, disorders of*). Dydrogesterone is also given together with an *oestrogen drug* as *hormone replacement therapy* to women after or during the menopause. Dydrogesterone may be prescribed to treat *endometriosis* or to prevent *miscarriage*. Possible side effects include swollen ankles, weight gain, breast tenderness, and nausea.

dying, care of the

Physical and psychological care that is given with the aim of making the final months or days of a dying person's life as free from pain, discomfort, and emotional distress as possible.

Carers may include doctors, nurses, and other medical professionals, counsellors, social workers, clergy, and the person's family and friends.

PHYSICAL CARE

Pain can be relieved by regular low doses of *analgesic drugs*. Opioid analgesics, such as *morphine*, may be given if pain is severe. Other methods of pain relief include *nerve blocks*, *cordotomy*, and *TENS*. Nausea and vomiting may be controlled by drugs. Constipation can be treated with *laxatives*. Breathlessness is another common problem in the dying, and this may be relieved by administering morphine.

Towards the end, the dying person may be restless and may suffer from breathing difficulty due to *heart failure* or *pneumonia*. These symptoms can be relieved by drugs and by placing the patient in a more comfortable position.

EMOTIONAL CARE

Emotional care is as important as the relief of physical symptoms. Many people who are terminally ill feel angry or depressed, and feelings of guilt or of regret are common responses. Loving, caring support from family, friends, and others is very important.

HOME OR HOSPICE?

Many terminally ill people would prefer to die at home, and few terminally ill patients need specialized nursing for a prolonged period. Specially trained nurses or health-care workers from a hospital, hospice, or charity may be able to provide additional support for the dying person and his or her carers.

Care in a hospice may be offered. Hospices are small units that have been established specifically to care for terminally ill people and their families.

dys-

A prefix meaning abnormal, difficult, painful, or faulty, as in dysuria (pain on passing urine).

dysarthria

A *speech disorder* caused by disease or damage to the physical apparatus of speech or to the nerves controlling this apparatus. Affected people can formulate, select, and write out words and sentences grammatically; the problem is with vocal expression only.

CAUSES

Dysarthria is common in many degenerative neurological conditions, such as *multiple sclerosis* and *Parkinson's disease*. It may also result from a *stroke*, *brain tumour*, or an isolated defect or damage to a particular nerve. Structural defects of the mouth, as occur in *cleft lip and palate*, can also cause dysarthria.

TREATMENT

Drug or surgical treatment of the underlying disease or structural defect may improve the person's ability to speak clearly. *Speech therapy* is also useful.

dyscalculia

A disorder in which there is difficulty in solving mathematical problems. (See also *learning difficulties*.)

dyschondroplasia

A rare disorder, also called multiple enchondromatosis or Ollier's disease, that is present from birth and characterized by the presence of multiple tumours of cartilaginous tissue within the bones of a limb. It is caused by a failure of normal *ossification* during bone development. The bones are shortened, resulting in deformity. Rarely, a tumour in the bone may become cancerous (see *chondrosarcoma*).

dysentery

An intestinal infection, causing diarrhoea (often mixed with blood, pus, or mucus) and abdominal pain. There are two distinct forms of dysentery: *shigellosis*, which is due to shigella bacteria; and *amoebic dysentery*, which is caused by the protozoan parasite ENTAMOEBA HISTOLYTICA. The main risk with dysentery is *dehydration* caused by loss of fluid in the diarrhoea.

dysfunction

An abnormality or impairment in the functioning of an organ or body system. (See also *bleeding, dysfunctional uterine*; *minimal brain dysfunction*; *psychosexual dysfunction*.)

The term "dysfunctional" may be used to describe a poor relationship between two or more people.

dysgraphia

Problems with writing (see *learning difficulties*).

dyskaryosis

Abnormal changes in the nuclei of cells, particularly in the early stages of *cancer*. Dyskaryosis may be detected by microscopic examination of cells in procedures such as a *cervical smear test*. (See also *cervical intraepithelial neoplasia*.)

dyskeratosis

An abnormality in keratinization (the deposition of the tough protein *keratin*) in the surface of the skin or nails. One form is due to a rare, inherited disorder that is most commonly caused by an X-linked recessive genetic trait, although autosomal dominant and autosomal recessive forms also exist (see *genetic disorders*). The condition affects more males than females and first becomes apparent in childhood.

Dyskeratosis is characterized by premature thickening of epithelial cells (see *epithelium*) in the skin; *leukoplakia* (raised white patches on the mucous membranes of the mouth or vulva); nail dystrophy (a disorder caused by inadequate nutrition); and *pancytopenia* (a decrease in the number of red cells, (*anaemia*), white cells (*neutropenia*), and platelets (*thrombocytopenia*) in the blood).

dyskinesia

Abnormal muscular movements. These uncontrollable twitching, jerking, or writhing movements cannot be suppressed, and they may affect control of voluntary movements. The disorder may involve the whole body or be restricted to a group of muscles.

Types of dyskinesia include *chorea* (jerking movements), *athetosis* (writhing movements), *choreoathetosis* (a combined form), *myoclonus* (muscle spasms), *tics* (repetitive fidgets), and *tremors*.

Dyskinesia may result from brain damage at birth or may be a side effect of certain drugs (see *tardive dyskinesia*), which often disappears when the drug is stopped. Otherwise, dyskinesia is difficult to treat. (See also *parkinsonism*.)

dyslexia

A reading disability characterized by difficulty interpreting written symbols.

CAUSE

Dyslexia is more common in males, and evidence suggests that a specific, sometimes inherited, neurological disorder underlies true dyslexia.

SYMPTOMS

A child with dyslexia has normal intelligence, but his or her attainment of reading skills lags far behind other scholastic abilities.

While many young children tend to reverse letters and words (for example, writing or reading p for q, or was for saw), most soon learn to correct such errors. Dyslexic children continue to confuse these symbols. Letters are often transposed (as in pest for step), and spelling errors are common. The children may even be unable to read words that they can spell correctly.

TREATMENT
It is very important to recognize the problem early to prevent added frustrations. Specific teaching can help an affected child develop "tricks" to overcome the deficit. Avoidance of pressure from parents combined with praise for what the child can do is equally important in helping progress.

dysmenorrhoea
Pain or discomfort experienced during or just before a menstrual period.
TYPES AND CAUSES
Primary dysmenorrhoea is common in teenage girls and young women. It usually starts two to three years after *menstruation* begins, but often diminishes after the age of 25. The exact cause is unknown. One possibility is excessive production of, or undue sensitivity to, *prostaglandins*, which are hormone-like substances that stimulate spasms in the uterus.

Secondary dysmenorrhoea is due to an underlying disorder, such as *pelvic inflammatory disease* or *endometriosis*, and usually begins in adult life.
SYMPTOMS
Cramp-like pain or discomfort is felt in the lower abdomen, sometimes accompanied by a dull ache in the lower back. Some women also have nausea and vomiting.
TREATMENT
Mild primary dysmenorrhoea is often relieved by *nonsteroidal anti-inflammatory drugs*. In severe cases, symptoms can usually be relieved by taking *oral contraceptives* or other hormonal preparations that suppress ovulation. The treatment of secondary dysmenorrhoea depends on the cause of the condition.

dysmorphia
An abnormality in the shape of a body tissue or structure.

dyspareunia
Painful sexual intercourse (see *intercourse, painful*).

dyspepsia
The medical term for *indigestion*.

dysphagia
The medical term for *swallowing difficulty*.

dysphasia
A disturbance in the ability to select the words with which to speak and write and/or to understand speech or writing.

It is caused by damage to speech and comprehension regions of the brain. (See also *aphasia*.)

dysphonia
Defective production of vocal sounds in speech, either as a result of disease or of damage to the larynx (voicebox) or to the nerve supply to the laryngeal muscles. (See also *larynx, disorders of*; *speech disorders*.)

dysphoria
A feeling of disquiet or restlessness. Dysphoria may be a side effect of certain drugs, or it may be a symptom of a psychiatric disorder.

Gender dysphoria is a persistent feeling that one has been born the wrong sex (see *gender identity*).

dysplasia
Any abnormality of growth. The term applies to deformities in structures such as the skull or hip (see *developmental dysplasia of the hip*) and to abnormalities of single cells. Abnormal cell features include the size, shape, and rate of multiplication of cells.

dyspnoea
The medical term for shortness of breath (see *breathing difficulty*).

dysrhythmia, cardiac
A medical term meaning disturbance of heart rhythm, sometimes used as an alternative to arrhythmia (see *arrhythmia, cardiac*).

dystocia
A term that means difficult or abnormal labour (see *childbirth*). Dystocia may occur, for example, if the baby is very large, or if the mother's pelvis is abnormally shaped or too small for the baby to pass through. (See also *childbirth, complications of*.)

dystonia
Abnormal muscle rigidity, which causes painful spasms, unusually fixed postures, or strange movement patterns. Dystonia may affect a localized area of the body, or may be more generalized. The most common types of localized dystonia are *torticollis* (painful neck spasm), and *scoliosis* (an abnormal sideways curvature of the spine), which is caused by an injury to the back that produces muscle spasm. Generalized dystonia may be caused by neurological

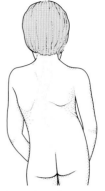

Scoliosis due to dystonia
Injury to the back may result in dystonia and abnormal spasm of the back muscles. This problem, in turn, may lead to scoliosis (abnormal sideways curvature of the spine).

disorders such as *Parkinson's disease*, or it may occur as a side effect of *antipsychotic drugs*.

Dystonia may be reduced by treatment with *anticholinergic drugs* or with *benzodiazepine drugs*. In some cases, *biofeedback training* may be helpful. Injections of botulinum toxin into the affected muscles are effective in treating some types of dystonia.

dystrophy
Any disorder in which the structure and normal activity of cells within a body tissue have been disrupted by inadequate nourishment of that part. The cause is usually unknown, but may be poor circulation of blood through the tissue, nerve damage or deficiency of a specific enzyme in the tissue.

Examples of dystrophy include *muscular dystrophies* and *leukodystrophies*. Corneal dystrophies, in which cells lining the cornea of the eye are damaged, are a rare cause of blindness.

dysuria
The medical term for pain, discomfort, or difficulty in passing urine (see *urination, painful*).

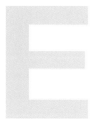

Eales' disease

A rare condition seen mainly in young men that is characterized by inflammation of the retinal veins and recurrent vitreous haemorrhage (leakage of blood into the *vitreous humour*, the gel-like substance that fills the rear chamber of the *eye*). The presence of blood in the vitreous humour may affect vision and lead to headaches. If vision is impaired, *laser treatment* may be performed to prevent further haemorrhage.

ear

The organ of hearing and balance. The ear consists of three parts: the outer ear, the middle ear, and the inner ear. The outer and middle ear are concerned mainly with the collection and transmission of sound. The inner ear is responsible for analysing sound waves; it also contains the mechanism by which the body keeps its balance.

OUTER EAR

The outer ear comprises the pinna (the visible part of the ear), which is composed of folds of skin and *cartilage*, and the ear canal, which is approximately 2.5 cm long in adults.

The outer part of the ear canal is composed of cartilage and produces *earwax*, which traps dust and foreign bodies. The canal is closed at its inner end by the eardrum, a thin, fibrous, circular membrane that is covered with a layer of skin. The eardrum vibrates in response to the changes in air pressure that constitute sound.

MIDDLE EAR

The middle ear is a small cavity between the eardrum and the inner ear that conducts sound to the inner ear by means of three tiny, linked, movable bones known as *ossicles*. The first bone, the malleus, is joined to the inner surface of the eardrum. The second, the incus, has one broad joint with the malleus (which lies almost parallel to it) and a delicate joint to the third bone, the stapes. The base of the stapes fills the oval window leading to the inner ear.

The middle ear is cut off from the outside by the eardrum. However, it is not completely airtight; a ventilation passage, called the *eustachian tube*, runs forwards and downwards into the back of the nose. The eustachian tube is normally kept closed, but it opens by muscular contraction when an individual yawns or swallows.

The middle ear acts as a transformer, passing the vibrations of sound from the air outside (which is a thin medium) to the fluid within the inner ear (which is a thicker medium).

INNER EAR

The inner ear is an intricate series of structures contained deep within the bones of the skull. It consists of a maze of winding passages, collectively known as the labyrinth. The front part, called the cochlea, is a tube that resembles a snail's shell, containing nerve fibres that detect different sound frequencies. (For more information about how this system works, see *hearing*.)

The rear part of the inner ear contains three semicircular canals and is concerned with balance. The semicircular canals are connected to a cavity called the vestibule and contain hair cells bathed in fluid. Some of these cells are sensitive to gravity and acceleration; others respond to the positions and movement of the head. Information from the inner ear is conducted to the brain via the *vestibulocochlear nerve*. (See also *disorders of the ear* box.)

earache

Pain in the *ear*, which may originate in the ear itself or may result from a disorder in one of the structures situated

---

ANATOMY OF THE **EAR**

The outer ear comprises the pinna and ear canal; the middle ear – the eardrum, malleus, incus, stapes, and eustachian tube; and the inner ear – the vestibule, semicircular canals, and cochlea. Sensory impulses from the inner ear pass to the brain via the vestibulocochlear nerve.

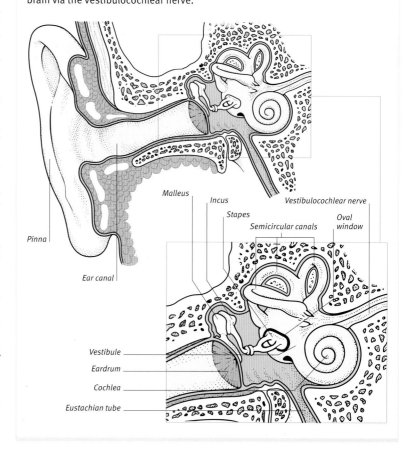

Pinna

Ear canal

Malleus

Incus

Stapes

Semicircular canals

Vestibulocochlear nerve

Oval window

Vestibule

Eardrum

Cochlea

Eustachian tube

near the ear. Earache is an extremely common symptom, especially in infancy and childhood.

CAUSES

A frequent cause of earache is acute *otitis media* (infection of the middle ear), which occurs most commonly in young children and results in severe, stabbing pain. There may also be loss of hearing and a raised temperature.

Another common cause of earache is *otitis externa* (inflammation of the ear canal), which is often caused by infection. Infection can affect the whole canal, or it may be localized, sometimes taking the form of a boil or abscess. The earache may be accompanied by irritation in the ear canal and a discharge of *pus*.

Intermittent earache may also occur in people with dental problems, *tonsillitis*, throat cancer (see *pharynx, cancer of*), pain in the jaw or neck muscles, and other disorders affecting areas near the ear. Earache in such cases occurs because the ear and nearby areas are supplied by the same nerves; the pain is said to be "referred" to the ear.

DIAGNOSIS AND TREATMENT

To determine the cause of earache, the ear is inspected (see *ear, examination of*). The mouth, throat, and teeth may also be examined.

Analgesic drugs (painkillers) may be prescribed to relieve the pain. Other treatment depends on the underlying cause of the earache. *Antibiotic drugs* may be prescribed for an infection. Pus in the outer ear may be removed by suction. Pus in the middle ear may be drained through a hole in the eardrum, a procedure known as *myringotomy*.

ear, cauliflower

See *cauliflower ear*.

ear, discharge from

Also called otorrhoea, emission of fluid from the ear. Not all discharge is the same; it may be watery or thick, clear or coloured, odourless or foul-smelling, and intermittent or continuous.

CAUSES

A discharge from the ear may be due to an outer-ear infection (see *otitis externa*). It may also follow perforation of the eardrum (see *eardrum, perforated*), which is usually due to a middle-ear infection (see *otitis media*). Rarely, after a skull fracture (see *skull, fracture of*), *cerebrospinal fluid* or blood may be discharged from the ear.

DISORDERS OF THE EAR

The *ear* is susceptible to many disorders, some of which can lead to *deafness*.

Congenital defects

In rare cases, the ear canal, *ossicles* (small bones in the middle ear), or *pinna* (visible part of the ear) are absent or deformed at birth. *Rubella* (German measles) in early pregnancy can damage the baby's developing ear, leading to deafness. Most cases of congenital *sensorineural deafness* (deafness due to problems with the inner ear, nerves, or the brain's auditory area) are genetic.

Infection

Infection is the most common cause of ear disorders. Infection in the ear canal leads to *otitis externa*; in the middle ear, it causes *otitis media*. This can lead to perforation of the eardrum (see *eardrum, perforated*). *Glue ear* (buildup of fluid in the middle ear), often due to infection, is the most common cause of childhood hearing difficulties. Viral infection of the inner ear may cause *labyrinthitis* with severe *vertigo* or sudden hearing loss.

Injury

Cauliflower ear occurs as the result of one major or several minor injuries to the pinna. Perforation of the eardrum can result from poking objects into the ear or from loud noise. Prolonged exposure to loud noise can cause *tinnitus* (noises within the ear) and/or deafness.

Pressure changes associated with flying or scuba diving can also cause minor damage (see *barotrauma*).

Tumours

Acoustic neuroma is a rare, noncancerous tumour of the *acoustic nerve* that may press on structures in the ear to cause deafness, tinnitus, and problems with balance. In *cholesteatoma*, skin cells accumulate in the middle ear.

Obstruction

Obstruction of the ear canal is often due to *earwax*, although in small children, an object may have been pushed into the ear (see *ear, foreign body in*).

Other disorders

In *otosclerosis*, a hereditary condition, a bone in the middle ear becomes immobilized, causing deafness. *Ménière's disease* is a rare condition in which deafness, vertigo, and tinnitus occur due to buildup of fluid in the inner ear. Progressive, age-related hearing loss is a condition known as *presbyacusis*.

Certain drugs, such as *aminoglycoside drugs* and some *diuretic drugs*, can also damage ear function.

INVESTIGATION

Hearing and balance are investigated using *hearing tests*, *caloric tests*, and *electronystagmography*. The ear canal and eardrum are viewed with an *otoscope*.

DIAGNOSIS AND TREATMENT

A swab of the discharge may be taken and sent to a laboratory for analysis to identify the cause of any infection. *Hearing tests* may also be performed. *X-rays* of the bones of the skull will be taken if there has been a *head injury* or if a serious type of middle-ear infection is suspected from the symptoms.

Treatment depends on the cause and usually includes *antibiotic drugs*.

eardrum

The circular membrane that separates the outer *ear* from the middle ear. The eardrum vibrates in response to sound waves, conducting the sound to the inner ear through the *ossicles* (the three small bones in the middle ear).

eardrum, perforated

The rupture or erosion of the *eardrum*. Perforation of the eardrum can cause brief, intense pain. There may also be slight bleeding, a discharge from the ear (see *ear, discharge from*), and a reduction in hearing.

CAUSES

Most commonly, perforation occurs as a result of buildup of pus in the middle ear due to acute *otitis media* (middle-ear infection). Perforation may also be associated with *cholesteatoma* (accumulation of skin cells and debris in the ear). Another cause is injury, for example from insertion of an object into the ear, a loud noise, *barotrauma* (damage caused by pressure changes) or a fracture to the base of the skull (see *skull, fracture of*).

E

In some cases, a doctor may deliberately puncture the eardrum to drain pus from the middle ear (see *myringotomy*).

DIAGNOSIS AND TREATMENT

Diagnosis is confirmed by examination of the ear (see *ear, examination of*). *Hearing tests* may also be performed to assess any hearing loss.

Analgesic drugs (painkillers) may help to relieve any pain and *antibiotic drugs* may be prescribed to treat or prevent infection. Most perforations heal very quickly, usually within a month. However, if the perforation fails to heal, *myringoplasty* (an operation to repair the eardrum) may be required.

ear, examination of

The *ear* may be examined to investigate the possible causes of *earache*, discharge from the ear (see *ear, discharge from*), hearing loss, a feeling of fullness in the ear, disturbed *balance*, *tinnitus* (noises within the ear), or swelling of lymph nodes (see *glands, swollen*) below or in front of the ear.

HOW IT IS DONE

The doctor begins by examining the pinna (the visible part of the outer ear) for any swelling, tenderness, ulceration, or deformity. To view the ear canal and eardrum, an *otoscope* may be used.

To obtain images of the middle and inner ears, *X-rays*, or *CT scanning* or *MRI* (techniques that produce cross-sectional or three-dimensional images of body structures), may be carried out. Hearing and balance can be assessed by means of *hearing tests* or *caloric tests*. *Electronystagmography* is a technique in which balance is assessed by observing the movements of the eye as water is poured into the ear.

ear, foreign body in

Foreign bodies can easily enter the ear canal. Children often insert small objects, such as peas or stones, into their ears, and insects may crawl or fly in.

If people try to remove objects from the ear themselves, they may push the items further into the ear canal and risk damaging the eardrum. Foreign bodies in the ear must always be removed by doctors. This can be done by syringing (see *syringing of ears*) or by using fine-toothed forceps. Insects can sometimes be floated out using warmed olive oil or lukewarm water.

ear, nose, and throat surgery

See *otorhinolaryngology*.

ear piercing

Making a hole in the earlobe or another, usually cartilaginous, part of the external ear to accommodate an earring. New ear piercings should be kept clean and dry to prevent infection. If a newly pierced ear becomes red, swollen, and painful and/or the hole discharges cloudy fluid or pus, the ear may be infected and medical advice should be sought.

ears, pinning back of

See *otoplasty*.

earwax

A yellow or brown secretion, also called cerumen, produced by glands in the outer ear canal. In most people, wax is produced in small amounts, comes out on its own, and causes no problems. However, some people produce so much wax that it regularly obstructs the canal. Excess earwax may produce a sensation of fullness in the ear and, if the canal is blocked completely, partial *deafness*. These symptoms are worsened if water enters the ear and makes the wax swell. Prolonged blockage may irritate the skin of the ear canal.

TREATMENT

Wax that causes blockage or irritation may come out after being softened with warmed olive oil or almond oil. Otherwise, the wax should first be softened and then removed by a doctor or nurse (see *syringing of the ears*).

eating disorders

Illnesses that are characterized by obsessions with weight and body image. Eating disorders are most common in young adolescent females, but they can also affect males.

In the eating disorder *anorexia nervosa*, patients, despite being painfully thin, perceive themselves as fat and starve themselves. Binge-eating followed by self-induced vomiting is one of the main features of *bulimia*, although in this disorder weight may be normal. The two conditions sometimes occur together. In morbid *obesity*, there is a constant desire to eat large quantities of food.

Ebola fever

A dangerous and highly contagious viral infection that causes severe haemorrhaging (see *bleeding*) from the skin and the *mucous membranes* (the thin, moist tissue that lines body cavities). Ebola fever

occurs predominantly in Africa. There is no specific treatment for the disease, which is fatal in many cases.

eburnation

The conversion of *bone* into an ivorylike mass. The *cartilage* that covers an articulating bone surface wears away, exposing the underlying bone tissue, which becomes increasingly dense and worn. Eburnation is a feature of *osteoarthritis*.

EB virus

See *Epstein–Barr virus*.

ecchymosis

The medical term for a *bruise* that is visible through the skin.

eccrine gland

A type of *sweat gland*.

ECG

The abbreviation for electrocardiography, a method of recording the electrical activity of the *heart* muscle. An ECG is useful for diagnosing heart disorders, many of which produce electrical patterns that deviate from normal. Electrodes connected to a recording machine are placed on the patient's chest, wrists, and ankles. The machine displays the heart's electrical activity on a screen or as a trace. (See also *ambulatory ECG*; *exercise ECG*.)

echinachea

A preparation of the plant genus ECHINACEA. Three species of echinacea are used in herbal medicine; they are believed to boost the body's *immune system* and therefore increase its resistance to infection.

echocardiography

A method of obtaining images of the structure and movements of the *heart* using *ultrasound* (inaudible, high-frequency sound waves).

WHY IT IS DONE

Echocardiography is an important diagnostic technique used to detect structural, and some functional, abnormalities of the heart wall, heart chambers, *heart valves*, and large *coronary arteries*.

The procedure is also used to diagnose congenital heart disease (see *heart disease, congenital*), *cardiomyopathy* (heart muscle disorders), *aneurysms* (ballooning of the heart or blood vessel walls), *pericarditis* (inflammation of the membrane that surrounds the heart), and blood clots in the heart.

ELECTROCARDIOGRAPHY

Electrocardiography causes no discomfort. Electrodes connected to a recording machine are applied to the chest, wrists, and ankles. The machine displays the electrical activity in the heart as a trace on a moving graph or a screen. Any abnormality is thereby revealed to the doctor, nurse, or paramedic. Normal and abnormal recordings are shown, below right.

An ECG can be taken at home, in the doctor's surgery, or in the hospital; a recording lasting 24 hours or longer can be obtained from a monitoring device worn by the patient.

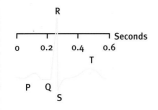

Normal ECG
This tracing shows the electrical activity associated with one normal heartbeat. The blue line shows the current flowing toward the recording lead. The rise at P occurs just before the atria (upper heart chambers) begin to contract, the QRS "spike" occurs just before the ventricles (lower chambers) begin to contract, and the rise at T occurs as the electrical potential returns to zero.

HOW ECG IS DONE

Small electrodes, connected by leads to the recording machine, are attached to the chest, wrists, and ankles using conducting jelly or pads. Signals from the electrodes produce a trace.

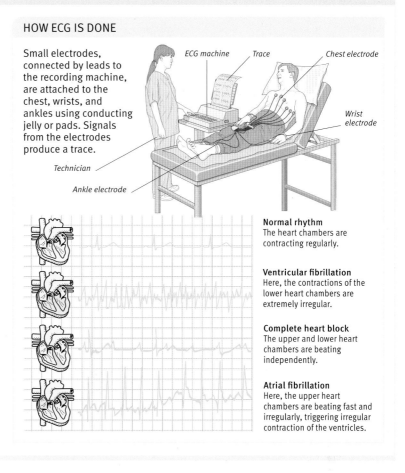

Normal rhythm
The heart chambers are contracting regularly.

Ventricular fibrillation
Here, the contractions of the lower heart chambers are extremely irregular.

Complete heart block
The upper and lower heart chambers are beating independently.

Atrial fibrillation
Here, the upper heart chambers are beating fast and irregularly, triggering irregular contraction of the ventricles.

HOW IT IS DONE

Echocardiography is harmless and causes no discomfort. A transducer is placed on the chest. It emits ultrasound waves and detects their echoes from the heart. The ultrasound waves are reflected differently by each part of the heart, resulting in a complex series of echoes, which are viewed on a screen and can be recorded or the results printed out. Developments such as multiple moving transducers and computer analysis give clearer anatomical pictures of the heart.

TYPES

In addition to standard echocardiography (as described above), several variants of the technique have been developed.

Transoesophageal echocardiography involves placing the transducer in the oesophagus using a flexible *endoscope* (viewing tube). This technique enables very detailed images to be obtained, as may be needed when planning heart valve surgery, for example.

Doppler echocardiography measures the velocity of blood flow through the heart, allowing assessment of structural abnormalitiess such as *septal defects*. Stress echocardiography can be used as an alternative to an *exercise ECG* in the assessment of *coronary artery disease*.

echo-free

A term used in *ultrasound scanning* to denote a structure that does not give rise to reflections (echoes) of ultrasound waves. A cyst filled with clear fluid, for example, is echo-free.

echogenic

A term used in *ultrasound scanning* to denote a structure that gives rise to reflections (echoes) of ultrasound waves.

echolalia

The compulsive repetition of something spoken by another person. The tone and accent of the speaker are copied as well as the words. Echolalia is sometimes a feature of *schizophrenia* and may occur in people with *learning difficulties* or *autism*.

ECHO virus

The name for a specific group of RNA *viruses*. There are 32 types of ECHO virus, and these cause a wide range of conditions, including skin rashes, colds (see *cold, common*), gastrointestinal disorders, and viral *meningitis*.

eclampsia

An uncommon but serious condition that develops in a woman in late *pregnancy*, during *childbirth*, or after delivery. Eclampsia is characterized by *hypertension* (high blood pressure), *proteinuria* (protein in the urine), *oedema* (accumulation of fluid in body tissues), and the development of *seizures*. The condition is life-threatening for both the mother and the baby.

Eclampsia occurs as a complication of moderate or severe, although not mild, *pre-eclampsia*.

SYMPTOMS

The warning symptoms of impending eclampsia include headaches, confusion, blurred or disturbed vision, and abdominal pain. If untreated, seizures may occur and may be followed by *coma*. Levels of blood *platelets* may fall severely, resulting in bleeding; liver and kidney function may also be affected.

TREATMENT AND OUTLOOK

Careful monitoring of blood pressure and proteinuria throughout pregnancy is required to enable prompt treatment of impending eclampsia, and immediate delivery, often by *caesarean section*, together with *antihypertensive drugs* and *anticonvulsant drugs* is needed. Patients may need intensive care to prevent the development of complications, such as kidney failure.

Blood pressure often returns to normal in the months following delivery, although it may remain high. There is a risk of a recurrence of eclampsia in subsequent pregnancies.

E.coli

See *Escherichia coli (E.coli)*.

econazole

An *antifungal drug* used as a cream in the treatment of fungal skin infections (such as *athlete's foot* and *tinea*), and in cream or pessary form to treat vaginal *candidiasis* (thrush). Skin irritation is a rare side effect.

Ecstasy

An illegal *designer drug*, related to the *amphetamine drugs*. Ecstasy has a mildly hallucinogenic effect and generates feelings of euphoria and sociability. In most people, the drug has no ill effects in the short-term, but repeated use carries a risk of liver damage. The most common side effect is *hyperthermia* (very high body temperature). The drug causes intense thirst; drinking large quantities of water to combat this may result in brain swelling, which may be fatal.

ECT

The abbreviation for electroconvulsive therapy, a treatment for very severe *depression* and some psychiatric conditions, such as *catatonia* and severe manic episodes (see *mania*). ECT is much less commonly used today than it was in the past, since the introduction of newer,

more effective drug treatment. However, ECT may be life-saving in severe cases of psychiatric illness that are resistant to other forms of treatment.

In this procedure, an electric current is passed through the brain in order to induce a *seizure*. ECT is administered under a short-lived general anaesthetic (see *anaesthesia, general*) and in combination with a *muscle-relaxant drug*, which reduces the physical effects of the induced seizure. Several treatments may be necessary. Temporary *amnesia* (memory loss) is a possible side effect.

ectasia

A term that means widening, usually used to refer to a disorder of a *duct*. For example, mammary duct ectasia is an abnormal widening of the ducts that carry secretions from the breast tissue to the nipple.

ectomorph

A term formerly used to describe an individual with a tall, thin body, a low level of body fat, slender limbs, small bones, and little muscle mass. (See also *endomorph*; *mesomorph*.)

-ectomy

A suffix that denotes surgical removal. For example, tonsillectomy is surgical removal of the tonsils.

ectoparasite

A *parasite* that lives in or on its host's skin. An ectoparasite derives nourishment from the skin or by sucking the host's blood. Various *lice*, *ticks*, *mites*, and some types of *fungi* are occasional ectoparasites of humans. By contrast, endoparasites live inside the body.

ectopic

A term used to describe a body structure that occurs in an abnormal location or position or a body function that occurs at an abnormal time.

ectopic heartbeat

A contraction of the heart muscle that is out of normal timing. An ectopic *heartbeat* occurs shortly after a normal beat and is followed by a longer-than-usual interval before the next one.

Ectopic beats can occur in a healthy heart and may be symptomless. Multiple ectopic beats can cause *palpitations* (awareness of a rapid or forceful heartbeat). When occurring after a *myocardial infarction* (heart attack), such multiple

beats are a sign of damaged heart muscle. They may lead to a condition called ventricular *fibrillation*, in which there is a rapid, uncoordinated heartbeat, which is potentially fatal.

Multiple ectopic beats that are causing palpitations, or those that occur after a myocardial infarction, are often treated with an *antiarrhythmic drug*. (See also *arrhythmia, cardiac*.)

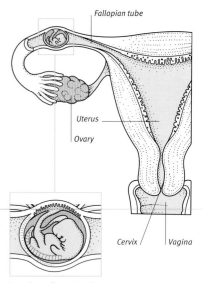

Location of an ectopic pregnancy
The pregnancy usually develops in the fallopian tube; occasionally it develops in the ovary, the abdominal cavity, or the cervix.

ectopic pregnancy

A *pregnancy* that develops outside the *uterus*, most commonly in a *fallopian tube*, but sometimes in an *ovary*, the abdominal cavity, or the *cervix* (neck of the uterus). As the pregnancy develops, it may damage surrounding tissues, causing serious bleeding. An ectopic pregnancy is potentially life-threatening and requires emergency treatment.

CAUSES

The fertilized ovum (egg) may become stuck in the fallopian tube if there is a *congenital* abnormality of the tube or if the tube has been damaged in any way. Damage is most commonly due to a pelvic infection (see *pelvic inflammatory disease*) or from surgery on the fallopian tubes. Ectopic pregnancy has also been associated with the use of some types of *IUD* (intrauterine contraceptive device) and progestogen-only *oral contraceptives*.

SYMPTOMS

The majority of ectopic pregnancies are discovered in the first two months, often before the woman even realizes that she is pregnant. Symptoms usually include severe pain in the lower abdomen and bleeding from the vagina. Internal bleeding may cause symptoms of *shock*, which include pallor, sweating, and faintness.

DIAGNOSIS AND TREATMENT

A blood test may be done to measure levels of human chorionic gonadotrophin (HCG); this hormone is produced naturally in pregnancy but in lower than normal amounts if the pregancy is ectopic. A transvaginal *ultrasound* examination may also be done, which involves inserting an ultrasound probe through the vagina, and, in some cases, a *laparoscopy* (internal examination using a viewing instrument).

If the diagnosis is made early on, treatment using the drug *methotrexate* may be considered. In most cases, surgery, usually *minimally invasive surgery*, is carried out to remove the embryo (which is usually already dead), the placenta, and any damaged tissue at the site of the pregnancy. If blood loss is severe, *blood transfusions* and/or a *laparotomy* may be necessary. An affected fallopian tube is removed if it cannot be repaired.

OUTLOOK

It is still possible to have a normal pregnancy even if one fallopian tube has been removed, although the chances of conception are slightly reduced. Women with two damaged tubes may require *in vitro fertilization* to achieve an intrauterine pregnancy.

ectopic testis

See *testis, ectopic*.

ectropion

A turning outwards of the *eyelid* so that the inner surface is exposed. It is most common in elderly people, in whom it usually affects the lower lid and is due to weakness of the muscle surrounding the eye. Ectropion may also be caused by the contraction of scar tissue in the skin near either lid. Ectropion often follows *facial palsy*, which causes paralysis of the muscles around the eye.

Even slight ectropion interferes with normal tear drainage by distorting the opening of the tear duct. Chronic *conjunctivitis* may result, causing redness, discomfort, and overflow of tears so that the skin becomes damp and inflamed. Constant wiping tends to pull the lid farther from the eye. Surgery to tighten the affected eyelid may be required.

eczema

An inflammation of the skin, usually causing itching and sometimes scaling or blisters. There are several different types of eczema and some forms are better known as *dermatitis* (such as contact dermatitis and photodermatitis). Eczema is sometimes the result of an *allergy*, but is often of unknown cause.

TYPES

Atopic eczema This is a chronic, superficial inflammation that occurs in people who have an inherited tendency towards allergy. The condition is common in babies. An intensely itchy rash occurs, usually on the face, in the elbow creases, and behind the knees. The skin often scales and small red pimples may appear. Infection may occur if the rash is scratched, breaking the skin.

For mild cases, *emollients* (such as petroleum jelly) help to keep the skin soft. In severe cases, ointments containing *corticosteroid drugs* may be used. *Antihistamine drugs* may be prescribed to reduce itching. Excluding certain foods from the diet may help to control the condition. Atopic eczema often clears up on its own as a child grows older. Severe atopic eczema that occurs in adults may be treated with *immunosuppressant drugs* such as oral ciclosporin or topical tacrolimus.

Nummular eczema This usually occurs in adults and is of unknown cause. It produces round, itchy, scaling patches on the skin that are similar to those of *tinea* (ringworm). Topical corticosteroids may reduce inflammation, but the eczema is often persistent.

Hand eczema This is usually caused by irritant substances such as detergents, but it may occur for no apparent reason. Itchy blisters develop, usually on the palms, and the skin may become scaly and cracked. Hand eczema usually improves if emollients are used and if

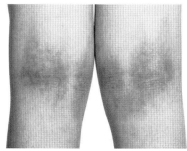

Atopic eczema
In this example of atopic eczema, the skin on the backs of the knees is raw and inflamed.

cotton gloves with rubber gloves over them are worn when coming into contact with irritants. If the eczema is severe, corticosteroids may be prescribed.

Stasis eczema This occurs in people with *varicose veins*. The skin on the legs may become irritated, inflamed, and discoloured. The swelling of the legs may be controlled with compression bandages or stockings. Corticosteroids ointments may give temporary relief.

GENERAL TREATMENT

To reduce irritation, a soothing ointment should be applied to the affected areas; these may then be covered with a dressing to prevent scratching. Absorbent, non-irritating materials (such as cotton) should be worn next to the skin; irritants (such as wool, silk, and rough synthetics) should be avoided.

EDD

The abbreviation for expected date of delivery, the date on which a baby is due to be born. The EDD is calculated as 40 weeks from the first day of the woman's last menstrual period (see *period, menstrual*). In practice, babies are rarely born exactly on their EDD.

edentulous

A term meaning without *teeth*, a condition arising either because the teeth have not yet grown or because they have fallen out or been removed by a dentist.

Edwards' syndrome

A *genetic disorder*, also known as trisomy 18 syndrome, that is associated with the presence of a third copy of chromosome 18. Edwards' syndrome affects about three times as many girls as boys.

Characteristics of the syndrome include a low birth weight, severe *learning difficulties*, low-set and malformed ears, a small jaw, hand abnormalities, opacities in the cornea, congenital heart disease (see *heart disease, congenital*), hernias, *ventricular septal defect* (a hole between the lower heart chambers), and kidney abnormalities.

About half the babies born with the syndrome do not survive beyond the first week of life. Very few infants live longer than a year. People with a family history of the syndrome should consider *genetic counselling* before starting a family.

EEG

The abbreviation for electroencephalography, a method of recording the electrical activity of the *brain*. A trace of

E

HOW **ELECTROENCEPHALOGRAPHY** IS DONE

A number of small electrodes are attached to the scalp. Shaving of the scalp is unnecessary. The electrodes are connected to an instrument that measures the brain's impulses in microvolts and amplifies them for recording purposes. The technique is painless, produces no side effects, and takes about 45 minutes. Recordings are taken while the subject is at rest, with the eyes open and then shut, during and after hyperventilation (overbreathing), and while looking at a flashing light. Electroencephalography is also helpful for recording activity as the patient goes to sleep, especially when epilepsy is suspected.

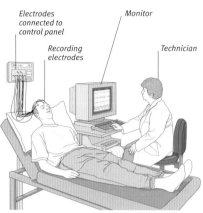

Electrodes connected to control panel

Recording electrodes

Monitor

Technician

EEG WAVE PATTERNS

α

β

δ

θ

Alpha waves
The prominent pattern of an awake, relaxed adult whose eyes are closed.

Beta waves
The lower, faster oscillation of a person who is concentrating on an external stimulus.

Delta waves
The typical pattern of sleep, also found in young infants; rarely, delta waves indicate the presence of a brain tumour.

Theta waves
The dominant waves of young children. In adults, they may indicate an abnormality of the brain.

the activity is displayed on a monitor or printed out on a moving strip of paper.

In EEG, small electrodes are attached to the scalp and connected to an instrument that records minute electrical impulses produced by the brain's activity. By revealing characteristic wave patterns, an EEG can help in diagnosing different types of epilepsy and identifying areas in the brain where abnormal electrical activity develops. (See also *How electroencephalography is done* box, above.)

effusion

The process by which fluid escapes. The term effusion also describes an abnormal collection of fluid (such as blood, *pus*, or *plasma*) in the tissues or a body cavity. An effusion can form as a result of inflammation or changes in pressure within blood vessels; alternatively, it can be due to changes in the blood constituents, such as in *nephrotic syndrome* (a kidney disorder). Effusion commonly occurs around the lung (see *pleural effusion*) or heart (see *pericardial effusion*) or within joints, causing swelling (see *effusion, joint*).

effusion, joint

The accumulation of fluid in the space around a *joint*, resulting in swelling, limitation of movement, and usually also pain and tenderness. All joints are

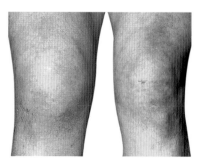

Location of knee joint effusion
Excessive production and accumulation of fluid within the right knee joint (left in image) as a result of injury or inflammation.

enclosed by a capsule lined with a membrane called the *synovium*. The synovium normally secretes small amounts of fluid (known as synovial fluid) to lubricate the joint. However, if the synovium is damaged or inflamed (for example, as a result of *arthritis*), it produces excessive fluid.

The pain and inflammation may be relieved by *analgesic drugs* and *nonsteroidal anti-inflammatory drugs* and by having injections of *corticosteroid drugs*. The swelling usually reduces if the affected joint is rested, bandaged firmly, cooled with ice-packs, and kept elevated. In some cases, the excess fluid is drawn out of the joint using a needle and syringe.

egg

See *ovum*.

ego

The conscious sense of oneself. In Freudian *psychoanalytic theory*, the ego maintains a balance between the primitive, unconscious instincts of the *id*, the controls of the *superego*, and the demands of the outside world.

Ehlers–Danlos syndrome

An inherited disorder of *collagen*, the most important structural protein in the body. Individuals with Ehlers–Danlos syndrome have abnormally stretchy, thin skin that bruises easily. Wounds are slow to heal and leave paper-thin scars, and the joints are loose and prone to recurrent dislocation. Sufferers bleed easily from the gums and digestive tract.

Ehlers–Danlos syndrome is most commonly inherited in an autosomal dominant pattern (see *genetic disorders*). There is no known specific treatment for the condition, although unnecessary accidental injury, as may occur in contact sports, should be avoided.

Eisenmenger complex

A condition in which deoxygenated blood flows directly back into the circulation rather than through the lungs. This is due to an abnormal connection between the left and right sides of the *heart* and to *pulmonary hypertension* (in which there is abnormally high blood pressure in the arteries supplying the lungs). The resultant *hypoxia* (lack of oxygen in the blood) causes *cyanosis* (bluish coloration of the skin), fainting, and difficulty in breathing.

Eisenmenger complex occurs most commonly in people who have certain uncorrected congenital heart defects (see *heart disease, congenital*), such as ventricular *septal defect*.

The diagnosis of Eisenmenger complex may be confirmed by cardiac *catheterization* (the insertion, under X-ray control, of a thin tube into the heart via a blood vessel). Once the condition has developed, surgical correction of the original defect will not help. Drug treatment may help control the symptoms but ultimately a *heart–lung transplant* may be needed.

ejaculation

The emission of *semen* from the penis at *orgasm*. Just before ejaculation, muscles around the epididymides (ducts in which *sperm* are stored; see *epididymis*), the *prostate gland*, and the *seminal vesicles* contract rhythmically, forcing the sperm from the epididymides to move forwards and mix with secretions from the seminal vesicles and the prostate. At ejaculation, this fluid is propelled out of the body through the *urethra*.

Because both semen and urine leave the body by the same route, the bladder neck closes during ejaculation. This not only prevents ejaculate from going into the bladder but also stops urine from contaminating the semen. (See also *reproductive system, male*.)

ejaculation, disorders of

Conditions in which the normal process or timing of *ejaculation* is disrupted.

TYPES

Premature ejaculation In premature ejaculation, semen emission occurs before or almost immediately following penetration. Premature ejaculation is the most common sexual problem in men, particularly in young men who have only recently become sexually active. It is often due to overstimulation or to anxiety about sexual performance. If the problem occurs frequently, sexual counselling and techniques for delaying ejaculation may help (see *sex therapy*).

Inhibited ejaculation This is a rare condition in which erection is normal, or even prolonged, but ejaculation is abnormally delayed or fails to occur. The problem may be psychological in origin, in which case counselling may help, or it may arise as a complication of a disorder such as *diabetes mellitus* or *alcohol dependence*. In some cases, inhibited ejaculation occurs as a side effect of certain drugs, such as some *antihypertensive drugs* and *antidepressant drugs*.

The cause is treated where possible; if drug treatment is thought to be the cause, a change to another drug may resolve the problem.

Retrograde ejaculation In retrograde ejaculation, the neck of the *bladder*, which normally closes during ejaculation, stays open. As a result, semen is forced backwards into the bladder and none is expelled from the penis.

Retrograde ejaculation may be due to a neurological disease, surgery on the bladder, or *prostatectomy* (removal of the prostate gland). There is no treatment, but sexual intercourse with a full bladder can sometimes result in normal ejaculation. If an affected man and his partner wish to have a baby, it is sometimes possible to harvest sperm from the bladder for use in *in vitro fertilization*. (See also *azoospermia*; *erectile dysfunction*; *psychosexual dysfunction*; *sexual problems*.)

elasticated bandage

A stretchable *bandage* that is useful in the treatment of *joint* injuries and for swelling of the legs due to *varicose veins*. It helps to minimize swelling while not impeding movement.

elbow

The hinge joint formed where the lower end of the *humerus* (upper-arm bone) meets the upper ends of the

ANATOMY OF THE **ELBOW**

The elbow is a hinge joint between the lower end of the humerus and the upper ends of the radius and ulna. The biceps muscle bends and rotates the arm at the elbow.

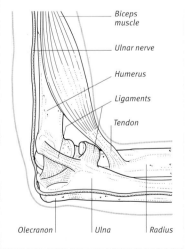

- Biceps muscle
- Ulnar nerve
- Humerus
- Ligaments
- Tendon
- Olecranon
- Ulna
- Radius

radius and *ulna* (the forearm bones). The elbow is stabilized by *ligaments* at the front, the back, and the sides. The elbow joint enables the arm to be bent and straightened, and the forearm to be rotated through almost 180 degrees around its long axis without more than a very slight movement of the upper arm.

DISORDERS

Disorders of the elbow include *arthritis* and various injuries to the joint and its surrounding muscles, tendons, and ligaments. Repeated strain on the tendons of the forearm muscles, where they attach to the elbow, can result in inflammation that is known as *epicondylitis*. There are two main types of epicondylitis: *tennis elbow* and *golfer's elbow*. Alternatively, a *sprain* of the ligaments around the elbow joint may occur.

Olecranon *bursitis* develops over the tip of the elbow in response to local irritation. Strain on the elbow joint can produce an *effusion* (the accumulation of fluid in a joint) or traumatic *synovitis* (inflammation of the membranes that line the joint capsule).

A sharp blow on the olecranon process (the bony tip of the elbow, also known as the "funny bone") may impinge on the *ulnar nerve* as it passes in a groove in this area, causing temporary discomfort: a pins-and-needles sensation and lancing pains that shoot down the arm into the fourth and fifth fingers.

A fall on to an outstretched hand or on to the tip of the elbow can cause a fracture or dislocation of the elbow.

elderly, care of the

Appropriate care to help minimize physical and mental deterioration in the elderly. For example, failing vision and hearing are often regarded as inevitable in old age, but removal of a *cataract* or use of a *hearing-aid* can often improve quality of life.

Isolation or inactivity leads to *depression* in some elderly people. Attending a day-care centre can provide social contact and introduce new interests.

Many elderly people are cared for by family members. Voluntary agencies can often provide domestic help to ease the strain on carers. Sheltered housing allows independence while providing a degree of supervision and assistance when it is needed. Elderly people with *dementia* or a physical disability may require more supervision, in a residential care or hospital setting. (See also *geriatric medicine*.)

E

elective

A term used to describe a procedure, usually a surgical operation, that is not urgent and can be performed at a scheduled time.

electrical injury

Damage to tissues caused by an electric current passing through the body and the associated heat release. The internal tissues of the body, being moist and salty, are good conductors of electricity. Dry skin provides a high resistance to current flow, but moist skin has a low resistance and thus allows a substantial current to flow into the body. Serious injury or death from domestic voltage levels is therefore more likely to occur in the presence of water.

PHYSICAL EFFECTS

All except the mildest electric shocks may result in unconsciousness. Alternating current (AC) is more dangerous than direct current (DC): it causes sustained muscle contractions, which may prevent the victim from releasing the source of the current. A current as small as 0.1 amp passing through the heart can cause a fatal *arrhythmia* (irregular heartbeat). The same current passing through the *brainstem* may cause cessation of the heartbeat and breathing.

Larger currents may cause charring of tissues, especially where the current enters and exits the body.

electric shock treatment

See *ECT*.

electrocardiography

See *ECG*.

electrocautery

A technique for destroying tissue using heat produced by an electric current. Electrocautery is used to remove skin blemishes such as *warts*. (See also *cauterization*; *diathermy*; *electrocoagulation*.)

electrocoagulation

Use of a high-frequency electric current to seal blood vessels by heat, stopping *bleeding*. Electrocoagulation is used in surgery; the current is delivered through a surgical knife, enabling the surgeon to make bloodless incisions. The procedure is also used to stop nosebleeds and to destroy abnormal blood vessel formations, such as *spider naevi*.

electroconvulsive therapy

See *ECT*.

electrode

A device through which an electrical current is transmitted or received. In *ECG*, for example, electrodes are applied to the chest wall to detect electrical impulses from the heart. Other procedures using electrodes include certain types of *physiotherapy*, in which electrodes are attached to the skin and emit electrical impulses to stimulate the underlying muscles. (See also *ECT*; *electrocautery*; *electrocoagulation*; *electrolysis*; *electronystagmography*.)

electroencephalography

See *EEG*.

electrolysis

Permanent removal of unwanted hair by introducing a short-wave electric current into the hair *follicle*. The current destroys the hair root either by causing a chemical reaction (a process that is called galvanism) or by generating heat, which seals off the blood vessels supplying the hair (see *diathermy*).

WHY IT IS DONE

Hair on the face and body can be removed temporarily by shaving or plucking or by the use of depilatory creams, abrasives, or wax preparations. However, electrolysis is the only method of permanent hair removal.

AREAS THAT CAN BE TREATED

With a few exceptions, electrolysis can be safely used on any part of the body. Its use should be avoided on the lower margins of the eyebrows because the skin above the eyelids is very delicate and easily damaged. It is also question-

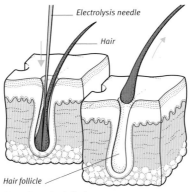

Electrolysis needle

Hair

Hair follicle

How electrolysis is done
To remove each hair, a fine needle is inserted into the follicle and a small electric current is passed through it. The current destroys the root of the hair and the hair is then pulled out. The procedure may cause some pain, but, in skilled hands, it is harmless. If the treatment is successful, there should be no further hair growth from that follicle.

able whether the technique should be used on the armpits due to the risk of bacterial infection. Electrolysis has no harmful effect on the breasts (where hair sometimes grows around the areola, the pigmented area surrounding the nipple) and does not affect *breast-feeding*. The legs are not well suited to electrolysis because treatment of this extensive area requires so many sessions that the procedure would be very time-consuming and expensive.

NEWER TREATMENTS

Alternative methods of hair removal, which are faster and less painful than electrolysis, are now available.

One new method is a form of *laser treatment* in which hair follicles are destroyed by a laser beam. The treatment can be used on several hundred hair follicles simultaneously. It works best on people with pale skin and dark hair, because the melanin (dark pigment) in the hair absorbs energy from the laser, while the skin (which has little melanin) is relatively unaffected.

Another new technique, known as photo-epilation, involves the use of intense pulsed light to disable hundreds of hair follicles at the same time, with minimal side effects.

electrolyte

A substance whose molecules dissociate (split) into its constituent *ions* (electrically charged particles) when dissolved or melted. For example, sodium chloride (table salt) dissociates into sodium cations (positively charged ions) and chloride anions (negatively charged ions) when dissolved in water.

electromyography

See *EMG*.

electronystagmography

A method of recording types of *nystagmus* (abnormal, jerky movements of the eye) in order to investigate their cause. In electronystagmography, electrical changes caused by eye movements are picked up by *electrodes* that are placed near the eyes and are recorded on a graph.

electrophoresis

The movement of electrically charged particles that are suspended in a *colloid* solution under the influence of an electric current. The direction, distance, and rate of movement of the particles vary according to their size, shape, and electrical charge.

Electrophoresis is used to analyse mixtures (to identify and quantify the proteins in blood, for example), and it may be used as a diagnostic test for *multiple myeloma*, a bone marrow tumour that produces abnormally high blood levels of a specific *antibody* (a protein manufactured by the immune system).

elephantiasis

A disease that occurs in the tropics and is characterized by massive swelling of the legs, the arms, and, in men, the scrotum (the pouch behind the penis that contains the testes). There is also thickening and darkening of the skin. Most cases of elephantiasis are due to chronic lymphatic obstruction caused by *filariasis* (a worm infestation).

elimination diet

A dietary programme used to identify a *food allergy* or *food intolerance*. Test foods, such as milk, are gradually omitted from the diet one at a time to see if they are responsible for the symptoms. (See also *exclusion diet*.)

ELISA test

A laboratory blood test used in the diagnosis of infectious diseases. ELISA stands for enzyme-linked immunosorbent assay. (See also *immunoassay*.)

elixir

A clear, sweetened liquid, which often contains alcohol, that forms the basis of many liquid medicines, such as *cough remedies*.

ellipsoidal joint

A type of mobile *joint*, such as the wrist joint, that allows all types of movement except full rotation.

emaciation

Abnormal thinness or wasting away of the body, which may be the result of a variety of conditions including *malnutrition*, *worm infestation*, or diseases such as *tuberculosis* or *cancer*.

embolectomy

Surgical removal of an embolus (a fragment of material, often a blood clot, that is carried in the bloodstream and has blocked an *artery*; see *embolism*).

There are two methods of embolectomy. In one procedure, an incision is made in the affected artery and the embolus is removed through a suction tube. In balloon embolectomy, a *balloon*

catheter (a flexible tube with a balloon at its tip) is passed into the affected blood vessel, to just beyond the embolus. The balloon is inflated and the catheter is withdrawn from the body, bringing the embolus out with it.

embolism

Blockage of an *artery* by an embolus (a fragment of material carried in the bloodstream). An embolus may consist of various substances. It is usually formed from a blood clot (thrombus). Other substances that may form an embolism include a bubble of air or other gas; a piece of tissue or tumour; a clump of bacteria, bone marrow, cholesterol, or fat; or, rarely, amniotic fluid forced into a woman's circulation during *childbirth*.

TYPES

A blood clot that has broken off from a larger clot elsewhere in the circulation is the most common type of embolus.

Pulmonary embolism is a disorder that may be due to a blood clot. The condition is usually the result of a fragment breaking off from a deep vein thrombosis (see *thrombosis, deep vein*) and being carried via the heart to block an artery supplying the lungs. Pulmonary embolism may cause sudden death. Blood clots may form inside the heart after a

myocardial infarction (heart attack), or in the atria (upper chambers of the heart) in *atrial fibrillation*, and then travel to the brain. This results in a cerebral embolism, which is an important cause of *stroke* (damage to part of the brain due to interruption to its blood supply).

Air embolism, in which a small artery is blocked by an air bubble, is rare. Fat embolism, in which a vessel is blocked by fat globules, is a possible complication of a major *fracture* of a limb; it occurs when fat is released from the marrow of the broken bone. Amniotic fluid embolism occurs during labour or immediately after delivery of the baby. This rare complication of childbirth is often fatal.

SYMPTOMS

Symptoms of an embolism depend on the site of the embolus. Pulmonary embolism can lead to breathlessness and chest pains. If the embolus lodges in the brain, a stroke may occur, affecting speech, vision, or movement. If an embolism blocks an artery to the leg, the limb will become painful and turn pale. If left untreated, *gangrene* (tissue death) may develop.

In serious cases of fat embolism, heart and breathing rates rise dramatically and there may be restlessness, confusion, and drowsiness.

TYPES OF **EMBOLISM**

Embolisms are named after the part of the circulation affected by the embolus involved (for example, a cerebral embolism affects an artery supplying the brain). When an embolus is released, it is carried through branches of an artery until it becomes lodged. Blood is prevented from reaching parts of the body beyond.

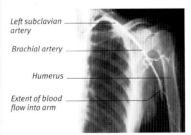

Left subclavian artery

Brachial artery

Humerus

Extent of blood flow into arm

Angiogram of embolism in the arm
This X-ray was taken after injection of a contrast medium into the blood vessel. It shows the obstruction, by an embolus, of the normal flow of blood through the subclavian artery and the brachial artery beside the humerus.

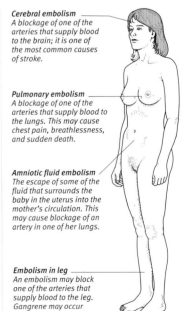

Cerebral embolism
A blockage of one of the arteries that supply blood to the brain; it is one of the most common causes of stroke.

Pulmonary embolism
A blockage of one of the arteries that supply blood to the lungs. This may cause chest pain, breathlessness, and sudden death.

Amniotic fluid embolism
The escape of some of the fluid that surrounds the baby in the uterus into the mother's circulation. This may cause blockage of an artery in one of her lungs.

Embolism in leg
An embolism may block one of the arteries that supply blood to the leg. Gangrene may occur below the blockage.

E

TREATMENT

If a severe embolism causes the person to collapse, emergency life-saving measures are undertaken to maintain the breathing and circulation (see *cardiopulmonary resuscitation*).

Embolectomy (surgical removal of the blockage) may be possible. If the embolus is formed from a blood clot and surgery is not possible, *thrombolytic drugs* (drugs that dissolve blood clots) and *anticoagulant drugs* (drugs that prevent clot formation) may be given.

embolization

Deliberate obstruction of a blood vessel using an artificial embolus (a fragment of material carried in the bloodstream) made of material such as gel foam, PVA (resin), liquid sclerosants (hardeners), or medical glue. Embolization is carried out to stop uncontrollable internal bleeding or to cut off the blood supply to a *tumour*, especially a *fibroid*. In the latter case, embolization can relieve pain; cause the tumour to shrivel, making surgical removal easier; or stop the tumour from spreading. Embolization can also be used to block flow through vascular abnormalities such as *haemangiomas*, in both the skin and internal organs.

A *catheter* (flexible tube) is introduced into a blood vessel near the one to be blocked. An embolus is released through the catheter; it lodges inside the vessel, blocking blood flow to the affected area.

embolus

A fragment of material, usually a blood clot, that is carried in the bloodstream and obstructs an *artery*. An embolus is life-threatening if it blocks blood flow through a vital artery (see *embolism*).

embrocation

A medication rubbed into the skin in order to relieve muscular or joint pain.

embryo

The unborn child during the first eight weeks of its development following *conception*; for the rest of the pregnancy it is known as a *fetus*.

Development of the embryo is governed internally by *genes* inherited from the parents and externally by factors such as the mother's diet and any drugs taken during pregnancy.

THE FIRST TWO WEEKS

The embryo develops from an *ovum* (egg) that has been fertilized by a *sperm* (see *fertilization*). It starts as a single cell, but divides several times as it travels along the *fallopian tube* to the *uterus* (womb) to form a spherical mass of cells.

About six days after conception, this mass becomes embedded in the uterus lining. At the site of attachment, the outer layer of cells obtains nourishment from the woman's blood; this part will later become the *placenta*. In the cell mass, a flat disc forms, consisting of layers of cells from which all the baby's tissues will form. The *amniotic sac* develops around the embryo.

THE THIRD WEEK

Early in the third week, the disc of cells becomes pear-shaped. The head of the embryo forms at the rounded end and the lower spine at the pointed end. A group of cells develops along the back of the embryo to form the notochord, a rod of cells that constitutes the basis for the spine. From this time onwards, the embryo has two recognizable halves that develop more or less symmetrically.

The notochord then furrows and the edges grow towards each other before fusing to form the neural tube. Later, the neural tube will develop into the *brain* and *spinal cord*.

THE FOURTH WEEK

During the fourth week, the embryo's back grows more rapidly than its front, giving it a C-shape. The neural tube extends towards the embryo's head, where a fold that will eventually form the brain becomes visible.

Developing ears appear as pits and rudimentary eyes form as stalks. Within the embryo, buds of tissue form that will become the lungs, pancreas, liver, and gallbladder. A heart starts to develop in the form of a tube. Outer layers of the embryo begin to form the limb buds and paired bulges appear on the sides of the neural tube that will eventually become the cartilage, bone, and muscle of the back.

THE FIFTH WEEK

During the fifth week of pregnancy, the embryo's external ears become visible; pits mark the position of the nose; the jaws form; and the limb buds extend, becoming flattened at the ends where the hands and feet will develop. Folds of tissue fuse to form the front wall of the chest and abdomen. The *umbilical cord* develops.

THE SIXTH TO EIGHTH WEEKS

During weeks six to eight, the embryo's face becomes recognizably human, the neck forms, the limbs become jointed, and fingers and toes appear.

After eight weeks, the embryo is about 2.5 cm long. Most of the internal organs have formed and all the external features are present.

embryo diagnosis

Also called preimplantation diagnosis, a procedure carried out on *embryos* at an early stage of development to determine whether they are affected by a *genetic disorder*. Embryo diagnosis may be carried out following *in vitro fertilization* (IVF) if the parents are known to be carriers of a specific disorder.

Several eggs are fertilized; they are grown for a few days in specialized laboratories until the first two or three cell divisions have taken place and the clusters contain approximately eight cells. One cell from each cluster is removed in order for its *DNA* to be analysed. Embryos that are found to be healthy can then be implanted in the mother's uterus (womb).

embryology

The study of the development and growth of the *embryo* and then the *fetus* from *conception* through the months of gestation until birth.

Embryology is an essential part of a medical student's training because it leads to a greater understanding of the anatomy of an adult and of the ways in which structural defects in the body may arise. For example, the occurrence of congenital heart defects is easier to understand when the stages of fetal heart development are explained. (See also *embryo diagnosis*.)

embryoma of the kidney

An alternative name for *Wilms' tumour*.

emergency

Any condition requiring urgent medical treatment, such as *cardiac arrest* (a halt in the pumping action of the heart), or any procedure that must be performed immediately, such as *cardiopulmonary resuscitation*.

emergency contraception

See *contraception, emergency*.

emesis

The medical term for *vomiting*.

emetic

A substance that causes *vomiting*, used to treat some types of poisoning and drug overdose. Emetics act by stimulating the

THE DEVELOPING **EMBRYO**

From the time of conception until the eighth week, the developing baby is known as an embryo. At conception, the fertilized egg consists of a single cell, the zygote, which contains genetic material from the sperm and the ovum. The zygote divides several times to form a ball of cells, which then implants into the lining of the uterus. At the point of attachment, the outer layer of cells forms the placenta, while a group of cells within one area of the cell ball develops into the embryo. A sac filled with amniotic fluid forms around the embryo to protect it. As the embryo grows, it begins to form features and, by the fifth week, it has developed a recognizable head and limb buds.

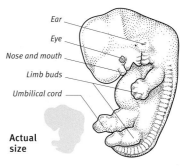

Embryo at about six weeks
The embryo is floating in the amniotic sac. The smaller sac above (the yolk sac) provides nourishment for the early embryo.

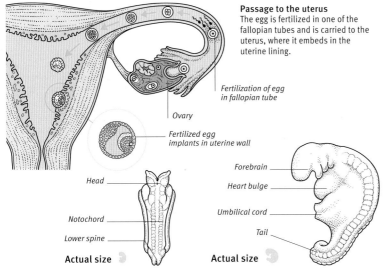

Passage to the uterus
The egg is fertilized in one of the fallopian tubes and is carried to the uterus, where it embeds in the uterine lining.

Fertilization of egg in fallopian tube

Ovary

Fertilized egg implants in uterine wall

Head

Notochord

Lower spine

Actual size

Three weeks
The embryo now becomes pear-shaped, with a rounded head, pointed lower spine, and notochord running along its back.

Forebrain

Heart bulge

Umbilical cord

Tail

Actual size

Four weeks
The embryo now becomes C-shaped and a tail is visible. The umbilical cord forms and the forebrain enlarges.

Ear

Eye

Nose and mouth

Limb buds

Umbilical cord

Actual size

Six weeks
Eyes are visible and the mouth, nose, and ears are forming. The limbs grow rapidly from initial tiny buds.

INTERNAL ORGANS AT FIVE WEEKS

All the internal organs (such as the liver, pancreas, stomach, kidneys, heart, lungs, and sex organs) have begun to form by the fifth week. During this critical stage of development, the embryo is highly vulnerable to harmful substances that are consumed by the mother (such as alcohol and some medications), which may cause birth defects.

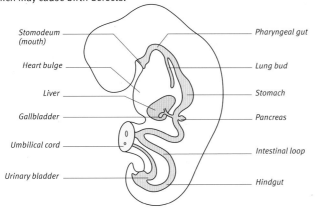

Stomodeum (mouth)

Heart bulge

Liver

Gallbladder

Umbilical cord

Urinary bladder

Pharyngeal gut

Lung bud

Stomach

Pancreas

Intestinal loop

Hindgut

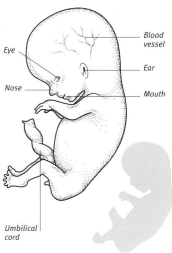

Eye

Nose

Umbilical cord

Blood vessel

Ear

Mouth

Actual size

Eight weeks
The face is more "human", the head is more upright, and the tail has gone. Limbs become jointed and digits appear.

part of the brain that controls vomiting and/or by directly irritating the lining of the stomach. The most widely used emetic is *ipecacuanha*.

EMG

The abbreviation for electromyogram, a recording of the electrical activity within a *muscle*.

WHY IT IS DONE

An EMG can help to diagnose muscle disorders, such as *muscular dystrophy*, or conditions in which the nerve supply to the muscle is impaired, such as *neuropathy*, *radiculopathy*, or *motor neuron disease*. In cases of nerve injury, the actual site of the nerve damage can often be located.

HOW IT IS DONE

Electrical activity is measured during muscle contraction and at rest. Small disc electrodes are attached to the skin over the muscle; alternatively, needle electrodes are inserted into the muscle. The impulses from the muscle are displayed on an oscilloscope screen, which shows muscle contraction and relaxation in the form of a wave pattern and reveals whether or not the muscle activity is normal. A permanent record can be made of the EMG. The procedure has no side effects.

EMLA

An acronym for "eutectic mixture of local anaesthetics". (The word "eutectic" means "easily melted".) EMLA is a brand-named cream applied to the skin to produce local anaesthesia (see *anaesthesia, local*). It is used to reduce discomfort before intravenous injection and *venepuncture*, particularly in children, and before treating localized skin conditions such as genital warts (see *warts, genital*).

emollient

A substance, such as lanolin or petroleum jelly, that has a soothing and softening effect when applied to the skin. Emollients have a moisturizing effect on the skin because they form an oily film on its surface, which prevents loss of water. Emollients are used in creams, ointments, lotions, and bath additives.

emotional deprivation

A lack of sufficient loving attention and of warm, trusting relationships during early childhood, causing normal emotional development to be inhibited. Emotional deprivation may result if

bonding does not occur in the early months of life or if a child is frequently separated from his or her parents for long periods during the first five years.

Emotionally deprived children may be impulsive, unable to cope with frustration, hungry for attention, and may have impaired intellectual development.

emotional overlay

A term used by some doctors to describe physical symptoms that they feel have been worsened by emotional difficulties. For example, it is common for symptoms of a condition to worsen when an individual is unhappy or worried. (See also *pain*.)

emotional problems

A common term for a range of psychological difficulties, often related to *anxiety* or *depression*. Emotional problems may have various causes.

empathy

The ability to understand and share the thoughts and feelings of another person. In *psychoanalysis*, the therapist partly relies on empathy to establish a relationship with a patient.

emphysema

A disease in which the walls of the alveoli (see *alveolus, pulmonary*) are progressively destroyed, thereby reducing the area of lung available for exchange of gases. The alveoli, of which there are many millions in each lung, are groups of air sacs at the end of bronchioles (tiny air passages). Through their thin walls, inhaled oxygen is passed into the bloodstream and carbon dioxide is removed from the capillaries to be breathed out.

Emphysema usually develops along with chronic *bronchitis* in a condition known as chronic obstructive pulmonary disease, also known as COPD (see *pulmonary disease, chronic obstructive*).

CAUSES

In almost all cases, emphysema is a direct result of smoking. In rare cases, an inherited deficiency of a chemical called alpha$_1$-antitrypsin in the body results in emphysema and, in a minority of people, also affects the liver (see *alpha$_1$-antitrypsin deficiency*).

Tobacco smoke and other air pollutants are believed to cause emphysema by provoking the release of chemicals within the alveoli that cause damage to the alveolar walls. Alpha$_1$-antitrypsin is

thought to protect against this chemical damage; therefore, people with a deficiency of this substance are particularly badly affected by emphysema.

The damage is slight at first, but in heavy smokers it becomes progressively worse; the alveoli burst and merge to form fewer, larger sacs with less surface area, which consequently impairs oxygen and carbon dioxide exchange. Over the years the lungs become increasingly less elastic, which further reduces their efficiency.

SYMPTOMS AND SIGNS

Initially, there are no symptoms, but as the disease progresses and the lungs suffer damage, there is an increasing shortness of breath. In some people, the chest becomes barrel-shaped as air is trapped in the lungs. There may also be a chronic cough (caused by the accompanying bronchitis) and a slight wheeze.

Eventually (sometimes after many years) the level of oxygen in the blood starts to fall. In some cases, *pulmonary hypertension* (raised blood pressure in the pulmonary artery) develops, leading to *cor pulmonale* (enlargement and strain on the right side of the heart). Affected people start to turn blue due to a lack of oxygen in the blood; their legs subsequently swell as a result of *oedema* (accumulation of fluid in the tissues). Other sufferers are able to compensate for oxygen deficiency to some extent by breathing faster, thereby retaining their normal colouring. Many people show signs falling somewhere between these two extremes.

DIAGNOSIS

A diagnosis is made from the patient's symptoms and signs, from a chest examination, and from various tests. A blood sample from an artery may be analysed to measure the concentration of oxygen and carbon dioxide in the blood; blood oxygen levels may alternatively be measured using an *oximeter*. A blood test for alpha$_1$-antitrypsin deficiency may be performed if there is a family history of the disorder. Chest *X-rays* are taken to exclude the possibility of another lung disease being responsible for the symptoms and to determine how great an area of the lungs has been affected. *Pulmonary function tests* are carried out to assess breathing capacity and the efficiency of the alveoli in exchanging gases.

TREATMENT AND PREVENTION

Once the damage to the lungs has occurred, there is no treatment that can reverse it. However, giving up smoking will greatly reduce the rate at which the lungs deteriorate. The efficiency of the remaining lung tissue may be improved in various ways. For example, *bronchodilator drugs* may be given to widen the bronchioles. A corticosteroid inhaler may be prescribed to help prevent flare-ups of the symptoms of COPD, and patients who are deficient in alpha$_1$-antitrypsin may be given replacement alpha$_1$-antitrypsin therapy.

If an infection develops, *antibiotic drugs* may be prescribed, and if there is oedema, *diuretic drugs* may help to reduce the volume of fluid in the body by promoting its output through increased urine production. If the blood oxygen level is continually low, *oxygen therapy* at home may be needed.

People who have a localized area of emphysema in one lung may be offered surgery to remove the affected area of tissue, which will allow the remaining lung tissue to re-expand. A single lung transplant operation (see *transplant surgery*) may be considered if respiratory failure is life-threatening.

emphysema, surgical

The abnormal presence of air in tissues under the skin following surgery or injury. Surgical emphysema most commonly occurs as a complication of *pneumothorax* (the abnormal presence of air in the pleural cavity between the lung and the chest wall).

empirical treatment

Treatment that is given simply on the grounds that its effectiveness has been observed in previous, similar cases. Empirical treatment is different to treatment that is based on an understanding of the nature of a disorder and the way in which the particular method of treatment works.

empyema

An accumulation of *pus* in a body cavity or an internal organ. Empyema can occur around a lung as a rare complication of an infection such as *pneumonia* or *pleurisy*. The main symptoms are chest pain, breathlessness, and fever. Treatment is generally by *aspiration* (removal of the pus by suction) and the injection of *antibiotic drugs*. An operation to open the chest cavity and drain the pus may sometimes be performed.

Empyema of the *gallbladder* is a complication of *cholecystitis* (inflammation of the gallbladder), causing abdominal pain, fever, and *jaundice* (yellowing of the skin and the whites of the eyes). This type of empyema is treated by surgical removal of the gallbladder.

EMU

An abbreviation for early morning urine, a specimen of urine collected on the patient's first visit to the toilet after waking up.

emulsifying ointment

A type of *emollient* containing emulsifying wax, white soft paraffin, and liquid paraffin. Emulsifying ointment is used to smooth, soothe, and hydrate the skin in all dry or scaling conditions. Rarely, ingredients such as preservatives may result in skin sensitization.

enalapril

An *ACE inhibitor drug* that is used in the treatment of *hypertension* (high blood pressure) and *heart failure* (a reduced pumping efficiency of the heart). The drug inhibits a chemical reaction that causes blood vessels to constrict, and thus allows vessels to dilate (widen); as a result, it lowers blood pressure and reduces the workload of the heart.

One side effect of enalapril is a sudden drop in blood pressure on taking the first dose. For this reason, the patient should rest while the dose is taken and for two or three hours afterwards. More common adverse effects of the drug include headaches and dizziness; these effects should diminish with continued treatment.

enamel, dental

The hard outer layer of a tooth (see *teeth*) that protects the inner structures.

encephalitis

Inflammation of the *brain*, and sometimes also the *meninges* (the three membranes that cover and protect the brain and the spinal cord), usually due to a viral infection. Encephalitis varies in severity from a mild problem, in which symptoms are barely noticeable, to a serious and potentially life-threatening disorder.

CAUSES
Mild cases of encephalitis may be due to glandular fever (see *mononucleosis, infectious*) or may be a complication of viral diseases such as *mumps* or *measles*.

In Europe (including the UK), the most common cause of life-threatening encephalitis is *herpes simplex*. In Southeast Asia, *Japanese B encephalitis*, due to a virus spread by mosquitoes, is the most dangerous type. Occasionally, outbreaks of viral encephalitis occur elsewhere in the world; for example, an outbreak of *West Nile virus*, another mosquito-borne form of the disease, occurred in New York in 1999.

People with *HIV* are particularly at risk from severe viral encephalitis, and may also develop cerebral abscesses (collections of pus in the brain tissue).

SYMPTOMS
Mild cases of encephalitis usually develop over several days and may cause only a slight fever and mild headache. In serious cases of encephalitis, the symptoms develop rapidly and include weakness or *paralysis*; speech, memory, and hearing problems; and a gradual loss of consciousness. *Coma* (a state of unconsciousness and unresponsiveness to external stimuli) and *seizures* may also occur. If the meninges are inflamed, certain other symptoms (for example, a stiff neck and abnormal sensitivity to light) may develop (see *meningitis*).

DIAGNOSIS AND TREATMENT
Diagnosis is based on results of blood tests; *CT scanning* or *MRI* (techniques that produce cross-sectional or three-dimensional images of the brain); *EEG* (a method of recording the electrical activity of the brain); *lumbar puncture* (taking a sample of fluid from the spinal canal for analysis); and, very occasionally, a brain *biopsy* (removal of a small sample of tissue for analysis).

Encephalitis due to herpes simplex is treated with *intravenous infusion* of the antiviral drug *aciclovir*, but there is no known treatment for encephalitis caused by other viral infections.

encephalitis lethargica

An epidemic form of *encephalitis* (brain inflammation). There have been no major outbreaks of the condition since the 1920s, but rare sporadic cases still occur. Symptoms of encephalitis lethargica are those of encephalitis, with additional lethargy and drowsiness.

Many survivors of the initial illness during the major epidemics developed a movement disorder that became known as post-encephalitic *Parkinson's disease*.

encephalocele

A type of *neural tube defect* resulting in defects of the brain rather than of the spinal cord, as occurs in *spina bifida*.

E

encephalomyelitis

Inflammation of the *brain* and *spinal cord*, resulting in damage to the *nervous system*, usually due to a viral infection.

CAUSES

Encephalomyelitis develops as a rare complication of *measles* or, less commonly, of other viral infections, such as *chickenpox*, *rubella* (German measles), or glandular fever (see *mononucleosis, infectious*). It may also occasionally follow vaccination against *rabies*.

SYMPTOMS

Symptoms of encephalomyelitis include fever, drowsiness, headache, seizures, partial *paralysis* or loss of sensation, and, in some cases, *coma* (a state of unconsciousness and unresponsiveness).

DIAGNOSIS AND TREATMENT

Diagnosis is based on the results of blood tests; *CT scanning* or *MRI* (techniques that produce cross-sectional or three-dimensional images of the body structures); *EEG* (a method of recording the electrical activity of the brain); *lumbar puncture* (taking a sample of fluid from the spinal canal for analysis); and, rarely, a brain *biopsy* (removal of a small sample of brain tissue for microscopic analysis).

There is no cure for the disease, but *corticosteroid drugs* are given to reduce inflammation and *anticonvulsant drugs* to control seizures.

OUTLOOK

The disease is often fatal; those who survive may suffer permanent damage to the nervous system.

encephalomyelitis, myalgic

Another term for the disorder *chronic fatigue syndrome*.

encephalopathy

Any disorder affecting the *brain*, especially chronic degenerative conditions.

TYPES AND CAUSES

Wernicke's encephalopathy is a degenerative condition of the brain caused by a deficiency of vitamin B$_1$ (see *Wernicke–Korsakoff syndrome*).

Hepatic encephalopathy is caused by the effect on the brain of *toxins* that have built up in the blood as a result of *liver failure*. It may lead to impaired consciousness, memory loss, a change in personality, tremors, and *seizures*.

In spongiform encepalopathy, the brain tissue shrinks and spaces develop within it; this leads to severe problems, such as paralysis and *dementia*. Bovine spongiform encephalopathy (BSE) is a disorder contracted by cattle after they

are given feed containing material from sheep or cattle. The cause of BSE is believed to be an infective agent that is known as a *prion*. Some cases of variant *Creutzfeldt–Jakob disease* in humans have been attributed to infection with the prions responsible for BSE, which were probably transmitted to humans via consumption of meat products.

Encephalopathy may also occur as a result of *HIV* infection, *chickenpox*, and *Reye's syndrome*.

Treatment of encephalopathy depends on the cause. (See also *hypertensive encephalopathy*.)

enchondroma

A noncancerous bone tumour that originates in cartilage in the *metaphysis* (the area in which new tissue is added as the bone grows).

encoding

The first stage in the *memory* process, also called registration. In this stage, information received by one of the senses is registered and then modified ready for storage by the brain.

encopresis

A type of *soiling* in which children pass normal faeces in unacceptable places after the age at which bowel control has been achieved. There is usually an underlying behavioural problem (see *behavioural problems in children*).

endarterectomy

An operation to remove the lining of an *artery* affected by *atherosclerosis*. Removing the diseased lining restores normal blood flow to the part of the body supplied by the artery.

WHY IT IS DONE

Endarterectomy is most commonly performed to treat carotid artery stenosis (narrowing or blockage of the carotid artery, usually due to fatty deposits called plaques), *transient ischaemic attack*, or *stroke*. The procedure may also sometimes be performed to treat *peripheral vascular disease*.

HOW IT IS DONE

Endarterectomy is a delicate procedure that may take several hours. The operation may be performed endoscopically (see *endoscopy*) or by open surgery. In open surgery, the artery is exposed, clamps are applied, an incision is made, and the diseased lining, as well as any thrombi (blood clots) that may have formed, are removed.

RESULTS

New lining grows in the artery within a few weeks of surgery. When narrowing of the arteries is widespread (that is, not confined to a single artery), *arterial reconstructive surgery* may be necessary.

endarteritis

Inflammation of the inner (intimal) layer of an *artery* wall. Endarteritis most commonly occurs as a result of a bacterial infection such as *syphilis*. The causative infection is treated with *antibiotic drugs*, such as penicillin.

end artery

An *artery*, or the final branch of an artery, that does not communicate with any other arteries. An end artery is therefore the sole supplier of blood to its surrounding tissues. If an end artery is damaged and can no longer supply blood to an area, the tissues of that area may die. End arteries are found in the *brain*, heart, retina, kidneys, and spleen.

endemic

A term applied to a disease or disorder that is constantly present in a particular region or in a specific group of people. *AIDS*, for example, has become endemic in central Africa. An endemic disease contrasts with an *epidemic*, which is not generally present but occasionally affects large numbers of people.

endemic goitre

A type of *goitre* (a swelling of the neck due to enlargement of the *thyroid gland*) that occurs in certain parts of the world due to a deficiency of *iodine* in the diet. Iodine is necessary for the production of the *thyroid hormones* triiodothyronine (T_3) and thyroxine (T_4). If there is too little iodine in the diet, the thyroid gland compensates for the deficiency by enlarging in order to produce sufficient amounts of thyroid hormones.

Endemic goitre is rare in the developed world. It may be treated using dietary measures alone.

endocarditis

Inflammation of the endocardium (the membrane that lines the inside of the heart), particularly the endocardium lining the *heart valves*.

CAUSES AND INCIDENCE

Endocarditis is most often caused by infection with *bacteria*, *fungi*, or other microorganisms, which may be introduced into the body during surgery (including dental procedures); by *intravenous* injection using dirty needles; or through breaks in the skin or mucous membranes. The organisms travel in the bloodstream to the heart. As a result, the lining of the valves becomes inflamed, the valves may be damaged, and blood clots may form on the affected areas.

People whose endocardium has previously been damaged by disease are particularly vulnerable to endocarditis, as are those with artificial heart valves or some forms of congenital heart disease. This is because clots that form on the injured surface trap the causative microorganisms, which then multiply rapidly at the site of damage.

Intravenous drug users are vulnerable to endocarditis, even if their hearts are healthy, because microorganisms from a dirty syringe or from unclean skin at the site of injection can be introduced into the bloodstream.

Those with a suppressed immune system are at increased risk of endocarditis due to a lowered resistance to infection; organisms that would normally be harmless can cause serious infection.

SYMPTOMS

Endocarditis may be either *subacute* or *acute*. In the subacute form, symptoms are often general and nonspecific; they may include fatigue, feverishness, and vague aches and pains. On physical examination, the only evident abnormality may be a heart *murmur*.

Acute endocarditis, which occurs less frequently, develops suddenly and causes shortness of breath, severe chills, high fever, and a rapid or irregular heartbeat. The infection quickly progresses and may destroy the heart valves, leading to *heart failure*.

DIAGNOSIS AND TREATMENT

Endocarditis is diagnosed by physical examination and analysis of blood samples, including *blood cultures*. Tests on the heart may include *ECG* (measurement of the heart's electrical activity), *chest X-ray*, and *echocardiography* (an ultrasound technique that produces detailed images of the heart). Echocardiography shows the structure and movement of the heart and can reveal any collections of infected material on the valves or in a chamber of the heart.

Treatment is with high doses of *antibiotic drugs*, usually given intravenously. Antibacterial drugs are given as preventive treatment for those people at risk. *Heart-valve surgery* may be needed to replace a damaged valve.

endocardium

The innermost of the three layers of the *heart* wall. The endocardium is formed of *endothelial* cells and is continuous with the linings of the blood vessels.

endocervix

The *mucous membrane* (layer of thin, moist tissue) that lines the cervical canal. The cervical canal connects the *uterus* to the vagina and runs through the centre of the *cervix* (the neck of the womb). (See also *endometrium*.)

endocrine gland

A type of *gland* that secretes *hormones* directly into the bloodstream rather than through a duct. The *thyroid gland*, *pituitary gland*, *ovaries*, testes (see *testis*), and *adrenal glands* are all endocrine glands. The endocrine glands in the body make up the *endocrine system*. (See also *exocrine gland*.)

endocrine system

The collection of glands around the body that produce *hormones* (chemical substances necessary for normal body functioning). These glands include the *pituitary gland*, *thyroid gland*, *parathyroid glands*, *pancreas*, testes (see *testis*), *ovaries*, and *adrenal glands*. Hormones that are produced by these glands are responsible for numerous bodily processes, including growth, metabolism, sexual development and function, and response to stress.

Any increase or decrease in the production of a specific hormone interferes with the process it controls. To prevent under- or overproduction, hormone secretion from many endocrine glands is regulated by the *pituitary gland*; the pituitary gland is, in turn, influenced by the *hypothalamus* in the brain according to a *feedback* mechanism (see *Control of hormone production* box, overleaf).

ENDOCRINE DISORDERS

In all endocrine disorders, there is either deficient or excess production of a hormone by a gland. Common causes of abnormal hormone production include a tumour or an autoimmune disease affecting a gland, or a disorder of the pituitary or the hypothalamus, which control many other glands. Abnormal hormone production often has a feedback effect on the secretion of trophic (stimulating) hormones by the pituitary and the hypothalamus, as in Addison's disease and Cushing's disease (shown below). The blood levels of different hormones may need to be measured in order to pinpoint the cause of a disorder.

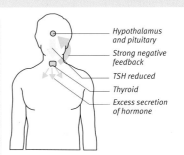

Thyrotoxicosis
This disorder is usually due to an autoimmune disease of the thyroid gland. Excess thyroid hormones cause the symptoms; the output of TSH and its hypothalamic-releasing hormone is reduced, but the thyroid gland continues to overproduce hormones.

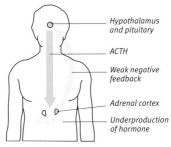

Addison's disease
Symptoms result from reduced hormone production by the defective adrenal cortices (outer zones of the adrenal glands). Feedback is weak, so the pituitary gland pours out adrenocorticotrophic hormone (ACTH), but it fails to stimulate the adrenals.

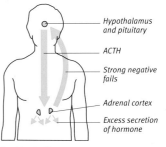

Cushing's disease
This disorder results from excess ACTH secretion by a pituitary tumour. The excess amounts of ACTH stimulate the adrenal cortices to make excess hydrocortisone, which causes the symptoms of the syndrome. Feedback fails to suppress ACTH secretion.

ENDOCRINE SYSTEM

The system consists of a collection of hormone-producing glands. Many of these glands are regulated by trophic (stimulating) hormones secreted by the pituitary. The pituitary is itself influenced by hormones secreted by the hypothalamus in the brain. Shown here are the principal glands, with a note on the hormones they produce.

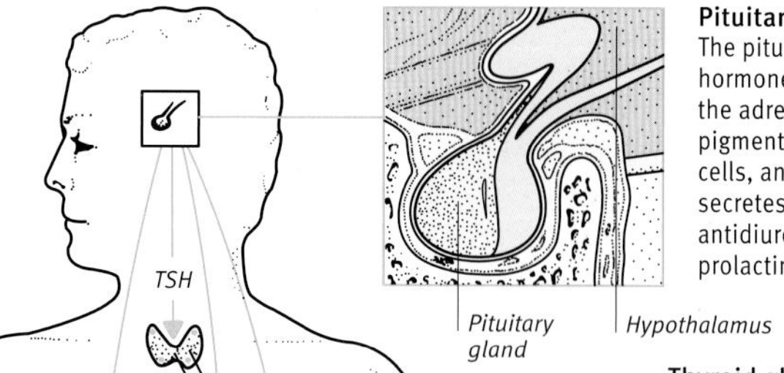

Pituitary gland
The pituitary gland secretes hormones that stimulate the adrenals, the thyroid, pigment-producing skin cells, and the gonads; it also secretes growth hormone, antidiuretic hormone, prolactin, and oxytocin.

Pituitary gland   *Hypothalamus*

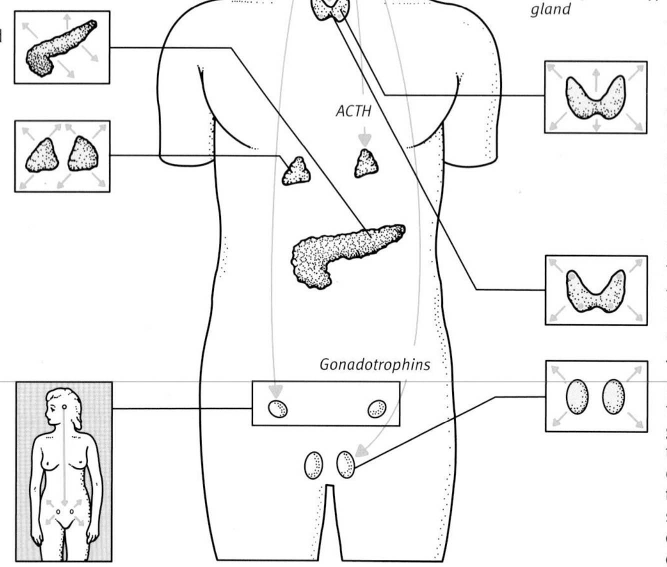

Pancreas
This gland secretes insulin and glucagon, which control the body's utilization of glucose.

Adrenal cortex
When stimulated by ACTH (adrenocorticotrophic hormone), the adrenal cortex produces hydrocortisone, which has widespread effects on metabolism; it also produces androgen hormones and aldosterone, which maintains blood pressure and the body's salt balance.

Thyroid gland
This gland produces the hormones thyroxine, triiodothyronine, and calcitonin, which stimulate metabolism, body heat production, and bone growth. Thyroid activity is controlled by TSH (thyroid-stimulating hormone), secreted by the pituitary.

Parathyroid glands
These glands, at the back of the thyroid, secrete parathyroid hormone, which maintains the calcium level in the blood.

Ovaries
In females, the ovaries produce oestrogen and progesterone, which influence many aspects of female physiology. This hormone production is controlled by gonadotrophin hormones, secreted by the pituitary.

Testes
In males, the testes produce testosterone in response to gonadotrophins secreted by the pituitary. A combination of gonadotrophins and testosterone stimulates sperm production and the development of other male characteristics.

TSH

ACTH

Gonadotrophins

CONTROL OF HORMONE PRODUCTION

Production of too much or too little hormone by a gland is prevented by feedback mechanisms. Variations in the blood level of the hormones are detected by the part of the brain known as the hypothalamus, which prompts the pituitary to modify its production of the appropriate trophic (gland-stimulating) hormones accordingly.

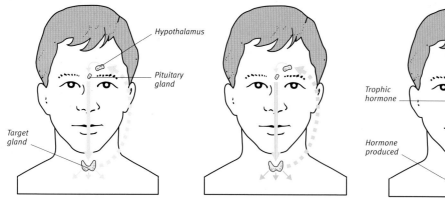

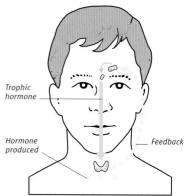

Hypothalamus

Pituitary gland

Target gland

Trophic hormone

Hormone produced

Feedback

1 The production of hormone by the target gland (in this illustration, the thyroid gland) and of trophic hormone by the pituitary gland is normal.

2 If hormone production by the target gland rises, the feedback effect causes less trophic hormone to be produced, which tends to return the situation to normal.

3 If hormone production by the target gland drops, the feedback lessens and more trophic hormone is produced, which tends to return the situation to normal.

endocrinology

The study of the *endocrine system*, or hormonal system, including the investigation and treatment of its disorders.

endodontics

A branch of *dentistry* concerned with the causes, prevention, diagnosis, and treatment of disease and injury that affect the nerves and pulp in *teeth* and the supportive tissues in the *gum*. Common endodontic procedures are *root-canal treatment* and *pulpotomy*.

endogenous

A term that refers to a disease or disorder that arises within the body. For example, an endogenous infection may occur if bacteria from the anus invade the urinary tract. Most disorders are *exogenous* (caused by external factors).

endogenous depression

A term formerly used for a type of *depression* (feelings of sadness, hopelessness, and a lack of interest in life) originating from biological factors in an individual. In contrast, "reactive depression" was seen to result from a stressful or emotional event or period of life. In many cases, however, depression is a combination of both of these types.

endolymph

The fluid contained within the membranous *labyrinth* (the structures in the inner *ear* that help to control *balance*).

Endolymph flows around the labyrinth as the body moves, causing nerve receptors in the labyrinth to send signals to the brain about the motion of the body. A significant increase in the volume of endolymph in the labyrinth may occur in *Ménière's disease*.

endometrial ablation

A treatment for persistent *menorrhagia* (heavy menstrual bleeding) involving removal of the *endometrium* (the inner lining of the uterus). In this procedure, *endoscopy* is used to view the interior of the uterus, while the endometrium is removed by *diathermy* (heat treatment), laser, or a microwave probe (MEA). Endometrial ablation can only be carried out if the woman has no desire to become pregnant in the future.

endometrial biopsy

A procedure in which a small sample of tissue is taken from the *endometrium* (the inner lining of the uterus) for microscopic analysis. Endometrial biopsies are used to detect areas of abnormal tissue such as tumours (see *uterus, cancer of*). Samples may be taken during hysteroscopy (examination of the interior of the uterus with a viewing instrument) or collected using a small vacuum device introduced through the cervix. Mild cramping pains may be a side effect.

endometrial cancer

See *uterus, cancer of*.

endometriosis

A condition in which fragments of the *endometrium* (the lining of the inside of the uterus) are found in other parts of the body, usually in the pelvic cavity. Endometriosis can cause *infertility* in up to two in five affected women.

INCIDENCE AND CAUSES

Endometriosis most commonly occurs in women who are aged between 25 and 40. The cause of the disorder is not clear. In some cases, it is thought to be due to the failure of certain fragments of the endometrium, shed during *menstruation*, to leave the body. Instead, they travel up the fallopian tubes and into the pelvic cavity, where they can adhere to and grow on any pelvic organ. These displaced patches of endometrium continue to respond to hormones that are produced in the menstrual cycle and bleed each month.

SYMPTOMS

The symptoms of endometriosis vary greatly. Some women have no symptoms, but the disorder most commonly causes abnormal or heavy menstrual bleeding. There may be severe abdominal pain and/or lower back pain during menstruation. Other possible symptoms include dyspareunia (see *intercourse, painful*), diarrhoea, constipation, and pain during defaecation.

The internal bleeding causes pain and is followed by healing, which produces internal scarring. Bleeding into an ovary may result in a blood-filled ovarian cyst

---

SITES OF **ENDOMETRIOSIS**

Fragments of the *endometrium* may travel from the uterus into the pelvic cavity via the fallopian tubes. They then implant on parts of the pelvic organs (such as the ovaries, vagina, cervix, bladder, and rectum) or on the peritoneum. The patches of endometrium continue to respond to the menstrual cycle and bleed every month. This causes the formation of painful cysts, which can be very small or may be as large as a grapefruit.

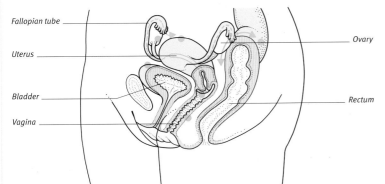

Fallopian tube
Uterus
Bladder
Vagina
Ovary
Rectum

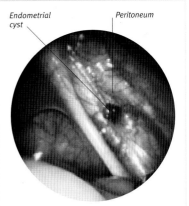

Endometrial cyst — Peritoneum

Peritoneal endometriosis
In this endoscopic view of the pelvic cavity, a fragment of endometrium has attached itself to the peritoneum (the membrane that lines the inside of the pelvic cavity) and a cyst has formed.

(known as a "chocolate cyst" because of its appearance). Endometrial tissue may be deposited in the muscular wall of the uterus (*myometrium*); this condition is called adenomyosis. In rare cases, there is bleeding from the rectum during menstruation.

DIAGNOSIS AND TREATMENT

Laparoscopy (examination of the abdominal cavity with a viewing instrument) confirms the diagnosis. Certain drugs (including *danazol*, *progestogen drugs*, *gonadorelin* analogues, or the combined *oral contraceptive* pill) may be given to prevent menstruation. Local ablation of the endometrial deposits, using either *laser treatment* or *electrocautery* (the application of heat produced by an electric current), may sometimes be needed.

If the woman is fertile, pregnancy often results in significant improvement. A *hysterectomy* (surgical removal of the uterus) and *oophorectomy* (surgical removal of the ovaries) may be offered if the woman does not have plans to have children.

endometritis

Inflammation of the *endometrium* (the inner lining of the uterus) resulting from infection. Endometritis is a feature of *pelvic inflammatory disease* (PID). It may also be a complication of *abortion* or childbirth, occur after insertion of an *IUD*, or be the result of a *sexually transmitted infection* such as a *chlamydial infection*.

Symptoms of endometritis include fever, vaginal discharge, and lower abdominal pain. Treatment includes removing any foreign body (such as an IUD or retained placental tissue) and *antibiotic drugs*.

endometrium

The inner lining of the *uterus*. The endometrium contains numerous *glands* and gradually increases in thickness during the menstrual cycle (see *menstruation*) until *ovulation* (release of an egg from the ovary) occurs. The surface layers of the endometrium are shed during menstruation if *conception* does not take place.

endomorph

A term formerly used to describe an individual with a round head and a large abdomen; short arms and legs with slender wrists and ankles; weak muscular and skeletal development; and a large proportion of body fat. (See also *ectomorph*; *mesomorph*.)

end organ

The specialized structure occurring at the end of a peripheral *nerve* that acts as a receptor for a particular *sensation*. An example of an end organ is one of the taste buds in the tongue.

endorphins

A group of pain-relieving *protein* molecules that are produced by the body. Endorphins relieve pain by activating *opiate* receptors in the *nervous system*. They have a similar chemical structure to the pain-relieving drug *morphine*. In addition, endorphins are thought to be involved in the body's response to stress, as well as in regulating intestinal contractions, determining mood, and controlling the release of certain hormones from the *pituitary gland*. (See also *enkephalins*.)

endoscope

A tubelike viewing instrument, with lenses and a light source attached, that is inserted into a body cavity for the purposes of investigating or treating disorders (see *endoscopy*). Endoscopes are named according to their use, and they can be flexible or rigid, depending on the part of the body to be examined. A selection of the common types of endoscope and their uses are shown in the illustrated box opposite.

endoscopy

Examination of a body cavity by means of an *endoscope* (a rigid or flexible viewing tube) for the purposes of diagnosis and/or treatment. The technique makes use of both *fibre-optics* and video technology and enables almost any hollow structure in the body to be inspected directly. Many procedures that formerly required major surgery can now be performed much more simply and safely by endoscopy.

USES

Endoscopes are named according to the part of the body for which they are being used (see *endoscopes* box). The endoscope is inserted via a natural body opening, such as the mouth or vagina, or into a small incision. Endoscopy is also used in diagnosis to inspect hollow organs. The organ may be photographed and a *biopsy* (removal of a small sample of tissue for microscopic analysis) may be performed. Endoscopy can be repeated safely at frequent intervals to allow monitoring the progress of a condition and the response to treatment.

Many operations are now performed by passing surgical instruments down an endoscope. The procedure is valuable in the treatment of acute emergencies, such as bleeding from the stomach or the removal of foreign bodies from the lungs. Operations such as female sterilization, the treatment of torn ligaments or cartilage within the knee joint, and the treatment of chronic infections of the nasal sinuses, are all routine endoscopic procedures. (See also *minimally invasive surgery*.)

endothelium

The layer of *cells* that lines the heart, blood vessels, and lymphatic ducts (see *lymphatic system*). Endothelial cells are squamous (thin and flat), providing a smooth surface that aids the flow of blood and lymph and helps to prevent the formation of thrombi (blood clots). (See also *epithelium*.)

endotoxin

A *poison* produced by certain *bacteria* that is not released until the death of those bacteria. Endotoxins cause fever when they are released in infected people. They also make the walls of the *capillaries* (the smallest blood vessels) more permeable, causing fluid to leak into the surrounding tissue. This sometimes results in a reduction in blood pressure, a condition called endotoxic shock. (See also *enterotoxin*; *exotoxin*.)

endotracheal tube

A tube that is passed into the *trachea* (windpipe) through the nose or mouth to enable delivery of oxygen during artificial *ventilation* or anaesthetic gases (see *anaesthesia*) during surgery. An inflatable cuff around the lower end of the endotracheal tube prevents any secretions or stomach contents from entering the lungs.

end stage

The most advanced stage of a disease, in which an affected organ or system is no longer able to carry out its normal functions. In these circumstances, the damage done to the body cannot be reversed; therefore, treatment is aimed at improving the patient's condition whenever possible and at relieving the symptoms (see *palliative care*). In some cases, a machine may be able to take over the function; for example, in end-stage kidney failure, filtering of the blood may be carried out by a dialysis

ENDOSCOPES

A typical flexible *fibre-optic* endoscope consists of a bundle of light-transmitting fibres. At one end is the head (featuring a viewing lens and steering device) and a power source. The tip has a light, a lens, and an outlet for air or water. Side channels enable attachments to be passed to the tip. In some endoscopes the tip may contain a camera that transmits a picture electronically to a screen. A rigid endoscope is a straight, narrow viewing tube that has a light source attached to it.

SOME COMMON TYPES OF ENDOSCOPE AND THEIR USES

Instrument	Region	Endoscope type
Cystoscope	Bladder	Flexible or rigid
Bronchoscope	Bronchi (main airways of the lungs)	Flexible or rigid
Gastroscope	Oesophagus, stomach, and duodenum	Flexible
Colonoscope	Colon (large intestine)	Flexible
Laparoscope	Abdominal cavity	Rigid
Arthroscope	Knee joint	Rigid

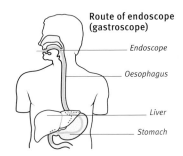

Route of endoscope (gastroscope)

- Endoscope
- Oesophagus
- Liver
- Stomach

FLEXIBLE ENDOSCOPE

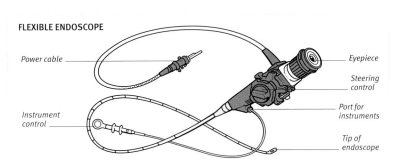

- Power cable
- Instrument control
- Eyepiece
- Steering control
- Port for instruments
- Tip of endoscope

Procedure for endoscopy

The patient may be sedated or given a local or general anaesthetic, depending on the operation. The endoscope is inserted through a natural opening (here, the mouth during gastroscopy). A camera at the tip of the endoscope relays images to a monitor and eyepiece. Minor procedures such as biopsy (removal of a tissue sample) may be carried out using very fine instruments passed down the endoscope.

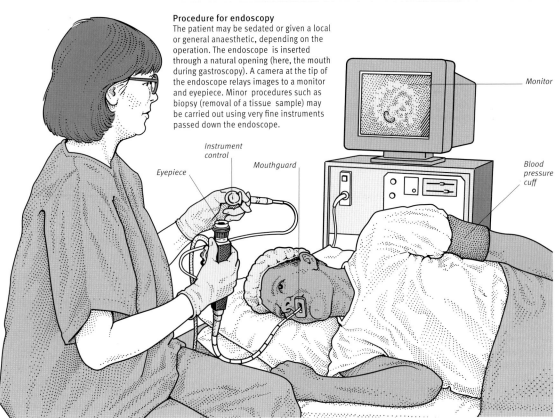

- Instrument control
- Eyepiece
- Mouthguard
- Monitor
- Blood pressure cuff

machine. The term "end stage" is used in relation to many conditions, including cancer, advanced kidney failure, and chronic lung diseases.

enema

A procedure in which fluid is passed into the *rectum* through a tube that has been inserted into the *anus*. An enema may be performed as a treatment, to prepare the intestine for surgery, or as an aid to diagnosis.

WHY IT IS DONE

An enema may be given to clear the intestine of faeces; for example, to relieve constipation, in preparation for intestinal surgery, or immediately prior to childbirth. Enemas may also be used to administer medicine, such as *corticosteroid drugs* in the treatment of the inflammatory bowel condition *ulcerative colitis*. A barium enema (see *barium X-ray examinations*) is used to diagnose disorders of the large intestine such as *diverticular disease*.

HOW IT IS DONE

Anaesthesia is not required, although the procedure may cause slight discomfort because the fluid stretches the intestine. The patient lies on his or her side with the hips raised on a pillow. A catheter (flexible tube) with a soft, well-lubricated tip is gently inserted into the rectum and the enema fluid is slowly introduced through it. The fluid is warmed first to prevent a sudden contraction of the intestine. Treatment doses are often packaged with their own applicators.

energy

The capacity to do work or effect physical change. Nutritionists use the term to refer to the fuel content of a food.

There are many different forms of energy, including light, sound, heat, chemical, electrical, and kinetic, and most of them play a role in the body. For instance, the *retina* (the light-sensitive inner layer at the back of the eye) converts light energy to electrical nerve impulses, making vision possible. The body's *muscles* use chemical energy obtained from food to produce kinetic energy (movement) and heat.

MEASUREMENT

Energy is measured in units called *calories* and *joules*. Because these units are extremely small, more practical units used in *dietetics* (nutritional science) are the kilocalorie (kcal, 1,000 calories) and kilojoule (kJ, 1,000 joules). *Carbohydrates*

and *proteins* provide about 4 kcal per gram (g), whereas *fats* provide about 9 kcal per g (see *metabolism*).

ENERGY STORAGE AND USE

In general, the energy liberated from the breakdown of food is stored as chemical energy in *ATP* (adenosine triphosphate) molecules. The stored energy is then available to power processes that consume energy, such as muscle contraction or the repair and maintenance of body structures.

energy requirements

The amount of *energy* that is needed by an individual for cell *metabolism*, muscular activity, and growth. This energy is provided by the chemical breakdown of *fats*, *carbohydrates*, and *proteins*, which are supplied by food in the diet and by *nutrients* that are stored in the liver, muscles, and *adipose tissue*.

ENERGY EXPENDITURE

Energy is needed to maintain the heartbeat, lung function, and constant body temperature. The rate at which these processes use energy, while the body is at rest, is called the basal metabolic rate (BMR). Any actions, such as movement or food digestion and absorption, increase energy expenditure above the BMR.

An individual's energy requirement increases during periods of growth and during *pregnancy* and *breast-feeding*.

ENERGY AND BODY WEIGHT

When more energy is ingested (in the form of food) than is used by the body, the surplus is stored and there is usually a gain in weight. When less energy is consumed than is spent, weight is usually lost as the stores are used up. (See also *nutrition*; *obesity*.)

engagement

The descent of the head of the *fetus* into the mother's *pelvis*. In a woman's first pregnancy, engagement has usually occurred by the 37th week, but in subsequent pregnancies it may not occur until *labour* begins. Rarely, engagement fails to occur. This may happen if, for example, the baby's position in the uterus is abnormal; if the baby's head is too big for the mother's pelvis; or if a condition known as *placenta praevia* (an abnormal positioning of the placenta across the opening of the uterus) has occurred.

Engelmann's disease

A rare, progressive, inherited form of bone *dysplasia* (a growth abnormality).

In affected individuals, the bones become abnormally long and thick, which usually results in abnormal stature and, sometimes, in delayed walking (see *walking, delayed*). There may also be muscle wasting, pain or weakness in affected limbs, delayed *puberty*, and *hypogonadism* (underactivity of the testes or ovaries).

The disease is inherited in an autosomal dominant pattern (see *genetic disorders*) and affects more males than females. It is usually diagnosed in the first few years of life. There is no specific treatment available, although *nonsteroidal anti-inflammatory drugs* may be given to relieve pain.

engorgement

Overfilling of the breasts with *milk*. Engorgement is common a few days after childbirth, when the milk supply arrives quickly and forcibly. Engorgement causes the breasts and nipples to become swollen and tender, and can make *breast-feeding* difficult. The problem can be relieved by *expressing milk*.

enhancement

The process of augmentation. The term may be used to describe improvements made to body structures or functions, or it may mean increasing the clarity of images in diagnostic imaging methods. For example, immunoenhancement is the process by which the body's *immune response* is increased by the use of antibodies (proteins made by the immune system).

enkephalins

A group of small *protein* molecules that are produced in the *brain* and by nerve endings elsewhere in the body (in the digestive system and adrenal glands, for example). Enkephalins have an analgesic (painkilling) effect and are also thought to affect mood, producing a sense of wellbeing. They are similar to *endorphins*, but they have a slightly different chemical composition and are released by different nerve endings.

enlarged prostate gland

See *prostate, enlarged*.

enophthalmos

A sinking inwards of the eyeball. Enophthalmos is most commonly caused by fracture of the eye socket or shrinkage of the eye due to the formation of scar tissue following injury.

ENT

The abbreviation for ear, nose, and throat (see *otorhinolaryngology*).

Entamoeba

A genus of amoebae (see *amoeba*), some of which are parasites of the human digestive tract.

Worldwide, ENTAMOEBA HISTOLYTICA is the most serious cause of amoebic disease, particularly in tropical areas. It is responsible for *amoebiasis* (amoebic dysentery), a disease in which the tissues of the intestinal lining are destroyed, causing the formation of *ulcers* in the intestines; *abscesses* may also form in the liver.

ENTAMOEBA GINGIVALIS is found in the mouths of humans and is associated with periodontal disease (any disorder of the tissues that surround and support the teeth) and *gingivitis* (inflammation of the gums). ENTAMOEBA COLI is a harmless intestinal parasite.

enteral feeding

A type of feeding that involves introducing nutrients directly into the intestines via a tube passed either through the abdominal wall or through a nostril and down the throat. Food may be provided in a partially broken-down form so that it does not need to be digested before being absorbed in the intestines. Enteral feeding is a useful method of feeding people with intestinal disorders, particularly inflammatory bowel disorders such as *Crohn's disease*. (See also *feeding, artificial*.)

enteric

Relating to or affecting the *intestine* (the main part of the digestive tract, which extends from the exit of the stomach to the anus).

enteric-coated tablet

A tablet whose surface is covered with a substance that is resistant to the action of *stomach* juices. Enteric-coated tablets pass undissolved through the stomach into the small intestine, where the covering dissolves and the contents are absorbed. Such tablets are used either when the drug might harm the stomach lining (as may occur with certain corticosteroid drugs) or when the stomach juices may affect the efficacy of the drug (as with sulfasalazine).

enteric fever

An alternative name for *typhoid fever* or *paratyphoid fever*.

enteritis

Inflammation of any part of the *intestine*, particularly the small intestine. Enteritis may be due to infection, particularly *giardiasis* and *tuberculosis*, or to *Crohn's disease*. Enteritis usually causes diarrhoea. (See also *colitis*; *gastroenteritis*.)

enteritis, regional

Another name for *Crohn's disease*.

enterobacteria

A group of rod-shaped, gram-negative (see *Gram's stain*) *bacteria* that live in the human or animal *intestine* (the principal part of the digestive tract, which extends from the exit of the stomach to the anus).

Some types of enterobacteria live harmlessly in the intestine. Several other types, however, cause intestinal diseases, with symptoms of diarrhoea and/or vomiting. Certain types are also responsible for urinary infections such as cystitis, which may occur when bacteria from the intestines gain access to the urethra. Examples of common enterobacteria include ESCHERICHIA COLI, SALMONELLA, YERSINIA, ENTEROBACTER, and SHIGELLA.

enterobiasis

The medical term for *threadworm infestation* of the intestines.

enterocele

A type of *hernia* in which part of the small intestine protrudes through a weakened area of the upper vaginal wall. An enterocele may develop when the muscles in a woman's vaginal canal become stretched, damaged, or weakened by any of the following: pregnancy, childbirth, surgery, or aging.

Pelvic floor exercises may help to improve the condition, but surgery may be needed to tighten the muscles. In some cases, *hysterectomy* (removal of the uterus) may be the best treatment. (See also *hernia repair*.)

Enterococcus

A genus of gram-positive (see *Gram's stain*) *bacteria* of the Streptococcaceae family. Enterococci are normally found in the human or animal *intestine* (the principal part of the digestive tract, which extends from the exit of the stomach to the anus).

They rarely cause problems in the intestine, but *urinary tract infections*, caused by enterococci entering the urethra, are common. If the bacteria spread in the bloodstream they can cause *septicaemia* (blood poisoning) and infective *endocarditis* (inflammation of the membrane lining the inside of the heart). The infections are usually treated with *antibiotic drugs*.

enterocolitis

A combination of *enteritis* (inflammation of the small intestine) and *colitis* (inflammation of the colon). Possible causes include inflammatory bowel disorders such as *Crohn's disease*.

enteropathic

A term used to describe any condition or organism related to disease of the *intestine* (the main part of the digestive tract, extending from the exit of the stomach to the anus). Enteropathic bacteria, for example, are species that may cause intestinal disease; enteropathic arthritis is joint inflammation associated with *inflammatory bowel disease*.

enteropathy, gluten

See *coeliac disease*.

enterostomy

An operation in which a portion of small or large *intestine* is joined to another part of the gastrointestinal tract or to the abdominal wall. For example, when part of the colon (large intestine) is brought through an incision in the abdominal wall to allow the discharge of faeces into a bag attached to the skin, the operation is called a *colostomy*; when the ileum (the last section of the small intestine) is used, the procedure is called an *ileostomy*.

enterotoxin

A type of *toxin* released by certain *bacteria* that inflames the intestinal lining, leading to diarrhoea and vomiting. Enterotoxins cause the symptoms of *cholera* and staphylococcal *food poisoning* (see *staphylococcal infections*). (See also *endotoxin*; *exotoxin*.)

Entonox

A brand name for a mixture of *nitrous oxide* and oxygen used to produce pain relief without loss of consciousness.

entrapment neuropathy

A condition, such as *carpal tunnel syndrome*, in which local pressure on a *nerve* causes muscle pain, numbness, and weakness in the area of the body supplied by that nerve.

E

E

entropion

A defect of the *eyelids* in which the edges of the lids turn inwards, causing the lashes to rub against the *cornea* (the transparent dome that forms the front of the eyeball) and the *conjunctiva* (the membrane that covers the white of the eye and the inside of the eyelid).

CAUSES

Entropion may be congenital (present from birth), especially in overweight babies. In addition, it is common in elderly people, due to weakness of the muscles around the lower eye, allowing the lower lid plate to turn inwards. Entropion of the upper or lower lid may also be caused by scarring, such as that due to *trachoma*.

COMPLICATIONS AND OUTLOOK

Entropion in babies does not disturb the eye and usually disappears within a few months. In later life, entropion can cause irritation, *conjunctivitis*, damage to the cornea, or problems with vision. Surgery to correct entropion can prevent such conditions.

ENT surgery

The abbreviation for ear, nose, and throat surgery (see *otorhinolaryngology*).

enucleate

To remove an organ, a tumour, or another structure surgically in such a way that it comes out cleanly and completely. An example of enucleation is the removal of an eyeball while leaving the other structures (such as muscles) in place in the eye socket.

enuresis, nocturnal

The medical term for bedwetting. It is a common condition in children, and boys are slightly more likely than girls to be affected. The problem tends to run in families.

CAUSES

Usually, enuresis results from slow maturation of nervous system functions concerned with bladder control. It may also result from, or worsen after, psychological stress. In a small number of bedwetters, there is a physical cause, such as a structural abnormality of the *urinary tract*. *Diabetes mellitus* or a *urinary tract infection* may cause bedwetting in a child who was previously dry. In cases due to physical problems, the child also has difficulty with daytime bladder control (see *incontinence, urinary*).

INVESTIGATION AND TREATMENT

If a child wets the bed persistently, tests, including *urinalysis*, may be performed to rule out a physical cause. For bedwetting that is not caused by a physical disorder, treatment starts with training the child to pass urine regularly during the day. Systems such as rewarding the child for each dry night (for example, by putting stars on a chart) are often successful. Getting the child to go to the toilet just before bed may be helpful.

Punishing a child for bedwetting, however, will not help, and may actually worsen the problem by making the child anxious.

Alarm systems, known as buzzer and pad systems, that involve placing a humidity-sensitive pad in the child's bed are available. The child is woken by the alarm if urine is passed and eventually learns to wake before starting to pass urine.

The drug desmopressin is a synthetic form of antidiuretic hormone (see *ADH*) that may occasionally be given to reduce the amount of water that is excreted by the kidneys. Desmopressin is useful on the occasional nights when a child needs to stay dry, such as when staying overnight with friends.

environmental medicine

The study of the effects on health of natural environmental factors, such as climate, altitude, sunlight, and the presence of various minerals. Environmental medicine overlaps to some extent with *occupational medicine*, in which the effects on people of their working environments are studied.

CLIMATE

The symptoms of particular types of illness may be affected by certain climates. For example, sufferers from chest disorders, such as chronic *bronchitis* and *asthma*, usually obtain some relief from their symptoms in a warm, relatively

THE IMPORTANCE OF **ENVIRONMENTAL MEDICINE**

Large areas of the world are naturally hostile to humans and were, in the past, avoided. Today, exploitation of natural resources has lured people into these regions and has highlighted the importance of environmental medicine.

Key

Desert regions

Cold regions with average winter temperature below −23°C

Mountain regions above 3,000 m

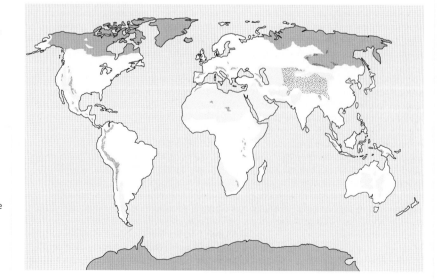

dry climate. Most respiratory complaints, in contrast, are more common during the winter.

ALTITUDE

Although mountainous regions have much less atmospheric pollution, they are not necessarily beneficial to health because the air becomes thinner as altitude increases. People with a chest condition who ascend in a few days from sea level to 1,500 m may find that their breathing difficulty worsens. Above about 3,000 m, breathing becomes difficult even for healthy people. Rapid ascent from sea level to 3,500 m or higher carries a risk of altitude sickness (see *mountain sickness*), which can cause sleeplessness, nausea, *pulmonary oedema* (fluid on the lungs), *cerebral oedema* (fluid on the brain), *coma*, or death. At high altitudes, blood cells become more numerous in an attempt to compensate for the lack of oxygen. This increase puts strain on the heart and causes a predisposition to *thrombosis* (abnormal blood clotting). Above about 6,000 m, sustained life seems to be impossible.

SUNLIGHT

Fair-skinned people who live in sunny climates may suffer ill effects from repeated exposure to sunlight (see *sunlight, adverse effects of*), including premature wrinkling of the skin and an increased risk of *cataract* (loss of transparency of the lens of the eye). There is also an increased risk of developing *skin cancers*, such as malignant melanoma (see *melanoma, malignant*) and *basal cell carcinoma*, as well as the precancerous condition solar *keratosis*. These risks have been increased by damage caused by environmental pollutants to the protective layers of ozone in the upper atmosphere. Health risks from sunlight may be reduced by protection of the skin, such as by using *sunscreens*.

MINERALS

Variations in the distribution of certain *minerals* in the environment are known to have an effect on health. For example, there is a higher-than-average incidence of cancer in areas where the radioactive gas *radon* is emitted from granitic rocks. In contrast, there is a lower-than-average incidence of tooth decay (see *caries, dental*) in populations in regions where the water has a high *fluoride* content.

enzyme

A *protein* that regulates the rate of a chemical reaction in the body. There are thousands of enzymes, each with a different chemical structure. It is this structure that determines the specific reaction regulated by the enzyme.

Every cell in the body produces various types of enzymes; different sets of enzymes occur in different tissues, reflecting their specialized functions. For example, the *pancreas* produces the digestive enzymes lipase, protease, and amylase, and among the numerous enzymes produced by the *liver* are some that metabolize drugs.

In order to function properly, many enzymes need an additional component, known as a coenzyme, which is often derived from a *vitamin* or *mineral*.

INDUCTION AND INHIBITION

Enzyme activity is influenced by many factors. One of these factors is the action of drugs. Liver enzyme activity is increased by certain drugs, such as *barbiturate drugs*, which affect the rate at which other drugs are metabolized by the liver cells. This effect, which is called enzyme induction, is responsible for a variety of important drug interactions (see *drug*).

Conversely, many drugs inhibit or block enzyme action. Some *antibiotic drugs* destroy bacteria by blocking bacterial enzymes while leaving human enzymes unaffected. Similarly, some *anticancer drugs* act by blocking enzyme activity in tumour cells, affecting normal body cells to a lesser degree.

ENZYMES AND DISEASE

Measuring enzyme levels in the blood can be useful in diagnosing certain disorders. For example, the level of heart muscle enzymes is raised following a *myocardial infarction* (heart attack) because the damaged heart muscle releases enzymes into the bloodstream, and muscle enzyme levels are raised in *muscular dystrophy*.

Many inherited metabolic disorders, including *phenylketonuria*, *galactosaemia*, and *G6PD deficiency*, are caused by defects in, or deficiencies of, enzymes. Abnormal enzymes or levels can be detected in tests on blood or other body fluids.

ENZYMES AND TREATMENT

Enzymes can play a valuable role in treating certain conditions. Pancreatic enzymes may be given to aid digestion in people who have *malabsorption* related to pancreatic disease.

Enzymes such as *streptokinase* and alteplase (see *tissue-plasminogen activator*) are used to treat acute *thrombosis* and *embolism* (conditions that cause blockage of blood vessels) by dissolving clots.

THE ACTION OF ENZYMES

An enzyme is a protein that acts as a catalyst for a chemical change in the body (that is, it greatly speeds up the rate at which the change occurs). The change may be a small modification to the structure of a substrate (the particular chemical on which the enzyme acts) in a body tissue, the splitting of a substrate, or the joining of two substrates.

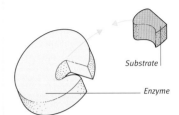

Substrate

Enzyme

1 The shape of an enzyme determines its activity. Each enzyme molecule will combine only with a particular substrate that has molecules of a complementary shape.

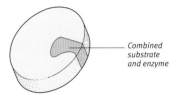

Combined substrate and enzyme

2 When the enzyme and substrate combine, their interaction causes a chemical change within the substrate. In the example shown here, the chemical is split into two products.

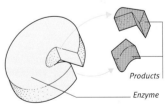

Products

Enzyme

3 After the chemical reaction has ended, the enzyme molecule remains unchanged and can move on to combine with another substrate molecule and repeat the process.

eosinophil

A type of leukocyte (*white blood cell*) that plays a role in allergic responses (see *allergy*) and fighting parasitic infections.

ependymoma

A rare *brain tumour* of the *glioma* type (arising from supporting glial cells in the *nervous system*) that occurs most commonly in children.

ephedrine

A drug that mimics the effects of the neurotransmitter *noradrenaline* (norepinephrine). Ephedrine is prescribed as a *decongestant drug* to treat nasal congestion. It may also be used to treat some cases of low blood pressure that are due to drug actions or disease, and, rarely, to treat asthma.

epicanthic fold

A vertical fold of skin extending from the upper eyelid to the side of the nose. Epicanthic folds are common in East Asian people but rare in other races, except in babies, in whom they usually disappear as the nose develops. Abnormal epicanthic folds are a feature of *Down's syndrome*. In some cases, the folds can be removed by cosmetic surgery.

epicardium

The outermost of the three layers that form the wall of the *heart*. The epicardium is a smooth membranous structure that envelops the *myocardium* (the muscle layer of the heart).

epicondyle

Any bony outgrowth to which *tendons* are attached (for example, at the lower end of the *humerus* where it forms part of the *elbow* joint). Overuse of muscles, leading to repeated tugging on the tendons, can result in pain and inflammation at an epicondyle (see *epicondylitis*).

epicondylitis

Painful inflammation of an *epicondyle*, and specifically one of the bony prominences of the *elbow* at the lower end of the *humerus*. Epicondylitis is the result of overuse of the forearm muscles, which causes repeated tugging on the tendons at their point of attachment to the bone.

Epicondylitis that affects the prominence on the outer elbow is called *tennis elbow*. When the prominence on the inner elbow is affected the condition is called *golfer's elbow*.

epidemic

A term applied to a disease that for the majority of the time is rare in a community but that suddenly spreads rapidly to affect a large number of people. A widespread epidemic is known as a *pandemic*.

Epidemics of new strains of *influenza* are common, occurring periodically when the influenza virus changes to a form to which the population has no resistance. (See also *endemic*.)

epidemiology

The branch of medicine concerned with the occurrence and distribution of disease, including *infectious diseases* (such as influenza) and noninfectious diseases (such as cancer and heart disease).

In epidemiological studies, the members of a population are counted and described in terms of such variables as race, sex, age, social class, and occupation. The *incidence* and *prevalence* of the disease of interest are then determined. These observations may be repeated at regular intervals in order to detect changes over time. The result is a statistical record that may reveal links between particular variables and distribution of disease.

In comparative epidemiological studies, two or more groups are chosen. For example, in a study of the link between smoking and lung cancer, one group may consist of smokers and the other of nonsmokers; the proportion with cancer in each group is calculated. In such cases, the epidemiologist is careful to make the two groups as identical as possible in all other relevant respects, and will match factors such as age and sex.

epidermis

The thin outermost layer of the *skin*.

epidermoid cyst

A harmless nodule under the skin's surface that contains yellow, cheesy material. The terms epidermoid cyst and *sebaceous cyst* are often used interchangeably.

epidermolysis bullosa

A group of rare, inherited conditions, varying widely in severity, in which blisters appear on the skin after minor injury or occur spontaneously.

CAUSES

Epidermolysis bullosa is caused by a genetic defect that may show either an autosomal dominant or an autosomal recessive pattern of inheritance (see *genetic disorders*).

DIAGNOSIS AND TREATMENT

The conditions can be diagnosed by a skin *biopsy* (removal of a small sample of tissue for microscopic analysis).

There is no specific treatment for the condition, but injury to the skin should be avoided and protective measures should be taken to prevent the rubbing of affected areas when blisters appear.

The outlook varies from gradual improvement in mild cases to progressive disease in the most severe cases.

epididymal cyst

A harmless, usually painless, swelling in the *epididymis* (the coiled tube that runs along the back of the testis). Small cysts are fairly common in men over the age of 40 and need no treatment. Rarely, the cysts may enlarge or become tender, causing discomfort. In such cases, it may be necessary for the cysts to be surgically removed.

epididymis

A long, coiled tube that runs along the back of the *testis* and connects the vasa efferentia (small tubes leading from the testis) to the *vas deferens* (the sperm duct that leads to the urethra). Sperm cells, which are produced in the testis, mature as they pass slowly along the epididymis, until they are capable of fertilizing an egg, and they are then stored until *ejaculation* takes place.

Disorders of the epididymis include *epididymal cysts* (fluid-filled swellings in the epididymis) and *epididymo-orchitis* (inflammation of the testis and epididymis). Infection or injury can block the epididymis; if both testes are affected, *infertility* may result.

epididymitis

See *epididymo-orchitis*.

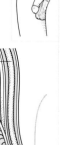

LOCATION OF THE **EPIDIDYMIS**

The epididymis runs along the back of the testis and links the vasa efferentia to the vas deferens.

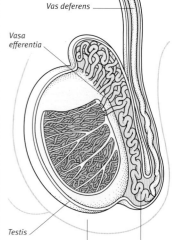

Vas deferens

Vasa efferentia

Testis

Scrotum

Epididymis

epididymo-orchitis

Acute inflammation of a *testis* and *epididymis* (coiled tube that runs along the back of the testis). Epididymo-orchitis causes acute pain and swelling at the back of the testis, and, in severe cases, swelling and redness of the *scrotum*.

The inflammation is caused by infection. Often, there is no obvious source of the infection, but sometimes the cause is a bacterial *urinary tract infection* (due to E.COLI or chlamydia, for example) that has spread via the *vas deferens* (the sperm duct leading to the urethra) to the epididymis.

Treatment is with *antibiotic drugs*. If there is an underlying urinary tract infection, its cause needs to be investigated. (See also *orchitis*.)

epidural anaesthesia

A method of administering pain relief in which a local anaesthetic (see *anaesthesia, local*) is injected into the epidural space (the space around the membranes that surround the spinal cord) in the middle and lower back. Epidural anaesthesia numbs the nerves that supply the chest (when injected into the middle back) and lower body. (when injected into the lower back) It is widely used to relieve pain during and after surgery, as well as during *childbirth*.

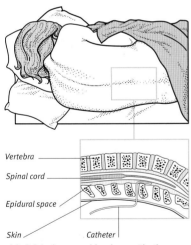

Administering an epidural anaesthetic
The anaesthetic is injected into the epidural space (the region surrounding the spinal cord within the spinal canal).

Vertebra
Spinal cord
Epidural space
Skin
Catheter

epidural space

The space between the outer membrane of the *spinal cord* and the walls of the vertebral canal that surround it. (See also *epidural anaesthesia*.)

epigastric hernia

A *hernia* (protrusion of an organ or tissue) through a weakened area in the upper central abdominal wall. The hernia may appear as a lump in the centre of the upper abdomen, between the base of the sternum (breastbone) and the navel. (See also *hernia repair*.)

epiglottis

The flap of *cartilage* lying behind the tongue and in front of the entrance to the *larynx* (voicebox). The epiglottis is usually upright to allow air to pass through the larynx and into the rest of the respiratory system. During swallowing, it tilts downwards to cover the entrance to the larynx, preventing food and drink from being inhaled into the trachea (windpipe).

epiglottitis

A potentially life-threatening infection causing inflammation and swelling of the *epiglottis* (the flap of cartilage at the back of the tongue that closes off the windpipe during swallowing). The swollen epiglottis obstructs breathing and can cause death by suffocation if the condition is not treated promptly.

Epiglottitis is now rare due to the routine *immunization* of infants with the *Hib vaccine* against HAEMOPHILUS INFLUENZAE, the causative bacterium.

epilepsy

A tendency to have recurrent *seizures*. Seizures are defined as transient neurological abnormalities that are caused by abnormal electrical activity in the brain. Human activities, thoughts, and emotions are normally the result of the regulated and orderly electrical excitation of nerve cells in the brain. During a seizure, a chaotic and unregulated electrical discharge causes various physical and mental symptoms.

CAUSES

In many people with epilepsy, the cause is unclear, although a genetic factor may be involved. In other cases, seizures may be the result of brain damage from a head injury; birth trauma; brain infection (such as *meningitis* or *encephalitis*); *brain tumour*; *stroke* (damage to part of the brain caused by an interruption to its blood supply); drug or alcohol intoxication; or a *metabolic disorder*.

SYMPTOMS

Many people who suffer from epilepsy do not have any symptoms between seizures. Some people experience an *aura* (a peculiar "warning" sensation) shortly beforehand. In some cases, a seizure may be triggered by flashing lights, stress, or lack of sleep. Epileptic seizures may occur more frequently during times of illness.

TYPES

Epileptic seizures can be classified into two broad groups: generalized and partial seizures.

Generalized seizures These seizures cause loss of consciousness and may affect all areas of the brain. There are two main types of generalized seizure: tonic–clonic (formerly grand mal) and absence (petit mal) seizures.

During a tonic–clonic seizure, there may initially be an aura, then the body becomes stiff and consciousness is lost. Breathing may be irregular or may stop briefly, then the body jerks uncontrollably. The episode usually ends spontaneously after a few minutes. The person may be drowsy and disorientated for a few hours afterwards, however, and may have no memory of the event. Prolonged tonic–clonic seizures are potentially life-threatening.

Absence seizures occur mainly in children. Periods of altered consciousness last for only a few seconds and there are no abnormal movements of the body. This type of seizure may occur hundreds of times daily.

Partial seizures These seizures are caused by abnormal electrical activity in a more limited area of the brain. They may be simple or complex.

In simple partial seizures, consciousness is not lost and an abnormal twitching movement, tingling sensation, or *hallucination* of smell, vision, or taste occurs, lasting several minutes.

In one type of partial seizure, called *temporal lobe epilepsy*, conscious contact with the surroundings is lost. The sufferer becomes dazed and may behave oddly. Typically, the person remembers little, if anything, of the event.

DIAGNOSIS

In order to make a diagnosis, a doctor needs as much information as possible about the seizures. The patient may not be able to recall the events, so an accurate account from a witness may be necessary. Examination of the nervous system is normally carried out between seizures. An *EEG* (a method of recording the activity of the brain), *CT scanning* or *MRI* of the brain, and blood tests may also be carried out.

E

TREATMENT

While a seizure is happening, any witnesses should make the surrounding area safe (for example, by removing hazardous objects) and ensure that the person can breathe while unconscious. Clothing around the neck should be loosened, and a soft item, such as a folded piece of clothing, should be placed under the head. Otherwise, witnesses should simply let the attack run its course. Once the convulsions have stopped, the person should be placed in the *recovery position*. A person having a seizure should never be restrained, and should never have anything put into his or her mouth.

Anticonvulsant drugs usually stop or reduce the frequency of recurrent seizures. The drugs may have unpleasant side effects, however, so the doctor will take care to find the drug that works best for that patient. With severe epilepsy, a combination of drugs may be needed to control seizures. If no seizures occur after two or three years of treatment, and depending on their cause, the doctor may suggest reducing or stopping the drug treatment.

Women who are taking anticonvulsant drugs and are planning a pregnancy will need to have their treatment reviewed before conceiving. They may need to change to another drug to reduce the risk of a fetal abnormality. Stopping treatment is not usually an option because seizures can be profoundly damaging to the fetus.

Surgery may be considered if a single area of damage to the brain is causing the seizures and drug treatment has not proved effective.

OUTLOOK

Epilepsy that develops during childhood may sometimes disappear soon after adolescence.

Affected adults can enjoy relatively normal lives, but may be restricted in their choice of work. For example, it is inadvisable for people with epilepsy to have occupations involving heights or operating dangerous machinery. In addition, there are certain restrictions on driving vehicles (see *driving, health and*). People with epilepsy are legally required to contact their vehicle licensing agency, who will explain the relevant restrictions.

Many people with epilepsy carry a special card, tag, or bracelet, such as those produced by *Medic-Alert*, which states that they have the condition.

Affected people should also advise their family, friends, and colleagues what to do if a seizure occurs.

epiloia

See *tuberous sclerosis*.

epinephrine

An alternative name for *adrenaline*.

EpiPen

A brand name for an assembled needle and syringe containing a dose of *adrenaline* (epinephrine) that is used for rapid administration to prevent or treat life-threatening allergic reactions (see *anaphylactic shock*). The EpiPen is designed for people who are prone to such reactions to use on themselves; it delivers the adrenaline directly into a muscle, usually a thigh muscle.

Anyone known to be at risk of an anaphylactic reaction should carry an EpiPen with them at all times and be taught how to administer it. An affected person's family, as well as other close contacts, such as teachers, colleagues, and friends, should also be aware of how to use the EpiPen.

epiphora

See *watering eye*.

epiphyseal fracture

A fracture (break) at the point where the epiphysis (the end section of a long bone) meets the diaphysis (the main shaft of the bone). This type of break may affect the subsequent growth of the fractured bone.

epiphyseal plate

The disc that separates the *epiphysis* (the end section of a long bone) from the *diaphysis* (the main shaft of the bone). During the period of growth, the epiphyseal plate is composed of *cartilage* (connective tissue formed of collagen). This cartilage is gradually replaced by bone as a result of *ossification*, a process by which cartilage cells multiply and absorb *calcium* to develop into bone.

epiphysis

The end section of a long bone (such as the femur in the legs, or the humerus in the arms) that is separated from the diaphysis (the main shaft of the bone) by the *epiphyseal plate*.

Problems that affect the epiphysis or the epiphyseal plate during the period of growth, such as inflammation (a

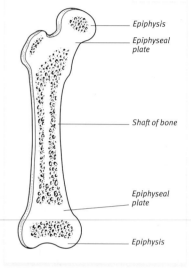

LOCATION OF **EPIPHYSES**

Each epiphysis is situated at an end of a long bone of the body and is separated from the shaft of the bone by an area called the epiphyseal plate.

Epiphysis
Epiphyseal plate

Shaft of bone

Epiphyseal plate

Epiphysis

condition called epiphysitis), may retard the growth of the affected bone and cause it to become deformed.

epiphysis, slipped

See *femoral epiphysis, slipped*.

episcleritis

A localized patch of inflammation that affects the outermost layers of the *sclera* (the white of the eye) in an area immediately underneath the *conjunctiva* (the transparent membrane that covers the sclera). Episcleritis mainly affects middle-aged men and is usually of unknown cause, although in some cases it may occur as a complication of *rheumatoid arthritis, herpes zoster,* or *gout*. The inflammation may cause a dull, aching pain and there may be *photophobia* (abnormal sensitivity of the eyes to light).

The disorder usually disappears by itself within a week or so, but it may recur. Symptoms may be relieved by using *eye-drops* or ointment containing a *corticosteroid drug*.

episiotomy

A surgical procedure in which an incision is made in the *perineum* (the tissue between the vagina and the anus) in order to facilitate the delivery of a baby. After delivery, the severed tissues are stitched back together.

WHY IT IS DONE

An episiotomy is advisable if the perineum fails to stretch over the baby's head and/or a large perineal tear is likely. The procedure prevents ragged tears that would be more painful, more difficult to repair, and more likely to lead to complications. Episiotomy is usually necessary in a *forceps delivery*, because the instruments occupy additional space in the vagina, and in a *breech delivery*, in which there is little opportunity for gradual stretching of the perineal tissues.

In many cases, however, the naturally elastic vagina should not have to be cut to allow a normal delivery.

epispadias

A rare congenital (present from birth) abnormality in which the opening of the *urethra* (the tube through which urine is excreted from the bladder) is not in the glans (head) of the *penis* but is on its upper surface. In some cases, the penis also curves upwards. Surgery is carried out during infancy, using tissue from the *foreskin* to reconstruct the urethra. (See also *hypospadias*.)

epistaxis

A medical term for *nosebleed*.

epithelioma

A noncancerous tumour arising from the *epithelium*, the tissue that covers the outer surface of the body and forms the membranous lining of internal organs). In some cases, an epithelioma may become cancerous, in which case it is known as a *carcinoma*.

epithelium

The layer of *cells* that covers the entire surface of the body and lines most of the structures within it. Epithelial cells vary in shape according to their function. There are three basic shapes: squamous (thin and flat), cuboidal, and columnar. These structures may vary further. For example, in the respiratory tract, epithelial cells bear brushlike filaments called cilia that create a current in the surrounding fluid. This current propels dust particles from inhaled air back up the bronchi (the large air passages in the lungs) and the trachea (windpipe).

Most internal organs lined with epithelium are covered with only a single layer of cells, but the skin, which is subjected to more trauma, consists of many layers including a dead outer layer of cells that is constantly being shed. Structures that are not lined with epithelium are the blood vessels, the lymph vessels (see *lymphatic system*), and the inside of the heart, which are lined with *endothelium*, and the chest and abdominal cavities, which are lined with *mesothelium*.

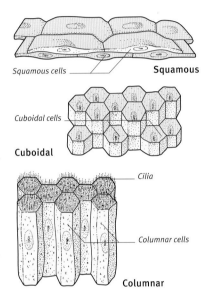

Types of epithelium
The cells of the epithelium vary in shape and size according to function. The three basic types are squamous, cuboidal, and columnar.

epoetin

A genetically engineered preparation of the *hormone* erythropoietin, which is produced by specialized cells in the kidneys and stimulates the *bone marrow* to produce *red blood cells*.

Epoetin may be used in the treatment of *anaemia* (reduced level of the oxygen-carrying molecule haemoglobin in the blood) in specific groups of patients: those with *kidney failure*, including people on *dialysis*; those receiving chemotherapy for cancer; and those with some types of *leukaemia* or certain other cancers. It may also be used to boost the level of red blood cells before surgery and sometimes as an alternative to blood transfusions in major orthopaedic (bone) surgery.

Epstein–Barr virus

A *virus* that belongs to the herpesvirus family. The Epstein–Barr virus (EBV) may cause glandular fever (see *mononucleosis, infectious*); after the initial infection, the virus remains dormant in the cells of the immune system and may later be reactivated. Epstein–Barr virus is one of the few viruses with a proven role in the development of cancerous tumours. In Africa, it is associated with *Burkitt's lymphoma*, and in Southeast Asia it is associated with cancer of the nasopharynx (see *nasopharynx, cancer of*). Epstein–Barr virus may also cause lymphomas to develop in patients who have undergone transplant surgery.

Other disorders that are associated with Epstein–Barr virus include some cases of acute *hepatitis*. In people with AIDS, the virus may lead to the development of a condition called oral hairy *leukoplakia*; this condition is characterized by roughened, white patches on the sides of the tongue.

Erb's palsy

Weakness or paralysis of the muscles in the upper arm and shoulder. Erb's palsy results from damage to the upper roots of the *brachial plexus* (a collection of nerve trunks formed from nerve roots near the top of the spine). Such an injury may occur during birth if excess pressure is applied to the baby's head during a difficult delivery, causing the fifth cervical root of the spinal cord to be damaged. It may also result from a road traffic accident, particularly in motorcycle riders, when an impact forces the head and neck to one side and severely strains the nerves on the opposite side. Erb's palsy is characterized by an arm that is rotated inwards at the shoulder and hangs limp down one side of the body.

ERCP

The abbreviation for endoscopic retrograde cholangiopancreatography, which is an *X-ray* procedure used for examining the *biliary system* and the pancreatic duct. ERCP is used mainly when other imaging techniques, such as *ultrasound scanning*, *CT scanning*, or *MRI*, fail to provide sufficiently detailed images.

HOW IT IS DONE

An *endoscope* (a flexible viewing tube with a lens and a light attached) is passed down the oesophagus, through the stomach, and into the *duodenum* (the upper part of the small intestine). A *catheter* (a fine, flexible tube) is passed through the endoscope into the common bile duct and pancreatic duct. Finally, a *contrast medium* (a substance opaque to X-rays) is introduced through the catheter to make

E

the pancreatic duct and the biliary system visible on X-rays. If disorder is detected during the procedure, it can sometimes be treated at the same time. For example, it may be possible to relieve a blockage due to a gallstone.

erectile dysfunction

The inability to achieve or maintain an erection, also sometimes known as impotence. Erectile dysfunction may be caused by psychological factors, including concerns about performance or relationship difficulties, or by physical disorders, such as *atherosclerosis*, *diabetes mellitus*, and neurological disorders including *multiple sclerosis* and damage to the spinal cord. Some drugs cause erectile dysfunction as a side effect but this reverses when the drugs are stopped. Erectile dysfunction also tends to be more common wth increasing age.

TREATMENT
Treatment depends on the cause but may include *counselling* or *sex therapy* for psychological problems. Drugs such as *sildenafil* or *tadalafil* may be used to treat both organic and psychological erectile dysfunction. Other treatments include the drug alprostadil, self-administered either by injection into the penis or as a gel applied to the urethra, or a surgical implant, which can produce a sustained erection.

erection

The hardness, swelling, and elevation of the *penis* that occurs in response to sexual arousal or physical stimulation. The erectile tissue of the penis becomes engorged with blood as the blood vessels within it dilate. Muscles around the vessels then contract and keep blood in the penis, thereby maintaining the erection.

erection, disorders of

Conditions in which the *erection* of the penis is disrupted. Such conditions include the inability to achieve or maintain an erection (see *erectile dysfunction*), persistent erection in the absence of sexual desire (see *priapism*), and curving of the penis during erection (see *chordee*).

ergocalciferol

An alternative name for vitamin D$_2$ (see *vitamin D*).

ergometer

A machine that measures and records the amount of physical work undertaken by the body and the body's response to a controlled amount of exercise. An ergometer makes continuous recordings, both during and after activity, of heart rate and rhythm (using an *ECG*); *blood pressure*; rate of breathing; and volume of oxygen taken in from the air.

ergometrine

A drug given after *childbirth*, *miscarriage*, or *abortion* to reduce the loss of blood from the *uterus* (womb). Ergometrine works by causing blood vessels in the uterine wall to contract, thereby reducing bleeding. The drug is often given in combination with *oxytocin*, which stimulates uterine contractions.

ergot

A product of CLAVICEPS PURPUREA, a *fungus* that grows on rye and various other cereals. Ergot contains poisonous *alkaloids* (nitrogen-containing substances), some of which have medicinal properties when taken in controlled doses. The drugs *ergotamine* and *ergometrine* are produced from ergot.

ergotamine

A drug used to treat *migraine* and sometimes also *cluster headaches*. It works by constricting the dilated blood vessels around the brain. Side effects of the drug include nausea, vomiting, muscle cramps, and abdominal pain. Ergotamine is now used infrequently, however, having been largely replaced by drugs such as *sumatriptan*.

erosion

The destruction and loss of surface tissue through physical or chemical processes (see *cervical erosion*; *erosion, dental*; *gastric erosion*).

erosion, dental

Loss of enamel from the surface of a tooth (see *teeth*) due to attack by *plaque* acids or other chemicals. The first sign of enamel loss is a dull, frosted appearance. As the condition progresses, smooth, shiny, shallow cavities form.

Erosion of the outer surfaces of the front teeth is most frequently caused by excessive intake of acidic fruit juices and carbonated drinks. Erosion of the inner surfaces of the molars may be a result of regurgitation of stomach acid, as occurs in people suffering from *gastro-oesophageal reflux disease* or *bulimia*. Erosion may be combined with, and may also accelerate, the processes of abrasion (mechanical wearing away of

teeth) and attrition (wearing down of the chewing surfaces). These problems may result in extensive damage to the teeth. (See also *caries, dental*.)

eruption

The process of breaking out, as of a skin rash or a new tooth. (See also *eruption of teeth*; *eruptive phase*.)

eruption of teeth

The process by which developing *teeth* grow from the jawbone, breaking through the *gum* to project into the mouth.

DECIDUOUS TEETH
Primary teeth (also known as deciduous or milk teeth) usually begin to appear at about six months of age. All 20 primary teeth have usually erupted by three years (see *teething*).

PERMANENT TEETH
Permanent teeth (which are also known as secondary teeth) usually begin to appear at about six years of age. The first permanent molars erupt towards the back of the mouth and appear in addition to the primary teeth. The eruption of permanent teeth nearer the front of the mouth is preceded by reabsorption of the roots of the primary teeth, which causes the teeth to become loose so that they fall out. Eventually, permanent teeth replace all of the primary teeth.

Wisdom teeth (the third molars) usually erupt between the ages of about 18 and 25. In some people, however, they never appear; in others, the wisdom teeth are impacted (blocked from erupting) because of insufficient space in the jawbone (see *impaction, dental*).

eruptive phase

The phase in the course of a condition such as *chickenpox* in which skin lesions, for example spots or blisters, break out.

erysipelas

A disorder, caused by a *streptococcal infection*, that produces inflammation and blistering of the face and is associated with a high fever and *malaise*. Erysipelas most often affects young children and elderly people. Treatment is with *penicillin drugs*. (See also *cellulitis*.)

erythema

A term meaning redness of the skin. Erythema can have many causes, such as *blushing*, *hot flushes*, *sunburn*, and inflammatory, infective, or allergic skin disorders such as *acne*, *dermatitis*, *eczema*, *erysipelas*, *rosacea*, and *urticaria*. Disorders

ERUPTION OF TEETH

The top diagrams show the approximate ages at which particular primary teeth usually appear. The ages at which specific types of permanent teeth usually appear are shown in the lower diagrams. Blue denotes erupting teeth; grey denotes erupted primary teeth; white denotes erupted permanent teeth.

 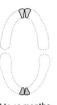 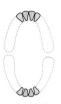 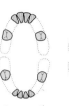 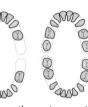

Primary teeth
The full primary set (left) consists of eight incisors, four canines, and eight molars. They usually start erupting at six months.

| 6 to 10 months: lower central incisors | 8 to 12 months: upper central incisors | 9 to 16 months: lateral incisors | 13 to 19 months: first molars | 16 to 23 months: canines | 23 to 33 months: second molars |

Permanent teeth
The full set of permanent teeth (below) consists of eight incisors, four canines, eight premolars, and twelve molars. They usually start erupting at six years.

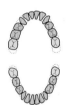 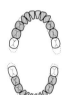 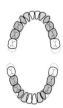 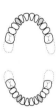 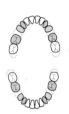 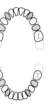 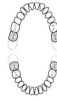 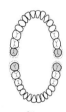

| 6 to 7 years: first molars | 6 to 8 years: central incisors | 7 to 9 years: lateral incisors | 9 to 12 years: canines | 10 to 12 years: first premolars | 10 to 12 years: second premolars | 11 to 13 years: second molars | 18 to 25: third molars |

in which redness of the skin is a feature include *erythema multiforme*, *erythema nodosum*, *erythema ab igne*, *lupus erythematosus*, and erythema infectiosum (also known as *fifth disease*).

erythema ab igne

Red, mottled skin that may also be dry and itchy. Erythema ab igne is caused by exposure to strong direct heat, such as when an individual has been sitting too close to a fire. The condition is most common in elderly women.

Dryness and itching can often be relieved by use of an *emollient* (soothing cream). The redness fades in time but may not disappear entirely.

erythema infectiosum

See *fifth disease*.

erythema marginatum

A pink rash that appears and disappears spontaneously and that may affect any area of the body except the face. Erythema marginatum is a characteristic sign of *rheumatic fever*.

erythema migrans

A red, circular rash that occurs as a result of infection with *Lyme disease*, a tick-borne bacterial disease. Erythema migrans first appears at the site of a bite from an infected tick. The rash then expands, over a period of days or weeks, to form a large, round patch. Erythema migrans is most commonly found on the thighs, groin, or trunk, or in the armpit.

erythema multiforme

Acute *inflammation* of the skin, and sometimes of the *mucous membranes* (the thin, moist tissue that lines body cavities), that is sometimes accompanied by generalized illness. Erythema multiforme means "skin redness of many varieties".

CAUSES

Erythema multiforme can develop as an adverse reaction to certain drugs, such as *aspirin* and *sulphonamides*, or it may

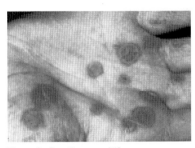

The rash of erythema multiforme
The spots of this rash are usually itchy. They may form into target lesions (concentric rings of different shades of red around a pale centre).

accompany certain viral infections (for example, *herpes simplex*) or bacterial infections (such as *streptococcal infections*). Other possible causes of erythema multiforme are pregnancy, *vaccination*, and *radiotherapy*. However, about half of all cases occur for no apparent reason.

SYMPTOMS

A symmetrical rash of red, frequently itchy, spots erupts on the skin of the limbs and, occasionally, on the face and the rest of the body. The spots may blister or form raised, pale-centred weals known as target lesions. People suffering from erythema multiforme may have a fever, sore throat, headache, and/or diarrhoea.

In a more severe form of erythema multiforme, known as *Stevens–Johnson syndrome*, the mucous membranes of the mouth, eyes, and genitals are all affected and become ulcerated.

TREATMENT

Treatment for erythema multiforme depends on the underlying cause. Any causative drug treatment will be withdrawn and any underlying condition will be treated if possible. *Corticosteroid drugs* may be given to reduce the inflammation. People suffering from Stevens–Johnson syndrome are also given *analgesic drugs* (painkillers) and may need intensive care.

erythema nodosum

A condition characterized by reddish-purple, tender swellings on the legs. Erythema nodosum is usually associated with another illness.

CAUSES

The most common cause of erythema nodosum is a *streptococcal infection* of the throat. However, the condition is also associated with other diseases, mainly *tuberculosis* and *sarcoidosis*, and may occur as a reaction to drugs, including *oral contraceptives*, *aspirin*, and *sulphonamide drugs*. Sometimes there is no apparent cause.

SYMPTOMS

The swellings, which may range from about 1 to 10 cm in diameter, are shiny and tender and occur on the fronts of the shins, the thighs, and, less commonly, the arms. Joint and muscle pains and fever also usually occur.

TREATMENT

Successful treatment of any underlying condition clears the swellings. Bed rest, *analgesic drugs* (painkillers), and, occasionally, *corticosteroid drugs* may also be necessary. The condition usually subsides within about a month.

erythematous

Characterized by *erythema* (redness of the skin).

erythrasma

A bacterial skin infection, caused by the organism CORYNEBACTERIUM, that affects the groin, armpits, and skin between the toes. Raised, irregularly shaped, discoloured patches appear in the affected areas. Erythrasma is most common in people who have *diabetes mellitus*. The condition generally clears up following a course of treatment with the antibiotic drug *erythromycin*.

erythrocyte

Another name for a *red blood cell*.

erythroderma

See *exfoliative dermatitis*.

erythrogenic toxin

A poisonous protein produced by streptococcal bacteria that causes the red rash in *scarlet fever*.

erythromelalgia

A rare condition, also known as Gerhardt–Mitchell disease, that principally affects the extremities of the body, most commonly the feet. It usually first appears in middle age, and may be associated with *polycythaemia* (an increase in the total red cell mass of the blood), *thrombocytosis* (an increase in the number of *platelets* in the blood), *gout* (a metabolic disorder that causes attacks of arthritis), and neurological disease.

Erythromelalgia is characterized by severe attacks of burning pain and mottled redness of the skin; it may be triggered by heat. Attacks of the condition can be relieved by elevating the affected limb and applying something cold, such as an ice-pack, to it. No specific treatment is available, but *aspirin* may relieve the condition in some cases.

erythromelia

Diffuse *erythema* (redness) and *atrophy* (wasting) of the skin of the lower limbs. The cause of erythromelia is unknown.

erythromycin

An *antibiotic drug* used in the treatment of skin, chest, throat, and ear infections. It may also be used in the treatment of *pertussis* (whooping cough), *legionnaires' disease*, some *chlamydial infections*, and some forms of *gastroenteritis*. Erythromycin is particularly useful as an alternative treatment for people who are allergic to *penicillin drugs*. Possible adverse effects include nausea, diarrhoea, and an itchy rash.

Erythrovirus

A genus of viruses that includes parvovirus, which causes *fifth disease* in humans.

escape beat

An automatic *heartbeat* that occurs after an abnormally long pause in the heart rhythm. An escape beat is therefore a delayed beat that terminates a longer cycle than normal.

eschar

A *scab* that forms on the surface of skin that has been subject to damage, for example by a *burn*.

Escherichia coli (E.coli)

A bacterium (see *bacteria*) that is normally found in the intestines but can cause illness under some circumstances.

Types of E.COLI are often the cause of traveller's diarrhoea, which is usually a mild illness, but some strains of the bacterium (such as strain 0157) can cause serious food-borne infections that result in *gastroenteritis* and *haemolytic–uraemic syndrome* (a condition in which red blood cells are destroyed and kidney funcion becomes impaired). Attention to good food hygiene and handwashing can help prevent the spread of food-borne E.COLI infections.

Esmarch's bandage

A broad rubber bandage that is wrapped around the elevated limb of a patient to force blood out of the blood vessels towards the heart. This action creates a blood-free area, so surgery on the limb can be performed more easily.

The patient is anaesthetized (see *anaesthesia*), then the Esmarch's bandage is wrapped from the fingers or toes upwards. An inflatable tourniquet (a device used to compress blood vessels) is then applied to the upper arm or thigh to stop blood from returning to the limb. The Esmarch's bandage is removed, leaving the inflated tourniquet in position during surgery.

esotropia

An alternative term for a convergent *squint*, in which one eye looks directly at an object while the other eye turns inwards. (See also *exotropia*.)

ESR

The abbreviation for erythrocyte sedimentation rate, which is the rate at which erythrocytes (*red blood cells*) sink to the bottom of a test tube.

WHY IT IS DONE

The ESR is increased if the level of *fibrinogen* (a type of protein) in the blood is raised. Fibrinogen is raised in response to a range of illnesses, including *inflammation*, especially when this is caused by infection or by an *autoimmune disease*. The ESR is also increased if levels of *antibodies* (proteins manufactured by the immune system) are very high, as occurs in *multiple myeloma*. ESR is therefore useful for helping to diagnose these conditions as well as in monitoring their treatment.

HOW IT IS DONE

Whole blood collected from the patient is mixed with anticoagulant (a chemical that prevents the blood from clotting) in a test tube. In one method, the blood is left undisturbed at a constant temperature for one hour. The red blood cells, which can be seen as a dark red clump, settle to the bottom of the test tube, leaving the clear, straw-coloured plasma at the top. The ESR is the number of millimetres the red blood cells fall in one hour.

essential amino acids

The eight *amino acids* required for protein synthesis, growth, and development, that cannot be made by the body and must be obtained in the diet.

essential fatty acids

The *fatty acids* that cannot be synthesized by the body and must therefore be obtained in the diet.

essential food factors

Any substances that are essential for normal functioning of the body but cannot be synthesized by the body itself so must be obtained through the diet. Examples of essential food factors are most *vitamins* and *minerals*, *essential amino acids*, and *essential fatty acids*.

essential hypertension

Hypertension (high blood pressure) that occurs without known cause.

estradiol

The most important *oestrogen hormone*, essential for the healthy functioning of the female reproductive system and for breast development. Synthetic estradiol is used to treat the symptoms and complications of the menopause (see *hormone replacement therapy*) and to stimulate sexual development in female *hypogonadism* (underactivity of the ovaries).

estriol

One of the *oestrogen hormones*. Estriol is the predominant oestrogen produced during pregnancy. Synthetic estriol is prescribed to treat the symptoms and complications of the menopause (see *hormone replacement therapy*) as well as to stimulate sexual development in female *hypogonadism* (underactivity of the ovaries).

estrone

An *oestrogen hormone*. Synthetic estrone is used to treat the symptoms and complications of the menopause (see *hormone replacement therapy*).

ESWL

The abbreviation for extracorporeal shock wave *lithotripsy*.

ethambutol

A drug used in conjunction with other drugs to treat *tuberculosis*. Ethambutol rarely causes side effects, but it may sometimes result in inflammation of the *optic nerve*, leading to blurred vision.

ethanol

The chemical name for the *alcohol* that is present in alcoholic drinks.

ether

A colourless liquid that produces unconsciousness when inhaled. Ether was the first general anaesthetic (see *anaesthesia, general*) to be introduced.

ethics, medical

See *medical ethics*.

ethinylestradiol

A synthetic form of the female sex hormone *estradiol*. Ethinylestradiol is most often used in *oral contraceptives*, in which it is combined with a *progestogen drug*. Rarely, it is used in *hormone replacement therapy*.

ethmoidal sinus

One of the air-containing spaces in the *ethmoid bone* behind the nose (see *sinus, facial*).

ethmoid bone

A *bone* that forms part of the floor of the cranium (skull) and contributes to the roof of the nasal cavity and to the orbits (eye sockets). The *olfactory nerves*, which are responsible for smell, pass through holes in part of the ethmoid bone called the cribriform plate.

ethosuximide

An *anticonvulsant drug* used in the treatment of absence (petit mal) seizures (see *epilepsy*). Ethosuximide may cause nausea and vomiting and, in rare cases, affects the production of blood cells in bone marrow (see *anaemia, aplastic*).

ethyl alcohol

Another name for ethanol, the *alcohol* in alcoholic drinks.

ethyl chloride

A colourless liquid that is applied to the skin as a spray to numb an area before minor surgical procedures or to relieve muscle pain.

etidronate, disodium

A *bisphosphonate drug* that is used to treat bone disorders (see *bone, disorders of*), such as *Paget's disease* and *osteoporosis*. Disodium etidronate works by reducing the activity of bone cells, thereby halting the progress of the disease. Side effects of the drug are generally mild.

etretinate

A *retinoid* drug, chemically related to *vitamin A*, that is used mainly in the treatment of severe *psoriasis* (a skin disease characterized by thickened patches of red, inflamed skin). Also known as acitretin, etretinate is also occasionally used in the treatment of other disorders that cause excessive skin thickening, such as *ichthyosis*. It reduces the production of keratin, the protein that forms the hard, outer layers of the skin.

Etretinate can cause liver damage and a rise in blood fats. The drug must not be taken during pregnancy because it can cause damage to the fetus.

eucalyptus oil

A substance distilled from the leaves of eucalyptus trees. Because of its aromatic smell and refreshing taste, it is used as a flavouring. It is also used in cough and cold remedies, when it may be applied as a rub, inhaled as vapour, or incorporated in tablets. There is little evidence that it has any curative properties, although it may relieve symptoms.

eugenics

The science based on improving the human race and the quality of human life through the principles of *genetics*. Modern eugenics is primarily concerned with the study (and, where possible, elimination) of *genetic disorders*.

eunuch

A man whose testes have been removed or destroyed so that he is sterile and lacks male hormones. A male castrated before *puberty* will have broad hips, narrow shoulders, and undeveloped male secondary *sexual characteristics* (such as a small penis, a feminine distribution of body hair, and a high-pitched voice).

euphoria

A state of confident wellbeing. It is a normal reaction to personal success but can also be induced by certain drugs, including prolonged use of *corticosteroid drugs*. Euphoria with no rational cause may be a sign of *mania*, damage from *head injury*, *dementia*, *brain tumours*, or *multiple sclerosis*.

eustachian tube

The passage that runs from the middle *ear* into the back of the nose, just above the soft *palate* (part of the roof of the mouth). The eustachian tube is lined with a smooth, moist, mucous membrane.

E

FUNCTION

The eustachian tube acts as a drainage channel from the middle ear and maintains hearing by opening periodically to regulate air pressure. The lower end of the tube opens during swallowing and yawning, allowing air to flow up to the middle ear, equalizing the air pressure on both sides of the *eardrum*.

DISORDERS

When a viral infection, such as a cold, causes blockage of the eustachian tube, equalization cannot occur, resulting in severe pain and temporary impairment of hearing. A person with a blocked eustachian tube who is subjected to rapid pressure changes may suffer from *barotrauma* (pressure damage to the eardrum and other structures). *Glue ear* (accumulation of secretions in the middle ear) or chronic *otitis media* (middle-ear infection) may occur if the tube is blocked, preventing adequate drainage from the middle ear.

These conditions, which often result in partial hearing loss, are much more common in children. This is because their *adenoids* are larger and more likely to cause a blockage if they become infected and because their eustachian tubes are shorter than those of adults.

euthanasia

The intentional act of ending a person's life painlessly in order to relieve suffering. In the UK, it is illegal to aid somebody to take their life. However, patients are legally entitled to refuse life-prolonging treatment, and doctors can legally give treatment to reduce pain and suffering even if such treatment unintentionally hastens death. In certain circumstances, it is also legal to withdraw treatment; for example, life-support for a patient who is brain-dead may be withdrawn.

euthyroid

A term used to describe a person whose *thyroid gland* is functioning normally. The term "euthyroid" is used especially to refer to someone who has been successfully treated for either *hypothyroidism* (underactivity of the thyroid) or *hyperthyroidism* (overactivity of the thyroid).

Evan's syndrome

An uncommon *autoimmune disorder* in which the body wrongly makes two *antibodies*: one attacks healthy red blood cells (see *anaemia, haemolytic*) and one destroys platelets (tiny blood cells involved in clotting). The spleen is usually the main site of cell destruction.

The anaemia can cause tiredness and pallor, and the deficiency of platelets may lead to bruising and a tendency to bleed easily. The haemolysis (red cell destruction) causes *jaundice* (yellowing of the skin and the whites of the eyes).

A blood transfusion may be needed in the early stages of the condition. *Corticosteroid drugs* may be prescribed to control haemolysis and platelet destruction. In severe cases, the spleen may be removed (see *splenectomy*). The antibodies may eventually disappear after several months or years.

evening primrose oil

An oil extracted from the seeds of the plant OENOTHERA BIENNIS, commonly called evening primrose. The oil contains an anti-inflammatory substance known as *gamolenic acid* and is believed by some to be of benefit in treating *eczema* and *premenstrual syndrome*.

eversion

Turning outwards. The term is used medically to describe a type of *ankle* injury or deformity in which the foot is turned outwards.

evidence-based medicine

Health care based on evidence, acquired through the evaluation of expert practice and research, that a particular test or treatment is appropriate for an individual patient.

Evista

A brand name for *raloxifene*, a drug that is prescribed for the prevention and treatment of *osteoporosis* in postmenopausal women.

evoked potential

The electrical signal generated when a sensory area, such as a *nerve*, a *muscle*, or the *retina* (the light-sensitive inner layer at the back of the eye), is stimulated. Tests to record evoked potentials are used to diagnose problems affecting the conduction of signals along sensory nerves. (See also *evoked responses*.)

evoked responses

The tracing of electrical activity in the brain in response to a specific external stimulus. The evoked responses procedure is similar to that for an *EEG* (electroencephalography).

The technique is used to check the functioning of various sensory systems (such as sight, hearing, or touch). The information obtained can be used to reveal abnormalities caused by inflammation, pressure from a tumour, or other disorders, and to help confirm a diagnosis of *multiple sclerosis*.

Ewing's sarcoma

A rare malignant form of *bone cancer*. Ewing's sarcoma arises in a large bone, usually the *femur* (thigh bone), *tibia*, (shin), *humerus* (upper-arm bone), or a pelvic bone, and spreads to other areas at an early stage. The condition is most common in children between ten and 15 years of age.

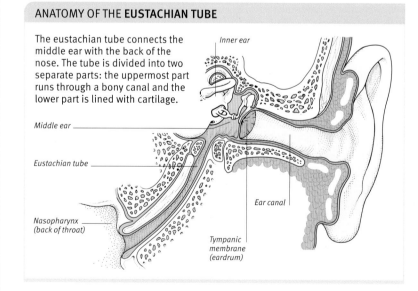

ANATOMY OF THE **EUSTACHIAN TUBE**

The eustachian tube connects the middle ear with the back of the nose. The tube is divided into two separate parts: the uppermost part runs through a bony canal and the lower part is lined with cartilage.

Inner ear

Middle ear

Eustachian tube

Nasopharynx (back of throat)

Ear canal

Tympanic membrane (eardrum)

SYMPTOMS

A bone affected by Ewing's sarcoma is painful and tender. It may also become weakened and fracture easily. Other symptoms include weight loss, fever, and *anaemia* (a reduced level of the oxygen-carrying pigment haemoglobin in the blood).

DIAGNOSIS AND TREATMENT

The sarcoma can be diagnosed by *X-rays* and bone marrow *biopsy* (removal of a sample of bone marrow for analysis). If cancer is found, the whole skeleton is examined by X-rays, r*adionuclide scanning*, *CT scanning*, or *MRI* (magnetic resonance imaging), and the lungs imaged by CT scanning to determine if, and how far, the cancer has spread.

Treatment of Ewing's sarcoma is with surgery, *radiotherapy*, and *anticancer drugs*. The outlook depends on how far the cancer has spread.

examination, physical

The part of a medical consultation in which the doctor looks at, feels, and listens to various parts of the patient's body. A physical examination is used to assess the patient's condition or to gather information to help the doctor make a *diagnosis*.

Most physical examinations include *palpation* (feeling with the hands), by which the doctor examines relevant areas of the body for signs such as swelling, tenderness, or enlargement of organs. In some cases, *percussion* of the chest, or other parts of the body, may be performed by tapping with the fingers and then listening to the sound produced. *Auscultation* (listening with a stethoscope) may be used to listen to blood flow through the arteries and sounds made by the heart and lungs. Other aspects of the examination may involve taking the patient's pulse or *blood pressure*, examining his or her eyes and ears, and assessing the strength and coordination of the muscles.

exanthema

A skin eruption or rash, or a disease in which a skin eruption or rash is a prominent feature, such as *measles*, *scarlet fever*, or *roseola infantum*.

exchange transfusion

A treatment for *haemolytic disease of the newborn*, a severe disorder that results from *rhesus incompatibility* between a pregnant mother and her baby and which causes destruction of red blood cells in the baby. This condition leads to dangerously high levels of the pigment *bilirubin* in the baby's blood as well as severe *anaemia* (a reduced level of the oxygen-carrying pigment haemoglobin in the blood). Exchange transfusion is used to treat both these symptoms by replacing the infant's blood with rhesus-negative donor blood.

excimer laser

A computer-controlled *laser* used to reshape the *cornea* (the transparent dome that forms the front of the eyeball). The laser removes very thin layers of tissue from the corneal surface (see *LASIK*; *PRK*). Corneal reshaping with a laser may be used to correct vision disorders including shortsightedness (*myopia*), longsightedness (*hypermetropia*), and *astigmatism* (unequal curvature of the cornea).

excision

The surgical cutting out of diseased tissue, such as a breast lump or gangrenous skin, from surrounding healthy tissue. (See also *excisional biopsy*.)

excisional biopsy

A type of *biopsy* that involves the removal of an entire area of affected tissue, together with a margin of adjacent healthy tissue, for microscopic analysis in a laboratory.

exclusion diet

A dietary programme that is used to identify a particular *food allergy* or *food intolerance*. Food is initially limited to a very restricted choice until symptoms improve; test foods, such as milk, are then reintroduced one at a time, at intervals of several days, to see if there is an adverse reaction. The reintroduction of such a test food is known as a food challenge.

Individuals on an exclusion diet are asked to keep a daily record of their symptoms from at least a week before starting the diet until the end of the programme. An exclusion diet should never be attempted without the advice of a doctor, dietitian, or nutritionist because it can result in serious nutritional deficiencies.

excoriation

Injury to the surface of the skin or to a *mucous membrane* (the thin, moist tissue that lines body cavities) caused by physical *abrasion*, such as scratching.

excrescence

Any abnormal raised growth on the surface of the body, such as a *wart*.

excretion

The discharge of any waste material from the body. Examples of such waste material are the by-products of digestion, waste products from the repair of tissues, and excess water.

ORGANS OF EXCRETION

The *kidneys* excrete urine, which contains excess nitrogen (as urea), together with excess water, salts, some acids, and most drugs. The *liver* excretes bile, which contains waste products and bile pigments formed from the breakdown of red blood cells. Some of the bile is passed from the body in the *faeces*. The large *intestine* excretes undigested food, some salts, and excess water in the form of faeces. The *lungs* discharge carbon dioxide and water vapour into the air. *Sweat glands* excrete salt and water onto the surface of the skin as a method of regulating the body's temperature.

exencephaly

A developmental defect of the cranium (skull) in which part of the bone is absent, leaving the brain exposed or allowing it to protrude. This defect is incompatible with survival.

exenteration

The surgical removal of all organs and soft tissue in a body cavity, usually to arrest growth of a *cancer*. Exenteration is sometimes used in *ophthalmology* when the eye and the contents of the eye socket are removed.

exercise

Physical activity performed to improve health. It may be taken for recreation, as part of a healthy lifestyle, to correct a physical injury or deformity (see *physiotherapy*), or as part of the treatment for some psychological problems.

TYPES OF EXERCISE

Different types of physical exercise have different effects on the body. Some forms (aerobic exercises) primarily improve the fitness of the cardiovascular and respiratory systems; some improve flexibility; some increase muscular strength; and some improve physical endurance.

During aerobic exercise, such as jogging or swimming, the heart and lungs work faster and more efficiently to meet the muscles' increased demand

E

for oxygen. Regular aerobic exercise improves the condition of both the cardiovascular and respiratory systems.

Exercises such as weight training increase muscle strength and endurance. Activities such as yoga and pilates improve flexibility. For further information on the effects of exercise, see the illustrated box below.

BENEFITS OF EXERCISE

Regular exercise is beneficial for both physical and psychological health. More specifically, regular aerobic exercise usually leads to reduced blood pressure and reduces the risk of *coronary artery disease*, *atherosclerosis* (accumulation of fatty deposits on artery walls), and *myocardial infarction* (heart attack). It can also help relieve the symptoms of *peripheral vascular disease*.

Exercise provides natural pain relief and a general feeling of wellbeing by increasing the secretion of *endorphins*, and can help relieve the symptoms of some psychological disorders, particularly *depression*. Regular exercise is also valuable in weight control, especially in combination with a healthy diet.

Regular weight-bearing exercise (such as running) increases bone density; hence *osteoporosis* is less common in people who have exercised throughout their adult lives. Such exercise also increases muscle mass and strengthens the muscles and ligaments, which may help to prevent or ease lower back pain and can make the ligaments less susceptible to strains.

RISKS

In some circumstances, vigorous exercise may pose a number of health risks. For example, people who are generally

---

THE EFFECTS OF EXERCISE

Exercise produces many changes in different body organs. Muscles receive an increased blood flow because of their greater energy needs, and the heart and lungs work faster and more efficiently to keep body tissues well supplied with blood. These changes are controlled by the chemicals adrenaline (epinephrine) and noradrenaline (norepinephrine) released from the sympathetic nervous system.

The lungs
The rate and depth of breathing increase to ensure a sufficient flow of oxygen from the lungs into the blood. This increase in breathing also helps to remove additional carbon dioxide produced by the muscle cells during exercise.

Bones
Regular exercise helps to maintain the strength and density of the bones and so prevents or slows the development of the bone disease osteoporosis.

The muscles
As the muscles flex and relax, there is a rise in the chemical activity within muscle cells. The rate at which the cells consume oxygen and glucose increases.

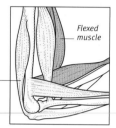

Flexed muscle

Relaxed muscle

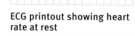

ECG printout showing heart rate at rest

Heart rate during exercise

The heart and circulation
The heart beats faster and more powerfully to increase the blood flow to the working muscles. Blood vessels in the intestines, liver, stomach, and kidneys narrow so that more blood is directed away from these areas and to the muscles.

COMMON TYPES OF EXERCISE

Aerobic

Aerobic exercise is activity in which the body continuously needs to take in additional oxygen to meet the muscles' increased demands. Regular aerobic exercise improves the performance of the cardiovascular and respiratory systems. Jogging, swimming, and cycling are examples of aerobic exercise.

Isometric

Isometric exercise is exercise without movement, in which one group of muscles exerts steady pressure against either an immovable object or an opposing group of muscles. It is an effective means of increasing muscle strength, but does not exercise the cardiovascular system or help in muscular endurance.

Isotonic

Isotonic exercise is exercise with movement, in which muscle tension is more or less constant and the body works against its own weight or external weights. Isotonic exercise includes weight training and calisthenics (repetitious movements with little or no equipment). It increases muscle strength, size, and endurance.

Isokinetic

Isokinetic exercise involves both isotonic and isometric exercise. The muscles move reasonably heavy loads, but are also put through their full range of movement. Isokinetics combines strength training with some aerobic exercise, but requires specialist equipment.

healthy but out of condition may suffer injury and put themselves at increased risk of a heart attack if they suddenly start exercising vigorously. Such people should therefore begin exercising gradually and slowly increase the amount and vigorousness of exercise. People who have not exercised regularly should consult a dictor first if they have *diabetes mellitus*, *hypertension* (high blood pressure), chest pains or any other discomfort on exertion, or get breathless with even slight exertion. Exercise should be avoided by people who have a high temperature or an injury that has not healed fully.

Professional sportspeople may have an increased risk of *osteoarthritis* in later life because of repeated minor damage to structures such as the knee and neck area of the spine.

exercise ECG

Also called a cardiac stress test, the use of electrocardiography (see *ECG*) to assess the function of the heart when it is put under the stress of exercise. Exercise ECG is usually carried out when a patient is suspected of having *coronary artery disease*. The procedure involves raising the heart rate by exercising, usually on a treadmill with an adjustable gradient or on an exercise bicycle. The heart's electrical activity is then recorded for analysis.

exercise tests

Tests in which exercise is used as a means of deliberately stressing the heart and the lungs. The use of exercise tests enables doctors to assess an individual's level of health and fitness. (See also *cardiac stress test*; *exercise ECG*.)

exfoliation

Flaking off, shedding, or peeling from a surface in scales or thin layers, as in *exfoliative dermatitis*.

exfoliative dermatitis

A skin disorder characterized by severe inflammation, redness, and scaling of the skin over most of the body. Exfoliative dermatitis may be the result of an allergic response to a drug (see *allergy*) or it may be due to worsening of a preexisting skin condition such as *psoriasis* or *eczema*. The condition sometimes occurs in *lymphoma* and *leukaemia*.

In exfoliative dermatitis, there is a widespread rash, accompanied by severe flaking of the skin, which results in increased loss of water and protein from the surface of the body. Protein loss may cause *oedema* (accumulation of fluid in tissues) and muscle wasting. Further possible complications include *heart failure* and infection. Treatment and outlook depend on the cause.

exhalation

The medical term for the process of breathing out (see *breathing*).

exhaustion

Extreme mental or physical *tiredness* in which a person lacks energy. It may result from overactivity or prolonged *insomnia* or it may be a symptom of a mental or physical disorder, such as *anxiety*, stress, severe *anaemia*, or prolonged *labour*. (See also *heat exhaustion*.)

exhibitionism

The habit of deliberately exposing the *genitalia* as a deviant sexual act. It is almost always confined to men. *Psychotherapy* or *behaviour therapy* may help to treat persistent offenders.

existential psychotherapy

An uncommon form of *psychotherapy* in which emphasis is placed on spontaneous interactions and feelings rather than on rational thinking. The psychotherapist is involved in the therapy to the same extent as the patient.

exocrine gland

A *gland* that secretes substances through a duct (a tube or passage) either on to the inner surface of an organ or the outer surface of the body. Examples of exocrine glands include the *salivary glands* and the *sweat glands*. The release of exocrine secretions can be triggered by a *hormone* or a *neurotransmitter*. (See also *endocrine gland*.)

exogenous

A term referring to a disease or disorder that has a cause external to the body. Examples are infection, poisoning, or injury. (See also *endogenous*.)

exomphalos

A rare *birth defect* in which a membranous sac containing part of the intestines protrudes through the *navel*. In mild cases of exomphalos, only one or two loops of intestine protrude; in severe cases, most of the abdominal organs are exposed. An affected infant may also have intestinal malformation.

Exomphalos is sometimes diagnosed before birth by *ultrasound* examination. The condition is treated using surgery.

exophthalmic goitre

An alternative name for *Graves' disease*, in which there is overproduction of thyroid hormones.

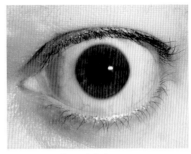

Appearance of exophthalmos
The staring appearance in exophthalmos is caused by swelling of the soft tissue in the eye socket, which pushes the eyeball forwards.

exophthalmos

Protrusion of one or both eyeballs caused by a swelling of the soft tissues within the *eye* socket.

CAUSES

Exophthalmos is most commonly associated with Graves' disease, which also causes *thyrotoxicosis* (overactivity of the thyroid gland). Other causes include an *eye tumour*, an *aneurysm* (ballooning of an artery), or inflammation behind the eye.

SYMPTOMS

Exophthalmos may restrict eye movement and cause *double vision*. In severe cases, increased pressure in the socket may restrict blood supply to the *optic nerve*, causing blindness. The eyelids may be unable to close, and vision may become blurred due to drying of the *cornea* (the transparent dome that forms the front of the eyeball).

TREATMENT AND OUTLOOK

In exophthalmos due to thyroid disease, treatment of the thyroid disorder may relieve the exophthalmos; however, exophthalmos may persist even if thyroid function returns to normal.

With early treatment, normal vision is usually restored. Occasionally, surgery may be required to relieve pressure on the eyeball and optic nerve.

exostosis

The most common type of noncancerous *bone tumour*, in which there is an outgrowth of bone tissue. Exostosis develops most commonly at one end of the *femur* (thigh bone) or the *tibia* (shin). The condition may be due to hereditary factors or to prolonged pressure on a particular bone.

SYMPTOMS

In most cases, exostosis produces no symptoms. Often it is recognized only after an injury, when it appears as a hard swelling. Occasionally, the tumour presses on a nerve, causing pain or weakness in the affected area.

DIAGNOSIS AND TREATMENT

Diagnosis can be confirmed by *X-rays*. The tumour may be surgically removed if it is causing symptoms or for cosmetic reasons.

exotoxin

A poison, released by certain types of *bacteria* (including *tetanus* bacilli and *diphtheria* bacilli), that enters the bloodstream and causes widespread effects around the body. Exotoxins are among the most poisonous substances known.

Infections by tetanus, diphtheria, and some other bacteria that release life-threatening exotoxins can be prevented by *immunization* with vaccines consisting of inactivated exotoxins. Treatment of such infections usually includes administration of *antibiotic drugs* and an *antitoxin* to neutralize the exotoxin. (See also *endotoxin*; *enterotoxin*.)

exotropia

An alternative term for a divergent *squint*, in which one eye is used for detailed vision and the other is directed outwards. (See also *esotropia*.)

expectorants

Cough remedies that encourage expectoration (the coughing up of *sputum*).

expectoration

The coughing up and spitting out of *sputum* (phlegm). (See also *cough*.)

expiratory reserve volume

The extra volume of air expired in the fullest possible exhalation; this amount is in addition to the volume that is normally expelled when a person is at rest. The expiratory reserve volume may be measured in pulmonary function tests.

expiratory stridor

An abnormal noise that is heard when a person exhales. Expiratory stridor may occur if the *vocal cords* are partially obstructing the flow of air or if there is an obstruction in the *trachea* (the wind-pipe) or bronchi (see *bronchus*), which are the main airways to the lungs. Expiratory stridor may occur either alone or with *inspiratory stridor*.

expire

To exhale (breathe out air from the lungs). The term also means "to die".

expired gas

Any gas that has been expelled from the lungs. Expired gas usually contains a high proportion of *carbon dioxide*. It may also contain other substances, such as *alcohol* and *carbon monoxide*, that are carried in the circulation.

exploratory surgery

Any operation carried out to investigate or examine part of the body to discover the extent of known disease or to establish a diagnosis. Advances in imaging, such as *MRI* (which produces cross-sectional or three-dimensional images of body structures), have reduced the need for exploratory surgery.

exposure

A term used to describe the effects on the body of being subjected to very low temperatures, or to a combination of low temperatures, wetness, and high winds. The primary danger in these conditions is *hypothermia* (a sharp fall in body temperature).

The term is also used to describe subjection to *radiation*, to environmental pollutants, or to infectious diseases.

expressing milk

A technique sometimes used by women who are *breast-feeding*, for removing milk from the breasts. The technique may be needed if the woman's breasts are overfull (see *engorgement*). A woman may also want to express milk so that it can be given to the baby in her absence or so that an infant who is unable to feed at the breast (due to prematurity, for example) can still benefit from breast milk. Milk can either be expressed by hand or using a *breast pump*. The milk may also be frozen for later use.

expressive dysphasia

A type of *dysphasia* (disturbance in the ability to use and/or understand words) in which the person can understand others and knows what he or she wishes to say, but has difficulty putting thoughts into words. (See also *aphasia*; *speech*; *speech disorders*; *speech therapy*.)

exsanguinate

To remove, withdraw, or deprive the body of circulating *blood*. Exsanguination usually results from severe internal or external bleeding. It can also be performed during surgery to create a blood-free area for the procedure. (See also *Esmarch's bandage*.)

exstrophy of the bladder

A rare *birth defect* in which the *bladder* is inside-out and is open to the outside of the body through a space in the lower abdominal wall. There are also usually other defects, such as *epispadias* in males (in which the opening of the urethra is on the upper surface of the penis) and failure of the pubic bones to join at the front. Untreated, an affected child constantly leaks urine.

Surgical treatment involves reconstructing the bladder and closing the abdominal wall. If the bladder is very small, it is removed and the urine diverted (see *urinary diversion*).

extensor

Any *muscle* that moves a *joint* in order to straighten a limb. An example of an extensor muscle is the *triceps muscle* in the arm, which straightens the elbow.

external cardiac massage

Rhythmic pressure applied to the chest to maintain circulation if a person's heart has stopped beating. In order to compress the heart (see *cardiac massage*), the centre of the chest is pressed repeatedly with the heels of both hands (for adults), or one hand (for children), or with two fingers (for babies). External cardiac massage may be used in first aid as part of *cardiopulmonary resuscitation*.

external fixation

The insertion of pins through the skin to hold together parts of a broken bone (see *fracture*). The pins are held in place by an external metal frame. Usually, the affected limb can be used within a few days; the frame and pins are removed under anaesthesia when the bone has healed. (See also *internal fixation*.)

external haemorrhoids

Haemorrhoids (dilated veins) that form around the outside of the *anus*. Haemorrhoids are commonly known as piles. The condition is sometimes associated with *internal haemorrhoids*, those that develop higher up inside the anal canal. If the blood in an external haemorrhoid clots, the resulting swelling is termed a thrombosed external haemorrhoid. This condition is very painful but usually subsides over several days, although urgent treatment may be needed in some cases. (See also *haemorrhoidectomy*; *internal haemorrhoids*.)

extracorporeal circulation

Circulation of blood outside the body through a machine that temporarily assumes an organ's functions. Examples of extracorporeal circulation include the use of a *heart–lung machine*, during open heart surgery, to keep blood moving around the body and carry out carbon dioxide–oxygen exchange, and *extracorporeal dialysis*.

extracorporeal dialysis

Haemodialysis performed through an artificial kidney to remove the substances that are normally excreted in the urine (see *dialysis*).

extracorporeal gas exchange

A technique in which blood is diverted out of the body and through an "artificial lung" to aid *respiration*. It involves a procedure called extracorporeal membrane oxygenation (ECMO), in which blood is passed over an artificial membrane and takes up oxygen, and the removal of waste carbon dioxide. Extracorporeal gas exchange is used to treat severe *respiratory failure*, in addition to mechanical *ventilation*.

extracorpuscular

A term meaning "situated or occurring outside the *corpuscles* (minute bodies or cells)". Extracorpuscular refers particularly to the environment outside the *blood cells* (for example, it may be used for agents that attack red blood cells from outside; see *anaemia, haemolytic*).

extraction, dental

The removal of one or more *teeth* by a dentist.
WHY IT IS DONE
Dental extraction may be performed when a tooth is severely decayed or too badly broken to be repaired or when an abscess (see *abscess, dental*) has formed. Teeth may also be removed if there is dental crowding or *malocclusion* (an incorrect bite); if they are loose due to severe gum disease (see *periodontitis*); or if they are preventing another tooth from erupting through the gum (see *eruption of teeth*).

HOW IT IS DONE
For most extractions, local anaesthesia is used (see *anaesthesia, dental*). A general anaesthetic (see *anaesthesia, general*) may be used to extract badly impacted wisdom teeth (see *impaction, dental*), to extract several teeth at once, or for extremely anxious or disabled patients or young children.

Teeth are usually extracted with dental forceps, which are designed to grasp the root of the tooth. When gentle but firm pressure is applied, the blades cut through the periodontal ligaments (the tough, fibrous membranes supporting the tooth in its socket), the socket is gradually expanded, and the tooth is removed. Occasionally the root fractures during this procedure and may need to be removed separately.

In difficult extractions, for example if the tooth is impacted, if the crown is missing, or if the roots are very curved, some gum and bone may need to be removed from around the tooth before the tooth is extracted and the gum is sutured (stitched).
COMPLICATIONS
Most extractions take place without complications. If bleeding does not stop after extraction of a tooth, suturing of the tissue around the socket may be necessary.

Occasionally, if a blood clot (see *blood clotting*) fails to form in the empty tooth socket or if the blood clot is dislodged, a condition called *dry socket* (infection in the tooth socket) develops.

extradural haemorrhage

Bleeding into the space between the inner surface of the skull and the external surface of the *dura mater* (the outer layer of the *meninges*, the protective covering of the brain).
CAUSE
Extradural haemorrhage most commonly occurs as a result of a blow to the side of the head that fractures the skull (see *skull, fracture of*) and ruptures an artery running over the dura mater.
SYMPTOMS
A *haematoma* (a collection of clotted blood) forms and enlarges, increasing pressure inside the skull. Symptoms result several hours or sometimes even days after the injury. These symptoms may include headache, drowsiness, vomiting, paralysis affecting one side of the body, and *seizures*. If left untreated, extradural haemorrhage may be life-threatening.

DIAGNOSIS AND TREATMENT
CT scanning or *MRI* (magnetic resonance imaging) are used to confirm the diagnosis. An X-ray may also be done if a skull fracture is suspected. Treatment may consist of *craniotomy* (drilling holes in the skull), draining the blood clot, and clipping shut the ruptured blood vessel.

extrapyramidal disease

Any of a group of disorders that are the result of damage to, or degeneration of, parts of the *extrapyramidal system* (nerve pathways that link motor nerve nuclei within the brain). Extrapyramidal diseases disrupt the execution of voluntary movements; these diseases are characterized by uncontrollable movements, changes in muscle tone, and postural disturbances. Examples of extrapyramidal diseases include *Huntington's disease, Parkinson's disease*, and some types of *cerebral palsy*.

extrapyramidal system

A network of *nerve* pathways that links the surface of the *cerebrum* (main mass of the brain) with motor nerve nuclei in the *basal ganglia*, and parts of the *brainstem*. This system influences and modifies electrical impulses sent from the brain to initiate movement in the skeletal muscles.

Damage or degeneration of components in the extrapyramidal system may be caused by *extrapyramidal disease*. It may also occur as a side effect of taking *phenothiazine drugs*.

extrasystole

A contraction of the heart that is independent of the heart's normal rhythm. Extrasystole arises in response to an electrical impulse in a part of the heart other than the sinoatrial node (see *ectopic heartbeat*).

extrauterine pregnancy

An alternative term for an *ectopic pregnancy*.

extravasation

The leakage and spread of fluid, usually from blood vessels or *lymph* vessels, into the surrounding tissues. Extravasation has a variety of causes, including injury, burns, and inflammation.

extravascular

Situated or occurring outside the vessels. The term refers particularly to the blood vessels (see *circulatory system*) and

E

the lymph vessels (see *lymphatic system*). Extravascular fluid is fluid that exists outside the blood and lymph circulations, in the body tissues.

extrinsic allergic alveolitis

Inflammation and thickening of the tiny air sacs in the lungs that is caused by an allergy to inhaled organic dusts (see *alveolitis*).

extrinsic asthma

Any form of *asthma* precipitated by an environmental factor. Extrinsic asthma is usually due to an *allergy* to a foreign substance, such as inhaled particles, certain foods, or a particular drug.

extrinsic factor

An alternative name for *vitamin B₁₂*.

extrovert

A person whose main interest is in other people and the outside world. Extroverts are active, sociable, and have many interests. (See also *introvert*; *personality*.)

exudation

The discharge of fluid from *blood vessels* into surrounding tissues. Exuded fluid (exudate) contains *cells* and *protein*. Most exudates are the result of inflammation. In inflamed tissue, the small bood vessels widen and tiny pores in the vessel walls enlarge, allowing fluid and cells (mainly *white blood cells*) to escape.

exudation cyst

A *cyst* (a fluid-filled lump or swelling) formed when an existing body cavity fills with fluid as a result of *exudation*.

An example is a *hydrocele* (fluid-filled swelling in the scrotum).

exudative retinitis

See *Coat's disease*.

eye

The organ of sight. The eye is a complex organ, consisting of a series of structures that focus an image on to the *retina* (the light-sensitive inner layer at the back of the eye) and nerve cells that convert this image into electrical impulses. These impulses are carried by the *optic nerve* to the visual cortex (an area on the back surface of the brain concerned with *vision*) for interpretation.

The eyes work in conjunction with one another, under the control of the brain. They align themselves on a particular

ANATOMY OF THE EYE

The eye is a complex organ that focuses light rays to form an image on the retina, the light-sensitive inner layer at the back of the eyeball. The cornea and lens focus the rays. The pupil controls the amount of light entering the eye and the ciliary body alters the shape of the lens to adjust the focus. The retina has millions of nerve cells that respond to light; they convert the image into a pattern of nerve impulses, which are transmitted to the brain via the optic nerve.

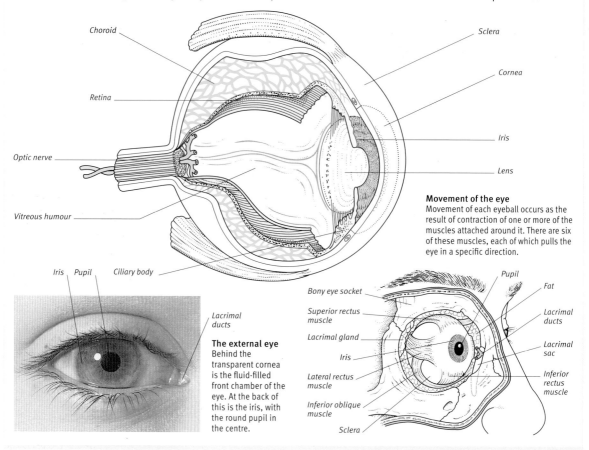

Choroid · Sclera · Retina · Cornea · Optic nerve · Iris · Lens · Vitreous humour · Iris · Pupil · Ciliary body

Movement of the eye
Movement of each eyeball occurs as the result of contraction of one or more of the muscles attached around it. There are six of these muscles, each of which pulls the eye in a specific direction.

The external eye
Behind the transparent cornea is the fluid-filled front chamber of the eye. At the back of this is the iris, with the round pupil in the centre.

Lacrimal ducts · Bony eye socket · Superior rectus muscle · Lacrimal gland · Iris · Lateral rectus muscle · Inferior oblique muscle · Sclera · Pupil · Fat · Lacrimal ducts · Lacrimal sac · Inferior rectus muscle object so that a clear image of the object is formed on each retina. If necessary, the eyes may sharpen the image by altering focus using an automatic process called *accommodation*, which changes the shape of the *lens*.

EYEBALL

The eyeballs lie in pads of fat within the bony *orbits* (eye sockets) that provide protection from injury. Each eyeball is moved by six delicate muscles. The eye has a tough, white outer layer known as the *sclera*. At the front of the sclera, the *cornea* (a transparent, thin-walled dome) serves as the main "lens" of the eye and does most of the focusing.

Behind the cornea is a shallow chamber filled with watery fluid (called the aqueous humour), at the back of which is the *iris* (the coloured part of the eye) with its *pupil* (circular opening), which appears black. Tiny muscles alter the size of the pupil in response to changes in light intensity in order to control the amount of light entering the eye.

Behind the iris, and in contact with it, is the crystalline lens, which is suspended by fibres from a circular ring of muscle: the *ciliary body*. Contraction of the ciliary body changes the shape of the lens, enabling fine focusing.

The main cavity of the eye contains a clear gel (the vitreous humour) and is located directly behind the lens. On the inside of the back of the eye is the retina, a complex structure of nerve tissue that is extremely sensitive to light. The retina requires a constant supply of oxygen and glucose. To meet this need, a thin network of blood vessels, the choroid plexus, lies immediately under it. The *choroid* is continuous at the front with the ciliary body and the iris; these three parts constitute the uveal tract.

CONJUNCTIVA AND EYELID

The eyeball is sealed off by a transparent, flexible membrane called the *conjunctiva*, which is attached to the skin at the corners of the eye and forms the inner lining of the eyelids. The conjunctiva contains mucus-secreting glands. These, together with the meibomian glands in the eyelids (which secrete an oily fluid), provide the tear film that protects the cornea and conjunctiva. Blinking, a protective *reflex*, helps to spread the tear film evenly over the cornea to enable clear vision.

eye, artificial

A *prosthesis* used to replace an *eye* that has been surgically removed. An artificial eye is worn purely for cosmetic and psychological reasons and fits neatly behind the eyelids into the cavity from which the natural eye was removed. Some movement of the artificial eye may be achieved by attaching the muscles that normally move the eye to the remaining conjunctival membrane (see *conjunctiva*) or to a plastic implant placed in the eye socket.

Often called "glass eyes", artificial eyes were once made of glass; now an easily mouldable plastic material is used.

eye-drops

Medication in solution that is used in the treatment of eye disorders or to aid in their diagnosis. Examples of drugs given in this form are *antibiotic drugs*, *antihistamine drugs*, drugs used either to dilate (widen) or constrict (narrow) the pupil, the circular opening in the centre of the iris, and *corticosteroid drugs*.

A specified number of eye-drops are applied to the inside of the lower eyelid after the lid has been drawn down using

E

DISORDERS OF THE EYE

Many *eye* disorders are minor, but some can cause loss of vision unless treated. (See also *disorders of the cornea* box; *disorders of the retina* box.)

Congenital defects

Squint (misalignment of the eyes) may be congenital (present at birth). Other examples of congenital defects are *nystagmus* (uncontrollable, jerky eye movements), *albinism* (absence of pigment in the iris), and developmental defects affecting the cornea and retina. A rare birth defect is *microphthalmos* (abnormally small size of one or both eyes). *Cataract* (opacity of the lens) can sometimes be seen in newborn infants.

Infection

Conjunctivitis (inflammation of the conjunctiva) is the most common eye infection. *Trachoma* (a persistent disease of the cornea or conjunctiva) or severe bacterial conjunctivitis can impair vision. Corneal infections can lead to blurred vision or corneal *perforation* if not treated early. Endophthalmitis (infection within the eye) can occur as a result of injury to the eye or infection elsewhere in the body.

Impaired blood supply

Narrowing, blockage, or *inflammation* of retinal blood vessels may cause visual loss.

Tumours

Malignant melanoma of the *choroid* is the most common cancerous tumour of the eye. *Retinoblastoma* (a cancer of the retina) most commonly affects children. *Basal cell carcinoma* affects the eyelid and may result from excessive exposure to sunlight.

Nutritional disorders

Various *vitamin* deficiencies affect the eyes. Vitamin A deficiency may lead to *xerophthalmia* (corneal and conjunctival dryness), *night blindness*, or, eventually, *keratomalacia* (corneal softening and disintegration).

Autoimmune disorders

Uveitis (inflammation of the iris, choroid, and/or ciliary body) may be caused by infection or an *autoimmune disorder* (in which the body's immune system attacks its own tissues), such as *ankylosing spondylitis* and *sarcoidosis*.

Degeneration

Macular degeneration of the retina is common in elderly people, as is cataract.

Focusing disorders

Myopia (shortsightedness), *hypermetropia* (longsightedness), and *astigmatism* are relatively common. *Presbyopia* is a progressive, age-related loss of the ability to focus at close range. *Amblyopia* (poor vision in one eye unrelated to structural abnormality) is often due to squint.

Other disorders

Glaucoma (increased pressure within the eyeball), can lead to permanent visual loss. In *retinal detachment*, the retina lifts away from the eye's underlying layer.

INVESTIGATION

An *ophthalmoscope* and *slit-lamp* are used to view the eye. Vision is evaluated using *Snellen charts* and *refraction* tests.

E

the tip of a clean finger. Blinking helps to spread the medicated solution evenly around the eyeball.

eye, examination of

An inspection of the structures of the *eyes*, either as part of a *vision test* or to make a diagnosis when an eye disorder is suspected.

WHY IT IS DONE

Eye examinations are used to determine the cause of visual disturbance or of other symptoms relating to the eye. They are also used to assess whether corrective devices, such as glasses or contact lenses, are necessary. Eye tests are essential to discover certain serious eye disorders, such as *glaucoma* (in which the fluid in the eye is at abnormally high pressure), because such disorders may be symptomless in the early stages and only detectable during an eye examination.

HOW IT IS DONE

An eye examination usually begins with a physical inspection of the eyes, the eyelids, and the surrounding skin. Eye movements are usually checked and the examiner looks for *squint* (misalignment of the eyes).

Visual acuity (sharpness of vision) in each eye is investigated using a *Snellen chart*, the standard eye test wall chart.

Refraction testing (using lenses of different strengths) may then be performed to determine precisely what glasses or contact lenses, if any, are required.

An investigation of the *visual fields* (the extent of peripheral vision) may also be carried out, especially in suspected cases of glaucoma or a variety of neurological conditions.

Colour vision is occasionally checked because loss of colour perception is a sign of certain disorders of the *retina* (the light-sensitive inner layer at the back of the eye) or of the *optic nerve* (which transmits impulses from the retina to the brain). In order to check for abrasions or ulcers, the *conjunctiva* (the transparent membrane covering the white of the eye and inside of the eyelids) and the *cornea* (the transparent dome that forms the front of the eyeball) may be stained with *fluorescein* (an orange dye).

Applanation *tonometry* (measurement of the pressure within the eye) is an essential test for glaucoma.

EQUIPMENT

The *ophthalmoscope* is an instrument used to examine the inside of the eye, particularly the retina.

The slit-lamp microscope, with its illumination and lens magnification, allows for examination of the conjunctiva, the cornea, the front chamber of the eye, the *iris* (the coloured part of the eye) and the *lens* (the component that is responsible for focusing).

To obtain a full view of the lens and the structures behind it, the *pupil* (the circular opening in the centre of the iris) must be widely dilated by using special *eye-drops*.

eye, foreign body in

Any material on the surface of the *eye* or under the eyelid, or an object that penetrates the eyeball.

CAUSES

Particles of dust are the most common type of foreign body to enter the eye. Occasionally, a fragment of metal, plastic, or wood may be deflected into the eye. Rarely, an object travelling at high speed may penetrate the eyeball.

SYMPTOMS AND COMPLICATIONS

A foreign body may cause irritation, redness, increased tear production, and *blepharospasm* (uncontrollable closure and squeezing of the eyelid). Some foreign bodies left within the eyeball may release damaging substances into the eye, resulting in blindness. Other foreign bodies may remain intact but cause infection that can lead to loss of sight. Sympathetic *ophthalmitis* is a rare condition that may threaten sight even in the uninjured eye.

TREATMENT

Foreign bodies on the surface of the *conjunctiva* (the transparent membrane covering the white of the eye and lining the inside of the eyelids) can usually be flushed out by gentle rinsing with water. Never try to remove a foreign body with a cotton bud or any other object. Medical attention is needed if the object has penetrated the eyeball. The doctor may drop *fluorescein* (an orange dye) into the eye to reveal the presence of any *corneal abrasions* or sites of penetration. *Ultrasound scanning, CT scanning,* or an *X-ray* of the eye may also be performed.

Anaesthetic *eye-drops* may be applied and a spatula used to remove an object from the *cornea* (the transparent dome that forms the front of the eyeball). The eye may then be covered with a patch. *Antibiotic drugs* may be prescribed to combat infection.

eye injuries

Eye injuries may be caused by a blow to the eye or penetration of a foreign body (see *eye, foreign body in*). However, the

---

CONDUCTING AN **EYE EXAMINATION**

In an eye examination, the ophthalmologist checks the external appearance, eye movement, visual acuity, visual field, and colour vision. The eyes are checked for the presence of a squint, abrasions, and ulcers. Applanation tonometry and a refraction test may also be carried out.

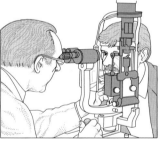

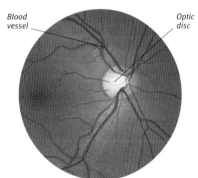

View of retina through ophthalmoscope
The retina (the inner back surface of the eye) is examined to assess its health and to detect the presence of disorders such as retinopathy.

Z
D A
F X H
P T N D
X A Z F N
H T X U D F
U Z N D F X T
A P H T X Z N U

Applanation tonometry
Measurement of the pressure within the eye is a test for glaucoma.

Snellen chart
This chart is used to check the visual acuity of each eye; the patient's ability to read letters of different sizes from the same distance is assessed.

eye often escapes serious injury because it is protected by the surrounding bone and the rapid blink reflex.

A blow to the eye may cause tearing of the *iris* (the coloured part of the eye) or the *sclera* (the white of the eye), with collapse of the eyeball and potential blindness. Minor injuries may lead to a *vitreous haemorrhage* (bleeding into the gel-filled cavity behind the lens); *hyphaema* (bleeding into the front chamber of the eye); *retinal detachment*; or injury to the trabeculum (the channel that drains fluid from the eye), which can lead to *glaucoma* (increase in fluid pressure in the eyeball).

Injuries to the centre of the *cornea* (the transparent dome that forms the front of the eyeball) impair vision by causing scarring. Damage to the *lens* (the component of the eye responsible for fine focusing) may cause a *cataract* (loss of transparency) to form.

eyelashes

Hairs that are arranged in rows at the edge of each eyelid and normally curve outwards. They prevent dust and debris from entering the eye. The lashes become finer and fewer with ages.

Growth in an abnormal direction may be due to injury to the eyelid or, more commonly, to an infection. Severe *blepharitis* (inflammation of the lid margins) may destroy the roots of the lashes. *Trachoma*, an infection in which the lid can be distorted by scarring, may lead to *trichiasis*, in which the lashes turn inwards and rub against the *cornea* (the transparent dome that forms the front of the eyeball).

eye, lazy

A popular term for *amblyopia* (in which normal vision has failed to develop in an otherwise healthy eye). The term "lazy eye" also refers to a convergent *squint* (in which one eye turns inwards).

eyelid

A fold of tissue at the upper or lower edge of an orbit (eye socket). The eyelids are held in place by *ligaments* attached to the socket's bony edges. They consist of thin plates of fibrous tissue (called tarsal plates) covered by muscle and a thin layer of skin. The inner layer is covered by an extension of the *conjunctiva* (the transparent membrane that covers the white of the eye). Along the edge of each lid is a row of *eyelashes*. Immediately behind the eye-lashes are the openings of ducts that lead from the meibomian glands, which secrete the oily fluid in tears.

The eyelids act as protective shutters, closing almost instantly as a *reflex* action if anything approaches the eye. They also spread the tear film across the *cornea* (the transparent dome that forms the front of the eyeball).

DISORDERS

Disorders affecting the eyelids include a *chalazion* (a swelling of a meibomian gland), *blepharitis* (inflammation of the edge of the eyelid), and a stye (a small abscess at the root of one of the lashes).

Certain disorders affect the shape and position of the eyelids. These include *entropion* (in which the eyelid margin turns inwards), *ectropion* (in which the eyelid margin turns outwards), and *ptosis* (in which the eyelid droops down).

Myokymia (twitching of the eyelid) is common, and usually caused by fatigue. *Blepharospasm* (prolonged contraction of the eyelid) is usually due to a condition such as photophobia (abnormal sensitivity of the eyes to light) or a foreign body. The skin of the eyelid is a common site for a *basal cell carcinoma*.

eyelid, drooping

See *ptosis*.

eyelid surgery

See *blepharoplasty*.

eye, painful red

A common combination of eye symptoms that may be due to any of various eye disorders.

Conjunctivitis (inflammation of the conjunctiva, the transparent membrane covering the white of the eye) is the most common cause of redness and irritation in the eye. *Uveitis* (inflammation of the iris, choroid, and/or ciliary body) is a common cause of dull, aching pain; this may be due to swelling in the front part of the eye and spasm in muscles around the iris. The redness is caused by widening of blood vessels around the iris.

Another cause of pain and redness in one eye is acute closed-angle *glaucoma* (a sudden increase in pressure within the eyeball). The pain is severe and may be accompanied by nausea, vomiting, and blurred vision. Increased blood flow in the surrounding blood vessels causes redness in the white of the eye.

Other causes of painful red eye include *keratitis* (inflammation of the cornea), which usually occurs as a result of a *corneal ulcer*, and a foreign body in the eye (see *eye, foreign body in*).

eye-strain

A common term used to describe aching or discomfort in or around the *eye*. Eye-strain is usually due to a headache caused by fatigue, tiredness of muscles around the eye, *sinusitis*, *blepharitis* (inflammation of the eyelid margins), or *conjunctivitis* (inflammation of the conjunctiva, the transparent membrane that covers the white of the eye).

eye teeth

A common name for the canine *teeth*.

eye tumours

Tumours of the eye are rare. However, when eye tumours do occur, they are usually painless and cancerous.

TYPES AND TREATMENT

Retinoblastoma This is a cancerous tumour of the *retina* (the light-sensitive inner layer at the back of the eye) that may occur in one or both eyes and most often affects children. Retinoblastoma may be treated by *radiotherapy*, *laser treatment*, or *cryosurgery* (freezing), but the eye may have to be removed to prevent spread of the tumour.

Malignant melanoma This form of cancer occurs in the *choroid* (the layer of tissue between the retina and the sclera, the white of the eye) and usually affects middle-aged or elderly people. There are no symptoms in the early stages, but the tumour eventually causes *retinal detachment* and distortion of vision. Small malignant melanomas can often be destroyed by laser treatment, but the eye may need to be removed to prevent spread of the tumour.

Secondary eye tumours If cancer elsewhere in the body spreads to the eye, secondary tumours develop. Symptoms depend on a tumour's location and growth rate. Secondary eye tumours may be controlled by radiotherapy; however, the primary tumour will need to be treated separately.

Basal cell carcinoma This is the most common type of tumour of the eyelid. It may be caused by excessive exposure to sunlight. The tumour usually has a crusty central crater and a hard rolled edge. In the early stages, a basal cell carcinoma of the eyelid may be treated by surgery, radiotherapy, or cryosurgery. If the tumour becomes large, the eyelid may need to be removed.

E

F

Fabry's disease

A rare inherited disorder caused by a deficiency of alpha-galactosidase A, an *enzyme* (a protein that acts as a catalyst) necessary for the metabolism of certain *lipids* (fats) in the body. Without the enzyme, lipid molecules accumulate in the tissues, especially in the nerves, heart, and kidneys.

Fabry's disease is inherited as an X-linked recessive trait (see *genetic disorders*) and therefore affects males more commonly than females.

SYMPTOMS
Among the first symptoms to develop, often in childhood, are pain and discomfort in the hands and feet as a result of damage to the peripheral nerves. As the condition progresses, heart and kidney function may become impaired. Female carriers usually show only mild symptoms.

TREATMENT AND OUTLOOK
Hand and feet pain is treated with *carbamazepine*. Sufferers usually survive into adulthood but are at risk from strokes, heart attacks, and kidney damage.

face-lift

A cosmetic operation to smooth out wrinkles and lift sagging skin on the face to make it look younger. The effect is achieved by making an incision near or along the hairline on each side of the face, lifting the skin off the face, and then removing the excess skin. The edges of skin are then stitched back together within the hairline.

Some bruising of the face is common following the procedure, and there may be some discomfort. Stitches are removed three to five days after the operation. In most cases, the scars, which fade within about a year, are hidden by natural crease lines or by the hair. The effect of a face-lift may last for up to ten years.

In a few cases, satisfactory healing does not occur because blood accumulates under the skin or because of infection that leads to severe scarring.

facet joint

A type of joint found in the *spine*, formed by the process (bony projection) of one vertebra fitting into a hollow in the vertebra above. Facet joints allow a degree of movement between vertebrae, which gives the spine its flexibility.

facial nerve

The seventh *cranial nerve*, which arises from structures in the *brainstem* and sends branches to the face, neck, salivary glands, and outer ear.

The facial nerve performs both motor and sensory functions. It controls the neck muscles and those of facial expression; it stimulates the secretion of saliva; and it conveys sensory information from the tongue and from the outer ear.

Damage to the facial nerve results in weakness of the facial muscles (see *facial palsy*) and, in some cases, loss of taste.

LOCATION OF THE FACIAL NERVE

Arising from the brainstem, the facial nerve has branches that connect to the outer ear, tongue, salivary glands, and muscles of facial expression in the neck and face.

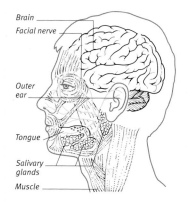

Brain
Facial nerve
Outer ear
Tongue
Salivary glands
Muscle

Such damage is probably most often due to a viral infection but may also occur in *stroke*.

facial pain

Pain in the face may be due to any one of a variety of causes or may occur for no known reason.

CAUSES
Injury to the face, such as by blows or cuts, is a common cause of facial pain. Facial pain is also commonly due to infection. *Sinusitis* (inflammation of the air spaces in the facial bones) can cause pain around the eyes and in the cheek bones. The onset of *mumps* can cause pain in the cheeks before swelling is apparent; the pain is in front of and/or below the ears. Pain from a *boil* in the nose or ear may also be felt in the face.

Problems with the teeth and jaws are another common cause of facial pain. Such problems include severe tooth decay (see *caries, dental*), an abscess (see *abscess, dental*), impacted wisdom teeth (see *impaction, dental*), or partial dislocation of the jaw (see *jaw, dislocated*).

Damage to one of the nerves that supply the face can also produce severe pain. Conditions resulting from nerve damage include the stabbing pain that precedes the rash of *herpes zoster* (shingles) and the intermittent shooting pain of *trigeminal neuralgia*, which usually affects the cheek, lip, gum, or chin on one side and is often brought on by touching the face or chewing.

A disorder elsewhere in the body may cause *referred pain* in the face. For example, in *angina pectoris* (chest pain due to impaired blood supply to the heart muscle), pain may also be felt in the jaw. During a *migraine* headache, pain may also occur on one side of the face. Facial pain that occurs for no apparent reason may occasionally be a symptom of *depression*.

TREATMENT
Treatment depends of the underlying cause. *Analgesic drugs* (painkillers) can provide temporary relief from pain, but severe or persistent facial pain requires medical attention.

facial palsy

Weakness of the facial muscles due to damage to, or inflammation of, the *facial nerve*. The condition is usually temporary and affects only one side of the face.

CAUSES
Facial palsy is most often due to Bell's palsy, which occurs for no known reason. Less commonly, the condition is associated with *herpes zoster* (shingles) affecting the ear and facial nerve. Facial palsy may also result from surgical damage to this nerve, or compression of the nerve by a tumour.

SYMPTOMS
Facial palsy usually develops suddenly. The eyelid and the corner of the mouth on one side of the face droop, and there may be pain in the ear on that side. The ability to wrinkle the brow or to close

the eye may be lost, and smiling is distorted. Depending on which nerve branches are affected, the sense of taste may be impaired or sounds may seem to be unnaturally loud.

TREATMENT
In many cases, facial palsy clears up without treatment. Pain can be relieved by taking *analgesics* (painkillers), and exercising the facial muscles may aid recovery. It may be necessary to tape the eyelid shut at bedtime in order to avoid the risk of *corneal abrasion*.

Bell's palsy may be treated with *corticosteroid drugs* to reduce inflammation and speed recovery. Re-routing or *grafting* of nerve tissue may help people suffering from palsy caused by an injury or a tumour.

facial spasm
An uncommon disorder in which the muscles that are supplied by the *facial nerve* twitch frequently. Facial spasm, which predominantly affects middle-aged women, is of unknown cause.

facial tic
See *facial spasm*.

facies
A term used to denote facial expression, which is often used as a guide to a person's health. For example, the typical facies seen in a child with enlarged adenoids is open-mouthed because of difficulty breathing through the nose.

The term "facies" may also be used to refer to a particular surface of a body structure, part, or organ.

facioscapulohumeral dystrophy
An autosomal dominant *genetic disorder* that causes muscle weakness and wasting. The condition first appears in childhood or adolescence. The muscle wasting chiefly affects the face, shoulder girdle, arms, and later the pelvis and legs.

factitious disorders
A group of disorders in which a patient's symptoms mimic those of a true illness but which have been invented by, and are under the control of, the patient. There is no apparent cause other than a wish for attention; the desire to assume the role of a patient may be an escape from everyday life in order to be cared for and protected.

The most common disorder of this type is *Munchausen's syndrome*, which is characterized by physical symptoms.

The sufferer may aggravate existing physical problems or even inflict self-injury. In *Ganser's syndrome*, symptoms are psychological. Factitious disorders differ from *malingering*, in which a person claims to be ill for a particular purpose (for example, in order to obtain time off work).

factor V
One of the blood proteins that maintains the balance between the blood clotting too easily or too slowly after an injury. About 5 per cent of the population have an inherited *mutation* in the gene controlling factor V production, known as factor V Leiden. They are at increased risk of deep-vein thrombosis (see *thrombophilia*), particularly if taking the oral contraceptive pill or going on long aircraft journeys.

factor VIII
One of the blood proteins involved in *blood clotting*. People with *haemophilia* have a reduced level of factor VIII in their blood and, consequently, have a tendency to abnormal bleeding and to prolonged bleeding when injured.

People with severe haemophilia require regular treatment with concentrates of factor VIII. This treatment reduces the bleeding tendency and allows the affected person a normal quality of life.

factor IX
A protein in blood that plays an important role in the clotting mechanism. A deficiency of factor IX causes a rare genetic *bleeding disorder* known as *Christmas disease*.

fad
See *food fad*.

faecal fistula
See *fistula*.

faecal impaction
A condition in which a large mass of hard *faeces* cannot be evacuated from the rectum. It is usually associated with long-standing *constipation*. Faecal impaction is most common in very young children and in elderly people, especially those who are bedridden.

The main symptoms are an intense desire to pass a bowel movement; pain in the rectum, anus, and centre of the abdomen; and, in some cases, watery faeces that are passed around the mass (and may be confused with diarrhoea).

Treatment of faecal impaction is with *enemas* or, if these are ineffective, by manual removal of the faecal mass.

faecal incontinence
See *incontinence, faecal*.

faecalith
A small, hard piece of impacted faeces that forms in a diverticulum (a sac in the wall of the intestine). A faecalith is harmless unless it forms a blockage at the entrance to the sac, which causes *diverticulitis*, or to the appendix, which causes *appendicitis*.

faecal occult blood test (FOBT)
A test used to check for the presence of hidden (occult) blood in the faeces (see *occult blood, faecal*). FOBT is a screening test that may be carried out because blood in the faeces may be one of the earliest indications of *polyps*, which may eventually develop into cancer, or colorectal cancer (see *colon, cancer of*; *rectum, cancer of*). People at high risk of bowel cancer are offered regular screening using the FOBT and *colonoscopy*. A general bowel cancer screening programme using FOBT is being phased in for everybody between the ages of 60 and 69; if the test is positive, further tests, including colonoscopy, will then be offered.

faecal vomiting
The vomiting of matter that resembles faeces, either in appearance or odour or both. Faecal vomiting is a symptom of serious intestinal obstruction (see *intestine, disorders of*).

faeces
Waste material from the digestive tract that is solidified in the large intestine and expelled through the *anus*. Faeces are composed of indigestible food residue (dietary *fibre*), dead bacteria, dead cells shed from the intestinal lining, intestinal secretions such as mucus, *bile* from the liver (which is the substance that gives faeces their brown colour), and water.

Examination of the faeces plays an important part in the diagnosis of disorders of the digestive tract, such as *malabsorption*. Samples of faeces may be examined for their colour, odour, consistency, or for the presence of blood. A test, known as a *faecal occult blood test (FOBT)*, is used to detect concealed blood in the faeces (see *occult blood, faecal*).

F

F

Microscopic examination may be carried out to detect pus, parasites, or microorganisms. Chemical tests may be performed to assess the excretion of fat. (See also *faeces, abnormal*.)

faeces, abnormal

Faeces that differ from normal in their colour, odour, consistency, or content. Abnormal faeces may be an indication of a disorder of the *digestive system* or a related organ, such as the *liver*. A change in the character of faeces, however, is most often due to a change in diet.

Diarrhoea (frequent passage of liquid or very loose faeces) may simply be due to anxiety. However, it may be the result of an intestinal infection (see *gastroenteritis*), an intestinal disorder (such as *ulcerative colitis* or *Crohn's disease*), or *irritable bowel syndrome*. Loose stools may also be an indication of *malabsorption* (impaired absorption of nutrients by the small intestine).

Constipation (infrequent passage of very hard faeces) is generally harmless. Constipation that develops unexpectedly, however, may be caused by a disorder of the large intestine, such as cancer (see *colon, cancer of*).

Pale faeces may be caused by diarrhoea, a lack of bile in the intestine due to *bile duct obstruction*, or a disease that causes malabsorption (such as *coeliac disease*). In malabsorption, the paleness is caused by the high fat content of the faeces. This type of faeces may be oily, foul-smelling, and difficult to flush away.

Dark faeces may result from taking iron tablets. If the faeces are black, however, there may be bleeding in the upper digestive tract.

Faeces that contain excessive mucus are sometimes associated with constipation or with irritable bowel syndrome. *Enteritis*, *dysentery*, or a tumour of the intestine (see *intestine, tumours of*) may also lead to the passage of excess mucus, often accompanied by blood.

Blood in the faeces differs in appearance depending on the site of bleeding. Bleeding from the stomach or duodenum is usually passed in the form of black, tarry faeces (see *melaena*). Blood from the colon is red and is usually passed at the same time as the faeces. Bleeding from the rectum or anus, which may be due to tumours or to *haemorrhoids* (piles), is usually bright red. Occasionally, however, it may not even be visible (see *occult blood, faecal*). (See also *rectal bleeding*.)

faeces, blood in the

See *faeces, abnormal*; *occult blood, faecal*; *rectal bleeding*.

Fahrenheit scale

A temperature scale in which the melting point of ice is 32° and the boiling point of water is 212°. On this scale, normal body temperature is 98.6°F, which is equivalent to 37° Celsius (C). To convert a temperature in Fahrenheit to its Celsius equivalent, subtract 32 and multiply by 0.56 (or 5/9). To convert a Celsius temperature to Fahrenheit, multiply by 1.8 (or 9/5) then add 32. (See also *Celsius scale*.)

Fahr's disease

A rare, degenerative neurological disorder that is characterized by the appearance of abnormal calcium deposits and is associated cell loss in certain areas of the brain. Fahr's disease may be *familial*, in which it shows either an autosomal recessive or autosomal dominant pattern of inheritance (see *genetic disorders*). In many cases, however, the cause of the disorder is unknown.

Symptoms of Fahr's disease include progressive *dementia* (deterioration in brain function) and the loss of acquired motor skills. Increased muscle stiffness and restricted movements may also develop. Possible complications include *athetosis*, characterized by slow, involuntary, writhing movements, or *chorea*, characterized by irregular, rapid, jerky movements. There may also be gradual deterioration of eyesight.

Individual symptoms of Fahr's disease are treated where possible, but there is no cure.

failure to thrive

Failure of expected growth in an infant or toddler, usually assessed by comparing the rate at which a baby gains weight with measurements on a standardized *growth chart*.

An undiagnosed illness such as a urinary tract infection may be the cause. In some cases, however, failure to thrive suggests a more serious disorder such as congenital *heart disease* or *kidney failure*. Emotional or physical deprivation can also result in failure to thrive, especially if the child is undernourished or neglected.

A child who fails to grow at the appropriate rate needs to undergo tests to determine the cause. (See also *growth, childhood*; *child development*.)

fainting

Temporary loss of consciousness due to reduced blood flow to the brain. The medical term is "syncope".

CAUSES

Episodes of fainting are often due to a *vasovagal attack* – an episode in which overstimulation of the *vagus nerve* (which controls vital organs such as the lungs and heart) causes slowing of the heartbeat and a fall in blood pressure, thereby reducing the flow of blood to the brain. Attacks are usually preceded by sweating, nausea, dizziness, and weakness, and are commonly the result of pain, stress, shock, a stuffy atmosphere, or prolonged coughing. Fainting may also result from postural *hypotension* (low blood pressure), which may occur when a person stands still for a long time or stands up suddenly. This problem is common in elderly people, in those with *diabetes mellitus*, and in those taking *antihypertensive drugs* or *vasodilator drugs*.

TREATMENT

In most cases, recovery from fainting occurs when normal blood flow to the brain is restored. This restoration usually happens within minutes because the loss of consciousness results in the person falling into a lying position, which restores the flow of blood to the brain. Medical attention is required in cases of prolonged *unconsciousness* or repeated attacks of fainting.

faith-healing

The supposed ability of certain people to cure disease by a healing force inexplicable to science.

falciparum malaria

The most severe form of *malaria*, which is caused by the parasitic protozoan PLASMODIUM FALCIPARUM.

fallen arches

One of the causes of *flat-feet*. Fallen arches can develop as a result of weakness of the muscles that support the arches of the foot.

fallopian tube

One of the two tubes that extend from the *uterus* to each *ovary*. The fallopian tube transports eggs and sperm and is where *fertilization* takes place.

STRUCTURE

The funnel-shaped fallopian tube is about 10 cm long. It opens into the uterus at one end. The other end, which

LOCATION OF THE FALLOPIAN TUBES

Situated in the pelvis, each tube extends from the upper part of the cavity of the uterus to an ovary.

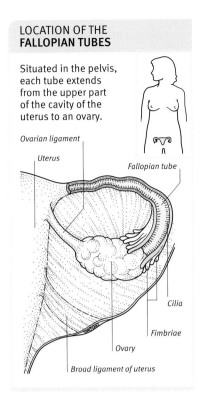

Ovarian ligament
Uterus
Fallopian tube
Cilia
Fimbriae
Ovary
Broad ligament of uterus

is divided into *fimbriae* (fingerlike projections), lies close to the ovary. The tube has muscular walls lined by cells with cilia (hairlike projections).

FUNCTION

The fimbriae take up the egg after it is expelled from the ovary. The beating cilia and muscular contractions propel the egg towards the uterus. After sexual intercourse, sperm swim up the fallopian tube from the uterus. The lining of the tube and its secretions sustain the egg and sperm, encouraging fertilization to take place, and nourish the egg until it reaches the uterus.

DISORDERS

The fallopian tube may become inflamed, usually as a result of a bacterial *sexually transmitted infection* (see *pelvic inflammatory disease*); this can, in some cases, lead to *infertility*. *Ectopic pregnancy* (development of an embryo outside the uterus) is another serious disorder that most commonly occurs in a fallopian tube. This arises when there is a delay in the passage of the fertilized egg along the tube, usually as a result of scarring or blockage. Implantation occurs in the fallopian tube wall, but it is too thin to sustain growth and may eventually rupture and cause internal bleeding. The pregnancy must be terminated.

Fallot's tetralogy

See *tetralogy of Fallot.*

fallout

See *radiation hazards.*

falls in the elderly

The tendency to fall over increases steadily with age, largely due to a gradual slowing down of *reflex* actions; an elderly person who trips is frequently too slow to prevent a fall.

CAUSES

Falls may simply be accidents, which are commonly the result of obstructions on the ground, or they may be caused by medical problems. Various medical conditions that are common in elderly people increase the likelihood of falls. Examples of such conditions are poor sight, *walking* disorders, cardiac *arrhythmia* (an irregular heartbeat), *hypotension* (low blood pressure), and *Parkinson's disease* (a movement disorder). Taking *sleeping drugs* or *tranquillizer drugs* may also increase the risk of falls. Falls sometimes herald the onset of a serious illness, such as *pneumonia.*

COMPLICATIONS

Broken bones (see *fracture*) are a common complication of falls, especially in women. Not only do women have more falls, but they are also more likely to suffer fractures because the strength of their bones may be reduced through *osteoporosis* (loss of bone density).

Falls may sometimes have serious indirect consequences in elderly people. Anyone who falls and lies on the floor for more than an hour, especially if it is cold, may develop *hypothermia.* A fall, or the fear of falling, can also have adverse psychological effects, causing a once active person to become demoralized and housebound.

PREVENTION

Falls may be prevented by taking common-sense measures such as ensuring that floors are free of clutter, good lighting is available, suitable footwear is worn, floor coverings and wiring are safe, and handrails are secure. For elderly people who live alone, personal alarms are available that can be worn round the neck at all times; in the event of a fall the alarm button can be pressed to summon help.

false negative

A test result that wrongly suggests that a particular disease or condition is not present. For example, a false negative

mammography result is one that suggests breast tissue is healthy when, in fact, breast cancer is present.

false positive

A test result that wrongly suggests that a certain disease or condition is present. For example, a false positive *mammography* result appears to reveal a breast cancer, but subsequent tests do not find any evidence of disease.

false pregnancy

See *pregnancy, false.*

false teeth

See *denture.*

false vocal cord

One of two folds of tissue in the *larynx* (voicebox) that are situated above the true *vocal cords* but which are not involved in the production of speech.

famciclovir

An *antiviral drug* used to treat viral infections such as *herpes zoster* (shingles) and genital *herpes simplex.* Minor side effects can include nausea, vomiting, and headache.

familial

A term applied to a characteristic or disorder that runs in families, that is, it occurs in more members of a particular family than would be expected from the occurrence in the population as a whole. An example of a familial characteristic is male-pattern baldness (see *alopecia*); an example of a familial disorder is *hyperlipidaemia* (abnormally high levels of fats in the blood).

familial adenomatous polyposis (FAP)

See *polyposis, familial adenomatous.*

familial cystinuria

See *cystinuria.*

familial goitre

See *goitre.*

familial hypercholesterolaemia

An inherited disorder of lipoprotein metabolism (see *fats and oils*) that is characterized by a high level of the fatty substance *cholesterol* in the blood. An individual suffering from familial hypercholesterolaemia lacks the *low density lipoprotein* receptors in the liver that remove excess cholesterol from the

F

F

blood. The condition shows an autosomal dominant pattern of inheritance (see *genetic disorders*). Because familial hypercholesterolaemia is inherited, if one member of the family has the condition, other members should be screened for it (see *familial screening*).

Raised levels of cholesterol in the blood lead to the early development of *atherosclerosis* (an accumulation of fatty deposits on the inner walls of the arteries), *coronary artery disease*, and other *vascular* diseases. Treatment, which must continue long term, is with *lipid-lowering drugs*, including *statins*, along with a diet that is low in cholesterol and a weight-reduction regime.

familial Mediterranean fever

An inherited condition that affects certain Sephardic Jewish, Armenian, and Arab families. The cause is unknown. Symptoms usually begin between the ages of five and 15 years, and include recurrent episodes of fever, abdominal and chest pain, and arthritis. Red skin swellings sometimes occur, and affected people may also suffer from psychiatric problems. Attacks usually last from 24 to 48 hours but may be longer. Between attacks there are usually no symptoms.

Although there is no specific treatment, those known to suffer from the condition can reduce the incidence of attacks by taking *colchicine*. Death may eventually occur from *amyloidosis*, a complication of the condition.

familial screening

Screening of a family in which one member is affected by an inherited disorder. Looking for evidence of increased susceptibility to a disorder may involve testing for a specific gene defect (as is the case for *cystic fibrosis*), which will also help specialists determine the chances of family members having an affected child.

Alternatively, tests may be carried out to detect a risk factor for a disorder; for example, if a person has a heart attack at an early age, his or her relatives may be tested for *hyperlipidaemia* (high levels of fats in the blood), which increases the risk of *coronary artery disease*.

In addition to being tested for a particular disorder, the relatives of an affected person may be offered regular check-ups so that any abnormal signs may be detected as early as possible and the necessary treatment started without any delay.

family planning

The deliberate limitation or spacing of births. Strategies for family planning include the different methods of *contraception*. (See also *birth control*.)

family therapy

A form of *psychotherapy*, designed to help someone with mental health problems, that is aimed at the whole family rather than just the individual sufferer. The therapist arranges regular meetings with the family to encourage discussion and understanding and to find out what feelings lie behind the way family members deal with each other in everyday life. The main theory behind family therapy is that improving the functioning of the family unit will benefit the individual's health.

famotidine

An *H₂-receptor antagonist* drug that promotes healing of *peptic ulcers* and reduces inflammation of the oesophagus (see *oesophagitis*). Famotidine acts by suppressing production of stomach acid. Side effects are uncommon, but may include headaches and dizziness.

Fanconi's anaemia

A rare type of aplastic anaemia (see *anaemia, aplastic*) in which the bone marrow, which normally makes all of the types of blood cells, produces abnormally low numbers of the cells.

Fanconi's syndrome

A rare kidney disorder that usually occurs in childhood. In Fanconi's syndrome, various important chemicals, such as *amino acids*, *phosphate*, *calcium*, and *potassium*, are lost in the urine. The results of these losses include failure to thrive, stunting of growth, and bone disorders such as *rickets*.

Possible causes include several rare inherited abnormalities of body chemistry and an adverse reaction to certain drugs, such as *tetracycline* that has passed its "use-by" date.

If an underlying chemical abnormality is detected and can be corrected, the affected child may resume normal growth. Alternatively, a *kidney transplant* may be possible.

fantasy

The process of imagining events or objects that are not actually occurring or present. The term also refers to the mental image itself.

Fantasy can give the illusion that wishes have been met. In this sense, it provides satisfaction and can be a means of helping people to cope when reality becomes too unpleasant. Fantasy can also stimulate creativity.

Psychoanalysts believe that certain fantasies are unconscious and represent primitive instincts; these fantasies are presented to the conscious mind in the form of symbols.

farmer's lung

An occupational disease affecting the lungs of farm workers. Farmer's lung is a type of allergic *alveolitis*, in which affected people develop *hypersensitivity* (an excessive reaction of the immune system) to certain moulds or fungi that grow on hay, grain, or straw. The causative organisms thrive in warm, damp conditions, and outbreaks are most common in areas of high rainfall.

SYMPTOMS
Symptoms typically develop about six hours after exposure to dust containing fungal spores. They include shortness of breath, headache, fever, and muscle aches. In acute attacks, the symptoms last for about a day. Repeated exposure to spores may lead to a chronic form of the disease, causing permanent scarring of lung tissues.

DIAGNOSIS AND TREATMENT
Diagnosis of farmer's lung may involve a *chest X-ray*; *pulmonary function tests*; and blood tests for a specific *antibody* to the fungus.

Corticosteroid drugs relieve the symptoms of the condition. Further exposure to the spores of the fungus should be avoided. Complete recovery is likely if the disease is diagnosed before permanent lung damage has occurred. (See also *fibrosing alveolitis*.)

farmer's skin

Premature aging of the skin caused by prolonged exposure to sunlight. Features of farmer's skin include a lack of elasticity, wrinkling, dryness, thinning (sometimes with thicker areas), and excessive skin pigmentation.

fascia

Fibrous *connective tissue* that surrounds many structures in the body. One layer of the tissue, known as the superficial fascia, envelops the entire body just beneath the skin. Another layer, the deep fascia, encloses muscles, forming a sheath for individual muscles and separating them into groups; it also holds in place soft organs such as the kidneys. Thick fascia in the palm of the hand and sole of the foot have a cushioning, protective function.

fasciculation

Spontaneous, irregular, and usually continual contractions of a muscle that is apparently at rest. Unlike the contractions of *fibrillation*, fasciculation is visible through the skin.

Minor fasciculation, such as that occurring in the eyelids, is common and is no cause for concern. However, persistent fasciculation with weakness in the affected muscle indicates damage to the nerve cells in the spine that control the muscle, or to the nerve fibres that connect the spinal nerves to the muscle; *motor neuron disease* is one such disorder.

fasciitis

Inflammation of a layer of *fascia* (fibrous connective tissue), causing pain and tenderness. It is usually the result of straining or injuring the fascia surrounding a muscle and most commonly affects the sole of the foot. Fasciitis may occur in people with *ankylosing spondylitis* (a rheumatic disorder affecting the spine) or those with *Reiter's syndrome* (inflammation of the urethra, conjunctivitis, and arthritis).

Treatment of fasciitis involves resting the affected area and protecting it from pressure. A local injection of a *corticosteroid drug* may be given. If fasciitis is part of a widespread disorder of the joints, treatment of this condition will generally improve symptoms. (See also *necrotizing fasciitis*.)

fascioliasis

A disease affecting the liver and bile ducts that is caused by infestation with the *liver fluke* species FASCIOLA HEPATICA. Fascioliasis is acquired through eating plant food (such as watercress) contaminated with the larvae of the fluke. Treatment is with *anthelmintic drugs*.

fasciotomy

An operation to relieve pressure on muscles by making an incision in the *fascia* (fibrous connective tissue) that surrounds them.

Fasciotomy is usually performed to treat *compartment syndrome*, a painful condition in which constriction of a group of muscles causes obstruction of blood flow; it gives the muscles space in which to expand. The procedure is also sometimes performed as a surgical emergency after an injury has resulted in muscle swelling or bleeding within a muscle compartment.

fasting

Abstaining from all food and drinking only water. In temperate conditions and at moderate levels of activity, a person can survive on water alone for more than two months; however, without consuming either food or drink, death usually occurs within about ten days.

EFFECTS ON THE BODY

In the absence of food, the energy needed to maintain essential body processes is supplied by substances stored in the body tissues. About six hours after the last meal, the body starts to use *glycogen* (a carbohydrate stored in the liver and muscles). This process continues for about 24 hours, after which time the body obtains energy from stored fat and by breaking down protein in the muscles. If fasting continues, the body's *metabolism* slows down in an attempt to conserve energy, and the fat and protein stores are consumed more slowly.

In the initial stages of fasting, weight loss is rapid. It then slows down, not only due to the slowing of the metabolism, but also because the body begins to conserve its salt supply, resulting in the retention of water in the tissues. This accumulated fluid causes *oedema* (swelling), which principally affects the legs and abdomen.

In prolonged fasting, the ability to digest food may be impaired because the stomach stops secreting digestive juices. Prolonged fasting also halts the production of sex hormones, causing *amenorrhoea* (the absence of menstruation) in women.

fat

A substance that is composed of one or more *fatty acids*. Fat is the main form in which energy is stored by the body. A layer of fat, known as *adipose tissue*, lies directly beneath the skin and surrounds various internal organs. Excess amounts of fat are deposited under the skin in *obesity*. (See also *fats and oils*.)

fat atrophy

Localized loss of fatty tissue beneath the skin. Fat atrophy can occur at injection sites in people with type 1 (insulin-dependent) *diabetes mellitus*. A particular pattern of fat atrophy also develops in some people being treated with *antiretroviral drugs* for *HIV* infection or *AIDS* (see *lipodystrophy*).

fatigue

See *tiredness*.

fat pad

A localized collection of fatty tissue. Fat pads are normally found in parts of the body that need cushioning and protection, such as behind the eyeballs, around the kidneys, behind the knees, under the heel bone, and in the cheeks (especially in infants). Abnormal fat pads may be noncancerous tumours (see *lipoma*) or may develop in certain disorders, such as *lipodystrophy*.

fats and oils

Nutrients that provide the body with its most concentrated form of *energy*. Fats are the largest group of *lipids*, and are compounds containing chains of carbon and hydrogen atoms with very little oxygen. Chemically, they consist mostly of *fatty acids* combined with *glycerol*. Fats are usually solid at room temperature, while oils are liquid. *Cholesterol* is not strictly a fat but a fatlike substance that is produced naturally in the body by the liver and also obtained from the diet; it is transported around the body in the blood in the form of lipoprotein.

TYPES

Fats and oils are divided into two main groups – saturated and unsaturated – depending on the proportion of hydrogen atoms they contain. If the fatty acids contain the maximum possible quantity of hydrogen, the fats are saturated. If some sites on the carbon chain are unoccupied by hydrogen, they are unsaturated. Monounsaturated fats are unsaturated fats with only one site that could take an extra hydrogen atom; if many sites are vacant, the fats are polyunsaturated. Animal fats, such as those in meat and dairy products, are largely saturated; vegetable fats tend to be unsaturated. Trans fats are unsaturated fats that are produced artificially by hydrogenating (chemically altering by adding hydrogens atoms) vegetable oils to turn them into solid fats.

FAT AND HEALTH

The amount and types of fat in the diet have important implications for health. A diet containing a large amount of fat, particularly saturated fat, is linked to obesity and an increased risk of *athero-*

F

F

sclerosis (deposition of fat on the walls of arteries) and of subsequent *coronary artery disease* and *stroke*. Trans fats, although they are unsaturated, seem to act like saturated fats in the body and are associated with the same health risks. Other serious disorders related to the consumption of excess fat include cancers of the breast, colon, and prostate and type 2 (non-insulin-dependent) *diabetes mellitus*.

USES IN THE BODY

Some dietary fats, mainly triglycerides (combinations of glycerol and three fatty acids), are sources of the fat-soluble vitamins A, D, E, and K and also of essential fatty acids.

Triglycerides are the main form of fat stored in the body. These stores act as an energy reserve; they also provide insulation and a protective layer for delicate organs such as the heart and kidneys. *Phospholipids* are structural fats found in cell membranes. Sterols, such as cholesterol, are found in animal and plant tissues; they have a variety of functions, and are essential for making hormones or vitamins. Phospholipids and sterols are made in the body from nutrients provided in the diet.

FAT METABOLISM

Dietary fats are first emulsified (reduced to microscopic particles) by *bile* salts before being broken down by lipase, a pancreatic *enzyme*. They are absorbed via the *lymphatic system* before entering the bloodstream.

To be carried in the blood, the lipids become bound to proteins; in this state, they are known as lipoproteins. There are four classes of lipoprotein: chylomicrons; high-density lipoproteins (HDLs); low-density lipoproteins (LDLs); and very low-density lipoproteins (VLDLs). LDLs and VLDLs contain large amounts of cholesterol, which they carry through the bloodstream and deposit in tissues; they are sometimes referred to as "bad fats". HDLs, commonly known as "good fats", pick up cholesterol and carry it back to the liver for processing and excretion. High levels of LDLs are associated with atherosclerosis, whereas HDLs have a protective effect. (See also *nutrition*.)

fatty acids

Organic acids, containing carbon, oxygen, and hydrogen, that are constituents of *fats and oils*. There are more than 40 fatty acids found in nature; they are differentiated by their constituent numbers of carbon and hydrogen atoms.

Certain fatty acids cannot be synthesized by the body and must be provided by the diet. These substances are collectively termed essential fatty acids. Nutritionally important essential fatty acids include the omega-3 fatty acids alpha-linolenic acid (ALA), eicosapentaenoic acid (EPA), and docosahexaenoic acid (DHA). Nutritionally important omega-6 fatty acids include gamma-linolenic acid (GLA), arachidonic acid (AA), and dihomo-gamma-linolenic acid (DGLA). (See also *nutrition*.)

fatty degeneration

A general term describing the accumulation of fat within the cells of tissues damaged by disease.

fatty diarrhoea

See *steatorrhoea*.

fatty liver

A condition in which fat accumulates within the liver cells. The most common cause of fatty liver is excessive consumption of alcohol which, if continued, eventually leads to *cirrhosis*. However, if the drinking of alcohol stops, the fat clears from the liver. Fatty liver can also occur in association with *obesity, diabetes mellitus*, starvation, and in some cases of chronic ill-health.

favism

A disorder that is characterized by an extreme sensitivity to the broad bean VICIA FABA (fava bean). If an affected person eats these beans, a chemical in the bean causes rapid destruction of red blood cells, leading to a severe type of anaemia (see *anaemia, haemolytic*).

Favism is uncommon except in some areas of the Mediterranean. It is a sex-linked *genetic disorder*. Affected people have *G6PD deficiency*, a defect in a certain chemical pathway in their red blood cells that normally helps protect the cells from injury.

Children with a family history of favism can be screened for the disorder at an early age. If the condition is found, they must avoid fava beans as well as certain drugs, including some *antimalarial drugs* and *antibiotic drugs*, that can have a similar effect on their red blood cells.

febrile

Feverish or related to *fever*. Febrile convulsions, for example, occur mainly in young children with high temperatures (see *convulsion, febrile*).

febrile convulsion

See *convulsion, febrile*.

feedback

A self-regulating mechanism that controls certain body processes, such as hormone and enzyme production. If, for example, levels of a hormone are too high, output of any substance that stimulates the hormone's release is inhibited; the result is reduced hormone production (negative feedback). The reverse process (positive feedback) restores the balance if levels of a hormone become too low. (See also *endocrine system*.)

feeding, artificial

The administration of nutrients other than by mouth, usually by way of a tube passed through the nose into the stomach or small intestine. If long-term artificial feeding is anticipated, a tube is inserted directly into the stomach or upper small intestine during endoscopic surgery (see *gastroscopy*). This is called *enteral feeding*. If the gastrointestinal tract is not functioning, nutrients must be introduced directly into the bloodstream (see *infusion, intravenous*). This type of feeding is known as *parenteral nutrition*.

TUBE FEEDING

Tube feeding may be necessary for people who have difficulty swallowing, or gastrointestinal disorders (for example, conditions resulting in *malabsorption*), or disorders affecting the nervous system or kidneys. Premature babies often require tube feeding if their *suckling reflexes* are undeveloped, as do critically ill patients due to their increased nutritional requirements.

Food mixtures, or preparations of nutrients, are given through a tube that is passed through the patient's nostril and down to the stomach or duodenum. There are two methods of feeding: continuous drip feeding, and bolus feeding (in which set amounts of nutrients are given at regular intervals throughout the day). In both methods, the rate of delivery of the food can be controlled by a pump.

INTRAVENOUS FEEDING

Intravenous feeding is usually given when large areas of the small intestine have been damaged by disease or have been surgically removed. Nutrient preparations are given and are inserted into a large central vein near the heart, via a *catheter* (a thin, flexible tube) that is buried under the skin.

feeding, infant

A person grows more rapidly in his or her first year than at any other time in life. A good diet is essential for healthy growth and development.

BREAST- OR BOTTLE-FEEDING

During the first six months, most nutritional requirements are satisfied by *milk* alone, whether by *breast-feeding* or by *bottle-feeding*. Both human milk and formula milk contain carbohydrate, protein, fat, vitamins, and minerals in similar proportions; human milk also contains *antibodies* and *white blood cells* that protect the baby against infection. From six months of age, supplementary *vitamins A, C,* and *D* should be given to breast-fed babies. (Formula milk already contains vitamin supplements.) Cows' milk should not be given in the first year of life. From one year, it is safe to feed with full-fat cows' milk.

FEEDING AN INFANT: INTRODUCING SOLIDS

Following concerns about increases in food allergies and childhood obesity, there have been changes in government guidelines on the age at which an infant is weaned on to solids. There is no need to feed solid foods to an infant below the age of six months. From this age, infants should, ideally, be placed in a highchair and encouraged to self-feed. The following is a flexible guide:

Age	Time	Food
6 months	Early morning	Breast- or bottle-feed.
	Breakfast	Cereal, followed by breast- or bottle-feed.
	Lunch	Offer minced or mashed, but not pureed, food. Give meat with vegetables. Offer water instead of milk.
	Mid-afternoon	Mashed banana or other soft fruit, followed by usual milk feed.
	Dinner	Breast- or bottle-feed if the baby is still hungry.
6 to 7 months	Early morning	Breast- or bottle-feed.
	Breakfast	Cereal with well-cooked scrambled egg. Offer breast- or bottle-milk from a cup.
	Lunch	Give meat or fish with some vegetables, then offer fruit. Give a drink of water.
	Late afternoon/dinner	Meat or cheese sandwich. Milk from a cup.
7 to 8 months	Early morning	Offer a drink of water instead of milk.
	Breakfast	Cereal and hard-boiled egg with wholemeal bread. A drink of milk.
	Lunch	Cheese, fish, or minced meat with some vegetables. Pudding or fresh fruit. A drink of water.
	Late afternoon/dinner	Meat or cheese sandwich. A drink of milk.
9 to 12 months	Early morning	A drink of water.
	Breakfast	Cereal, then well-cooked egg or fish with wholemeal toast and butter. A drink of milk.
	Lunch	Chopped meat, fish, or cheese, with vegetables. Pudding or fresh fruit. A drink of water.
	Late afternoon/dinner	Meat or cheese sandwich. A drink of milk.

WARNING Avoid eggs, fish, and citrus fruit (including juice) before six months. Nuts should not be given to babies under one year, and whole nuts should not be given under five years. Avoid gluten before six months. Parents should be especially careful about feeding their children foods containing gluten or peanuts because serious allergies to these products are common.

INTRODUCING SOLIDS

Solids should be introduced from six months of age. How they are introduced depends on the baby's birth weight, rate of growth, and contentment with feeding. From six months, the baby should be eating true solids, such as minced meat and vegetables, and at this stage can start eating well-cooked eggs. Vegetables, such as avocado, and wheat-based cereals can be introduced as soft finger foods. A baby under one year should not be given honey or products containing nuts. Salt and sugar used in home-prepared meals should be kept to a minimum to prevent kidney problems and dental decay, respectively. By the age of one year, three family-food meals and two milk feeds, one at breakfast and one at bedtime, would be the norm.

FEEDING PROBLEMS

A few babies have an intolerance to certain foods, such as lactose or cows' milk protein (see *food intolerance*; *nutritional disorders*). Reactions can include vomiting, diarrhoea, or rashes. Difficulties associated with milk usually appear within the first month; solids should be introduced one by one so that any foods that cause problems can be identified.

Prolonged crying after feeds may mean that the baby needs help bringing up wind, that artificial milk is not being digested properly, or that the baby has colic (see *colic, infantile*).

felbinac

A *nonsteroidal anti-inflammatory drug* (NSAID) that is used for the relief of pain and inflammation in injuries such as sprains or bruising. Felbinac is applied topically as a gel or aerosol foam. Rarely, it may cause localized skin irritation. As some of the drug is absorbed in the bloodstream, felbinac should not be taken by anyone with an adverse reaction to oral (taken by mouth) NSAIDs, such as worsening of asthma.

Felty's syndrome

A disorder that is characterized by an enlarged *spleen* and an abnormally low white *blood cell* count. Felty's syndrome occurs in some people with *rheumatoid arthritis*, but the exact cause is unknown.

Symptoms of Felty's syndrome may include general malaise, fatigue, loss of appetite, weight loss, *anaemia*, joint swelling and stiffness, and recurrent infections. Possible signs of the condition include an enlarged spleen and, in some cases, swollen *lymph nodes*.

F

F

Treatment is the same as for rheumatoid arthritis. *Splenectomy* (removal of the spleen) may be needed in some cases.

female

An individual with two X *sex chromosomes*. Females are also characterized by the presence of a vagina and vulva (see *sexual characteristics, primary*).

female catheter

A short *catheter* (flexible tube) that can be inserted into a woman's bladder through the *urethra* for the purpose of withdrawing *urine*.

feminization

Development of female secondary sexual characteristics in a male (such as breast enlargement and loss of facial hair). The condition is due either to a hormonal disorder or *hormone* therapy. (See also *demasculinization*; *intersex*; *masculinization*; *sex determination*; *sexual characteristics, secondary*; *testicular feminization syndrome*.)

femoral artery

A major blood vessel that supplies oxygenated blood to the leg. The femoral artery is formed in the pelvis from the iliac artery, which is the terminal branch of the *aorta*. It then runs from the groin down the front of the thigh, and passes behind the knee to become the popliteal artery, which branches again to supply the lower leg.

femoral epiphysis, slipped

Displacement of the upper *epiphysis* (growing end) of the *femur* (thigh bone). Such displacement is rare; it usually affects children between the ages of 11 and 13, and occurs more often in boys and obese children. The condition tends to run in families.

During normal growth, the epiphysis is separated from the shaft of the bone by a plate of *cartilage*. This area is relatively weak, so a fall or any other type of injury can cause the epiphysis to slip out of position. If this happens, a limp develops, and pain is felt in the knee or groin. The leg tends to turn outwards, and movements of the hip are restricted.

Surgery is needed to fix the epiphysis into its correct position; the procedure is usually successful, although following the injury and repair, the hip tends to be more susceptible than normal to *osteoarthritis*. In some cases, the other hip may also need to be stabilized.

femoral hernia

A type of *hernia* that occurs in the groin area, at the point where the *femoral artery* and femoral vein pass from the lower abdomen to the thigh. Women who are overweight or who have had several pregnancies are at risk of femoral hernia because their abdominal muscles are weakened.

femoral nerve

One of the main nerves of the leg. The nerve fibres that form the femoral nerve emerge from the lower spine and run down into the thigh, where they branch to supply the skin and front muscles of the thigh. The nerve branches supplying the skin convey sensation; the branches supplying the muscles stimulate contraction of the *quadriceps muscle*, thereby straightening the knee.

Damage to the femoral nerve (which impairs the ability to straighten the knee) is usually the result of a slipped disc in the lumbar region of the spine (see *disc prolapse*). Damage may also result from a dislocation of the hip or from a *neuropathy*.

femur

The medical name for the thigh bone, which is the longest bone in the body. The lower end of the femur hinges with the tibia (shin) to form the knee joint. The upper end is rounded into a ball (the head of the femur) that fits exactly into a socket in the pelvis to form the hip joint.

The head of the femur is joined to the bone shaft by a narrow piece of bone called the neck of the femur, which is a common fracture site (see *femur, fracture of*). At the lower end, the bone is enlarged to form two lumps (the condyles) that distribute the weight-bearing load through the knee joint. On the outer side of the upper femur is a protuberance called the greater trochanter.

The shaft of the femur is surrounded by muscles that move the hip and knee joints. The shaft is also well supplied with blood vessels; therefore, a fracture can result in considerable blood loss.

femur, fracture of

A break in the femur (the thigh bone). The symptoms, treatment, and possible complications of a fracture depend on whether the bone has broken across its neck (the short section between the top of the shaft and the hip joint) or across the shaft. The treatment also depends on the age of the patient and the condition of the bones.

FRACTURE OF NECK OF FEMUR

This type of fracture, which is often called a broken hip, is very common in elderly people, especially in women with the bone disorder *osteoporosis* (loss of bone density). It is usually associated with a fall. In a fracture of the neck of the femur, the broken ends are often considerably displaced; in such cases there is usually severe pain in the hip and groin, making standing impossible. Occasionally, the broken bone ends become impacted (pushed together). In this case, there is less pain, and walking may be possible.

The diagnosis is confirmed by *X-ray*. If the ends of the bone are displaced, an operation is necessary, either to realign the bone ends and fasten them together, or to replace the entire head and neck of the femur with an artificial substitute (see *hip replacement*). If the bone ends are impacted, the fracture may heal naturally, but surgery may still be recommended.

A possible complication is damage to the blood supply to the head of the femur, resulting in the disintegration of the bone in that area (see *avascular necrosis*). *Osteoarthritis* may develop in

LOCATION OF THE **FEMUR**

The femur extends from the hip joint, down the thigh, to the knee joint.

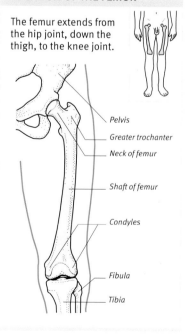

Pelvis

Greater trochanter

Neck of femur

Shaft of femur

Condyles

Fibula

Tibia

the hip joint after fracture of the femur neck. In elderly people, immobility and surgery may result in complications, such as *pneumonia*, that are not directly related to the fracture site.

FRACTURE OF SHAFT OF FEMUR
Fracture of the bone shaft usually occurs when the femur is subjected to extreme force, such as that occurring in a traffic accident. In most cases, the bone ends are considerably displaced, causing severe pain, tenderness, and swelling. With a fractured femoral shaft there is often substantial blood loss from the bone.

The diagnosis is confirmed by X-ray. The fracture is usually repaired by surgery in which the fractured ends of the bone are realigned and fastened together with a metal pin or a more extensive fixation device. Sometimes, however, the bone ends can be realigned by manipulation and surgery is unnecessary. After realignment, the leg is supported with a *splint* and put in *traction* to hold the bone while it heals.

Possible complications include failure of the bone ends to unite or fusion of the broken ends at the wrong angle; *osteomyelitis* (infection of the bone); or damage to a nerve or artery. A fracture of the lower shaft can cause permanent knee stiffness.

fenbufen

A *nonsteroidal anti-inflammatory drug* (NSAID) that is used to relieve pain and stiffness caused, for example, by *rheumatoid arthritis*, *osteoarthritis*, and *gout*. Fenbufen is also used to reduce pain and to help speed recovery following muscle and ligament sprains.

In common with many NSAIDs, fenbufen can cause irritation of the stomach lining (see *gastritis*) and may also cause a rash.

fenestration

A surgical procedure in which an artificial opening, or window, is created in a sheath or a membrane. For example, fenestration may involve removal of part of the wall of a *cyst* to prevent fluid from reaccumulating.

fenoprofen

A *nonsteroidal anti-inflammatory drug* (NSAID) that is used to relieve pain and stiffness caused, for example, by *rheumatoid arthritis*, *osteoarthritis*, and *gout*. Fenoprofen is also used to treat muscle and ligament sprains; it reduces pain and helps to speed recovery.

In common with many NSAIDs, fenoprofen may cause irritation of the stomach lining (see *gastritis*).

fentanyl

An *opioid* analgesic drug that is given by injection to provide pain relief during surgery and to enhance general anaesthesia (see *anaesthesia, general*). It is also used in the form of a skin patch to control the severe chronic pain of conditions such as cancer.

In common with other opioid drugs, fentanyl has side effects that include depressed breathing, constipation, nausea, and vomiting. The use of patches containing fentanyl may be associated with local irritation of the skin.

ferritin

A complex of *iron* and protein, found mainly in the liver and spleen. Ferritin is the principal form in which iron is stored in the body.

ferrous fumarate

A form of *iron* given in an oral preparation to treat iron-deficiency *anaemia*. Ferrous fumarate can cause diarrhoea, constipation, and abdominal pain.

ferrous sulphate

Another name for *iron* sulphate.

fertile period

The period during a woman's *menstrual cycle* when *conception* is most likely to occur. The fertile period is usually between three and five days in duration, beginning just before *ovulation*. Ovulation occurs about 14 days before a new menstrual cycle begins.

fertility

The ability to produce children without undue difficulty. Fertility depends on both male and female partners.

MALE FERTILITY
A man's fertility depends on the production of normal quantities of healthy *sperm* in the testes (see *testis*). This, in turn, depends on adequate production of *gonadotrophin hormones* by the *pituitary gland*. Male fertility also depends on being able to achieve an *erection* and to ejaculate *semen* into the vagina during *sexual intercourse*. Males become fertile at puberty and usually remain so, although to a lessening degree, well into old age.

FEMALE FERTILITY
A woman's ability to conceive depends on normal *ovulation* (the monthly pro-

duction of a healthy *ovum*, or egg, by an *ovary*) and the ovum's unimpeded passage down a *fallopian tube* towards the *uterus*; on thinning of the mucus surrounding the mouth of the *cervix*, to enable sperm to penetrate; and on changes in the lining of the uterus that prepare it for the implantation of a fertilized ovum.

These processes, in turn, depend on normal production of gonadotrophins by the pituitary gland, and of the sex hormones *oestrogen* and *progesterone* by the ovaries.

Women become fertile at puberty and remain so (although to a lessening degree as they become older) until the *menopause*, which usually occurs between 45 and 55 years of age. (See also *fertility drugs*; *infertility*.)

fertility drugs

COMMON DRUGS
• Clomifene • Follicle-stimulating hormone • Gonadorelin analogues • Human chorionic gonadotrophin • Luteinizing hormone • Metformin • Tamoxifen

A group of hormonal or hormone-related drugs that are used to treat some types of *infertility*.

In women, fertility drugs may be given when the abnormal production of hormones by the *pituitary gland* or ovaries (see *ovary*) disrupts *ovulation* (the release of an ovum, or egg, from an ovary) or causes mucus around the *cervix* to become so thick that sperm cannot penetrate it. Treatment with the drug *clomifene*, which may continue over a number of months, can help to bring about ovulation in women whose pituitary glands do not produce sufficient hormones for ovulation to occur naturally. If this treatment fails to produce ovulation, treatment with follicle-stimulating hormone (FSH), followed by an injection of human chorionic gonadotrophin (HCG; see *gonadotrophin hormones*), may be given in order to stimulate ripening of the ovum and ovulation. Women with *polycystic ovary syndrome* who have not responded to treatment with clomifene may be treated with metformin.

Treatment with fertility drugs must be monitored carefully to avoid overstimulation of the ovaries, symptoms of which may include nausea, vomiting, abdominal swelling, and the development of massive ovarian cysts. The condition is potentially life-threatening.

THE PROCESS OF **FERTILIZATION**

Fertilization occurs when the head of a sperm penetrates a mature ovum. After penetration, the nuclei (which contain the genetic material) of the sperm and ovum fuse and the body and tail of the sperm drop off. the newly fertilized ovum, called a zygote, then forms an outer layer that is impenetrable to other sperm. the zygote undergoes repeated cell divisions as it passes down the fallopian tube. By the time it reaches the uterus, it has grown into a solid ball of cells called a morula. it then develops an inner cavity with a small cluster of cells to one side; this is called a blastocyst.

F

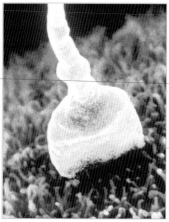

Sperm and ovum
A single sperm penetrates the ovum, thereby fertilizing it. To achieve this, the sperm releases enzymes that dissolve a path through the ovum's outer layers.

FERTILE PERIOD

Ovulation occurs halfway through the menstrual cycle (13 to 16 days before the start of a period), after which the released ovum is available for fertilization for about two days. Sperm can also live for about two days, so the peak fertile period is about four days (two pre- and two post-ovulation).

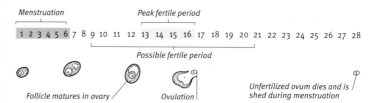

Peak and possible fertile periods
Although the peak fertile period is about four days, the possible fertile period may last seven to 12 days, due to variations in how long the ovum and sperm can survive and the timing of ovulation. The illustration shows the peak and maximum possible fertile periods in a 28-day cycle.

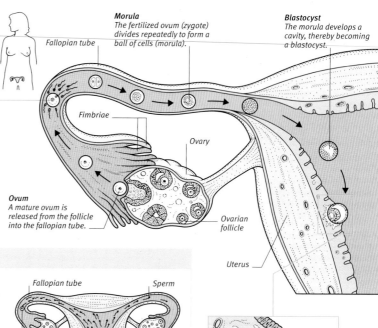

Morula
The fertilized ovum (zygote) divides repeatedly to form a ball of cells (morula).

Blastocyst
The morula develops a cavity, thereby becoming a blastocyst.

Fallopian tube

Fimbriae

Ovary

Ovum
A mature ovum is released from the follicle into the fallopian tube.

Ovarian follicle

Uterus

JOURNEY OF THE SPERM

When semen is ejaculated into the vagina, as many as 500 million sperm are released, most of which are capable of fertilizing an ovum. But, as they travel upwards (propelled by their whiplike tails), more than half are killed by acidic vaginal secretions; many more die during the journey up through the cervix and uterus and into the fallopian tubes. The journey can take from less than half-an-hour to five hours and, by the end, only a few thousand sperm have survived.

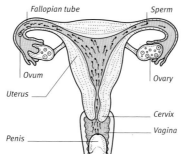

Lifespan of sperm
A sperm can survive in a fallopian tube for up to 48 hours, during which time it is capable of fertilizing an ovum.

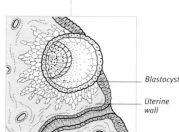

Blastocyst
The blastocyst embeds in the uterine wall (implantation), where it develops into an embryo and also forms the placenta.

Fertility drugs are generally less effective in men but may be used when abnormal hormone production by the pituitary gland or testes interferes with sperm production. Low sperm production may be treated with gonadotrophins (FSH or HCG). (See also *testosterone*.)

fertilization

The union of a *sperm* and an *ovum* (egg cell). In natural fertilization (see the illustrated box), the sperm and ovum unite in the woman's *fallopian tube* following *sexual intercourse*.

Fertilization may also occur as a result of semen being artificially introduced into the cervix (see *artificial insemination*) or it may take place in a laboratory (see *in vitro fertilization*).

festinating gait

An involuntary style of *walking* in which a person moves, often on tiptoe, with progressively shortening and accelerating steps. It is a feature of *parkinsonism*.

fetal alcohol syndrome

A rare combination of birth defects that occur as a result of continued, excessive *alcohol* consumption by the baby's mother during *pregnancy*.

The affected baby has diminished growth, a small head and brain, and small eyes. He or she may also have a cleft palate, a small jaw, heart defects, and joint abnormalities. As a newborn, the baby sucks poorly, sleeps badly, and is irritable due to alcohol withdrawal.

Some affected babies die during the first few weeks of life. Those who survive may experience delayed mental development and are, to some degree, mentally and physically disabled.

fetal circulation

Blood circulation in the fetus is different from the normal circulation after birth (see *circulatory system*). The fetus neither breathes nor eats, so oxygen and nutrients are obtained, via the *placenta* and *umbilical cord*, from the mother's blood. The other fundamental difference in circulation is that blood bypasses the lungs in the fetus.

Oxygen and nutrients enter the fetal blood through the placenta, an organ embedded in the wall of the uterus and connected to the fetus by the umbilical cord. The maternal and fetal circulations are separated by a thin membrane in the placenta, which allows the exchange of nutrients and waste products.

Before birth

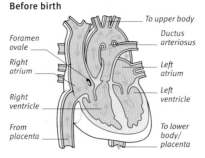

After birth

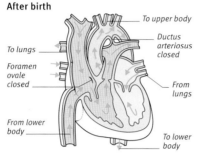

Fetal heart circulation
In the fetus, blood passes directly from the right atrium of the heart to the left atrium through the foramen ovale. Another channel, the ductus arteriosus, allows blood to pass from the pulmonary artery to the aorta. After birth, both channels close redirecting blood through the lungs.

Oxygenated and nutrient-rich blood flows from the mother to the fetus along a vein in the umbilical cord before entering the right atrium (upper chamber) of the heart. Then, instead of flowing to the lungs, it bypasses them by flowing into the left atrium via an opening known as the foramen ovale. From there, the blood passes to the left ventricle (lower chamber), where it is pumped to the upper parts of the body to provide the tissues with oxygen.

Blood returning to the heart flows into the right atrium and from there into the right ventricle. In the fetus, the blood is only partly deoxygenated at this stage and has more tissues to supply with oxygen. Bypassing the lungs again, it flows from the pulmonary artery into the aorta, through a channel called the ductus arteriosus. The aorta carries the blood to the lower parts of the body. From there, completely deoxygenated blood is carried via the umbilical cord to the placenta, where carbon dioxide and other waste products diffuse into the mother's blood.

After birth, the foramen and the ductus arteriosus normally close. Blood pumped from the right ventricle passes via the pulmonary artery to the lungs for reoxygenation and elimination of carbon dioxide and other wastes. In rare cases, the foramen ovale or ductus arteriosus fails to close after birth, causing a congenital heart disorder (see *heart disease, congenital*).

fetal death

See *stillbirth*.

fetal distress

The physical stress experienced by a fetus during *labour* as a result of not receiving enough oxygen. During each contraction, the uterus tightens and thus reduces the oxygen supply from the placenta to the fetus. If there are also problems, such as pressure on the *umbilical cord* or the mother losing blood, there may be an inadequate amount of oxygen reaching the fetus.

MONITORING

Various monitoring techniques may be used during childbirth to detect any signs of fetal distress. A cardiotocograph (see *fetal heart monitoring*) will record whether the baby's heart rate is slow or if it is failing to show normal variability. *Acidosis* (high acidity in the body), which indicates that the oxygen supply to the fetus is inadequate, can be detected in a sample of blood taken from the baby's scalp. Signs of *meconium* (fetal faeces) in the amniotic fluid can also be an indication of fetal distress.

DELIVERY

Fetal distress sometimes occurs as a temporary episode, but, if acidosis is severe, the distressed fetus may need to be delivered promptly by *caesarean section*, *forceps delivery*, or *vacuum extraction*. (See also *childbirth*.)

fetal heart monitoring

The use of an instrument to record and/or listen to an unborn baby's heartbeat during *pregnancy* and *labour*.

WHY IT IS DONE

The fetal heart is checked routinely during pregnancy with a fetal stethoscope or *Doppler ultrasound* scanning. Additional monitoring is carried out if tests indicate that the placenta is not functioning normally or if the baby's growth is slow. Uterine contractions or other stimuli, such as reflex kicking, increase the heart rate in a healthy fetus; the midwife or obstetrician can detect this using a fetal heart monitor. During labour, monitoring can detect *fetal distress*, in which oxygen deprivation causes abnormalities in the fetal heart rate.

F

F

HOW IT IS DONE

The most simple form of fetal heart monitoring involves using a special fetal stethoscope. Cardiotocography, a more sophisticated electronic version, is a procedure that produces a continuous paper recording of the heartbeat and a recording of the uterine contractions. The heartbeat is picked up either externally by an *ultrasound* transducer strapped to the mother's abdomen or, as an alternative during labour, internally by an electrode attached to the baby's scalp that passes through the vagina and cervix. The mother's uterine contractions are measured and recorded by an external pressure gauge strapped to the mother's abdomen, or by an internal plastic tube inserted through the vagina into the amniotic fluid.

fetal movement

Movements made by a developing fetus in the uterus, which can usually be detected by the mother from between about the 16th and 20th weeks of pregnancy. Fetal movement at this stage may feel like a gentle "flutter" to the mother; later in pregnancy the fetus becomes more vigorous in its movements and may kick as it moves around in the amniotic sac. Some fetuses are more active than others. In late pregnancy, to monitor fetal wellbeing, the number of movements may be recorded on a "kick chart".

fetishism

Reliance on special objects in order to achieve sexual arousal. The objects need not have an obvious sexual meaning; they may include shoes, rubber or leather garments, and parts of the body such as the feet or ears.

Fetishism usually has no obvious cause. According to psychoanalysts, the origin may be a childhood *fixation* of sexual interest upon some aspect of the mother's appearance. Treatment is necessary only if the behaviour leads to distress or is causing persistent criminal acts.

fetoscopy

A procedure for directly observing a fetus inside the uterus using a fetoscope, which is a type of *endoscope* (a tubelike viewing instrument). Fetoscopy allows a close-up look at the fetus, particularly the face, limbs, genitals, and spine, and is used to diagnose various *congenital* abnormalities before birth.

DEVELOPMENT OF THE **FETUS**

By the 32nd week of pregnancy, the internal organs of the fetus are almost fully mature and it is perfectly formed. In most cases, the fetus has turned to lie head-down in the pelvis.

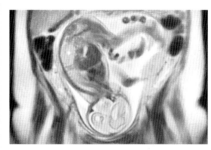

Fetus in sac
This MRI scan shows the developing fetus head-down in the mother's uterus during the 36th week of pregnancy. Internal organs (such as the brain) are fully formed.

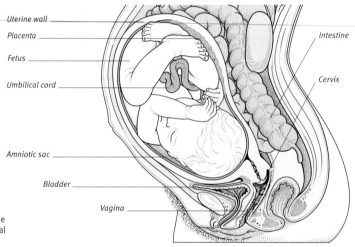

Uterine wall
Placenta
Fetus
Umbilical cord
Amniotic sac
Bladder
Vagina
Intestine
Cervix

GROWTH OF THE FETUS FROM 8 TO 40 WEEKS

Between the eighth week and term (the 40th week), the length of the fetus (from crown to rump) increases by 20 times and its weight increases by about 1,700 times.

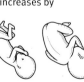

Week	8	12	16	20	24	28	32	36	40
Length	2.5 cm	7.5 cm	16 cm	25 cm	33 cm	37 cm	40.5 cm	46 cm	51 cm
Weight	2 g	18 g	135 g	340 g	570 g	900 g	1.6 kg	2.5 kg	3.4 kg

The technique carries some risks, so it is performed only when other tests, such as *ultrasound scanning*, detect an abnormality. By attaching additional instruments, doctors can use the fetoscope to take samples of fetal blood or tissue for analysis and to perform surgical procedures, such as insertion of a catheter into the fetal bladder. (See also *amniocentesis; chorionic villus sampling.*)

fetus

The unborn child from the end of the eighth week after conception until birth. For the first eight weeks, the unborn child is called an *embryo*.

The fetus develops in the mother's *uterus* in a sac filled with *amniotic fluid*, which cushions it against injury. The oxygen and nutrients required by the fetus are supplied via the *placenta*, an organ embedded in the inner wall of the uterus that is attached to the fetus by the *umbilical cord*.

FEV

See *forced expiratory volume*.

fever

Known medically as pyrexia, elevation of body temperature above the normal level of 37°C in the mouth and 0.6°C lower in the axilla (armpit). A fever may be accompanied by symptoms such as shivering, sweating, a headache, thirst, unusually rapid breathing, and a flushed face. *Confusion* or *delirium* sometimes occur with a fever, especially in elderly people. A high fever may cause seizures in a child under five years (see *convulsion, febrile*) or *coma*.

CAUSES

Most fevers are caused either by bacterial infections, such as *tonsillitis*, or by viral infections, such as *influenza*. In such cases, proteins called pyrogens are released when the white blood cells fight the microorganisms that are responsible for the infection (see *immune system*). Pyrogens act on the temperature-controlling centre in the brain, causing it to raise the temperature of the body in an attempt to destroy the invading microorganisms.

Fever may also occur in other conditions where infection is not present. Such conditions include *dehydration*, *thyrotoxicosis* (a condition that results from overactivity of the thyroid gland), *lymphoma* (a tumour of the lymphatic system), and *myocardial infarction* (heart attack).

TREATMENT

Drugs such as *aspirin*, other *nonsteroidal anti-inflammatory drugs*, or *paracetamol* may be given to reduce fevers due to infections. Aspirin should not be given to a child under the age of 16, except on the advice of a doctor, nor should it be taken by women who are pregnant or breast-feeding. Otherwise, treatment is directed at the underlying cause; for example, *antibiotic drugs* are given to treat a bacterial infection.

feverfew

The common name for the plant TANACETUM PARTHENIUM, which is used in herbal medicine for the treatment of headache and migraine.

fibrates

Types of *lipid-lowering drug*s that are used to treat high blood levels of *triglycerides* or *cholesterol*.

fibre, dietary

The indigestible plant material in food. Dietary fibre includes certain types of polysaccharide, cellulose, hemicellulose, lignin, and gums and pectins (see *carbohydrates*). Since humans do not have the enzymes necessary to digest these substances, the material passes through the digestive system virtually unchanged and cannot be used as a source of energy.

Some components of dietary fibre hold water, thereby adding bulk to the faeces and aiding bowel function. For this reason, dietary fibre can be effective in treating *constipation*, *diverticular disease*, and *irritable bowel syndrome*. A high-fibre diet can help to reduce blood cholesterol levels. Certain high-fibre foods, such as fruit and vegetables, are also beneficial in protecting against cancers. Unrefined carbohydrate foods, including wholemeal bread, cereals, and root vegetables, are very rich in dietary fibre. (See also *nutrition*.)

fibre-optics

The transmission of images through bundles of thin, flexible glass or plastic threads. Light from a powerful external source is conducted along the length of the fibre, without losing its intensity, by a process known as total internal reflection. Fibre-optics have led to the development of *endoscopes*, instruments that enable structures deep within the body to be viewed directly.

fibrillation

Localized, spontaneous, rapid contractions of muscle fibres that can affect both skeletal and heart muscle.

In skeletal muscle, fibrillation generally occurs when a nerve supplying a muscle is destroyed, causing the muscle to become weak and waste away. Unlike *fasciculation* (muscular quivering), fibrillation in skeletal muscle is not visible through the skin; instead, the contractions can be detected using an *EMG* (electromyogram).

Fibrillation in the heart muscle is caused by disruption to the spread of nerve impulses through the wall of one of the chambers of the heart. Either the upper chambers (see *atrial fibrillation*) or the lower chambers (see *ventricular fibrillation*) of the heart may be affected. The condition can be detected by the

GOOD SOURCES OF **FIBRE** (per 100g portion)

Essential for the efficient working of the digestive system, fibre is usually eaten as fruit or grains. Among the best sources are bran, apricots, prunes, and wholemeal bread. Eating sufficient fibre in food can reduce constipation. The recommended daily intake is 25 to 30 grams.

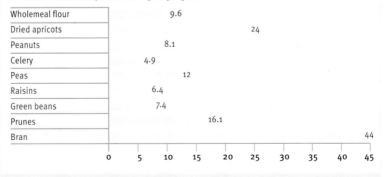

	value
Wholemeal flour	9.6
Dried apricots	24
Peanuts	8.1
Celery	4.9
Peas	12
Raisins	6.4
Green beans	7.4
Prunes	16.1
Bran	44

F

use of an *ECG* (electrocardiogram). Fibrillation in heart muscle has the potential to be serious because it impairs the ability of the chambers to contract efficiently.

fibrin

A substance that is produced in the blood during the process of *blood clotting*. Fibrin is formed from a dissolved protein called *fibrinogen*. It forms long filaments that bind clumps of *platelets* and other blood cells into a mass that plugs the bleeding point, thereby preventing further blood loss.

fibrinogen

A protein that is present in blood and which is converted into *fibrin* during the *blood clotting* process.

fibrinolysis

The breakdown of *fibrin*, the principal component of any blood clot. Fibrin is a stringy protein that is formed in blood as the end product of coagulation (see *blood clotting*).

Blood also contains a fibrinolytic system, which is activated in parallel with the coagulation system when a blood vessel is damaged. The fibrinolytic system prevents the formation of clots in undamaged blood vessels, thereby preventing a blockage in these vessels, and also acts to dissolve a clot once healing of a broken blood vessel wall has taken place.

Thrombosis (abnormal formation of blood clots) occurs when there is a disturbance in the normal balance between the coagulation and fibrinolytic mechanisms.

Drugs with a fibrinolytic effect (see *thrombolytic drugs*) can be used to treat certain disorders, such as *pulmonary embolism* and *myocardial infarction*, in which blood clots block the circulation.

fibrinolytic drugs

Another name for *thrombolytic drugs*, which are used to dissolve blood clots.

fibroadenoma

A noncancerous fibrous tumour most commonly found in the breast. Fibroadenomas occur most often in women under the age of 30 and in black women. Multiple tumours may develop in one or both breasts.

Fibroadenomas of the breast are painless, firm, round lumps that are usually between 1 and 5 cm in diameter

and movable. Although the cause of fibroadenomas is not fully understood, their development in the breast is believed to be linked to the sensitivity of breast tissue to female sex hormones. The lumps tend to grow more quickly during pregnancy, probably due to the increased levels of female sex hormones.

A sample of tissue from the lump is removed and examined to confirm the diagnosis (see *biopsy*). Fibroadenomas are harmless and do not require treatment unless they become very large or cause discomfort.

fibroadenosis

An outdated term for the general lumpiness that is a normal feature of some women's breasts. Cyclical changes in hormone levels often lead to the appearance of lumps in the breasts, and the lumpiness is more obvious before a menstrual period.

Lumpy breasts do not increase the risk of developing breast cancer. However, a new solitary, discrete *breast lump* should be assessed by a doctor to rule out the possibility of breast cancer. (See also *mammary dysplasia*.)

fibrocystic disease

A term that is used to refer either to the inherited disorder *cystic fibrosis* or to general lumpiness of the breasts (see *fibroadenosis*).

fibroid

A slow-growing and noncancerous tumour that develops in the wall of the *uterus*. A fibroid is composed of smooth muscle and *connective tissue*. There may be one or more fibroids, and they may range in size from as small as a pea to as large as a grapefruit. Fibroids are common, appearing most often in women between the ages of 35 and 45.

CAUSE

The cause of a fibroid is thought to be related to an abnormal response to *oestrogen hormones*. *Oral contraceptives* that contain oestrogen can cause enlargement of fibroids, as can *pregnancy*. Decreased production of oestrogen after the *menopause* usually causes any fibroids to shrink.

SYMPTOMS

In many cases, there are no symptoms. If a fibroid enlarges and projects into the cavity of the uterus, it may cause heavy or prolonged periods. A large

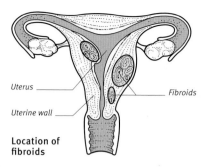

Uterus

Uterine wall

Fibroids

Location of fibroids

fibroid may exert pressure on the bladder, causing frequent passing of urine, or on the bowel, causing backache or constipation. Fibroids that distort the uterine cavity may cause recurrent *miscarriage* or *infertility*. Rarely, a fibroid may become twisted, resulting in sudden pain in the lower abdomen.

DIAGNOSIS AND TREATMENT

Fibroids that do not cause symptoms are often discovered during a routine pelvic examination. *Ultrasound scanning* can confirm the diagnosis. In some cases, a transvaginal ultrasound scan (in which a small probe is placed in the vagina) may be done to give a more accurate image.

Small, symptomless fibroids generally require no treatment, but regular examination may be needed to assess growth. For fibroids that are causing symptoms, drug treatment may be recommended. Such treatment may be with the hormone gonadotrophin releasing hormone agonist (GnRHa), which may be combined with low-dose *hormone-replacement therapy* to shrink the fibroids as well as relieve symptoms. Alternative drug treatments to relieve symptoms include *tranexamic acid*; *anti-inflammatory drugs*; the contraceptive pill (see *oral contraceptives*); or an *IUS*. If drug treatment is ineffective, surgery may be an option. Surgical procedures that may be used include myomectomy (removal of the fibroids), *endometrial ablation*, (removal of the lining of the uterus), or uterine artery embolization (cutting off the blood supply to the fibroids). Removal of fibroids usually results in regained fertility. Sometimes, however, a *hysterectomy* (removal of the uterus) is required.

fibroma

A noncancerous tumour of the cells that form *connective tissue*. For example, a neurofibroma is a tumour of the cells that surround nerve fibres (see *neurofibromatosis*). Treatment is only needed if there are symptoms.

fibromyalgia

Formerly known as fibrositis, fibromyalgia is a chronic condition in which there is muscle and ligament pain, often accompanied by localized areas of tenderness, tiredness, and sleep disturbance. It is most common in women aged 30 to 60. The cause is unknown.

Fibromyalgia can cause a wide range of symptoms, which may vary in severity from person to person and at different times in the same person. The main symptom is pain in muscles and ligaments, most commonly affecting the neck, shoulders, back, and feet. There may also be tender spots, typically at the elbows, neck, knees, and hip joints. Other symptoms may include tiredness, headache, sleep disturbances, diarrhoea, constipation, frequent urination, abnormal sensations in the hands and feet, painful periods, poor concentration, anxiety, and depression.

There is no cure for fibromyalgia and treatment is aimed at relieving symptoms. For many people, exercise is effective in alleviating pain, improving sleep, and increasing energy levels. Other treatments may include stress reduction, psychological therapies such as *cognitive–behavioural therapy*, painkillers, *antidepressant drugs*, and *antianxiety drugs*. However, fibromyalgia is often long-standing and full recovery is uncommon.

fibroplasia

The formation of fibrous tissue, which is a process that occurs normally during the healing of a wound, that may occur abnormally in some tissues. In one form of the condition, known as *retrolental fibroplasia*, fibrous tissue develops behind the lens of the eye and causes blindness. This type of fibroplasia is usually seen only in newborn premature babies and is the result of excessive treatment with oxygen.

fibrosarcoma

A rare, cancerous tumour of the cells that make up *connective tissue* (the material that surrounds body structures and holds them together). A fibrosarcoma may develop from a noncancerous *fibroma* or may be cancerous from the start.

Fibrosarcoma is treated by surgical removal and/or *radiotherapy*. However, this may be only temporarily successful if cells from the tumour have already spread through the bloodstream to initiate growths elsewhere in the body.

fibrosing alveolitis

Inflammation and thickening of the walls of the alveoli (the tiny air sacs in the lungs; see *alveolus, pulmonary*) that results in scarring of lung tissue (see *interstitial pulmonary fibrosis*). Fibrosing alveolitis most frequently occurs in people over the age of 60. Usually, fibrosing alveolitis is a long-term disorder that develops over months or years. Rarely, an acute form occurs that develops rapidly over a few days or weeks. Both forms tend to become progressively worse and are difficult to treat.

CAUSES

In some cases, fibrosing alveolitis is the result of an *autoimmune disorder* (in which the immune system attacks the body's own tissues) and may be associated with such conditions, particularly *rheumatoid arthritis* and systemic *lupus erythematosus*. Other causes may include *radiotherapy* of the organs in the chest and treatment with *anticancer drugs*. In many cases, however, the cause is unknown; the condition is then known as idiopathic pulmonary fibrosis.

SYMPTOMS

Symptoms include shortness of breath, a persistent dry cough, and joint pains. As the condition progresses, breathing becomes increasingly difficult, especially during vigorous exercise. In severe cases, there is increased risk of *respiratory failure* and chronic *heart failure*. Some people with the disorder are more susceptible to *lung cancer*.

TREATMENT

Treatment involves *corticosteroid drugs* combined with other *immunosuppressant drugs* to slow the progress of lung damage. Home oxygen therapy may be used to assist breathing. For some people, a lung transplant may be life-saving.

fibrosis

An overgrowth of scar tissue or *connective tissue*. It may occur as a result of an exaggerated healing response to infection, inflammation, or injury, or from lack of oxygen in a tissue, usually due to inadequate blood flow through it (in heart muscle damaged by a *myocardial infarction*, for example).

In fibrosis, specialized structures (for example, kidney or muscle cells) are replaced by fibrous tissue, which results in impaired function of the organ affected. An overgrowth of fibrous tissue can compress hollow structures, a situation that occurs in *retroperitoneal fibrosis*, in which the ureters (tubes draining urine

from the kidneys into the bladder) become blocked. Fibrous tissue formed within a muscle after a tear causes shortening of the muscle and disruption of the normal contraction of its fibres. The likelihood of further tears occurring is increased unless the muscle is stretched and exercised.

fibrositis

A former term for *fibromyalgia*.

fibula

F

The outer and thinner of the two long bones of the lower leg. The fibula is much narrower than the other lower leg bone, the *tibia* (shin), to which it runs parallel and to which it is attached at both ends by *ligaments*. The top end of the fibula does not reach the knee; the lower end extends below the tibia and forms part of the *ankle joint*.

The main function of the fibula is to provide an attachment for the muscles. It provides little supportive strength to the lower leg.

FRACTURE

The fibula is one of the most commonly broken bones. A fracture of the fibula just above the ankle may occur with a severe ankle sprain as a result of a violent twisting movement. *Pott's fracture* is a fracture at this location combined with dislocation of the ankle and sometimes with fracture of the tibia.

LOCATION OF THE FIBULA

The fibula lies beside the tibia on the outside of each lower leg.

Femur
Knee joint
Tibia
Fibula
Ankle joint

F

To confirm a fracture of the fibula, *X-rays* are taken. In some cases, the lower leg is immobilized in a plaster *cast* to allow the bone to heal. If a fracture occurs in the middle portion of the fibula, however, immobilization may not be needed. If the fracture is severe (especially if it is accompanied by dislocation of the ankle), surgery may be necessary to fasten the broken pieces of bone with pins. A fractured fibula may take up to six weeks to heal.

fifth disease

An infectious disease that often causes a widespread rash. Fifth disease, which is also known as slapped cheek disease or erythema infectiosum, mainly affects children and is caused by a strain of parvovirus (B19). It is usually transmitted in airborne droplets from the coughs and sneezes of infected individuals, but it may occasionally be transmitted through a blood transfusion or from mother to fetus.

Many children do not develop symptoms; in other children, the rash appears 13 to 18 days after infection. It starts on the cheeks as separate, rose-red, raised spots, which subsequently converge to give the characteristic appearance of the condition. Within a few days, the rash spreads to the trunk and limbs. The rash is frequently accompanied by mild fever and generally clears up after about ten days.

Adults, who contract the disease only rarely, tend to be more severely affected than children. They may have joint pain and swelling that lasts for up to two years. Infection may bring a temporary halt to the production of red blood cells in the bone marrow (known as an aplastic crisis); it can therefore have serious implications for people with *anaemia*. Infection during pregnancy (particularly during the first 20 weeks) may result in an increased risk of miscarriage and of the unborn baby developing *hydrops fetalis*.

The only treatment for the infection is with drugs to reduce the fever. In most cases, the condition clears up within two weeks. However, people at risk of anaemia may need hospital treatment. One attack of parvovirus confers lifelong immunity.

fight-or-flight response

The arousal of the sympathetic part of the *autonomic nervous system*, generally in response to fear. *Adrenaline* (epinephrine), *noradrenaline* (norepinephrine), and other hormones are released from the adrenal glands and nervous system, leading to a raised heart rate, pupil dilation, and increased blood flow to the muscles. These responses make the body more efficient in either fighting or fleeing the apparent danger. Prolonged or excessive fight-or-flight responses occur as part of *anxiety disorders*.

figure-of-eight bandage

A *bandage* that is wrapped over itself a number of times to resemble the figure eight. A figure-of-eight bandage is often used in first aid to support the elbows, wrists, knees, and ankles.

filariasis

A group of tropical diseases, caused by various parasitic worms or their larvae, which are transmitted to humans by insect bites. Adult female worms, which may measure anything between 2 cm and 50 cm long, produce thousands of larvae, which are carried through the body in the bloodstream. Bloodsucking insects (primarily certain species of mosquito) ingest the larvae while feeding on blood from infected people and transmit them by biting others.

Filariasis is prevalent in tropical Africa, Indonesia, the South Pacific, coastal Asia, southern Arabia, Mexico, and Guatemala.

TYPES AND SYMPTOMS

Some species of worm live in the lymphatic vessels. Swollen *lymph nodes* and recurring fever are early symptoms of the disease. Inflammation of lymph vessels results in localized *oedema* (accumulation of fluid in the tissues). After repeated infections, the affected area, which is commonly a limb or the scrotum, becomes very enlarged; in addition, the skin becomes thick, coarse, and fissured, resulting in a condition known as *elephantiasis*.

The larvae of another type of worm invade the eye, causing blindness (see *onchocerciasis*). A third type of larva, which may sometimes be seen and felt moving beneath the skin, causes *loiasis*, characterized by irritating and sometimes painful areas of oedema called calabar swellings.

DIAGNOSIS AND TREATMENT

Diagnosis is confirmed by microscopic examination of the blood (see *blood tests*). The *anthelmintic drugs* diethylcarbamazine or ivermectin generally cure the infection, but they may also cause side effects such as fever, sickness, muscle pains, and increased itching.

PREVENTION

In addition to being used for treatment, diethylcarbamazine can also be given as a preventive measure; and insecticides and protective clothing help protect against insect bites. (See also *insects and disease*; *roundworms*.)

THE CYCLE OF FILARIASIS

Filariasis is caused by parasitic worms and/or their larvae. There are several stages in the development of this infection as it spreads through the body.

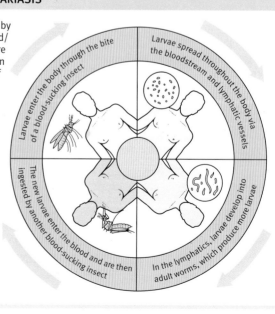

Larvae enter the body through the bite of a blood-sucking insect

Larvae spread throughout the body via the bloodstream and lymphatic vessels

In the lymphatics, larvae develop into adult worms, which produce more larvae

The new larvae enter the blood and are then ingested by another blood-sucking insect

filling defect

An abnormal finding on *contrast X-rays* occurring as a result of a lesion occupying space within a hollow organ. Normally, in contrast X-rays, a radiopaque dye (a contrast medium) is introduced into a hollow body structure, such as the intestine, and X-rays are taken; the dye outlines the shape of the structure. Anything that protrudes into the cavity of a body structure, such as *polyps* in the large intestine or a tumour in the bladder, will prevent the cavity from filling with the contrast medium and will therefore produce a distorted shape on the X-ray image.

filling, dental

The process of replacing a chipped or decayed area of tooth with an inactive material. The term may also be used to describe the restorative material itself.

Amalgam, a hard-wearing mixture of silver, mercury, and other metals, is often used for back teeth.

If a front tooth is chipped, bonding (see *bonding, dental*), in which plastic or porcelain tooth-coloured material is attached to the surface of the tooth, may be used.

WHY IT IS DONE

When enamel is damaged, bacteria can invade the dentine beneath and eventually attack the pulp (inner tissue containing blood vessels and nerves), causing the tooth to die. Teeth are therefore repaired, where possible, at the first signs of damage to prevent decay. Filling also restores a tooth's original shape, which is important for appearance and also for a correct bite.

HOW IT IS DONE

If the filling required is large or in a sensitive area, the dentist numbs the surrounding gum with a local anaesthetic (see *anaesthesia, dental*). Any soft, decayed material is removed with sharp instruments. A high-speed drill is used to remove harder material and to shape a hole that will hold the filling securely. While the dentist works, a suction tube placed in the patient's mouth draws away saliva and produces water to cool the end of the drill.

If the pulp is almost exposed, the bottom of the cavity is lined with a sedative paste to protect the sensitive pulp from pressure and temperature changes. If one or more of the walls of the tooth is missing through extensive decay, a steel band may be placed around the tooth to support the filling. The dentist then mixes the filling material, and packs it into the cavity, smoothing the surface and checking that the bite is correct. The filling material then hardens.

OUTLOOK

Amalgam fillings have a limited life and may need to be replaced after about ten years. Occasionally, a filling needs to be replaced sooner if decay has spread under the filling or the filling has become dislodged or fractured.

film

A thin, transparent sheet of cellulose acetate or similar material, coated with a light- or *radiation*-sensitive emulsion, on which images such as *X-rays* are produced. The term is also used to describe any thin layer or coating, such as the covering of *tears* on the eyeball. (See also *blood film*.)

film badge

A device that enables hospital staff who work in *X-ray* and *radiotherapy* departments to monitor their exposure to *radiation*. The badge consists of a piece of photographic film in a holder, which is worn on the clothing. The film has a fast (sensitive) emulsion on one side and a slow emulsion on the other. Small doses of radiation blacken only the fast emulsion; higher doses start to blacken the slow emulsion and make the fast emulsion turn opaque.

fimbriae

A fringe of threadlike or fingerlike filaments, such as those that make up the ends of the *fallopian tubes* that open on to the ovaries (see *ovary*). During *ovulation*, the fimbriae guide the egg (see *ovum*) into the tube.

finasteride

A specific *enzyme* inhibitor drug that prevents the conversion of *testosterone* into the more potent male hormone dihydrotestosterone. Finasteride is used in the treatment of benign (noncancerous) enlargement of the prostate (see *prostate, enlarged*); it shrinks the gland, thereby improving urine flow. It is also used to treat male pattern baldness in men. Side effects of finasteride include *erectile dysfunction* and reduced *libido* and *semen* volume.

fine tremor

A *tremor* (an involuntary trembling or oscillating movement) characterized by very small and rapid vibrations.

finger

One of the digits of the *hand*. Each finger has three phalanges (finger bones), and the thumb has two. The phalanges join at hinge joints moved by muscle tendons that flex (bend) and extend (straighten) the finger. The tendons are covered by synovial sheaths that contain fluid, enabling the muscles to work without friction. A small artery, vein, and nerve run down each side of the finger. The entire structure is enclosed in skin with a *nail* at the tip.

DISORDERS

Finger injuries are common, especially *lacerations*, *fractures*, and ruptures of the tendons. *Mallet finger* occurs when the extensor tendon along the back of a finger is pulled away from its attachment after a blow to the fingertip.

Infections may occur in the finger pulp at the tip; *paronychia* (infection of the tissue around a nail) sometimes follows a minor cut. Inflammation that is due to *rheumatoid arthritis* or *osteoarthritis* may affect the joints of the fingers, causing stiffness, pain, swelling, and deformity. In addition, the flexor tendons, which run along the front of the fingers, may become inflamed and stuck in the tendon sheath, causing a condition known as *trigger finger*.

Altered control of the muscles in the walls of the blood vessels and impaired blood supply to the hands and fingers

STRUCTURE OF A **FINGER**

The phalanges (finger bones) are joined at hinge joints and moved by tendons.

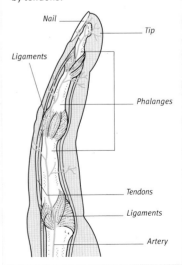

Nail
Tip
Ligaments
Phalanges
Tendons
Ligaments
Artery

may cause *Raynaud's disease*. Dactylitis is a spindle-shaped swelling of the fingers that occurs in *sickle-cell anaemia*. Swelling of the fingers is also a rare feature of tuberculosis and syphilis.

Clubbing of the fingers is a sign of chronic lung disease or of certain forms of congenital heart disease. Tumours of the finger are rare, but they may occur in *chondromatosis*, a condition that is characterized by multiple noncancerous tumours of the *cartilage*.

Congenital finger disorders include *syndactyly* (fused fingers), *polydactyly* (extra fingers), missing fingers, or a webbed appearance of the hand due to a deep membrane between the fingers.

finger-joint replacement

A surgical procedure in which one or more artificial joints (made of metal, plastic, or silicone rubber) are used to replace finger joints that have been destroyed by disease, usually by *rheumatoid arthritis* or *osteoarthritis*.

HOW IT IS DONE

Usually, several finger joints are treated at the same time. An incision is made to expose the joint; the ends of the two diseased bones in the joint are cut away, along with diseased cartilage. An artificial joint is then inserted into the bone ends. The finger is immobilized in a splint until the wound has healed. After about ten days, the dressings are removed and the patient is encouraged to exercise the fingers and resume normal activities.

RESULTS

Finger-joint replacement is usually successful in relieving arthritic pain and enabling the patient to use his or her hands again. However, it rarely restores normal movement.

fingerprint

An impression that is left on a surface by the pattern of fine curved ridges on the skin of the fingertip. These ridges occur in four patterns: loops, arches, whorls, and compounds (which are combinations of the other three). No two people (not even identical twins) have the same fingerprints.

first aid

The immediate treatment of any injury or sudden illness before professional medical care can be provided. Most first aid consists of treating minor injuries and *burns*, and *fractures*. Sometimes, however, emergency life-saving first aid treatment may be needed.

The aims of first-aid treatment in an emergency are to preserve life; to protect the individual from further harm; to provide reassurance; to make the victim comfortable; to arrange for medical help; and to find out as much as possible about the circumstances of the accident or injury.

Various techniques can be used to achieve these aims. For example, the *recovery position* helps to maintain an open airway in an unconscious person who is breathing; *rescue breathing* is necessary if a person is not breathing. *Cardiopulmonary resuscitation* is essential if a person is not breathing and has no heartbeat.

fish oil

A product occurring naturally in some species of oily fish, such as mackerel. Fish-oil preparations, which are rich in *omega-3 fatty acids*, are used as *lipid-lowering drugs*.

fissure

A cleft or groove, which can be either normal or abnormal. A dental fissure is a naturally occurring defect in the enamel of a tooth in which tooth decay (see *caries, dental*) commonly arises. The sylvian fissure is one of the deep folds that separate the temporal lobe of the *brain* from the frontal and parietal lobes. An *anal fissure* is a tear occurring in the anal canal.

fissure sealant

A substance that is bonded to the biting surface of a tooth to seal any naturally occurring *fissures* (clefts or grooves) in the enamel and to help prevent tooth decay (see *dental caries*). Treatment with fissure sealant may be offered as a preventive measure to children whose molar teeth have recently emerged (see *eruption of teeth*).

fistula

An abnormal passage leading from an internal organ to the body surface or connecting two organs. Fistulas may rarely be congenital (present from birth), or they may be acquired as a result of tissue damage.

Congenital types include *tracheoesophageal fistulas*, branchial fistulas (see *branchial disorders*), and thyroglossal fistulas (see *thyroglossal disorders*).

Acquired fistulas may result from infection, injury, or cancer. Fistulas between the *intestine* and the skin may

occur in the inflammatory bowel condition *Crohn's disease*; these fistulas may allow the intestinal contents to escape to the skin through an opening, in which case they are known as faecal fistulas. Fistulas of the urinary tract, which open from the *urethra* or *bladder* to the perineum (the area between the anus and genitals), may be the result of *radiotherapy* to the pelvis, or they may be caused by a difficult childbirth. Such fistulas may cause leakage of urine (see *incontinence, urinary*) or *urinary tract infection*.

Certain types of *arteriovenous fistula* (between an artery and a vein) are surgically constructed to provide ready access to the circulation in people who are having *dialysis*.

TREATMENT

Identifying the cause of a fistula, and treating it if possible, is the first line of action. Some types of fistula close spontaneously but most need surgery. In faecal fistulas, a temporary colostomy may be necessary to divert faeces away from the affected area.

fit

See *seizure*.

fitness

The capacity for performing physical activities without exhaustion. Fitness depends on strength (the ability to exert force for pushing, pulling, lifting), flexibility (the ability to bend, stretch, and twist through a full range of movements), and endurance (the ability to maintain a certain amount of effort for a certain period of time).

HOW FITNESS IS ACHIEVED

Cardiovascular fitness is the precondition for all other forms of fitness; for this reason, regular aerobic exercise (see *aerobics*), which makes the body's use of oxygen more efficient, is the basis of any fitness programme. Specific activities, such as weight training or yoga, can help to develop strength and flexibility when included in a programme (see *exercise*). Although fitness training has cumulative effects that build up over many months (provided that there is a sustained increase in activity levels), the effects are specific to the muscles used and the ways in which they are used. A variety of activities is therefore necessary to achieve overall fitness.

BENEFITS OF FITNESS

When the body is fit, the maximum work capacity and endurance are increased. A fit person has a better chance of avoiding *coronary artery disease* as well as of preventing the effects of aging and chronic disease.

The strength, endurance, and efficiency of the heart is also increased by exercise. A fit heart pumps 25 per cent more blood per minute when at rest, and over 50 per cent more blood per minute during physical exertion, than an unfit heart. A fit person's heart normally beats 60 or 70 times a minute; an unfit person's heart beats 80 to 100 times per minute.

fitness testing

A series of exercises designed to determine an individual's level of *fitness*, primarily his or her cardiovascular fitness and muscle performance. Fitness testing is often carried out before a person starts an exercise programme to evaluate its safety and suitability or to monitor progress thereafter.

A physical examination is usually performed, including measurement of body fat, height, and weight. Blood and urine tests may be done, including an analysis of blood *cholesterol*. The performance of the heart is measured by taking the pulse before, during, and after aerobic exercise such as step climbing, riding a stationary bicycle, or running on a treadmill. The more efficient the heart, the slower it works during exercise and the quicker it returns to normal afterwards.

Another test involves measuring a person's overall performance in a standard exercise. This is most suitable for monitoring progress through an exercise programme and for setting goals. The test may be based either on measuring the distance covered in a fixed time or the time needed to cover a fixed distance. (See also *aerobics*; *exercise*.)

fixation

In *psychoanalytic theory*, the process by which an individual becomes, or remains, emotionally attached to real or imagined objects or events that occurred during early childhood. If the fixations are powerful, resulting from traumatic events, they may lead to immature and inappropriate behaviour. Regression to these events is regarded by some analysts as the basis of certain emotional disorders.

The word "fixation" also describes the alignment and stabilization of fractured bones. Fixation may be external,

as with a plaster *cast*, or internal, using pins, plates, or nails introduced surgically into the injured area.

fixative

A chemical agent, such as *formaldehyde*, that is used for the hardening and preservation of tissue specimens prior to microscopic analysis (see *histology*).

fixed pupil

An abnormal *pupil* (the circular opening in the centre of the *iris*) that does not react to light or adjust on *accommodation* (the process by which the eye focuses on objects). A fixed pupil may be symptomatic of various eye disorders (see *eye, disorders of*), such as acute *glaucoma* and *uveitis*, or, rarely, of a *brain tumour* in which *brainstem* structures that control eye reflexes are compressed. Both pupils being fixed and dilated is a sign of brain death.

fixed-rate pacemaker

An artificial cardiac *pacemaker* (a device that sends electrical impulses to the *heart* to maintain a regular *heartbeat*) that is set to pace at a single rate regardless of the patient's own *heart rate*. Fixed-rate pacemakers are still used in some clinical and diagnostic settings, and may be appropriate for some elderly people. However, for active people rate-responsive pacemakers (see *demand pacemaker*) are often a better choice; these devices deliver electrical stimuli as required and at a rate that matches the patient's level of activity.

flaccid

Lacking in firmness or characterized by a loss of *muscle* tone.

flail chest

A type of chest injury that usually results from a traffic accident or from violence. In flail chest, several adjacent ribs are broken in more than one place, resulting in a segment of chest wall that moves in the opposite way to normal as the victim breathes: when the victim inhales and the ribcage expands, the flail segment moves inwards and during exhalation it moves outwards.

The injury may severely impair the efficiency of breathing and may lead to *respiratory failure* and *shock*. It makes breathing and coughing very painful, which can increase the risk of chest infection and lung collapse (see *atelectasis*).

flat-feet

A condition, usually affecting both feet, in which the arch of the foot is absent and the sole rests flat on the ground. The arches normally form gradually as the supportive ligaments and muscles in the soles of the feet develop; they are not usually fully formed until about the age of six. In some people, however, the ligaments are lax, or the muscles in the feet are weak, and the feet therefore remain flat. Less commonly, the arches of the feet may not form because of a hereditary defect in bone structure.

Flat-feet can be acquired in adult life because of fallen arches, sometimes as the result of a rapid increase in weight. Weakening of the supporting muscles and ligaments of the feet may occur in certain neurological or muscular diseases, such as *poliomyelitis*.

In most cases, flat-feet are painless and require no treatment, although in some cases the feet may ache on walking or standing for prolonged periods. Arch supports or orthotic insoles can be worn in the shoes for comfort and special exercises can be used to help strengthen weakened ligaments and muscles. A small number of affected children require an operation to correct the bones in the feet.

flatulence

Abdominal discomfort or fullness that is relieved by belching or by passing wind through the anus. Flatulence is a feature of many gastrointestinal conditions, such as *irritable bowel syndrome* and *gallbladder* disorders.

When an individual is in an upright position, most swallowed air passes back up the *oesophagus* to be expelled through the mouth. When a person is in a prone position, the air may pass through the intestine and anus instead. Gas formed in the intestine is passed only through the anus.

flatus

Gas, commonly known as "wind", that is passed via the anus. Gas is formed in the large intestine by the action of bacteria on *carbohydrates* and *amino acids* in food. The gas consists of hydrogen, carbon dioxide, and methane. Air may be swallowed while eating and enter the stomach or intestine.

Large amounts of gas may cause *flatulence* (abdominal discomfort), which may be relieved by the passage of wind or by *defaecation* (passing faeces).

F

flatworm

Any species of worm that has a flattened shape. Two types of flatworm are parasites of humans: cestodes (*tapeworms*) and trematodes (schistosomes, flukes; see *liver fluke*; *schistosomiasis*).

flea bites

See *insect bites*.

flecainide

An *antiarrhythmic drug* used in the treatment of *tachycardia*, *atrial fibrillation*, and *arrhythmias* associated with conditions such as Wolff–Parkinson–White syndrome (an abnormality of heart rhythm). Flecainide is given, in the form of tablets or injection, to people who are physically resistant to or intolerant of other treatments. The treatment is always started in hospital.

Side effects include dizziness, visual disturbances, and worsening of the existing arrhythmia or development of a new type. In rare cases, nausea, vomiting, *urticaria* (nettle rash), *vertigo*, and *jaundice* occur.

flexor

Any *muscle* that acts to flex a *joint*. An example of a flexor muscle is the *biceps muscle*, in the upper arm, which contracts to bend the elbow.

flies

See *insects and disease*.

floaters

Small fragments that are perceived to be floating in the field of vision. Floaters move rapidly with eye movement but drift slightly when the eyes are still. They do not usually affect vision.

The majority of floaters are the result of shadows cast on the *retina* by microscopic structures in the *vitreous humour* (the jellylike substance behind the lens of the eye). In older people, the vitreous humour tends to shrink slightly and detach from the retina, often resulting in conspicuous floaters, which usually decrease over time. The sudden appearance of a cloud of dark floaters, especially if they are accompanied by light flashes, suggests *retinal tear* or *retinal detachment*. A red floater that is large enough to obscure vision is usually caused by a *vitreous haemorrhage*.

floating kidney

A *kidney* that is more mobile within the body than usual.

HOW TO USE DENTAL **FLOSS**

Floss should be used as an adjunct to toothbrushing to remove plaque and food particles from gaps between teeth and around gums. Care should be taken to avoid damaging the gum margins, and floss should never be reused.

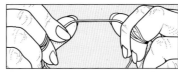

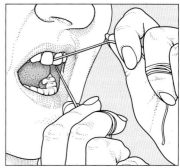

1 Break off a generous length of floss (about 50 cm) and wrap the ends around one finger of each hand.

2 Holding the floss taut, guide it gently into the gap between the teeth until it reaches the gum line. Then rub the sides of each tooth with the floss using an up-and-down motion.

floating ribs

The lowest two pairs of *ribs*, which are attached to the *spine* at the back but are not attached to the *sternum* (the breastbone) by cartilage in the same way as the other ribs.

flooding

A technique used in *behaviour therapy* for treating *phobias*. Flooding forces the patient to confront the focus of his or her fear directly and for prolonged periods. With the support of a therapist, the patient is repeatedly confronted with the object or situation that he or she is afraid of. The aim is that, through the process of flooding, the patient's distress should eventually be reduced.

floppy infant

A baby whose muscles lack normal tone, causing the limbs to be limp and floppy (see *hypotonia in infants*).

floppy valve syndrome

See *mitral valve prolapse*.

flossing, dental

The removal of plaque (see *plaque, dental*) and food particles from between the teeth using soft nylon or silk thread or tape. Dental floss may be waxed or unwaxed. Flossing should be carried out as an adjunct to toothbrushing.

flu

See *influenza*.

flucloxacillin

A *penicillin drug* usually used to treat *staphylococcal infections*.

fluconazole

An *antifungal drug* used in the treatment of *candidiasis* (thrush), a fungal infection that commonly affects the vagina or the mouth. Fluconazole may also be used to prevent fungal infections in immunocompromised people and to treat *cryptococcosis* (a fungal infection that can cause meningitis). Although generally well tolerated, fluconazole may sometimes cause nausea, vomiting, diarrhoea, flatulence, and abdominal discomfort.

fluctuant

A term used to describe the movement within a swelling when it is examined by touch. It is a sign that the swelling contains fluid. The term is often used to describe an *abscess*.

fluid retention

The excessive accumulation of fluid in body tissues. Mild fluid retention is a common feature of *premenstrual syndrome*, but it disappears with the onset of menstruation. A more severe case of fluid retention may be associated with an underlying heart, liver, or kidney disorder (see *ascites*; *nephrotic syndrome*; *oedema*). *Diuretic drugs* may be used to treat fluid retention.

fluke

A type of flattened worm, also known as a trematode, that may infest humans or animals. The two main diseases caused by flukes are *liver fluke* infestation, which occurs worldwide, and *schistosomiasis*, a debilitating disease that is common in tropical countries.

fluorescein

A harmless orange dye that is used in *ophthalmology* to aid the diagnosis of certain eye disorders. It can be applied to the front of the eye to detect abrasions of the *conjunctiva* or *cornea*. When fluorescein comes into contact with defective cells, and a blue light is then shone into the eye, the fluorescein glows green. Fluorescein is also given intravenously during fluorescein *angiography* in order to detect abnormalities of the blood vessels in the *retina* (the light-sensitive inner layer at the back of the eye), which occur in such conditions as *macular degeneration* and *diabetic retinopathy*.

fluoridation

The addition of *fluoride* to the water supply as a means of reducing the incidence of dental *caries* (tooth decay). Some areas have naturally high levels of fluoride in the drinking water; in other areas, however, fluoride may be added to bring the concentration up to the recommended level. In the UK, decisions to add fluoride to drinking water are made by the local authorities.

fluoride

A mineral that helps to prevent dental *caries* (tooth decay) by strengthening tooth enamel (see *teeth*), making it more resistant to acid attacks. Fluoride may also reduce the acid-producing ability of microorganisms in *plaque*.

Fluoride that is ingested during the formation of teeth has a lifelong beneficial effect because it is incorporated into the developing tooth substance. In the UK, fluoride is added to the water supply in some areas, and fluoridation has led to a decrease in the incidence of tooth decay among children in those areas.

Fluoride is also beneficial to both children and adults when it is applied directly to the teeth as part of dental treatment or used in the form of a mouthwash or toothpaste. However, the ingestion of excess fluoride as the teeth are forming can lead to *fluorosis* (staining of the tooth enamel).

fluorosis

Mottling or staining of the tooth enamel (see *teeth*) that is caused by the ingestion of excessive amounts of *fluoride* while the teeth are being formed. Mild fluorosis causes white lines or flecking on the surface enamel. In severe cases of fluorosis, brown stains develop on the tooth enamel. However, dental fluorosis is rare in the UK.

fluorouracil

An *anticancer drug* that is used in the treatment of cancers of the breast, bladder, ovaries, and intestine.

fluoxetine

An *antidepressant drug* that belongs to the group of drugs known as *selective serotonin reuptake inhibitors* (SSRIs). Fluoxetine is used to treat *depression*, to reduce binge eating and purging activity (*bulimia nervosa*), and to treat *obsessive–compulsive disorder*. The drug works by increasing the amount of *serotonin* that is available in the brain, thereby stimulating brain cells. Unlike many other SSRIs, fluoxetine is effective in treating depression in childen and adolescents. However, because it may be associated with a small risk of self-harm or suicide in such patients, it is usually prescribed with caution to those under 18 years old and such patients are carefully monitored.

The most common adverse effects of fluoxetine include restlessness, insomnia, headache, and diarrhoea.

flupentixol

An *antipsychotic drug* that is used to treat *schizophrenia* and similar illnesses. Flupentixol is also sometimes prescribed to treat *depression*. Side effects of the drug most commonly include weight gain, blurred vision, nausea, a rapid heartbeat, dizziness, and *parkinsonism*.

flurazepam

A type of *benzodiazepine drug* that is used as a sleeping drug in the short-term treatment of *insomnia*. The effects of flurazepam may persist the following day, causing drowsiness and lightheadedness. Prolonged use of the drug may result in dependence (see *drug dependence*).

flurbiprofen

A *nonsteroidal anti-inflammatory drug* that is used particularly to ease the symptoms of musculoskeletal disorders, such as *rheumatoid arthritis*.

flush

Reddening of the face, and sometimes of the neck, caused by dilation of the blood vessels near the skin surface.

Flushing may occur during *fever* or as a result of embarrassment. *Hot flushes* are common at the *menopause*.

fluticasone

A *corticosteroid drug* that is taken in the form of an inhaler to control *asthma*, as a nasal spray to relieve the symptoms of allergic rhinitis (see *rhinitis allergic*), and as an ointment or cream to treat *dermatitis* and *eczema*.

Side effects of fluticasone are rare, but they may include nosebleeds when the drug is taken as a nasal spray, *candidiasis* (thrush) of the mouth and throat when it is taken as an inhaler, and skin irritation when it is taken as an ointment or cream.

Flynn–Aird syndrome

A rare, inherited disorder characterized by *atrophy* (wasting away) of the muscles and skin, *ataxia* (incoordination and clumsiness), and dementia. Other symptoms include tooth decay (see *caries, dental*), stiffness in the joints, *retinitis pigmentosa* (degeneration of the rods and cones of the *retina*), peripheral *neuropathy* (a peripheral nerve disorder), *cataracts*, and progressive loss of hearing. Flynn–Aird syndrome has an autosomal dominant pattern of inheritance (see *genetic disorders*).

foam, contraceptive

See *spermicides*.

focal point

The point at which light rays converge after passing through a *lens*. In people with normal vision, light rays from a viewed object converge on the light-sensitive *retina* after passing through the cornea and lens, producing a clear image. In shortsightedness, the focal point occurs in front of the retina and the image is blurred; in longsightedness it occurs beyond the retina, with the same result.

foetus

An alternative spelling for *fetus*.

Foley catheter

A type of *catheter* (flexible tube) that is fed through the *urethra* into the *bladder* and used for the continuous drainage of *urine* (see *catheterization, urinary*). A Foley catheter is kept in place within the *bladder* by means of a balloon at its tip that is inflated with either air or liquid.

F

folic acid

A *vitamin* that is essential for the production of red *blood cells* by the *bone marrow*. Folic acid is contained in a variety of foods, particularly liver and raw vegetables; adequate amounts are usually included in a normal diet, but it is destroyed by prolonged cooking.

During pregnancy, folic acid is important for fetal growth, the development of the nervous system, and the formation of blood cells. To help prevent *neural tube defects* (such as *spina bifida*), women who are planning a pregnancy should take the recommended dose of folic acid supplement before conceiving and then during the first 12 weeks of pregnancy. If there is a family history of neural tube defects, a higher dose of folic acid supplement is recommended.

Folic acid deficiency is a cause of megaloblastic *anaemia*, which produces symptoms such as headaches, fatigue, and pallor. Deficiency can occur during any serious illness or can result from a nutritionally poor diet, especially in people who drink large amounts of alcohol.

folie à deux

A French term that is used to describe the unusual occurrence of two people sharing the same psychotic illness (see *psychosis*). Often the two people are closely related and share one or more paranoid *delusions*. If the sufferers become separated, one of them usually rapidly loses the symptoms, which have been imposed by the dominant, and genuinely psychotic, partner.

folk medicine

Any form of medical treatment that is based on popular tradition, such as the charming of warts or the use of copper bracelets to treat rheumatism.

follicle

A small cavity in the body. For example, a *hair* follicle is a pit in the skin from which a single strand of hair emerges. Another example is an ovarian follicle, which is a fluid-filled cavity in the *ovary* in which an *ovum* (egg) develops.

follicle-stimulating hormone

A *gonadotrophin hormone* that is produced by the *pituitary gland* and acts on the *ovary* or *testis*. In women, follicle-stimulating hormone (FSH) causes an egg follicle to start maturing in the ovary in the first week of the menstrual cycle, ready for *ovulation*. In men, FSH

stimulates *sperm* production in the testes. FSH is given medically to treat certain types of *infertility*.

folliculitis

Inflammation of one or more hair follicles as a result of a *staphylococcal infection*. Folliculitis can occur almost anywhere on the skin, but the condition most commonly affects the neck, armpits, thighs, or buttocks, causing a *boil*; it may also affect the bearded area of the face, producing pustules (see *sycosis barbae*). Treatment of folliculitis is with *antibiotic drugs*. Because the infection is easily spread, careful hygiene is important, and an affected individual should wash any clothes worn next to the skin daily in boiling water until the condition has cleared up.

fomites

Inanimate objects (for example, bed linen, clothing, books, or telephone receivers) that are not in themselves harmful but which may be capable of harbouring harmful microorganisms or parasites and, therefore, of conveying an infection from one person to another. Fomites principally transmit respiratory infections, such as *influenza*. The singular form of the word fomites is "fomes".

fontanelle

Either one of two membrane-covered spaces between the bones of a baby's skull. At birth, the skull bones are not yet fully fused, and two soft areas can be felt through the scalp. These are the anterior fontanelle, which is diamond-shaped and usually closes up by age 18 months, and the posterior fontanelle, which is triangular and closes up within the first two months.

It is normal for the fontanelles to become tense and bulge out when a baby cries. Persistent tension at other times, however, may indicate an abnormality, particularly *hydrocephalus* (the accumulation of fluid in the skull). A sunken fontanelle may be a sign of *dehydration*. If a fontanelle is abnormally large or takes a long time to close, the cause may be a brain abnormality or a disorder, such as *rickets*, affecting the skull bones. Early closure of the fontanelles results in a deformity called *craniosynostosis*.

Occasionally, a third fontanelle is present between the other two; this is a feature of *Down's syndrome*. Sometimes

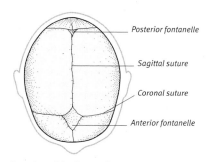

Location of the fontanelles
There are two soft areas on the baby's skull – the anterior fontanelle is diamond-shaped, the posterior fontanelle is triangular.

a baby may have extra bones in the anterior fontanelle, but this is not abnormal. These extra bones fuse into the skull when the gap between them closes.

food additives

Any substance that is added to food for the purposes of preservation or to improve its acceptability in terms of taste, colour, or consistency.

TYPES AND USES

Additives fall into five main groups: those that preserve food; those that affect texture; those that affect appearance and taste; added nutrients, such as vitamins; and miscellaneous additives, such as rising and glazing agents, flour improvers, and anti-foaming agents. For further information on the many different types of food additives, see the table opposite.

Preservatives, such as sodium nitrate, are added to food to control the growth of bacteria, moulds, and yeasts. Other additives, such as antioxidants, can improve the keeping quality of food by preventing any undesirable chemical changes within it; for example, antioxidants prevent rancidity in some foods containing fat.

Additives that improve the texture of food include thickeners, emulsifiers, stabilizers, and gelling agents. Lecithin, which occurs naturally in all animal and plant cells, is an emulsifier that is added to margarine to prevent separation.

The appearance and taste of many foods and drinks may be improved through the use of colourings, flavourings, sweeteners, and flavour enhancers. Artificial *sweeteners*, such as saccharin and aspartame, may be used instead of sugar, especially in products that are aimed at people trying to lose weight. Many colourings are natural (for example, beetroot red).

FOOD ADDITIVES

Most additives approved by the EU have been given an E number, which must be listed by type and name and/or by number on food labels. Some examples of food additives and foods in which they are used are shown below. Antioxidants improve the keeping qualities of certain foods by preventing undesirable chemical changes. Preservatives also improve keeping quality, but by inhibiting growth of microorganisms. Emulsifiers and stabilizers improve the texture of foods. Sweeteners improve palatability and reduce dental problems associated with excess sugar intake.

Additive	Comments	Often used in
Antioxidants		
E300–302	L-ascorbic acid/ascorbates (vitamin C)	Fruit drinks
E307	Synthetic alpha-tocopherol	Cereal-based baby foods
E322	Lecithins	Low-fat spreads
Colours		
*E102	Tartrazine (yellow/orange)Soft drinks	Soft drinks
*E104	Quinoline yellow (greenish/yellow)	Smoked fish
E160	Carotenes/Annatto (orange)	Cheese
Emulsifiers and stabilizers		
E406	Agar (extracted from seaweed)	Ice cream
E412	Guar gum (extracted from cluster beans)	Packet soups
E440	Pectin (occurs naturally in fruits and plants)	Jams, preserves
Preservatives		
*E210–219	Benzoic acid/benzoates	Fruit products
*E220–227	Sulphur dioxide/sulphites	Meat products
*E249–252	Nitrites/nitrates	Cooked and cured meats
Sweeteners		
*E950	Acesulfame-K	Baked goods, dairy products, confectionery
*E951	Aspartame	Carbonated drinks, sugar substitutes
*E954	Saccharin	Sugar substitutes, chewing gum

*Warning: may produce reactions in susceptible people

RISKS

Certain additives may produce an allergic reaction in some individuals, although this is relatively rare. Some substances, particularly food colourings such as tartrazine, may be a contributory factor in *behavioural problems in children*, but this is difficult to confirm.

food allergy

An inappropriate or exaggerated reaction of the *immune system* to a food. Sensitivity to cows' milk protein is a fairly common food allergy in young children. Other foods that are commonly implicated in food allergy are nuts (particularly peanuts), wheat, fish, shellfish, and eggs. Food allergy is more common in those who suffer from other forms of *allergy* or *hypersensitivity*, such as *asthma*, allergic *rhinitis*, and *eczema*.

Immediate reactions, which occur within an hour (or sometimes only minutes) of eating the trigger foods, include swelling of the lips, tingling in the mouth or throat, vomiting, abdominal distension, abnormally loud bowel sounds, and diarrhoea. Serious food allergies can cause *anaphylactic shock*, which requires immediate self-injection with *adrenaline* (epinephrine). The only effective treatment for food allergy is avoidance of the offending food. (See also *food intolerance*.)

food-borne infection

Any infectious illness caused by eating food contaminated with viruses, bacteria, worms, or other organisms.

There are two mechanisms by which food can become infected. Firstly, many animals that are kept or caught for food may harbour disease organisms; if meat or milk from such an animal is eaten without being thoroughly cooked or pasteurized, the organisms may cause illness in their human host. In the UK, the only common infection of this type is *food poisoning*. Secondly, food may be contaminated with organisms spread from an infected person or animal, usually by flies moving from faeces to food (see *Food poisoning* box overleaf).

Immunization is available against certain food- and *water-borne infections*, such as *typhoid fever*.

food challenge

The controlled reintroduction into the diet of a food suspected of causing symptoms. Food challenges are usually attempted after a person has already been following an *exclusion diet*.

food fad

A like or dislike of a particular food or foods that is taken to extremes. A food fad may lead to undue reliance on, or avoidance of, a particular food. Fads are common in toddlers, adolescents, and people who are under *stress*. When a food fad becomes obsessive or persistent, it may indicate a serious eating disorder. (See also *anorexia nervosa*; *bulimia*.)

food intolerance

An adverse reaction to a food or an ingredient of food that occurs each time an individual eats the substance.

F

FOOD POISONING

Some animals, including cows, pigs, poultry, and shellfish, harbour disease organisms (such as bacteria, viruses, worms, and parasites) in their tissues; these organisms may cause infection if meat, fish, or dairy products are consumed raw or are improperly cooked. Beef, pork, and fish tapeworm infestations, salmonella poisoning, and (rarely) brucellosis can be transmitted in this way. Adequate pasteurization of milk and the inspection of meat and fish before they go on sale prevent most infections and infestations of this type from occurring. Proper hygiene during food preparation and thorough cooking of meat, fish, shellfish, poultry, and eggs further reduce the risk of infection.

FOOD CONTAMINATION

Intestinal infections may be spread from person to person if organisms in faeces contaminate food, either directly or indirectly. Contamination can occur if vegetable crops are sprayed with sewage, if flies settle on faeces and then on food, or if food is handled by a person who has not washed his or her hands.

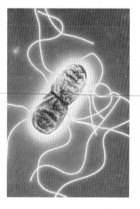

Contaminating organism
The photograph (left), taken through an electron microscope, shows a typical *Salmonella* bacterium. The organism uses its many flagellae (whiplike structures) to move. *Salmonella* is a common contaminant of poultry, eggs, and egg products and may cause severe food poisoning.

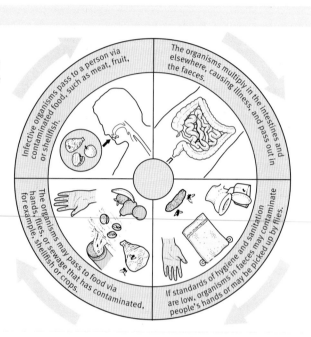

Food intolerance does not have a psychological cause; it is not the result of *food poisoning*; and it does not involve the *immune system*.

Food intolerance is commonly of unknown cause. Certain foods may be poorly tolerated as a result of impaired digestion and absorption, which may be associated with disorders of the *pancreas* or of the *biliary system* (which produce digestive juices to break down food). Some individuals have a genetic deficiency of a specific *enzyme*, such as *lactase* (which is required for the digestion of lactose, the sugar that occurs in milk); on drinking milk, those people with lactose intolerance develop abdominal cramps, flatulence, and loose stools.

food poisoning

A term used to describe any gastrointestinal illness of sudden onset that is likely to have been caused by contaminated food or water. Most cases of food poisoning are caused by contamination of food or water by bacteria, viruses, or parasites. The illness is more common in hot weather.

Food poisoning is usually suspected when, for example, several members of a household (or customers at a particular restaurant) become ill after eating the same food.

BACTERIAL CAUSES

The bacteria commonly responsible for food poisoning belong to the groups SALMONELLA, CAMPYLOBACTER, and E. COLI, certain strains of which are capable of multiplying rapidly in the intestines to cause widespread inflammation. Food poisoning may also be caused by LISTERIA (see *listeriosis*).

Certain farm animals, especially poultry, commonly harbour the bacteria that are responsible for food poisoning. If frozen poultry is incompletely thawed before being cooked, or if it is not cooked thoroughly, it is liable to cause food poisoning. Eggs laid by affected poultry may also contain disease-causing bacteria, although fresh eggs are unlikely to be heavily contaminated. Bacteria may also be transferred to food from the excrement of infected animals or people; the bacteria can be transmitted either by flies or through poor personal hygiene.

Some types of bacteria cause the formation of toxins, which may be difficult to destroy even after thorough cooking. For example, the organism CLOSTRIDIUM PERFRINGENS is resistant to heat, and it may survive in precooked foods, such as pies, that have been incorrectly stored. *Botulism* is an uncommon, life-threatening form of food poisoning that is caused by a bacterial toxin. The foods most likely to cause botulism are home-preserved fruit, vegetables, and fish.

VIRAL CAUSES

The viruses that are most commonly responsible for food poisoning are astrovirus, rotavirus, and a small round-structured virus (SRSV), which affects shellfish. This form of poisoning can occur when raw or partly cooked foods have been in contact with water contaminated by human excrement.

OTHER INFECTIVE CAUSES

The protozoan parasite CRYPTOSPORIDIUM (see *cryptosporidiosis*), which principally affects farm animals, can be passed on to humans through drinking water supplies, swimming pools, or by direct contact with infected animals. People with *HIV* infection or *AIDS* are particularly susceptible to contracting this type of food poisoning.

NONINFECTIVE CAUSES

Noninfective causes of food poisoning include poisonous mushrooms and toadstools (see *mushroom poisoning*), fresh fruit and vegetables contaminated with high doses of insecticide, and chemical poisoning from some foods, such as fruit juice, that are stored in containers made partly from zinc.

Certain foods, such as puffer fish, considered a delicacy in Japan, or cassava, a staple food in many tropical countries, can also cause moderate to lethal poisoning if improperly cooked or prepared.

SYMPTOMS

The onset of symptoms depends on the cause of poisoning. Symptoms usually develop within 30 minutes in cases of chemical poisoning, between one and 12 hours in cases of bacterial toxins, and between 12 and 48 hours with most bacterial and viral infections.

Symptoms of food poisoning usually include diarrhoea, nausea and vomiting, stomach pain, and, in severe cases, *shock* and collapse. Botulism affects the nervous system, causing visual disturbances, difficulty with speech, paralysis, and vomiting.

DIAGNOSIS

The diagnosis of bacterial food poisoning can usually be confirmed from examination of a sample of faeces. Chemical poisoning can often be diagnosed from a description of what the person has eaten, and from analysis of a sample of the suspect food.

TREATMENT

Mild cases can be treated at home. Lost fluids should be replaced by the intake of plenty of clear fluids (see *rehydration therapy*). In severe cases, or when the very young or elderly are affected, hospital treatment may be necessary. If poisoning by a bacterial toxin is suspected, the stomach may be washed out (see *lavage, gastric*).

Except for botulism and some cases of mushroom poisoning, most food poisoning is not serious; recovery usually occurs within about three days. Some strains of E. COLI can seriously damage red blood cells, causing *kidney failure* (see *haemolytic–uraemic syndrome*). (See also *cholera*; *dysentery*; *seafood poisoning*; *typhoid fever*.)

PREVENTION

Some simple measures can virtually eliminate the risk of food poisoning. Hands should always be washed before food is handled, and fresh fruit and vegetables should be rinsed in clean water. Cutting boards and implements that have been used for raw meat should be washed with hot water before being used for other foods. All packaged foods should be used by their "best before" dates. Meat, poultry, and eggs must be cooked thoroughly, until they are piping hot all the way through. Raw and cooked foods should be stored well apart in the refrigerator, and raw meat should be kept in the coldest part. Advice should be sought when preparing unfamiliar foods.

foot

The foot has two vital functions. The first of these functions is to support the weight of the body in standing or walking; the second function of the foot is to act as a lever that propels the body forwards.

STRUCTURE

The largest bone of the foot, the heelbone (see *calcaneus*), is jointed with the ankle bone (the talus). The tarsal bones are located in front of the talus and calcaneus and they are jointed to the five *metatarsal bones*. The bones of the toes are called the *phalanges*; the big toe has two phalanges and all the remaining toes have three.

Tendons passing around the ankle connect the muscles that act on the various bones of the foot and toe. The main blood vessels and nerves pass in front of and behind the inside of the ankle to supply the foot. The undersurface of a normal foot forms a natural arch that is supported by ligaments and muscles. Fascia (fibrous tissue) and fat form the sole of the foot, which is covered by a layer of tough skin.

DISORDERS

Injuries to the foot often result in *fracture* of the foot bones (the metatarsals and phalanges). The calcaneus may fracture following a fall from a height on to a hard surface.

Congenital foot abnormalities are fairly common and include club-foot (see *talipes*), *flat-feet*, and *claw-foot*. A *bunion* is a common deformity of the foot in which a thickened *bursa* (fluid-filled pad) lies over the joint at the base of the big toe.

Corns are small areas of thickened skin that are usually caused by tightly fitting shoes. Verrucas (see *plantar warts*) develop on the soles of the feet. *Athlete's foot* is a fungal infection that affects the skin between the toes, causing it to become very itchy, sore, and cracked.

Gout is a relatively common type of arthritis that often affects the joint at the base of the big toe or one of the joints in the foot. An ingrowing toenail (see *toenail, ingrowing*) commonly occurs on the big toe and may lead to inflammation and infection of the surrounding tissues (see *paronychia*).

Foot-drop is the inability to raise the foot properly causing it to drag along the ground when the person is walking. The condition may occur as a result of damage to the muscles in the leg that are responsible for performing this movement or, alternatively, to the nerves that supply these muscles.

ANATOMY OF THE FOOT

An adult has 26 bones (about one eighth of the total number in the entire skeleton) in each foot. The calcaneus is attached to the talus above. In front are the navicular, cuboid, and cuneiform bones, which are attached to the metatarsals. The phalanges form the toes.

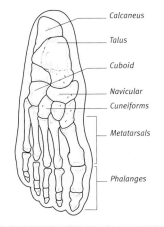

Calcaneus

Talus

Cuboid

Navicular

Cuneiforms

Metatarsals

Phalanges

F

foot-drop

A condition in which the foot cannot be raised properly and hangs limp from the ankle, causing it to catch on the ground when the affected person is walking along.

Neuritis (inflammation of a nerve) affecting the nerves that supply the foot muscles is a common cause. This condition may be due to *diabetes mellitus*, *multiple sclerosis*, or a *neuropathy* (nerve disease). Weakness in the foot muscles can also result from pressure on a nerve at the point where it leaves the spinal cord, due to a *disc prolapse* or a *tumour*. Damage to the muscles in the leg from an injury may also be a cause of foot-drop.

The underlying cause is treated, but in many people the weakness persists. A lightweight plastic *caliper splint* may be used to keep the foot in place when the person is walking.

foramen

A natural opening in a bone or other body structure, usually to allow the passage of nerves or blood vessels. For example, the foramen magnum is a hole in the base of the skull through which the *spinal cord* passes.

Forbes–Albright syndrome

A condition that is characterized by *amenorrhoea* (the absence of menstruation) and *galactorrhoea* (the production of breast milk) that is not associated with pregnancy. Forbes–Albright syndrome is usually the result of a *pituitary tumour* that secretes excessive amounts of the hormone *prolactin*. Treatment with the drug *bromocriptine* may suppress prolactin production. However, surgical removal of the tumour may be necessary in some cases.

forced expiratory volume

The maximum volume of air that can, over a given period of time, be forcibly exhaled from the lungs, usually over one second. Forced expiratory volume (FEV) tests are often carried out in conjunction with *forced vital capacity* (FVC) tests to check for a variety of lung disorders. (See also *pulmonary function tests*.)

A low result may indicate one of a variety of disorders, including chronic obstructive pulmonary disease (see *pulmonary disease, chronic obstructive*) and diminished lung volume, such as that found in *emphysema*.

forced vital capacity

The largest volume of air that can be expired following a deep inhalation. Forced vital capacity (FVC) is one of the variables measured in a lung function test (see *pulmonary function tests*), which is carried out to check for a variety of lung disorders.

forceps

A tweezerlike instrument that is used for handling tissues or equipment during surgical procedures. Various types of forceps have been designed for specific purposes. For example, forceps that are used for holding and removing wound dressings have scissor handles to make manipulation easier; tissue forceps have fine teeth at the tip of each blade so that body tissues can be handled delicately during surgery. (See also *forceps delivery*.)

forceps delivery

The use of specially designed forceps (see *forceps, obstetric*) to ease out the baby's head during a difficult birth (see *childbirth*).

WHY IT IS DONE

Forceps delivery is used if the mother is overtired or unable to push out her baby unaided, or if the baby is showing signs of *fetal distress*. Forceps are also used to control the baby's head once the body has been delivered in *breech delivery* to prevent an overly rapid birth. They may also be used if the baby's head is stuck in the middle of the mother's pelvis and needs to be rotated to make delivery possible.

HOW IT IS DONE

The mother is given a painkiller and either local or epidural *anaesthesia*. She lies on her back, with her legs raised in stirrups. Forceps can be applied only if the cervix (neck of the uterus) is fully dilated and the baby's head is engaged in the pelvis. An *episiotomy* (making a cut in the perineum) is usually needed for a forceps delivery. The forceps blades are placed on either side of the baby's head, just in front of the ears, and gentle traction is applied to bring about delivery of the baby.

Recovery and care for mother and child is usually the same as after a vaginal delivery.

forceps, obstetric

Surgical instruments that are used in *forceps delivery* to deliver the head of a baby in a difficult labour and birth.

OBSTETRIC FORCEPS

The two wide, blunt blades are designed to fit around the baby's head. The handles are inserted separately and lock together so that the blades are held apart. There are several different sizes and shapes, depending on the position of the baby.

FORCEPS

Positioning
The forceps blades lie along the sides of the baby's head just in front of the ears.

Obstetric forceps are of various types but basically consist of two blades that cup around the baby's head.

Fordyce's disease

A fairly common condition consisting of raised yellow patches on the lips and gums and in the lining of the mouth. The patches are composed of misplaced *sebaceous glands*. The disease is also known as Fordyce's granules. The condition is not serious and does not usually need treatment.

forebrain

The foremost, and largest, of the main divisions of the *brain*. The forebrain is responsible for controlling many of the brain's higher functions, including conscious thought.

foreign body

An object that is present in an organ or passage of the body but should not be there. A foreign body may enter the body accidentally (for example, by inhalation or swallowing), or it may be introduced deliberately (for example, a child pushing a bead into a nostril). The most common sites for foreign bodies include the airways (see *choking*), ears (see *ear, foreign body in*), eyes (see *eye, foreign body in*), rectum, and vagina.

foremilk

The breast milk that is produced at the beginning of a feed (see *breast-feeding*). Foremilk is bluish in appearance; it contains *lactose* and proteins, but little fat. (See also *hindmilk*.)

forensic medicine

The branch of medicine that is concerned with the law, especially criminal law. A forensic pathologist is a doctor who specializes in the examination of bodies when it appears that death was the result of unnatural causes. Forensic specialists may examine victims of alleged sexual assault.

Forensic scientists use laboratory methods to study body fluids (such as blood and semen) found on or near the victim and compare them with samples obtained from suspects. Forensic scientists are also trained in ballistics and in the identification of fibres from materials such as clothing. In addition, forensic scientists may advise on *blood groups* and *genetic fingerprinting* in certain legal investigations.

forensic psychiatry

A branch of *psychiatry* specializing in the diagnosis of mental illness related to criminal behaviour.

foreplay

A sexually stimulating activity that commonly precedes *sexual intercourse* but may also occur independently. Foreplay can involve any of a range of activities, including kissing, caressing, and oral sex.

foreskin

The popular name for the prepuce, which is the loose fold of skin that covers the glans (head) of the *penis* when it is flaccid and which retracts during erection.

At birth, the foreskin is attached to the glans and is not retractable. It separates from the glans during the first three to four years of life. The foreskin may be removed (see *circumcision*) for religious, medical, or social reasons.

DISORDERS

In *phimosis*, the foreskin remains persistently tight after the age of five, which causes difficulty in passing urine

and ballooning of the foreskin. There may also be recurrent *balanitis* (infection of the glans, causing pain and/or itchiness). Erection is frequently painful, which is why the condition is often discovered only at puberty.

In *paraphimosis*, the foreskin becomes stuck in the retracted position, causing painful swelling of the glans that requires emergency treatment.

forewaters

A term that is commonly used to refer to the *amniotic fluid* (the "waters") that is discharged from the uterus when the part of the *amniotic sac* in front of the presenting part of the fetus ruptures just before childbirth. This may happen before or after the onset of labour. (See also *hindwaters*.)

forgetfulness

The inability to remember (see *memory*). (See also *amnesia*.)

formaldehyde

A colourless, pungent, irritant gas. In medicine, a solution of formaldehyde and a small amount of alcohol in water, a preparation known as formalin, is used as a preserving medium for tissue specimens or to harden them before they are stained and examined.

forme fruste

The term that is used to describe any disease that does not follow its usual course. One example of forme fruste is when certain characteristic symptoms of the disease fail to appear; another example is when the progression of the disorder terminates at an earlier stage than expected.

formication

An unpleasant sensation, as though ants were crawling over the skin. This feeling may occur following abuse of certain drugs, such as *alcohol* or *morphine*. Scratching of the skin in an attempt to relieve the sensation can sometimes cause a rash to develop, which may result in an incorrect diagnosis of skin disease.

formula, chemical

A way of expressing the constituents of a chemical in symbols and numbers. Water, for example, has the formula H_2O, indicating that each molecule of water is composed of two atoms of hydrogen (H_2) and one of oxygen (O).

formulary

A book of formulae. The term "formulary" is commonly used to refer to a publication that lists drug preparations and their components and effects. The contents of a formulary may be decided by a group of medical professionals who are working together to ensure similar patterns of drug usage.

fornix

An archlike structure or the space encompassed by such a structure. The term is used to describe the fornix cerebri, a triangular structure of *white matter* in the *brain*, and also the recesses of the *vagina* around the *cervix*.

Fosamax

A brand name for alendronate sodium (see *alendronic acid*), a drug prescribed for certain bone disorders, such as *osteoporosis*. (See also *bone, disorders of*.)

fossa

A depression or hollow area. Examples include the posterior fossa, an area at the back of the base of the brain occupied by the *cerebellum*, and the cubital fossa, the hollow at the front of the elbow joint.

Fothergill's disease

An alternative name for *trigeminal neuralgia*, a disorder of the *trigeminal nerve* (the fifth cranial nerve, which supplies the facial muscles).

fovea

An area situated near the centre of the *retina* that has the highest concentration of light-sensitive cells. The fovea allows detailed vision. (See also *colour vision*.)

Foville's syndrome

A neurological condition that results from damage to tissue (usually *infarction* or a tumour) in the centre of the *brainstem*. The damage causes numbness and paralysis on one side of the face, together with impaired eye movement. There is also damage to the motor nerve fibres to the opposite side of the body, causing paralysis or weakness (see *hemiplegia*).

Fox–Fordyce disease

A chronic pruritic (itching) condition, found most commonly in women, that is characterized by small pimples in areas where apocrine glands (see *sweat glands*) are located.

F

The pimples of Fox–Fordyce disease are caused by the obstruction and rupture of apocrine ducts in the *epidermis* (the outermost layer of the skin). Treatment with topical retinoids (derivatives of *vitamin A*) and *antibiotic drugs* may help to relieve symptoms in patients who have suffered from the disease in the long term.

fracture

A break in a bone. Fractures most often occur across the width of a bone, but can be lengthwise, oblique, or spiral.

TYPES

There are two main types of fracture: closed (simple) or open (compound). In a closed fracture, the broken bone ends remain beneath the skin and little of the surrounding tissue is damaged; in an open fracture, one or both of the bone ends project through the skin. If the ends of the bone have moved out of alignment, which can occur in either a closed or an open fracture, the fracture is termed "displaced".

Fractures may be further divided according to the pattern of the break: for example, transverse or spiral fractures of long bones. In a greenstick fracture, the break is not through the full width of the bone. This type of fracture occurs only in children because their bones are more pliable. In an avulsion fracture, a small piece of bone is pulled off by a tendon.

CAUSES

Most fractures are the result of a sudden injury that exerts more force on the bone than it can withstand. The force may be direct, for example when a finger is hit by a hammer, or indirect, for example when twisting the foot exerts severe stress on the shin.

In some diseases, such as *osteoporosis* and certain cancers, the bone is weakened to such an extent that even a minor injury, or occasionally no injury at all, can cause the bone to break; this is known as a pathological fracture. Compression fractures of the vertebrae are common in people suffering from osteoporosis. Elderly people are most prone to fractures because they are more likely to fall and their bones are very fragile.

SYMPTOMS AND SIGNS

Common sites of fracture include the hand, wrist (see *Colles' fracture*), ankle joint, *clavicle* (collarbone), and the neck of the femur (see *femur, fracture of*). There is usually swelling and tenderness at the site of the fracture. The pain is often severe and is usually made worse by movement.

DIAGNOSIS AND TREATMENT

X-rays can confirm the presence of a fracture. Bone begins to heal soon after it has broken, so the first aim of treatment is to ensure that the bone ends are aligned. Displaced bone ends are moved back into position, under general anaesthesia, by manipulation either through the skin or through an incision. The bone is then immobilized. In some cases, the ends of the bone may be fixed with metal pins or plates.

RECOVERY AND COMPLICATIONS

Most fractures heal without any problems. Healing is sometimes delayed because the blood supply to the affected bone is inadequate (as a result of damaged blood vessels) or because the bone ends are not sufficiently close together. If the fracture fails to unite, internal fixation or a *bone graft* may be necessary. *Osteomyelitis* (infection of bone tissue) is a possible complication of an open fracture.

Physiotherapy plays an important part in rehabilitation following a fracture because complete immobility of a bone for a prolonged period can result in loss of muscle bulk in that area and stiffness in nearby joints.

(See also *fracture, dental*; *humerus, fracture of*; *jaw, fractured*; *march fracture*; *Pott's fracture*; *radius, fracture of*; *rib, fracture of*; *skull, fracture of*; *Smith's fracture*; *stress fracture*; *ulna, fracture of*.)

fracture, dental

A break in a tooth (see *teeth*) most commonly caused by falling onto a hard surface or by being hit in the mouth with a hard object. Fractures may involve the crown or the root of a tooth, or both.

Fractures of the enamel can usually be repaired by bonding (see *bonding, dental*); in some cases, a replacement crown may be fitted (see *crown, dental*). *Pulpotomy* (removal of part of the pulp of the tooth) may be performed in cases where the pulp is damaged. Root fractures may be treated by splinting (see *splinting, dental*), *root-canal treatment*, or removal of the tooth (see *extraction, dental*).

fragile X syndrome

An inherited defect of the *X chromosome* that causes learning difficulties. The disorder occurs within families according to an unusual X-linked recessive pattern of inheritance (see *genetic disorders*). Although fragile X syndrome principally affects males, females can also inherit the disorder. Both men and women can be carriers without having any signs of the disorder.

In addition to having learning difficulties, affected people may have a prominent nose and jaw, and increased ear length; they are also prone to epileptic seizures and behavioural difficulties. Affected males tend to have large testes. Some carriers may also show intellectual impairment.

The condition cannot be treated, but affected children may benefit from speech therapy, specialist education, and help from a psychologist for any accompanying behavioural problems. Life expectancy is normal, but affected boys usually need lifelong care. Couples who have a family history of fragile X syndrome may wish to seek genetic counselling when planning to have a child.

Fragmin

A brand name for dalteparin, which is a low molecular weight *heparin* (an *anticoagulant drug* that is used in the prevention and treatment of abnormal *blood clotting*).

Fraley's syndrome

A rare condition in which the uppermost renal calyces in the *kidney* (part of the central region where urine collects before passing out of the kidney) are compressed; this is usually caused by some of the blood vessels that supply the area. Abdominal pain, back pain in the area of the kidney, and blood in the urine are usually the main symptoms. Possible complications of this syndrome include recurrent urinary tract infections and kidney stones formation (see *calculus, urinary tract*).

Franceschetti's syndrome

A rare genetic disorder, also known as Treacher–Collins syndrome, that causes severe facial malformations. The condition is congenital (present from birth). The nose, cheek bones, lower jaw, and chin are deformed, and the child may have a receding chin (see *micrognathia*). There is a pronounced droop to the outer corners of the eyes. Surgery to reconstruct abnormal features results in significant improvement in appearance and function.

FRACTURES: TYPES AND TREATMENT

There are two main types of fracture: simple (closed) and compound (open). Within these two categories are several other types, three of which are illustrated to the right.

Compound fracture
A sharp piece of bone punctures the skin and is therefore exposed to organisms. There is a high risk of infection.

Simple fracture
The broken bone does not break the skin. Because organisms do not come into contact with the fracture, infection is rare.

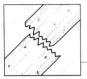

Transverse fracture
This may result from a sharp, direct blow or be a stress fracture caused, for example, by prolonged running.

Greenstick fracture
This type usually occurs in children. Sudden force causes only the outer side of the bent bone to break.

Comminuted fracture
The bone shatters into more than two pieces. This fracture is usually caused by severe force, such as in a car accident.

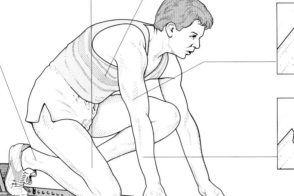

F

REPAIR OF FRACTURES

There are various ways of repairing fractures depending on the particular bone, the severity of the fracture, and the age of the patient.

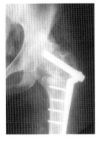

Internal fixation
The photograph (left) shows the repair of a fracture in the hip. A metal pin has been inserted through the neck of the femur and is held in place by a plate screwed to the shaft.

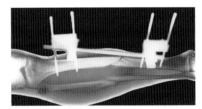

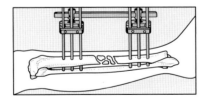

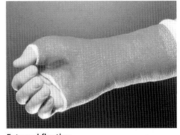

External fixation
Immobilization may be achieved by means of a plaster cast (above) or, in cases such as an unstable fracture of the tibia (left and above left), through the use of metal pins inserted into bone on either side of the break and locked into position on an external metal frame.

THE BONE HEALING PROCESS

After a fracture, the bone starts to heal immediately. Any displacement of the bone ends must therefore be corrected without delay to minimize deformity.

2 Macrophages (immune system cells) invade the fracture site to remove wound debris. Fibroblasts then create a mesh to form a base for new tissue.

4 Remodelling takes place, with denser, stronger bone being laid down. New blood vessels have formed.

1 A blood clot forms between the bone ends, sealing off the ends of the damaged vessels.

3 New bone (callus) is laid down between the ends of the bones and over the fracture line.

5 Over a period of weeks, the bone returns to its former shape.

F

Fraser's syndrome

An inherited condition in which there is cryptophthalmos (absence of the opening between the upper and lower *eyelids*) together with malformations of the ear; cleft palate (see *cleft lip and palate*); narrowing of the *larynx* (the voicebox); *syndactyly* (fusion of two or more fingers or toes); imperforate anus (see *anus, imperforate*); cardiac defects, kidney malformation; and genital *masculinization* in females. Fraser's syndrome is inherited as an autosomal recessive genetic trait (see *genetic disorders*).

Many babies born with Fraser's syndrome die within the first year of life. For those who survive, surgery to the eyelids and corneas may provide some degree of vision and eyelid movement. People with a family history of the condition may wish to seek *genetic counselling* before starting a family.

fraternal twins

An alternative term for dizygotic *twins*.

freckle

A tiny patch of *pigmentation* that occurs on sun-exposed skin. Freckles tend to become more numerous with continued exposure to sunlight. A tendency to freckling is inherited and occurs most often in fair and red-haired people. Freckles are harmless.

free-floating anxiety

An all-pervasive feeling of apprehension or tension with no apparent cause. Free-floating anxiety is often associated with *generalized anxiety disorder*.

Freeman–Sheldon syndrome

A rare *congenital* disorder with the following characteristics: sunken eyes; underdevelopment of the cartilage of the nose; pursed lips; various skeletal malformations; and muscle weakness. Intelligence and life expectancy are normal. The syndrome is usually inherited as an autosomal dominant genetic trait (see *genetic disorders*). Affected children may need corrective surgery to improve deformities of the face, hands, or feet. People with a family history of the condition may wish to seek *genetic counselling* before starting a family.

free radicals

Highly active molecules that bind to and destroy body cells. Free radicals can be formed as a result of the effects of external sources such as smoke, sunlight, and food. They are produced in the body principally as a result of the chemical reactions involved in metabolism. They are thought to contribute to the cumulative damage to body cells that occurs with aging and to the development of cancers and possibly heart disease. Free radicals and their effects may be neutralized by antioxidants, such as *vitamin C* and *vitamin E*.

frenulum

Any fold of tissue or *mucous membrane* that limits the movement of an organ or part of the body. One example of a frenulum is the fold of mucous membrane on the inside of the upper lip that connects the lip to the gum; another example is the attachment of the *foreskin* to the glans (head) of the penis.

frequency

See *urination, frequent*.

Freudian slip

A slip of the tongue or a minor error of action that could betray what the person really wanted to say or do.

Freudian theory

A discipline that was developed by the Viennese neurologist Sigmund Freud (1856–1939). The theory developed out of Freud's treatment of neurotic patients using *hypnosis* and, later, the interpretation of their dreams. Freudian theory formed the basis of the technique of *psychoanalysis*.

Freud believed that an individual's feelings, thoughts, and behaviour were controlled by unconscious wishes and conflicts originating in childhood. Problems are said to occur when the desires are not fulfilled or if conflicts remain unresolved into adulthood.

The essence of Freud's theory concerns early psychological development, particularly sexual development. Freud defined three developmental stages: oral, anal, and genital (representing the areas of the body on which the infant's attention becomes fixed at different ages). He also identified three components of personality: the *id*, the *ego*, and the *superego* (based respectively on pleasure, reality, and moral and social constraints). (See also *psychoanalytic theory*; *psychotherapy*.)

friar's balsam

A brand name for the aromatic liquid tincture of benzoin. Friar's balsam is used with hot water as a *steam inhalation* to help relieve nasal congestion, acute rhinitis, and sinusitis, as well as to loosen coughs. Friar's balsam is available over the counter.

Friedreich's ataxia

A rare inherited disease in which degeneration of nerve fibres in the spinal cord causes loss of coordinated movement and balance. The condition is inherited as an autosomal recessive trait (see *genetic disorders*).

SYMPTOMS

Symptoms tend to appear between the ages of five and 15 years. Early signs of the condition include difficulty in walking and deformities of the lower legs and feet, such as *claw-foot*. The difficulty in movement then extends to the arms and trunk. Once symptoms have developed, the disease becomes progressively more severe; the muscles then weaken and waste away. A gradual loss of sensation occurs in the extremities, which may eventually spread to other parts of the body; speech becomes slow and slurred; and *nystagmus* (involuntary, jerky eye movements) is common.

Other symptoms include chest pain, shortness of breath, and palpitations. Many people with Friedreich's ataxia develop heart problems, such as *cardiomyopathy* (disease of the heart muscle) and abnormalities of the heart rhythm (see *arrhythmia, cardiac*). Some people with the condition also develop *diabetes mellitus*.

TREATMENT AND OUTLOOK

Treatment can help with the symptoms but cannot alter the course of the disease. Braces or surgery may be used to correct deformities, physiotherapy may help to maintain movement for as long as possible, and drugs can be given for heart conditions. However, most affected people die in early adulthood. People with a family history of the condition may wish to seek *genetic counselling* before starting a family.

frigidity

A lack of desire for sexual contact or an inability to become aroused during stimulation (see *sexual desire, inhibited*). (See also *orgasm, lack of.*)

frontal

A term referring to the front part of an organ (for example, the frontal lobe of the *brain*).

frostbite

Damage to body tissues caused by extreme cold. Frostbite can develop at any temperature below freezing; the lower the temperature, the more rapidly frostbite will develop. The risk of frostbite is increased by windy conditions.

Frostbite can affect any part of the body, but the extremities (the nose, ears, fingers, and toes) are most susceptible and tend to be affected first. People who have impaired circulation, such as those with *diabetic vascular disease*, are at increased risk.

SYMPTOMS

The first symptom is a *pins-and-needles* sensation, followed by complete numbness in the affected region. The affected skin appears white, cold, and hard; it may then become red and swollen.

TREATMENT AND OUTLOOK

Treatment of frostbite involves slowly rewarming the affected areas by immersion in warm water (ensuring that it is not too hot to touch), then applying bandages. When warmed, mildly affected tissues become red, swollen, and sore. If frostbite is more severe, blisters appear, and the area becomes very painful.

If the damage is restricted to the skin and the tissues that immediately underlie it, rewarming may result in complete recovery of the tissues. Recovery from frostbite damage usually occurs within about six months, although some lasting sensitivity to extreme temperatures is common. Following severe frostbite, symptoms including stiffness, pain, and numbness may persist indefinitely.

If blood vessels are affected by frostbite, *gangrene* (tissue death) may follow. In such circumstances, amputation may be necessary.

frottage

A sexual *deviation* in which an individual rubs his or her body against another person in order to achieve sexual arousal. Typically, this activity is carried out in a crowd of people where a man rubs his (clothed) genitals against a woman's buttocks or thigh.

frozen section

A method of preparing a *biopsy* specimen (a sample of tissue removed for microscopic analysis) that can provide a rapid indication of whether or not a tissue is cancerous.

WHY IT IS DONE

Frozen section may be used to determine whether *breast lumps* are cancerous. It can also be used to check whether thyroid or intestinal tumours are cancerous and to diagnose *lymphomas* (cancerous tumours of lymphoid tissue).

HOW IT IS DONE

Frozen section may be done during an operation so that the results can be used to determine the appropriate surgical treatment. The surgeon removes a sample of tissue and sends it to the pathology laboratory for analysis. The sample is quickly frozen in liquid nitrogen, cut into very thin sections, placed on a glass slide, and stained so that the cells can be examined under a microscope. The entire process takes about 20 minutes. Information about the sample is then conveyed to the operating theatre.

frozen shoulder

Increasing stiffness and pain in the *shoulder* that limits normal movement of the joint. In severe cases of frozen shoulder, the shoulder may be completely rigid, and pain may be intense.

CAUSES

Frozen shoulder is caused by inflammation and thickening of the lining of the joint capsule. In some cases, it occurs following a minor injury to the shoulder. Frozen shoulder can also occur if the shoulder is immobilized for a long period, such as following a *stroke*. In many cases, however, the disorder develops for no apparent reason.

The condition is more common in people over the age of 40. People with *diabetes mellitus* are also more susceptible to developing frozen shoulder.

TREATMENT

Moderate symptoms of frozen shoulder can be eased by exercise, and by taking *analgesic drugs* (painkillers) and *nonsteroidal anti-inflammatory drugs* to relieve pain and inflammation. In severe cases, *corticosteroid drugs* may need to be injected into the affected joint.

Manipulation of the joint under general anaesthesia can restore mobility. However, this treatment carries the risk of increasing pain initially.

OUTLOOK

Recovery is often slow, and the shoulder may remain stiff for some months, but it is usually back to normal and pain-free within two years.

fructose

A simple sugar (monosaccharide) that is naturally present in honey and certain fruits. Fructose and *glucose* are the two components of *sucrose* (table sugar).

Fructose can be converted into energy as easily as glucose but, unlike glucose, fructose metabolism is not dependent on *insulin*. For this reason, fructose can be a useful element in the diet of people suffering from *diabetes mellitus*.

frusemide

An alternative name for *furosemide*, a *diuretic drug*.

frustration

A deep feeling of discontent and tension as a result of unresolved problems or unfulfilled needs, or because the individual's path to a goal is blocked. In some people, frustration can lead to *regression* (childlike behaviour), *aggression*, or *depression*.

FSH

An abbreviation for *follicle-stimulating hormone*, a *gonadotrophin hormone* produced by the *pituitary gland*.

FTT

The abbreviation for *failure to thrive* in infants and children. A child who fails to grow at the appropriate rate needs tests to determine the cause.

Fuchs' spots

Pigmented spots that develop on the *retina* (the light-sensitive inner layer at the back of the eye). The condition sometimes occurs in people who suffer from a severe degree of *myopia* (shortsightedness).

Fuchs' syndrome

A slowly progressing disease that usually affects both eyes and which may be hereditary. It is also known as Fuchs' corneal dystrophy. The condition occurs when cells in the innermost layer of the *cornea* (the transparent front part of the eye) gradually deteriorate. Fuchs' syndrome may result in pain and severe visual impairment. There is no preventive treatment for the disease. In some cases, a corneal transplant may eventually be necessary to restore sight.

Fucithalmic eye drops

A brand of eye drops containing *fusidic acid*, an *antibiotic drug*. The drops are used for bacterial conjunctivitis.

fugue

An episode of altered consciousness in which a person purposefully wanders away from home or work and, in some cases, adopts a new identity. Afterwards, the person has no recollection of what has occurred.

Fugues may last for hours or days. During a short fugue, the sufferer may be confused and agitated. During a fugue lasting for days, behaviour may appear normal but there may be accompanying symptoms, such as hallucinations, feelings of unreality, and unstable mood.

Fugues are rare. Possible causes include *dissociative disorders*, *temporal lobe epilepsy*, *depression*, *head injury*, and *dementia*. (See also *amnesia*.)

fulminant

A term used to describe a disorder that develops and progresses suddenly and with great severity. A virulent infection, a severe form of arthritis, or a cancer that has spread rapidly is often described as being fulminant.

fumes

See *pollution*.

functional disorders

Illnesses in which there is no evidence of organic disturbance even though physical performance is impaired.

functional endoscopic sinus surgery (FESS)

Surgery that is carried out in order to improve the drainage of the facial sinuses or to clear a blockage in them. The procedure, which involves the use of an endoscope, enlarges the drainage holes leading to the nose.

fundus

The bottom or base of an organ, or the part that is farthest away from the organ's opening. The optic fundus is the back of the retina as viewed through an ophthalmoscope.

fungal infections

A wide range of diseases that are caused by the multiplication and spread of *fungi*. Fungal infections, which are also known as mycoses, range from mild and barely noticed to severe and sometimes even fatal. (In addition to infections, fungi are also responsible for some allergic disorders, such as allergic *alveolitis* and *asthma*.)

CAUSES

Some fungi are harmlessly present all of the time in areas of the body such as the mouth, skin, intestines, and vagina.

Usually, however, they are prevented from multiplying by competition from bacteria. Other fungi are kept from multiplying to a harmful degree by the body's *immune system*.

Fungal infections are therefore more common in people who are taking *antibiotic drugs* (which destroy the bacterial competition) and in those whose immune systems are suppressed by *immunosuppressant drugs*, *corticosteroid drugs*, by a disorder such as *AIDS*, or by chemotherapy. Such serious fungal infections are described as *opportunistic infections* because they take advantage of the body's lowered defences. Some fungal infections are more common in people with *diabetes mellitus*.

Fungi that cause skin infections thrive in warm, moist conditions, such as those that occur between the toes and in the genital area.

TYPES

Fungal infections can be broadly classified into three categories: superficial (affecting the skin, hair, nails, inside of the mouth, and genital organs); subcutaneous (beneath the skin); and deep (affecting internal organs).

The main superficial infections are *tinea* (including ringworm and athlete's foot) and *candidiasis* (thrush), both of which are common. Tinea affects external areas of the body. Candidiasis is caused by the yeast CANDIDA ALBICANS and usually affects the genitals or inside of the mouth.

Subcutaneous fungal infections are rare. The most common is *sporotrichosis*, which may follow contamination of a scratch. Most other conditions of this type, the most important of which is *mycetoma*, occur mainly in tropical countries.

Deep fungal infections are uncommon, but they can present a serious threat to people who have an immune deficiency disorder or those who are taking immunosuppressant drugs. Fungal infections of this sort include *aspergillosis*, *histoplasmosis*, *cryptococcosis*, and *blastomycosis*, all of which are caused by different species of fungi. The fungal spores enter the body through inhalation into the lungs. Candidiasis can also spread from its usual sites of infection to affect the oesophagus, the urinary tract, and other internal tissues.

TREATMENT

Treatment of fungal infections is with *antifungal drugs*, either used topically

on the infected area, or given by mouth or intravenously for generalized infections. (For further information, see *Fungal diseases* box, opposite.)

fungi

Simple parasitic life-forms that include yeasts, moulds, mushrooms, and toadstools. The fungi that are responsible for causing disease can be divided into two groups: filamentous fungi and yeasts. Filamentous fungi are made up of branching threads known as hyphae, which form a network called a mycelium. Mushrooms and toadstools are the reproductive structures (known as fruiting bodies) of a filamentous fungus that has spread in dead matter or soil. Yeasts are single-celled organisms.

FUNGI AND DISEASE

The majority of fungi are either completely harmless or actually beneficial to human health. However, there are a number of fungi that can cause illness and disease.

The fruiting bodies of some fungi contain toxins that may cause poisoning if they are eaten (see *mushroom poisoning*). Certain other fungi infect food crops and also produce toxins that may cause food poisoning. The best known of these fungi is a species that infects cereals and produces *ergot*, a toxin that constricts blood vessels. Another fungus that sometimes grows on peanuts and produces *aflatoxin*, a poison and *carcinogen*.

The inhaled spores of some fungi can cause allergic *alveolitis*, a persistent allergic reaction in the lungs. Farmer's lung, which is caused by spores from mouldy hay, is an example of such a reaction. Fungal spores are sometimes responsible for various other allergic disorders, such as allergic *rhinitis* (hay fever) and *asthma*.

Some fungi are capable of invading the body and forming colonies in various parts of the body such as the lungs, the skin, or sometimes in a variety of tissues throughout the body, leading to conditions that range from mild irritation to severe, sometimes even fatal, widespread infection (see *fungal infections*) and illness. For further information, see *Fungal diseases* box, opposite. (See also *candidiasis*.)

fungicidal

A term used to describe the ability to kill fungi (see *antifungal drugs*).

FUNGAL DISEASES

The skin, genitals, and nails are common sites of fungal infection. Examples include *tinea* (ringworm) and *candidiasis* (thrush). Fungi may rarely infect the lungs and other internal organs, causing a more serious disease. They may also cause allergic lung disease, such as farmer's lung.

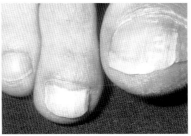

Fungal nail infection
This condition can affect toenails or fingernails. It is liable to last for years. Antifungal medications are of benefit to some people.

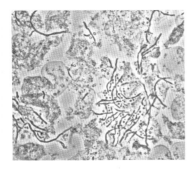

Colony of fungal cells
The microscope photograph (left) shows a colony of yeast cells in a skin fragment.

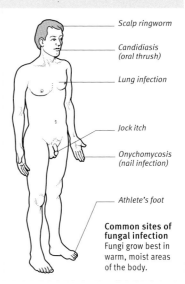

Scalp ringworm

Candidiasis (oral thrush)

Lung infection

Jock itch

Onychomycosis (nail infection)

Athlete's foot

Common sites of fungal infection
Fungi grow best in warm, moist areas of the body.

FUNGAL GROWTH

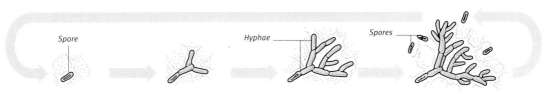

Spore

Hyphae

Spores

1 Many fungal colonies originate from spores that have been carried in the air and have settled at a suitable site for growth.

2 If nutrients are available and other conditions (such as temperature) are favourable, a spore starts to divide.

3 The cells of many fungi divide to form a network consisting of branched chains of tubular filaments called hyphae.

4 Eventually, a colony may start to form its own spores. These spores may be carried to new sites to set up new growths.

funny-bone

A popular term for the small area at the back of the *elbow* where the ulnar nerve passes over a prominence of the *humerus* (upper-arm bone).

A blow to the nerve causes acute pain, numbness, and a tingling sensation in the forearm and hand.

furosemide

A *diuretic drug* used in the treatment of *oedema* (the accumulation of fluid in body tissues) and *heart failure*. Furosemide belongs to a group of drugs known as loop diuretics, which cause a rapid, temporary increase in the output of urine. When given by injection, furosemide has a very rapid effect; it may therefore be used in emergencies to relieve *pulmonary oedema* (a buildup of fluid around the lungs).

Furosemide increases the rate at which potassium is excreted from the body, which may cause headaches, dizziness, and muscle cramps. In order to prevent excessive potassium loss, doctors frequently give potassium supplements, or alternatively potassium-sparing diuretics, in combination with the drug.

furuncle

An alternative term for a *boil*.

fusidic acid

A type of *antibiotic drug* that is used in the treatment of a variety of bacterial infections that are resistant to *penicillin drugs*. Fusidic acid is commonly used in preparations applied to localized areas of skin in conditions such as impetigo. The drug is also used in various eye and ear preparations.

fusion inhibitors

A group of *antiretroviral drugs* (drugs used to treat HIV infection and AIDS) that work by interfering with the entry of the virus into cells. Enfuvirtide is the main fusion inhibitor drug. It is used in combination with other antiretrovirals to treat resistant strains of HIV.

FVC

The abbreviation for *forced vital capacity*. (See also *forced expiratory volume*.)

Fybogel

A brand name for a bulk-forming *laxative drug*.

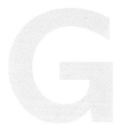

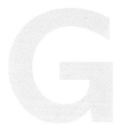

G6PD deficiency

An *X-linked disorder* in which an abnormal gene causes a deficiency of G6PD (the *enzyme* glucose 6 phosphate dehydrogenase) in red blood cells. In a healthy person, this enzyme contributes to a chemical process that protects the cells from damage. G6PD deficiency makes the red cells prone to damage or destruction by infectious illness or by certain drugs or foods.

The disorder most commonly affects southern European and black men. Women are unaffected but they can carry the abnormal gene and are at risk of passing it on to their sons.

Some drugs, such as certain *antimalarial drugs* and *antibiotics*, may precipitate haemolysis (destruction of red cells) in people who have the abnormal gene; see the table below for important drugs that may pose this risk. In one form of G6PD deficiency, called *favism*, haemolysis may be triggered by a chemical in broad beans, and affected people must avoid eating them.

After taking a precipitating drug or food, or during an infectious illness, an affected person develops symptoms of anaemia (see *anaemia, haemolytic*), such as *jaundice*, fatigue, headaches, and shortness of breath (which may occur even after mild exertion).

G6PD deficiency is diagnosed with a blood test. There is no specific treatment, but symptoms provoked by a drug or food can be prevented by avoiding that substance.

GABA

The abbreviation for gamma-aminobutyric acid, a *neurotransmitter* (a chemical released from nerve endings that relays messages in the *nervous system*). GABA controls the flow of nerve impulses by blocking the release of other neurotransmitters, such as *noradrenaline* and *dopamine*, that stimulate electrical activity in the nerve cells; as a result, this activity is inhibited.

The action of GABA is enhanced by *benzodiazepine drugs*, *anticonvulsant drugs*, and possibly *alcohol*. In contrast, it has been suggested that people with *Huntington's disease* (an inherited disorder that causes a loss of brain function and abnormal movements) suffer degeneration of GABA-secreting brain cells, leading to overstimulation of the *basal ganglia* (an area of the brain that helps coordinate movement) and producing the typical symptoms.

gabapentin

An *anticonvulsant drug* used either alone or with other anticonvulsants to treat some types of *epilepsy*. It is also used to treat neuropathic pain, such as that from an attack of shingles (see *herpes zoster*). Common side effects include drowsiness, dizziness, unsteadiness, and fatigue.

gag reflex

An automatic impulse to retch, brought about by the *autonomic nervous system* in response to a particular stimulus, such as a foreign object touching the back of the throat. The reflex protects the airway from becoming blocked by debris. If a person becomes unconscious, however, the gag reflex may be lost, and the person may be at risk of choking.

gait

A term used to describe the manner or style of *walking*. Gait varies from one person to another. An abnormal gait, or an unusual change in the gait, may indicate a neuromuscular or brain disorder (such as *Parkinson's disease*). (See also *festinating gait*.)

galactocele

A *breast cyst* that contains milk or a milky substance. A galactocele can be caused by obstruction of a milk duct in the *breast* during *breast-feeding*. In most cases, it occurs at the end of breast-feeding when milk is allowed to stagnate in the breast. The swelling may occasionally become infected, leading to a *breast abscess*. Usually, no treatment is needed; the fluid is reabsorbed, or can be expelled by massaging the breast towards the nipple.

galactokinase deficiency

A rare, inherited condition in which there is a deficiency of galactokinase, an *enzyme* involved in the breakdown of galactose (a simple sugar derived from the milk sugar *lactose*). Galactokinase deficiency is an autosomal recessive *genetic disorder*. The condition leads to a form of *galactosaemia* (the inability to convert galactose into *glucose*, another simple sugar). The only manifestation of galactokinase deficiency galactosaemia is *cataracts*, which usually become apparent within the first few weeks of life.

galactorrhoea

The spontaneous, persistent production of breast milk by a woman who is not pregnant or *breast-feeding*, or, very rarely, by a man. Lactation (milk production) is initiated by a rise in the level of *prolactin*, a hormone produced by the *pituitary gland*. Galactorrhoea is caused by excessive secretion of prolactin due either to a *pituitary tumour* or to another endocrine disorder, such as *hypothyroidism*. Less commonly, it may also be caused by certain drugs, including *antidepressant drugs*, combined *oral contraceptives*, and some *antipsychotic drugs*.

As well as triggering breast milk production, excess prolactin may adversely affect the *ovaries*, causing *amenorrhoea*

SELECTED DRUGS TO BE AVOIDED BY PEOPLE WITH **G6PD DEFICIENCY**	
Class	**Drugs to avoid**
Antimalarial drugs	Primaquine, chloroquine, quinine, quinidine, dapsone
Antibacterial and antibiotic drugs	Nitrofurantoin, sulphonamides (such as co-trimoxazole), quinolone drugs (such as ciprofloxacin and nalidixic acid)
Analgesics (painkillers)	Aspirin
Miscellaneous	Probenecid

(absence of menstrual periods) or *infertility*. If the underlying cause is a pituitary tumour, there may be symptoms associated with the tumour, such as headaches and visual disturbances.

Treatment with *bromocriptine* suppresses prolactin production, but the underlying cause of the disorder may also require treatment. Bromocriptine is not suitable for treating galactorrhoea due to drug treatment. In such cases, use of the causative drug should be reviewed as there may be a suitable alternative.

galactosaemia

A rare, inherited condition in which the body is unable to convert galactose (a simple sugar derived from the milk sugar *lactose*) into *glucose* (another simple sugar) due to the absence of a particular *enzyme* in the liver and in red blood cells.

Galactosaemia causes no symptoms at birth, but *jaundice*, diarrhoea, and vomiting may develop after a few days, and the baby fails to gain weight. If untreated, the disorder may result in liver disease, *cataracts* (opacities in the lenses of the eyes), and *learning difficulties*.

The diagnosis is confirmed by urine and blood tests. An affected person must avoid milk products, and use lactose-free milk, throughout life.

gallbladder

A small, muscular, pear-shaped sac, situated just beneath the *liver*, in which *bile* is stored and concentrated.

Bile, which is produced by the liver, enters the gallbladder via the hepatic and cystic ducts. When food passes from the *stomach* into the *duodenum* (the first part of the small intestine), gastrointestinal hormones make the gallbladder contract. This causes it to release the bile, via the common bile duct, into the duodenum, where it aids the breakdown of fats contained in the food. (See also *biliary system*.)

gallbladder cancer

A rare cancer that occurs mainly in the elderly. It is usually associated with *gallstones*, but affects only a tiny proportion of those people with gallstones.

Gallbladder cancer may cause *jaundice* and tenderness in the abdomen, but it is sometimes symptomless.

ANATOMY OF THE GALLBLADDER

The gallbladder receives bile from the liver via the common hepatic duct. It expels bile into the small intestine via the cystic duct and the common bile duct.

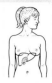

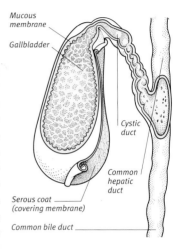

Mucous membrane

Gallbladder

Cystic duct

Common hepatic duct

Serous coat (covering membrane)

Common bile duct

G

DISORDERS OF THE **GALLBLADDER**

The gallbladder rarely causes problems in childhood or early adulthood but, from middle age onwards, an increasing occurrence of *gallstones* may sometimes give rise to symptoms.

The digestive system can function normally without a gallbladder, and its removal has few known long-term adverse effects.

Metabolic disorders

The principal disorder, with which most other gallbladder problems are associated, is the formation of gallstones. Every year thousands of people develop gallstones. Women are affected up to four times as often as men, depending on their age and ethnicity.

The formation of gallstones results from a metabolic problem in which the chemical composition of bile (the digestive juice stored in the gallbladder) is altered. There are three main types of gallstone: stones formed from the fatty substance *cholesterol*; stones made from *bile* pigments; and mixed gallstones, which contain both cholesterol and pigments. The great majority are mixed.

Only about 20 per cent of affected people experience symptoms or complications; many carry "silent" gallstones, producing no symptoms. Attempts by the gallbladder to expel the stone or stones, however, can cause severe *biliary colic* (abdominal pain).

Infection and inflammation

If a gallstone lodges in the gallbladder outlet, trapped bile may irritate and inflame the lining, and bile may become infected. This disorder is called acute *cholecystitis*. The first symptom may be biliary colic, followed by fever and abdominal tenderness.

Repeated attacks of biliary colic and acute cholecystitis can lead to chronic cholecystitis, in which the gallbladder becomes shrunken and thick-walled and ceases to function. Rarely, it may become inflamed when no gallstones are present: a condition called acalculous cholecystitis.

Cholecystitis can proceed to *empyema*, in which the gallbladder fills with pus; a high fever and severe abdominal pain may result.

Congenital and genetic defects

Abnormalities that may be present from birth include absence of the gallbladder,

an oversized gallbladder, or two gallbladders. These defects, however, rarely cause problems.

Tumours

Gallbladder cancer usually occurs in a gallbladder that contains gallstones. This cancer is, however, extremely uncommon compared to the high prevalence of gallstones.

Other disorders

In rare cases where the gallbladder is empty and a stone obstructs its outlet, the gallbladder may become distended and filled with mucus secreted by its lining. A gallbladder with this problem is known as a *mucocele*.

INVESTIGATION

Investigations may include a physical examination; imaging techniques such as plain abdominal *X-rays*, *ultrasound scanning*, *radionuclide scanning*, *ERCP*, and *cholecystography*; and blood tests.

The cancer is usually diagnosed by *ultrasound scanning*. Treatment is by surgical removal of the tumour and, for advanced cases, *radiotherapy* and *chemotherapy*. However, if the cancer has spread to the liver by the time it is detected, the outlook is poor.

gallium

A metallic element whose radioactive form is used in *radionuclide scanning* (a technique using a tiny amount of a radioactive substance to obtain images of internal organs). Gallium is injected into the bloodstream before a scan in order to reveal areas of inflammation, such as those that occur in cancers, *abscesses*, *osteomyelitis*, and *sarcoidosis*.

gallstone ileus

See *ileus, gallstone*.

gallstones

Lumps of solid matter found in the *gallbladder* (the sac under the liver where bile is stored) or in the *bile ducts* (which connect the gallbladder and liver to the duodenum). Most gallstones are made of *cholesterol* and bile pigments from the breakdown of red blood cells.

CAUSES AND INCIDENCE

Gallstones develop due to a disturbance in the chemical composition of *bile*. They are rare in childhood and become increasingly common with age. Women are affected more than men. Risk factors for developing gallstones include a high-fat diet and being overweight.

SYMPTOMS

Most gallstones cause no symptoms. Any symptoms often begin when a stone lodges in the gallbladder outlet. This problem causes *biliary colic* (intense pain in the upper right area of the abdomen or between the shoulderblades), nausea, and sometimes indigestion and flatulence. Possible complications include *cholecystitis* (inflammation of the gallbladder), *pancreatitis* (inflammation of the pancreas), and *bile duct obstruction*.

DIAGNOSIS AND TREATMENT

Diagnosis may be by *ultrasound scanning*, X-ray oral *cholecystography*, *ERCP* (an endoscopic X-ray procedure that may also be used for treatment), or *cholangiography*.

Stones that are not causing symptoms are usually left alone. In other cases, it may be possible to remove the stones during ERCP. Alternatively, the stones may be shattered using ultrasonic shockwaves (see *lithotripsy*); the frag-

ments pass into the intestine and then out of the body in the faeces. Some gallstones can be dissolved slowly (over several months) with drugs such as *ursodeoxycholic acid*; these drugs may also be given after other types of treatment to prevent further stones from forming. In some cases, it may be necessary to surgically remove the gallbladder and stones by *cholecystectomy*.

gambling, pathological

A chronic inability to resist impulses to gamble, resulting in personal, social, and/or financial problems.

gamete

A sex cell. Gametes are found in the reproductive systems of adults: *sperm* are formed in the testes in males, and an *ovum* (egg cell) is released approximately every month from the ovaries in females. Sperm and ova come together during *fertilization* to create offspring. (See also *meiosis*.)

gamete intrafallopian transfer (GIFT)

A technique for assisting *conception* (see *infertility*) in women. It can only be used if a woman has functioning *fallopian tubes*. In GIFT, ova (eggs) are removed from the woman's *ovary* during *laparoscopy* (viewing of the interior of the abdomen) and mixed with *sperm* in the laboratory. The mixed eggs and sperm are introduced into one of the fallopian tubes, where *fertilization* takes place. A fertilized egg may then become implanted in the *uterus*.

Gamgee tissue

The brand name for a material consisting of a thick layer of highly absorbent cotton wool enclosed in gauze. Gamgee tissue may be used for padding and compression of soft-tissue injuries, but may also be used on open wounds, such as *ulcers*, to aid healing by applying compression and absorbing body fluids.

gamma aminobutyric acid

See *GABA*.

gamma camera

A piece of equipment used to generate diagnostic images in *radionuclide scanning*. A tiny amount of a radioactive substance is introduced into the body (usually by injection) and taken up in variable amounts by the tissues to be examined. The gamma camera detects

radiation emitted from the tissues and displays its pattern of distribution as an image on a monitor.

gamma-globulin

A substance that contains *antibodies* against a specific infection. Injections of gamma-globulins provide temporary protection against diseases such as *chickenpox* and *tetanus*. (See *immunization*; *immunoglobulin injections*.)

gamolenic acid

A *fatty acid* that is found in evening primrose oil and starflower (borage) oil.

ganciclovir

An *antiviral drug* used to treat severe *cytomegalovirus* infection. This condition occurs in individuals whose *immune system* is impaired or suppressed, for example, because they have *AIDS* or are taking *immunosuppressant drugs* (such as after an organ transplant).

Because ganciclovir is toxic, it produces a range of side effects, including nausea, diarrhoea, dyspepsia, abdominal pain, weakness, and suppression of blood cell formation in the bone marrow. For this reason, the drug is used only when the benefits are likely to outweigh the risks.

ganglion

A group of *nerve* cells that have a common function; for example, the *basal ganglia* in the brain are concerned with the control of muscular movements.

The term is also used to describe a fluid-filled swelling associated with the sheath of a *tendon*. A ganglion may disappear spontaneously; if necessary, it may be drained or removed surgically.

gangrene

Death of tissue, usually caused by loss of the blood supply. Gangrene may affect a small area of skin or a large portion of a limb.

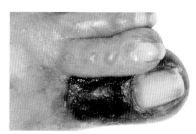

Gangrene of the foot
This shows a gangrenous foot, with areas of dead tissue and blackening of the skin on the big toe.

SYMPTOMS AND TYPES

Pain is felt as the tissues are dying, but once dead they become numb. The affected tissue turns black. There are two types of gangrene: dry and wet.

In dry gangrene, there is usually no infection and the tissue dies because it has no blood supply. This type of gangrene does not spread. It may be caused by *arteriosclerosis*, *diabetes mellitus*, *thrombosis*, frostbite, or an *embolism*.

Wet gangrene develops when an area of dry gangrene or a wound becomes infected by *bacteria*. Redness, swelling, and oozing pus may occur around the blackened tissues. The gangrene spreads, and the area gives off an unpleasant smell. A virulent type called *gas gangrene* is due to a bacterium that destroys muscles and produces a foul-smelling gas.

TREATMENT

Treatment of dry gangrene involves attempting to improve the circulation to the affected area before the tissues die. *Antibiotic drugs* can prevent wet gangrene from setting in. To treat wet gangrene, *amputation* of the affected part and surrounding tissue may be necessary.

Ganser's syndrome

A rare *factitious disorder* in which an individual seeks, either consciously or unconsciously, to mislead others about his or her mental state and may simulate symptoms of *psychosis*.

Gardnerella vaginalis

A *bacterium* that is often found in the vaginal discharge of women who have *bacterial vaginosis*.

gargle

A liquid preparation to wash and freshen the mouth and throat. Some gargles contain *antiseptics* or local *anaesthetics* to relieve sore throats.

gargoylism

Another name for *Hurler's syndrome*.

gas-and-air

A mixture of *nitrous oxide* and *oxygen* that is mainly used for temporary pain relief in emergencies or during *labour*.

gas gangrene

A rare but life-threatening form of *gangrene* (tissue death), usually due to infection by the bacterium CLOSTRIDIUM PERFRINGENS. This organism thrives in *anaerobic* environments, where there is little or no oxygen, such as dying tissue.

Gas gangrene develops suddenly and normally occurs at the site of a recent serious wound. The bacteria multiply in the damaged tissue, producing toxins that release a gas, and spread incredibly rapidly to healthy tissue.

The affected area is swollen and painful, and pale or reddish-brown in colour. Gas collects in the tissues, causing a crackling sensation if the area is pressed. Other symptoms that develop early in the infection include sweating, fever, and anxiety. If left untreated, the condition may lead to *shock* (failure of blood circulation), *kidney failure*, *coma*, and even death.

Penicillin drugs destroy the bacteria at the edges of the gangrene, but all of the diseased tissue needs to be surgically removed. *Amputation* of an affected limb may be required, in some cases, to control the spread of infection. *Hyperbaric oxygen treatment*, in which the patient is exposed to oxygen at high pressure, may help to kill the bacteria.

gastrectomy

Removal of the whole *stomach* (total gastrectomy) or of part of the stomach (partial gastrectomy). Total gastrectomy is used to treat some *stomach cancers*. Partial gastrectomy used to be a treatment for *peptic ulcers* (ulcers of the stomach or duodenum) but has largely been replaced by drug treatment.

A person who has had a gastrectomy may experience fullness and discomfort after meals. Possible postoperative complications include the regurgitation or vomiting of *bile*, which may lead to inflammation of the stomach or the oesophagus; diarrhoea; and *dumping syndrome* (sweating, nausea, dizziness, and weakness after meals, due to food leaving the stomach too quickly). Other complications include *malabsorption* (a reduced ability to absorb nutrients), which may lead to *anaemia* or *osteoporosis* (loss of bone density). After a total gastrectomy, patients cannot absorb vitamin B_{12} and need injections of the vitamin for the rest of their lives.

gastric erosion

A break in the surface layer of the membrane that lines the *stomach*. Gastric erosions occur in some cases of *gastritis* (inflammation of the stomach lining). Many result from ingestion of irritants, *alcohol*, *nonsteroidal anti-inflammatory drugs* (such as *aspirin* and *ibuprofen*), or *corticosteroid drugs*. The physical stress

of serious illness, injuries such as *burns*, or major surgery may also cause erosions to develop.

Often there are no symptoms, but erosions may bleed, causing *vomiting of blood* or blood in the faeces. Persistent loss of blood may lead to *anaemia*.

Gastric erosions are diagnosed by *gastroscopy* (examination of the stomach with a flexible viewing instrument). They usually heal in a few days when treated with antacid drugs, H_2-receptor antagonists, or proton pump inhibitors (see *ulcer-healing drugs*). Drugs that block the production of stomach acid are often given to people who are at high risk of developing erosions, such as those receiving *intensive care*.

gastric lavage

See *lavage, gastric*.

gastric ulcer

A raw area in the *stomach* wall caused by a breach of the lining (see *gastric erosion*) that penetrates into the tissues. A gastric ulcer is a type of *peptic ulcer* (ulcer of the stomach or duodenum).

gastrin

A *hormone* produced by cells in the *stomach* lining. Gastrin causes the stomach to produce more acid and helps to propel food through the digestive tract. (See also *gastrointestinal hormones*.)

gastritis

Inflammation of the *stomach* lining due to irritation of the tissues. The condition may be *acute* or *chronic*.

Acute gastritis may be due to infection with the HELICOBACTER PYLORI bacterium. It may also be caused by drugs, usually *nonsteroidal anti-inflammatory drugs* such as *aspirin*; *alcohol*; or severe physical stress, such as *burns* or major surgery.

Chronic gastritis is most often due to H. PYLORI infection but may be due to prolonged irritation by *smoking*, alcohol, or *bile*; by an *autoimmune disorder* that damages the stomach lining (see *anaemia, megaloblastic*); or by degeneration of the lining with age.

Symptoms include discomfort in the upper abdomen, nausea, and vomiting. In acute gastritis, the faeces may be blackened by blood lost from the stomach (see *melaena*); in chronic gastritis, slow blood loss may lead to anaemia (see *anaemia, iron-deficiency*), resulting in symptoms such as pallor, tiredness and breathlessness.

Diagnosis may be made by *gastroscopy* (examination of the stomach with a flexible viewing instrument), during which a *biopsy* (removal of a tissue sample for analysis) may be performed. Treatment is usually with *ulcer-healing drugs*, which may be combined with *antibiotics* if H. PYLORI is the cause.

gastroenteritis

Inflammation of the *stomach* and intestines, usually causing sudden upsets that last for two or three days. *Dysentery, typhoid fever, cholera, food poisoning*, and *travellers' diarrhoea* are all forms of gastroenteritis. It may be caused by a variety of *bacteria*, bacterial *toxins*, *viruses*, and other organisms in food or water. There are also a number of noninfectious causes, such as *food intolerance* and certain irritant drugs.

The usual symptoms are appetite loss, nausea, vomiting, cramps, and diarrhoea. Their onset and severity depend on the cause; symptoms may be mild, or may be so severe that *dehydration*, *shock*, and collapse occur.

Mild cases usually require rest and *rehydration therapy* only. For severe illness, treatment in hospital may be necessary, with fluids given by *intravenous infusion*. *Antibiotic drugs* may be given for some bacterial infections, but others need no specific treatment.

gastroenterology

The study of the *digestive system* and the diseases and disorders that affect it.

gastroenterostomy

Surgery to create a connection between the *stomach* and the *jejunum* (the middle two-thirds of the small intestine), sometimes combined with a partial *gastrectomy* (removal of the lower part of the stomach). The operation, formerly carried out to treat duodenal ulcer (see *peptic ulcer*), is now rarely performed.

gastrointestinal hormones

A group of *hormones* released from specialized cells in the *stomach*, *pancreas*, and small intestine that control various functions of the digestive organs. *Gastrin, secretin, cholecystokinin*, and *vasoactive intestinal polypeptide* are the best known of these hormones (see *Hormones in the digestive tract*).

gastrointestinal tract

The part of the *digestive system* consisting of the *mouth, oesophagus, stomach,*

HORMONES IN THE DIGESTIVE TRACT

Hormones released from endocrine cells in the stomach, pancreas, and intestine aid digestion by stimulating the release of bile from the gallbladder and enzymes from the pancreas into the duodenum.

Cholecystokinin
Released by the duodenum in response to fats and acid, cholecystokinin causes the gallbladder to squeeze bile into the duodenum and stimulates the production of pancreatic enzymes, which pass into the duodenum through the pancreatic duct.

Gastrin
Secreted mainly by cells in the stomach in response to eating food (especially protein), gastrin causes the stomach to produce more acid and stimulates contraction of muscle in the wall of part of the stomach, ileum, and colon. This contraction propels food through the digestive tract.

Secretin
Secreted by the lining of the duodenum in response to acid entering from the stomach, secretin acts on the pancreas to increase the output of bicarbonate, which neutralizes acid from the stomach. It also increases the release of enzymes from the pancreas.

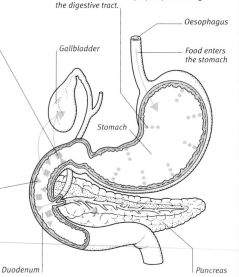

Gallbladder

Oesophagus

Food enters the stomach

Stomach

Duodenum

Pancreas

---

and *intestines*. These structures together form a long tube through which food passes as it is digested.

gastro-oesophageal reflux disease (GORD)

Also sometimes known as acid reflux, GORD is regurgitation of acidic fluid from the stomach into the *oesophagus* (the tube that connects the throat to the stomach), which may inflame the oesophagus and result in *heartburn* due to *oesophagitis*.

Mild GORD is common but is not usually serious. It is often the result of leakage of the lower oesophageal sphincter (the muscular valve between the oesophagus and stomach), which may occur during pregnancy and often affects overweight people. However, repeated episodes of discomfort may indicate a *hiatus hernia* (in which part of the stomach protrudes into the chest). Possible complications of GORD include *oesophageal stricture* (narrowing), oesophageal ulcers, *Barrett's oesophagus*, or, rarely, oesophageal cancer (see *oesophagus, cancer of*).

GORD may be treated with drugs, including *antacids, alginates, proton pump inhibitors*, or H_2-*receptor antagonists*.

If drug treatment is ineffective, surgery to tighten the lower oesophageal sphincter or correct a hiatus hernia may be recommended.

gastroscopy

Examination of the *stomach* via a flexible *endoscope* (a viewing instrument) inserted through the mouth. The *oesophagus* and *duodenum* (the first part of the small intestine) are also inspected; for this reason, the procedure is more accurately called an oesophagogastroduodenoscopy. The patient is often sedated throughout.

Gastroscopy is used to investigate bleeding, or other disorders, of the oesophagus, stomach, or duodenum. Attachments to the gastroscope enable a *biopsy* (removal of a tissue sample for analysis) to be carried out, as well as treatments such as *laser treatment*. A gastroscope may also be used to ease the passage of a gastric feeding tube through the skin (see *gastrostomy*).

gastrostomy

A surgically created opening in the *stomach*. It is usually made to connect the stomach to the outside of the body, so that a feeding tube can be passed into the stomach or small intestine.

Gastrostomy may be performed on people who cannot eat properly due to oesophageal cancer (see *oesophagus, cancer of*) or who are unable to chew and swallow due to a *stroke*.

Gaucher's disease

A *genetic disorder* in which lack of the *enzyme* glucocerebrosidase leads to build up of a fatty substance, glucosylceramide, in the liver, spleen, bone marrow, and, sometimes, in the brain. It is treated by injections of the missing enzyme.

gauze

An absorbent, open-weave fabric, usually made of cotton. Sterilized gauze is often used to clean wounds, or applied as a *dressing* to soak up fluids from wounds. It is not used on areas of damaged tissue such as burns or ulcers, because it may stick to the surface and dislodge new tissue when it is removed.

gavage

Feeding of liquids through a *nasogastric tube* (see *feeding, artificial*). Gavage can also refer to *hyperalimentation* (feeding beyond appetite requirements).

gel

A jelly-like suspension consisting of small, insoluble particles that are dispersed through a liquid. Gels are often used as bases for *topical* skin treatments, particularly those that are used on the face and scalp.

gemfibrozil

A drug that lowers the level of fats in the blood. Gemfibrozil is usually given to people with *hyperlipidaemia* after dietary measures have failed to reduce blood fat levels. It may cause nausea and diarrhoea, and should not be taken by people with liver disease.

gender identity

An individual's inner feeling of maleness or femaleness. Gender identity is not necessarily the same as biological sex. It is fixed within the first two to three years of life and is reinforced during puberty; once established, it cannot usually be changed.

A minority of people have persistent feelings of discomfort about their sexual identity. This condition is called gender dysphoria; in the most severe cases, a person may feel that he or she is the wrong sex (see *transsexualism*).

gene

A particular area of *DNA*, the material within cells that governs the physical characteristics, development, and functioning of an individual. DNA is a very long, chain-like molecule that exists in the *chromosomes* in the nuclei of cells. The *nucleus* of each non-dividing cell (except egg and sperm cells) contains 23 pairs of chromosomes that collectively contain about 20,000 to 25,000 genes. All body cells (except egg and sperm cells) contain identical sets of genes because they are all derived, by a process of division, from a single fertilized egg.

During growth and cell repair, cells divide to form two identical new cells, each containing a full set of genes (see *mitosis*). *Gametes* (cells involved in reproduction), however, undergo a different form of division, called *meiosis*; as a result, they contain just one gene from each pair, so that each parent contributes half of the genetic material used to form an offspring.

GENE FUNCTION

Each gene controls or influences a specific feature or process in the body. Genes act by directing the manufacture of specific *proteins* (see *What genes are and what they do*, following page). Many proteins are involved in forming body structures, or in regulating particular chemical processes (see *enzyme*). Certain proteins, however, are produced solely to influence other genes by switching them "on" or "off". The genes that make these regulatory proteins are known as control genes.

G

WHERE DO YOUR **GENES** COME FROM?

A person's genes are inherited from his or her parents. Half come from the mother and half from the father via the egg and sperm cells. Each parent provides a different selection, or "mix", of his or her genes to each child; this accounts for the marked differences in appearance, health, and personality among most brothers and sisters. Everyone holds a copy of his or her genes within each body cell.

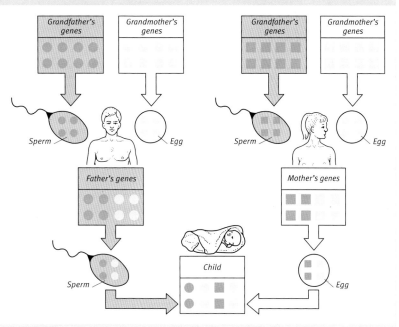

Gene transmission
In this diagram, only eight genes are shown – in reality, each cell in the body contains about 20,000–25,000 genes. Half of them come from the mother and half from the father – thus a quarter of the genes originate from each of the four grandparents.

WHAT **GENES** ARE AND WHAT THEY DO

G

Genes are units of DNA (the material that controls the body's growth, structure, and functions) contained in every cell. They exert their effects by directing the manufacture of proteins. All of a person's genes come from his or her parents. The physical differences between people, such as in eye, hair, and skin colour, arise from slight differences in gene structure.

DNA PRINTOUT

Through painstaking laboratory research, the exact structure of many genes is now known.

```
TTC-GAG-CAT-CTG-GGG-ATG-
TCA-TGT-CCT-TCA-TCG-TTT-
TGA-TTA-CCG-ACC-CCA-TCG-
TAT-GAC-ACG-CAA-GTT-CCG-
CGG-TCA-CGC-ACG-TCA-TGT-
GGG-GAC-TCG-TAA-TCA-CGT-
CAA-GCG-AGT-TTA-AAT-AGA-
CGA-CGC-AGC-TTT-GAA-TTC-
TAT-ACC-TAC-TAA-CTG-TTA-
TTG-TTA-TGT-GAT-GGG-TTA-
ATG-AGC-GGA-GTG-CAT-TAT-
```

DNA base sequence
This printout shows a small part of the sequence in the gene that codes for the protein trypsin, a digestive enzyme.

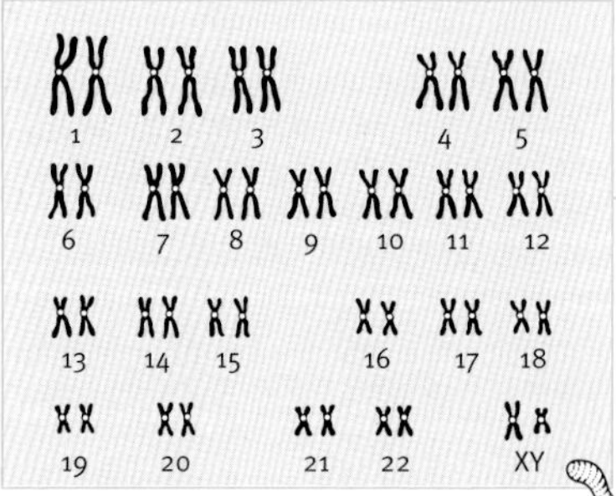

Chromosomes
Genes are contained in the chromosomes within the nuclei of a person's cells. Each chromosome contains a long strand of DNA (deoxyribonucleic acid).

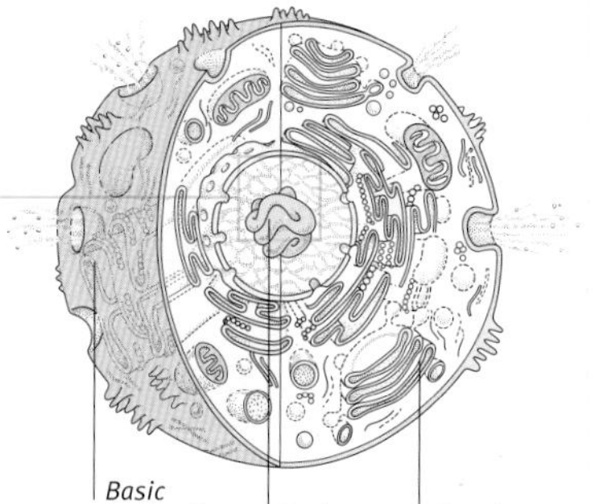

Basic body cell
Nucleus
Cytoplasm

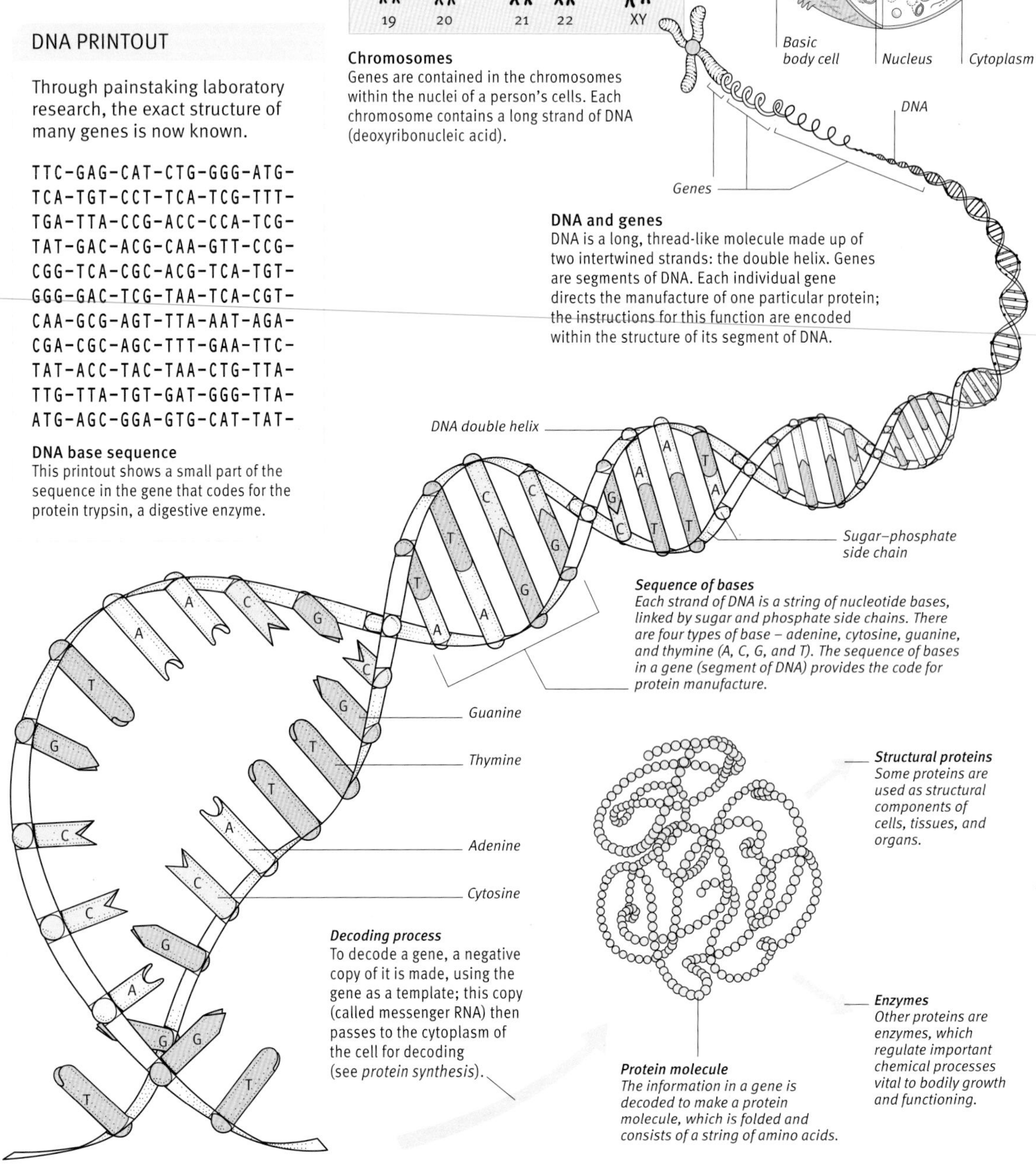

DNA

Genes

DNA and genes
DNA is a long, thread-like molecule made up of two intertwined strands: the double helix. Genes are segments of DNA. Each individual gene directs the manufacture of one particular protein; the instructions for this function are encoded within the structure of its segment of DNA.

DNA double helix

Sugar–phosphate side chain

Sequence of bases
Each strand of DNA is a string of nucleotide bases, linked by sugar and phosphate side chains. There are four types of base – adenine, cytosine, guanine, and thymine (A, C, G, and T). The sequence of bases in a gene (segment of DNA) provides the code for protein manufacture.

Guanine

Thymine

Adenine

Cytosine

Structural proteins
Some proteins are used as structural components of cells, tissues, and organs.

Enzymes
Other proteins are enzymes, which regulate important chemical processes vital to bodily growth and functioning.

Decoding process
To decode a gene, a negative copy of it is made, using the gene as a template; this copy (called messenger RNA) then passes to the cytoplasm of the cell for decoding (see *protein synthesis*).

Protein molecule
The information in a gene is decoded to make a protein molecule, which is folded and consists of a string of amino acids.

DISORDERS DUE TO SINGLE GENE DEFECTS

Autosomal dominant

In these disorders, only one copy of the defective gene needs to be present in order to cause an abnormality. Each child of an affected person usually has a 1 in 2 chance of inheriting the defective gene and being affected, and a 1 in 2 chance of being unaffected.

Examples
- Achondroplasia
- Familial polyposis
- Hereditary spherocytosis
- Huntington's disease
- Marfan syndrome
- Neurofibromatosis
- Polycystic kidney disease (adult type)
- Tuberous sclerosis

Key Defective gene ● Normal gene

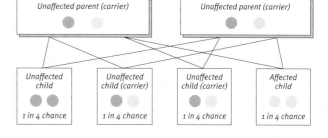

Autosomal recessive

In this group, the disorder occurs when a pair of abnormal genes is inherited. Usually, both parents of an affected person are unaffected carriers of the defective gene. Each of their children has a 1 in 4 chance of being affected and a 2 in 4 chance of being a carrier.

Examples
- Albinism (oculocutaneous)
- Cystic fibrosis
- Friedreich's ataxia
- Galactosaemia
- Hurler's syndrome
- Phenylketonuria
- Sickle cell anaemia
- Tay–Sachs disease

Key Defective gene ● Normal gene

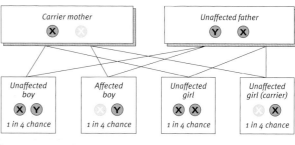

X-linked recessive

These conditions are caused by defects on the X chromosome. They usually cause abnormalities only in males, in whom the defect cannot be masked by the equivalent gene on a second, normal X chromosome. Women may be carriers of the defect. There is a 1 in 2 chance of their sons having the disorder and a 1 in 2 chance that their daughters will be carriers.

Examples
- Christmas disease
- Colour blindness (most types)
- Fragile X syndrome
- G6PD deficiency
- Haemophilia
- Muscular dystrophy (Duchenne)

Key Defective X chromosome Normal X chromosome Y chromosome

The whole complex process of development and growth is regulated by the sequential switching "on" and "off" of particular genes. The activities of control genes also determine the specialization of cells. Within any cell, some genes are active and others are idle, according to the cell's particular function; for example, nerve cells and liver cells will have different sets of active and idle genes. If the control genes are disrupted, however, cells lose their specialist abilities and can multiply out of control; this is the probable mechanism by which cancers develop (see *carcinogenesis*; *oncogenes*).

GENE MUTATION

Occasionally, when new cells are formed, a fault occurs in the copying process, leading to a *mutation* (change). The mutant gene is then passed on each time the cell subsequently divides. Disorders that result from such mutant genes are known as *genetic disorders*.

ALLELES

The gene at any particular location on a chromosome can exist in any of various forms, called *alleles*. If the effects of a specific allele mask those of the allele at the same location on its partner chromosome, that allele is described as *dominant*; the masked allele is *recessive*. (See also *genetic code*; *inheritance*.)

gene mapping

A process by which the location of particular *genes* on each *chromosome* is determined. In some cases, gene location gene can be found by certain tests. Alternatively, the positions of genes that are close to one another on one chromosome (and so are usually passed on together) may be found by a process called linkage analysis. The information is shown as a diagram of a chromosome with the gene locations marked on it.

general anaesthetic

See *anaesthesia, general*.

generalized anxiety disorder

A psychiatric illness characterized by chronic and persistent apprehension and tension that has no particular focus. There may also be various physical symptoms such as trembling, sweating, lightheadedness, and irritability. The condition can be treated with *psychotherapy* (such as *cognitive–behavioural therapy*), *antidepressants*, or drugs such as *beta blockers* or *sedatives* that relieve symptoms but do not treat the underlying condition. (See *anxiety*; *anxiety disorders*.)

general practice

The term used in the UK for the provision of personal medical care outside a hospital setting. Doctors who provide it are called general practitioners (GPs). This form of health-care is now more commonly known as *primary care*.

generic drug

A medicinal drug that is marketed under its official medical name (its generic name) rather than under a patented name (its brand name). Most drugs are now prescribed under their generic names.

gene therapy

An experimental treatment in which copies of a normal *gene* are inserted into the *DNA* of a person's cells to counter the effects of a faulty gene or to help fight certain types of cancer in which genes play a role. Gene therapy is still in its infancy and there remain many technical, ethical, and religious problems to be resolved.

TYPES

Broadly, there are two main types of gene therapy: somatic (body) cell therapy and germ-line (egg or sperm) therapy. In somatic therapy, a normal gene is inserted only into body cells, not germ cells. This treats the symptoms of a disease but does not affect its heritability. In germ-line therapy, a normal gene is inserted into the germ cells and would be passed on to future generations. However, germ-line therapy in humans is currently prohibited.

METHODS

Copies of a normal gene can be introduced into body cells in various ways. In one method, a virus (inactivated to prevent it from causing disease) is modified so that it contains the normal human gene and used to carry the gene into the patient's cells. In another method, naked DNA with the normal gene is injected directly into the patient. Other methods that have been tried include packaging normal DNA in tiny liposomes or attaching normal DNA to macromolecules (very large molecules); these liposomes or macromolecules may then be introduced into the body in various ways, such as by inhalation.

PROBLEMS

Theoretically, gene therapy could provide an effective treatment for various serious conditions, particularly single-gene, autosomal recessive diseases such as cystic fibrosis, phenylketonuria, and sickle-cell anaemia (see *Disorders due to single gene defects*, previous page). However, in many common disorders, such as diabetes mellitus, coronary artery disease and hypertension, several genes are involved and the genes themselves are not the sole causative factors. In addition, current gene therapy techniques do not provide a long-term cure and patients need regular repeat treatments. However, repeat treatments may stimulate an immune response against the treatment. Gene therapy also carries the risk of inducing tumours and, if an inactivated virus is used to insert the normal gene, there is the risk that the virus may revert to a disease-causing form. Furthermore, there are concerns about whether it is ethically or theologically acceptable to alter something as fundamental as a person's genes.

genetically modified foods

Commonly known as GM foods, these are foods or food constituents – most commonly plants or plant derivatives – whose *DNA* (genetic material) has been deliberately altered to modify certain characteristics. In genetic modification, DNA is isolated from one organism and inserted into the DNA of another.

The procedure is intended to be beneficial; for example, GM plants may be more resistant to pests. However, there are continuing concerns about the safety of GM foods – although there have been no proven major health hazards since GM foods were introduced – and over environmental and ecological aspects.

genetic code

The inherited instructions, contained in *genes*, that specify the activities of cells and thereby the development and functioning of the body. Each gene in a *chromosome* contains the coded instructions for a cell to make a *protein* that has a specific function in the body.

The DNA that makes up genes consists of two long, intertwined strands, each comprising a sequence made up of four chemicals called nucleotide bases (see *nucleic acids*). These four bases are adenine, thymine, cytosine, and guanine (often abbreviated to A, T, C, and G). They are joined in pairs (base-pairs), thus linking the two strands of the DNA molecule. The sequence of these bases along the DNA strands makes up the genetic code. During *protein synthesis*, *RNA* (ribonucleic acid) is used to help read this code and create the protein.

genetic counselling

Medical guidance offered to people who have a known risk of having a child with a *genetic disorder*, such as cystic fibrosis, or who are at increased risk of developing a genetic disorder themselves. The counsellor will examine individual and family medical histories and, in some cases, arrange for tests such as *chromosome analysis* and *genetic probes*.

Genetic counselling enables people to make informed decisions about their future, particularly parenthood. If there is a significant risk of a couple having an affected child, doctors may be able to offer pre-implantation genetic testing with *in vitro fertilization* (see *embryo diagnosis*), or antenatal diagnosis, to optimize the chances of their having a healthy child. If parents already have an affected child, genetic counselling will provide information on the outlook for that child.

genetic disorders

Any disorder caused, wholly or partly, by one or more faults in a person's *DNA*. Genetic disorders may be *congenital* (present at birth) or may become apparent later in life. Many of them are *familial* (shared by various people in the same family). A child may, however, be born with a genetic disorder when there is no previous family history.

A genetic disorder can occur in two different ways: one or both parents have a defect in their own genetic material that is then inherited by the child, or a *mutation* occurs during the formation of the *ovum* or *sperm* cell.

The disorders fall into three broad categories: *chromosomal abnormalities*, single gene (unifactorial) defects, and multifactorial defects. Chromosomal abnormalities involve a child having an abnormal number of whole *chromosomes* (as in *Down's syndrome*), or extra or missing bits of chromosomes. Single gene defects are caused by one abnormal gene or pair of genes. Multifactorial disorders are due to the effects of several genes, usually combined with lifestyle and/or environmental influences.

SINGLE GENE DEFECTS

There are two main forms of single gene defect. In sex-linked disorders, the defective gene is carried on one of the sex chromosomes – almost always the X chromosome. In autosomal disorders, the defective gene is carried on one of the other 44 chromosomes. These disorders are subdivided into autosomal dominant and autosomal recessive disorders. See *Disorders due to single gene defects* (p.335) for examples.

Another, rare group of single gene defects involves the *mitochondrial DNA*, which exists outside the nuclei.

X-linked recessive disorders The most common type of sex-linked disorder, X-linked recessive disorders are caused by a defective gene on an X chromosome.

Women have two X chromosomes; men have only one, inherited from their mothers. When a woman inherits one defective gene, its effect is masked by the normal gene on her other X chromosome and she has no outward abnormality. She is, however, capable of passing the gene on to her children and is called a carrier. On average, carriers transmit the defective gene to half their sons, who are affected, and to half their daughters, who become carriers in turn. When a male inherits the defective gene from his mother, he has no normal gene on a second X chromosome to mask it, so he displays the abnormality. Affected males therefore greatly outnumber affected females. The males pass the defective gene to none of their sons but to all of their daughters, who become carriers. *Haemophilia* is a disorder of this type.

Autosomal dominant disorders In these conditions, the defective gene is *dominant* in relation to the equivalent normal gene, so only one copy needs to be present in order to cause an abnormality. People who have an autosomal dominant disorder carry one normal copy and one defective copy of the affected gene, and are termed *heterozygotes*. Affected people have a 50 per cent chance of passing the defective gene on to their children. *Huntington's disease* is a disorder of this type.

Autosomal recessive disorders The defective gene that causes an autosomal recessive disorder is *recessive* in relation to the normal gene, so two faulty copies of the gene are required to cause an abnormality. People who have the disorder carry two identical defective copies of the gene, and are called homozygotes. In most cases, both parents of an affected individual are heterozygotes: they carry one copy of the defective gene and one copy of the normal gene. *Cystic fibrosis* is a disorder of this type.

MITOCHONDRIAL DISORDERS

In rare cases, a defect in a specific area of mitochondrial DNA causes diseases. Such disorders include certain myopathies (muscle disorders), neuropathies (nerve disorders), and some cases of degeneration of the retina, and *deafness*. These disorders are always passed on from the mother, because sperm cells have very few or no mitochondria.

MULTIFACTORIAL DISORDERS

These disorders are inherited but the pattern of inheritance is complicated and such disorders are often influenced not only by genes but also by environmental and/or lifestyle factors, as in some cases of *asthma*, *diabetes mellitus*, and *schizophrenia*.

genetic drift

Chance fluctuation in *gene* frequency within a finite, isolated sample of a population over a number of generations. The chance of random variation increases as the population size decreases because, in a large population, the random nature of the transmission of *alleles* (various forms of a gene at a particular location) tends to average out.

genetic engineering

A branch of *genetics* concerned with the alteration of genetic material in an organism in order to produce a desired change in the organism's characteristics. Genetic engineering has been used to mass-produce a variety of substances that are useful in medicine.

A *gene* responsible for making a useful substance is identified and inserted into the *DNA* of another cell (most often a bacterium or yeast); this altered DNA is called recombinant DNA. The altered cell reproduces rapidly to form a colony of cells containing the gene. This colony produces the substance in large amounts. Some human hormones (notably *insulin* and *growth hormone*) and proteins such as *factor VIII* (used to treat *haemophilia*), are made in this way. Vaccines against infectious diseases and some drugs can also be produced by genetic engineering.

genetic fingerprinting

A technique that can be used to demonstrate relationships between people (for example in *paternity testing*) or, in forensic investigations, to identify a suspect.

DNA contains a *genetic code* ("genetic fingerprint") that is unique to each individual, except in the case of identical twins. DNA can be extracted from any material containing body cells, such as blood, semen, hair, or saliva. Its genetic code can then be analysed and compared with that from a sample obtained from another person, or from the scene of a crime.

genetic probe

A specific fragment of *DNA* used in laboratory tests to determine whether a particular genetic defect is present in a person's DNA. The probe contains the same structure as the abnormal gene and, when added to a sample of the person's DNA, will bind to that gene if it is present. A radioactive or fluorescent marker may be added to the probe so that it can easily be detected.

Genetic probes are used in antenatal diagnosis of *genetic disorders*, and in determining whether people with a family history of a genetic disorder carry the defective gene themselves (see *familial screening*). Genetic probes are also sometimes used for the rapid identification of infectious microorganisms.

genetics

The study of *inheritance* (transmission of characteristics from one generation to the next). Genetics involves determining the chemical basis for inheritance of particular characteristics, and investigating the causes of similarities and differences between individuals of a species or between different species.

Branches of human genetics include population genetics, which studies the relative frequency of various *genes* in different human races; molecular genetics, which is concerned with the structure, function, and copying of *DNA*; and clinical genetics, which is concerned with the study and prevention of *genetic disorders*.

genetic screening

See *familial screening*.

genital herpes

See *herpes, genital*.

genitalia

The reproductive organs, especially those that are external. Male genitalia include the *penis*, *testes* (situated in the *scrotum*), *prostate gland*, *seminal vesicles*, and associated ducts, such as the *epididymis* and *vas deferens*. Female genitalia include the *ovaries*, *fallopian tubes*, *uterus*, *vagina*, *clitoris*, *vulva*, and *Bartholin's glands*.

genitalia, ambiguous

A group of conditions, also known as intersex, in which an individual's external sex organs are not clearly male or

G

female, or in which the organs appear to be those of the opposite chromosomal sex. Cases of ambiguous genitalia may result from an abnormality of the *sex chromosomes* or a *hormonal disorder* (see *hermaphroditism*; *sex determination*; *adrenal hyperplasia, congenital*).

genital phase

A term used in *psychoanalytic theory* to refer to a stage of a person's psychosexual development. The genital phase begins at around the ages of 3–5 years. (See also *anal phase*; *oral phase*.)

genital ulcer

An eroded area of skin on the *genitalia*. There are various possible causes. The most common cause of genital ulcers is a *sexually transmitted infection*, particularly genital herpes (see *herpes, genital*) or *syphilis*. *Chancroid* and *granuloma inguinale* are tropical bacterial infections that cause genital ulcers. *Lymphogranuloma venereum* is a *chlamydial infection* that produces genital blisters. *Behçet's syndrome* is a rare condition that causes tender, recurrent ulcers in the mouth and on the genitals. Cancer of the penis or vulva may first appear as a painless ulcer with raised edges.

genital warts

See *warts, genital*.

genito-urinary medicine

The branch of medicine concerned with *sexually transmitted infections* and their effects on the body.

genome, human

The complete set of human genetic material. The human genome consists of 23 *chromosomes*, which, together, contain about 20,000–25,000 *genes*. All cells (except for egg and sperm cells) contain two sets of the 23 chromosomes, one inherited from the father and the other from the mother.

The Human Genome Project, an international research programme, was launched in 1990 with the aim of identifying all the genes in the human body. The project was finally completed in the year 2003.

genotype

The entire genetic makeup of an individual, or group of related individuals, as opposed to the individual's observable characteristics (see *phenotype*). The term is also used to describe the set of

alleles (any of various forms of a *gene*) at a specific location within a *chromosome*; the genetic information carried by alleles determines a particular characteristic of that organism.

gentamicin

An *antibacterial drug* given by injection to treat serious infections such as *meningitis* and *septicaemia* (blood poisoning). Gentamicin can result in damage to the kidneys or the inner ear if the dosage is not carefully controlled.

The drug is also used in various eye-drops and ear-drops but is unlikely to cause serious side effects when taken in these types of preparation.

genu valgum

The medical term for *knock-knee*.

genu varum

The medical term for *bowleg*.

geriatric medicine

The medical speciality concerned with the care of elderly people, also known as "care for the elderly". This group require specialist medical care because they respond to illness and treatment in a different way from younger people. Physical and mental decline due to *aging* can mean that illnesses are more severe in older people, and people may have two or more diseases at once. In addition, the liver and kidneys become less efficient at breaking down and excreting drugs, so drug dosages for elderly people must be carefully controlled to avoid dangerous side effects.

Geriatric medicine relies on an integrated team of healthcare workers, including a doctor (or a specialist called a geriatrician or care-of-the-elderly physician), nurse, physiotherapist, and occupational therapist. This team helps older people to maintain independence and health, and to cope after illness or injury. (See also *rehabilitation*.)

germ

The popular term used to describe any microorganism that causes disease, such as *viruses* and *bacteria*.

German measles

The common name for the viral infection *rubella*.

germ cell

An embryonic *cell* with the potential to develop into a *spermatozoon* or *ovum*.

The term also describes a *gamete* (mature sex cell) or any cell that is undergoing gametogenesis (the process by which gametes are formed).

germ cell tumour

A growth comprised of immature *sperm* cells in the male *testis* or of immature egg cells (see *ovum*) in the female *ovary*. A *seminoma* is one type of germ cell tumour (see *testis, cancer of*).

gerontology

The study of developmental, biological, medical, psychological, and sociological *aging*. (See also *geriatric medicine*.)

Gerstmann's syndrome

A neurological disorder involving a writing disability such as *agraphia*, together with the inability to understand mathematical calculations, to distinguish right from left, and to identify the fingers (a type of *agnosia*). Many sufferers also experience *aphasia* (complete loss of language skills). The syndrome may occur after a *stroke* or damage to the left parietal lobe of the *brain*, but the precise cause is unknown.

Gestalt theory

A school of *psychology* that emphasizes the viewing of personal experiences as a whole rather than breaking them down into collections of stimuli and responses. Gestalt therapy aims to increase self-awareness by looking at all aspects of a person in his or her environment.

gestation

The period between the *conception* and birth of a baby; it is the time during which the infant develops in the *uterus*. Gestation typically lasts about 40 weeks (counted from the first day of the pregnant woman's last menstrual period), although any duration between 37 and 42 weeks is considered normal. (See also *embryo*; *fertilization*; *fetus*; *pregnancy*.)

gestational diabetes

Diabetes mellitus that develops during pregnancy, usually clearing up after delivery (see *diabetic pregnancy*).

gestodene

A *progestogen drug* that is used with the oestrogen drug *ethinylestradiol* in combined *oral contraceptives*. Gestodene is reported to carry a slightly increased risk of venous *thromboembolism* in comparison with older drugs.

Ghon's tubercle

An abnormal area in the lung, also known as a Ghon's focus, that is produced by infection with *tuberculosis* in a person who has not previously been exposed to the disease. Often, a Ghon's tubercle heals without causing symptoms, but in some cases it may result in tuberculosis that spreads via the *lymphatic system*, in the bloodstream, or in the air sacs of the lungs. A healed tubercle may become calcified, and may be discovered during a routine *chest X-ray*.

Gianotti–Crosti syndrome

A characteristic, harmless response of the skin to certain viral infections, including *hepatitis B* infection, *Epstein Barr virus* (see *mononucleosis, infectious*), and *coxsackievirus*. In this condition, a papular (lumpy) rash develops on the face, buttocks, and limbs and lasts for several weeks. The condition mainly affects children between the ages of six months and twelve years.

SYMPTOMS AND SIGNS

There may be no noticeable symptoms. Alternatively, there may be a mild temperature, and swelling of the *lymph nodes* in the armpits and groin that persists for some months. The liver may become enlarged.

DIAGNOSIS AND TREATMENT

Blood tests and *liver function tests* are carried out to investigate liver function and detect possible causative viruses. There is no specific treatment, but a mild, topical *corticosteroid* cream may be prescribed for itching. The rash usually fades in two to eight weeks.

giant cell arteritis

An alternative name for *temporal arteritis*.

giardiasis

An infection of the small intestine caused by the *protozoan* (single-celled) parasite GIARDIA LAMBLIA. Giardiasis is spread by eating or drinking contaminated food or water or through direct contact with an infected person.

SYMPTOMS

Most of those infected have no symptoms. If, however, symptoms do occur, they begin between one and three weeks after infection. They include diarrhoea, and wind, as well as faeces that are foul-smelling, greasy, and tend to float in the toilet. Abdominal discomfort, cramps, and swelling, loss of appetite, and nausea may also occur. In some cases, giardiasis may become *chronic*.

HOW **GIARDIASIS** IS SPREAD

Giardiasis is spread by contaminated water or food, or by personal contact. This parasitic infection is most common in the tropics, but it has become a more frequent occurrence in developed countries, especially among groups of preschool children.

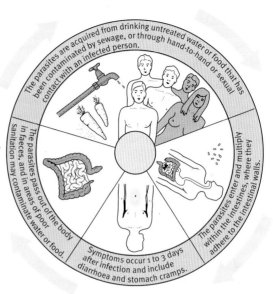

The parasites are acquired from drinking untreated water or food that has been contaminated by sewage, or through hand-to-hand or sexual contact with an infected person.

The parasites pass out of the body in faeces, and in areas of poor sanitation may contaminate water or food.

Symptoms occur 1 to 3 days after infection and include diarrhoea and stomach cramps.

The parasites enter and multiply within the intestines, where they adhere to the intestinal walls.

DIAGNOSIS AND TREATMENT

The infection is diagnosed from microscopic examination of a faecal sample or by a *jejunal biopsy* (removal of a small sample of tissue from the middle section of the small intestine for analysis).

Acute giardiasis usually clears up without treatment but the drug *metronidazole* quickly relieves symptoms and helps to prevent the spread of infection. Infection can be prevented in the first place by avoiding food or water that could possibly be contaminated.

gibbous

A term meaning "humped", as in a gibbous *spine*, which curves outwards (see *kyphosis*).

giddiness

See *dizziness*.

GIFT

See *gamete intrafallopian transfer*.

gigantism

Excessive growth (especially in height) during childhood or adolescence that results from overproduction of *growth hormone* by a tumour of the pituitary gland (see *pituitary tumours*). If untreated, the tumour may compress other hormone-producing cells in the gland, causing symptoms of hormone deficiency (see *hypopituitarism*).

People with gigantism may be treated with a drug that blocks the release of growth hormone, such as *bromocriptine*, or they may have to have surgery or *radiotherapy* to remove or destroy the pituitary tumour. (See also *acromegaly*.)

Gilbert's disease

A common inherited condition that affects the way in which *bilirubin* is processed by the *liver*. Usually there are no symptoms, but *jaundice* may be brought on by unrelated illnesses. Sufferers are otherwise healthy and no treatment is necessary.

Gilles de la Tourette's syndrome

A rare, inherited neurological disorder that is transmitted by an autosomal dominant gene (see *genetic disorders*).

Gilles de la Tourette's syndrome is more common in males and starts in childhood with repetitive grimaces and tics. Involuntary barks, grunts, or other noises may appear as the disease progresses. In some cases, the sufferer has episodes of compulsively using foul language (a condition called coprolalia).

People with Tourette's syndrome usually have it their whole lives; in some sufferers *antipsychotic drugs* may help to relieve some of the symptoms.

gingiva

The Latin name for the *gums*.

gingival hyperplasia

See *hyperplasia, gingival*.

gingival pocket

A feature of chronic *periodontitis*.

gingivectomy

The surgical removal of part of the *gum* margin. Gingivectomy may be used to treat severe cases of gingival *hyperplasia* (thickening of the gums) or to remove pockets of infected gum in advanced cases of *periodontitis* (gum disease). Gingivectomy is usually performed by a dentist under local anaesthesia.

gingivitis

Inflammation of the *gums*. Gingivitis is usually due to a buildup of *plaque* around the base of the teeth. *Toxins* produced by bacteria in the plaque irritate the gums, causing them to become infected, tender, swollen, and reddish-purple in colour. Gingivitis may also result from injury to the gums, usually through rough tooth-

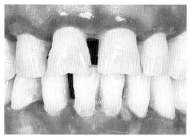

Example of gingivitis
The gums around the bases of the upper teeth are puffy, shiny, and tender and overhang the teeth margins. Affected gums often bleed when brushed.

brushing or flossing. Pregnant women and people with diabetes are especially susceptible to the disorder.

Gingivitis can be reversed; good *oral hygiene* is the main method of preventing and treating it. If left untreated, however, it may lead to damage of the gum tissue, which may in turn lead to chronic *periodontitis* (an advanced stage of gum disease). Acute ulcerative gingivitis (see *gingivitis, acute ulcerative*) may develop in people who have chronic gingivitis, particularly those with a lowered resistance to infection.

gingivitis, acute ulcerative

Painful infection and ulceration of the *gums*. Acute ulcerative gingivitis is uncommon, primarily affecting people aged between 15 and 35. It is caused by abnormal overgrowth of bacteria that

usually exist harmlessly in small numbers in gum crevices. Predisposing factors include poor *oral hygiene*, smoking, throat infections, and *stress*. In many cases, the disorder is preceded by *gingivitis* or *periodontitis*.

The gums become sore and bleed easily. Craterlike ulcers, which bleed spontaneously, develop on the gum tips between teeth. There may be a foul taste in the mouth, bad breath, and swollen lymph nodes (see *glands, swollen*). The infection may spread to the lips and the insides of the cheeks (see *noma*).

A *hydrogen peroxide* mouthwash can relieve the inflammation. *Scaling* is then performed to remove plaque. In severe cases, *antibiotic drugs* may be given to control infection.

gingivostomatitis

Inflammation of the gums and mouth. Gingivostomatitis is often due to a viral infection, particularly *herpes simplex*. The condition can also be due to a bacterial infection or an adverse reaction to a prescribed drug. (See also *cold sore*.)

ginkgo

An extract from the maidenhair tree, GINKGO BILOBA. Preparations containing ginkgo are claimed to help treat circulatory disorders, reduced circulation in the brain, *senility*, *depression*, and *premenstrual syndrome*. Possible side effects include muscle spasms and cramps.

gland

A group of specialized *cells* that manufacture and release chemical substances, such as *hormones* and *enzymes*.

There are two main types of gland: endocrine and exocrine. *Endocrine glands* do not have ducts and release their secretions directly into the bloodstream; examples include the pituitary, thyroid, and adrenal glands. *Exocrine glands* have ducts and release their secretions to the surface or interior of the body. Examples include the sebaceous glands, which secrete sebum on to the surface of the skin, and the salivary glands, which secrete saliva into the mouth. The pancreas releases endocrine and exocrine secretions (for example *insulin* and *cholecystokinin*, respectively).

Lymph nodes are sometimes called glands, particularly when they are enlarged due to infection (see *glands, swollen*). Strictly speaking, this is incorrect usage because lymph nodes do not secrete chemicals.

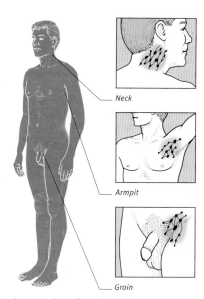

Neck

Armpit

Groin

Common sites of swollen glands
The three most common sites where swollen lymph nodes (glands) can be felt are in the neck, armpit, and groin.

glands, swollen

Enlargement of the *lymph nodes* (which are commonly called "glands"), due to inflammation and/or proliferation of white blood cells within them. Swollen lymph nodes are a common symptom, especially in children. They are usually caused by a minor infection or an allergic reaction (see *allergy*).

Rare causes include cancer affecting the lymph nodes (see *Hodgkin's disease*; *lymphoma*) or cancer of the white blood cells (see *leukaemia*).

glandular fever

See *mononucleosis, infectious*.

glans

The head of the *penis*. The glans is covered by a loose fold of skin called the *prepuce* (foreskin), which retracts when the penis becomes erect; in some males, this skin is removed by *circumcision*. The term "glans" may also be applied to the tip of the *clitoris* in females.

glasses

Devices, worn on the face, that contain lenses to correct focusing errors in the eyes and thereby achieve clear vision.

Lenses are made of glass or plastic, and the shape and thickness of a lens are chosen during a *vision test*. Convex lenses (which curve outwards) are needed for *hypermetropia*, or longsightedness, and concave lenses (which curve inwards) for *myopia*, or shortsightedness (see *Why glasses are used* box, right). Most lenses are single-vision, but bifocal, trifocal, and varifocal lenses are available. Tinted lenses protect the eyes from sunlight. (See also *bifocal*; *contact lenses*.)

glass eye

See *eye, artificial*.

glass test

A test for *meningitis* that involves pressing a clear glass against a rash. If the rash remains visible through the glass, it may be a form of *purpura* (leaking of blood beneath the skin), which sometimes occurs in meningitis.

glaucoma

A condition in which the *intraocular pressure* (fluid pressure inside the *eyes*) causes impaired vision. *Aqueous humour* (watery fluid) is secreted into the front of the eye by the *ciliary body* (a structure behind the *iris*) to maintain the eye's shape and nourish the tissues. Excess fluid drains away at the edge of the iris. In glaucoma, however, this excess fluid may not be able to escape. It causes compression and obstruction of the blood vessels that supply the *retina* and the *optic nerve*. This, in turn, may destroy nerve fibres and cause gradual loss of vision.

TYPES, CAUSES, AND SYMPTOMS

The most common form of glaucoma is chronic simple (open-angle) glaucoma. It rarely occurs before the age of 40, and tends to run in families. In this condition, the outflow of aqueous humour is gradually blocked over a period of years, causing a slow rise in pressure. There are often no symptoms until visual loss is advanced.

In acute (closed-angle) glaucoma, the outflow of aqueous humour is rapidly blocked, and the pressure rises suddenly. This may cause a severe, dull pain in and above the eye, fogginess of vision, and the perception of haloes around lights at night. Nausea and vomiting may occur, and the eye may become red with a dilated pupil.

Congenital glaucoma is due to an abnormality in the drainage angles of the eyes that develops before birth. Glaucoma can also be caused by injury or an eye disease such as *uveitis* or *lens dislocation*.

A less common form, called normal-pressure or low-tension glaucoma, occurs in people whose intraocular pressure is normal or only slightly raised but causes the same damage to the retina and optic

WHY **GLASSES** ARE USED

Glasses compensate for certain visual defects in which the lens of the eye does not focus light correctly on to the retina, at the back of the eyeball. For *hypermetropia* (longsightedness) or *presbyopia*, convex (or plus) lenses are needed. *Myopia* (shortsightedness) requires concave (or minus) lenses.

LONGSIGHTEDNESS

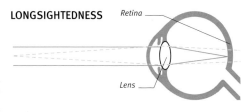

Before correction
Longsightedness occurs when focusing power is inadequate. Light from distant objects is focused on to the retina, but light from close objects is focused behind it.

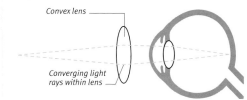

After correction
Convex magnifying (or plus) lenses cause light rays to converge (bend together). As a result, they focus the light from close objects correctly on to the retina.

SHORTSIGHTEDNESS

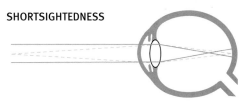

Before correction
The focusing power of the eye is too great. Light from close objects is focused correctly; however, light from distant objects is focused in front of the retina, and the objects appear blurred.

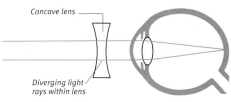

After correction
Concave weakening (or minus) lenses cause light rays to diverge (bend apart). As a result, they focus the light from distant objects correctly on to the retina.

ASTIGMATISM

In astigmatism, the surfaces of the cornea, rather than being a hemisphere as normal, are steeper in one direction than in the others; as a result, the light rays in one meridian (plane) are out of focus. Lenses to correct astigmatism are designed with additional curvature in one meridian, then set accurately in the frame of the glasses so that the steepest curves correspond to the flattest meridian of the cornea. As a result, they cancel out the effects of the distortion in the cornea. Both concave and convex lenses can be designed to correct astigmatism.

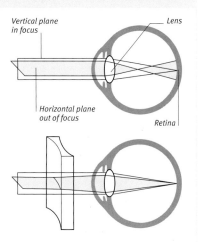

G

Ciliary body

Blocked drainage channel

Cornea

Iris

Aqueous humour

Lens

Acute closed-angle glaucoma
This type of glaucoma is caused by an unduly narrow angle between the iris and the back of the peripheral cornea. Dilation of the pupil may therefore lead to a sudden complete blockage of the outflow, which, in turn, causes a rapid increase in pressure in the eyeball.

nerve as excessively high fluid pressure. This condition is not well understood; and it seems that the pressure, although not considered to be excessive, is too high for the tissues to withstand, and thus causes damage.

DIAGNOSIS AND TREATMENT
Tonometry is used to check for glaucoma by measuring the pressure in the eye. *Ophthalmoscopy* may show depression of the head of the optic nerve due to the increased pressure. Tests of the *visual field* are needed to assess whether vision has already been impaired, because longstanding or severe glaucoma can result in loss of peripheral vision (see *tunnel vision*). Early detection is important, before there are any symptoms, and people with a family history of glaucoma should have regular eye tests and tonometry.

Prompt treatment is essential to prevent permanent loss of vision. Chronic simple glaucoma can usually be controlled with eye-drops (for example, *timolol* or *prostaglandin drugs* such as *latanoprost*), or tablets that reduce pressure in the eye. Treatment needs to be continued for life. If drugs are ineffective, surgery or *laser treatment* can unblock the drainage channel at the edge of the iris or create an artificial channel (see *trabeculectomy*).

Acute glaucoma requires emergency drug treatment, often in hospital. Surgery or laser treatment may be needed in order to prevent a further attack. Such treatment may consist of removing a small part of the iris (a procedure called *iridectomy*) or making one or more holes in the iris (*iridotomy*) to enable the aqueous humour to drain more easily.

Treatment for normal-pressure glaucoma is the same as for open-angle glaucoma, but is aimed at reducing the intraocular pressure to an even lower level than normal.

Gleason's score

A system of grading prostate cancer cells (see *prostate, cancer of*) to determine the most appropriate treatment and the patient's outlook.

Several tissue samples are taken and are assigned a score between 1 and 5. The lowest and highest scores are added together to give the Gleason's score, which is a number between 2 and 10. A low Gleason's score indicates that the cancer cells are very similar to normal prostate cells; a high score means that the cancer cells are very different. In general, the more the cancerous cells diverge from the normal prostate cells, the more serious the cancer.

glenoid

A term meaning "resembling a pit or socket". For example, the glenoid fossa (depression) is the cavity at the top of the scapula (shoulderblade) into which the head of the humerus (the bone of the upper arm) fits.

glibenclamide

An oral hypoglycaemic drug (see *hypoglycaemics, oral*) used to treat type 2 (non-insulin-dependent) *diabetes mellitus*. In this form of diabetes, body cells are resistant to the action of the hormone *insulin*, and absorb insufficient glucose. The drug causes the pancreas to increase insulin secretion thereby compensating for the resistance.

gliclazide

An oral hypoglycaemic drug (see *hypoglycaemics, oral*) used, along with dietary measures, to treat type 2 *diabetes mellitus*. The drug causes the pancreas to increase insulin secretion.

glimepiride

An oral hypoglycaemic drug (see *hypoglycaemics, oral*) that is used to treat

type 2 *diabetes mellitus*. The drug causes the pancreas to increase insulin secretion. Side effects are infrequent but may include mild nausea and diarrhoea. Low blood sugar (see *hypoglycaemia*) may occur if the drug is not taken with sufficient food.

glioblastoma multiforme

A fast-growing and highly cancerous type of primary *brain tumour*. Glioblastoma multiforme is a type of *glioma* that often develops in the *cerebrum* (the main mass of the brain). The cause is unknown. Treatment may include surgery, *radiotherapy*, and/or *chemotherapy*.

glioma

A type of *brain tumour* arising from connective tissue (glial cells) in the brain. Types of glioma include *astrocytoma*, *glioblastoma multiforme*, *ependymoma*, *medulloblastoma*, and *oligodendroglioma*. Symptoms, diagnosis, and treatment are as for other types of brain tumour.

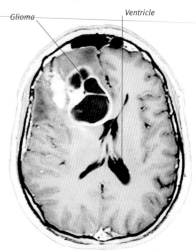

Glioma   Ventricle

Brain scan of a glioma
In this scan, taken from below, a glioma (a type of brain tumour) is visible as a dark area in the right hemisphere (on the left of the image).

glipizide

An oral hypoglycaemic drug (see *hypoglycaemics, oral*) used to treat type 2 *diabetes mellitus*. Glipizide acts by stimulating the pancreas into increasing its production of *insulin*. Side effects are usually mild and infrequent, but dizziness and drowsiness may occur. Rarely, glipizide can cause an abnormal reaction of the skin to sunlight and can reduce blood sodium levels. Low blood sugar (see *hypoglycaemia*) may occur if the drug is not taken with sufficient food.

global

A term used of a disorder affecting an entire body function or system. For example, global aphasia (see *aphasia*) is the loss of all ability to speak, write, or understand language; global paralysis is extreme weakness of the muscles in every part of the body, which may result in a complete inability to move.

globin

The protein that combines with certain iron-containing compounds to form the oxygen-carrying pigments *haemoglobin*, which is found in *red blood cells*, and *myoglobin*, which is present in muscle.

globulin

Any of a group of proteins that are insoluble in water but soluble in dilute salt solutions. There are many globulins in the blood, including *immunoglobulins* (also called antibodies).

globus hystericus

A condition in which there is an uncomfortable feeling of a "lump in the throat". This lump is felt to interfere with swallowing and breathing; however, there is no physical basis for the condition. In severe cases, *hyperventilation* (rapid breathing) and symptoms of a *panic attack* ensue.

Globus hystericus occurs most commonly in people who are anxious or depressed. Treatment is by reassurance, breath-control training, or *psychotherapy*.

glomerulonephritis

Inflammation of the filtering units (see *glomerulus*) in both kidneys. Damage to the glomeruli impairs the removal of waste products, salt, and water from the bloodstream, which may cause serious complications. Glomerulonephritis is one of the most common causes of chronic *kidney failure*.

CAUSES

Some types of glomerulonephritis are caused by the *immune system* making *antibodies* to eliminate microorganisms (usually infectious bacteria, such as those that cause *streptococcal infections* of the throat). The antibodies combine with bacterial *antigens* to form particles called immune complexes. These particles circulate in the bloodstream and become trapped in the glomeruli, triggering an inflammatory process that may damage the glomeruli and prevent them from working normally. Glomerulonephritis also occurs in certain *autoimmune disorders*, such as systemic *lupus erythematosus*. Infectious diseases such as *malaria* and *schistosomiasis* are causes in tropical countries.

SYMPTOMS

Mild glomerulonephritis may cause no symptoms, and it may only be discovered during routine urine testing; alternatively, the condition may remain undetected until the kidney damage has reached an advanced stage and accumulated waste products have started to produce symptoms.

Some people develop symptoms suddenly. They may experience a dull ache over the kidneys. The urine may become bloodstained because, when damaged, the glomeruli allow red blood cells to escape into the urine. Protein may also be lost into the urine, causing *oedema* (see *nephrotic syndrome*); this is a common condition in affected children. *Hypertension* (high blood pressure) is a potentially serious complication. Long-term glomerulonephritis is a common cause of chronic kidney failure.

DIAGNOSIS AND TREATMENT

Diagnosis involves *kidney function tests*, *urinalysis* (the microscopic and chemical analysis of urine), *ultrasound scanning* of the kidneys and, in most cases, *kidney biopsy* (removal of a small tissue sample for microscopic analysis).

Treatment for glomerulonephritis is usually given in hospital, and depends on the cause and the severity of the disease. Children with nephrotic syndrome usually respond to *corticosteroid drugs*. Glomerulonephritis caused by a streptococcal infection usually clears up after the infection is successfully treated with *antibiotic drugs*.

Adults tend to respond less well to treatment, but kidney failure may sometimes be prevented or delayed. Drugs may be prescribed to control hypertension, and a special diet may be given to reduce the workload on the kidneys. Temporary *dialysis* may be necessary to help remove waste products from the blood, and *diuretic drugs* may be given to help treat any oedema.

A few people with severe glomerulonephritis respond to treatment with *immunosuppressant drugs* (which reduce the activity of the immune system); others may undergo *plasmapheresis* (a procedure that removes immune complexes and other harmful substances from the bloodstream).

THE EFFECTS OF **GLOMERULONEPHRITIS**

Normally, the glomeruli retain red cells and protein molecules in the blood while filtering out salts and waste. If they are damaged, however, they allow blood cells and protein to leak into the urine, causing characteristic symptoms.

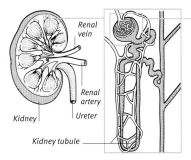

Renal vein

Renal artery

Kidney

Ureter

Kidney tubule

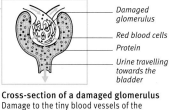

Damaged glomerulus

Red blood cells

Protein

Urine travelling towards the bladder

Cross-section of a damaged glomerulus
Damage to the tiny blood vessels of the glomerulus causes red blood cells and protein to pass into the urine. As a result, the urine may be bloodstained.

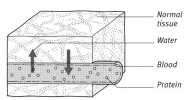

Normal tissue

Water

Blood

Protein

Healthy tissue
Through *osmosis*, protein molecules in the blood draw back water that has been lost to surrounding tissues.

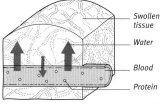

Swollen tissue

Water

Blood

Protein

Oedema
If protein is lost into the urine, there is a fall in osmotic pressure and more water escapes into surrounding tissues, causing swelling.

G

glomerulosclerosis

Scarring caused by damage to the glomeruli (see *glomerulus*), the filtering units of the kidney.

Mild glomerulosclerosis occurs as a normal part of the aging process. The condition may also occur in some severe types of *glomerulonephritis*. In addition, it may be associated with *diabetes mellitus*, *hypertension* (high blood pressure), *AIDS*, or intravenous *drug abuse*.

glomerulus

A filtering unit in the *kidney*. Each glomerulus consists of a cluster of capillaries (tiny blood vessels) enclosed in a capsule and supplied with blood from the renal artery; it forms part of a larger filtering unit called a *nephron*. Filtered blood eventually leaves the kidney via the renal vein. (See also *glomerulonephritis*; *glomerulosclerosis*.)

glomus tumour

A small, bluish swelling in the skin, usually on a finger or toe near or under the nail. The swelling feels tender and is more painful if the limb is hot or cold. Glomus tumours are caused by an overgrowth of the nerve structures that normally control blood flow and temperature in the skin. They are harmless but can be surgically removed.

glossectomy

Removal of all or part of the *tongue*. Glossectomy may be performed to treat *tongue cancer*. If a large part of the tongue is removed, speech is impaired and eating is difficult.

glossitis

Inflammation of the *tongue*. The tongue feels sore and swollen and looks red and smooth; adjacent parts of the mouth may also be inflamed.

Glossitis occurs in various forms of *anaemia* and in *vitamin B* deficiency. Other causes include infection of the mouth (especially by *herpes simplex*), irritation by dentures, and excessive use of alcohol, tobacco, or spices.

Treatment is for the underlying cause. Rinsing of the mouth with a salt solution and good *oral hygiene* may help to relieve the soreness.

glossodynia

A painful, burning sensation in the *tongue*, often with no known cause. Glossodynia tends to disappear of its own accord over time.

glossolalia

Speaking in an imaginary language that has no actual meaning or syntax. (See also *neologism*.)

glossopharyngeal nerve

The ninth *cranial nerve*. This nerve supplies the tongue and the throat, and performs both sensory and motor functions. It conveys sensations, especially taste, from the back of the *tongue*, regulates the secretion of saliva by the *parotid gland*, and controls movement of the throat muscles.

glottis

The part of the *larynx* (voicebox) that consists of the *vocal cords* and the slit-like opening between them.

glucagon

A *hormone* that stimulates the breakdown of stored *glycogen* into *glucose* (a simple sugar). Glucagon is released by the *pancreas* when the blood level of glucose is low (see *feedback*).

Glucagon is used as an injected drug in the emergency treatment of people with *diabetes mellitus* who are unconscious as a result of *hypoglycaemia* (low blood glucose). Nausea and vomiting are occasional adverse effects.

glucagonoma

A tumour of the *pancreas* that secretes *glucagon* (the hormone responsible for raising blood sugar levels). Glucagonomas, which can be cancerous or noncancerous, may lead to attacks of *hyperglycaemia* (high blood glucose) due to excess glucagon production.

glucocorticoids

A group of *corticosteroid hormones*, produced by the cortex (outer layer) of the *adrenal glands*, that affect the chemical breakdown of *carbohydrates* by increasing both the blood sugar level and the amount of *glycogen* stored in the liver. Glucocorticoids also enable the body to respond effectively to physical stress. Both natural and synthetic glucocorticoids are used to treat inflammatory conditions (see *corticosteroid drugs*). The main glucocorticoid is *hydrocortisone*, also called cortisol.

gluconeogenesis

A process in which *glucose* (a simple sugar) is synthesized from sources other than *carbohydrates*, such as *amino acids* and *glycerol*. The process, which

The nerve arises from the medulla oblongata and branches to the lower jaw and the throat.

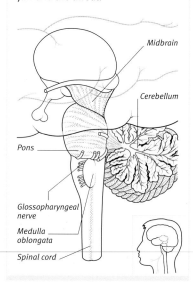

Midbrain

Cerebellum

Pons

Glossopharyngeal nerve

Medulla oblongata

Spinal cord

occurs mainly in the *liver* and muscles, is an important source of energy when insufficient amounts of carbohydrate are available (for example, between meals or when a person is fasting).

glucosamine

A molecule that occurs naturally as a component of various substances in the body, including *cartilage* and *collagen*. Glucosamine may be prescribed to relieve symptoms of *arthritis*. It is also sold as a food supplement.

glucose

A simple *sugar* (monosaccharide) that is naturally present in fruits and is also a product of the digestion of *starch* and *sucrose*. Glucose is the chief source of energy for the body and is carried to all tissues in the circulation. (The term "blood sugar" refers to levels of glucose in the bloodstream.)

The level of glucose in the blood is normally kept fairly constant by the actions of various *hormones*, notably *insulin*, *glucagon*, *adrenaline*, *corticosteroid hormones*, and *growth hormone*. An abnormally high level of glucose in the blood (known as *hyperglycaemia*) may cause glucose to be lost into the urine. An abnormally low blood glucose level is called *hypoglycaemia*.

glue ear

Accumulation of fluid in the cavity of the *middle ear*, causing impaired hearing. Persistent glue ear is most common in children. It is often accompanied by enlarged *adenoids* and frequently occurs with viral respiratory tract infections, such as the common *cold*. It is usual for both ears to be affected.

In glue ear, the lining of the middle ear becomes overactive, producing large amounts of a sticky fluid, and the *eustachian tube* (which links the middle ear to the back of the nose and throat) becomes blocked so that the fluid cannot drain away. The accumulated fluid interferes with the movement of the delicate bones of the middle ear.

Glue ear is sometimes first detected by *hearing tests*. Examination with an *otoscope* (viewing instrument) can confirm the diagnosis.

Mild cases of the condition often clear up without specific treatment. If symptoms persist, the insertion of *grommets* (small tubes) may be necessary, which allows air into the middle ear and encourages fluid to drain away. *Adenoidectomy* (removal of the adenoids) may also be required.

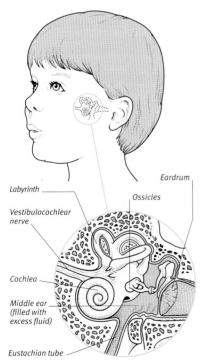

Effects of glue ear
In this condition, sticky fluid in the middle ear prevents free movement of the eardrum and ossicles, causing deafness.

glue-sniffing

See *solvent abuse*.

glutaraldehyde

A topical preparation for the treatment of *warts*, especially *plantar warts* (verrucas). It may cause a rash or irritation and may stain the skin brown.

gluteal

A term meaning "relating to the buttocks", as in the gluteal muscles.

gluten

A combination of gliadins and glutenins (types of proteins) formed when certain cereal flours (notably wheat, rye, and barley) are mixed with water. Sensitivity to gluten causes *coeliac disease*.

gluten enteropathy

See *coeliac disease*.

gluten intolerance

See *coeliac disease*.

gluteus maximus

The large, powerful *muscle* in each of the buttocks that gives them their rounded shape. The gluteus maximus is responsible for moving the thigh sideways and backwards.

glycerol

A colourless, syrupy liquid with a sweet taste. It is an essential constituent of *triglycerides* (simple fats) in the body. It may also be prepared commercially from *fats and oils*. Glycerol is added to moisturizing creams to help prevent dryness and cracking of the skin. It is also used in ear-drops to help soften earwax, and in *cough remedies* to help soothe a dry, irritating cough. Glycerol is also added to rectal *suppositories*; it relieves *constipation* by softening hard faeces.

glyceryl trinitrate

A *vasodilator drug* used for the treatment and prevention of symptoms of *angina pectoris* (chest pain due to inadequate blood supply to the heart). *Sublingual* or *buccal* sprays and tablets are available for rapid pain relief and slow-release tablets or skin patches for sustained pain relief. Possible side effects include headaches, dizziness, and flushing. A topical preparation of glyceryl trinitrate is available to treat anal fissures. Additional side effects of this preparation include anal irritation and rectal bleeding.

LOCATION OF THE GLUTEUS MAXIMUS

The top of the muscle is attached to the sacrum, coccyx, and pelvis. The lower part is attached to the femur (thigh bone).

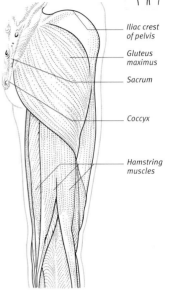

Iliac crest of pelvis

Gluteus maximus

Sacrum

Coccyx

Hamstring muscles

glycogen

The main form of *carbohydrate* stored in the body. Glycogen is a polysaccharide, consisting of chains of *glucose* molecules, and is found mainly in the liver and in muscles.

When there is excess glucose in the blood, it is converted to glycogen by the action of *insulin* and *glucocorticoids* (a class of *corticosteroid hormones*). When the blood glucose level is low, glycogen is converted back to glucose (regulated by *adrenaline* and *glucagon*) and released into the bloodstream.

glycogen storage diseases

A group of rare *genetic disorders* characterized by an absence or deficiency of certain *enzymes* (proteins that act as catalysts) responsible for the metabolism of *glycogen*. These enzyme defects may lead to abnormal concentrations of glycogen in the tissues, insufficient *glucose* (a simple sugar) in the blood, or the inability of the body to use glucose as energy. Also known as glycogenoses or GSDs, these diseases may affect the liver, the muscles, or both.

G

TYPES AND CAUSES

There are several types of GSD. One is glycogen storage disease type I. This condition is caused by a defect in glucose-6-phosphatase, an enzyme that aids *gluconeogenesis* in the liver. The majority of GSDs have an autosomal recessive pattern of inheritance: they occur when a child inherits the affected *gene* from parents who are carriers.

SYMPTOMS AND SIGNS

These features vary according to the particular type of GSD. Symptoms and signs may include failure to grow normally during childhood; muscle cramps and wasting; an enlarged liver; and low blood glucose levels.

DIAGNOSIS, TREATMENT, AND OUTLOOK

Diagnosis may involve biochemical tests (see *biochemistry*) on tissue samples from a muscle or a liver *biopsy*.

Some types of GSD can be controlled by management of symptoms, including by diet control. In certain cases a *liver transplant* is an option, but in other cases no treatment is possible and death occurs in the first few years of life.

glycosuria

The presence of *glucose* in the urine. Glycosuria results from failure of the *kidneys* to reabsorb glucose back into the bloodstream after the blood has been filtered to remove waste products.

Failure to reabsorb sufficient glucose may be due to *hyperglycaemia* (an abnormally high blood glucose level), as in *diabetes mellitus*. It may also occur if the kidney tubules have been damaged (for example, as a result of drug poisoning) and thus cannot reabsorb even normal amounts. In addition, glycosuria may occur during pregnancy, but is usually not serious provided that the blood glucose level is normal and there are no other symptoms.

Glycosuria is diagnosed by testing the urine (see *urinalysis*). The treatment depends on the cause.

glycosylated haemoglobin

A form of *haemoglobin* that is bound to the sugar glucose. Measurement of the blood level of glycosylated haemoglobin (known as the HbA1C test) is useful in monitoring *diabetes mellitus* because glycosylated haemoglobin levels indicate blood glucose levels over the preceding three months. In most people, about four to seven per cent of haemoglobin is glycosylated. In people with diabetes, the level of glycosylated haemoglobin may be raised if treatment has not kept the blood glucose level within the normal range. However, in people with abnormal haemoglobin, such as those with *sickle cell anaemia*, glycosylated haemoglobin cannot be used to monitor blood glucose levels.

GM foods

See *genetically modified foods*.

gnathic

Pertaining to the *jaw*, as in gnathitis (inflammation of the jaw).

goitre

Enlargement of the *thyroid gland*, visible as a swelling at the base of the neck.

CAUSES

The thyroid gland may enlarge (without any disturbance of its function) at *puberty*, during pregnancy, or in women taking *oral contraceptives*. In many parts of the world the main cause of a goitre is a dietary deficiency of *iodine*, an element needed by the thyroid to produce thyroid hormone. This form of the condition is called *endemic goitre*.

A condition called toxic goitre develops as a result of *thyrotoxicosis* in *Graves' disease* and in certain other forms of *hyperthyroidism* (overactivity of the thyroid). A goitre is also a feature of various types of *thyroiditis* (inflammation of the thyroid), including *Hashimoto's thyroiditis* and *De Quervain's thyroiditis*. Other causes include a tumour or nodule in the gland and, in rare cases, *thyroid cancer*.

There are also various types of familial goitre. This kind of goitre is caused by an inherited thyroid disorder; it appears during childhood and is often associated with signs of *hypothyroidism*, such as learning difficulties.

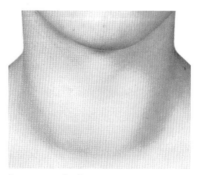

Appearance of goitre
The thyroid gland can become enlarged for a variety of reasons, including dietary deficiency of iodine, inflammation, or an autoimmune disorder affecting the gland.

SYMPTOMS

A goitre can range in size from a barely noticeable lump to a large swelling, depending on the cause. Large goitres may press on the *oesophagus* or the *trachea* and therefore make swallowing or breathing difficult.

DIAGNOSIS AND TREATMENT

Diagnosis may involve various *thyroid-function tests*, including blood tests and *radionuclide scanning*, to determine the activity of the thyroid gland.

A goitre that is not due to disease may eventually disappear of its own accord. Goitre due to iodine deficiency can be treated by iodine-rich foods. When a goitre is the result of disease, treatment is for the underlying disorder. Large goitres can be surgically removed (see *thyroidectomy*).

gold

A *disease-modifying antirhematic drug* used to treat active, progressive *rheumatoid arthritis* and, occasionally, arthritis arising as a complication of *psoriasis*. It is given either by injection (as sodium aurothiomalate) or orally (as auranofin). Adverse effects include *dermatitis*, loss of appetite, nausea, and diarrhoea. Gold may also damage the kidneys, liver, and bone marrow, and therefore regular monitoring with blood tests is necessary for people taking the drug.

Goldberg–Maxwell syndrome

A common form of male pseudohermaphroditism (a biological *intersex* condition in which the external genitalia of a genetic male resemble those of a female). Affected individuals have testes but have a small penis and a divided scrotum that resembles labia. (See also *sex determination*.)

Goldenhar's syndrome

A rare, *congenital* type of *dysplasia* (growth abnormality) in which the head and face fail to develop normally before birth. Common features include missing or abnormally developed ears and malformations of the jaw, mouth, palate, eyes, and vertebrae.

golfer's elbow

A condition caused by overuse of the forearm muscles that bend the wrist and fingers, usually due to activities such as using a screwdriver or playing golf with a faulty grip. The injury leads to inflammation of the *epicondyle* (bony prominence) on the inner part of the elbow, where the affected muscles are attached. Symptoms include pain and tenderness of the elbow and sometimes also the forearm.

Treatment consists of resting the elbow and taking *analgesic drugs* (painkillers). Severe or persistent pain may be relieved by applying topical anti-inflammatory creams or gels or by local injections of a *corticosteroid drug*.

gonadal dysgenesis

Defective development of the *gonads* (the testes and ovaries). Gonadal dysgenesis is a feature of *Turner's syndrome*.

gonadorelin

A medicinal version of gonadotrophin-releasing hormone (GnRH), which is naturally released by the *hypothalamus*. GnRH stimulates the nearby pituitary gland to secrete the two *gonadotrophin hormones* follicle-stimulating hormone (FSH) and luteinizing hormone (LH).

Gonadorelin can be given by injection. It is used to investigate suspected disease of the hypothalamus.

Gonadorelin analogues are synthesized forms of, and closely resemble, gonadorelin. They cause the hypothalamus to release less GnRH, and this effect leads to a reduction in the levels of FSH and LH. Gonadorelin analogues are used to counter the effects of natural hormones during gonadorelin treatment of *infertility*. The drugs are also used to treat *endometriosis* and hormone-dependent cancers including *breast cancer* and *prostate cancer*.

gonadotrophin hormones

Hormones that stimulate cell activity in the *ovaries* and *testes*. Gonadotrophins are essential for fertility. The most important are follicle-stimulating hormone (FSH) and luteinizing hormone (LH), secreted by the *pituitary gland*. Another gonadotrophin, HCG (see *gonadotrophin, human chorionic*), is produced by the placenta in pregnancy.

Certain gonadotrophins are used as drugs in the treatment of *infertility*.

gonadotrophin, human chorionic

A *hormone* produced by the *placenta* in early *pregnancy*. Human chorionic gonadotrophin (HCG) stimulates the *ovaries* to produce *oestrogen* and *progesterone*, which are necessary for a healthy pregnancy. HCG may also be produced in nonpregnant women by a

choriocarcinoma (a cancerous tumour of the uterus), and by some testicular tumours (see *testis, cancer of*) in men.

HCG is excreted in the urine; the detection of HCG levels in urine forms the basis of *pregnancy tests*. HCG extracted from the urine of pregnant women is given by injection to treat certain types of *infertility*. It may help to induce *ovulation* in women who have not been ovulating, and, in men, it may increase *sperm* production. HCG is occasionally given to prevent *miscarriage* in women whose production of progesterone is deficient.

gonads

The sex glands: the testes (see *testis*) in men and the ovaries (see *ovary*) in women. The activities of the gonads, both male and female, are regulated by *gonadotrophin hormones*, which are released by the pituitary gland.

gonorrhoea

One of the most common *sexually transmitted infections*. Gonorrhoea is widespread throughout the world.

CAUSES AND INCIDENCE

Gonorrhoea, which is caused by the bacterium NEISSERIA GONORRHOEAE, is most often transmitted during sexual activity, including oral and anal sex. An infected woman may also transmit the disease to her baby during *childbirth*.

SYMPTOMS AND SIGNS

Gonorrhoea has an incubation period of between two and ten days. In men, symptoms include a discharge from the *urethra* and pain on passing urine. Many infected women have no symptoms; if symptoms are present, they usually consist of a vaginal discharge or a burning sensation on passing urine.

Infection acquired through anal sex can cause gonococcal *proctitis* (inflammation of the rectum and anus). Oral sex with an infected person may lead to gonococcal *pharyngitis*, which sometimes causes a sore throat. A baby exposed to the infection during birth may acquire the eye infection gonococcal *ophthalmia*.

COMPLICATIONS

Untreated gonorrhoea may spread to other parts of the body. In men, it may cause *prostatitis* (inflammation of the prostate) or *epididymo-orchitis* (inflammation of a testis and the chamber where sperm mature), affecting fertility. In women, it causes *pelvic inflammatory disease*, which may damage the *fallopian*

tubes. This problem increases the risk of later *ectopic pregnancy* and may lead to *infertility*. Gonococcal bacteria in the bloodstream may result in *septicaemia* or *septic arthritis*.

DIAGNOSIS AND TREATMENT

Tests are performed on a sample of discharge or on swabs taken from the urethra, *cervix*, or *rectum* in order to confirm the diagnosis.

Gonorrhoea is treated with *antibiotic drugs*. Treatment is effective but does not protect against reinfection; in addition, bacterial resistance to antibiotics is an increasing problem. The patient's recent sexual contacts will need to be tested to establish whether or not they are also infected (see *contact tracing*).

Goodpasture's syndrome

A rare *autoimmune disorder* (in which the body's immune system attacks its own tissues) causing *inflammation* of the glomeruli (see *glomerulus*) in the kidneys and the alveoli (tiny air sacs) in the lungs, as well as *anaemia*. Goodpasture's syndrome is a serious disease; unless treated early it may lead to life-threatening bleeding into the lungs and progressive *kidney failure*. It is most common in young men, but can develop at any age and in women.

Goodpasture's syndrome may respond to treatment with *immunosuppressant drugs* and *plasmapheresis* (a procedure for removing unwanted antibodies from blood plasma). People who have severe or repeated attacks of the disorder require *dialysis* (a technique for removing waste products from the blood) and, ultimately, a *kidney transplant*.

GORD

The abbreviation for *gastro-oesophageal reflux disease*.

goserelin

A synthetic drug chemically related to the hypothalamic hormone *gonadorelin*. Goserelin is used to treat *breast cancer*, *prostate cancer*, *fibroids*, *infertility*, and *endometriosis*. Adverse effects of goserelin include loss of bone density following prolonged use.

gout

A common *metabolic disorder* that causes attacks of *arthritis*, usually in a single joint (often the base of the big toe). Gout is due to high levels of uric acid in the blood (see *hyperuricaemia*); these high levels of uric acid result in the deposition of uric acid crystals in joint tissue, which causes the arthritis. The affected joint is red, swollen, and extremely tender. Attacks last for a few days and often recur. They are sometimes accompanied by fever. With recurrent attacks, more joints may be involved, and there may be constant pain due to joint damage from chronic inflammation. In addition, gout may be associated with kidney stones (see *calculus, urinary tract*) or, rarely, with kidney damage due to the deposition of crystals in kidney tissue.

The diagnosis is confirmed by tests on blood or fluid from the affected joint to measure uric acid levels.

The pain and inflammation of acute (of sudden onset) attacks can be controlled by *nonsteroidal anti-inflammatory drugs* or *colchicine*. If these drugs are ineffective, a *corticosteroid drug* may be injected into the joint. Many people require no further treatment. Long-term treatment with drugs that help to lower urate levels, such as *allopurinol*, can stop or reduce the frequency of recurrent attacks. However, allopurinol should not be started during an attack because it may worsen or prolong the symptoms.

Graefe's sign

Lagging of the upper eyelid (see *lid lag*) as it follows the downward rotation of the eyeball in *Graves' disease*.

grafting

Transplanting healthy tissue from one part of the body to another (autografting) or from one person to another (allografting). Tissue transplants from an animal to a person (xenografting) are also carried out.

Grafting is used to repair or replace diseased, damaged, or defective tissues or organs. Common operations are *skin graft, bone graft, stem cell* or *bone marrow transplant, corneal graft, kidney transplant, heart transplant, liver transplant, heart–lung transplant, heart-valve surgery*, and *microsurgery* on blood vessels and nerves.

COMPLICATIONS

With autografting, the grafted tissue is usually assimilated well into the surrounding tissue at the new site. There is a risk of tissue rejection following other forms of grafting. Exceptions are grafts between identical twins, because their tissue matches exactly, and corneal grafting, because the cornea has no blood supply and therefore no white blood cells and antibodies to act as a defence system against the foreign cells.

GOUT

Gout is a common joint disease, affecting 10 times more men than women. In men it may occur at any time after puberty; in women it usually occurs only after the menopause. There is often a family history of the disorder. Hyperuricaemia (excess uric acid in the blood) leads to the formation of uric acid crystals inside joints. Crystals may also be deposited in the soft tissues in the ears and around tendons.

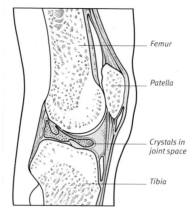

Crystal precipitation
Crystals of uric acid precipitate (solidify) into the joint space and surrounding tissues of the knee, causing intense inflammation and extreme pain.

Labels: Femur, Patella, Crystals in joint space, Tibia

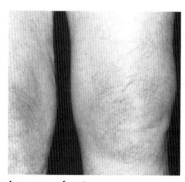

Appearance of gout
Deposition of uric acid crystals in the joint space has caused inflammation and swelling of the patient's affected left knee.

DIAGNOSIS

Gout is suspected if an attack of arthritis affects a single joint. A blood test is usually performed; a high level of uric acid will suggest gout. Examination of fluid from the joint may confirm the diagnosis.

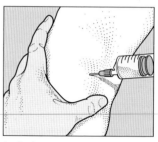

Aspiration
Fluid is aspirated (removed through a needle into a syringe) from the swollen joint and examined under a microscope to detect any uric acid crystals.

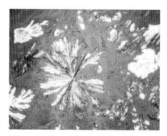

Microscopic evidence
The presence of uric acid crystals in the fluid confirms the diagnosis of gout.

To overcome rejection, as close a match as possible between the tissues of recipient and the tissues of donor is sought (see *tissue-typing*). The recipient is given *immunosuppressant drugs* to suppress the body's natural defences. (See also *transplant surgery*.)

graft-versus-host disease

A complication of some *stem cell* or *bone marrow transplants* in which certain *immune system* cells (killer T-*lymphocytes*) in the transplanted stem cells or marrow attack the tissues of the recipient.

Graft-versus-host (GVH) disease may occur soon after transplantation or may take some months to appear. The first sign is usually a skin rash. This may be followed by diarrhoea, abdominal pain, *jaundice*, *inflammation* of the eyes and mouth, and breathlessness. Most people with GVH recover within a year, but about one in five may eventually develop fatal complications.

GVH disease can usually be prevented by giving *immunosuppressant drugs* to all transplant patients. If, in spite of prophylactic treatment, the disease develops, it can be treated with *corticosteroid drugs* and immunosuppressant drugs such as *ciclosporin*. In some cases, however, it can be difficult to control.

Gram's stain

An *iodine*-based stain used to differentiate between types of *bacterium*.

A specimen of bacteria is stained with gentian violet and a solution of Gram's stain. It is then treated with a decolorizing agent, such as acetone, before being counterstained with a red dye. Bacteria that retain the dark violet stain are known as Gram-positive; those that lose the violet stain after decolorization and take up the counterstain (so that they appear pink) are known as Gram-negative.

Examples of Gram-positive bacteria include STREPTOCOCCUS and CLOSTRIDIUM. Gram-negative bacteria include VIBRIO CHOLERAE, which causes *cholera*, and various species of SALMONELLA.

grand mal

The former name for tonic–clonic seizures, which occur in *epilepsy*. The episode may start with warning sensations, such as unease or fear. This so-called aura lasts for a few seconds. The person then loses consciousness and collapses, and may briefly stop breathing. During the seizure there are generalized, jerky muscle contractions. As it finishes, the muscles relax and bowel and bladder control may briefly be lost. This type of seizure usually lasts for only a few minutes; the person may have no recall of it on awakening.

grand multipara

A term relating to a pregnant woman who has had five or more previous pregnancies that have resulted in *delivery*. During any subsequent pregnancy, a grand multipara woman is considered to be at increased risk of a variety of conditions including *anaemia*, *hypertension* (high blood pressure), *diabetes mellitus*, *placenta praevia*, *malpresentation*, prolonged labour, delivery by *caesarean section*, ruptured *uterus*, and *postpartum haemorrhage*.

granulation tissue

Red, moist, granular tissue that develops on the surface of an ulcer or an open *wound* during the process of *healing*.

granulocyte

A type of white *blood cell*.

granuloma

A growth comprising cells of a type associated with chronic *inflammation*. Granulomas usually occur as a reaction to certain infections, such as *tuberculosis*, or to a foreign body, such as a suture (stitch), but they may also develop for unknown reasons in conditions such as *sarcoidosis*.

A pyogenic granuloma is an excess of *granulation tissue* developing at the site of an injury to the skin or mucous membrane. (See also *granuloma annulare*; *granuloma inguinale*.)

granuloma annulare

A harmless skin condition characterized by circular, raised areas of skin that spread outwards, forming rings. It occurs mostly in children and young adults, usually on the backs of the hands and feet. The cause is unknown.

The diagnosis of granuloma annulare is often made simply from its appearance, but may be confirmed by a skin *biopsy* (removal of a tissue sample for analysis). No treatment is necessary. In most cases, the skin heals fully over several months or years.

granuloma inguinale

A *sexually transmitted infection* that causes ulceration of the genitals. The infection is caused by the bacterium CALYMMATOBACTERIUM GRANULOMATIS, also known as Donovan's bodies. It is common in parts of the tropics but rare in temperate countries.

The first symptoms are painless, raised nodules on the penis or labia (external female genitals) or around the anal area. The nodules gradually ulcerate forming red, raised areas, which may contain pus. Left untreated, the affected areas may eventually heal but there will be extensive scarring.

A *biopsy* (removal of a tissue sample for microscopic analysis) is performed on a sore in order to confirm diagnosis. The antibiotic drug *tetracycline* is an effective treatment.

granulomatosis

Any condition marked by the formation of multiple *granulomas* (collections of inflamed tissue), such as *Hodgkin's disease* and *Wegener's granulomatosis*.

granulomatous lung disease

A condition in which one or more *granulomas* (collections of inflamed tissue) develop within the lungs. In certain diseases, such as *Churg–Strauss syndrome* and *Wegener's granulomatosis*, granulomas and vasculitis (an inflammation of the blood vessels) develop at the same time.

Other conditions result from an *immune system* response to a foreign substance or infectious organism. Causes include *tuberculosis*, fungal infections, and inhaled rock or mineral dusts. In some diseases, however, such as *sarcoidosis*, the cause is unknown.

grasp reflex

A primitive reflex (see *reflex, primitive*) in which the fingers or toes curl when the palm or sole is touched or stroked. The grasp reflex is normal in babies, but if it continues into later life or appears in an adult, it may indicate a disorder of the frontal lobe of the brain.

Graves' disease

An *autoimmune disorder* (in which the *immune system* attacks the body's own tissues) that affects the *thyroid gland*. Graves' disease is characterized by toxic *goitre* (an overactive and enlarged thyroid gland); overproduction of thyroid hormones (*hyperthyroidism*), which leads to *thyrotoxicosis*; and *exophthalmos* (bulging eyeballs).

gravida

The medical term for a pregnant woman. The term "gravida" is often combined with a prefix to indicate the number of pregnancies that a woman has had (including the current one); for example, a primigravida is a woman who is pregnant for the first time.

gravitational ulcer

A form of skin ulcer that occurs in the lowermost parts of the body. The usual site is the lower leg (see *leg ulcer*), and a common cause is *varicose veins*.

gray

An SI unit (part of the International System of Units) of radiation dosage (see *radiation unit*).

graze

See *abrasion*.

greenstick fracture

A type of *fracture* that occurs when a long bone in the arm or leg bends and cracks on one side only. This type of fracture occurs only in children, whose bones are still growing and flexible.

grey baby syndrome

A rare but potentially fatal condition in newborn, and particularly premature, babies. Grey baby syndrome is caused by the antibiotic drug *chloramphenicol*, which is not usually prescribed for newborns but may be passed to a baby via the mother's bloodstream. Newborn babies' bodies cannot process or excrete the drug effectively, so very high levels build up. An affected infant is cold and has grey skin (see *cyanosis*) due to circulatory collapse (see *shock*).

If the condition is detected early, and the drug is discontinued, the infant may recover fully. Treatment with chloramphenicol should be avoided in late pregnancy and during breast-feeding.

grey matter

Regions of the *central nervous system* consisting mainly of closely packed and interconnected *nerve* cell bodies and their branching dendrites. (In contrast, the nerve cells' *axons*, which conduct nerve impulses, make up the *white matter* of the central nervous system.)

Grey matter is found mostly in the outer layers of the *cerebrum* (the main mass of the *brain* that is responsible for advanced mental functions) and in deeper regions of the brain, such as the *basal ganglia*. Grey matter also makes up the core of the *spinal cord*.

grief

A painful emotion, usually caused by loss of a loved one. (See *bereavement*.)

grip

The ability of the *hand* to hold objects firmly. The hand has an opposable thumb (which can touch each of the fingers), specialized skin on the palm and fingers to give adhesion, and a complex system of muscles, tendons, joints, and nerves that enables precise movements of the *digits*. The hand is capable of performing two types of grip: grasping, in which the whole hand is used, and pinching, a precise hold using the thumb and one finger.

Gripping ability is greatly reduced by conditions that cause muscular weakness or impairment of sensation in the hands. Such conditions include *stroke* or *nerve injury*, and disorders that affect the bones or joints of the hand or wrist, such as *arthritis* or a *fracture*.

gripe

Severe abdominal pain (see *colic*).

griseofulvin

An *antifungal drug*. Griseofulvin is particularly useful for infections affecting the scalp, beard, palms, soles of the feet, and nails. Common side effects are headache, dry mouth, abdominal pain, and *photosensitivity* (increased sensitivity of the skin to sunlight). Long-term treatment with the drug may cause liver or bone marrow damage

Groenouw's corneal dystrophy

An inherited disorder of the eye. There are two forms of the condition: type I (granular) and type II (macular).

Granular corneal dystrophy is an autosomal dominant disorder (see *genetic disorders*) characterized by small granular opacities in the top layers of the *cornea*. It develops in the first ten years of life. Macular corneal dystrophy is an autosomal recessive disorder typified by a diffuse haze with areas of dense corneal opacity. It develops in young people up to the age of 20.

Treatment for discomfort associated with the disorder may include *antibiotic* eye-drops. Severe cases may require laser surgery or a corneal transplant.

groin

The hollow between the lower abdomen and the top of the thigh.

groin, lump in the

A swelling in the *groin*. The most common cause is enlargement of a lymph node due to an infection (see *glands, swollen*). Another common cause is a *hernia*, in which the abdominal contents protrude through a weak area in the abdominal wall. Rarely, in males, an undescended testis may lead to a lump in the groin (see *testis, undescended*). Treatment depends on the cause.

groin strain

Pain and tenderness in the *groin* as a result of overstretching a *muscle*, typically while running or playing sport. The muscles commonly affected are the adductors (on the inside of the thigh) and the rectus femoris (at the front of the thigh). Groin strain is most often treated with *physiotherapy*, but recovery may be slow.

grommet

A small tube that may be inserted through an incision in the *eardrum* during surgery to treat *glue ear*, usually in children (see *myringotomy*). The grommet equalizes the pressure on both sides of the eardrum, permitting mucus to drain down the *eustachian tube* into the back of the throat.

Grommets are usually allowed to fall out as the hole in the eardrum closes; this generally occurs six to 12 months after insertion.

group therapy

Any treatment of psychological problems in which a group of patients is given therapy together. The group meets regularly, under the guidance of a therapist, in order to discuss their problems. Interaction between the members of the group is thought to be beneficial.

Group therapy may be useful for people with personality problems and for those who are suffering from *alcohol dependence*, *drug dependence*, *anxiety disorders*, and *eating disorders*.

growing pains

Vague aches and pains that occur in the limbs of children aged between six and 12 years old. Pains are usually felt at night, often in the calves. The cause is unknown, but the pains seem to be unrelated to the growing process itself.

Growing pains are of no medical significance and need no treatment. In contrast, pains that occur in the morning, cause a limp, or prevent normal use of a limb are not growing pains and should be assessed by a doctor.

growth

An abnormal proliferation of cells in a localized area (see *tumour*). Growth is also increase in size, usually as a result of increasing age (see *growth, childhood*).

growth, childhood

The increase in size that occurs as a child develops. Growth is usually monitored by measuring height, weight, and, in babies, head circumference.

The period of fastest growth occurs before birth. Growth is still rapid in the first few years of life, especially in the first year, but the rate decreases during childhood. *Puberty* marks another major period of growth, which continues until adult height and weight are reached, usually at age 16 to 17 in girls and between 19 and 21 in boys. See *growth charts* (p.352).

The body shape changes during childhood because different areas grow at different rates. For example, at birth, the head is already about three-quarters

CHANGES IN BODY PROPORTIONS BETWEEN BIRTH AND ADOLESCENCE

As a child grows, the body proportions change radically in relation to the body's overall length (see right). For example, a newborn baby's legs account for only three eighths of the body length, while before adolescence legs account for one half. A newborn's head accounts for as much as a quarter of the total body length, while an adolescent's head accounts for only one eighth.

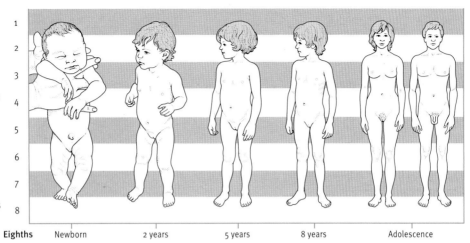

Eighths   Newborn   2 years   5 years   8 years   Adolescence

of its adult size; it grows to almost full size in the first year. Thereafter, it becomes proportionately smaller because the body grows at a much faster rate than that of the head.

Growth can be influenced by *heredity* and by environmental factors, such as nutrition and general health. *Hormones* also play an important role, particularly *growth hormone*, *thyroid hormones*, and, at puberty, the *sex hormones*.

A chronic illness, such as *cystic fibrosis*, may retard growth. Even a minor illness can slow the growth rate briefly, although the rate usually catches up when the child recovers. In some cases, slow growth is the only sign that a child is ill, malnourished, or emotionally distressed, when it is known as *failure to thrive*. However, *short stature* does not always indicate poor health.

Abnormally rapid growth is rare. Usually, it is a familial trait, but it may occasionally indicate an underlying disorder, such as a pituitary gland tumour causing *gigantism*. (See also *age*; *child development*.)

growth, excessive

See *gigantism*.

growth factor

Any of various chemicals that are involved in stimulating new cell growth and maintenance. Some growth factors, such as vascular endothelial growth factor, which stimulates the formation of new blood vessels, are significant in the growth and spread of cancers.

growth hormone

A substance produced by the *pituitary gland* that stimulates normal body growth. Growth hormone increases the production of protein in muscle cells and the release of energy from the breakdown of fats.

Oversecretion of the hormone leads to *gigantism* if it occurs before puberty or *acromegaly* if it occurs afterwards. A deficiency of the hormone may result in *short stature*. Synthetic growth hormone may be given by injection to treat short stature that is caused by pituitary or genetic disorders.

growth rate

The increase in size of an individual over a given period of time. Growth rate may be expressed in absolute terms or relatively, as a percentage of the average growth rate. (See also *growth, childhood*; *height velocity*.)

growth, restricted

See *short stature*.

GTN

The commonly used abbreviation for *glyceryl trinitrate*.

guaiac

A chemical used to detect haemoglobin (the oxygen-carrying pigment in red blood cells) in faeces. Tests using guaiac, known as *faecal occult blood tests*, are performed in order to detect hidden bleeding in the digestive tract (see *occult blood, faecal*).

Guillain–Barré syndrome

A rare condition affecting the *peripheral nervous system* that causes weakness, usually in the limbs.

CAUSES

The cause of Guillain–Barré syndrome is believed to be an allergic reaction to an infection, usually viral; the nerves are damaged by *antibodies* produced against the virus. Most cases develop two or three weeks after the infection.

SYMPTOMS

Weakness, which is often accompanied by numbness and tingling, usually starts in the legs and spreads to the arms, and may result in *paralysis*. The muscles of the face and those controlling speech, swallowing, and breathing may also be affected.

DIAGNOSIS AND TREATMENT

Diagnosis is confirmed by electrical tests to measure how fast nerve impulses are conducted, and by a *lumbar puncture*, in which a sample of cerebrospinal fluid is taken from the spinal canal for analysis.

Most people recover fully with only supportive treatment. Severe cases may need treatment with *plasmapheresis* (in which blood is treated to remove antibodies) or *immunoglobulin*. Mechanical *ventilation* may be used to aid breathing if the chest muscles and *diaphragm* are severely affected.

Some people are left with a permanent weakness, others may have further attacks of the disease, and a number may be left with weakness and also suffer further attacks.

GROWTH CHARTS

Growth charts are used to record the growth of children from the age of two to 18 years. Recording of a child's weight and height are carried out as part of a routine health check. The doctor or health visitor measures the child's weight and height and plots them against age on a chart. The growth curve is compared with the typical range, represented by the shaded area on the chart, for all children of the same age and gender.

The vertical axis on the charts show the weight, in kilograms and pounds, and the height in centimetres and inches; the horizontal axis shows the age range from two to 18 years. About 98 per cent of children fall below the line of the 98th percentile; the 50th percentile is the average, and 50 per cent fall below this line; only 2 per cent of children fall below the line of the 2nd percentile.

BOYS' WEIGHT (2–18 YEARS)

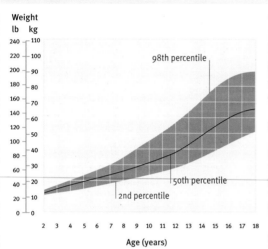

GIRLS' WEIGHT (2–18 YEARS)

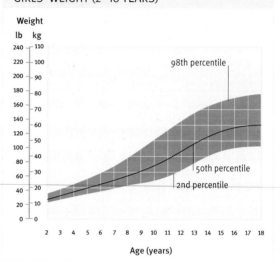

BOYS' HEIGHT (2–18 YEARS)

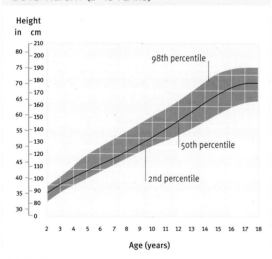

GIRLS' HEIGHT (2–18 YEARS)

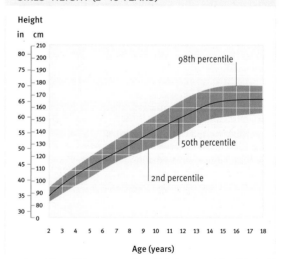

Growth in boys

Normally, there is a steady increase in height and weight until the onset of puberty. A sudden spurt in growth occurs during puberty (between the ages of 13 and 16). This chart was constructed using the height and weight of thousands of children; it is used by doctors to check whether growth of a particular boy is significantly above or below average.

Growth in girls

Normally, there is a steady increase in height and weight until the onset of puberty. A sudden spurt in growth occurs during puberty (between the ages of 11 and 14). These charts were constructed using the height and weight of thousands of children; it is used by doctors to check whether growth of a particular girl is significantly above or below average.

guilt

A painful emotion that arises from the awareness of having broken a moral code. Guilt (unlike shame, which depends on how other people view the transgression) is self-inflicted. Some psychoanalysts view it as a result of the prohibitions of the *superego* (conscience) that are instilled in early life, while others see guilt as a conditioned response to actions that on previous occasions have led to punishment. Feeling guilty for no reason, or for an imagined crime, is one of the main symptoms of *depression*.

Guinea worm disease

Also known as dracunculiasis, a tropical disease caused by the parasitic worm DRACUNCULUS MEDINENSIS, a type of roundworm that can grow to about 1 m long. Formerly widespread throughout tropical regions, the disease now occurs only in parts of Africa as a result of various eradication programmes.

Infection results from drinking water containing the water flea CYCLOPS, which harbours the worm larvae. Once consumed in a drink, the larvae pass through the intestine and mature in body tissues. After about a year, the adult female worm, now pregnant, reaches the skin surface and creates an inflamed blister that bursts, exposing the end of the worm. *Urticaria* (nettle rash), nausea, vomiting, and diarrhoea often develop during the formation of the blister.

The traditional remedy for the disease is to gradually wind the worm from the skin on to a small stick, a process that may take weeks or months. There is no medication to eradicate or prevent infection but the worm can often be removed surgically. *Anthelmintic drugs* may be given to facilitate removal of the worm, *nonsteroidal anti-inflammatory drugs* may be used to reduce inflammation, and *antibiotic drugs* may be given to control secondary infection; the patient may also be immunized against *tetanus*.

Gulf War syndrome

A term that has been used to describe a wide range of debilitating symptoms first reported by Gulf War veterans. Common symptoms include headaches, chronic fatigue, limb pains, difficulty concentraing, and memory problems. Exposure to chemicals, intensive vaccination programmes, and combat stress have all been implicated as possible causes of the syndrome.

gullet

The common name for the *oesophagus*.

gum

The soft tissue surrounding the *teeth* that protects underlying structures and keeps the teeth in position in the *jaw*.

Healthy gums are pink or brown and firm. Careful *oral hygiene* helps to keep the gums clean and prevent disease. *Gingivitis* (an early, reversible stage of gum disease characterized by inflammation of the gums) may occur if *plaque* is allowed to accumulate around the base of the teeth. If untreated, gingivitis may lead to chronic *periodontitis*, advanced gum disease in which infected pockets form between the gums and teeth and which is a major cause of tooth loss in adults

Bleeding gums are nearly always a symptom of gingivitis; rarely, they are due to *leukaemia* or *scurvy* (vitamin C deficiency). Gingival *hyperplasia* (fleshy thickening of the gums) occurs most commonly as a side effect of treatment with *phenytoin* (an anticonvulsant drug). (See also *receding gums*.)

gumboil

See *abscess, dental*.

gumma

A soft tumour that may develop in the late stages of untreated *syphilis*. Gummas are rare in developed countries.

gustatory

Related to the organs or sense of *taste*.

gut

A common name for the *intestine*.

Guthrie test

The former term for the *blood spot screening tests* performed routinely on newborn babies.

guttate psoriasis

A form of *psoriasis* (a skin disease characterized by patches of inflamed skin) that is found mainly in children and young adults, especially following *streptococcal infections*. A particular feature of guttate psoriasis is the formation of multiple small, teardrop-shaped skin blemishes. When it occurs in children following a streptococcal infection, guttate psoriasis usually clears up completely. However, affected children are at a higher risk of developing plaque psoriasis (which is the more common form of psoriasis) in later life.

gynaecology

The medical speciality concerned with the female *reproductive tract*. Gynaecology deals with *contraception*; the investigation and treatment of menstrual problems (see *menstruation, disorders of*); *sexual problems*; *infertility*; problems relating to the *menopause*; and disorders such as uterine *fibroids* and *ovarian cysts*. Gynaecologists also deal with disorders in the early stages of pregnancy, such as recurrent *miscarriage*.

gynaecomastia

Enlargement of one or both *breasts* in men or boys. The condition is sometimes due to an excess of the female sex hormone *oestrogen*.

CAUSES AND INCIDENCE

Mild, temporary gynaecomastia can occur in boys at birth due to maternal hormones, and the condition is also common at *puberty*.

Gynaecomastia that develops in later life may be due to a chronic liver disease, such as *cirrhosis*, in which the liver is unable to break down oestrogen. Hormone-secreting tumours, such as pituitary or testicular tumours, may also be responsible for the condition.

Adult gynaecomastia, which sometimes occurs in only one breast, can also occur when synthetic hormones and some drugs, such as *digoxin*, *spironolactone*, and *cimetidine*, cause a change to the balance of sex hormones. Very rarely, a discrete lump that develops on one breast may be a male breast cancer.

DIAGNOSIS AND TREATMENT

Investigation may involve *blood tests*. If cancer is suspected, a *biopsy* (removal of the lump or a piece of tissue for analysis) will be performed.

Treatment depends on the cause. If a drug is responsible, an alternative will be given if possible. If there is no underlying disease, the swelling usually subsides over a period of time. In severe cases, however, cosmetic surgery (see *mammoplasty*) may be considered.

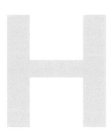

H₁-receptor antagonists

An abbreviation for histamine₁-receptor antagonists (a type of *antihistamine drug*), a group of drugs used in the treatment of allergic reactions.

H₂-receptor antagonists

An abbreviation for histamine₂-receptor antagonists, a type of *ulcer-healing drug*. (See also *cimetidine*; *famotidine*; *ranitidine*.)

H5N1 virus

A virus that causes a virulent strain of *avian influenza*.

habit tic

A type of *tic* (repetitive, involuntary movement of a muscle) that has a psychological cause and does not result from damage to or disease of the nervous system.

habitual miscarriage

Also known as recurrent pregnancy loss or recurrent miscarriage, the spontaneous abortion (see *miscarriage*) of a fetus in three or more consecutive pregnancies, after less than 24 weeks' gestation. Habitual miscarriages may be caused by defects or disorders of the uterus, such as *fibroids*, or of the cervix (see *cervical incompetence*). Certain conditions affecting the mother, such as systemic *lupus erythematosus* or *Hughes' syndrome*, may also cause habitual abortion.

habituation

The process of becoming accustomed to an experience. In general, the more a person is exposed to a stimulus, the less he or she is affected by it. People can become habituated to certain drugs and develop a reduced response to their effects (see *tolerance*).

haem

An iron-bearing pigment that combines with globin (a protein) to form *haemoglobin*, the main component of *red blood cells*. The haem binds with *oxygen* to transport it from the lungs to the tissues.

haem-

A prefix that is placed before a variety of words (for example, *haemoglobin*) to indicate *blood*.

haemangioblastoma

A rare type of brain tumour consisting of blood-vessel cells. Haemangioblastomas develop slowly as cysts, often in the *cerebellum*, and are mostly noncancerous. Symptoms include headache, vomiting, *nystagmus* (abnormal jerky eye movements) and, if the tumour is in the cerebellum, *ataxia* (lack of muscle coordination). Most haemangioblastomas can be removed surgically.

haemangioma

A birthmark caused by an abnormal distribution of blood vessels. Haemangiomas may be flat or raised.

TYPES

Port-wine stains are large, flat, purplered marks, which are permanent and can be unsightly. In rare cases, port-wine stains are associated with abnormalities in the blood vessels of the brain (see *Sturge-Weber syndrome*).

Small, flat marks, often known as stork marks or stork bites, are common in newborn babies, particularly on the back of the neck. Most begin to fade about three weeks after birth.

Raised bright red haemangiomas, often called strawberry marks, usually enlarge rapidly during the first few weeks after birth. They generally disappear without leaving a scar by the time a child is five to seven years old.

COMPLICATIONS AND TREATMENT

Haemangiomas do not usually require treatment. However, a haemangioma that bleeds persistently or that looks unsightly may need to be removed by *laser treatment*, *cryosurgery* (destruction of tissue by extreme cold), *radiotherapy*, *embolization* (obstruction of blood flow to tissue), or *plastic surgery*.

haemarthrosis

Bleeding into a *joint*, causing the capsule that encloses the joint to swell, and resulting in pain and stiffness.

CAUSES

Haemarthrosis is usually the result of severe injury to a joint, such as a torn capsule, torn ligaments, or fracture of a bone forming part of the joint. Often the cause is a sports injury to the knee.

Less common causes are *bleeding disorders*, such as *haemophilia* (in which failure of the blood-clotting mechanism causes abnormal bleeding). Any joint may be affected and bleeding into the joint may occur spontaneously or be caused by even a minor knock. Excessive amounts of *anticoagulant drugs* can also cause haemarthrosis.

Repeated haemarthrosis may damage joint surfaces, causing *osteoarthritis*.

SYMPTOMS AND SIGNS

Haemarthrosis causes a joint to swell immediately after injury. The joint may gradually stiffen into a fixed position as a result of spasm in surrounding muscles.

TREATMENT

Ice-packs may reduce swelling and pain. Fluid may be withdrawn from the joint in order to relieve pain and for diagnosis. Haemophiliacs are given *factor VIII* to promote blood clotting. Resting the joint in an elevated position can prevent further bleeding.

haematemesis

The medical term for *vomiting blood*.

haematocolpos

The accumulation of menstrual blood in the vagina due to blockage of the vaginal opening. This rare condition occurs either when the *hymen* (the membrane around the vaginal opening) lacks the perforation that would normally allow the blood to leave the body or as a result of developmental abnormalities of the vagina. Haematocolpos requires surgical treatment to drain the blood and, if necessary, to reconstruct the vagina.

haematology

The study of *blood* and its formation, as well as the investigation and treatment of disorders that affect the blood and the *bone marrow*.

Microscopic examination and counting of blood and bone marrow cells are essential procedures in diagnosing types of blood disorder, such as *anaemia* or *leukaemia*. Analysis of blood is used in the diagnosis of a range of disorders as well as specific blood disorders.

haematoma

A localized collection of *blood* (usually clotted) that is caused by bleeding from a ruptured blood vessel. Haematomas can occur almost anywhere in the body and vary from a minor to a potentially fatal condition.

Less serious types of haematoma include those that develop under the nails or in the tissues of the outer ear (see cauliflower ear). Most haematomas disappear without treatment in a few days, but if they are painful they may need to be drained. More serious types include extradural and subdural haematomas, which press on the brain (see *extradural haemorrhage*; *subdural haemorrhage*).

haematoma auris

The medical term for *cauliflower ear*.

haematospermia

An alternative term for haemospermia, the medical term for blood in the semen (see *semen, blood in the*).

haematuria

Blood in the *urine*, which may or may not be visible to the naked eye. In small amounts, the blood may give the urine a smoky appearance.

Almost any *urinary tract* disorder can cause haematuria. *Urinary tract infection* is a common cause; *prostatitis* may be a cause in men. *Cysts*, *kidney tumours*, *bladder tumours*, stones (see *calculus, urinary tract*), and *glomerulonephritis* (inflammation of the filtering units of the kidney) may cause haematuria. *Bleeding disorders* may also cause the condition.

Blood that is not visible to the naked eye may be detected by a dipstick *urine test* or microscopic examination. *CT scanning*, *ultrasound scanning*, or intravenous *urography* can help to determine the cause. If bladder disease is suspected, *cystoscopy* is performed.

haemochromatosis

An inherited disease in which too much dietary iron is absorbed. Excess iron gradually accumulates in the liver, pancreas, heart, testes, and other organs. Men are more frequently affected than women because women regularly lose iron in menstrual blood.

SYMPTOMS AND COMPLICATIONS

Haemochromatosis rarely causes problems until middle age. Loss of sex drive and a reduction in the size of the testes are often the first signs. Excess iron over a period of time causes enlargement of the liver and *cirrhosis* (chronic liver damage) and can lead to *diabetes mellitus*, bronzed skin coloration (due to iron pigment deposition in the skin), cardiac *arrhythmia*, and, eventually, *liver failure* and *liver cancer*.

DIAGNOSIS AND TREATMENT

Diagnosis is based on *blood tests* and a *liver biopsy* (removal of a small sample of tissue for analysis). Treatment is by

venesection (withdrawal of blood from a vein). Initially, the procedure is performed every week. After iron levels have returned to normal, however, the process of venesection is required less often. (See also *haemosiderosis*.)

haemodialysis

One of the two means of *dialysis* (artificial filtration of the blood) used to treat *kidney failure*.

haemoglobin

The oxygen-carrying pigment that is present in red *blood cells*. Haemoglobin molecules, which are produced by *bone marrow*, are made up of four protein chains (two alpha- and two beta-globin chains) and four haem (a red pigment that contains iron).

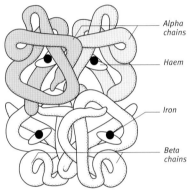

Structure of haemoglobin
Each molecule contains four globin chains –
two alpha and two beta. Each chain carries
a haem component capable of binding oxygen.

Oxygen from the lungs enters red blood cells in the bloodstream. The oxygen then combines chemically with the haem in the haemoglobin to form oxyhaemoglobin, which gives blood in the *arteries* its bright red colour. In this medium, oxygen is carried around the body and delivered to the areas that need it. When the oxyhaemoglobin has released its oxygen it reverts to haemoglobin, giving the blood in the *veins* its distinctive darker colour.

DISORDERS

Some defects in haemoglobin production are the result of a *genetic disorder*; defects such as these are subdivided into two types, namely errors of haem production, which are known as *porphyrias*, and errors of globin production, known as *haemoglobinopathies*. Other defects, such as some types of *anaemia*, have a nongenetic cause.

haemoglobinopathy

A term used to describe the *genetic disorders* in which there is a fault in the production of the globin chains of *haemoglobin* (the oxygen-carrying substance in the blood). Examples of haemoglobinopathies include *sickle cell anaemia* and the *thalassaemias*.

haemoglobinuria

The presence of *haemoglobin* in urine. Haemoglobin is an oxygen-carrying substance mainly contained in red blood cells, but a small amount is free in the blood plasma. Excessive breakdown of red blood cells, due to heavy exercise, cold weather, falciparum *malaria*, or haemolytic *anaemia*, increases the concentration of free haemoglobin in the plasma. The body excretes the excess haemoglobin in the urine.

haemolysis

The destruction of red *blood cells*. Haemolysis is the normal process by which old red blood cells are destroyed, mainly in the *spleen*. Bilirubin, a waste product of haemolysis, is excreted into the *bile* by the liver. Abnormal haemolysis, in which red blood cells are destroyed prematurely, may cause anaemia and jaundice (see *anaemia, haemolytic*).

haemolytic anaemia

See *anaemia, haemolytic*.

haemolytic disease of the newborn

Excessive *haemolysis* (destruction of red blood cells) in the fetus and newborn by *antibodies* produced by the mother. Haemolytic disease of the newborn is most often caused by *rhesus incompatibility*. This occurs when a mother with Rh-negative type blood, who has previously been exposed to Rh-positive blood through birth, miscarriage, abortion, or *amniocentesis*, is pregnant with a baby that has Rh-positive blood. Haemolytic disease has become uncommon since the introduction of routine preventive treatment for Rh-negative women during pregnancy (see *anti-D (Rh₀) immunoglobulin*).

SYMPTOMS AND SIGNS

In mild cases of the disease, the newborn baby becomes slightly jaundiced during the first 24 hours of life (due to an excess of the bile pigment *bilirubin* in the blood) and slightly anaemic. In more severe cases, the level of bilirubin in the blood may increase to a dangerous level,

Alpha chains

Haem

Iron

Beta chains

H

H

causing a risk of *kernicterus* (a type of brain damage). Severely affected babies have marked anaemia while still in the uterus. They become swollen (*hydrops fetalis*) and are often stillborn.

TREATMENT

In mild cases, no treatment is necessary. In other cases, the aim is to deliver the baby before the anaemia becomes too severe, usually by *induction of labour* at 35–39 weeks' gestation. If the baby is too young to be delivered safely, fetal blood transfusions may be necessary.

After birth, *phototherapy* (light treatment that converts bilirubin in the skin into a water-soluble form that is more easily excreted from the body) can help to reduce *jaundice*. An exchange blood transfusion may be needed.

haemolytic–uraemic syndrome

A rare disease in which red *blood cells* are destroyed prematurely and the *kidneys* are damaged, causing acute *kidney failure*. *Thrombocytopenia* (reduction of *platelets* in the blood) can also occur. haemolytic–uraemic syndrome most commonly affects young children.

CAUSES

The precise cause of haemolytic–uraemic syndrome is uncertain, but the disorder may be triggered by a serious bacterial or viral infection. It is thought that the lining of small blood vessels in the kidneys becomes damaged, causing small clots to form. These clots cause *haemolysis* (breakdown of red cells) as blood flows past them.

SYMPTOMS

The onset of the disease is sudden; symptoms include weakness, lethargy, and a reduction in the volume of urine. Severe *hypertension* (high blood pressure) is common and may cause *seizures*.

DIAGNOSIS AND TREATMENT

Blood and urine tests can determine the degree of kidney damage. *Dialysis* (artificial filtration of the blood) may be needed until the kidneys have recovered. Most patients recover normal renal function.

haemophilia

An inherited *bleeding disorder* caused by deficiency of a blood protein, *factor VIII*, which is essential for blood clotting. Haemophiliacs (who are almost always male) suffer recurrent bleeding, usually into their joints, which may occur spontaneously or after injury.

INCIDENCE AND CAUSES

The lack of factor VIII is due to a defective gene, which shows a pattern of *sex-linked inheritance*. Affected males pass on the gene not to their sons but to their daughters, who are carriers of the condition. Some of the sons of carrier females may be affected, and some of the daughters of carriers may themselves be carriers. Many haemophiliacs have an uncle, brother, or grandfather who is also affected. However, in about one third of cases there is no family history of haemophilia.

SYMPTOMS

The severity of the disorder differs markedly among individuals. However, episodes of bleeding are painful and, unless treated promptly, can lead to deformity of the knees, ankles, and other joints. Injury, and even minor operations such as tooth extraction, may lead to profuse bleeding. Internal bleeding can lead to blood in the urine or extensive bruises.

DIAGNOSIS AND TREATMENT

Haemophilia is diagnosed by *blood-clotting tests* and by *amniocentesis* or *chorionic villus sampling* in a fetus. Bleeding can be controlled by infusions of factor VIII concentrates. People with a severe form of the disorder may need regular intravenous injections of factor VIII as a preventive measure.

OUTLOOK

Most people with haemophilia can lead an active life but should avoid the risk of injury. Contact sports, such as football, are not advisable but other forms of exercise, such as swimming and walking, can be beneficial. The female relatives of anyone with haemophilia should obtain genetic counselling before planning a pregnancy.

Haemophilus influenzae

A bacterium that causes various infectious diseases in humans. There are several types of HAEMOPHILUS INFLUENZAE; type b (Hib) causes infections such as *meningitis*, *epiglottitis*, *septicaemia*, and *pneumonia*. Infants are routinely immunized against HAEMOPHILUS INFLUENZAE type b as part of the childhood immunization schedule (see *Hib vaccine*).

haemoptysis

The medical term for *coughing up blood*.

haemorrhage

The medical term for *bleeding*. (See also *haematoma*.)

haemorrhagic fever

See *viral haemorrhagic fever*.

haemorrhagic shock

Physiological *shock* (a dangerous reduction of blood flow throughout the body tissues), which is caused by severe blood loss. (See also *hypovolaemia*.)

haemorrhoidectomy

Surgical removal of *haemorrhoids*. The procedure is used to treat large, prolapsing, or bleeding haemorrhoids, if other simpler methods such as *banding* have not been successful.

Complete healing after a haemorrhoidectomy takes three to six weeks. *Laxative drugs* are usually given during this period to soften faeces and make them easier to pass.

haemorrhoids

Swollen veins in the lining of the *anus*. Haemorrhoids may occur close to the anal opening, when they are called external haemorrhoids, or higher in the anal canal, in which case they are called internal haemorrhoids. Sometimes these veins protrude outside the anal canal, in which case they are called prolapsing haemorrhoids.

CAUSES

Haemorrhoids are caused by increased pressure in the veins of the anus, most commonly through straining repeatedly to pass hard faeces. Such faeces may result from a diet that is too high in refined foods and too low in fibre (see *constipation*). Haemorrhoids are also common during pregnancy, when the weight of the fetus exerts pressure on blood vessels.

SYMPTOMS

Rectal bleeding and discomfort on defaecation are the most common features. Prolapsing haemorrhoids often produce a mucous discharge and itching around the anus. A complication of prolapse is *thrombosis* and *strangulation*. This occurs when a blood clot forms in the vein, preventing it from returning to its position in the anus and restricting its blood supply. The condition can cause extreme pain.

DIAGNOSIS AND TREATMENT

Diagnosis is usually by *proctoscopy* (inspection of the rectum with a viewing instrument). Mild cases are controlled by drinking plenty of fluids, eating a high-fibre diet, and establishing regular bowel movements. Rectal suppositories and creams that contain *corticosteroid drugs* and local *anaesthetics* reduce pain and swelling. More troublesome haemorrhoids may be treated by *sclerotherapy* (injection of an irritant liquid), *cryosurgery* (application of extreme cold),

TREATING **HAEMORRHOIDS**

In the procedures shown below, the patient will usually have been given a laxative so that the lower bowel is clear of faeces. Banding requires no anaesthesia; either general or epidural anaesthesia is given before a haemorrhoidectomy is performed.

BANDING HAEMORRHOIDS

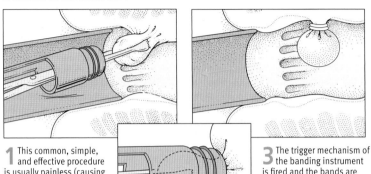

1 This common, simple, and effective procedure is usually painless (causing no more than a mild ache afterwards) and no anaesthesia is required. The patient lies on one side, the proctoscope (instrument for examining the rectum) is positioned, and the haemorrhoid is grasped with forceps.

2 The banding instrument is inserted and pressed into the anal wall. Gentle traction is applied to draw the mass into the drum of the instrument.

3 The trigger mechanism of the banding instrument is fired and the bands are squeezed on to the neck of the mass. The proctoscope is withdrawn, leaving the haemorrhoid with its base tightly constricted by the bands. The haemorrhoid then withers and drops off painlessly within a few days of the operation.

HAEMORRHOIDECTOMY

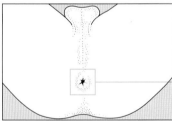

Stages of the procedure
Under general or epidural anaesthesia, the patient's rectum is examined with a proctosigmoidoscope to exclude a diagnosis

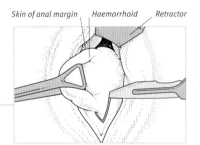

Skin of anal margin *Haemorrhoid* *Retractor*

of tumour. The patient is then placed in the lithotomy position. The haemorrhoid is clamped, placed under traction (as shown above), secured with a suture, and then removed with a scalpel.

or by banding, in which a band is tied around the haemorrhoid, which causes it to wither and drop off. A *haemorrhoidectomy* (surgical removal of the haemorrhoids) is generally required for prolapsing haemorrhoids.

haemosiderosis

A general increase in *iron* stores in the body. Haemosiderosis may occur after repeated blood transfusions or, more rarely, as a result of excessive iron intake.

haemospermia

The medical term for blood in the semen (see *semen, blood in the*).

haemostasis

The arrest of *bleeding*. There are three main natural mechanisms by which bleeding is stopped after injury. First, small blood vessels constrict. Second, small *blood cells* called platelets aggregate and plug the bleeding points. Third, the blood plasma coagulates, forming filaments of a substance called *fibrin*, which help seal the damaged blood vessel (see *blood clotting*). Defects in any of these mechanisms can cause a *bleeding disorder*.

haemostatic drugs

A group of drugs to treat bleeding disorders and to control bleeding. Haemostatic

preparations that help blood clotting are given to people with clotting factor deficiencies. For example, *factor VIII* is used for *haemophilia*. Drugs that prevent the breakdown of fibrin in clots, such as *tranexamic acid*, can also help stop bleeding.

haemothorax

A collection of blood in the pleural cavity (the space between the chest wall and the lung). Haemothorax is most commonly caused by chest injury, but it may arise spontaneously in people with defects of blood coagulation or as a result of cancer.

Symptoms of haemothorax include pain in the affected side of the chest and upper abdomen, and breathlessness. If extensive, there may be partial lung collapse. Blood in the pleural cavity is withdrawn through a needle.

Hailey–Hailey disease

Also known as benign familial *pemphigus*, a form of pemphigus (a blistering skin disease) that mainly affects the neck, armpits, and groin. Hailey–Hailey disease tends to run in families.

hair

A threadlike structure composed of dead cells containing *keratin*, a fibrous protein.
STRUCTURE AND FUNCTION
The root of each hair is embedded in a tiny pit in the dermis (inner) layer of the *skin* called a hair *follicle*. Each shaft of hair consists of a spongy semihollow core (the medulla), a surrounding layer of long, thin fibres (the cortex), and, on the outside, several layers of overlapping cells (the cuticle).

While a hair is growing, the root is enclosed by tissue called a bulb, which supplies the hair with keratin. The bulb is the pale swelling that sometimes can be seen when a hair is pulled out. The upgrowth of dead cells and keratin from the root forms the hair. Once the hair has stopped growing, the bulb retracts from the root and the hair eventually falls out.

Hair is involved in the regulation of body temperature (known as thermoregulation). If the body is too cold, arrector pili muscles in the skin contract, pulling the hairs upright to form goose pimples. Erect hairs trap an insulating layer of air next to the skin.
TYPES
There are three types of human hair. From the fourth month of gestation, the fetus is covered with downy hair called

H

H

THE STRUCTURE OF A **HAIR**

The hair shaft consists of dead cells and keratin. It has three layers: the medulla (core), the cortex, and the cuticle (covering).

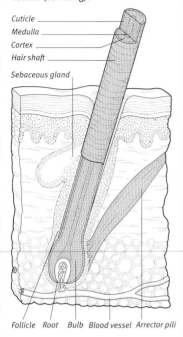

Cuticle
Medulla
Cortex
Hair shaft
Sebaceous gland

Follicle   Root   Bulb   Blood vessel   Arrector pili

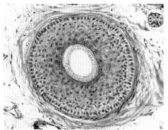

Cross-section through a hair
In this light micrograph, the medulla, the cortex, and the outer cuticle of the hair can all be clearly differentiated.

lanugo, which is shed during the ninth month. After birth and until puberty, vellus hair, which is fine, short, and colourless, covers most of the body. The third type, terminal hair, is thicker, longer, and often pigmented; it grows on the scalp, the eyebrows, and the eyelashes. At puberty, terminal hair replaces vellus in the pubic area and the armpits. In most men and some women the process continues on the face, limbs, and trunk.

COLOUR AND TEXTURE
Hair colour is determined by the amount of pigment called melanin that is present in the hair shaft. Melanin is produced by cells called melanocytes at the base of the hair follicle. Red melanin is responsible for red and auburn hair, black melanin for all other colours. If cells receive no pigment, the cortex of each hair becomes transparent and the hair appears white. The degree of curliness of a hair depends on the cross-section shape of its follicle.

DISORDERS
Brittle hair may be due to excessive styling, *hypothyroidism* (underactivity of the thyroid gland), or severe vitamin or mineral deficiency. Very dry hair can be caused by malnutrition. Ingrown hairs occur when the free-growing end of the hair penetrates the skin near the follicle, which may cause inflammation. (See also *hirsutism*; *hypertrichosis*.)

hairball

A ball of hair in the stomach, found in people who nervously suck or chew their hair (see *bezoar*).

hair cycle

The alternating phases of activity in a *hair* follicle. There are two main phases: an active phase, when new hair forms in the follicle, and a resting phase, when cell activity slows down and stops. The active phase lasts for several years, until a hair has reached its maximum length. During the resting phase, that hair dies. In the next growth phase, a new hair is formed and pushes the dead one out of the follicle. The growth cycles of hairs may be disrupted by various factors, including hormonal or immune system disorders; pregnancy; adverse reactions to drugs; and *radiotherapy*.

hairiness, excessive

See *hirsutism*; *hypertrichosis*.

hair removal

Hair is usually removed from the body purely for cosmetic reasons. It may also be shaved from around an incision site before a surgical operation. Methods of temporarily removing hair include shaving, *depilatory* creams, waxing, and sugaring. Methods of permanently removing hair include *electrolysis*, laser treatment, and photo-epilation.

hair transplant

A cosmetic operation in which hairy sections of scalp are removed and transplanted to hairless areas in order to treat *alopecia* (baldness).

HOW IT IS DONE
There are several different hair transplant techniques. In strip grafting, a strip of skin and hair is taken from a donor site, usually at the back of the scalp or behind the ears. The removed hairs and their follicles are then inserted into numerous incisions made in a bald area, known as the recipient site. The procedure usually takes 60–90 minutes. The patient is given a mild sedative and the donor and recipient sites are anaesthetized. The donor site heals in about five days. Although transplanted hairs fall out shortly afterwards, new hair growth appears from the follicles between three weeks and three months later.

Other transplant techniques include punch grafting, in which a punch is used to remove small areas of bald scalp, which are replaced with areas of hairy

SCALP HAIR GROWTH

There are about 100,000 hairs on the scalp, although there is considerable individual variation. The exact number depends on the number of hair follicles, which is established before birth. Scalp hair grows about one centimetre per month. Each hair goes through alternating periods of growth and rest. On average, a person sheds about 100 scalp hairs a day.

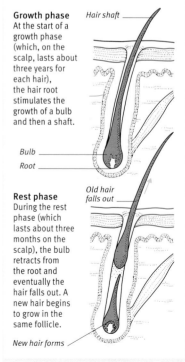

Growth phase
At the start of a growth phase (which, on the scalp, lasts about three years for each hair), the hair root stimulates the growth of a bulb and then a shaft.

Hair shaft

Bulb
Root

Rest phase
During the rest phase (which lasts about three months on the scalp), the bulb retracts from the root and eventually the hair falls out. A new hair begins to grow in the same follicle.

Old hair falls out

New hair forms

scalp; flap grafting, in which flaps of hairy skin are lifted, rotated, and stitched to replace bald areas; and male pattern baldness reduction, which involves cutting out areas of bald skin and stretching surrounding areas of hair-bearing scalp to replace them.

hairy cell

A large, abnormal white blood cell with numerous hairlike projections. Hairy cells occur with a rare form of *leukaemia*, known as hairy cell leukaemia, when they proliferate in the blood, bone marrow, liver, and spleen.

Haldol

A brand name for the antipsychotic drug *haloperidol*.

half-life

The time taken for the activity of a substance to reduce to half its original level. The term is usually used to refer to the time taken for the level of *radiation* emitted by a radioactive substance to decay to half its original level. The concept is useful in *radiotherapy* for assessing how long material will stay radioactive in the body. Half-life is also used to refer to the length of time taken by the body to eliminate half the quantity of a drug.

halitosis

The medical term for bad breath. Halitosis is usually the result of smoking, drinking alcohol, eating onions or garlic, or poor oral hygiene. Persistent bad breath not caused by any of these may be a symptom of mouth infection, *sinusitis*, or certain lung disorders, such as *bronchiectasis*.

Hallervorden–Spatz syndrome

A very rare disorder thought to be caused by a buildup of iron in certain areas of the brain. The symptoms, which are progressive, usually appear in early childhood and include abnormal muscle rigidity and spasms (see *dystonia*).

Hallgren's syndrome

A *congenital* disorder (present at birth) that is characterized by *deafness*; congenital *cataract* (opacity of the lens of the eye); and *ataxia* (clumsiness and incoordination) due to brain damage.

hallucination

A perception that occurs when there is no external stimulus. Auditory hallucinations (the hearing of voices) are a major symptom of *schizophrenia* but may also be caused by *bipolar disorder* and certain brain disorders. Visual hallucinations most often occur in states of *delirium* brought on by a physical illness or alcohol withdrawal (*delirium tremens*). *Hallucinogenic drugs* are another common cause of visual hallucinations. Hallucinations of smell are associated with *temporal lobe epilepsy*. Those of touch and taste are rare, however, and occur mainly in people with *schizophrenia*. People who are subjected to *sensory deprivation* or overwhelming physical stress sometimes suffer from temporary hallucinations.

hallucinogenic drug

A drug that causes *hallucination*. Hallucinogens include certain drugs of abuse, such as *LSD*, *marijuana*, *mescaline*, and *psilocybin*. Some prescription drugs, such as *anticholinergic drugs* and *levodopa*, occasionally cause hallucinations.

hallux

The medical name for the big *toe*.

hallux rigidus

Loss of movement in the large joint at the base of the big *toe* as a result of *osteoarthritis*. The joint is usually tender and swollen. Treatment comprises resting the toe and wearing a support insert in the shoe. Surgery may be required.

hallux valgus

A deformity of the big *toe* in which the joint at the base projects out from the foot, and the top of the toe turns inwards. The condition is more common in women, because it is usually associated with wearing narrow, pointed, high-heeled shoes, but it may be caused by an inherited weakness in the joint. A hallux valgus often leads to formation of a *bunion* or to osteoarthritis in the joint, causing pain and limiting foot movement. Severe deformity may be corrected by *osteotomy* (removal of part of a bone) or *arthrodesis* (fusion of bones in a joint).

haloperidol

An *antipsychotic drug* used to treat mental illnesses such as *schizophrenia* and *mania*. Haloperidol is also given to control the symptoms of *Gilles de la Tourette's syndrome* (a rare neurological disorder) and, in small doses, to treat agitation and restlessness in the elderly. Rarely, it may be used to treat intractable hiccups. Possible side effects of the drug include drowsiness, lethargy, weight gain, dizziness, involuntary movements (tardive dyskinesia) and *parkinsonism*.

hamartoma

A noncancerous mass, resembling a tumour, which consists of an overgrowth of tissues that are normally found in the affected part of the body. Hamartomas are common in the skin (the most common is a *haemangioma*), but they also occur in the lungs, heart, or kidneys.

hammer-toe

A deformity of the toe (usually the second toe) in which one of the joints remains in a bent position due to a *tendon* abnormality. A painful *corn* often develops on this joint. A protective pad can ease pressure on the joint and relieve pain, but surgery may be needed if the pain is persistent.

Hammer toe

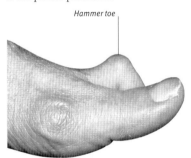

Appearance of hammer-toe
This photograph shows the typical appearance of a hammer-toe, in which one of the joints of the second toe is fixed in a bent position.

hamstring muscles

A group of *muscles* at the back of the thigh. The upper ends of the hamstring muscles are attached by *tendons* to the *pelvis*; the lower ends are attached by tendons called hamstrings to the *tibia* and *fibula*. The hamstring muscles bend the knee and swing the leg backwards from the thigh.

Tearing of the hamstring muscles is common in sports. The injury happens suddenly and is very painful. Bruising over the area develops several days later. Repeated strenuous exercise may sprain the muscles (see *overuse injury*). Both types of injury can often be prevented by warming-up exercises.

Painful spasms of the hamstring muscles can also sometimes occur as a protective response to a knee injury; by restricting movement of the damaged knee joint, the muscle spasms help to limit further injury.

H

hand

The hand, which is the most versatile part of the body, allows humans (and other primates) to hold and manipulate objects. This ability is primarily due to the fact that the fingers and thumb can move independently and can grip.

STRUCTURE

The hand is made up of the *wrist*, palm, and fingers. Movement of the hand is achieved mainly by *tendons* that attach the muscles of the forearm to the bones of the hand (the carpals, metacarpals, and phalanges). These tendons are surrounded by synovial sheaths containing a lubricating fluid that prevents friction. Other movements are controlled by short muscles in the palm of the hand; some of these muscles make up the prominent areas along the sides of the hand from the bases of the thumb and little fingers to the wrist.

Blood is supplied to the hand by two arteries (the radial on the thumb side of the wrist and the ulnar on the little finger side). Prominent veins on the back of the hand drain blood away. Sensation and movement in the hand are controlled by the radial, ulnar, and median nerves.

DISORDERS

The hands are highly susceptible to injury, including cuts, burns, bites, fractures, and tendon injuries. *Dermatitis* is also common, since the hands are exposed to a considerable variety of irritating substances.

Other hand disorders include *Dupuytren's contracture*, which causes shrinkage of tissues in the palm, and *Volkmann's contracture*, in which damage to muscles in the forearm causes wrist and finger deformities. Degeneration of a tendon sheath on the upper side of the wrist may cause a harmless swelling called a *ganglion*. *Osteoarthritis* commonly affects the joint at the base of the thumb. *Rheumatoid arthritis* may cause deformity of the hands by attacking the joints at the base of the fingers and rupturing tendons.

hand–arm vibration syndrome

Also known as vibration white finger, hand–arm vibration syndrome is *Raynaud's phenomenon* due to prolonged use of vibrating tools. The main symptom is pain and numbness in the hand and arm but there is often also blue or white coloration of the fingers and a tingling sensation in affected areas. In some cases, symptoms may affect both hands even though only one has been exposed to vibration. The syndrome tends to develop slowly over years and is the result of repeated damage to blood vessels and nerves. Exposure to cold tends to aggravate the condition.

There is no specific treatment, but avoiding vibrating tools is essential to prevent the disease progressing. In certain cases, *calcium channel blockers* may help to relieve some symptoms.

handedness

Preference for using the right or left hand. Some 90 per cent of adults use the right hand for writing; about two-thirds prefer the right hand for most activities that require coordination and skill. The remainder are either left-handed or ambidextrous (able to use both hands equally well).

It is uncertain why all humans are not simply ambidextrous. Up to the age of about 12, it is possible to switch handedness if, for example, the dominant hemisphere of a person's brain has been damaged.

Handedness is related to the division of the brain into two hemispheres, each of which controls movement and sensation on the opposite side of the body. In most right-handed people the speech centre is in the left hemisphere of the brain. *Inheritance* is probably the most important factor in determining an individual's handedness.

hand-foot-and-mouth disease

An infectious disease that mainly affects young children and which is caused by *coxsackievirus*. Hand-foot-and-mouth disease may occur in small epidemics, usually in the summer.

The illness is usually mild and lasts for only a few days. Symptoms include blistering of the palms, soles of the feet, and inside of the mouth, and a slight fever. There is no treatment other than mild *analgesic drugs*. This infectious disease is not related to foot-and-mouth disease, which occurs in cattle.

handicap

The extent to which a physical or mental *disability* interferes with a person's normal functioning and causes him or her to be disadvantaged.

Hand–Schuller–Christian disease

A form of *histiocytosis X* that affects children. Problems include patchy bone loss, loose teeth, exophthalmos (protruding eyeballs), and swollen *lymph nodes*. Involvement of the pituitary gland can result in *diabetes insipidus* and *growth hormone* deficiencies.

hangnail

A strip of skin torn away from the side or base of a fingernail, exposing a raw, painful area. Hangnails usually occur when frequent immersion in water has dried the skin on the fingers. Biting the nails is another common cause. Unless it is trimmed away and covered until healed, a hangnail may develop into *paronychia* (infection of the skin fold around the nail).

THE SKELETAL STRUCTURE OF THE **HAND** AND WRIST

Four of the eight wrist bones (carpals) articulate with the radius and ulna. The rest are connected to the five bones of the palm (metacarpals). Each metacarpal, in turn, articulates with a phalanx (a finger bone).

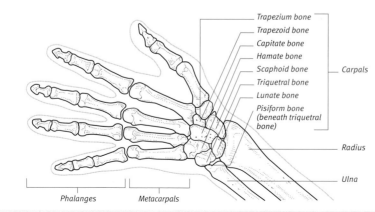

Trapezium bone
Trapezoid bone
Capitate bone
Hamate bone
Scaphoid bone
Triquetral bone
Lunate bone
Pisiform bone (beneath triquetral bone)
Carpals
Radius
Ulna
Phalanges
Metacarpals

hangover

The unpleasant effects that are commonly experienced after overindulgence in *alcohol*, characterized by headache, nausea, *vertigo*, and depression. Alcohol increases production of urine, and some of the symptoms of a hangover are a result of mild dehydration. (See also *alcohol intoxication*.)

Hanhart's syndrome

A *birth defect* in which there are severe physical deformities, including underdevelopment of the lower jaw (see *micrognathia*) and tongue, misshapen and missing teeth, and malformations of the limbs.

Hansen's disease

A chronic bacterial infection, also called leprosy, that damages nerves, mainly in the limbs and facial area, and may also cause skin damage.

CAUSE

The disease is caused by a bacterium, MYCOBACTERIUM LEPRAE, which is spread in droplets of nasal mucus. Hansen's disease is not highly contagious; a person is infectious only in the early stages. Prolonged close contact puts people at risk. The disease is most prevalent in Asia, Central and South America, and Africa.

SYMPTOMS AND SIGNS

Hansen's disease has a long incubation period – about three to five years. There are two main types: the lepromatous type, in which damage is widespread, progressive, and severe; and the tuberculoid type, which is milder. Damage is initially confined to the skin or to peripheral nerves supplying the skin and muscles. Skin areas supplied by affected nerves become lighter or darker and sensation and sweating are reduced. As the disease progresses, the peripheral nerves swell and become tender. Hands, feet, and facial skin eventually become numb and muscles become paralysed, leading to deformity. Other possible features include blindness, destruction of bone, and sterility.

DIAGNOSIS AND TREATMENT

Diagnosis is made from the symptoms and the presence of the causative bacteria in a *skin biopsy* sample. Drug treatment may be with a combination of *dapsone*, *rifampicin*, and clofazimine, which kills most of the bacteria in a few days. Drug treatment stops further progression of the disease but does not reverse any damage that has already occurred. *Plastic surgery* may be needed to correct deformities; and nerve and tendon transplants may improve the function of damaged limbs.

hantavirus

A viral infection that is transmitted to humans through the urine or faeces of infected rodents, such as rats. Symptoms range from a minor flu-like illness with headache and a sore throat to high fever, nausea and vomiting, and abnormal bleeding. Some strains of hantavirus can cause severe infections that may lead to *kidney failure*, serious lung damage, and death.

Harada's syndrome

A combination of certain eye and brain disorders that occurs in the Far East, particularly in Japan. The condition usually affects young adults.

The eye problems, which affect both eyes, include severe inflammation of the *iris*, the *ciliary body*, or the *choroid*; oedema (a buildup of fluid) in the *retina*; and *retinal detachment*. These problems are associated with *meningoencephalitis* (inflammation of the brain tissue and the membranes surrounding it). Other conditions that occur with Harada's syndrome include deafness, alopecia (hair loss), and patchy loss of pigmentation in the skin, eyes, and ends of the hair.

hardening of the arteries

The popular term for *atherosclerosis*.

harelip

A common term for the *birth defect* in which there is a split in the upper lip due to failure of the two sides to fuse during fetal development. A harelip is often associated with a similar failure of the two halves of the palate to join. (See also *cleft lip and palate*.)

Harrison's sulcus

A depression seen at the lower part of the ribcage of a child that is usually caused by exaggerated suction of the *diaphragm muscle* in respiratory conditions such as severe *asthma*. Harrison's sulcus may also be the result of the normal pull of the diaphragm on ribs that have been weakened – for example, in conditions such as *rickets*.

Hartnup disease

A rare disorder, inherited in an autosomal recessive manner (see *genetic disorders*), in which the body does not absorb and process sufficient amounts of certain *amino acids* (chemicals that make up proteins), particularly tryptophan (see *metabolism, inborn errors of*).

A deficiency of tryptophan may result in episodes of various symptoms, in particular *cerebellar ataxia* (a poorly co-ordinated, unsteady gait); symptoms similar to those of *pellagra*: a red, scaly rash on skin exposed to the sun; depression; and thought disorders. There may also be headaches and diarrhoea. Symptoms can be triggered by infections, stress, or exposure to sunlight and last for up to four weeks. Flare-ups are often followed by long periods of remission.

The diagnosis can be confirmed by testing the urine for abnormally high levels of amino acids. Treatment with nicotinic acid and a high-protein diet often offers a good prognosis. The frequency of attacks usually decreases with increasing age.

Hashimoto's thyroiditis

An *autoimmune disorder* in which the body's immune system develops *antibodies* against its own thyroid gland cells. As a result, the thyroid gland cannot produce enough *thyroid hormones*, a condition known as *hypothyroidism*. Hashimoto's thyroiditis is eight times more common in women than men. The principal symptoms of Hashimoto's thyroiditis are tiredness, muscle weakness, and weight gain, and the thyroid gland becomes enlarged (see *goitre*).

A positive diagnosis is confirmed by *blood tests* indicating the presence of antithyroid antibodies and low levels of thyroid hormones. Treatment is by life-long thyroid hormone replacement therapy. In some cases, other autoimmune disorders (such as systemic *lupus erythematosus*) may also develop.

hashish

Sometimes shortened to "hash", this is another name for *marijuana*.

Haverhill fever

A form of rat-bite fever (see *rats, diseases from*) caused by infection with the bacterium STREPTOBACILLUS MONILIFORMIS. Unlike other forms of the disease, Haverhill fever can not only be transmitted through the bite of a rodent but can also be passed on indirectly, in contaminated water or milk products.

Havrix

The brand name for one form of a *vaccine* against *hepatitis A*.

hay fever

The popular name for the seasonal form of allergic rhinitis (see *rhinitis, allergic*) that is often combined with another condition, allergic *conjunctivitis*.

Hb

The abbreviation for *haemoglobin*, an oxygen-carrying component of the red blood cells.

HbA1C test

A test that measures the level of *glycosylated haemoglobin* in the blood. The test is useful for monitoring control of blood glucose levels in *diabetes mellitus* because it reflects blood glucose levels over the preceding three months.

HCG

The abbreviation for the hormone human chorionic gonadotrophin (see *gonadotrophin, human chorionic*).

HDL

The abbreviation for the lipoprotein known as *high-density lipoprotein*.

head

The part of the body that contains the *skull*, the *brain*, and the organs of sight, hearing, smell, and taste. The term head is also used to refer to the uppermost part of any structure and to the rounded portion of a *bone* that slots into an area of another bone to form a *joint*.

headache

One of the most common types of pain. A headache is only rarely a symptom of a serious underlying disorder. The pain arises from tension in the *meninges* (the membranes around the brain), and in the blood vessels and muscles of the scalp.

Headache may be felt all over the head or may occur on only one side, or in the forehead or the back of the neck. Sometimes the pain shifts from one area to another. The pain of headache may be superficial, throbbing, or sharp and may be accompanied by nausea, vomiting, and visual or other sensory disturbances.

TYPES

Many headaches are simply a response to some adverse stimulus, such as hunger. Headaches such as these usually clear up quickly. Tension headaches, due to tightening in the face, neck, and scalp muscles as a result of stress or poor posture, are also common, and may last for days or weeks. *Migraine* can be a severe,

incapacitating headache that is preceded or accompanied by visual and/or stomach disturbances. *Cluster headaches* cause intense pain behind one eye.

CAUSES

Common causes of headache include *hangover* and noisy or stuffy environments. Some headaches are caused by the overuse of painkillers (see *analgesic drugs*). Other possible causes include *sinusitis*, *toothache*, *cervical osteoarthritis*, and *head injury*. *Food additives* may also be a cause. Among the rare causes of headache are a *brain tumour*, *hypertension* (high blood pressure), *temporal arteritis* (inflammation of arteries in the face, neck, and scalp), an *aneurysm* (ballooning of a blood vessel), and increased pressure within the skull.

TREATMENT

Most headaches can be relieved by painkillers and rest. If a neurological cause is suspected, *CT scanning* or *MRI* (magnetic resonance imaging) may be performed.

head-banging

The persistent, rhythmic banging of the head against a wall or hard object. Head-banging is seen in some people with severe *learning difficulties*, particularly those who lack stimulation. It also occurs in some normal toddlers, often when they are frustrated or angry; most children grow out of the behaviour.

head injury

Injury to the head may occur as a result of traffic accidents, sports injuries, falls, assault, accidents at work and at home, or bullet wounds. Most people suffer a minor head injury at least once in their lives, but very few of the injuries are severe enough to require treatment.

A head injury can damage the scalp, skull, or brain. Minor injuries usually cause no damage to the underlying brain. Even when there is a *skull fracture*, or the scalp is split, the brain may not be damaged. However, a blow to the head may severely shake the brain, and this can sometimes cause *brain damage* even when there are no external signs of injury.

A blow often bruises the brain tissue, causing death of some of the brain cells in the injured area. When an object actually penetrates the skull, foreign material and dirt may be implanted in the brain and lead to infection. A blow or a penetrating injury may also tear blood vessels causing *brain haemorrhage* (bleeding in or around the brain). Head injury may cause

swelling of the brain; this is particularly evident after bullet wounds because their high velocity causes extensive damage. If the skull is fractured, bone may be driven into the underlying brain.

SYMPTOMS AND SIGNS

If the head injury is mild, there may be no symptoms other than a slight headache. In some cases there is *concussion*, which may cause confusion, dizziness, and blurred vision (sometimes persisting for several days). More severe head injuries, particularly blows to the head, may result in unconsciousness that lasts longer than a few minutes, or *coma*, which may be fatal.

Post-concussive *amnesia* (loss of memory of events that occurred after an accident) may occur, especially if the skull has been fractured. This amnesia usually lasts more than an hour after consciousness is regained. There may also be pretraumatic amnesia (loss of memory of events that occurred before the accident). The more serious the injury to the brain, the longer unconsciousness and amnesia are likely to last.

After a severe brain injury, a person may suffer some muscular weakness or paralysis and loss of sensation.

Symptoms such as persistent vomiting, pupils of unequal size, double vision, or a deteriorating level of consciousness suggest progressive brain damage.

DIAGNOSIS AND TREATMENT

Investigations may include *skull X-rays* and *MRI* or *CT scanning*. A blood clot inside the skull may be life-threatening and requires surgical removal. Severe skull fractures may also require surgery.

OUTLOOK

Recovery from concussion may take several days. There may be permanent physical or mental disability if the brain has been damaged. Recovery from a major head injury can be very slow and there may be signs of progressive improvement for several years afterwards.

head lag

The backward flopping of the head that occurs when an infant is placed in a sitting position. Head lag is obvious in a newborn because the neck muscles are still weak, but by four months the baby can hold his or her head upright (see *child development*).

head lice

Tiny, wingless insects (*PEDICULUS HUMANUS CAPITIS*) that live on the human scalp and feed by sucking blood. Infestation with

H

head lice is extremely common, especially among young school children, and is not caused by poor hygiene. An affected child may often pass head lice on to other family members.

The insects do not fly or jump but are spread through head-to-head-contact or shared combs, hairbrushes, and hats. Female lice stick their eggs (known as nits) to hair shafts, close to the scalp. The nits may be seen as small, white specks; often, however, the first sign of infestation is intense itching due to an *allergy* to lice bites.

TREATMENT

Infestations of head lice can be treated using medicated lotions containing insecticides, which kill the lice. Because head lice can develop resistance to particular chemicals, a pharmacist should be consulted about local patterns of resistance. For children under two years of age, or those with eczema or asthma, treatment should be discussed with a doctor or pharmacist. To avoid the risk of reinfestation, it is important to treat all family members at the same time.

Some people are reluctant to use insecticides repeatedly. An alternative method of ridding the scalp of head lice is to apply liberal amounts of hair conditioner and comb through the hair carefully with a special fine-tooth comb to remove the insects and nits. This procedure (known as the wet combing method) needs to be repeated every few days in order to be effective and to prevent recurrences. Whichever method is used, frequent inspection of a child's head is the key to controlling head lice.

healing

The process by which the body repairs bone, tissue, or organ damage caused by injury, infection, or disease.

The initial stages of healing are the same in all parts of the body. After injury, *blood clots* form in damaged tissues. White *blood cells*, *enzymes*, *histamine*, other chemicals, and *proteins* from which new cells can be made accumulate at the site of damage. Fibrous tissue is laid down in the blood clot to form a supportive structure, and any dead cells are broken down and absorbed by the white blood cells. Some tissues, such as bone and skin, can then regenerate by the proliferation of new cells around the damaged area. In skin injuries, the fibrous tissue shrinks as new skin forms underneath. The tissue hardens to form a scab, which falls off when new skin

growth is complete. A scar may remain. An inadequate blood supply or persistent infection prevents regeneration, and some tissues, such as nerve tissue, may be unable to regenerate. In these cases, the fibrous tissue may develop into scar tissue, which keeps the tissue structure intact but may impair its function.

health

At its simplest, a term that is used to describe the absence of physical and mental disease. A wider concept promoted by the World Health Organization is that all people should have the opportunity to fulfil their genetic potential. This includes their ability to develop without the impediments of poor nutrition, environmental contamination, or infectious diseases. (See *diet and disease*; *health hazards*.)

health centre

Premises in which healthcare professionals, such as health visitors, district nurses, and general practitioners, work together.

health food

A term applied to any food products thought to promote health.

health hazards

Environmental factors that are known to cause, or are suspected of causing, disease. The major types of health hazard are the numerous infectious diseases that are transmitted by contact or by insects or other animals (see *bacteria*; *fungal infections*; *insects and disease*; *viruses*; *zoonosis*); an insufficient supply, or the contamination, of food and water (see *food additives*; *food-borne infection*; *food poisoning*); work-related hazards (see *occupational disease and injury*); hazards associated with domestic and social life, including driving; *smoking* and *alcohol* consumption; and global environmental hazards (see *radiation hazards*; *sunlight, adverse effects of*).

health promotion

The work of healthcare professionals in encouraging people to adopt a healthier lifestyle and so reduce their risk of developing various diseases. The print and broadcast media, internet-based resources, and patient self-help or campaigning groups also have a role to play in health promotion.

Health promotion involves the recommendation of specific tests as appropriate. Examples include encouraging women

to undergo regular *cervical smear tests* and mammograms (see *mammography*) to detect early signs of cervical or breast cancer, and advising people at increased risk of coronary heart disease to have their blood *cholesterol* levels checked.

Health promotion may also involve a formal individual consultation to review a person's health and make appropriate recommendations for him or her, for example, regarding diet and exercise.

hearing

The sense that enables sound to be perceived. The *ear* transforms the sound waves it receives into nerve impulses that pass to the *brain*.

Each ear has three distinct regions: the outer, middle, and inner ear. Sound waves are channelled through the ear canal to the middle ear, from where a complex system of membranes and tiny bones conveys the vibrations to the inner ear. The vibrations are converted into nerve impulses in the *cochlea*. These impulses travel along the auditory nerve to the medulla of the brain. From there, they pass via the *thalamus* to the superior temporal gyrus, part of the cerebral cortex involved in perceiving sound. For further details, see *Hearing* box, overleaf. (See also *deafness*.)

hearing aids

Electronic devices that improve hearing in people with certain types of *deafness*. A hearing aid consists of a tiny microphone (to pick up sounds), an amplifier (to increase their volume), and a speaker (to transmit sounds). Newer devices are small enough to be hidden in the ear canal. The particular device required depends on the type and cause of the hearing loss. (See also *cochlear implant*.)

hearing loss

A deterioration in the ability to perceive sound. (See also *deafness*.)

hearing tests

Tests carried out to assess *hearing*. All newborn babies are given a hearing screening test using *otoacoustic emission* to check for a normal response of the inner ear to sound. Hearing tests are also performed as part of a routine assessment of *child development* and whenever hearing impairment is suspected. They are sometimes included in a general medical examination. Hearing tests may also be used in the investigation of *tinnitus* or dizziness.

H

HEARING

The ears are the organs of hearing. Each ear has three regions: the outer ear, middle ear, and inner ear. The outer ear channels sound vibrations through the eardrum to the middle ear. The eardrum has to have equal air pressure on each side so that it can vibrate freely; the pressure is equalized via the eustachian tube, which runs from the back of the throat to the middle ear. Inside the middle ear, a complex system of membranes and tiny bones conveys the vibrations to the inner ear via a membrane called the oval window. In the inner ear, the vibrations are converted to nerve impulses and sent to the brain via the vestibulocochlear nerve.

Structure and function of cochlea

Running the length of the cochlea is a fluid-filled tube called the cochlear duct. It contains several membranes and a structure called the organ of Corti. Tiny hairs on the organ of Corti brush against a membrane called the tectorial membrane, producing electrical signals. These signals are detected by nerve fibres.

ROUTE TO THE BRAIN

Electrical signals are picked up by nerve fibres in the cochlea and pass along the vestibulocochlear nerve to the medulla. From there, they pass via the thalamus to the superior temporal gyrus – the part of the cerebral cortex (see *brain*) involved in receiving and perceiving sound.

Malleus (hammer) and incus (anvil)
The malleus, attached to the eardrum, transmits vibration to the incus.

Stapes (stirrup) and oval window
The stapes transmits vibrations from the incus to the oval window, the membrane between the middle and inner ear.

Vestibulocochlear nerve
Tiny nerve fibres from the cochlea join up to form the vestibulocochlear nerve, which carries impulses from the cochlea to the brain.

Outer ear
The pinna (the visible part of the ear) channels sound waves into the ear canal towards the eardrum.

Eardrum
The eardrum separates the outer and middle ear. Sound waves of different frequencies cause the eardrum to vibrate at different speeds.

Cochlea
The cochlea consists of a hollow spiral passage. It picks up sound vibrations transmitted through the oval window and converts them into nerve impulses.

Eustachian tube
This tube allows air to pass into and out of the middle ear.

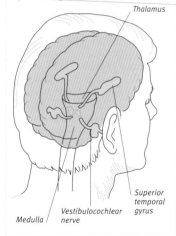

Thalamus

Medulla

Vestibulocochlear nerve

Superior temporal gyrus

Oval window

Normal coiled shape of cochlea

Cochlear duct

Nerve fibres

Cochlea
(shown uncoiled)

COMPARISON OF FREQUENCY RANGES

The frequency of a sound (how high or low it is) is measured in Hertz (Hz). Different animals can hear different ranges of sound frequencies. The diagram shows the normal ranges that can be heard by a human, a bat, a dolphin, and a dog. Humans can hear a range between about 20 and 20,000 Hz.

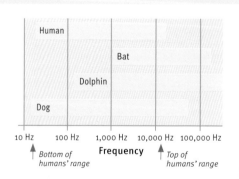

Human

Bat

Dolphin

Dog

| 10 Hz | 100 Hz | 1,000 Hz | 10,000 Hz | 100,000 Hz |

↑ *Bottom of humans' range*

Frequency

↑ *Top of humans' range*

Electron micrograph of inner ear
This image shows four rows of hair cells (centre) in the organ of Corti. On their surfaces are sensory hairs (top right), which convert sound waves into electrical impulses; these are picked up by the vestibulocochlear nerve (bottom right).

In the otoacoustic emission test, a probe is inserted into the ear canal. The probe produces soft clicks and also detects any sounds emitted by the ear in response to the clicks. If the ear does not emit any sounds, this indicates hearing impairment. An audiometer (an electrical instrument) is used to test the ability of an individual to hear sounds at different frequencies and volumes. The lowest level at which a person can hear and repeat words (the speech reception threshold) is tested in each ear, as is the ability to hear words clearly (speech discrimination). Tuning fork tests (see *Rinne's test*) can be used to determine whether hearing loss is conductive or sensorineural (see *deafness*).

heart

The muscular pump in the centre of the chest that beats continuously and rhythmically to send *blood* to the lungs and the rest of the body. During an average lifetime, the heart contracts more than 2,500 million times.

STRUCTURE

Much of the heart consists of myocardium, a type of muscle, which, when given oxygen and nutrients, contracts rhythmically and automatically without any other stimulus. The internal surface of the heart is lined with a smooth membrane called endocardium, and the entire heart is enclosed in a tough, membranous bag, the *pericardium*.

Inside the heart there are four chambers. A thick central muscular wall, the septum, divides the heart cavity into right and left halves. Each half consists of an upper chamber, called an *atrium* (plural: atria), and a larger lower chamber, called a *ventricle*. (See *Structure of the heart* box, overleaf.)

The body's principal blood vessels emerge from the top and sides of the heart. The superior and inferior venae cavae (see *vena cava*), the largest veins, deliver deoxygenated blood from the body to the heart. The *aorta*, which is the main artery, carries oxygen-rich blood to be circulated around the body. The pulmonary vessels carry blood to and from the lungs, where the blood absorbs oxygen and releases the waste product carbon dioxide.

FUNCTION

The two sides of the heart have distinct, though interdependent, functions. The right atrium receives deoxygenated blood from the entire body via the two venae cavae. This blood is transferred to

SELECTED **HEARING TESTS**

Tests	Function	
Tuning fork tests	These basic tests are used to determine whether hearing loss is conductive or sensorineural. In Rinne's test, the patient is asked whether the sound is louder with the vibrating tines held near the opening of the ear canal (air conduction) or with the base of the fork held against the mastoid bone (bone conduction). In a normal ear or one with sensorineural loss, air	conduction is greater than bone conduction. In conductive hearing loss, bone conduction is greater than or equal to air conduction. Weber's test, in which the base of the fork is placed on the forehead, is useful for diagnosing unilateral hearing loss. If the hearing loss is conductive, the patient hears the tuning fork better in the ear with the poorer hearing.
Pure-tone audiometry	This is a test in which an audiometer is used to generate sounds of different frequencies and intensities and a person's ability to hear these sounds is measured. Hearing is first assessed by transmitting the sounds through one earphone while the other ear is prevented from hearing them. The sound frequencies range from 250 to 8,000 Hertz; for each	frequency, the sound is increased in intensity until it can be heard. The patient gives a signal at the moment when he or she detects each sound and the results are recorded on a graph called an audiogram. Bone conduction is then assessed in the same way but the signal is transmitted through a rubber pad held against the bone behind the ear.
Auditory brainstem response (ABR)	This test may be used to evaluate the presence of hearing in someone who cannot cooperate with other tests (such as a very young baby). The brain's response to sound stimulation produced by an audiometer is	analysed by means of electrodes placed on the scalp. Auditory brainstem response can also help to rule out acoustic neuroma (a benign tumour affecting the auditory nerve, part of the vestibulocochlear nerve).
Impedance audiometry	Also known as tympanometry, this test is used to assess middle-ear damage occurring in cases of conductive deafness or to detect the effects of fluid within the middle ear. A probe is fitted tightly into the entrance of the ear canal, thereby sealing off the outside air pressure and sound. The probe emits a continuous sound. Air is pumped	through the probe at varying pressures and, at the same time, a microphone in the probe registers the differing reflections of sounds from the eardrum as pressure changes in the ear canal. The reflections are recorded on a graph known as a tympanogram. The pattern of differing reflections relates to the type of disease that is causing the deafness.

the right ventricle, then pumped to the lungs via the pulmonary artery to be oxygenated and lose carbon dioxide. The left atrium of the heart receives oxygenated blood from the lungs (via the pulmonary veins); this oxygenated blood is transferred to the left ventricle, which pumps it through the aorta to all body tissues. One-way valves at the chamber exits ensure that blood flows in one direction (see *heart valves*).

THE CARDIAC CYCLE

The pumping action of the heart consists of three phases, which together make up a cycle corresponding to one heartbeat (see *Heart cycle* box, p.367). These phases are called diastole, atrial systole, and ventricular systole. In diastole, the heart muscle relaxes and the heart fills with blood. In atrial systole, the two atria contract, sending blood

into the ventricles. In ventricular systole, the two ventricles contract, pumping blood into the blood vessels.

For the heart to function efficiently, the muscular contractions must occur in a precise sequence. This sequence is regulated by electrical impulses that emanate from the *sinoatrial node* (an area of specialized muscle at the top of the right atrium), which is the heart's natural pacemaker. The electrical impulses are carried to the atria and ventricles partly by the heart muscle itself and partly by nerve fibres.

In order to prevent bottlenecks from developing in the blood circulation, the volume that is pumped at each beat by the two sides of the heart must be balanced exactly. Resistance to blood flow through the general circulation is much greater than resistance through the

STRUCTURE OF THE **HEART**

The heart is positioned centrally in the chest, with its right margin directly underneath the right side of the sternum (breastbone). The rest of the heart points to the left, with its lowest point (the apex) located underneath the left nipple.

The heart acts as a dual pump. Deoxygenated blood from the body arrives, via the two venae cavae, in the right atrium (upper heart chamber), is transferred to the right ventricle (lower chamber), and is then pumped via the pulmonary artery to the lungs. There it is reoxygenated and returns, via the pulmonary veins, to the left side of the heart. It enters the left atrium, is transferred to the left ventricle, and is then pumped, via a large vessel (the aorta), to all parts of the body.

Trachea
Superior vena cava
Pulmonary artery
Right bronchus
Right atrium
Tricuspid valve
Right ventricle
Inferior vena cava

Aorta
Left atrium
Aortic valve
Pulmonary valve
Mitral valve
Left ventricle
Septum
Aorta

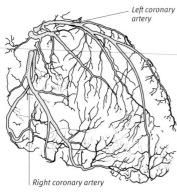

Left coronary artery

Right coronary artery

Blood supply
Although the heart muscle is continually pumping blood, it cannot obtain much oxygen from this flow, so it needs its own blood supply. This is provided by the two coronary arteries, which arise from the aorta. These arteries, with their branches, supply the entire heart muscle. A network of veins, called coronary veins (not shown), drains blood back into the right atrium.

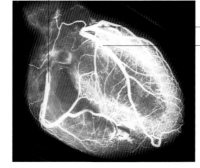

Right coronary artery

Circumflex artery
Left anterior descending artery

Angiogram of coronary arteries
This image (left) gives a view of the heart from the rear and clearly shows the coronary arteries. The image was achieved by angiography: an X-ray of the heart was taken after the coronary arteries had been injected with a contrast medium (a fluid that shows up on X-rays).

lungs. Therefore, the left side of the heart must contract more forcibly than the right; for this reason, the left side has greater muscular bulk.

heart, artificial

An implantable mechanical device that takes over the action of the *heart* or assists the heart in maintaining the blood circulation. Problems that may occur with artifical hearts include the formation of blood clots in the mechanical device and infection. Artificial hearts are therefore used only as a temporary measure until a *heart transplant* can be performed.

heart attack

See *myocardial infarction*.

heartbeat

A contraction of the *heart* that pumps blood to the lungs and the rest of the body. The different parts of the heart contract in a precise sequence that is regulated by electrical impulses from the *sinoatrial node*, at the top of the right *atrium*. Each heartbeat consists of three phases, which occur in a cycle: diastole (resting phase), atrial systole (contraction of the heart's upper chambers), and ventricular systole (contraction of the lower chambers). The rate at which con-

tractions occur is called the *heart rate*. The term *pulse* refers to the character and rate of the heartbeat when felt at a point on the body, such as the wrist.

heart block

A disorder of the *heartbeat* caused by an interruption to the passage of electrical impulses through the heart's conducting system. Heart block may be congenital or may be due to heart disease, such as *coronary artery disease*, disorders of the heart valves, or heart muscle disease. Other causes include overdose of a *digitalis drug* (used in the treatment of heart disease) and *rheumatic fever*.

TYPES

There are two main types of heart block: *atrioventricular block*, a blockage in the heart's conducting system between an *atrium* (upper chamber of the heart) and a *ventricle* (lower chamber of the heart); and *bundle branch block*, in which the block is confined to conduction within the ventricles.

Atrioventricular block There are three degrees of atrioventricular heart block. In first degree block, there is an increased delay between contraction of the atria and that of the ventricles. In second degree block, some atrial beats fail to reach the ventricles. In complete heart block, there is a total blockage in the heart's conducting system that prevents atrial beats from being conducted to the ventricles. The two chambers therefore beat at their own intrinsic rate, with the ventricles beating very slowly and independently of the atria.

Bundle branch block Each ventricle has its own conduction system, known as the right and left bundle branches. These work together. Blockage in one or other of the bundle branches (or, less commonly, both) leads to an abnormal pattern of conduction through the ventricles.

Right bundle branch block can sometimes be seen in a healthy heart. It may also be due to certain conditions, such as congenital heart disease (see *heart disease, congenital*). Left bundle branch block is more serious and is always a sign of an underlying cardiac disorder. It is usually caused by *coronary artery disease* but may also occur as a result of *hypertension* (high blood pressure) or *aortic stenosis*.

SYMPTOMS

First degree heart block and left or right bundle branch block alone usually cause no symptoms. However, in more severe atrioventricular heart block, the rate of ventricular contraction does not increase in response to exercise. This may cause breathlessness as a result of *heart failure* (reduced pumping efficiency) or chest pains due to *angina pectoris* (caused by reduced blood supply to the heart muscle). If the ventricular beat becomes very slow, or if it stops altogether for a few seconds, episodes of loss of consciousness may occur.

DIAGNOSIS AND TREATMENT

Both types are usually diagnosed by *ECG* (electrocardiography), which may be performed at rest and while exercising on a treadmill (see *exercise ECG*); 24-hour ECG heart monitoring may also be done (see *Holter monitor*). *Echocardiography*

HEART CYCLE

There are three main phases in each heartbeat. The beat is generated by electrical waves that emanate from the heart's own pacemaker, the sinoatrial node. The images in this box show blood flow, an electrocardiogram tracing, and the direction of electrical impulses at each stage of the cycle.

Diastole
In this resting phase, the heart fills with blood. Deoxygenated blood flows into the right side of the heart; at the same time, oxygenated blood flows into the left side.

Atrial systole
In this second phase, the two atria (upper chambers of the heart) contract, squeezing more blood into the ventricles (lower chambers) and filling them completely.

Ventricular systole
The two ventricles contract to pump deoxygenated blood into the pulmonary artery and oxygenated blood into the aorta. Once the heart is empty, diastole begins again.

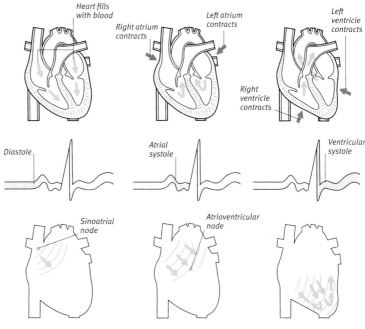

In diastole, the heart muscle is at rest. Towards the end of this phase, the sinoatrial node emits an electrical impulse, which starts to spread through the heart muscle.

As the electrical impulse spreads through the two atria, it causes them to contract. By the end of atrial systole, the impulse reaches another node, the atrioventricular node.

After a momentary pause, waves of electrical activity from the atrioventricular node pass along special fibres to all parts of the ventricles, producing ventricular systole.

(ultrasound scanning of the heart) may be carried out to investigate the condition of the heart muscle and valves.

Heart block with no symptoms may not require any treatment. Heart block causing symptoms is usually treated by fitting a permanent artificial *pacemaker*. Drugs to increase the heart rate and the strength of the heart's contractions may be given temporarily. Any underlying heart disease is treated as necessary.

heartburn

A burning pain in the centre of the chest, which may travel from the tip of the breastbone up to the throat.

Heartburn is often brought on by lying down or bending forwards. It may be caused by overeating, eating rich or spicy food, or by drinking alcohol. Recurrent heartburn is a symptom of *oesophagitis* (inflammation of the oesophagus), which is usually caused by *gastro-oesophageal reflux disease*.

heart disease, congenital

A term used to describe any *heart* abnormality that is present from birth. Congenital defects (see *Types of congenital heart disease* box, p.369) may affect different parts of the heart, including the chambers, *valves*, or main blood vessels.

H

Developmental errors leading to defects arise early in the life of the *embryo*. *Rubella* (German measles) in the mother is the most common known cause, but in most cases the reasons for the defects are not known.

Hereditary factors do not seem to be significant. If a couple have an affected child, there is little increased risk of a second child being affected. People born with heart defects have little increased risk of having an affected child.

SYMPTOMS AND COMPLICATIONS

Symptoms of congenital heart disease arise from either insufficient or excessive circulation of blood to the lungs or the body. Defects in heart anatomy can also cause some deoxygenated blood to be pumped to the body instead of the lungs or some oxygenated blood to the lungs instead of the body. Some heart anomalies cause *cyanosis* (blueness of the skin) and breathlessness, but others may go undetected.

Possible complications resulting from an untreated heart defect include underdevelopment of the limbs and muscles, and *pneumonia* after even mild respiratory infections. With prolonged cyanosis, *clubbing* (thickening and broadening) of the ends of fingers and toes may develop. If there is insufficient capacity in the heart to increase blood flow on effort, the child may rapidly tire during physical exercise. In some untreated cases, a serious complication called *Eisenmenger complex* (increased resistance of the lungs to blood flow) develops.

DIAGNOSIS AND TREATMENT

Antenatal diagnosis, using specialized *ultrasound scanning*, is possible for most defects. After birth, any suspected defect is investigated using *chest X-rays*, *ECG*, or *echocardiography*.

Oxygen and various drug treatments may improve the symptoms. Some conditions, such as small septal defects or patent ductus arteriosus, may become smaller or may disappear of their own accord. Other defects will require surgical correction. Narrowed heart valves can often be treated by balloon *valvuloplasty*. In other cases, *open heart surgery* or a *heart transplant* may be required.

OUTLOOK

Following successful surgery, the child's health often improves dramatically, with resumed growth, increased activity, and a near-normal life expectancy.

Children and adults with heart defects (corrected or uncorrected) are at an increased risk of bacterial *endocarditis*, a potentially dangerous infection of the heart lining and heart valves. To prevent this, they are given *antibiotic drugs* before all surgical procedures, including dental treatments.

heart disease, ischaemic

The most common form of heart disease. In ischaemic heart disease, there is narrowing or obstruction of the coro-

DISORDERS OF THE HEART

Heart disorders are by far the most common cause of death in developed countries. They also affect the quality of life of millions of people. A wide range of conditions can affect the heart's structure and/or disrupt its action.

Congenital defects

Structural abnormalities in the heart are among the most common birth defects. They result from errors of development in the fetus and include *septal defects* ("holes in the heart") and some types of *heart valve* abnormalities (see *heart disease, congenital*).

Genetic disorders

Genetic factors do not usually play a large part in directly causing heart disorders. They do, however, contribute to *hyperlipidaemias*, which predispose affected people to *atherosclerosis* and *coronary artery disease*.

Infection

Infection of the lining of the heart and of the heart valves (see *endocarditis*) can result in malfunction of the heart valves. Viral infections can lead to some types of *cardiomyopathy* (malfunctioning of the heart muscle) or *myocarditis* (inflammation of the heart muscle).

Tumours

Tumours arising in the heart tissues are rare. The main types are noncancerous *myxomas*, which develop inside the heart chambers, and cancerous *sarcomas*. Secondary tumours, spreading from elsewhere in the body, are more common than primary tumours.

Arterial disorders

The coronary arteries (supplying blood to the heart) may become narrowed due to atherosclerosis. Areas of heart muscle may be starved of oxygen, and *angina pectoris* or, eventually, *myocardial infarction* may result.

Nutritional disorders

Obesity is an important factor in heart disease, probably through its effect on other risk factors, such as *hypertension*, *diabetes mellitus*, and *cholesterol*. Malnutrition may cause the heart muscle to become thin and flabby from lack of protein and calories. *Thiamine* (vitamin B_1) deficiency, common in alcoholics, causes *beriberi* with congestive *heart failure*.

Poisoning

The most common toxin affecting the heart is alcohol. Excessive drinking over many years may cause a type of cardiomyopathy. Another common source of toxins is smoking; nicotine and carbon monoxide in tobacco smoke are thought to encourage the development of atherosclerosis, which can lead to coronary artery disease.

Drugs

Certain medications, such as the anticancer drug *doxorubicin*, *tricyclic antidepressants*, and even drugs used to treat heart disease, may disturb the heartbeat or damage the heart muscle.

Other heart disorders

Many disorders may be complications of an underlying condition, such as cardiomyopathy or a congenital defect. they include cardiac *arrhythmia*; some cases of *heart block*; heart failure; and *cor pulmonale*, which is a failure of the right side of the heart due to lung disease.

INVESTIGATION

Investigative techniques include auscultation (listening to the heart); *ECG* (electrocardiography); imaging techniques such as *chest X-ray*, *echocardiography*, coronary *angiography*, *CT scanning*, and *MRI*; cardiac catheterization (see *catheterization, cardiac*); *blood tests*; and, rarely, *biopsy* of the heart muscle.

TYPES OF **CONGENITAL HEART DISEASE**

The major malformations are atrial and ventricular *septal defects*; *coarctation of the aorta*; *transposition of the great vessels*; *patent ductus arteriosus*; *tetralogy of Fallot*; *hypoplastic left heart syndrome*; *pulmonary stenosis*; and *aortic stenosis* (not shown). Affected areas are shown in bold colour.

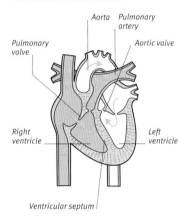

Aorta *Pulmonary artery*

Pulmonary valve *Aortic valve*

Right ventricle *Left ventricle*

Ventricular septum

How blood circulates
Deoxygenated blood (grey) is pumped from the right ventricle through the pulmonary arteries into the lungs, where it exchanges carbon dioxide for oxygen. Oxygenated blood (blue) enters the left side of the heart; it is pumped from the left ventricle through the aorta to the body tissues.

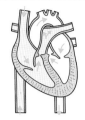

5%

Pulmonary stenosis
This is a narrowing of the pulmonary valve, or (rarely) of the upper right ventricle, and reduces the blood flow to the lungs.

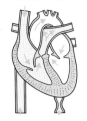

10%

Coarctation of the aorta
In this disorder, localized narrowing of the aorta reduces the supply of blood to the lower part of the body.

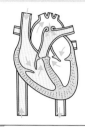

8%

Patent ductus arteriosus
The ductus arteriosus fails to close after birth and blood from the aorta continues to flow through it into the pulmonary artery.

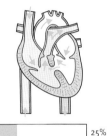

25%

Ventricular septal defect
This is a hole in the wall (septum) between the ventricles, causing blood to flow from the left ventricle to the right and into the lungs.

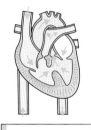

7%

Tetralogy of Fallot
This defect includes a hole in the ventricular septum, pulmonary stenosis, a displaced aorta, and a thickened right ventricle.

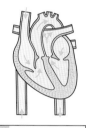

14%

Transposition of the great vessels
Oxygenated blood passes back to the lungs, instead of through the aorta to the body tissues.

H

nary arteries, usually due to *atherosclerosis*, that results in a reduced blood supply to the heart (see *coronary artery disease*).

heart failure

Inability of the *heart* to cope with its workload of pumping blood to the lungs and to the rest of the body. Heart failure can primarily affect either the right or the left side of the heart; however, it most commonly affects both sides. Heart failure can be acute or chronic (congestive).

TYPES AND CAUSES

Left-sided heart failure This may be due to *hypertension* (high blood pressure), *anaemia*, *hyperthyroidism* (overactivity of the thyroid), a *heart valve* defect (such as *aortic stenosis*, *aortic incompetence*, or *mitral incompetence*), or a congenital heart defect (see *heart disease, congenital*). In all of these conditions, the left side of the heart must work harder than normal to pump the same amount of blood. Sometimes, the heart can compensate for the extra workload by an increase in the size of the left side and in the thickness of its muscular walls, or by an increase in the *heart rate*. This compensation is only temporary, however, and heart failure eventually follows.

Other causes of left-sided heart failure include *coronary artery disease*, *myocardial infarction* (heart attack), *cardiac arrhythmias* (irregularities of heart rhythm), and *cardiomyopathy* (disease of the heart muscle). In cardiomyopathy, the pumping power of the heart is reduced to a point where it can no longer deal with its normal workload.

Whatever the underlying cause, in left-sided heart failure the left side of the heart fails to empty completely with each contraction, or has difficulty in accepting blood that has been returned from the lungs. The retained blood creates a back pressure that causes the lungs to become congested with blood. This condition leads to *pulmonary oedema* (excess fluid in the lungs), of which the main symptom is shortness of breath, eventually even when at rest. The patient may awaken at night with attacks of breathlessness, wheezing, and sweating.

Right-sided heart failure This is most often caused by *pulmonary hypertension* (raised blood pressure in the arteries supplying the lungs). This is itself caused by left-sided heart failure, or a lung disease such as chronic obstructive pulmonary disease (see *pulmonary disease, chronic obstructive*). Right-sided failure can also be due to a heart valve defect, such as *tricuspid incompetence*, or to a congenital heart defect.

In all types of right-sided heart failure, there is back pressure in the circulation from the heart into the venous system, causing swollen neck veins, enlargement of the liver, and *oedema* (excess fluid in body tissues), especially swelling of the legs and ankles. In addition, the intestines may become congested, causing discomfort and indigestion.

INVESTIGATION AND TREATMENT

Investigation of suspected heart failure may involve a physical examination, *X-ray*, *ECG*, and *echocardiography*.

H

Attacks of acute heart failure may subside of their own accord or may require urgent, life-saving treatment. Immediate treatment of heart failure consists of bed rest, with the patient sitting up. *Diuretic drugs* are given to increase the output of urine from the kidneys, thereby ridding the body of excess fluid and reducing blood volume. *Morphine* and *oxygen* may be given as emergency treatment in acute left-sided heart failure. Long-term drug treatment usually involves the use of *ACE inhibitor drugs* and diuretics. *Angiotensin-II ant-agonists*, other *vaso-dilator drugs*, and *beta-blocker drugs* may also be required. If heart failure is associated with *atrial fibrillation*, *digoxin* will most likely be prescribed to control the heart rate.

Other possible treatments of heart failure include fitting a *pacemaker*, *coronary artery bypass*, and *heart transplant*.

heart imaging

Any technique that provides images of heart structure. Imaging is used to detect disease or abnormalities.

TYPES

A *chest X-ray*, the simplest and most widely used method of heart imaging, shows heart size and shape, and the presence of abnormal *calcification*. *Pulmonary oedema* (excess fluid in the lungs) and engorgement of the vessels connecting the heart and lungs are also usually detectable with X-rays.

Echocardiography is useful for investigating congenital heart defects and abnormalities of the valves or heart wall. An ultrasound technique that uses the *Doppler effect*, known as Doppler echocardiography, allows measurement of blood flow through valves. *Angiography* may be used to assess the condition of the coronary arteries and valves.

Radionuclide scanning can be used to detect *myocardial infarction* (heart attack), to measure heart muscle function and its blood supply, or to determine the viability of the heart muscle following disruption to the blood supply. The information obtained from the scan depends on the radioisotope used; for example, thallium-201 may be used to investigate if heart muscle is still viable. Radionuclide scans can also be used to produce images of ventricular function. For example, a *MUGA scan* is used to determine how much blood the heart can pump with each heartbeat and whether different parts of the heart wall are contracting properly.

CT scanning and *MRI* (magnetic resonance imaging) can be used to produce detailed cross-sectional or three-dimensional images of heart structure.

heart–lung machine

A machine that temporarily takes over the function of the *heart* and *lungs* in order to facilitate operations such as *open heart surgery*, *heart transplant*, and *heart–lung transplant*.

A heart–lung machine consists of a pump (to replace the heart's function) and an oxygenator (to replace the lungs' function). It bypasses the heart and lungs. Once the machine is in operation, the patient's heart can be stopped while surgery is carried out.

The use of a heart–lung machine tends to damage red blood cells and to cause blood clotting. These problems can be minimized by the administration of *heparin*, which is an anticoagulant drug.

heart–lung transplant

A procedure in which the *heart* and *lungs* of a patient are removed and replaced by donor organs. This surgery is used to treat diseases in which lung damage has affected the heart, or vice versa. Such diseases include *cystic fibrosis*, *fibrosing alveolitis*, and some severe congenital heart defects (see *heart disease, congenital*). A *heart–lung machine* takes over the function of the patient's heart and lungs during the operation. A heart–lung transplant is no more dangerous than a *heart transplant* and is technically more straightforward because blood vessels to the lungs need not be disturbed.

heart rate

The rate at which the *heart* contracts to pump blood around the body. In most people, heart rate is between 60 and 100 beats per minute at rest. It tends to be faster in childhood and to slow slightly with age. Very fit people may have a rate below 60 beats per minute.

CHANGES IN HEART RATE AND OUTPUT

The rate at which the heart beats, and the amount of blood pumped out with each contraction, can vary considerably according to the body's demands for oxygenated blood. At rest, the heart contracts at 60 to 80 beats per minute and each ventricle puts out about 80 ml of blood at each beat (about six litres per minute). During vigorous exercise, the heart rate may increase to 200 contractions per minute; the output may increase to almost 250 ml per beat, producing a total output of 50 litres per minute. Such changes in heart rate and output are brought about by the action of heart muscle and by the involvement of the *autonomic nervous system* (the part of the nervous system concerned with automatic control of body functions).

First, the heart muscle responds automatically to any increase in activity by increasing its output. This increase occurs because active muscles squeeze the veins that pass through them, pushing the blood back towards the heart. The more the ventricles are filled with blood during diastole (the filling phase of the heart's cycle), the more forcibly they contract during ventricular systole to expel the blood.

Second, the heart rate is under the control of the autonomic nervous system. The parts of the system concerned with heart action are a nucleus of nerve cells called the cardiac centre, in the *brainstem*, and two sets of nerves called parasympathetic and sympathetic nerves, whose activities, controlled by the cardiac centre, exert opposing effects on the heart.

When a person is at rest, the parasympathetic nerves (particularly the *vagus nerve*) are active. Signals carried along the vagus nerve act on the sino-atrial node to slow the heart rate from its inherent rate of about 140 impulses per minute to around 70 impulses per minute (a process called vagal inhibition). During or in anticipation of muscular activity, vagal inhibition lessens and the heart rate speeds up. The speed may increase even more when the sympathetic nerves come into action. These nerves release the hormone *noradrenaline* (norepinephrine) which increases heart rate and the force of contractions. The release of *adrenaline* (epinephrine) and noradrenaline by the adrenal glands also acts to increase the heart rate.

The switch from parasympathetic to sympathetic activity is triggered by any influence on the cardiac centre that signals a need for increased blood output from the heart. Such influences may include fear or anger, low *blood pressure*, or a reduction of oxygen in the blood.

MEASURING HEART RATE

Doctors can measure the rate and rhythm of the heart by feeling the *pulse* or by listening to the heart with a *stethoscope*. A more accurate record can be obtained by *ECG* (a test in which the electrical activity of the heart is measured). A resting heart rate that is above 100 beats per minute is termed a

HEART–LUNG TRANSPLANT

In this procedure, both the heart and the lungs of a patient have to be removed and are replaced with organs taken from a brain-dead donor. The donor organs are then inserted into the patient. The removed heart can sometimes be given to another patient. A heart–lung transplant is more straightforward than a *heart transplant* because blood vessels to the lungs need not be disturbed.

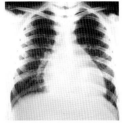

Chest X-ray

1 The donor heart and lungs must be healthy. The lungs must also match the size of the patient's chest, as measured by means of chest X-rays.

2 In both donor and patient, the heart and lungs are reached via an incision in the sternum (breastbone), and the chest is opened up.

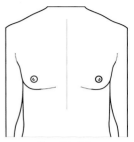

Site of incision

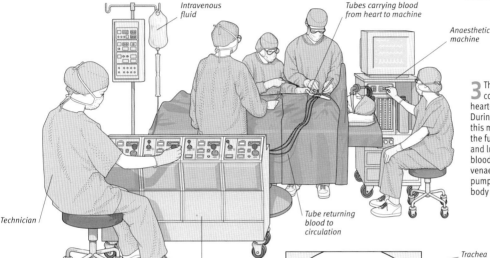

Intravenous fluid

Tubes carrying blood from heart to machine

Anaesthetic machine

Technician

Tube returning blood to circulation

Heart–lung machine

3 The patient is connected to a heart–lung machine. During the operation, this machine takes over the function of heart and lungs, oxygenating blood taken from the venae cavae and pumping it back to the body via the aorta.

WHY IT IS DONE

Subject to the availability of a donor, a heart–lung transplant can offer hope to someone who is dying of a terminally chronic lung disease, whether or not he or she is also suffering from heart disease. The range of diseases that can be treated with this operation include *emphysema*, *cystic fibrosis*, *sarcoidosis*, and *interstitial pulmonary fibrosis*. The record of success for the heart–lung transplant operation is better than that for lung transplant alone.

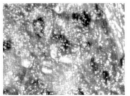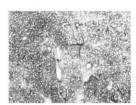

Healthy and diseased lung
These images are of a healthy lung (left) and a lung damaged by emphysema (right), in which the alveoli (tiny air sacs) have become greatly enlarged and the walls surrounding them are damaged.

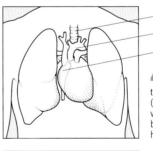

Trachea

Aorta

Right atrium/vena cava

4 In both patient and donor, the heart and lungs are removed through cuts in the aorta, trachea (windpipe), and the area where the venae cavae join the heart. The blood vessels linking the donor heart and lungs are left intact.

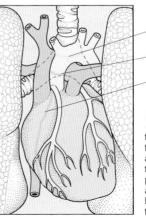

Tracheal reconnection

Aortic reconnection

Right atrium/vena cava reconnection

5 The donor heart and lungs are inserted into the patient. The trachea and aorta are joined to those of the patient, and the right atrium of the donor heart is joined to the patient's venae cavae. (This procedure is simpler than attaching a donor heart in a heart transplant, because fewer connections have to be made.)

H

H

tachycardia, and a rate that is less than 60 beats per minute is called a *bradycardia*. (See also *arrhythmia, cardiac*.)

heart sounds

The sounds made by the *heart* during each *heartbeat*. In each heart cycle, there are two main heart sounds that can clearly be heard through a *stethoscope*. The first is like a "lubb". It results from closure of the *tricuspid* and *mitral valves* at the exits of the atria (upper heart chambers), which occurs when the ventricles (lower heart chambers) begin contracting to pump blood out of the heart. The second sound is a higher-pitched "dupp" caused by closure of the pulmonary and aortic valves at the exits of the ventricles when the ventricles finish contracting.

Abnormal heart sounds may be a sign of various disorders. For example, high-pitched sounds or "clicks" are due to the abrupt halting of valve opening, which can occur in people with certain *heart valve* defects. Heart *murmurs* are abnormal sounds caused by turbulent blood flow. Murmurs may be due to heart valve defects or to congenital heart disease.

heart surgery

Any operation performed on the *heart*. *Open heart surgery* allows the treatment of most types of heart defect that are present at birth (see *heart disease, congenital*) as well as various disorders of the *heart valves*. *Coronary artery bypass* is performed to redirect blood away from a blocked coronary artery. Narrowing of the coronary arteries can be treated by balloon angioplasty (see *angioplasty, balloon*) and insertion of a *stent* (rigid tube). Balloon angioplasty may also be used to open up narrowed heart valves when the patient is unsuitable for open heart surgery (see *valvuloplasty*). *Heart transplant* surgery may be used to treat progressive, incurable heart disease.

heart transplant

Replacement of a patient's damaged or diseased *heart* with a healthy heart taken from a donor who has just died. Typically, a transplant patient has advanced *coronary artery disease* or *cardiomyopathy* (disease of heart muscle). During the operation, the function of the heart is taken over by a *heart–lung machine*. Most of the diseased heart is removed, but the back walls of the atria (upper chambers) are left in place. The ventricles (lower chambers) are then attached to the remaining areas of the recipient's

heart. Because the transplanted heart has no nerve supply, patients tend to have a high resting heart rate and no variation in blood pressure from day to night.

After the immediate postoperative period, the outlook is good. Patients do, however, face the long-term problems associated with other forms of *transplant surgery*, including *rejection* and infection. (See also *heart–lung transplant*).

HEART-VALVE REPLACEMENT

Any one of the four heart valves (aortic, pulmonary, mitral, or tricuspid) may be replaced by a natural or an artificial valve. The procedure shown in the steps below is for replacement of the aortic heart valve.

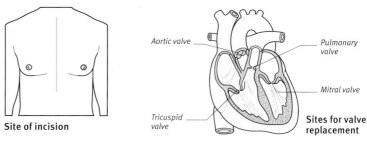

Site of incision

Aortic valve
Pulmonary valve
Mitral valve
Tricuspid valve

Sites for valve replacement

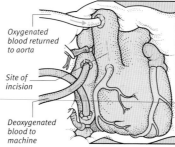

Oxygenated blood returned to aorta

Site of incision

Deoxygenated blood to machine

1 In nearly all heart-valve surgery, an incision is made through the breastbone (sternum) into the chest cavity. The patient is put on a heart–lung machine, the beating of the heart is stopped, and the heart is opened.

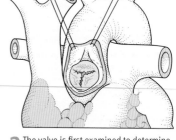

2 The valve is first examined to determine whether it can be repaired or whether it must be replaced. If the latter is necessary (as here), the valve is excised. (The dotted line in this picture shows where the incision is made.)

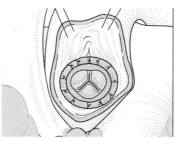

3 The replacement valve is sutured into position and the aorta is closed. The patient is disconnected from the heart–lung machine and the chest wall is sewn up. The operation takes between two and four hours.

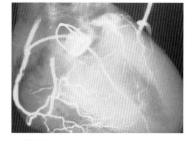

Artificial heart valve in place
This chest X-ray shows the metal components of an artificial heart valve. A ball-and-cage valve has been used to replace the patient's diseased valve.

heart valve

A structure at the exit of a *heart* chamber, consisting of two or three cup-shaped flaps, that allows blood to flow out of the chamber but prevents it from flowing back in. There are four heart valves: aortic, pulmonary, mitral, and tricuspid. The opening and closing of the heart valves during each heart cycle produces *heart sounds*.

DISORDERS

Heart valves may be affected by *stenosis* (narrowing), in which the heart must work harder to force blood through, or by incompetence or insufficiency (leakiness), which makes the valve unable to prevent *regurgitation* (backwash) of blood. These defects cause heart *murmurs*.

Defects of the heart valves may be present from birth (see *heart disease, congenital*) or acquired later in life. The most common congenital valve defects are *aortic stenosis* and *pulmonary stenosis*. Acquired heart-valve disease is usually the result of degenerative changes or *ischaemia* (reduced blood supply) affecting part of the heart and leading to aortic stenosis or *mitral incompetence*. *Rheumatic fever* can cause *mitral stenosis*, mitral incompetence, defects of the aortic valve, *tricuspid stenosis*, and *tricuspid incompetence*. Heart valves may also be damaged by bacterial *endocarditis*.

Heart-valve disorders commonly lead to *heart failure*, *arrhythmias*, or symptoms that arise from reduced blood supply to the tissues.

Heart-valve defects may be diagnosed by *auscultation*, *chest X-ray*, *ECG*, or *echocardiography* and may be corrected by *heart-valve surgery*.

heart-valve surgery

An operation to correct a *heart valve* defect or to remove a diseased or damaged valve. A heart valve may have to be repaired, widened, or replaced because it is either incompetent (leaky), stenotic (narrowed), or both. Widening of a valve may involve *valvotomy* or *valvuloplasty*. A damaged valve can be replaced by a mechanical one (fashioned from metal and plastic), a valve constructed from human or animal tissue, a pig valve, or a valve taken from a human donor after death. A *heart–lung machine* is used during valve replacement.

After heart-valve surgery, there may be symptoms of breathlessness for several weeks that require continued medication. Some people require long-term treatment with *anticoagulant drugs* to prevent the formation of blood clots around the new valve. Certain types of replacement heart valve, such as mechanical valves, are more likely to cause blood clots than other types.

heat cramps

Painful muscle contractions caused by salt loss through profuse *sweating*. Heat cramps are usually brought on by strenuous activity in extreme heat. They may develop independently or may occur as a symptom of *heat exhaustion* or *heatstroke*. Prevention and treatment consist of drinking plenty of fluids, although heat cramps often resolve themselves.

heat disorders

The body functions most efficiently at a temperature of about 37°C, and any major deviation from this temperature disrupts body processes. The body has special mechanisms for keeping its internal temperature constant; any malfunctioning or overloading of these mechanisms may cause a heat disorder.

The mechanisms by which the body loses excess heat are controlled by the part of the brain called the *hypothalamus*.

H

HEART-VALVE REPLACEMENT TYPES

There are three main types of replacement heart valve: bioprostheses (such as the Carpentier–Edwards valve, right), mechanical valves (such as the tilting-disc valve, centre right), and homografts (valves taken from a human donor, far right). A valve is replaced only if it cannot be repaired. Heart-valve replacement (see previous page) is carried out by open surgery, which requires a *cardiopulmonary bypass*. The most frequently replaced valves are the aortic and mitral valves.

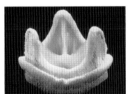

Bioprostheses
These are taken from pigs (as above) or can be made from porcine or bovine tissue and used with or without a stent (a tube to help the valve to hold its shape).

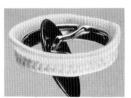

Mechanical valves
There are two main types: those with one (as above) or more tilting-discs, and ball-and-cage. Mechanical valves are made from carbon fibre, metal, and plastic.

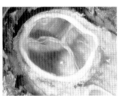

Homografts
These are healthy valves taken from a person who has died of a disease that does not affect the heart. Homografts are a type of bioprosthesis.

Examples	Bioprosthesis (xenograft)	Mechanical	Homograft
Made from	Bovine or porcine tissue with or without a stent (rigid tube)	Metal and plastic	Human valve
Availability	Readily available	Readily available	Limited availability
Suitable age group	Over 60	All ages	All ages
Duration	Up to 15 years	Lifetime	Up to 15 years
Post-operative drug therapy	Three months' treatment with anticoagulant drugs	Lifelong treatment with anticoagulant drugs	Three months' treatment with anticoagulant drugs
Possible complications	Infection; stroke; tendency to become calcified	Infection; stroke; calcification; leakage around base of valve	Less prone to infection

When blood temperature rises, the hypothalamus sends out nerve impulses to stimulate the *sweat glands* and dilate blood vessels in the skin. These changes in the skin cool the body down, but excessive sweating may result in an imbalance of salts and fluids in the body, leading to *heat cramps* or *heat exhaustion*. When the hypothalamus is disrupted (for example, by *fever*), the body may overheat, leading to *heatstroke*. Excessive external heat may cause *prickly heat*.

Most heat disorders can be prevented by gradual acclimatization to hot conditions and taking salt tablets or solution. A light diet and frequent cool baths or showers may also help. Alcohol and strenuous exercise should be avoided.

heat exhaustion

Fatigue, leading to collapse, that is caused by overexposure to heat. The principal causes of heat exhaustion are insufficient water intake, insufficient salt intake, and a deficiency in *sweat* production. In addition to fatigue, symptoms may include faintness, dizziness, nausea and vomiting, headache, and, when salt loss is heavy, *heat cramps*. The skin is usually pale and clammy, breathing is fast and shallow, and the pulse is rapid and weak. Unless it is treated, heat exhaustion may develop into *heatstroke*.

Treatment of heat exhaustion involves rest and replenishing lost water and salt. Prevention is usually by gradual acclimatization to hot conditions.

heat, prickly

See *prickly heat*.

heatstroke

A life-threatening condition in which overexposure to heat, coupled with a breakdown of the body's mechanisms for regulating temperature, cause the body to become overheated. A common cause is prolonged, unaccustomed exposure to the sun in a hot climate. Unsuitable clothing, strenuous activity, overeating, and overconsumption of alcohol can also be contributory factors.

Heatstroke is often preceded by *heat exhaustion*, which consists of fatigue and profuse *sweating*. With the onset of heatstroke, the sweating diminishes and may stop entirely. The skin becomes hot and dry, breathing is shallow, and the pulse is rapid and weak. Body temperature rises dramatically and, without treatment, the victim may lose consciousness and even die.

Heatstroke can be prevented by gradual acclimatization to hot conditions (see *heat disorders*). If it does develop, emergency treatment is needed. This consists of cooling the victim by wrapping him or her in a cold, wet sheet, fanning the body, sponging with water, and giving the person a rehydrating solution to drink (see *rehydration therapy*).

heat treatment

The use of heat to treat disease, aid recovery from injury, or to relieve pain. Heat treatment is useful for certain conditions, such as ligament *sprains*, because it stimulates blood flow and promotes healing of tissues.

Moist heat may be administered by soaking the affected area in a warm bath, or by applying a hot *compress* or *poultice*. Dry heat may be administered by a heating pad, a hot-water bottle, or a heat lamp that produces *infra-red* rays. More precise methods of administering heat to tissues deeper in the body include *ultrasound treatment* and *short-wave diathermy*.

hebephrenia

A form of *schizophrenia* that usually becomes evident in adolescence. It is characterized by inappropriate and disorganized behaviour, withdrawal from social contact, and changes in mood.

Heberden's node

A bony enlargement affecting the joint at the end of the finger, adjacent to the nail. The tendency to develop Heberden's nodes is a feature of *osteoarthritis* and is usually inherited.

heel

The part of the *foot* below the *ankle* and behind the arch. It consists of the *calcaneus* (heel bone), an underlying pad of fat that acts as a cushion, and a layer of skin, which is usually thickened and hardened due to pressure from walking.

heel, cracked

Painful cracks that develop in the thickened skin over the heels. Regular removal of any hard skin using a file or pumice stone, combined with the use of moisturizing cream, can reduce the frequency of such cracks and the severity of the pain. Cracked heels may also be caused by a bacterial infection of the skin on the soles of the feet, also known as pitted keratolysis. The disorder causes small, round pits to develop in the skin; these pits eventually join together to form cracks.

heel, painful

Discomfort resulting from disorders of the *calcaneus* (heel bone) or the soft tissues around it. Pain in the heel may result from fracture of the calcaneus; a spur (bony growth on the calcaneus); inflammation of the pad cushioning the back of the heel (see *calcaneal bursitis*); or inflammation of the tissues at the bottom of the heel (called plantar *fasciitis*), which, in some cases, is a feature of *ankylosing spondylitis*. In addition, the skin over the heel may become blistered as a result of walking long distances and/or wearing ill-fitting shoes.

heel prick blood test

See *blood spot screening tests*.

height chart

A chart used by a doctor or health visitor to record a child's growth and to compare his or her height with the typical range in a particular age group. (See also *growth, childhood*.)

height velocity

The rate of children's increase in height at a particular age.

Heimlich manoeuvre

A first-aid treatment for *choking* in adults and children over one year old. The aim of the Heimlich manoeuvre is to dislodge the material that is causing the blockage.

The first aider stands behind the victim and places one fist, covered by the other, centrally just below the victim's ribcage and pulls sharply inwards and upwards to give an abdominal thrust. This action forces air out of the airways and should help to dislodge any blockage.

Helicobacter pylori

A bacterium (see *bacteria*) now known to be the cause of most *peptic ulcers* as well as a factor in *stomach cancer*. The infection is probably acquired during childhood through person-to-person spread. There is an extremely high worldwide incidence of HELICOBACTER PYLORI infection, with higher rates in developing countries. Of those infected, only about 15 per cent develop peptic ulcer, although 95 per cent of people with duodenal ulcers are found to be infected with HELICOBACTER PYLORI. The bacterium is thought to damage the mucus-producing layer of the stomach and duodenum, bringing gastric acid into contact with the linings of these structures and causing ulceration.

INVESTIGATION AND TREATMENT

There are several different ways of diagnosing HELICOBACTER PYLORI infection. A *breath test* relies on the ability of the bacterium to split molecules of radio-tagged *urea*, releasing labelled carbon dioxide, which can then be detected in the breath. Tests to check for the presence of *antibodies* (proteins produced by the immune system) to the bacterium may be useful, but they cannot confirm that infection has been eradicated. A *biopsy* sample taken from the stomach or duodenal lining can be used to conduct chemical tests, for microscopic analysis, or *cultured* for the organism.

Treatment to eradicate the infection with a combined course of acid-suppressing *ulcer-healing drugs* and *antibiotic drugs* has proved successful in achieving long-term recovery from peptic ulcers. Reinfection is rare. (See also *gastritis*.)

heliotherapy

A form of *phototherapy* involving exposure to sunlight.

helminth infestation

Infection by any parasitic worm. (See *worm infestation*.)

helper T-cell

A type of white blood cell, also known as a helper T-lymphocyte (see *lymphocyte*), that has an important role in the *immune system*. Helper T-cells assist in the destruction of abnormal cells (such as cancer cells) in the body by recognizing foreign *antigens* on the surface of the abnormal cells and subsequently stimulating the production of *killer T-cells*.

Helweg–Larsen's syndrome

An autosomal dominant *genetic disorder*, affecting both sexes, that is chiefly characterized by a reduced ability to lose body heat through sweating. Affected individuals have anhidrosis (inability to sweat) from birth; they have a very small number of sweat glands, and those that do exist are abnormally enlarged. This defect leads to disturbances in body temperature. There are also malformations in the skin and nail tissues. In addition, affected people develop *deafness* due to inner ear problems in their 30s or 40s.

hemianopia

Loss of half of the *visual field* in each eye. Hemianopia may be "homonymous" (in which the same side of both eyes is affected) or "heteronymous" (in which the loss occurs in opposite sides of the eyes). The visual loss can be either temporary or permanent.

Hemianopia results from damage to the *optic nerves* or the brain. Transient homonymous hemianopia in young people is usually caused by *migraine*. In older people, it occurs in *transient ischaemic attacks* (brief interruptions of blood supply to the brain). Permanent homonymous hemianopia is usually caused by a *stroke*, but it may result from brain damage by a tumour, injury, or infection. Hemianopia may also be caused by pressure on the optic nerve from a *pituitary tumour*.

hemiballismus

Irregular and uncontrollable flinging movements of the arm and leg on one side of the body, caused by disease of the *basal ganglia* (nerve cell clusters in the brain concerned with muscular coordination). (See also *athetosis*; *chorea*.)

hemicolectomy

The surgical removal of half, or a major portion, of the *colon*. (See also *colectomy*.)

hemiparesis

Muscular weakness or partial *paralysis* in one side of the body (see *hemiplegia*).

hemiplegia

Paralysis or weakness on one side of the body, caused by damage or disease affecting the motor nerve tracts in the opposite side of the brain. A common cause is a *stroke*. Other causes include *head injury*, *brain tumour*, *brain haemorrhage*, *encephalitis* (brain inflammation), *multiple sclerosis*, complications of *meningitis*, or a *conversion disorder* (a type of psychological disorder). Treatment is for the underlying cause, and is carried out in conjunction with *physiotherapy*.

hemivertebra

A *birth defect* in which half of a vertebra (spinal bone) fails to develop fully.

Hemoccult

A brand name for a type of *faecal occult blood test* that uses guaiac to screen for gastrointestinal bleeding, a possible sign of colorectal cancer (see *colon, cancer of*; *rectum, cancer of*).

Henoch–Schönlein purpura

Inflammation of small blood vessels, causing the leakage of blood into the skin, joints, kidneys, and intestine. The disease is most common in young children, and may occur after an infection such as a sore throat. Henoch–Schönlein purpura may also be due to an abnormal allergic reaction.

The main symptom is a raised purplish rash on the buttocks and backs of the limbs. The joints are swollen and often painful, and colicky abdominal pain may occur. In some cases, there is intestinal bleeding, leading to blood in the faeces. The kidneys may become inflamed, resulting in blood and protein in the urine.

The only treatment usually required is bed rest and *analgesic drugs* (painkillers). Complications may arise if kidney inflammation persists. In severe cases, *corticosteroid drugs* may be given.

heparin

An *anticoagulant drug* used to prevent and treat abnormal *blood clotting*. Heparin is given by injection and is used as an immediate treatment for *deep vein thrombosis* or for *pulmonary embolism*; it may also be given as a preventive measure to people immobilized as a result of illness or surgery. Low molecular weight heparins, such as *tinzaparin*, which only need to be injected once a day, are now widely used and can be self-administered at home.

Adverse effects of heparin include rash, aching bones, and abnormal bleeding in different parts of the body. Long-term use may cause *osteoporosis*.

hepatectomy, partial

Surgical removal of part of the *liver*. This procedure may be needed to remove a damaged area of liver following injury, or to treat noncancerous liver tumours and *hydatid disease*. Rarely, *liver cancer* is treated in this way.

hepatectomy, total

Surgical removal of the *liver*. A hepatectomy is the first stage in an operation to perform a *liver transplant*.

hepatic

Relating to the *liver*.

hepatic encephalopathy

A brain disorder caused by a buildup of toxins in the body as a result of *liver failure*. (See also *encephalopathy*.)

hepatic failure

This is the medical term for *liver failure*, in which the function of the liver is severely impaired.

hepatitis

Inflammation of the *liver*, with accompanying damage to liver cells. The condition may be acute (see *hepatitis, acute*) or chronic (see *hepatitis, chronic*) and may have various causes. (See also *hepatitis A*; *hepatitis B*; *hepatitis C*; *hepatitis D*; *hepatitis E*; *hepatitis, viral*.)

hepatitis A

A disorder caused by the hepatitis A virus, which is in the urine and faeces of infected people and is transmitted in contaminated food (commonly shellfish) or drink. The incubation period is 15–40 days, after which nausea, fever, and *jaundice* develop. Recovery usually occurs within three weeks. Serious complications are rare. Active *immunization* protects against hepatitis A, and may be advised for people travelling to Mediterranean or developing countries. An attack of the disease can confer immunity against subsequent infection.

hepatitis, acute

Short-term inflammation of the *liver*. Acute hepatitis usually clears up in one to two months. In some cases, the disorder may progress to chronic hepatitis (see *hepatitis, chronic*), but it rarely leads to acute *liver failure*.

Acute hepatitis is fairly common. The most frequent cause is infection with a hepatitis virus (see *hepatitis, viral*), but it can also be due to other infections, such as *cytomegalovirus* infection. It may also occur as a result of *paracetamol* overdose or exposure to toxic chemicals, including alcohol (see *liver disease, alcoholic*). However, in some cases no cause can be found. Symptoms of acute hepatitis range from mild to severe. They include tiredness; fever; nausea and vomiting; pain in the upper right side of the abdomen; and *jaundice*.

Blood tests, including *liver function tests*, may be used for diagnosis. In most cases, natural recovery occurs within a few weeks. If the disorder is caused by exposure to a chemical or drug, detoxification using an *antidote* may be possible. *Intensive care* may be required if the liver is badly damaged. Rarely, a *liver transplant* is the only way of saving life. In all cases, alcohol should be avoided after the illness.

hepatitis B

A disorder caused by the hepatitis B virus. The infection is transmitted in blood, blood products, or other body fluids (often through contact with used needles and syringes); blood transfusions; or sexual contact. After an incubation period of one to six months, the onset of symptoms, such as headache, fever, and *jaundice*, may be sudden or gradual; sometimes, there are no symptoms. Most affected people recover, but hepatitis B can be fatal. A vaccine is available; it is usually given to people at high risk of coming into contact with the virus, such as healthcare workers or people visiting areas where the disease is common.

In some cases, the virus continues to cause inflammation and can still be detected in the blood for longer than six months after infection. People who suffer from persistent infection are at long-term risk of *liver cancer* and *cirrhosis* and may need to be treated with *interferon*.

hepatitis C

Caused by the hepatitis C virus and formerly known as non-A non-B *hepatitis*, this infection is often transmitted through sharing needles. Blood transfusions no longer pose a significant risk in the UK because all blood used for transfusions is now routinely screened for the virus.

Hepatitis C has an incubation period of six to 12 months. It begins as a mild illness, which may go undetected. In about three in four patients, chronic hepatitis develops (see *hepatitis, chronic*), which can progress to *cirrhosis* of the liver and an increased risk of *hepatoma* (a type of liver cancer). There is no vaccine against hepatitis C.

hepatitis, chronic

Inflammation of the *liver* that persists for a prolonged period. Eventually, chronic hepatitis causes scar tissue to form and may lead to the development of *cirrhosis* and *portal hypertension*. The disorder may develop following an attack of acute hepatitis (see *hepatitis, acute*) or *hepatitis C*. It may also occur as the result of an *autoimmune disorder*, a viral infection (see *hepatitis, viral*), a reaction to certain types of prescribed drugs or, more rarely, to a *metabolic disorder* such as *haemochromatosis* or *Wilson's disease*. In some cases, no obvious cause can be found.

Symptoms of chronic hepatitis, such as *jaundice* and slight fatigue, may alternate with periods in which there are no symptoms at all. If left untreated, the condition may progress to *liver failure*.

Chronic hepatitis is diagnosed by *liver biopsy*. Autoimmune hepatitis is treated with *corticosteroid drugs* and *immunosup-pressants*. Viral infections often respond to *interferon*. In the drug-induced type of chronic hepatitis, withdrawal of the medication can lead to recovery. For metabolic disturbances, treatment is for the underlying disorder.

hepatitis D

An infection of the liver caused by the hepatitis D virus, which occurs only in people who already have *hepatitis B* infection. People who develop hepatitis D will usually suffer from severe chronic liver disease. Hepatitis D is also known as delta hepatitis.

hepatitis E

A type of *hepatitis* caused by the hepatitis E virus, which is transmitted in contaminated food or drink. The disease is similar to *hepatitis A*.

hepatitis, serum

The former name for *hepatitis B*.

hepatitis, viral

Any type of *hepatitis* caused by a viral infection. Five viruses that attack the liver as their primary target have been identified. They cause *hepatitis A*, *hepatitis B*, *hepatitis C*, *hepatitis D*, and *hepatitis E*.

hepatocele

Protrusion of part of the *liver* through the wall of the abdomen.

hepatocellular carcinoma

The most common type of primary *liver cancer* that arises from within mature liver cells. Hepatocellular carcinoma may develop in people who are suffering from *cirrhosis* of the liver, especially following infection with *hepatitis B* or *hepatitis C*. Incidence of hepatocellular carcinoma is far greater in tropical areas of the world. Symptoms of the condition include hepatomegaly (enlargement of the liver), *jaundice*, and weight loss.

hepatoma

A tumour of the *liver*. A cancerous hepatoma is also known as a *hepatocellular carcinoma*.

hepatomegaly

Enlargement of the *liver*, which may occur as a result of any liver disorder (see *liver, disorders of*).

hepatotoxic

A term for substances, such as certain drugs, that cause damage to liver cells.

MAIN TYPES OF VIRAL **HEPATITIS**

	Viral hepatitis type A	Viral hepatitis types B and C
Transmission of infection	The virus is present in the faeces of infected people and is transmitted by faecal contamination of water and food (such as through poor hygiene in food handling). Faeces are infective from two to three weeks before until about eight days after the onset of jaundice. Local epidemics can occur.	These viruses are present in the blood and other body fluids of infected people, many of whom appear to be in normal health. Infection is spread sexually or by sharing hypodermic needles; in the past it was spread by use of contaminated blood and blood products.
Groups at particular risk	Travellers to areas where hygiene standards are poor and prevalence of the virus is high (such as parts of Asia, Africa, or South America) are most at risk.	Risk groups include intravenous drug users, people with multiple sexual partners, recipients of unscreened blood transfusions, babies born to mothers with the virus, and healthcare workers who come into contact with blood or blood products.
Incubation period	This lasts for 15–40 days after the virus has entered the body.	This lasts for 1–6months (type B) and 6–12 months (type C) after infection.
Symptoms and outlook	In many cases there are no symptoms. There may be nausea, vomiting, malaise, and a mild flulike illness with jaundice, lasting about two to three weeks. The condition never progresses to chronic hepatitis.	Symptoms are similar to those of the type A virus, although they may be more severe. About ten per cent of adults with type B and about 70 per cent with type C develop chronic hepatitis, with continuing illness and eventual cirrhosis of the liver.
Preventive measures	Travellers should take advice about the need for immunization for travel to a given destination. Active immunization involves two doses of the hepatitis A vaccine, given six to 12 months apart; this provides immunity for up to ten years.	Measures include the screening of blood donors, treatment of donated blood, and safer sex. Intravenous drug users should not share needles. Immunization against hepatitis B may be offered to people at high risk of contracting the virus (such as babies of infected mothers, healthcare workers, and drug users). Travellers should take advice about the need for immunization for their destination. The vaccine is given in three doses; the second dose is given one month after the first, and the third six months after the first.

herald patch

A single pink patch with a scaly edge that appears on the skin of the trunk. A herald patch develops about a week before the full rash of the skin disorder *pityriasis rosea* breaks out.

herbal medicine

Systems of medical treatment in which various parts of different plants are used to promote health and to treat symptoms of illness. Herbal medicine is a form of *complementary medicine*. Herbal remedies are also used in treatments such as *homeopathy* and *Chinese medicine*.

Although herbal medicine is thought by some to be harmless because it is natural, some herbal remedies contain significant amounts of pharmacologically active substances that may interact with other drugs or affect other medical conditions. Herbal remedies should only be used on the advice of an approved practitioner; a patient should always inform his or her doctor of any herbal medicine he or she is using.

herd immunity

Protection of a whole community from an infectious disease as a result of immunity in a majority, but not all, of that community. Such immunity may be naturally acquired or may be induced by *immunization*. For example, vaccination of more than 85 per cent of a population against diphtheria will prevent the spread of the disease, should it occur, due to an insufficient number of susceptible people who could catch it and pass it on to others. As a result, even those people without immunity receive a degree of protection from being part of an immune population.

hereditary haemorrhagic telangiectasia

An inherited condition in which capillaries (tiny blood vessels) in the skin and in the mucous membranes of areas such as the nose, mouth, and gastrointestinal tract are distended and prone to recurrent bleeding. The condition can result in iron deficiency anaemia (see *anaemia, iron deficiency*). Hereditary haemorrhagic telangiectasia shows an autosomal dominant pattern of inheritance (see *genetic disorders*). (See also *telangiectasia*.)

hereditary spherocytosis

See *spherocytosis, hereditary*.

heredity

The transmission of traits and disorders through genetic mechanisms. Each individual inherits a combination of *genes* via the sperm and egg cells from which he or she is derived. The interaction of the genes determines inherited characteristics, including, in some cases, disorders or susceptibility to disorders. (See also *genetic disorders*; *inheritance*.)

heritability

A measure of the extent to which a disease or disorder is the result of inherited factors, as opposed to environmental influences such as diet and climate. Certain disorders (such as *haemophilia* and *cystic fibrosis*) are known to be caused entirely by hereditary factors. In contrast, other disorders are caused wholly by environmental factors. However, between these two extremes are many disorders (such as *schizophrenia*) in which both inheritance and environment probably play a part.

A rough estimate of heritability can be obtained from the known incidence of a disorder in the first-degree relatives (parents or siblings) of affected people compared with the incidence of the disorder in a population exposed to similar environmental influences. Estimates of heritability are useful in *genetic counselling*. (See also *genetic disorders*.)

hermaphroditism

A *congenital* disorder in which *gonads* (testes or ovaries) of both sexes are present within one individual, and in

H

which the external genitalia are not clearly male or female. True hermaphroditism is extremely rare and its cause is unknown. A more common condition is *pseudohermaphroditism*, in which the gonads of only one sex are present, but the external genitalia are not clearly either male or female, or are those of the opposite sex.

hernia

Protrusion of an organ or tissue through a weak area in the muscle or tissue that normally contains it. The term is usually applied to a protrusion of the intestine through the abdominal wall. In a *hiatus hernia*, the stomach protrudes through the diaphragm, into the chest.

CAUSES

Abdominal hernias may be caused by a *congenital* weakness in the wall of the abdomen. Hernias may also be the result of damage caused by lifting heavy objects, persistent coughing, or straining to defaecate, or they may develop following an operation.

TYPES

There are several types of abdominal hernia, which are classified according to their location in the body. The most important are inguinal hernias, which mainly affect men; femoral hernias, which are more common in overweight women; and umbilical hernias, which occur in babies.

SYMPTOMS AND TREATMENT

The first symptom of an abdominal hernia is usually a bulge in the abdominal wall. There may also be some abdominal discomfort.

Sometimes the protruding intestine can be pushed back into place (known as a reducible hernia). In other cases, however, the hernia bulges out and cannot be put back (an irreducible hernia). This condition is painful, and surgery is usually necessary to repair the weakened area (see *hernia repair*).

If the trapped portion of intestine becomes twisted, the blood supply to that area of the intestine will be impaired or may be cut off entirely. This problem, known as a strangulated hernia, needs urgent treatment, otherwise *gangrene* of the bowel may develop.

Umbilical hernias in babies can usually be left untreated as they tend to disappear naturally by age five.

hernia repair

Surgical correction of a *hernia*. Surgery is usually performed to treat a hernia of the abdominal wall that is painful or cannot be pushed back into place. A strangulated hernia (in which the blood supply to a trapped portion of intestine is cut off) requires emergency surgery.

Hernia repair is often performed as day surgery, and may be done under local or general anaesthesia. Either open or *minimally invasive surgery* (using an endoscope to repair the hernia from within the abdominal cavity) may be used. During surgery, the hernia is repositioned and the defect in the overlying muscle is repaired. Often, the defect is repaired using a synthetic mesh, which significantly reduces the chance of the hernia recurring.

herniated disc

See *disc prolapse*.

herniorrhaphy

See *hernia repair*.

heroin

A *narcotic drug* similar to *morphine*. When used for medical purposes, it is generally known as *diamorphine*. Heroin may also be abused for its mood-altering effects (see *heroin abuse*).

MAIN TYPES OF ABDOMINAL **HERNIA**

Inguinal hernia	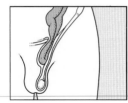	At least 2 per cent of adult males in the UK suffer at some time from this kind of hernia, in which part of the intestine bulges through the inguinal canal (the passage through which the testes descend into the scrotum). The hernia is detected as a bulge in the groin or scrotum; untreated, the hernia may become stuck, so early surgery is generally recommended.
Femoral hernia	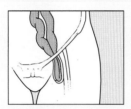	This type of hernia occurs most commonly in obese women; part of the intestine emerges where the femoral vein and artery pass from the abdomen to the thigh. A femoral hernia is noticed as a swelling of the top front of the thigh. Although the hernia itself may be large, its neck is narrow, and the condition can only be corrected by surgery.
Epigastric hernia	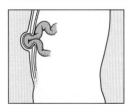	Also called a ventral hernia, an epigastric hernia is caused by a weakness in the muscles of the central upper abdomen; the intestine bulges out at a point between the navel and the breastbone. This form of hernia is three times more common in men than in women and is most likely to occur in people between 20 and 50 years old.
Umbilical hernia	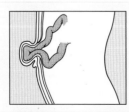	This occurs when part of the intestine protrudes through the abdominal wall at the navel. Babies are the most common sufferers; the hernia can be repaired surgically or it may disappear naturally by about the age of five. A similar problem, a parumbilical hernia, occurs mostly in obese, middle-aged women who have had several children.
Incisional hernia	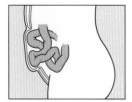	An area of weakness may occasionally develop following a surgical incision in the wall of the abdomen. This area may then develop into an incisional hernia. The defect may become so severe that a large amount of intestine bulges through the abdominal wall; if this happens, a repair using a piece of mesh may be necessary.

HERNIA REPAIR

During surgery the hernia is removed or repositioned and the weakened abdominal wall is reinforced with stitching or mesh.

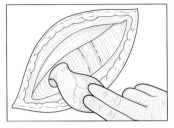

1 The protruding sac of intestine is pushed back into the abdomen or, in some cases (such as strangulation), the sac is removed surgically.

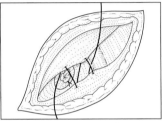

2 The muscular wall of the abdomen may then be repaired by overlapping the edges of the weakened area and securing them with rows of stitching.

ALTERNATIVE METHOD

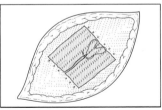

Mesh repair
Synthetic mesh may be used to reinforce the abdominal wall; two mesh leaves are secured by stitching, then joined at the centre.

heroin abuse

Nonmedical, illicit use of heroin. The heroin taken by drug abusers is a white or brownish powder that can be smoked, sniffed, or dissolved in water and injected. Heroin has an analgesic (painkilling) effect and produces sensations of calmness, warmth, drowsiness, and a loss of concern for outside events. Long-term use of heroin causes *tolerance* and psychological and physical dependence (see *drug dependence*). The sudden withdrawal of the drug produces shivering, abdominal cramps, diarrhoea, vomiting, and restlessness.

Heroin addiction has many adverse effects on the user, including injection scars, skin abscesses, weight loss, *erectile dysfunction*, and the risk of infection with *hepatitis B*, *hepatitis C*, and *HIV* through sharing needles. Death commonly occurs from accidental overdose.

herpangina

A throat infection that is caused by *coxsackievirus*. Herpangina most commonly affects young children. The virus is usually transmitted via infected droplets coughed or sneezed into the air. Many people harbour the virus but do not have symptoms.

SYMPTOMS

After an incubation period of two to seven days, there is a sudden onset of fever, accompanied by a sore throat and sometimes also headache, abdominal discomfort, and muscular pains. The throat becomes red and a few small blisters appear, which enlarge and burst, forming shallow ulcers. These symptoms usually clear up within a week, without specific treatment

herpes

Any of a variety of conditions that are characterized by an eruption of small, usually painful, blisters on the skin. The term "herpes" usually refers to an infection with the *herpes simplex* virus. Two forms of this virus, called HSV1 and HSV2, are generally responsible for *cold sores* and genital herpes (see *herpes, genital*), respectively. A closely related organism, the varicella–zoster virus, is responsible for two other conditions in which skin blisters are a feature: *chickenpox* and *herpes zoster* (shingles).

herpes, genital

A *sexually transmitted infection* caused mainly by HSV2, one form of the *herpes simplex* virus. Genital infections can also be due to HSV1 that has been transmitted by oral contact with the genitals. After an incubation period of about a week, the virus produces soreness, burning, itching, and small blisters in the genital area. The blisters burst to leave small, painful ulcers, which heal in 10 to 14 days. The lymph nodes in the groin may become enlarged and painful, and the person may develop other symptoms such as a headache, fever, and aching muscles.

TREATMENT

Genital herpes cannot be cured, but early treatment can reduce the severity of symptoms. *Antiviral drugs*, such as *aciclovir* make the ulcers less painful and also encourage healing. Other measures include taking *analgesic drugs* and bathing the genital area in a salt solution.

OUTLOOK

Once the virus has entered the body, it stays there for the rest of the person's life. Recurrent attacks may occur, usually during periods when the person is feeling run down, anxious, or depressed, or, in some cases, a few days before menstruation. The virus may be shed continuously and can be transmitted to others through sexual intercourse, even when the infected person has no symptoms. Recurrent attacks tend to become less frequent and less severe over time.

Genital herpes may be passed from a pregnant woman to her baby during delivery. If the genital herpes develop in late pregnancy, delivery by *caesarean section* is usually recommended.

herpes gestationis

A rare skin disorder of pregnant women that produces crops of tense, itchy blisters on the legs and abdomen. Herpes gestationis is an *autoimmune disorder* that is essentially a type of *pemphigoid* triggered by pregnancy.

Severe cases are treated with *corticosteroid drugs*. An affected woman may need to be monitored as there is an increased risk of fetal *prematurity* and low *birthweight*. The disorder may initially worsen after delivery but then clears up. It tends to recur in subsequent pregnancies.

herpes simplex

A common viral infection that is characterized by small, fluid-filled blisters. Herpes simplex infections are *contagious* and are usually spread by direct contact. Most infections are quite mild.

TYPES

There are two forms of the virus: HSV1 (herpes simplex virus, type 1) and HSV2 (herpes simplex virus, type 2). Most people are infected with HSV1 at some time in their lives, usually during childhood. HSV1 is usually associated with infections of the lips, mouth, and face; HSV2 is often associated with infections of the genitals and infections acquired by babies at birth. There is considerable overlap between the two types; sometimes, conditions usually due to HSV1 are caused by HSV2, and vice versa.

H

Type 1 virus The initial infection may be symptomless; alternatively, it may cause a flulike illness with mouth ulcers. Thereafter, the virus remains dormant in nerve cells in the facial area. In many people, the virus is periodically reactivated, causing *cold sores* that invariably erupt in the same site (usually around the lips).

Sometimes the virus can infect a finger after touching a cold sore, causing a painful eruption called a *herpetic whitlow*. HSV1 may also produce eczema herpeticum (an extensive rash of skin blisters) in a person with a pre-existing skin disorder, such as *eczema*. Eczema herpeticum may require hospital admission. If the virus gets into an eye it may cause *conjunctivitis*, which usually lasts only a few days; more seriously, it may cause a *corneal ulcer*.

Rarely, HSV1 spreads to the brain, leading to *encephalitis*. The virus may cause a potentially fatal generalized infection in a person with an *immunodeficiency disorder* or in someone taking *immunosuppressant drugs*.

Type 2 virus HSV2 is the usual cause of sexually transmitted genital herpes (see *herpes, genital*), in which painful blisters erupt in the genital area. In some people, the blisters tend to recur.

TREATMENT

Treatment of herpes simplex depends on its type, site, and severity of symptoms. *Antiviral drugs*, such as *aciclovir*, may be helpful, particularly if used early in an infection.

herpes zoster

An infection of the *nerves* supplying certain skin areas that is characterized by a painful rash of small crusting blisters. Also called shingles, herpes zoster is especially common among older people.

TYPES

Herpes zoster usually affects only one side of the body, and follows the path of a nerve. It commonly develops on a strip of skin over the ribs, although the rash may also appear on the neck, arm, or lower part of the body. Sometimes the infection involves the face and eye; this form of the disorder is called herpes zoster ophthalmicus.

CAUSES

Herpes zoster is caused by the *varicella–zoster* virus, which also causes *chickenpox*. After an attack of chickenpox, some of the viruses survive and lie dormant for many years in the nerve cells near the spinal cord. In some people, a decline in the efficiency of the

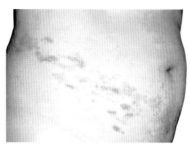

Example of herpes zoster
An extensive rash of blisters has spread around one side of the body, just under the ribs, and on to the front of the abdomen.

immune system – especially in old age – because of disease or severe stress, allows the viruses to re-emerge and cause herpes zoster. The disorder is also common in people whose immune system is weakened by stress or by certain drugs, such as *corticosteroid drugs* or *anticancer drugs*.

SYMPTOMS

The first indication of herpes zoster is excessive sensitivity in the skin, followed by pain, which is often severe. The infection can be difficult to diagnose at this stage and may be mistaken for a different condition; for example, pain in the chest wall may be mistaken for angina pectoris. After about five days, the rash appears as small, raised, red spots that soon turn into blisters. Within a few days, the blisters dry, flatten, and develop crusts. Over the next two weeks, the crusts drop off, sometimes leaving small pitted scars.

The most serious feature of herpes zoster is pain after the attack, known as postherpetic neuralgia, which affects about a third of all infected people. This pain is caused by nerve damage, and may last for months or years. Herpes zoster ophthalmicus may cause a *corneal ulcer* or *uveitis* (inflammation of the uvea: the iris, ciliary body and its muscle, and the choroid).

TREATMENT

If treatment is begun soon after the rash appears, *antiviral drugs*, such as *aciclovir*, will reduce the severity of the symptoms and minimize nerve damage. *Analgesic drugs* (painkillers) may also be helpful in relieving pain. If *postherpetic neuralgia* is a problem, *anticonvulsant drugs*, such as *gabapentin*, may be helpful.

herpetic whitlow

A painful swelling on the finger caused by infection with the *herpes simplex* virus. (See also *whitlow*.)

heterosexuality

Sexual attraction of an individual to members of the opposite sex. (See also *bisexuality*; *homosexuality*.)

heterozygote

A term used to describe a person whose cells contain two different *alleles* (forms of a particular gene) controlling a specified inherited trait. A *homozygote* has identical alleles controlling that trait. (See also *inheritance*; *genetic disorders*.)

hiatus hernia

A condition in which part of the *stomach* protrudes upwards into the chest through an opening in the *diaphragm* called the hiatus, which is normally occupied by the *oesophagus*. The cause is unknown, but hiatus hernia is more common in obese people. In some cases, it is present at birth.

Many people have no symptoms. In some people, however, the hiatus hernia impairs the efficiency of the oesophageal sphincter, the muscle at the junction between the oesophagus and the stomach. Weakness in this muscle allows acid reflux as the stomach acid escapes into the oesophagus (see *gastro-oesophageal reflux disease*). This problem may lead to *oesophagitis* (inflammation of the oesophagus) or to *heartburn*, which produces pain or discomfort in the centre of the chest.

Alginates, *antacid drugs*, H_2-receptor antagonists, or proton-pump inhibitors (see *ulcer-healing drugs*) may be helpful in reducing acid reflux and/or stomach acidity. In severe cases, surgery may be required to return the stomach to its

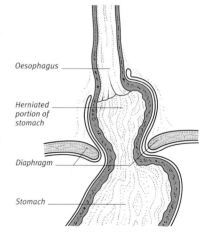

Oesophagus

Herniated portion of stomach

Diaphragm

Stomach

Common type of hiatus hernia
Part of the stomach slides into the chest through the oesophageal hiatus (opening).

normal position and to tighten the oesophageal sphincter. This can now be carried out by *minimally invasive surgery*.

Hib vaccine

A vaccine administered routinely at two, three, and four months of age, and with a booster at 12 months, to provide immunity to the bacterium HAEMOPHILUS INFLUENZAE type b (Hib). Before the vaccine was generally available, Hib infection was a common cause of bacterial *meningitis* and *epiglottitis* in children.

hiccup

A sudden, involuntary contraction of the *diaphragm* followed by rapid closure of the *vocal cords*. Most attacks of hiccups last only a few minutes, and are not medically significant. Rarely, they may be due to a condition, such as *pneumonia* or *pancreatitis*, that causes irritation of the diaphragm or *phrenic nerves*. *Chlorpromazine*, *haloperidol*, or *diazepam* may be prescribed for frequent, prolonged attacks.

Hickman catheter

A flexible plastic tube, also known as a skin-tunnelled catheter, that is passed through the chest and inserted into the subclavian vein, which leads to the heart. It is often used in people who have *leukaemia* or other cancers and need regular *chemotherapy* and blood tests. The catheter allows drugs to be injected directly into the bloodstream and blood samples to be obtained easily. It is inserted under local *anaesthesia*. A Hickman catheter can remain in position for months; the external end is plugged when not in use.

hidradenitis suppurativa

Inflammation of the *sweat glands* in the armpits and groin due to a bacterial infection. Abscesses develop beneath the skin; the affected area becomes reddened and painful and may ooze pus. The condition tends to recur and can eventually cause scarring. *Antibiotic drugs* may help reduce the severity of an outbreak.

hidrosis

The medical term for *sweating*. (See also *hyperhidrosis*; *hypohidrosis*.)

high-density lipoprotein

A type of lipoprotein, made up of protein and *lipid* (fat), that transport lipids in the blood. High levels of high-density lipoprotein (HDL) can help to protect against *atherosclerosis* (fatty deposits on artery walls) because it removes cholesterol from the circulation and takes it to the liver for processing. (See also *fats and oils*; *low-density lipoprotein*.)

high-dependency unit

A level of hospital inpatient care intermediate between that of a general ward and that of an *intensive care* unit. Also known as a "step-down" facility, staff in a high-dependency unit provide monitoring and support for acutely ill patients. It also has facilities for short-term *ventilation* and emergency resuscitation.

hilum

The term used to describe a small indentation on the surface of an internal organ where blood vessels, nerve fibres, or other similar structures enter or leave the organ. For example, the hilum of the lung is its junction with the main bronchus and the major vessels. A commonly used alternative term is "hilus".

hindmilk

The breast milk that is produced at the end of a feed. Hindmilk contains more fat than *foremilk* and therefore provides the baby's main source of energy. (See also *breast-feeding*.)

hindwaters

A term for the *amniotic fluid* that is discharged behind the presenting part of the baby (usually the head) during pregnancy and delivery. In contrast, the forewaters (the "waters") precede the presenting part of the baby and may rupture (or "break") before or after the onset of labour.

hinge joint

A type of mobile *joint* that allows movement in one plane only (forwards and backwards). Examples of hinge joints are the knee joint and the elbow joint.

hip

The *joint* between the *pelvis* and the upper end of the *femur* (thigh bone). The hip is a ball-and-socket joint; the smooth, rounded head of the femur fits securely into the acetabulum, a cup-like cavity in the pelvis. Tough ligaments attach the femur to the pelvis, further stabilizing the joint and giving it the necessary strength to support the weight of the body and take the strain of leg movements. The structure of the hip allows a considerable range of leg movement.

LOCATION OF **HIP**

The hip is a ball-and-socket joint comprising the dome at the top of the femur (thigh bone) and the cup-shaped depression in the pelvic bone.

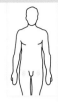

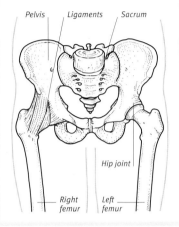

Pelvis   Ligaments   Sacrum

Hip joint

Right femur   Left femur

DISORDERS

Injuries to the hip joint, such as dislocation of the joint, are usually caused by extreme force, as in a road traffic accident. Fractures may also occur in the hip joint, due to breaks in the head or neck of the femur (see *femur, fracture of*). This type of injury is more common in elderly people, whose bones are weakened by *osteoporosis* (loss of bone density).

Osteoarthritis (degeneration of bone ends within a joint) is a common disorder of the hip. It causes symptoms such as pain and stiffness (particularly during activity), swelling, and restricted movement of the joint.

Certain forms of hip disorder occur in babies and children. *Developmental dysplasia of the hip* is a condition that is present at birth; in this disorder, the hip socket is malformed and the head of the femur does not fit correctly into it. *Perthes' disease* is a rare condition affecting young children, in which the head of the femur breaks down; it causes limping, pain in the hip, and restricted movement of the joint.

hip, clicking

A relatively common condition in adults in which a characteristic dull clicking can be heard and felt during certain movements of the hip joint. Clicking hip is caused by a tendon slipping over

H

the bony prominence on the outer side of the *femur* (thigh bone) and is not an indication of disease.

Clicking of the hip may sometimes be heard during examination of newborn babies; in this instance, it indicates possible dislocation of the hip (see *developmental dysplasia of the hip*).

hip, congenital dislocation of

See *developmental dysplasia of the hip*.

hip dysplasia, developmental

See *developmental dysplasia of the hip*.

hippocampus

A structure in the *limbic system* of the brain. The hippocampus, consisting of a band of *grey matter*, is involved with some learning processes and long-term memory storage.

Hippocratic oath

A set of ethical principles that are derived from the writings of the Greek physician Hippocrates that is concerned with a doctor's duty to work for the good of the patient.

hip replacement

A surgical procedure to replace all or part of a diseased *hip* joint with an artificial substitute. The replacement is most often carried out in older people whose joints are stiff and painful as a result of *osteoarthritis*. It may also be needed if *rheumatoid arthritis* has spread to the hip joint or if the top end of the femur (thigh bone) is badly fractured (see *femur, fracture of*).

Hirschsprung's disease

A *congenital* disorder in which the *rectum*, and sometimes the lower part of the *colon*, lack the ganglion cells that control the intestine's rhythmic contractions. The affected part of the colon becomes narrowed and blocks the movement of faecal material.

The disease is rare and tends to run in families. It occurs about four times more often in boys. Symptoms, which include constipation and bloating, usually develop in the first few weeks of life. The child usually has a poor appetite and may fail to grow properly.

A *barium X-ray examination* can show the narrowed segment of the intestine. A *biopsy* may also be taken. Treatment involves removing the narrowed segment of intestine and rejoining the normal part to the anus.

PERFORMING A **HIP REPLACEMENT**

In this operation, the surgeon pushes aside or cuts through the surrounding muscles to expose the hip joint. The femur (thigh bone) is cut and the pelvis is drilled to make room for the two components of the artificial joint. These parts are secured in place, the femur is repaired, and the muscles and tendons are replaced and repaired.

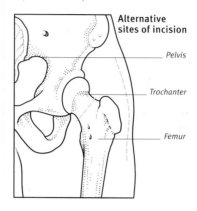

Alternative sites of incision
Pelvis
Trochanter
Femur

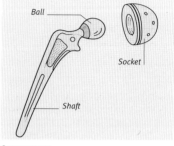

Ball
Socket
Shaft

Components
An artificial hip joint has two parts. The ball and shaft are metal; the socket may be metal or plastic.

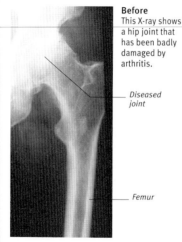

Before
This X-ray shows a hip joint that has been badly damaged by arthritis.

Diseased joint

Femur

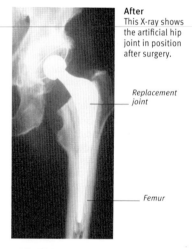

After
This X-ray shows the artificial hip joint in position after surgery.

Replacement joint

Femur

---

hirsutism

Excessive hairiness, which particularly appears in women. The additional hair is coarse in texture and grows in a male pattern on the face, trunk, and limbs. Hirsutism can be a symptom of certain conditions, such as *polycystic ovary syndrome* and congenital *adrenal hyperplasia*, in which the level of naturally occurring male hormones in the blood is abnormally high. Hirsutism can also be a result of taking anabolic steroids (see *steroids, anabolic*). More commonly, however, hirsutism is not a sign of any disorder at all; it occurs mildly in many normal women, especially after the *menopause*, in which hormone balance is upset (See also *hypertrichosis*.)

hirudin

An anticoagulant contained in the saliva of leeches (see *leech*) that prevents blood from clotting.

histamine

A chemical present in cells (mainly *mast cells*) throughout the body that is released during an allergic reaction (see *allergy*). Histamine activates two main types of receptors: H_1 and H_2. H_1 activation is responsible for the swelling and redness that occur in *inflammation*. It also narrows the airways in the lungs and causes itching. H_2 activation stimulates acid production by the stomach, but in large amounts it can irritate the stomach lining, causing *gastritis* or *peptic ulcers*.

Allergic reactions caused by H_1 can be controlled by *antihistamine drugs*. Overproduction of stomach acid due to H_2 can be counteracted by H_2-receptor antagonists (see *ulcer-healing drugs*).

histamine₁-receptor antagonists

See *H₁-receptor antagonists*.

histamine₂-receptor antagonists

See *H₂-receptor antagonists*.

histiocytosis X

A rare childhood disease, now more commonly known as Langerhans cell histiocytosis, in which there is an overgrowth of a type of tissue cell called a histiocyte. The cause is unknown, but the condition probably results from a disturbance of the *immune system*. In the mildest form, rapid cell growth occurs in one bone only, usually the skull, a *clavicle*, a rib, or a *vertebra*, causing swelling and pain. In the most severe, and least common, form, there is a rash and enlargement of the *liver*, *spleen*, and *lymph nodes*, as well as lung involvement. In these cases, treatment is with *anticancer drugs*, but the outlook is poor.

histocompatibility antigens

A group of proteins that have a role in the *immune system*. Certain types of histocompatibility antigen are present on every cell in the body; they are essential for the immunological function of *killer T-cells*, which help to defend the body against disease. The antigens act as a guide enabling the killer T-cells to distinguish between self and nonself and to kill abnormal or foreign cells.

The main group of histocompatibility antigens is the human leukocyte antigen (HLA) system, which consists of several series of antigens. There are six different *genes* known as HLA-A, HLA-B, HLA-C, HLA-DP, HLA-DQ, and HLA-DR. Each of these has many different forms, or *alleles*; for example, HLA-B has over 40 different numbered alleles. A person's tissue type (the particular set of HLAs in the body tissues) is unique, except in the case of identical twins, who have identical sets of HLAs.

HLA analysis has some useful applications. Comparison of HLA types may show that two people are related, and it has been used in *paternity testing*. The HLA system is also used in *tissue-typing* to help match recipient and donor tissues before *transplant surgery*. Certain HLA types occur more frequently in people with particular diseases. For example, HLA-B27 is associated with several forms of arthritis, particularly *ankylosing spondylitis*, and HLA-DR2 and an HLA-DQ type with *narcolepsy*. HLA testing can help to confirm the diagnosis in someone who may have one of these conditions.

histology

The study of tissues, including their cellular structure and function. The main application of histology in medicine is in the diagnosis of disease. This process often involves obtaining a sample of tissue (see *biopsy*) and examining it under a microscope to detect any abnormalities, such as cancerous cells or areas of scar tissue. Examination of tissue samples may also be performed to determine the extent of a disease, such as cancer, once it has been detected. If a cancerous tumour is found, for example, it may be removed, together with an area of surrounding tissue; by examining this material, doctors can tell whether the whole of the diseased area has been removed or whether cancerous cells have spread beyond the edges of the tumour.

histopathology

A branch of *histology* concerned with the effects of disease on the microscopic structure of tissues.

histoplasmosis

An infection caused by inhaling spores of the fungus HISTOPLASMA CAPSULATUM, which is found in soil contaminated with bird or bat droppings. Histoplasmosis occurs in parts of the Americas, the Far East, and Africa. Treatment is by intravenous infusion of *antifungal drugs*.

history-taking

The process by which a doctor gathers information from patients regarding the symptoms of their illnesses and details of any previous disorders. (See also *diagnosis*.)

histrionic personality disorder

A psychiatric disorder characterized by exaggerated emotional reactions and attention-seeking behaviour. Affected people also constantly demand praise or reassurance, and require immediate satisfaction of their demands. The disorder usually first appears in early adulthood, and is more common in women.

HIV

The abbreviation for human immunodeficiency virus. HIV is a *retrovirus* that infects and gradually destroys cells in the immune system and may eventually lead to *AIDS* (acquired immunodeficiency syndrome). There are two closely related viruses: HIV-1, which is the most common cause of AIDS throughout the world; and HIV-2, which is largely confined to West Africa.

METHODS OF TRANSMISSION

HIV is transmitted in body fluids, such as blood, semen, and vaginal secretions. It most commonly gains access to the body during sexual activity (vaginal, anal, or oral), particularly when contaminated body fluids come into contact with broken skin. Other sources of infection are nonsterile needles (for example, among people who abuse intravenous drugs and share needles and syringes) and, in some parts of the world, contaminated blood transfusions. In addition, if a pregnant women is infected, the virus can pass to the fetus via the *placenta*. It is not transmitted by everyday physical contact such as shaking hands or hugging.

EFFECTS OF THE VIRUS

HIV infects cells that have a special structure, called a CD4 receptor, on their surface. These include immune system cells called CD4 lymphocytes, which defend the body against cancerous and infected cells, as well as certain cells in other tissues, such as the brain. The virus multiplies in the cells, killing them in the process; the dead cells then release more virus particles into the blood. If the virus is untreated, the number of CD4 lymphocytes falls. This results in a reduced ability to fight off infections and certain types of cancer.

HIV is extremely successful at withstanding attempts by the body to destroy it. Every time HIV replicates, it changes its *antigen* makeup, thereby ensuring that it is difficult for the body to mount an effective immune response to it.

SYMPTOMS

Initially, some people infected with HIV may have no symptoms. However, in the first couple of months after exposure many people develop a flulike illness similar to glandular fever (see *mononucleosis, infectious*), with symptoms that may include fever, fatigue, sore throat, aching muscles, headache, nausea, vomiting, diarrhoea, and a rash. These symptoms usually clear up after a few weeks but may last for several months. Subsequently, there may be period, which may last for

H

H

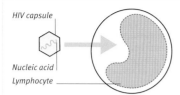

HIV capsule

Nucleic acid

Lymphocyte

1 HIV (human immunodeficiency virus), like any virus, consists of some nucleic acid inside a capsule made of protein. The virus invades a lymphocyte (a type of white blood cell).

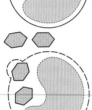

2 The strand of nucleic acid escapes from the capsule and uses the host cell's resources to make copies of itself.

3 Each copy forms a capsule and leaves the host cell, which eventually ceases to function efficiently in fighting disease.

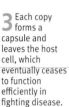

several years, during which there are no symptoms, although some people have swollen lymph nodes, muscle pain, and/ or night sweats during this time. Even though there may be no symptoms, the virus continues to multiply in the body and can be passed on to others.

Later, various vague complaints such as weight loss, fever, sweats, or unexplained diarrhoea (known as *AIDS-related complex*) may herald the development of AIDS. There may also be skin disorders such as seborrhoeic *dermatitis*; various viral, fungal and bacterial infections, such as persistent *herpes simplex* infections, oral *candidiasis*, *tuberculosis*, and *shigellosis*; and a variety of neurological disorders, including *dementia*.

The development of full-blown AIDS is marked by the occurrence of certain specific conditions, which are known as AIDS-defining illnesses. These include cancers (*Kaposi's sarcoma* and lymphoma of the brain), and various infections (*pneumocystis pneumonia*, tuberculosis, *human papillomavirus*, *cytomegalovirus* infection, *toxoplasmosis*, diarrhoea due to CRYPTOSPORIDUM or ISOSPORA, candidiasis, disseminated *strongyloidiasis*, and *cryptococcosis*), many of which are described as *opportunistic infections*.

DIAGNOSIS, TREATMENT, AND OUTLOOK

HIV is diagnosed through an *HIV test*, a blood test that detects the presence of *antibodies* (proteins manufactured by the immune system) to HIV in the blood.

People infected with HIV should have regular monitoring to determine when specific treatments, such as *antiretroviral drugs*, are necessary. The main types of antiretroviral used are *protease inhibitors*, such as indinavir and ritonavir, and *reverse transcriptase inhibitors*, such as *zidovudine*. There is also a new group of drugs, called fusion inhibitors, that may be used to treat resistant strains of HIV. Drug therapy, which usually involves a combination of drugs, can slow the progress of the disease and may prevent the development of full-blown AIDS.

In wealthier countries, HIV infection is no longer necessarily a fatal disease. It remains life-threatening, however, and the most effective strategy for defeating it is prevention of infection.

PREVENTION

The risk of infection with HIV can most easily be reduced by practising *safer sex*. Intravenous drug users should take care not to share needles. Others who may be at risk, such as healthcare workers who may come into contact with infected body fluids or needles, should observe recommended safety regulations. (See also *needlestick injury*.)

hives

An alternative name for *urticaria*.

HIV test

A *blood test* that is used to detect the presence in the blood of *antibodies* to *HIV*, the virus that can lead to AIDS. Antibodies are proteins made by the *immune system* in response to a foreign protein (antigen) in the body, although they may not develop for three months after initial infection with HIV. A positive result, in which these antibodies are detected, indicates the presence of HIV. As well as diagnosis, the HIV test can also be used for screening.

HLA

Abbreviation for *human leukocyte antigen*.

HLA types

See *histocompatibility antigens*.

hoarseness

A rough, husky, or croaking voice. Hoarseness is usually due to irritation of, or strain on, the *larynx* (voicebox).

CAUSES

Short-lived hoarseness is often due to overuse of the voice, which strains the muscles in the larynx. It is also commonly caused by inflammation of the vocal cords in acute *laryngitis*.

Persistent hoarseness may be due to chronic irritation of the larynx, which can be caused by smoking, excessive alcohol consumption, chronic *bronchitis*, or constant dripping of mucus from the nasal passages. *Polyps* (harmless growths) on the vocal cords may also cause hoarseness. In people with *hypothyroidism* (underactivity of the thyroid), hoarseness can result from formation of tissue on the vocal cords. In young children, it may be a symptom of *croup*.

Occasionally, persistent hoarseness in adults has a more serious cause, such as cancer of the larynx (see *larynx, cancer of*), *thyroid cancer*, or *lung cancer*.

TREATMENT

In cases where voice strain or laryngitis is the cause, resting the voice often helps recovery. If hoarseness persists for more than two weeks, a doctor should be consulted. A *laryngoscopy* (direct examination of the larynx) may be performed to exclude any serious underlying causes.

Hodgkin's disease

An uncommon cancerous disorder in which there is a proliferation of cells in lymphoid tissue (which is found mainly in the *lymph nodes* and *spleen*). This is also known as a lymphoma. Men are affected more commonly than women. The cause is unknown.

SYMPTOMS AND SIGNS

The most common sign is the painless enlargement of lymph nodes, typically in the neck or armpits. There may be a general feeling of illness, with fever, weight loss, and night sweats. There may also be generalized itching and, rarely, pain in the swollen lymph nodes after drinking alcohol. As the disease progresses, the *immune system* becomes increasingly impaired.

DIAGNOSIS AND TREATMENT

A diagnosis of Hodgkin's disease is usually made by performing a *biopsy* (removal of a sample of tissue for microscopic analysis) of an enlarged lymph node. The identification of characteristic cells, called Reed–Sternberg cells, in the biopsy confirm the diagnosis. The extent of the disease (its *stage*) can be assessed by chest X-ray, *CT scanning*, or *MRI* of the abdomen and a *bone marrow biopsy*.

If the disease is localized to a small area, treatment with *radiotherapy* is curative in many cases. If the disease has spread to involve many organs, long-term *chemotherapy* is necessary. In some cases, a *bone marrow transplant* may bring about prolonged remission. (See also *lymphoma, non-Hodgkin's*.)

hole in the heart

The common term for a *septal defect*.

holistic medicine

A form of therapy that treats the whole person rather than the specific disease symptoms. A holistic approach is emphasized by many practitioners of *complementary medicine*.

Holmes–Adie pupil

Also known as Adie's syndrome, a dilated *pupil*, usually only in one eye, that may be irregular in shape. The pupil does not respond, or may respond only very slowly, to bright light; in addition, it responds only partially when focusing on different distances. The condition, which is most common in young women, is of unknown cause and has no detrimental effects.

Holmes–Rahe questionnaire

A survey, devised in the 1960s, that is used to determine the comparative stress levels caused by certain common life events, such as the death of a partner, changes in financial or social circumstances, and serious illness.

Each potentially stressful event on the scale is allotted a specific score, with the death of a partner given the maximum (100) and the other stressors ranked in order of their scores. People undergoing the test select all of the stressful events that apply to them from the scale, then add together the scores for these stressors to determine their overall stress level.

Holter monitor

A wearable device used in *ambulatory electrocardiography* (ECG) to record the heart's electrical activity continuously for 24 hours or longer. The monitor records this activity by means of electrodes attached to the chest and allows the detection of intermittent *arrhythmias* (irregularities in the heartbeat).

Holt–Oram syndrome

A genetic disorder in which there is an atrial septal defect (a hole in the wall dividing the upper two heart chambers) together with various malformations of the upper limbs, particularly of the hands and forearms.

homeopathy

A system of *complementary medicine* that involves administering minute doses of a substance that in larger doses would be capable of inducing or worsening symptoms of the condition being treated.

homeostasis

The automatic processes by which the body maintains a constant internal environment despite changes within or outside it. Homeostasis is vital for the body, because tissues and organs can only function efficiently within a narrow range of conditions. The body regulates conditions such as temperature and acidity by means of negative *feedback*; for example, when the body overheats, *sweating* is stimulated until the temperature returns to normal. Homeostasis also involves the regulation of *blood pressure* and the levels of substances such as hormones and *glucose*.

homocystinuria

A rare, inherited condition caused by an *enzyme* deficiency. Homocystinuria is a type of inborn error of metabolism (see *metabolism, inborn errors of*) in which there is an abnormal presence of homocystine (an *amino acid*) in the blood and urine. People with homocystinuria may be very tall, with long limbs and fingers. Some have skeletal deformities and abnormalities of the eye *lens*. The condition is incurable, but it may be improved by a special diet.

homosexuality

Sexual attraction to people of the same sex. (See also *bisexuality; heterosexuality*.)

homozygote

A term used to describe a person whose cells contain two identical *alleles* (forms of a gene) controlling a specified inherited trait. The cells of a *heterozygote* contain two different alleles controlling that trait. (See also *inheritance; genetic disorders*.)

hookworm infestation

Infestation of the small intestine by small, round, bloodsucking worms of the NECATOR AMERICANUS or ANCYLOSTOMA DUODENALE species. Infestation with hookworm occurs mainly in tropical countries, particularly in areas where sanitation is poor or where human faeces is used to fertilize crops.

H

HOOKWORM LIFE-CYCLE

Infestation begins with larvae that penetrate the skin or are ingested and enter the bloodstream. They migrate throughout the body, particularly to the small intestine. Adult worms develop and lay eggs, which leave the body in faeces and eventually hatch into larvae.

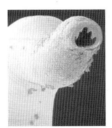

Head of hookworm
The hookworm uses its sharp, curved, tooth-like structures to cling to the bowel wall.

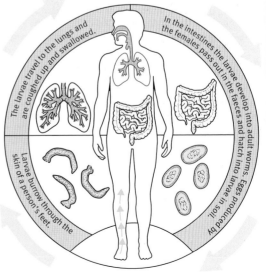

The larvae travel to the lungs and are coughed up and swallowed.

In the intestines the larvae develop into adult worms. Eggs produced by the females pass out in the faeces and hatch into larvae in soil.

Larvae burrow through the skin of a person's feet.

The worm larvae enter the body by penetrating the skin of the feet or by ingestion. They migrate through the body and mature into adults in the small intestine. Adult worms are about 12 mm long and have mouths with hooked teeth; they feed by attaching to the intestinal wall and sucking blood. The female worms lay eggs, which then pass out in the faeces.

When the larvae penetrate the skin, a red, itchy rash may develop on the feet. In light infestations, there may be no further symptoms. In heavier infestations, migration of the larvae through the lungs may produce coughing and, in some cases, *pneumonia*; adult worms in the intestines may cause abdominal discomfort. However, the most important problem of hookworm infestation is *anaemia* due to loss of blood.

Diagnosis is made by microscopic examination of the faeces for worm eggs. *Anthelmintic drugs* kill the worms. (See also *larva migrans*.)

hordeolum

The medical name for a *stye*.

hormonal contraception

See *contraception, hormonal methods of*.

hormonal disorders

Conditions caused by malfunction of an *endocrine gland*.

hormone

A hormone is a chemical messenger that is released into the bloodstream by a gland or tissue in order to have a specific effect on tissues elsewhere in the body, altering their activity. Hormones control a wide variety of body functions, including *metabolism* of cells, growth, sexual development, and the body's response to stress or illness.

Many hormones are produced by *endocrine glands*. The primary function of the major endocrine glands (the pituitary, thyroid, parathyroid, and adrenal glands and the pancreas, ovaries and testes) is the production of various hormones. Hormones are also secreted by other organs (see *Sources and effects of particular hormones* table, opposite), including the brain, kidneys, intestines, and, in pregnant women, the *placenta*.

hormone antagonist

A drug that is used to block the action of a *hormone*.

hormone replacement therapy (HRT)

COMMON DRUGS

OESTROGEN DRUGS	• Conjugated oestrogens • Estradiol • Estriol • Estrone • Estropipate
PROGESTOGEN DRUGS	• Dydrogesterone • Levonorgestrel • Medroxyprogesterone • Norethisterone • Norgestrel
OTHERS	• Tibolone

The use of a synthetic or natural *hormone* to treat a hormone deficiency. Most commonly, the term HRT refers to the use of female hormones to replace those lost after the *menopause*. This loss may occur naturally or as a result of treatment such as *radiotherapy* or the removal of the ovaries.

BENEFITS AND RISKS

HRT relieves symptoms of oestrogen withdrawal, particularly night sweats, *hot flushes*, and vaginal dryness. Minor adverse effects of HRT include nausea, breast tenderness, fluid retention, and leg cramps.

HRT for menopausal symptoms is given only for short-term use around the menopause. It is no longer recommended for long-term use because of the increased risk of developing disorders such as *breast cancer*, *stroke*, and *thromboembolism*; it may also increase the risk of *coronary artery disease*. The increased risk of breast cancer is related to the duration of HRT use; the risk reduces to its previous level within about five years of stopping HRT.

In the long term, HRT may give protection against *osteoporosis* (loss of bone density that can lead to fractures). However, it is now only used for this purpose in women who are unable to take other treatments, such as *bisphosphonate drugs*; when other treatments have been unsuccessful; or in women who have gone through a premature menopause (before the age of 40).

Whether or not HRT is appropriate depends on the individual woman concerned. Women who are considering HRT should consult their doctor, who will discuss their specific circumstances. Once it has been started, hormone replacement therapy should be reviewed regularly by a doctor.

TYPES OF HRT

In women with a uterus, HRT involves taking a continuous dose of an *oestrogen drug*, which is combined with an additional *progestogen drug* for 10 to 13 days of the 28-day cycle. The progestogen drug provokes bleeding which is similar to that of menstruation. This is necessary to prevent excessive thickening of the lining of the uterus and the risk of it becoming cancerous.

Alternatively, in cases in which more than one year has passed since the woman's last menstrual period, continuous bleed-free HRT, or a single drug with both oestrogenic and progestogenic effects (such as *tibolone*), can be used. Women who have had a *hysterectomy* need only take oestrogen drugs.

Oestrogen drugs can be administered in the form of tablets, skin patches, gels, or implants; progestogen drugs are administered as tablets, skin patches, or vaginal gel.

horn, cutaneous

A hard, noncancerous protrusion that can occasionally be found on the skin of elderly people. Caused by overgrowth of *keratin*, cutaneous horns vary in colour from yellow to brown or black. They may develop where there was previously a wart and may grow slowly. Left untreated, a cutaneous horn can grow considerably, and surgical removal may be advised.

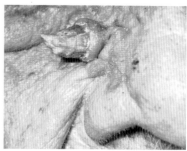

Appearance of cutaneous horn
The horny protuberance that has developed on this woman's face results from an overgrowth of keratin (a skin protein).

Horner's syndrome

A group of physical signs (such as narrowing of the eye pupil, drooping of the eyelid, and absence of *sweating*) affecting one side of the face that indicates damage to part of the sympathetic nervous system (see *autonomic nervous system*).

horseshoe kidney

A *congenital* abnormality in which the two kidneys are fused at the base, forming a so-called horseshoe shape. The joined kidneys usually function normally, but this condition may be associated with other kidney problems, such as urinary tract infection.

SOURCES AND EFFECTS OF PARTICULAR **HORMONES**

The various glands of the hormonal system constitute a control and communications network that is complementary to the nervous system. However, instead of using nerve impulses, the glands secrete chemical messages (in the form of hormones) to affect other glands and tissues in various parts of the body. Hormones are carried in the bloodstream to their targets, where they exert their specific effects. The table below lists the hormones that are secreted by different parts of the body and gives a description of their wide-ranging actions.

Gland or hormone-secreting tissue	Hormone secreted	Effects
Hypothalamus	Releasing or inhibiting hormones	Stimulate or suppress hormone secretion by pituitary gland
Pituitary gland	Growth hormone	Stimulates growth and metabolism
	Prolactin	Stimulates milk production after childbirth
	ACTH (adrenocorticotrophic hormone)	Stimulates hormone production by adrenal glands
	TSH (thyroid-stimulating hormone)	Stimulates hormone production by thyroid gland
	FSH (follicle-stimulating hormone); LH (luteinizing hormone)	Stimulate gonads (ovaries or testes)
	ADH (antidiuretic hormone)	Acts on kidneys to conserve water
	Oxytocin	Stimulates contractions of uterus during labour and milk let-down reflex in breast-feeding
	MSH (melanocyte-stimulating hormone)	Acts on skin to promote production of skin pigment (melanin)
Brain	Endorphins; enkephalins	Alleviate pain; boost mood
Thyroid gland	Thyroid hormones	Increase metabolic rate; affect growth
	Calcitonin	Lowers level of calcium in blood
Parathyroid glands	Parathyroid hormone	Increases level of calcium in blood
Thymus	Thymic hormone	Stimulates lymphocyte development
Heart	Atrial natriuretic factor	Lowers blood pressure
Adrenal glands	Adrenaline (epinephrine); noradrenaline (norepinephrine)	Prepare body for physical and mental stress
	Hydrocortisone	Affects metabolism
	Aldosterone	Regulates sodium and potassium excretion by kidneys
	Androgens	Affect growth and sex drive (in both males and females)
Kidneys	Renin	Regulates blood pressure
	Erythropoietin	Stimulates production of red blood cells
Pancreas	Insulin	Lowers blood sugar level
	Glucagon	Raises blood sugar level
Placenta	Chorionic gonadotrophin (HCG); oestrogens; progesterone	Maintain pregnancy
Gastrointestinal tract	Gastrin; secretin; cholecystokinin	Regulate secretion of some digestive enzymes
Testes	Testosterone	Affects development of male secondary sexual characteristics and genital organs
Ovaries	Oestrogens; progesterone	Affect development of female secondary sexual characteristics and genital organs; control menstrual cycle; maintain pregnancy

H

hospice

A hospital or part of a hospital devoted to the care of patients who are terminally ill (see *dying, care of the*).

hospitals, types of

Most of the hospitals in the UK are part of the National Health Service. Each NHS district has a general hospital providing services that include medicine, surgery, *gynaecology*, *obstetrics*, and *paediatrics*. Increasingly, more specialist services are concentrated in fewer centres. Many of the UK's private hospitals cater for non-emergency surgery, obstetric care, or inpatient care for the mentally ill.

host

In medical terminology, an organism, either animal (including human) or plant, in which a parasite lives for part or all of its life-cycle.

hot abscess

An *abscess* (a collection of pus) that is of relatively brief duration, but which causes severe, painful inflammation that is red, swollen, and hot to the touch. (See also *cold abscess*.)

hot flushes

Temporary reddening of the face, neck, and upper trunk that is accompanied by a sensation of heat and is often followed by *sweating*. Hot flushes are usually the result of decreased *oestrogen* production during or following the *menopause*, and they sometimes occur following the removal of the ovaries (see *oophorectomy*). If they are severe, hot flushes can often be alleviated by *hormone replacement therapy (HRT)*, but this is not advised in the long term. Alternatively, they can be treated with *clonidine*, an antihypertensive drug.

hot spot

An area of increased radionuclide uptake as seen on a *radionuclide scan*. A hot spot usually indicates an abnormal area in which there is increased activity in the tissue. The term may be used in relation to any radionuclide scan, but it is commonly applied to a bone scan in which the hot spot may indicate an abnormality such as an infection or a tumour.

house-dust mite

A microscopic organism commonly found in homes that may cause a variety of allergic reactions. Inhalation of dust containing the faeces of the house-dust mite is a common cause of *asthma*, *eczema*, and allergic rhinitis (see *rhinitis, allergic*) in susceptible people.

The mites are most abundant in warm, humid conditions. Effective control of mites involves lowering air humidity; increasing ventilation; and limiting the habitats of mite colonies by frequent and thorough cleaning of critical areas, including carpets, mattresses, and bed frames. Placing soft toys and furnishings in the freezer or tumble drier is another effective method of destroying the mites. (See also *mites and disease*.)

household poisons

Toxins that are commonly found and used in the home. Accidental *poisoning* with such chemicals accounts for about one in 50 of all serious domestic injuries. The most frequent victims are young children.

Swallowed household poisons commonly include cleaning products such as detergents, bleach, and stain removers; prescription and over-the-counter medicines (see *drug poisoning*); cosmetics, including nail varnish, perfumes, and skin lotions; paints, paint strippers, and varnishes; and rodent bait and insecticides. Powerful domestic chemicals, such as oven cleaner, can cause poisoning when absorbed through the skin.

Vapour from aerosol sprays and fumes from many cleaning and DIY products can be poisonous if they are inhaled, especially if they are concentrated in a confined space. Improperly maintained fuel-burning appliances, such as hot-water heaters, can produce *carbon monoxide*, a poisonous gas that is potentially fatal if inhaled.

All drugs, cleaning materials, and other household chemicals should be kept well out of the reach of children. Chimneys and flues, as well as heating systems and gas appliances, should be checked annually for carbon monoxide buildups. For extra protection, carbon monoxide alarms can also be fitted.

In the event of ingestion of a household poison, an ambulance should be called, the victim's breathing and pulse should be monitored continuously and emergency first aid given if necessary (see *rescue breathing*; *cardiopulmonary resuscitation*). Even if there are no symptoms, a doctor should always be consulted and given as much information as possible about the ingested substance. The victim should be given nothing to drink, and vomiting should not be induced unless trained medical personnel instruct otherwise.

housemaid's knee

Also known as prepatellar *bursitis*, inflammation of the fluid-filled sac that acts as a cushion over the kneecap.

HPV

The abbreviation for *human papillomavirus*.

HRT

See *hormone replacement therapy*.

5HT₁ agonists

Another name for *serotonin agonists*.

5HT₃ antagonists

Another name for *serotonin antagonists*.

HTLV

The abbreviation for *human T-cell lymphotropic virus*.

Hughes' syndrome

A potentially serious condition, also called antiphospholipid syndrome, that is characterized by an increased tendency for the blood to clot inside the blood vessels (see *thrombosis*). The syndrome is sometimes referred to as "sticky blood".

CAUSE
Hughes' syndrome is thought to be an *autoimmune disorder*, in which the immune system attacks fatty molecules called phospholipids, which are found throughout the body (particularly in cell membranes). The condition may occur alone or with another autoimmune disease, such as systemic *lupus erythematosus*. It is most common in women.

SYMPTOMS AND COMPLICATIONS
Thrombi (clots) may form in both arteries and veins anywhere in the body. The legs are most commonly affected (see *thrombosis, deep vein*). In the brain, a clot can cause areas of tissue to be starved of blood, leading to headaches, migraines, and memory loss. In the lungs, they can cause shortness of breath, chest pain, or coughing up blood. Other possible symptoms include dizziness or disturbances in balance; visual disturbances; and a pins-and-needles sensation. The blood vessels under the skin may also be affected, particularly on the wrists and knees, causing a red, lacy rash called *livedo reticularis*.

Clotting within an artery may lead to life-threatening complications such as *myocardial infarction* (heart attack), *pulmonary embolism*, *transient ischaemic attack*, or *stroke*. These disorders may occur at an unusually young age (under age 45). In pregnant women, clots may develop in the placenta, disrupting the blood supply to the fetus and causing *miscarriage*; affected women may have several consecutive miscarriages.

TREATMENT AND OUTLOOK
Hughes' syndrome is treated with drugs that reduce the tendency of the blood to clot: aspirin, heparin, or warfarin. Treatment is long-term or even lifelong, but greatly improves the outlook. It enables people to lead a completely normal life and, in women of childbearing age, drastically reduces the risk of miscarriage.

human chorionic gonadotrophin

See *gonadotrophin, human chorionic*.

human gamma-globulin

See *gamma-globulin*.

human genome

See *genome, human*.

human leukocyte antigen (HLA)

A protein that belongs to the group of proteins called *histocompatibility antigens*, which play a role in the *immune system*.

human papillomavirus (HPV)

A type of *virus* that is responsible for *warts* and *genital warts*. There are more than 100 strains of HPV, and infection with some of these strains is thought to be a causative factor in some cases of cervical cancer (see *cervix, cancer of*), oropharyngeal cancer (see *mouth cancer*), and anal cancer (see *anus, cancer of*). A vaccine has been developed that protects against the two strains of HPV associated with cervical cancer, and a vaccination programme is being introduced for girls aged 12 to 13.

human T-cell lymphotropic virus

A type of retrovirus, also called human T-cell leukaemia virus or HTLV. There are several types of HTLV, the most common of which is HTLV-1, which is endemic in tropical regions, including southern Japan, the Caribbean, South America, and West Africa. The virus can be transmitted by sexual contact, breast-feeding, a transfusion of contaminated blood, or by intravenous drug users who share contaminated needles.

SYMPTOMS AND TREATMENT
Most people infected with HTLV-1 have no symptoms, but a small proportion (less than one in 20) may develop serious disorders. One such disorder is the cancerous condition adult T-cell leukaemia, which may appear up to 20 years after infection. In this disease, there is

rapid and abnormal turnover of white blood cells in the bone marrow and of lymphoid tissue cells. Typically, the *lymph nodes*, *liver*, and *spleen* are enlarged. *Anticancer drugs* may halt the condition temporarily, but people tend to survive for only a few months to a few years.

Another condition associated with HTLV-1 is *myelopathy* (spinal cord disease). This condition causes pain in the lower back and legs, together with progressively worsening weakness of the legs and difficulty in walking.

humerus

The bone of the upper arm. The dome-shaped head of the bone lies at an angle to the shaft and fits into a socket in the *scapula* (shoulderblade) to form the *shoulder* joint. Below its head, the bone narrows to form a cylindrical shaft, which has a spiral groove housing the *radial nerve* (one of the main nerves in the arm, running from the shoulder to the hand). It flattens and widens at its lower end, forming a prominence on each side called an *epicondyle*. At its base, it articulates with the *ulna* and the *radius* (the bones of the forearm) to form the *elbow*.

humerus, fracture of

The *humerus* (upper-arm bone) is most commonly fractured at its neck (the upper end of the shaft, below the head), particularly in elderly people. Fractures of the shaft occur in adults of all ages. Fractures at the lower end of the humerus occur most commonly in children.

COMPLICATIONS
Certain complications may arise if the broken bone ends are displaced and damage surrounding tissues. A fracture in the shaft of the humerus can result in damage to the radial nerve; in severe cases, this damage may lead to wrist-drop. Fractures may also be associated with damage to the brachial artery, which runs down the inner side of the upper arm. If such damage goes undetected, the blood circulation to the forearm and hand may be impaired, resulting in a deformity called Volkmann's contracture.

Some supracondylar fractures (breaks just above the elbow) fail to heal properly despite treatment. As a result, the elbow may be deformed and there is an increased risk that *osteoarthritis* may subsequently develop in the joint.

DIAGNOSIS AND TREATMENT
An *X-ray* can show a fracture of the humerus. A fracture at the neck of the bone usually requires only a *sling* to

LOCATION OF **HUMERUS**

The humerus is the bone of the upper arm, located between the shoulder and elbow joints.

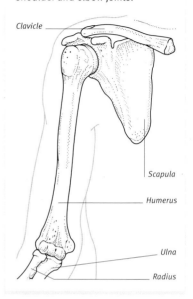

Clavicle

Scapula

Humerus

Ulna

Radius

immobilize the bone; a fracture of the shaft or lower bone normally needs a plaster *cast*. Most fractures of the humerus heal in six to eight weeks.

humoral immunity

A state of protection against disease that is brought about by the production of antibodies by the immune system to combat infection. In contrast, cellular immunity is the direct response of lymphocytes (a type of white blood cell) to infection and abnormal cells in the body.

humours

A term that describes any liquid or jelly-like substance in the body. The term usually refers to the *aqueous humour* and *vitreous humour* in the *eye*.

hunger

A disagreeable feeling caused by the need for food; it is different from *appetite*, which is a pleasurable sensation caused by the presence of food. Hunger occurs when the stomach is empty and the blood *glucose* level is low, which may occur several hours after the last meal or following strenuous exercise. In response to these stimuli, messages from the *hypothalamus* in the brain cause the muscular stomach wall to contract rhythmically; these contractions, if they

H

are pronounced enough, can produce hunger pains. Hunger can also occur in *thyrotoxicosis* (a disorder of the thyroid gland), and in *diabetes mellitus* when there is an incorrect balance between insulin and carbohydrate intake that causes abnormally low blood glucose levels (see *hypoglycaemia*).

Huntington's disease

An uncommon disease that causes degeneration of the *basal ganglia* (paired nerve cell clusters in the brain). The disease is due to a defective *gene* and is inherited in an autosomal dominant manner (see *genetic disorders*).

Symptoms of Huntington's disease do not usually appear until between about 35 and 50, although they can sometimes develop in childhood. The main symptoms are *chorea* (rapid, jerky, involuntary movements) and *dementia* (progressive mental impairment). The chorea usually affects the face, arms, and trunk, resulting in random grimaces and twitches, and clumsiness. Dementia takes the form of irritability, personality and behavioural changes (including outbursts of aggressive, antisocial behaviour), loss of memory (especially short-term memory), and apathy. The disease progresses slowly; affected people live for about ten to 20 years after the onset of symptoms.

At present, there is no cure for Huntington's disease and treatment is aimed at alleviating symptoms with drugs. Speech therapy and occupational therapy may also be of benefit. Genetic testing is available for people with family members affected by the condition. However, because there is no effective treatment for Huntington's disease, this may raise difficult ethical questions.

Hurler's syndrome

A rare, inherited condition caused by an *enzyme* defect. The syndrome is a type of inborn error of metabolism (see *metabolism, inborn errors of*) in which there is an abnormal accumulation of substances called mucopolysaccharides in the body tissues (see *mucopolysaccharidosis*).

Affected children may appear normal at birth; however, at six to 12 months of age, they develop cardiac abnormalities, umbilical *hernia*, skeletal deformities, and enlargement of the tongue, *liver*, and *spleen*. Growth is limited and mental development slows. If the condition is diagnosed in early infancy, a *bone marrow transplant* may be curative.

hyaline cartilage

The most common type of *cartilage*. Hyaline cartilage is also known as intra-articular cartilage. This type of cartilage is a smooth, tough, connective tissue that covers and protects the bone surfaces that are in contact with each other within a *joint*.

hyaline casts

Cylinders of semi-transparent matter that may be seen in urine viewed under a microscope. Hyaline casts are moulded in the same shape as the kidney tubules and are composed of protein derived from the breakdown of cells. Although they may be present in people with *kidney disease*, hyaline casts may also be a normal finding, particularly if an individual has exercised prior to giving the urine sample.

hyaline membrane disease

A lung condition affecting premature babies that is more commonly known as *respiratory distress syndrome*.

hyaluronic acid

A component of connective tissue and the fluid surrounding most joints (see *synovium*). Synthetic hyaluronic acid can be injected into joints affected by *osteoarthritis* and may help to relieve pain for up to six months.

hyaluronidase

A type of *enzyme* (a protein that regulates a chemical reaction in the body) that occurs naturally in the *testes*, the *spleen*, and certain other body tissues. Hyaluronidase increases tissue permeability and is used in pharmaceutical preparations to enhance the body's absorption of injected fluids.

HyCoSy

See *hysterocontrast sonography*.

hydatid disease

A rare infestation that is caused by the larval stage of the small tapeworm ECHINOCOCCUS GRANULOSUS (see *tapeworm infestation*). Tapeworm larvae usually

ORIGINS OF **HYDATID** DISEASE

The infestation is generally confined to dogs and sheep, but occasionally a child swallows eggs from dog faeces. The worm eggs hatch into larvae, which migrate through the body, especially to the liver or lungs, to form slow-growing cysts. Symptoms may not appear until years later.

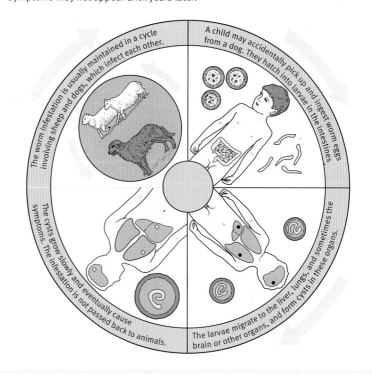

The worm infestation is usually maintained in a cycle involving sheep and dogs, which infect each other.

A child may accidentally pick up and ingest worm eggs from a dog. They hatch into larvae in the intestines

The larvae migrate to the liver, lungs, and sometimes the brain or other organs, and form cysts in these organs.

The cysts grow slowly and eventually cause symptoms. The infestation is not passed back to animals.

settle in the liver, lungs, or muscle, causing the development of cysts. In rare cases, the brain is affected.

The infestation is generally confined to dogs and sheep, but may be passed on to humans through accidental ingestion of worm eggs from materials contaminated with dog faeces.

SYMPTOMS, DIAGNOSIS, AND TREATMENT
The cysts grow slowly, and symptoms may not appear for some years. In many cases, there are no symptoms.

Cysts in the liver may cause a tender lump or lead to *bile duct obstruction* and *jaundice*. Cysts in the lungs may press on an airway and cause inflammation; rupture of a lung cyst may cause chest pain, the coughing up of blood, and wheezing. Cysts in the brain may cause *seizures*. Ruptured cysts may, rarely, cause *anaphylactic shock*, a severe allergic reaction that can be fatal.

Diagnosis of hydatid disease is by *CT scanning* or *MRI* (magnetic resonance imaging). The cysts are usually drained or removed surgically.

hydatidiform mole

An uncommon noncancerous tumour that develops from placental tissue early in a pregnancy in which the *embryo* has failed to develop normally. A hydatiform mole is thought to be the result of a chromosomal abnormality that occurs at conception. A pregnancy in which a hydatiform mole occurs is known as a *molar pregnancy*.

The mole, which resembles a bunch of grapes within the uterus, is caused by degeneration of the *chorionic villi* – minute, finger-like projections in the *placenta*. The cause of the degeneration is unknown. In a small number of affected pregnancies, the mole develops into a *choriocarcinoma*, a cancerous tumour that can invade the walls of the uterus if left untreated.

SYMPTOMS, DIAGNOSIS, AND TREATMENT
Vaginal bleeding and severe morning sickness generally occur in early pregnancy and the uterus may be larger than expected for the duration of the pregnancy. There is no viable fetus.

Diagnosis of a hydatiform mole is by *ultrasound scanning*, which will reveal the tumour, and urine and by blood tests to detect excessive amounts of human chorionic gonadotrophin, or HCG (see *gonadotrophin, human chorionic*), a hormone that is produced by the tumour. The mole is removed by emptying the uterus using suction. This procedure is carried out under general anaesthetic (see *anaesthesia, general*).

There is a small risk that the condition may occur in a subsequent pregnancy. Women who have had a hydatidiform mole should have their levels of HCG monitored for at least two years, and should not conceive again until their HCG levels have been normal for at least one year.

hydralazine

An *antihypertensive drug* that is used principally as an emergency treatment for *hypertension* (high blood pressure). Hydralazine may cause nausea, headache, dizziness, irregular heartbeat, loss of appetite, rash, and joint pain. Taken long term and in high doses, it may cause *lupus erythematosus*.

hydramnios

See *polyhydramnios*.

hydration

In medical terms, either the ingestion of water or the amount of water present in an individual or a tissue. (See also *dehydration*; *rehydration therapy*.)

hydrocele

A soft, painless swelling in the *scrotum* caused by the space around a *testis* filling with fluid. A hydrocele may be caused by inflammation, infection, or injury to the testis; occasionally, the cause is a tumour. More often, there is no apparent cause. Hydroceles commonly occur in middle-aged men, and treatment is rarely necessary. If the swelling is uncomfortable or painful, however, the fluid may be withdrawn through a needle. Recurrent swelling may be treated by surgery.

hydrocephalus

An excessive buildup of *cerebrospinal fluid* within the skull. The condition occurs either because too much cerebrospinal fluid is produced or because the fluid does not drain away normally. The excess fluid causes an increase in pressure within the skull, which may lead to brain damage.

Hydrocephalus may be *congenital* (present at birth), when it is often associated with other abnormalities, such as *spina bifida*. Or it may be a result of major *head injury*, brain *haemorrhage*, infection (such as *meningitis*), or tumour.

With congenital hydrocephalus, the main feature is an enlarged head that continues to grow rapidly. Other features

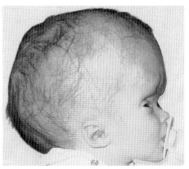

Baby with hydrocephalus
The skull enlargement is due to pressure from excess fluid within the cavities of the brain. To prevent brain damage, the fluid must be drained by means of a tube inserted into the skull.

H

include rigidity of the legs, vomiting, *epilepsy*, irritability, lethargy, and the absence of normal reflex actions. If it is not treated, hydrocephalus progresses to severe brain damage, which may result in death within weeks.

If hydrocephalus occurs later in life, when the skull bones have fused, the skull is unable to expand to accommodate the extra fluid. In this situation, the raised pressure within the skull causes symptoms including headache, vomiting, loss of coordination, and the deterioration of mental function.

In most cases, treatment of hydrocephalus involves a surgical procedure in which a tube called a shunt is inserted into the skull. This tube enables the fluid from the brain to drain into another part of the body, for example, the abdominal cavity, where it can be absorbed. In older children and adults, treatment is given for any underlying cause of the condition, such as a brain tumour.

hydrochloric acid

A strong acid released by the stomach lining. This acid forms part of the stomach juices and helps in the digestion of proteins. Excessive production of hydrochloric acid, which may be triggered by smoking or stress, can lead to irritation of the stomach lining, and is an important factor in the development of *peptic ulcers*. If the acid escapes from the stomach into the oesophagus (see *gastro-oesophageal reflux disease*), it can irritate the tissues, causing *oesophagitis* and *heartburn*.

hydrochlorothiazide

A thiazide *diuretic drug* used in various combined preparations to treat *hypertension* (high blood pressure) and also to reduce *oedema* (fluid retention) in people with *heart failure* or liver *cirrhosis*. Adverse effects include leg cramps, dizziness, rash, and *erectile dysfunction*. The drug may rarely cause *gout* and may aggravate *diabetes mellitus*.

hydrocortisone

Also called cortisol, a *hormone* produced naturally by the *adrenal glands*. Synthetic hydrocortisone is used as a *corticosteroid drug* to treat severe allergic conditions; for example, it is given by injection to treat *anaphylactic shock*. It is also used as a replacement treatment when the adrenal glands fail to function (see *Addison's disease*). Hydrocortisone is widely given in the form of a cream or ointment, to treat inflammatory skin conditions, such as heat rash, and is effective at reducing itching; however, used to excess, hydrocortisone creams may cause thinning of the skin, wrinkles or loss pigmentation.

hydrogen peroxide

A substance used as mild *antiseptic* solution or cream to treat infections of the skin or mouth, or used to bleach hair. Hydrogen peroxide combines with catalase, an enzyme present in the skin and mouth, to release oxygen. This reaction kills bacteria. Solutions used to treat the skin and mouth usually contain three per cent hydrogen peroxide; those used for bleaching hair are stronger. Occasionally, solutions containing hydrogen peroxide may irritate the skin.

hydronephrosis

A condition in which a *kidney* becomes swollen with urine due to an obstruction in the *urinary tract*. The excess urine causes pressure to build up inside the kidney and prevents it from functioning normally. Hydronephrosis may affect one or both kidneys.

In some cases, hydronephrosis may be due to a *congenital* narrowing of the *ureter*. In other cases, the obstruction of a ureter may be caused by a stone (see *calculus, urinary tract*), a *kidney tumour*, or a blood clot. Occasionally, hydronephrosis is caused by obstruction to the outflow of urine from the bladder by an enlarged prostate gland (see *prostate, enlarged*) in men, or by enlargement of the uterus in pregnant women. In such cases, both kidneys are affected.

Acute hydronephrosis, in which there is a sudden blockage of the ureter, causes severe pain in the abdomen and the small of the back. Chronic hydronephro-

sis, in which the obstruction develops slowly, may cause no symptoms until total blockage results in *kidney failure*. Hydronephrosis also increases the risk of kidney infection because bacteria can multiply more easily in stagnant urine.

Hydronephrosis can be diagnosed using X-rays (see *intravenous urography*), *CT scanning*, or *MRI* (techniques that produce cross-sectional or three-dimensional images of body structures). Following diagnosis, it is usually possible to relieve pressure by draining urine through a tube either directly onto the surface of the skin or by bypassing the blockage. Further treatment will then be needed to treat the cause of the blockage.

If the blockage can be removed surgically, the kidney is likely to function normally again. Occasionally, however, a kidney is so badly damaged that it requires removal (see *nephrectomy*).

hydrophobia

A popular term, now almost obsolete, for *rabies*.

hydrops

An abnormal accumulation of fluid in a body tissue (see *oedema*), cavity, or sac (a baglike body structure).

hydrops fetalis

Serious *oedema* (swelling of the body tissues) that occurs in a *fetus* before birth. Hydrops fetalis is often the result of rhesus incompatibility (see *haemolytic disease of the newborn*). In pregnant women who are affected by rhesus incompatibility, additional *ultrasound scanning* may be carried out to detect any swelling and help doctors to determine whether any treatment will be necessary for the fetus.

hydrotherapy

A form of *physiotherapy* in which exercises are performed in water to aid recovery from injury or to improve mobility. Hydrotherapy includes the use of exercise pools, whirlpool baths, and showers.

People who cannot bear their full body weight on a limb (such as people with arthritis or those who have fractured a limb) may undergo exercises in a hydrotherapy pool. The buoyancy of the water supports the person's body; in addition, the water provides gentle resistance that helps to improve muscle strength. Warm whirlpool baths can also provide a gentle massage to stimulate areas of the body and relieve stiffness.

hydrous ointment

An oil-and-water based greasy skin preparation that is used to treat dry or scaling skin conditions such as *eczema* and *psoriasis*. Hydrous ointment hydrates the affected area and can provide relief from itching.

hydroxocobalamin

A long-acting synthetic preparation of *vitamin B_{12}*. Hydroxocobalamin is given by injection to treat disorders involving vitamin B_{12} deficiency, particularly pernicious anaemia (see *anaemia, megaloblastic*), in which vitamin B_{12} cannot be absorbed from the intestines.

hydroxyapatite

A complex crystalline form of calcium phosphate that occurs naturally in the body as a major component of bones and teeth. A synthetic form of hydroxyapatite is used as a *calcium* supplement to reduce bone loss when the intake of dietary calcium is inadequate.

5-hydroxytryptamine

Another name for *serotonin*.

hydroxyzine

A sedating *antihistamine drug* used to relieve itching and, occasionally, in the treatment of *anxiety*.

hygiene

The science and practice of preserving health. The word "hygiene" is commonly used of personal cleanliness. It can also refer to *public health* – the scientific study of various environmental influences on health, such as safe sanitation and good housing. The terms "industrial hygiene" and "occupational hygiene" refer to the scientific discipline of assessing and regulating the work environment in order to prevent *occupational disease and injury*.

hygiene, oral

See *oral hygiene*.

hygroma, cystic

A *lymphangioma* (a type of noncancerous tumour) that occurs around the head and neck, the armpits, or the groin and contains clear fluid. Cystic hygromas are usually present from birth, reach their maximum size by the time the child is about two years old, then gradually disappear. The tumour may be surgically removed if it is obstructing the airway, but the final appearance is usually better if surgery can be avoided.

LOCATION OF **HYMEN**

The membrane that forms the hymen surrounds the opening to the vagina, inside a woman's labia minora.

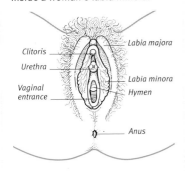

Clitoris
Urethra
Vaginal entrance
Labia majora
Labia minora
Hymen
Anus

hymen

The thin membrane around the vaginal opening. The hymen has a central perforation which is usually stretched or torn by the use of tampons or during first sexual intercourse.

Imperforate hymen is a rare condition in which the hymen has no perforation; as a result, at the onset of menstruation, menstrual blood collects in the *vagina*, causing lower abdominal pain. The condition is easily corrected by a minor operation.

hyoid

A small, U-shaped bone that is situated centrally in the upper part of the neck. The hyoid is not joined to any other bone but is suspended by ligaments from the base of the skull. It provides an anchor point for the muscles of the tongue and for the muscles of the upper front part of the neck. The hyoid may be fractured as a result of *strangulation*.

hyoscine

An *anticholinergic drug* prescribed in two distinct forms: hyoscine butylbromide, used to relieve the symptoms of *irritable bowel syndrome*, and hyoscine hydrobromide, used to control *motion sickness*. An injection of hyoscine hydrobromide may be given as part of a *premedication* because it dries secretions in the mouth and lungs. Possible adverse effects of both forms include a dry mouth, blurred vision, drowsiness, and constipation.

hyper-

A prefix that is placed before a word to mean "above", "excessive", or "greater than normal".

hyperacidity

A condition in which excess acid is produced by the *stomach*. Hyperacidity is often confused with *acid reflux* or *waterbrash*. It occurs in people who have a duodenal ulcer (see *peptic ulcer*) or *Zollinger–Ellison syndrome*.

hyperactivity

A behaviour pattern in which children are overactive and have difficulty in concentrating. The occasional occurrence of such behaviour in small children is considered to be normal. If a child exhibits persistent hyperactivity, however, and other possible causes (such as a stressful home environment or physical illness) have been eliminated, he or she may have a condition known as *attention deficit hyperactivity disorder (ADHD)*. Assessment by a paediatrician is needed before a decision on treatment is made.

hyperacusis

An excessively sensitive sense of hearing. In people who have hyperacusis, exposure to loud noises may cause pain or discomfort in the ears.

hyperaemia

Excess blood in part of the body. Hyperaemia can occur if the outflow of blood from an area is blocked. The condition more commonly arises due to an inflammatory reaction in which the flow of blood to a particular area increases; for example, around a wound or an insect bite. The skin over the affected area may be warm and red.

LOCATION OF **HYOID** BONE

The U-shaped hyoid bone provides an anchor for the muscles at the back of the tongue.

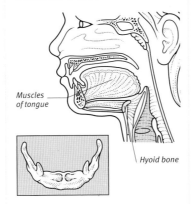

Muscles of tongue
Hyoid bone

hyperaesthesia

The medical term for an extreme sensitivity of the skin to normal stimuli, such as touch.

hyperaldosteronism

An alternative term for *aldosteronism*, a metabolic disorder caused by overproduction of the hormone *aldosterone* by the *adrenal glands*.

hyperalimentation

Administration of increased amounts of *nutrients*. Hyperalimentation is usually given intravenously or through a stomach tube (see *feeding, artificial*).

hyperbaric oxygen treatment

A procedure designed to increase the amount of *oxygen* in the tissues. This increase is achieved by placing a person in a special chamber and exposing him or her to oxygen at a much higher atmospheric pressure than normal.

Hyperbaric oxygen treatment is used to treat any condition in which the body tissues are deprived of oxygen. For example, it is used to treat *carbon monoxide* poisoning; in this condition, carbon monoxide attaches to *haemoglobin* (the oxygen-carrying pigment in red blood cells), preventing the blood from carrying sufficient oxygen to the tissues. The treatment is also used for people with *decompression sickness* due to activities such as diving. In addition, the treatment may be used for people who have suffered severe soft tissue injuries, such as deep *burns* and *crush injury*, in which *oedema* (a buildup of fluid in the tissues) hinders the passage of oxygen from the blood to the tissues.

Another use for hyperbaric oxygen treatment is to treat *gas gangrene*. This condition is caused by bacteria that thrive in an oxygen-free environment; the bacteria cannot survive once oxygen is supplied to the affected tissues.

hyperbilirubinaemia

A raised level of *bilirubin* (a breakdown product of red blood cells) in the blood. Mild hyperbilirubinaemia may be undetectable except by a blood test, but if the blood bilirubin rises to twice the normal level, *jaundice* develops.

hypercalcaemia

An abnormally high level of *calcium* in the blood. Hypercalcaemia may occur as a result of *hyperparathyroidism* (overproduction of parathyroid hormone, a

H

substance that normally helps to control the level of calcium in the blood). Cancer may also cause hypercalcaemia, either by spreading to the bones or by producing abnormal hormones that cause the bones to release calcium. Less commonly, the condition occurs as a result of intaking excessive amounts of *vitamin D* or of certain inflammatory disorders, such as *sarcoidosis*.

SYMPTOMS

Hypercalcaemia causes nausea, vomiting, lethargy, depression, thirst, and excessive urination. Higher blood levels of calcium produce confusion, extreme fatigue, and muscle weakness. If the disorder is left untreated and the calcium levels continue to rise, hypercalcaemia can be extremely serious, causing cardiac *arrhythmias* (irregularities of the heartbeat), *kidney failure*, *coma*, and may even lead to death.

Long-standing hypercalcaemia may cause *nephrocalcinosis* (calcification of the kidney) or kidney stones (see *calculus, urinary tract*).

DIAGNOSIS, AND TREATMENT

Diagnosis is by *blood tests* to measure the blood level of calcium and further tests to help reveal the cause. Treatment involves rehydration and, if necessary, reduction of dangerously high calcium levels with drugs such as *bisphosphonates* or *corticosteroids*. The underlying cause is also treated if possible.

hypercapnia

An excess of carbon dioxide in the blood. The condition is caused by failure of internal mechanisms, such as *breathing* rate, that normally control blood carbon dioxide levels. Hypercapnia leads to respiratory *acidosis*.

hypercholesterolaemia

A condition in which there is an increased concentration of *cholesterol* in the blood. Hypercholesterolaemia is thought to be associated with high levels of *low-density lipoprotein* (LDL) in the blood; the condition may be caused by a genetic defect in which there is a lack of LDL receptors, which remove cholesterol from the bloodstream. (See also *hyperlipidaemias*.)

hyperemesis

The medical term for excessive *vomiting*. Hyperemesis may cause dehydration and weight loss. The condition may occur during pregnancy, when it is known as hyperemesis gravidarum.

Unlike morning sickness, the vomiting is so severe that the affected woman cannot keep down any food or fluid. The cause is not known, but a contributing factor is thought to be an excess of the hormone *human chorionic gonadotrophin (HCG)*, which may be due to the existence of more than one fetus or to a *hydatidiform mole*. Stress may aggravate the symptoms. If left untreated, hyperemesis gravidarum may be life-threatening for the mother and fetus. (See also *vomiting in pregnancy*.)

hyperglycaemia

An abnormally high level of *glucose* in the blood that occurs in people with untreated or inadequately controlled *diabetes mellitus*. Hyperglycaemia may also occur in people with diabetes as a result of an infection, stress, or surgery.

Features of hyperglycaemia include the passing of large amounts of urine, thirst, *glycosuria* (glucose in the urine), and *ketosis* (accumulation in the body of organic substances called ketones). If it is severe, hyperglycaemia can lead to confusion and *coma*, which requires emergency treatment with *insulin* and *intravenous infusion* of fluids.

hypergonadism

Overactivity of the gonads (*testes* or *ovaries*) that results in overproduction of *androgen hormones* or *oestrogen hormones*. Hypergonadism may be caused by disorders of the gonads or a disorder of the *pituitary gland* that results in overproduction of *gonadotrophin hormones*. If hypergonadism develops during childhood, it results in premature sexual development (see *precocious puberty*) and excessive growth.

hyperhidrosis

The medical term for excessive *sweating*. It may be localized (affecting only the armpits, feet, palms, or face) or it may affect all areas with *sweat glands*. The condition may be caused by hot weather, exercise, or anxiety. In some cases it is due to an infection, *thyrotoxicosis*, *hypoglycaemia*, or a nervous system disorder. Usually, however, it has no known cause and begins at puberty, disappearing by the person's mid-20s or early 30s.

If hyperhidrosis is severe, persistent, and cannot be controlled by antiperspirants, injections of *botulinum toxin* into the skin may be used. In extreme cases, surgery may be considered to destroy the nerve centres that control sweating.

hyperkalaemia

Abnormally high blood levels of *potassium*, often due to failure of the kidneys to excrete it. Hyperkalaemia can lead to a fatal heart irregularity if severe.

hyperkeratosis

Thickening of the skin's outer layer due to an increased amount of *keratin*, a tough protein that is the major component of the outer skin layer. The most common forms of hyperkeratosis affect small, localized areas of skin and include *corns*, *calluses*, and *warts*. A rare, inherited form of the condition affects the whole of the soles and palms. The term "hyperkeratosis" may also be used to describe thickening of the nails.

hyperlipidaemias

A group of *metabolic disorders* that are characterized by high levels of *lipids* (fats) in the blood.

CAUSES

Some hyperlipidaemias are due to the inheritance of an abnormal *gene*. They may also be associated with another disorder, such as *hypothyroidism* (underactivity of the thyroid), *diabetes mellitus*, *kidney failure*, or *Cushing's syndrome* (high levels of corticosteroid hormones in the blood). Sometimes hyperlipidaemias may result from the use of *corticosteroid drugs*.

Hyperlipidaemias are classified according to which forms of lipids have elevated blood levels. Lipids are carried in the blood in several forms, principally *cholesterol* and *triglycerides* in the form of lipoproteins (lipids linked to proteins). Lipoproteins are classified according to their density, which depends on their relative proportions of cholesterol and protein: the higher the proportion of cholesterol, the lower the density of the lipoprotein. Elevated levels of *low-density lipoproteins* (LDLs) and very low-density lipoproteins (VLDLs) contribute to hyperlipidaemias. *High-density lipoproteins* (HDLs) are not involved.

RISKS AND SYMPTOMS

Hyperlipidaemias are associated with an increased risk of *atherosclerosis* (narrowing of the arteries as a result of fatty deposits) and *coronary artery disease*.

The symptoms depend on the particular type of hyperlipidaemia; they may include fatty yellow nodules in the skin on the back of the hands, on the tendons around the ankles and on the wrist joints; a white line around the rim of the *cornea*; and abdominal pain.

DIAGNOSIS AND TREATMENT

A diagnosis is made using *blood tests*. If hyperlipidaemia is confirmed, screening of close relatives and children of the affected person is also usually done.

Treatment is designed to reduce blood lipid levels, usually by means of weight loss, a low-fat diet, and *lipid-lowering drugs*. It is also very important to minimize any other risk factors for coronary artery disease, by stopping smoking, for example. With early medical treatment and, if necessary, appropriate lifestyle changes, the risk of a heart attack can be reduced. There is no known cure for inherited hyperlipidaemias. (See also *hypercholesterolaemia*.)

hypermagnesaemia

An abnormally high level of *magnesium* in the blood. The most common cause of hypermagnesaemia is *kidney failure*, although the condition may also be caused by excessive magnesium intake;

hypothyroidism (underactivity of the thyroid gland); *Addison's disease*; and it may be associated with *hypercalcaemia*. Hypermagnesaemia may lead to lethargy, weakness, and irregularities with the electrical activity of the heart. As levels of magnesium increase, the condition may result in *coma*. Treatment of hypermagnesaemia is of the underlying cause.

hypermetropia

Commonly known as longsightedness, hypermetropia is an error of *refraction* (the focusing of light rays within the eye) that initially causes difficulty in seeing near objects and goes on to affect distance vision. The condition tends to run in families.

Hypermetropia is caused by the eye being too short from front to back, which results in images not being clearly focused on the *retina*. This refractive error is present from birth, but symptoms do not generally appear until later

life because the focusing power of *accommodation*, which compensates for hypermetropia, declines with age.

Hypermetropia is corrected by wearing *glasses* or *contact lenses* with convex lenses, which reinforce focusing power.

hypernephroma

A type of *kidney cancer*, also known as renal cell carcinoma.

hyperparathyroidism

Overproduction of parathyroid hormone (PTH) by the *parathyroid glands*. Normally, PTH, together with *vitamin D* and another hormone called *calcitonin*, controls the level of *calcium* in the body. An excess of PTH raises the level of calcium in the blood (see *hypercalcaemia*) by removing calcium from bones. This effect can lead to bone disorders, such as *osteoporosis* (thinning of bones). In an attempt to bring the high calcium level back to normal, the kidneys excrete

H

HYPERPARATHYROIDISM

In this disorder, the parathyroid glands produce excessive amounts of parathyroid hormone. As a result of the hormone overproduction, there is an increased level of calcium in the blood and urine, a loss of cacium from the bones, and the

formation of calcium deposits (a condition known as calcinosis) in various tissues throughout the body. Surgical removal of abnormal parathyroid tissue is carried out to prevent complications from developing.

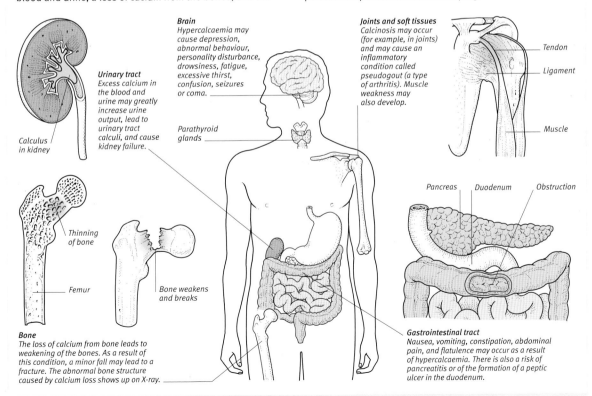

Calculus in kidney

Urinary tract
Excess calcium in the blood and urine may greatly increase urine output, lead to urinary tract calculi, and cause kidney failure.

Brain
Hypercalcaemia may cause depression, abnormal behaviour, personality disturbance, drowsiness, fatigue, excessive thirst, confusion, seizures or coma.

Parathyroid glands

Joints and soft tissues
Calcinosis may occur (for example, in joints) and may cause an inflammatory condition called pseudogout (a type of arthritis). Muscle weakness may also develop.

Tendon

Ligament

Muscle

Thinning of bone

Femur

Bone weakens and breaks

Pancreas   **Duodenum**   **Obstruction**

Bone
The loss of calcium from bone leads to weakening of the bones. As a result of this condition, a minor fall may lead to a fracture. The abnormal bone structure caused by calcium loss shows up on X-ray.

Gastrointestinal tract
Nausea, vomiting, constipation, abdominal pain, and flatulence may occur as a result of hypercalcaemia. There is also a risk of pancreatitis or of the formation of a peptic ulcer in the duodenum.

large amounts of calcium in the urine, which can lead to the formation of kidney stones (see *calculus, urinary tract*).

CAUSES

Hyperparathyroidism is most often caused by a small noncancerous tumour of one or more of the parathyroid glands, in which case it is known as primary hyperparathyroidism. This usually develops after the age of 40 and is twice as common in women as in men. Hyperparathyroidism may also occur when all the glands become enlarged for no known reason. It may also develop in response to a condition that causes abnormally low levels of calcium in the body, such as chronic *kidney failure*, in which case it is known as secondary hyperparathyroidism.

SYMPTOMS

Hyperparathyroidism may cause muscle aches and pains, depression, and pain in the abdomen. Often however, the only symptoms are those that are caused by kidney stones. If hypercalcaemia is severe, there may be nausea, tiredness, excessive urination, confusion, and muscle weakness.

DIAGNOSIS AND TREATMENT

The condition is diagnosed by *X-rays* of the hands and skull and by *blood tests* to measure levels of calcium and PTH. An *ultrasound scan* of the neck may also be performed to check for the presence of parathyroid tumours.

If the hyperparathyroidism is only mild, no treatment may be needed; instead, the affected person's blood calcium levels and kidney function will be monitored annually. More serious cases may need treatment with drugs to lower the blood calcium levels. If a parathyroid tumour is found, the affected gland will be surgically removed; this usually cures the condition. If the remaining tissue cannot produce enough PTH, treatment for *hypoparathyroidism* (underactivity of the parathyroid glands) is required.

hyperphosphataemia

An abnormally high level of *phosphates* in the blood. Hyperphosphataemia is usually caused by decreased phosphate excretion as a result of impaired kidney function or *kidney failure*. It may also be associated with *hypoparathyroidism* (underactivity of the parathyroid gland) or *hypocalcaemia* (low blood calcium levels). A side effect of hyperphosphataemia is the formation of calcium phosphate crystals in the blood and soft tissues. This can cause *arteriosclerosis*,

which may lead to *myocardial infarction* (heart attack) or *stroke*. Treatment is of the underlying cause.

hyperpigmentation

Abnormally dark coloration of the skin. Hyperpigmentation is usually seen in scar tissue and damaged areas of skin, such as in areas affected by *acne*. The condition results in permanent changes in skin colour and is more obvious in darker skin. Hyperpigmentation is also a feature of *Addison's disease*.

hyperplasia

Enlargement of an organ or tissue due to an increase in the number of its cells. However, unlike the cells of a tumour, the new cells are normal. Hyperplasia is usually the result of hormonal stimulation. It may occur normally (such as in the enlargement of breast tissue in pregnancy) or it may indicate a disorder. (See also *hypertrophy*.)

hyperplasia, gingival

Abnormal enlargement of the gums. Causes include *gingivitis* (inflammation of the gums), ill-fitting dentures, persistent breathing through the mouth, and taking the anticonvulsant drug *phenytoin*. Surgical treatment may be needed.

hyperpyrexia

A term used to refer to extremely high body temperature (see *hyperthermia*).

hypersensitivity

Overreaction of the *immune system* (defence against infection) to an *antigen* (a protein that is recognized as foreign). Hypersensitivity reactions occur only on second or subsequent exposures to particular antigens, after the first exposure has sensitized the immune system. Such reactions have the same mechanisms as those of protective *immunity*; however, while the latter may protect against disease, hypersensitivity reactions lead to tissue damage and disease.

There are four main types of hypersensitivity reaction.

TYPE I

Type I is associated with *allergy*. After first exposure to an antigen (which may be a harmless substance such as grass pollen), *antibodies* (substances that can recognize and bind to the antigen) are formed. These antibodies coat mast cells in various tissues. On second exposure, the antigen and antibodies combine, causing the mast cells to disintegrate and

release chemicals that cause the symptoms of *asthma*, allergic *rhinitis* (hay fever), *urticaria* (nettle rash), *anaphylactic shock* (a severe allergic reaction), or other allergic illnesses.

TYPE II

In type II reactions, antibodies bind to antigens on the surfaces of cells in particular tissues, leading to possible destruction of those cells. Type II reactions may lead to certain *autoimmune disorders* (in which antibodies attack the body's own tissues). They may also be responsible for some cases of *haemolysis* (destruction of red blood cells) triggered by certain drugs.

TYPE III

In type III reactions, antibodies combine with antigens to form particles known as immune complexes. These particles lodge in various tissues and activate further responses form the immune system, leading to tissue damage. This type of reaction is responsible for *serum sickness*, allergic *alveolitis* (a lung disease caused by exposure to the spores of certain fungi), and the large swellings that sometimes form after a person has a booster vaccination.

TYPE IV

In type IV reactions, sensitized *T-lymphocytes* (a class of white *blood cell*) bind to antigens and release chemicals known as lymphokines, which promote an inflammatory reaction. Type IV reactions are responsible for *contact dermatitis* and the rash that occurs in *measles*; they may also play a part in some "allergic" reactions to drugs.

TREATMENT

Treatment of hypersensitivity depends on the type, cause, and severity. When possible, exposure to the offending antigen should be avoided.

hypersplenism

Overactivity of the *spleen* that results in, and which is associated with, blood disease. One of the functions of the spleen is to break down *blood cells* as they age and wear out. An overactive spleen may begin to destroy cells regardless of their age and condition, causing a deficiency of any of the types of blood cell. In most cases, the spleen will also be enlarged.

If the condition occurs for no reason it is called primary hypersplenism. More commonly, however, it is secondary to another disorder, such as *Hodgkin's disease* or *malaria*, in which the spleen has become enlarged.

Signs of hypersplenism include *anaemia* and *thrombocytopenia* (deficiency of platelets). There may also be decreased resistance to infection. Primary hypersplenism is treated with *splenectomy* (removal of the spleen). Treatment of secondary hypersplenism is aimed at controlling the underlying cause.

hypertension

Persistently raised *blood pressure* (the pressure of blood in the main arteries). Blood pressure goes up temporarily as a normal response to stress and physical activity, and it rises naturally with increasing age and weight. A person with hypertension, however, has persistently high blood pressure even when at rest. Because the condition itself causes no symptoms, a large number of people have hypertension without realizing it; however, because hypertension causes the risk of developing serious cardiovascular disorders to increase, regular medical checks are advised in order to detect the condition at an early stage. Hypertension is very common, particularly in men, and its incidence is highest in the middle-aged and elderly.

Blood pressure is measured as two values, each expressed as millimetres (mm) of mercury (chemical symbol Hg) or mmHg. The systolic value (the higher value) is the pressure when blood surges into the aorta from the heart; the diastolic value is the pressure when the ventricles (lower chambers of the heart) relax between beats. A blood pressure consistently exceeding about 140 mmHg (systolic) and 90 mmHg (diastolic) at rest is defined as hypertension.

SYMPTOMS AND COMPLICATIONS
Hypertension is usually symptomless, and generally goes undiscovered until detected during a routine physical examination. However, if it is severe or accelerated (see *malignant hypertension*) it may cause headaches, breathlessness, and visual disturbances. The condition puts considerable strain on the heart and blood vessels, increasing the risk of *stroke*, *coronary artery disease*, and *heart failure*. Hypertension may eventually lead to kidney damage and *retinopathy* (damage to the retina at the back of the eye).

CAUSES
In many cases, there is no obvious cause, in which case the condition is called essential hypertension. Genetic factors are important, although hypertension is not attributed to a specific

HYPERTENSION

Hypertension (high blood pressure) affects 10 to 20 per cent of adults in the UK. It is diagnosed if a person's resting *blood pressure* is persistently raised. Blood pressure is expressed by two values – the systolic and diastolic pressures – and measured in millimetres of mercury.

Although hypertension rarely causes symptoms, it is a serious condition. It may cause excessive strain on the arteries. Left untreated, it increases the risk of stroke and other disorders. In most cases there is no obvious cause for hypertension, but in some people there is a specific cause, such as a kidney disorder, pregnancy, or the use of oral contraceptives. Hypertension is linked to obesity and, in some people, to a high salt intake. Smoking compounds the risks of the condition.

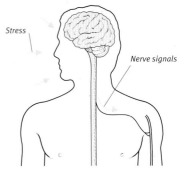

Stress and hypertension
Acute stress or pain act on the nervous system, causing blood vessels to constrict and the heart to work harder. Both lead to a brief rise in blood pressure. Hence, pressure should be measured when a person is relaxed. It is possible (but unproven) that frequent stress may eventually cause hypertension.

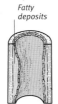

Atheroma
Hypertension and atherosclerosis, in which arteries are narrowed by fatty deposits called atheroma (left), are closely linked both to each other and to obesity.

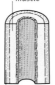

Constriction
Factors such as nicotine in tobacco cause constricted arteries (left) and a short-term rise in blood pressure that may worsen hypertension.

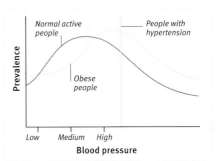

Variation in blood pressure
In any population, blood pressure varies over a wide range in the same way as height. Many people are considered to be hypertensive because they are at the top end of this range (see above). In obese people, the range is similarly wide but shifted towards the top end: hence, more obese people are hypertensive.

COMMON FACTORS AND PREVENTIVE MEASURES

Factors associated with essential hypertension	• Age (incidence higher in the elderly) • Family history of the condition • Gender (incidence higher in men than in women)
Factors that may aggravate hypertension	• Smoking • Obesity • Excess alcohol intake • Diabetes mellitus • High salt intake
Self-help and treatment	• Regular screening of blood pressure is important for early diagnosis and can help to prevent complications. • Sufferers from essential hypertension should: reduce weight; not smoke; reduce or stop alcohol intake; reduce salt intake; take regular exercise; learn relaxation. • Antihypertensive drugs, prescribed by a doctor, can usually keep high blood pressure under control.

gene. Other factors that are associated with hypertension include high alcohol intake, a high-salt diet, obesity, *diabetes mellitus*, a sedentary lifestyle, and smoking. There is also evidence that low birth weight increases the risk of developing hypertension in later life.

If hypertension results from a specific disorder, the condition is known as secondary hypertension. Causes include various *kidney* disorders; certain disorders of the *adrenal glands*; *pre-eclampsia* (a complication of pregnancy); *coarctation of the aorta* (a congenital heart defect); and the use of certain drugs. Taking the combined contraceptive pill (see *oral contraceptives*) can lead to hypertension in susceptible women.

DIAGNOSIS

The patient's blood pressure is measured at rest on several occasions in order to make a diagnosis. If there is any doubt, an ambulatory blood pressure device is fitted to monitor blood pressure over a 24-hour period. This may detect a condition known as white coat hypertension, in which blood pressure is raised during a test by a doctor but is otherwise normal and does not require treatment. The eyes may also be examined for evidence of longstanding hypertension. If hypertension is confirmed, other tests will be performed, both to investigate possible causes and to detect any early signs of complications or associated conditions, such as coronary artery disease. These tests may include *X-rays*, blood tests (including blood glucose and lipids), urine tests, and *ECG* (electrocardiography).

TREATMENT

With mild to moderate hypertension, if no underlying cause is found, lifestyle changes are recommended as the first line of treatment. For example, a low-fat, low-salt diet should be adopted; regular exercise should be taken; smokers should stop smoking; and drinkers should reduce their alcohol consumption. Anybody with hypertension who is overweight should try to lose weight by modifying the diet and introducing gradually increasing amounts of exercise into the daily routine. *Biofeedback training* and relaxation techniques can also help to reduce blood pressure.

If self-help measures have no effect, or if hypertension is severe, *antihypertensive drugs* may be given. There is a large range of drug treatments available and the treatment chosen depends on the presence of other disorders, such as

diabetes mellitus. The response of the condition to treatment, as well as any side effects it has provoked, may prompt a change of treatment. Usually, the patient is monitored by having regular blood pressure checks, so that adjustments to drug type or dosage can be made if necessary. It may be possible for the patient to monitor his or her own blood pressure at home, but the individual's machine should be checked regularly and calibrated against the doctor's machine.

In many cases, drug treatment must continue for life, but this may help to extend life expectancy significantly. (See also *intracranial hypertension, benign*; *portal hypertension*; *pulmonary hypertension*.)

hypertension, malignant

See *malignant hypertension*.

hypertensive arteriosclerosis

Thickening and loss of flexibility in the walls of arteries (see *arteriosclerosis*) as a result of persistent *hypertension* (high blood pressure).

hypertensive encephalopathy

A variety of symptoms, including headache, *seizures*, and loss of consciousness, caused by malignant, or accelerated, *hypertension* (high blood pressure). (See also *encephalopathy*.)

hypertensive retinopathy

Damage to the *retina* (the light-sensitive layer at the back of the eye) caused by persistent *hypertension* (high blood pressure) affecting the blood vessels in the eyes. Any changes visible in the retina reflect those occurring in small blood vessels throughout the body. Examination of the retina is therefore important in the assessment of hypertension. (See also *retinopathy*.)

hyperthermia

The medical term for very high body temperature.

hyperthermia, malignant

Also known as malignant hyperpyrexia, a sudden rise in body temperature to a dangerously high level, which is brought on by general anaesthesia (see *anaesthesia, general*). The condition is caused by exposure to inhaled anaesthetics or to the *muscle-relaxant drug* succinylcholine. In most cases, susceptibility to malignant hyperthermia is inherited, with an autosomal dominant pattern of inherit-

ance (see *genetic disorders*). People with certain muscle disorders may also be at risk. The condition is rare.

The patient's body temperature rises soon after the anaesthetic is given, sometimes as high as 42°C (107.6°F). At the same time, large amounts of *lactic acid* pass from the muscles into the blood, causing *acidosis* and possibly leading to kidney damage. There are signs of greatly increased *metabolism*, such as an increase in heart rate and breathing rate. The muscles stiffen and the patient turns blue (see *cyanosis*). Without emergency treatment, *seizures* and death may follow rapidly.

Malignant hyperthermia may be suspected if a patient does not relax normally in the early stages of anaesthesia. If it occurs, the anaesthetic is stopped immediately and the patient's body is cooled with ice-packs. Oxygen and repeated intravenous injections of dantrolene sodium are given until the patient's body temperature returns to normal. The patient will also receive care in an intensive care unit.

If a person is known to be susceptible to malignant hyperthermia, or has a family history of the condition, the anaesthetist must be informed before any surgical procedure, even if the patient has previously undergone general anaesthesia with no problems. The patient may be given dantrolene sodium before surgery to prevent hyperthermia.

hyperthyroidism

Production of excess *thyroid hormones* by an overactive *thyroid gland* (speeding up body functions). The most common form of hyperthyroidism is *Graves' disease*, which is an *autoimmune disorder*. Less commonly, hyperthyroidism is associated with enlarged nodules in the thyroid gland.

SYMPTOMS AND SIGNS

The characteristic signs of hyperthyroidism include increased appetite, weight loss, increased *sweating*, heat intolerance, rapid *heart rate*, and protruding eyes (in people with Graves' disease). In severe cases, the thyroid gland often becomes enlarged (see *goitre*) and there is physical and mental hyperactivity and muscle wasting (see *Symptoms and signs of hyperthyroidism* box, opposite).

DIAGNOSIS, TREATMENT, AND OUTLOOK

The diagnosis of hyperthyroidism is confirmed by measuring the level of thyroid hormones present in the blood. The condition can be treated with drugs

SYMPTOMS AND SIGNS OF **HYPERTHYROIDISM**

Hyperthyroidism (oversecretion of thyroid hormones) produces a range of symptoms associated with overactivity of the body's metabolism. Early signs of the condition include weight loss, increased appetite, intolerance to heat, and increased sweating; there may also be tremors and a rapid heart rate.

One form of the condition, called Graves' disease, may cause bulging eyes. In severe cases of hyperthyroidism, the thyroid gland is often enlarged, causing a visible swelling (goitre) in the neck, and there tends to be physical and mental hyperactivity and muscle wasting.

Protruding eyes
This symptom (known as exophthalmos) affects 30–50 per cent of people with Graves' disease.

Thyroid gland enlargement
This symptom (known as goitre) may be due to hyperthyroidism; however, it may also be associated with hypothyroidism (underactivity of the thyroid gland).

Muscle wasting
Severe hyperthyroidism may cause wasting of both skeletal and heart muscle.

Increased appetite
This symptom is a result of metabolic overactivity, causing increased energy use. Despite increased appetite, the affected person may lose weight.

HYPERTHYROID HEART RATE

Excessively high levels of thyroid hormones may speed up the heart rate and may also cause an irregular heart rhythm.

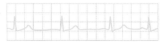

Healthy heartbeat
This diagram of an *ECG* trace shows a normal heart rate and rhythm.

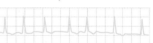

Hyperthyroid heartbeat
This trace shows the fast, irregular rate and rhythm seen in hyperthyroidism.

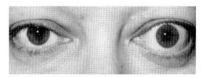

Appearance of exophthalmos
In people with Graves' disease, overactivity of the thyroid may cause swelling of the tissues around one or both eyes, resulting in a staring appearance.

H

---

that inhibit the production of thyroid hormones (see *antithyroid drugs*), by removing part of the thyroid gland, or by radioactive iodine to destroy part of the thyroid tissue.

Many people recover fully after treatment, but their hormone levels need to be monitored regularly so that any further abnormal changes can be detected and treated. Treatment with radioactive iodine may result in *hypothyroidism* (underactivity of the thyroid gland).

hypertonia

Increased rigidity in a muscle. Hypertonia may be caused by damage to the nerves supplying the muscle or by changes within the muscle itself. The condition causes episodes of continuous muscle spasm. Persistent hypertonia in limb muscles following a *stroke* or *head injury* leads to *spasticity*.

hypertonic solution

A fluid that is more concentrated than blood plasma or the fluid within cells. If a hypertonic solution is introduced into the body, water will pass from the cells

into the solution (see *osmosis*). If the solution is too concentrated, the body's cells may lose too much water. Fluids used for intravenous infusion are usually *isotonic* (having the same concentration as the fluids in cells); if they are being used to treat dehydration, infused fluids are mildly *hypotonic*.

hypertrichosis

Growth of excessive *hair*, all over the body, even in places that are not normally hairy. Hypertrichosis often occurs as a result of taking certain drugs (including *ciclosporin* and *minoxidil*). It may also be associated with *anorexia nervosa*. In addition, the term "hypertrichosis" is used to describe hair growth in a mole (see *naevus*).

Hypertrichosis is not the same as *hirsutism*, which is excessive hair growth (particularly in women) due to abnormal levels of male hormones.

hypertrophic cardiomyopathy

A disease of the heart muscle (see *cardiomyopathy*) in which the walls of the left *ventricle* (the heart's lower chamber)

become abnormally thickened, preventing the heart from pumping efficiently. This may lead to breathlessness, chest pain, and *palpitations*.

Hypertrophic cardiomyopathy is most commonly inherited, and it shows an autosomal dominant pattern of inheritance (see *genetic disorders*). Family members can be screened (see *familial screening*) by means of *echocardiography*, although the condition may not become apparent until after puberty. Hypertrophic cardiomyopathy is sometimes a cause of sudden death (see *death, sudden*) in young people.

Treatment is with *antiarrhythmic drugs* and, in some cases, an implantable defibrillator (see *defibrillation*).

hypertrophic pulmonary osteoarthropathy

A condition in which severe pain and swelling of the wrists and ankles is associated with *clubbing* of the ends of the fingers and toes. The most common cause of the condition is *lung cancer*. *X-rays* of the affected bones show new bone formation in the long bones near

H

the painful joints. Hypertrophic pulmonary osteoarthropathy may sometimes improve with treatment of the underlying lung cancer.

hypertrophy

Enlargement of an organ or tissue due to an increase in the size, rather than number, of its constituent cells. For example, skeletal muscles enlarge in response to increased physical demands. (See also *hyperplasia*.)

hyperuricaemia

An abnormally high level of *uric acid* in the blood. Hyperuricaemia may lead to *gout* due to the deposition of uric acid crystals in the joints; it may also cause kidney stones (see *calculus, urinary tract*) and collections of crystals in other body tissues (see *tophus*).

CAUSES

Hyperuricaemia may be caused by an inborn error of metabolism (see *metabolism, inborn errors of*), by the rapid destruction of cells in a disease such as *leukaemia*, or by any medication that reduces the excretion of uric acid by the kidneys, such as *diuretic drugs*. Large amounts of *purine* (a nitrogen-containing substance) in the diet may also cause hyperuricaemia.

TREATMENT

Drugs such as *allopurinol* or *sulfinpyrazone* may be prescribed for the duration of the patient's life. Purine-rich foods, such as liver, poultry, and dried pulses, should be avoided.

hyperventilation

The term used to describe abnormally deep or rapid breathing. Hyperventilation is usually caused by *anxiety*. It may also develop as a result of uncontrolled *diabetes mellitus* or *kidney failure*; oxygen deficiency; some lung disorders; or abuse of *stimulant drugs*.

Hyperventilation causes an abnormal loss of carbon dioxide from the blood, which can lead to an increase in blood alkalinity (see *alkalosis*). Symptoms of hylperventilation include numbness of the extremities, faintness, *tetany* (painful muscle cramps and twitches, especially in the hands and feet), and a sensation of not being able to take a full breath.

If the hyperventilation is due to anxiety, the affected person may find it helpful to breathe in and out of a paper bag. This action reduces the loss of carbon dioxide and may help to relieve the symptoms of alkalosis.

Controlled hyperventilation of patients, using mechanical *ventilators*, is often part of the treatment for *cerebral oedema* (swelling of the brain) after injury or surgery to the brain.

hypervigilance

A feature of *post-traumatic stress disorder*, hypervigilance is a continuously heightened state of arousal and an exaggerated startle reaction.

hypervitaminosis

Any condition caused by an excess intake of one or more *vitamins* (usually from unnecessary use of vitamin supplements). Hypervitaminosis is most likely to arise with *vitamin A* and *vitamin D* because excess amounts of these vitamins are stored in the body rather than excreted.

hyphaema

Blood in the front chamber of the *eye*, usually caused by an injury that ruptures a small blood vessel in the *iris* or *ciliary body*. Initially, there may be blurred vision, but the blood usually disappears completely within a few days and normal vision is restored.

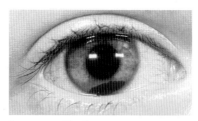

Appearance of hyphaema
Blood that has collected in the front chamber of the eye is clearly visible in front of the iris. This case, like most instances, was caused by injury.

hypnagogic

A term that refers to the state of transition between wakefulness and sleep. Hypnagogic images are vivid mental pictures that occur just before sleep. Distressing hypnagogic hallucinations may feature in *narcolepsy* (a sleep disorder).

hypnosis

A trance-like state of altered awareness characterized by extreme suggestibility. Some psychoanalysts induce a hypnotic state as a means of helping patients remember and come to terms with disturbing events. More often, hypnosis is used to help patients to relax. It may be useful in people suffering from *anxiety*, *panic attacks*, or *phobias*, or in those wishing to correct addictive habits.

hypnotherapy

The use of *hypnosis* as part of a psychological therapy.

hypnotic drugs

A term sometimes used for drugs that induce sleep (see *sleeping drugs*).

hypo-

A prefix meaning "under", "below", or "less than normal".

hypoaldosteronism

A rare condition that is characterized by a deficiency of the hormone *aldosterone*, which is produced by the *adrenal glands*. The condition may be caused by damage or disease affecting the adrenal glands. It may occur in *Addison's disease*, in which the adrenal glands are damaged, often as a result of an autoimmune process. Hypoaldosteronism may produce muscle weakness. It is treated by the drug fludrocortisone.

hypocalcaemia

An abnormally low level of *calcium* in the blood. The most common cause is *vitamin D* deficiency. More unusual causes include chronic *kidney failure* and *hypoparathyroidism* (underactivity of the parathyroid glands).

In mild cases, hypocalcaemia is symptomless; in severe cases, it leads to *tetany* (painful muscle spasms and twitches, especially in the hands and feet). It may also result in bone softening, causing *rickets* in children and *osteomalacia* in adults.

hypocapnia

Abnormally low *carbon dioxide* levels in the blood. Hypocapnia may be caused by *hyperventilation* (abnormally deep or rapid breathing); it can result in a pins-and-needles sensation and painful muscle cramps and spasms.

hypochondriasis

A disorder that is characterized by a person's unrealistic belief that he or she is suffering from a serious illness, despite medical reassurance to the contrary. In its mildest form, hypochondriasis causes people to worry constantly about their health and interpret any symptom, however trivial, as evidence of disease. In its most severe form, hypochondriasis may dominate the person's life; he or she may constantly seek medical advice and may undergo numerous tests and treatments for disease.

The likelihood of hypochondriasis is increased in people who have had past experience of a serious disorder (particularly during childhood) or have seen such disorders in relatives. Other predisposing factors include social stresses and personality type. Hypochondriasis may also be a complication of other psychological disorders such as *phobia*, *obsessive–compulsive disorder*, *generalized anxiety disorder*, and brain diseases such as *dementia*.

Where possible, treatment is of the underlying mental health problem. Hypochondriasis without an identifiable underlying cause is difficult to treat.

hypochondrium

The area on each side of the upper abdomen, below the lower ribs.

hypodermic

A term that means "under the skin". The word is usually used to describe injections that are delivered into the layer of fat beneath the skin, as well as for the needles and syringes used to administer these injections.

hypogammaglobulinaemia

An abnormally low blood level of *immunoglobulins* (proteins that are produced by immune system cells to fight infection; also called antibodies) that belong to the group called *gammaglobulins*. Hypogammaglobulinaemia is associated with an increased susceptibility to infections. The condition may be either inherited or acquired.

Inherited hypogammaglobulinaemia is an X-linked disorder (see *genetic disorders*) that results in susceptibility to infections from approximately three to six months of age. This condition requires repeated treatment with intravenous immunoglobulin.

There are several types of acquired hypogammaglobulinaemia. Common variable hypogammaglobulinaemia may appear during childhood or it may occur later in adult life; it requires regular immunoglobulin replacement therapy. Immunoglobulin A (IgA) deficiency is a very common form of hypogammaglobulinaemia that may produce no symptoms and may carry no heightened risk of infection. Secondary hypogammaglobulinaemia occurs in association with a number of other diseases, including *multiple myeloma* and chronic lymphocytic leukaemia (see *leukaemia, chronic lymphocytic*).

hypoglossal nerve

The 12th *cranial nerve*, which controls movement of the tongue.

LOCATION OF HYPOGLOSSAL NERVE

The hypoglossal nerve arises in the medulla oblongata (part of the brainstem), passes through the base of the skull, and runs around the throat to the tongue.

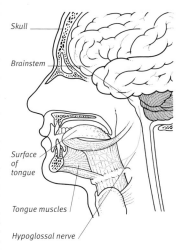

Skull

Brainstem

Surface of tongue

Tongue muscles

Hypoglossal nerve

hypoglycaemia

An abnormally low level of *glucose* in the blood. Almost all cases of hypoglycaemia occur in people with Type 1 *diabetes mellitus*, in whom the *pancreas* fails to produce enough *insulin*, resulting in an abnormally high glucose level. To lower the level, insulin is given. Too high a dose of insulin can reduce the blood glucose to an excessively low level. Hypoglycaemia can also occur if a diabetic person misses a meal or takes strenuous exercise.

Less commonly, the condition may occur in people with Type 2 diabetes mellitus (in which body cells are resistant to the effects of insulin). Rarely, the condition can result from drinking too much alcohol or from an insulin-producing pancreatic tumour.

Symptoms include *sweating*, hunger, dizziness, trembling, headache, *palpitations*, confusion, and sometimes double vision. The person's behaviour is often irrational and aggressive. *Coma* may occur in severe cases. Hypoglycaemia may also be the cause of seizures and jittery behaviour in newborn babies (see *neonatal hypoglycaemia*).

At the first sign of a hypoglycaemic attack, an affected person should consume a sugary food or drink. If the person has lost consciousness, emergency medical help is required; the patient must receive an injection of glucose solution or the hormone glucagon. (See also *reactive hypoglycaemia*.)

hypoglycaemics, oral
COMMON DRUGS

SULPHONYLUREA DRUGS •Chlorpropamide •Glibenclamide •Gliclazide •Glimepiride •Glipizide •Gliquidone •Tolbutamide
OTHERS •Acarbose •Metformin •Pioglitazone •Repaglinide •Rosiglitazone

A group of *antidiabetic drugs* that are used to reduce the level of glucose in the blood of an individual with type 2 *diabetes mellitus*.

Oral hypoglycaemics have many different modes of action. Sulphonylurea drugs act by increasing the body's *insulin* production. *Metformin* increases the uptake of glucose into body tissues and increases its use by the body, thereby helping to reduce blood glucose levels. Other oral hypoglycaemics work in a variety of ways. For example, *acarbose* reduces or slows the absorption of carbohydrate from the intestines after meals; *repaglinide* stimulates the release of insulin from the pancreas; and *rosiglitazone* and *pioglitazone* reduce resistance to the effects of insulin in the tissues.

Too high a dose of hypoglycaemic drugs may provoke the onset of *hypoglycaemia* (abnormally low blood sugar levels), causing symptoms such as dizziness, nausea, and sweating. The use of metformin or acarbose does not usually result in this condition.

hypogonadism

Underactivity of the gonads (*testes* or *ovaries*). Hypogonadism may be caused by disorders of the gonads or a disorder of the *pituitary gland* that causes deficient production of *gonadotrophin hormones*. In men, hypogonadism causes the symptoms and signs of *androgen hormone* deficiency; in women, it causes those of *oestrogen* deficiency.

hypohidrosis

Reduced activity of the *sweat glands*. Hypohidrosis is a feature of hypohidrotic ectodermal dysplasia, a rare, inherited, incurable condition that is characterized by reduced sweating and is accompanied

H

by dry, wrinkled skin, sparse hair, small, brittle nails, and conical teeth. Other causes of hypohidrosis include *exfoliative dermatitis* and some *anticholinergic drugs*.

hypokalaemia

A deficiency of *potassium* in the blood. Hypokalaemia is usually caused by excess fluid loss due, for example, to severe diarrhoea, but may be the result of treatment with *diuretic drugs*.

hypomagnesaemia

An abnormally low level of *magnesium* in the blood. Hypomagnesaemia may result from malabsorption, malnutrition, alcohol abuse (see *alcohol-related disorders*), severe diarrhoea, or some *kidney* diseases. Magnesium deficiency causes impaired nerve and muscle function and may lead to *seizures*. Treatment of hypomagnesaemia is by injection of magnesium salts.

hypomania

A mild degree of *mania*.

hypoparathyroidism

Insufficient production of *parathyroid hormone* by the *parathyroid glands*. A deficiency of this hormone results in low levels of *calcium* in the blood (see *hypocalcaemia*).

The most common cause of hypoparathyroidism is damage to the parathyroid glands during surgery. Occasionally, the glands are absent from birth or may cease to function for no apparent reason.

A low level of calcium in the blood may lead to *tetany* (increased excitability of the nerves, causing uncontrollable, painful, cramplike spasms, especially in the hands and feet). Occasionally, *seizures* similar to those of an epileptic attack may occur.

The condition is diagnosed by *blood tests*. To relieve an attack of tetany, calcium may be injected slowly into a vein. To maintain the blood calcium at a normal level, a lifelong course of calcium and *vitamin D* tablets is necessary.

hypophosphataemia

An abnormally low level of *phosphates* in the blood. Hypophosphataemia may be associated with *hyperparathyroidism*, *osteomalacia*, *rickets*, and certain kidney abnormalities, such as *Fanconi's syndrome*. It may cause symptoms such as fatigue, muscle weakness, *haemolysis* (premature breakdown of red blood cells), confusion, and *seizures*. Treatment

of hypophosphataemia involves replacement of phosphates and, if possible, treatment of the underlying cause.

hypophysectomy

The surgical removal or destruction (by radiotherapy) of the *pituitary gland*. Hypophysectomy may be performed to treat a *pituitary tumour*. Lifelong hormone treatment is necessary following hypophysectomy because *hypopituitarism* is an inevitable result.

hypopigmentation

A lack or absence of normal colour in the skin. The condition is due to underproduction of *melanin*, the brown pigment in skin, hair, and eyes. It may be the result of inflammation, scarring, or the skin condition *vitiligo*.

hypopituitarism

Underactivity of the *pituitary gland*, resulting in inadequate production of one or more pituitary *hormones*. The effects depend on which hormones are affected. Possible causes are a *pituitary tumour*, an abnormality affecting the *hypothalamus* (part of the brain), or injury to the pituitary gland. Hypopituitarism may also follow surgery or radiotherapy of the pituitary gland (see *hypophysectomy*). Treatment involves replacing the deficient hormones.

hypoplasia

The failure of an organ or a body tissue to develop fully and to reach its normal adult size.

hypoplasia, enamel

A defect in tooth enamel (see *enamel, dental*), sometimes due to *amelogenesis imperfecta*. It may also be caused by vitamin deficiency, injury, or infection of a primary tooth that interferes with enamel maturation.

hypoplastic left-heart syndrome

A very serious form of congenital heart disease (see *heart disease, congenital*), in which a baby is born with a poorly formed left *ventricle* (lower heart chamber), often associated with other heart defects. The *aorta* is malformed and blood can reach it only via a duct (the ductus arteriosus) that links the aorta to the pulmonary artery.

At birth, the baby may seem healthy. However, within a day or two the ductus arteriosus naturally closes off, as a result of which the baby becomes pale

and breathless and collapses. Hypoplastic left-heart syndrome can be treated surgically, sometimes by heart transplant.

hyposensitization

A preventive treatment of *allergy* to specific substances, such as grass pollens and insect venom. Hyposensitization involves giving gradually increasing doses of the allergen (substance to which the person is allergic) so that the *immune system* becomes less sensitive to that substance. The treatment may need to be repeated annually for a few years. Increasing concerns about the risk of *anaphylactic shock*, which may be life-threatening, have severely restricted the use of hyposensitization.

hypospadias

A *congenital* defect of the *penis*, in which the opening of the *urethra* is on the underside of the *glans* (head of the penis) or shaft. In some cases, the penis curves downwards, a condition that is known as *chordee*. Hypospadias can usually be corrected by surgery.

hyposplenism

A condition characterized by diminished functioning of the *spleen*. If the spleen suffers a loss of function, there is a resultant reduction in production of the *antibodies*, *lymphocytes*, and *phagocytes* that act to destroy invading microorganisms. Hyposplenism therefore results in increased susceptibility to certain severe infections. Those people whose spleen has been removed (see *splenectomy*) or is failing to function normally are advised to have pneumococcal immunization and long-term *antibiotic drugs*.

hypostasis

The pooling of blood in the lowest areas of limbs or organs, due to gravity. Hypostasis usually occurs as a result of poor circulation. The condition also occurs after death, when blood settles in the parts of the body that were lowest at the time of death.

hypotension

The medical term for low *blood pressure*. In its most common form, known as postural hypotension, symptoms occur when a person abruptly stands or sits up. Normally, blood pressure is maintained with changes in posture; in people with postural hypotension, it falls. Postural hypotension may be a side effect of *antidepressant drugs* or *antihypertensive drugs*.

HYPOPLASTIC LEFT-HEART SYNDROME

The heart defects associated with this syndrome are shown on the right and compared with those of the normal heart, on the left. Neither the left ventricle (pumping chamber) nor the aorta is properly formed.

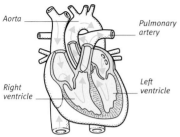

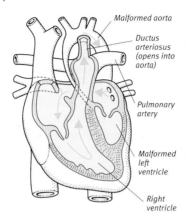

Aorta

Pulmonary artery

Right ventricle

Left ventricle

Malformed aorta

Ductus arteriosus (opens into aorta)

Pulmonary artery

Malformed left ventricle

Right ventricle

Defect of the heart
In a normal heart, blood is pumped by the left ventricle to the body via the aorta. If the left ventricle is poorly formed, blood can reach the body only via the ductus arteriosus, which closes soon after birth.

It may also occur in people with *diabetes mellitus*. Acute hypotension is a feature of *shock*, and may be caused by serious injury or a disease such as *myocardial infarction* (heart attack) or *adrenal failure*.

Treatment depends on the cause. In the absence of serious disease, low blood pressure is associated with a decreased risk from *cardiovascular disorders* and *stroke*. Symptomless hypotension does not require treatment.

hypothalamus

A region of the *brain*, roughly the size of a cherry, situated behind the eyes and under another area of the brain called the thalamus. The hypothalamus has nerve connections to most other regions of the nervous system and plays a role in regulating many body functions.

FUNCTION

The hypothalamus controls the sympathetic nervous system (part of the *autonomic nervous system*). In response to sudden alarm or excitement, signals are sent from higher regions of the brain to the hypothalamus, initiating sympathetic nervous system activity. This causes a faster *heartbeat*, widening of the pupils, an increase in breathing rate and blood flow to muscles (which collectively are known as the "fight or flight" response).

Other groups of nerve cells in the hypothalamus are concerned with the control of body temperature. When blood flowing to the brain is hotter or cooler than normal, the hypothalamus switches on mechanisms that regulate body temperature (including sweating and shivering). It receives information from internal sense organs regarding the body's water content and the level of glucose in the blood; if these are too low, the hypothalamus stimulates thirst and appetite for food (see *feedback mechanism*). The hypothalamus is also involved in regulating sleep, motivating sexual behaviour, and determining mood and emotions.

LOCATION OF THE HYPOTHALAMUS

This small area of the forebrain is situated under the thalamus and above the pituitary gland.

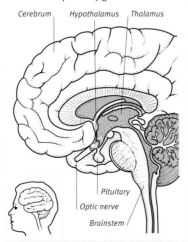

Cerebrum *Hypothalamus* *Thalamus*

Pituitary

Optic nerve

Brainstem

A further role of the hypothalamus is to coordinate the functions of the nervous and endocrine (hormonal) systems. The area connects with the *pituitary gland* through a short stalk of nerve fibres and controls hormonal secretions from this gland. One form of control is through direct nerve connections. The other is through specialized nerve cells, which secrete hormones called releasing factors; these enter specialized blood vessels and pass to the pituitary gland. In this way, the hypothalamus converts nerve signals into hormonal signals; therefore, it indirectly controls many *endocrine glands*, including the *thyroid gland*; the cortex of the *adrenal glands*; and the *ovaries* or *testes*.

DISORDERS

Disorders of the hypothalamus are usually due to an *intracerebral haemorrhage* or a hypothalmic or *pituitary tumour*. They have diverse effects, ranging from hormonal disorders to disturbances in temperature regulation, and increased or decreased need for food and sleep.

hypothermia

A fall in body temperature to below 35°C. Hypothermia most often occurs in sick, elderly people who are exposed to low temperatures. The body loses its sensitivity to cold as it ages, becoming less able to reverse a fall in temperature. Hypothyroidism (underactivity of the thyroid gland) also predisposes an individual to hypothermia. Babies may also have an increased risk of hypothermia because they lose heat rapidly and cannot easily reverse a fall in temperature. The condition is also common in climbers and walkers who are inadequately dressed for cold weather.

SYMPTOMS AND SIGNS

A person suffering from hypothermia is usually pale and listless. The *heart rate* is slow, the body is cold, and the victim is often drowsy and confused. In severe hypothermia, breathing becomes slow and shallow, the muscles are stiff, the victim may become unconscious, and may actually appear dead. Eventually, the heart may stop beating.

TREATMENT

Hypothermia is a medical emergency and requires hospital admission. In most cases, it can be prevented by self-help measures such as dressing warmly and keeping moving in cold weather. Most people with hypothermia make a full recovery; the outlook is best for young, otherwise healthy people.

H

hypothermia, surgical

The deliberate reduction of body temperature to prolong the period for which the vital organs can safely be deprived of their normal blood supply during *open heart surgery*. Cold reduces the rate of metabolism in tissues and thus increases their tolerance to lack of oxygen. Cooling may be achieved by continuously instilling cold saline at about 4°C into the open chest cavity.

hypothyroidism

The underproduction of *thyroid hormones* due to underactivity of the *thyroid gland*. These hormones are important in *metabolism* and a deficiency therefore causes many of the body's functions to slow down. Most cases of hypothyroidism are caused by an *autoimmune disorder* (a disorder in which the immune system attacks the body's own tissues) such as *Hashimoto's thyroiditis*. Hypothyroidism may also result from removal of part of the thyroid gland to treat *hyperthyroidism* (overactivity of the thyroid gland). In rare cases, babies are born with an underactive thyroid gland (congenital hypothyroidism).

SYMPTOMS AND SIGNS

In adults, symptoms include tiredness, lethargy, cold intolerance, muscle weakness, cramps, a slow heart rate, dry skin, hair loss, constipation, a deep and husky voice, and weight gain. Women may also experience heavy menstrual periods. A syndrome called *myxoedema*, in which the skin and other tissues thicken, may develop. Enlargement of the thyroid gland may also occur (see *goitre*). Babies with congenital hypothyroidism may have feeding difficulties, constipation, jaundice (see *jaundice, neonatal*), and excessive sleepiness.

DIAGNOSIS AND TREATMENT

Hypothyroidism is diagnosed by measuring the level of thyroid hormones in the blood. Babies are screened for the condition shortly after birth as part of the *blood spot screening tests*.

In all cases, treatment consists of replacement therapy with the thyroid hormone *thyroxine*, usually for life. Hormone treatment is monitored regularly so that the correct dosage is maintained.

hypotonia

Abnormal *muscle* slackness. Normally, a muscle that is not being used has a certain inbuilt tension, but in a number of disorders affecting the nervous system this natural tension is reduced.

hypotonia in infants

Also known as floppy infant syndrome, excessive limpness in infants. Hypotonic babies cannot hold their limbs up against gravity and therefore tend to lie flat with their arms and legs splayed.

Hypotonia may be caused by *Down's syndrome* or *hypothyroidism* (underproduction of thyroid hormones) and may be an early feature of *cerebral palsy*. It occurs in disorders of the spinal cord, such as *Werdnig–Hoffman disease*, and in some children with *muscular dystrophy*.

hypotonic solution

A fluid that is less concentrated than blood plasma or the fluid within cells. If a hypotonic solution is introduced into the body, the water in the fluid will pass through cell walls and into the cells (see *osmosis*). If the solution is too weak (for example, if it is pure water), the body's cells will become overfilled with water and will rupture. Fluids used for intravenous infusion are *isotonic* (having the same concentration as the fluids in cells), except when they are being used to treat dehydration, in which case they are mildly hypotonic. (See also *hypertonic solution*.)

hypoventilation

A condition in which too little air enters the alveoli (tiny air sacs) in the lungs. Hypoventilation is due to breathing that is too shallow or slow, or to a reduction in lung function (for example, from a disorder such as *emphysema*). The inadequate air supply leads to insufficient oxygen passing from the alveoli into the bloodstream (see *respiration*), and as a result, too little oxygen reaches the body tissues (see *hypoxia*) and carbon dioxide builds up.

hypovitaminosis

A general term for any condition that results from the deficiency of one or more *vitamins*. Hypovitaminosis may be due to an inadequate dietary intake of vitamins or to a digestive disorder that causes *malabsorption*.

hypovolaemia

An abnormally low volume of blood in the circulation. Hypovolaemia is most commonly the result of blood loss due to injury, internal bleeding, or surgery but it may also occur as a result of loss of fluid from *diarrhoea* and *vomiting*. Without treatment, hypovolaemia can lead to *shock*.

hypoxaemia

An abnormally low level of oxygen in the arterial blood (the blood that carries oxygen to the body tissues). This condition may lead to *hypoxia*.

hypoxia

An inadequate supply of *oxygen* to the tissues. Temporary hypoxia may result from strenuous exercise. More serious causes include impaired breathing (see *respiratory failure*), *ischaemia* (reduced blood flow to part of the body), and severe *anaemia*. A rare cause is *carbon monoxide* poisoning. Hypoxia also occurs in unacclimatized people at high altitude. Severe, prolonged hypoxia may lead to tissue death.

Hypoxia in muscles forces the muscle cells to produce energy by *anaerobic* processes, which can lead to cramps. In heart muscle, it may cause *angina pectoris*. In the brain, it causes confusion, dizziness, and loss of coordination; and may lead to unconsciousness and death if it is persistent.

Hypoxia can be assessed by using an *oximeter* to measure the oxygen concentration of blood in the tissues. Severe hypoxia may require *oxygen therapy* or artificial *ventilation*.

hypromellose

A substance that is included in artificial tears (see *tears, artificial*).

hysterectomy

Surgical removal of the *uterus*. Hysterectomy may be performed to treat *fibroids* (noncancerous tumours of the uterus), and cancer of the uterus (see *uterus, cancer of*) or cervix (see *cervix, cancer of*). It may also be performed to treat *endometriosis* (displaced fragments of the uterine lining) and to remove a prolapsed uterus (see *uterus, prolapse of*). Hysterectomy used to be performed frequently to relieve heavy menstrual bleeding, but alternative treatments, such as *endometrial ablation* or insertion of a progestogen *IUD*, are now increasingly used in these instances.

TYPES

The most common type of hysterectomy is a total hysterectomy, in which both the uterus and cervix are removed. Occasionally, the fallopian tubes and ovaries are removed as well. For the treatment of cervical cancer, a radical hysterectomy (in which the uterus, cervix, and pelvic lymph nodes are removed) is performed.

PERFORMING A **HYSTERECTOMY**

Hysterectomy may be performed through the abdomen or the vagina. For an abdominal hysterectomy, the incision is made in the lower abdomen (see below). In vaginal hysterectomy, the uterus is removed through an incision at the top of the vagina.

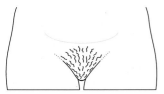

Site of incision for abdominal hysterectomy
The incision is made in the lower abdomen (in this case horizontally) level with the top of the pubic hair.

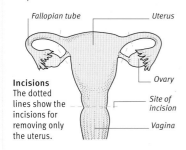

Incisions
The dotted lines show the incisions for removing only the uterus.

Fallopian tube
Uterus
Ovary
Site of incision
Vagina

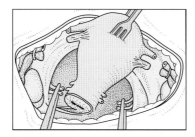

Abdominal hysterectomy
The uterine vessels are clamped. Traction is placed on the top of the uterus and the vessels are tied and then divided. In some cases, the fallopian tubes are cut and the tubes and ovaries left in place.

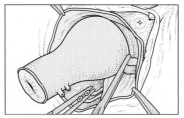

Vaginal hysterectomy
After a vaginal incision is made, the uterus and cervix are removed. (The ovaries cannot be removed in a vaginal hysterectomy.) The upper end of the vagina is repaired by stitching.

A hysterectomy may be performed through the vagina or through an incision in the abdomen. A procedure known as laparoscopically assisted vaginal hysterectomy is carried out partly through the vagina and partly using *minimally invasive surgery*. A vaginal hysterectomy has the advantage of needing no external incision, and, as a result, the patient usually makes a more rapid recovery. However, a vaginal hysterectomy cannot be performed if the uterus is significantly enlarged or if the hysterectomy is being carried out as a treatment for cancer.

RECOVERY AND OUTLOOK
After the operation, a drainage tube may be inserted at the site of the incision to aid healing. For a few days there may be some vaginal bleeding and discharge, as well as tenderness and pain. A vaginal hysterectomy requires a short hospital stay; any further stay depends on the age and health of the woman and whether or not there are any postoperative problems. Full recovery from a vaginal hysterectomy usually takes between three and six weeks. The recovery period

after an abdominal hysterectomy may be longer and may also require a longer stay in hospital. Sexual intercourse can usually be resumed about six to 12 weeks after surgery.

Following a hysterectomy, a woman is unable to bear children; she does not have menstrual periods and does not need to use contraception. If a woman's ovaries have also been removed before or around the woman's menopause, *hormone replacement therapy* (HRT) may be given. It is not uncommon for a woman to suffer from depression after a hysterectomy if she has not not adequately counselled beforehand.

hysteria

An old-fashioned term encompassing a wide range of physical or mental symptoms that are attributed to mental stress. Symptoms formerly grouped under this term are now included in the more specific diagnostic categories of *conversion disorder*; *somatization disorder*; *dissociative disorders*; and *factitious disorders*. The term is still used loosely to describe irrational behaviour.

hysterocontrast sonography (HyCoSy)

Ultrasound examination of the uterine cavity and the fallopian tubes. A *contrast medium* visible on ultrasound is introduced into the uterine cavity through the vagina and the cervix. Hysterocontrast sonography is a technique that is used to investigate *infertility*; the main advantage that this method has over *hysterosalpingography* is that it does not involve *X-rays*.

hysterosalpingography

An *X-ray* procedure in which a dye (*radiopaque* contrast medium) is introduced into the cavity of the *uterus* through the *cervix* in order to make the uterus and *fallopian tubes* visible on X-rays. Hysterosalpingography is used to investigate *infertility*.

H

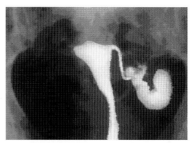

Hysterosalpingography
This image shows the uterus (centre) and fallopian tubes. The right tube (left on image) is blocked near the uterus, allowing no contrast medium into it; the other is obstructed further down and has dilated.

hysteroscopy

A technique that uses a hysteroscope (a type of *endoscope*) to view the inside of the *uterus* and *fallopian tubes* for the purposes of diagnosing disorders and, if necessary, taking *biopsy* samples. Hysteroscopy can be performed under local *anaesthesia*. Minor surgery, such as the removal of *fibroids* (noncancerous tumours of the uterus), may also be performed using a hysteroscope.

iatrogenic

A term meaning "physician-produced". It may be applied to any medical condition, disease, or adverse event resulting from medical treatment.

IBS

See *irritable bowel syndrome*.

Ibugel

A brand name for a topical gel containing *ibuprofen* that is used for relieving muscle pain.

ibuprofen

A *nonsteroidal anti-inflammatory drug* (NSAID) used as a painkiller to treat conditions such as headache, menstrual pain, and injury to soft tissues. The anti-inflammatory effect of ibuprofen also helps to reduce the joint pain and stiffness that occurs in types of *arthritis*.

Side effects may include abdominal pain due to inflammation of the stomach lining; nausea; heartburn; and diarrhoea. Ibuprofen should not be used by people who have had a previous reaction to it (for example, *asthma*, *rhinitis*, or rash) or to any other NSAID, including aspirin. Ibuprofen should also not be used by people who have, or have ever had, a peptic ulcer. To minimize any risk of adverse effects, it is recommended that the lowest effective dose of ibuprofen should be taken for the shortest duration.

ICD

The commonly used abbreviation for International Classification of Diseases, a list of all known diseases that is published by the *World Health Organization*. An updated version is produced approximately every ten years. ICD enables countries and organizations to gather statistical information on the frequency of a disease and causes of death.

ice-packs

A means of applying ice (wrapped in a towel or other material) to the skin in order to reduce inflammation or swelling, relieve pain, or stem bleeding. The low temperature causes the blood vessels to constrict (narrow), thus reducing the blood flow.

Ice-packs are used to relieve pain in a variety of disorders, including severe *headache*. They are used on sports injuries to minimize swelling and bruising, and they can also be used to help stop bleeding from small vessels, as in a nosebleed.

ichthammol

A drug used in skin preparations for the treatment of *eczema*, to reduce itching.

Ichthopaste

A brand name for a medicated bandage that is impregnated with the drug *ichthammol* and *zinc* paste. Ichthopaste is used in the treatment of chronic *eczema*, to reduce itching.

ichthyosis

A rare, inherited condition in which the skin is dry, thickened, scaly, and darker than normal due to abnormal production of *keratin*. Ichthyosis usually appears at, or shortly after, birth and usually improves during childhood. Commonly affected areas are the thighs, arms, and backs of the hands.

Lubricants and emulsifying ointments may be applied to help relieve the dryness, and bath oils may also be used to moisten the skin. Ichthyosis may also be treated with the retinoid drug *acitretin*.

ICP

The abbreviation for *intracranial pressure*.

ICSI

See *intracytoplasmic sperm injection*.

icterus

A term for *jaundice*.

ICU

The abbreviation for *intensive care unit*.

id

One of the three constituents of the personality (together with the *ego* and *superego*) described by Sigmund Freud. The id is defined as the primitive, unconscious energy store from which come the instincts for food, love, sex, and other basic needs. It thus guides behaviour and also fuels the turmoil leading to the conflict and guilt of neurosis. The id seeks simply to gain pleasure and avoid pain. (See also *psychoanalytic theory*.)

IDDM

The abbreviation for insulin-dependent *diabetes mellitus* (type 1 diabetes).

ideas of reference

An individual affected by ideas of reference finds personal significance in casual remarks made or action taken by other people. The individual may feel that people in public places are talking about, or laughing at, him or her. The condition falls short of a *delusion* because affected individuals are aware that they are not actually noticed more than others; however, they may be unable to discuss these feelings.

identical twins

Two offspring, also known as *monozygotic twins*, who develop from a single fertilized *ovum* (egg) and share identical *genes*. (See also *twins*.)

identification

A term used in *psychology* to refer to the process of unconsciously taking on another person's traits or behaviour. In children, identification with an older person, usually a parent, is considered a normal part of development.

identity crisis

A colloquial term used to describe feelings of uncertainty about one's own personality. Experiencing an "identity crisis" is common in periods of emotional turmoil, such as *adolescence*.

idiopathic

A term that is used to refer to a medical condition that has no known cause.

idiopathic epilepsy

A term used to describe *epilepsy* that has no known physical cause (such as brain injury, for example).

idiopathic hypertension

See *essential hypertension*.

idiopathic thrombocytopenic purpura (ITP)

An *autoimmune disorder* in which *platelets* are destroyed, leading to bleeding beneath the skin (see *purpura*).

ITP may be acute or chronic. Acute ITP mainly affects children, is usually mild, and disappears without treatment.

Chronic ITP generally affects adults and is much more serious. Initial treatment is with *corticosteroid drugs*; if this is unsuccessful, a *splenectomy* (surgical removal of the spleen) is required. *Immunosuppressant drugs* may be given if all other treatment fails.

idoxuridine

An *antiviral drug* used in skin preparations to treat the blistering rashes caused by *herpes simplex* and *herpes zoster* (shingles) infections. Recently developed antiviral drugs, such as *aciclovir*, are more effective and idoxuridine is now used less often.

Ig

The abbreviation for *immunoglobulin*.

IgA nephropathy

A kidney disease that causes *haematuria* (passage of blood in the urine) and in which deposits of IgA *immunoglobulins* (certain proteins produced by the *immune system* to combat infection) are found within the kidneys. Excessive amounts of IgA are sometimes produced in response to a throat infection. In such cases, IgA complex collects in the filtering units of the kidneys. IgA nephropathy is the most common form of *glomerulonephritis*.

The condition mainly affects children and young men. It may cause either microscopic haematuria (in which blood is passed in the urine but cannot be seen by the naked eye) or episodes of macroscopic haematuria (in which blood can be seen in the urine). In some cases, *nephrotic syndrome* develops; in this condition, large amounts of protein are passed in the urine, leading to raised blood pressure and *oedema* (swelling of the tissues).

Treatment of IgA nephropathy may involve *corticosteroid drugs* and *immunosuppressant drugs*, in addition to treatment to relieve any symptoms. Overall, the prognosis for IgA nephropathy is good. In some cases, however, kidney function deteriorates and, in up to one in five people, *kidney failure* develops after many years.

ileal conduit

A section of the *ileum* (the final part of the small intestine) used by a surgeon to provide a substitute channel for urine outflow when the bladder has been removed. (See *urinary diversion*; see also *cystectomy*.)

ileal pouch

A reservoir constructed from loops of the *ileum* (lower part of the small intestine) to replace a rectum that has been surgically removed. If an ileal pouch cannot be created, a permanent *ileostomy* will be required.

ileitis, regional

An outdated name for *Crohn's disease*.

ileostomy

An operation in which the *ileum* (lower part of the small intestine) is cut and the end brought through the abdominal wall and formed into an artificial opening called a *stoma*. Waste is discharged from the remaining part of the ileum into a disposable bag (stoma bag) or drained into a pouch made from the end of the ileum and situated beneath the skin (a procedure called a continent ileostomy). In the latter situation, faeces draining into the pouch are emptied regularly through a soft catheter. An ileostomy may be either permanent or temporary.

WHY IT IS DONE

Permanent ileostomy is usually performed on people who have severe,

---

PROCEDURE FOR **ILEOSTOMY**

Two incisions are made in the abdominal wall (usually on the right side): a small circular cut for the stoma (usually sited about 5 cm below the waist and away from the hip bone and groin crease) and a vertical cut to give access to the intestine and the *mesentery*. The site of the stoma is discussed with the patient prior to surgery.

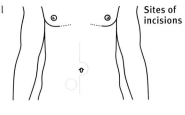

Sites of incisions

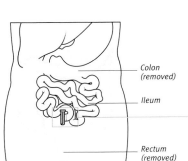

Colon (removed)

Ileum

Rectum (removed)

1 After removal of the colon, the cut end of the ileum is clamped and part of the mesentery is cut to free a short length of ileum for the stoma.

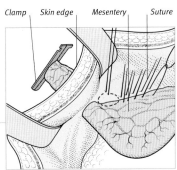

Clamp   Skin edge   Mesentery   Suture

2 The free end of the ileum is pushed out through the circular incision in the abdomen; the mesentery is then stitched to the inner abdominal wall.

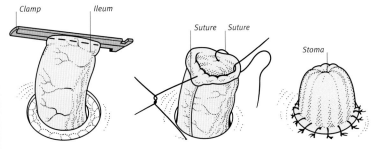

Clamp   Ileum

Suture   Suture

Stoma

3 The main vertical incision is closed, and the clamp is removed from the protruding end of the ileum (left). This end is then turned back and attached to the abdominal surface with sutures (middle). When completed, it forms a protruding spout of ileum (right). After the intestine begins to function normally, an ileostomy bag is fitted around the stoma. The bag is attached to the skin by adhesive seals.

uncontrolled *ulcerative colitis*. The operation is done after a total *colectomy* (removal of the colon and rectum).

Temporary ileostomy is sometimes performed at the same time as partial *colectomy* (removal of part of the colon) to allow the colon to heal before waste material passes through it. It may also be done as an emergency treatment for an obstruction in the intestine. The stoma is created from a loop of the intestine that is brought to the skin surface. Once the intestine has healed, a second operation is carried out to close the temporary ileostomy.

RECOVERY PERIOD

During convalescence, patients are given counselling and are taught the practical aspects of stoma care or drainage of continent ileostomies. Full recovery from the operation takes about six weeks.

ileum

The final, longest, and narrowest section of the small intestine. It is joined at its upper end to the *jejunum* and at its lower end to the large intestine (caecum, colon, and rectum). The ileum's function is to absorb nutrients from food that has been digested in the stomach and the first two sections of small intestine (the *duodenum* and jejunum).

LOCATION OF THE ILEUM

The ileum is situated between the jejunum (the middle part of the small intestine) and the caecum (the first part of the large intestine).

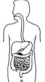

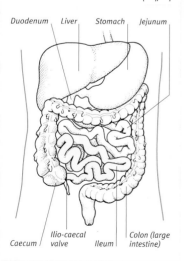

Duodenum Liver Stomach Jejunum

Caecum Ilio-caecal valve Ileum Colon (large intestine)

DISORDERS

Occasionally, the ileum becomes obstructed – for example, by pushing through a weakness in the abdominal wall (see *hernia*) or by becoming caught up with scar tissue following abdominal surgery (see *adhesion*). Other disorders of the ileum include *Meckel's diverticulum* (a pouch in the ileum wall that may become ulcerated) and diseases in which the absorption of nutrients is impaired, such as *Crohn's disease*, *coeliac disease*, tropical *sprue*, and *lymphoma*.

ileus, gallstone

The blockage of the small intestine by a *gallstone* that has travelled from the biliary tract. Gallstone ileus is sometimes a complication of *cholecystitis* (inflammation of the gallbladder). Symptoms may include severe abdominal pain and bloating, vomiting, and lack of bowel movements. Surgery is usually needed to remove the stone. The gallbladder is generally removed at the same time.

ileus, paralytic

A disorder in which the muscles of the intestines are unable to contract normally, and as a result the intestinal contents cannot pass out of the body. Paralytic ileus is usually a temporary condition. It commonly follows abdominal surgery and may also be induced by severe abdominal injury, *peritonitis* (inflammation of the membrane lining the abdomen), acute *pancreatitis* (inflammation of the pancreas), major disturbances in blood chemistry (such as *diabetic ketoacidosis*), or interference with the blood or nerve supply to the intestine. Symptoms include a swollen abdomen, vomiting, and failure to pass faeces.

The condition is treated by resting the intestine. A tube passed through the nose or mouth into the stomach or intestine removes accumulated fluids and keeps the stomach empty. Body fluid levels are maintained by *intravenous infusion* (drip).

ilium

The largest of the hip bones that form part of the *pelvis*.

illness

Perception by a person that he or she is not well. Illness is a subjective sensation; it may have both physical and psychological causes. The term "illness" is also used to mean disease or disorder.

illusion

A distorted sensation that is based on the misinterpretation of a real stimulus (for example, a pen is seen as a dagger). Illusion differs from a *hallucination*, in which a perception occurs without any stimulus. Usually, illusions are brief and can be understood when they are explained. They may be caused by tiredness or anxiety, to drugs, or to forms of brain damage. *Delirium tremens* (a condition usually arising from alcohol withdrawal in alcoholics) often brings on illusions.

image, body

See *body image*.

imaging techniques

Techniques that produce images of structures within the body (see *Imaging the body* box, opposite).

X-RAY TECHNIQUES

The most commonly used and simplest techniques are the *X-rays* (sometimes called plain X-rays) used to view dense structures such as bone. Simple X-ray examinations include those of the chest, skull, and limbs following injury.

Contrast X-rays involve the introduction into the body of a medium that is opaque to X-rays. The techniques include *barium X-ray examinations* (used to examine the oesophagus, the stomach and the intestine); *cholecystography* (used to visualize the gallbladder and common bile duct); *bronchography* (to view the airways connecting the windpipe to the lungs); *angiography* and *venography* (to provide images of the blood vessels); *intravenous urography* (to visualize the kidneys and urinary tract); and *ERCP* (in which the pancreatic duct and biliary system are examined after introducing a contrast medium through an *endoscope*).

Many X-ray techniques have now been superseded by newer procedures that are simpler to perform and safer and more comfortable for the patient.

ULTRASOUND TECHNIQUES

Ultrasound scanning involves the passing of high-frequency sound waves through the body using a transducer placed against the skin. The waves are reflected to varying degrees by structures of different density; the pattern of echoes is recorded electronically on a screen. Ultrasound scanning can now be used to produce three-dimensional images as well as moving images to show, for example, the opening and closing of a valve or blood flow within a vessel.

IMAGING THE BODY

Over the past two decades many methods of imaging the body have been developed and are now widely used. These techniques have made it possible to visualize internal structures in a variety of ways. Today, in addition to conventional X-rays (which primarily show bones), techniques such as CT scanning, radionuclide scanning, ultrasound scanning, MRI, and PET scanning are used to provide detailed diagnostic pictures of soft tissues and organs. The examples given here show some of the different ways in which the kidneys can be imaged.

X-RAYS

Radiopaque contrast media may be utilized to give distinct X-ray images of soft tissues, as in intravenous urography, which is used to give clear images of the kidneys and urinary tract.

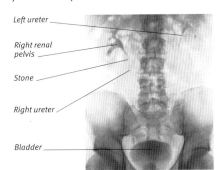

Left ureter

Right renal pelvis

Stone

Right ureter

Bladder

Intravenous urogram
This intravenous urogram shows the renal pelvises (urine-collecting areas of the kidneys) and the ureters, which have been filled with contrast medium. In the right-hand renal pelvis and ureter (on the left of the urogram), the medium has been retained due to a kidney stone blocking the ureter; the stone appears as a small gap in the ureter.

SCANNING TECHNIQUES

The body, particularly the soft tissues, can be imaged using a variety of modern techniques. Some of these techniques, such as CT scanning and MRI, rely on computers to process the raw imaging data and produce the actual image.

Others, such as ultrasound scanning and radionuclide scanning, can produce images without the need of a computer for image processing, although one may be used for image enhancement.

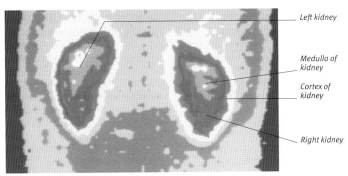

Left kidney

Medulla of kidney

Cortex of kidney

Right kidney

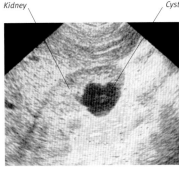

Kidney

Cyst

Radionuclide scanning
A radioactive substance is introduced into the body, and the radiation emitted is detected by a gamma camera, which then converts it into an image. Active or overactive cells will take up more of the substance, and will appear brighter, than underactive cells. This scan (taken from the back) shows healthy kidneys. In each kidney, the medulla (central part) has absorbed more of the radioactive substance than the cortex (outer part).

Ultrasound scanning
Ultra-high-frequency sound waves reflected from tissues in the body are converted into an image by special electronic equipment. This scan shows a fluid-filled cyst inside a kidney; the cyst appears as a dark area on the image.

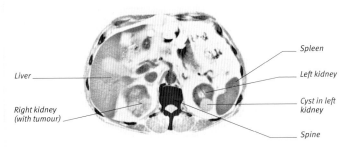

Liver

Right kidney (with tumour)

Spleen

Left kidney

Cyst in left kidney

Spine

CT scanning and MRI
These techniques produce cross-sectional images (slices) or three-dimensional images of body structures. This CT scan shows a cross-section through the body, as seen from below; the front of the body is at the top of the image. The right kidney (shown on the left of the image) is enlarged and distorted by a tumour. The left kidney has a cyst.

COMPUTER-ASSISTED SCANNING

Many scanning techniques use computers to process the raw imaging data and produce the actual image. In *CT scanning* (computed tomography scanning), X-rays are passed through the body at different angles. The computer analyses the data to produce cross-sectional images ("slices") of the tissues that are being examined. Newer CT scanners can use a spiral technique to produce three-dimensional images of structures.

In *MRI* (magnetic resonance imaging), the patient is placed in a strong magnetic field within the scanner and radiofrequency waves are passed through the body. A computer analyses changes in the magnetic alignment of hydrogen nuclei in the cells to give a cross-sectional or three-dimensional image of the tissues. This technique provides greater contrast between normal and abnormal tissues than that given by CT scanning.

PET scanning (positron emission tomography scanning) involves introducing very short-lived radioisotopes into the tissues of the brain. A computer analyses the paths of the gamma rays emitted by these radioisotopes, thereby providing information about both the structure and function of the brain.

In *radionuclide scanning*, a gamma camera records radiation emitted from tissues into which a radioactive substance has been introduced. A computer transforms the recordings into images and may be used to obtain more information from the results. Certain radioactive substances are taken up, to varying degrees, by different tissues, allowing specific organs to be studied in isolation.

Imdur

A brand name for a slow-release preparation of *isosorbide* mononitrate, a drug used in the treatment of *angina pectoris* (chest pain caused by an inadequate blood supply to the heart).

imidazole drugs

A specific group of *antifungal drugs* used for the treatment of fungal infections such as *candidiasis* (vaginal thrush) and *tinea* (ringworm). Examples include *clotrimazole* and *ketoconazole*.

Imigran

A brand name for *sumatriptan*, a *serotonin agonist* drug that is used to treat *migraine* or cluster headaches. Imigran is available in different forms, including tablets, injection, and nasal spray.

imipramine

A tricyclic *antidepressant drug* that is most commonly used in treatment of *depression*. It is also used to treat nocturnal bed-wetting (see *enuresis, nocturnal*) in children. Possible adverse effects of imipramine include excessive sweating, blurred vision, dizziness, dry mouth, constipation, nausea, and, in older men, difficulty passing urine.

immersion foot

A type of *cold injury*, also called trench foot, occurring when the feet are wet and cold for a long time. Initially, the feet turn pale and have no detectable pulse; later, they become red, swollen, and painful. If the condition is ignored, muscle weakness, skin ulcers, or *gangrene* may develop.

immobility

Reduced physical activity, for example through disease, injury, or following major surgery. Immobility is particularly harmful in elderly people because it causes muscle wasting and progressive loss of function.

COMPLICATIONS

Total immobility can produce various complications including *bedsores*, *pneumonia*, or *contractures* (deformity caused by the shrinkage of tissue). A common complication that occurs with partial immobility is *oedema* (fluid retention), which causes swelling of the legs. Rarely, sluggish blood flow encourages formation of a *thrombus* (abnormal blood clot) in a leg vein.

TREATMENT

Regular *physiotherapy* and adequate nursing care are important for any person who is totally immobile.

immobilization

An orthopaedic term that describes techniques that are used to prevent movement of joints or displacement of fractured bones. Immobilization is performed so that fractured bones can reunite properly (see *fracture*).

immune complex

A combination of an *antigen* (any substance that the body identifies as foreign and that provokes an immune response) and an *antibody* (a protein produced by the immune system for the purpose of attacking foreign substances). Immune complexes are normally removed from the circulation by the liver and spleen. However, they may sometimes continue to circulate and eventually become trapped in organs or other tissues, causing inflammation, tissue damage, and specific immune complex diseases (which are also known as type III *hypersensitivity* reactions).

One example of an immune complex disease is extrinsic allergic *alveolitis*. In this disorder, immune complexes form after exposure to allergens such as fungal spores; the immune complexes then collect in the lungs, causing inflammation of the *alveoli* (tiny air sacs). Other conditions caused by immune complexes include some forms of *glomerulonephritis* (inflammation of the glomeruli, tiny structures in the kidneys that help to filter blood); certain connective tissue diseases, including systemic *lupus erythematosus* and *rheumatoid arthritis*; and adverse reactions to the thrombolytic drug *streptokinase*.

immune response

The body's defensive reaction to microorganisms, cancer cells, transplanted tissue, and other substances or materials that are recognized as antigenic or "foreign". The immune response consists of the production of cells called *lymphocytes*; substances called *antibodies* or *immunoglobulins*; and other substances and cells that act to destroy the antigenic material. (See also *immune system*).

immune system

A collection of cells and proteins that works to protect the body from harmful microorganisms, such as *bacteria*, *viruses*, and *fungi*. The immune system plays a role in the control of *cancer* and is responsible for the phenomena of *allergy*, *hypersensitivity*, and rejection after *transplant surgery*.

NATURAL IMMUNITY

The term "natural (or innate) immunity" is given to the protection every individual is born with, such as the skin and mucous membranes that line the mouth, nose, throat, intestines, and vagina. Natural immunity also includes *antibodies*, or *immunoglobulins* (protective proteins), that are passed to the child from the mother via the placenta. If microorganisms penetrate these defences, they encounter "cell-devouring" white blood cells called phagocytes, and other types of white cells, such as cell-killing (cytotoxic) cells.

Microorganisms may also encounter substances that are naturally produced within the body (such as *interferon*) or a

THE **INNATE IMMUNE SYSTEM**

Each of us has many inborn defences against infection. These defences include external barriers such as the skin and eye surfaces (below), the inflammatory response (right), and the action of white blood cells called phagocytes (below right). Others include a substance called complement (which is activated by and attacks bacteria) and another called *interferon* (which has antiviral effects).

All of these defences are nonspecific and quick-acting. By contrast, the adaptive immune system (see overleaf) mounts specific attacks against particular microbes. These cells are most effective on second exposure to the organisms.

The two parts of the immune system work together; antibodies produced by the adaptive immune system assist phagocyte action.

THE INFLAMMATORY RESPONSE

If microbes break through the body's outermost barriers, inflammation is the second line of defence. Chemicals such as histamine are released, prompting the effects shown below, including the attraction of phagocytes to the microorganisms and the release of substances such as complement. The symptoms of inflammation are redness, pain, swelling, and heat.

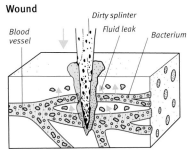

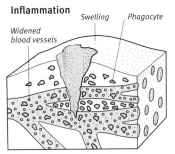

Inflammatory process
Following tissue injury (here due to a splinter in the skin) and the entry of bacteria or other microbes, blood vessels in the area widen and there is an increased leakage of fluid from the

blood into the tissues. These reactions allow easier access for immune system components that will fight the invaders, including phagocytes and soluble factors (such as the group of substances known as complement).

Physical and chemical barriers
These barriers, briefly described below, provide the first line of defence against harmful microbes (bacteria, viruses, and fungi).

Eyes
Tears produced by the lacrimal apparatus help to wash away microorganisms; tears contain an enzyme called lysozyme, which can destroy bacteria.

Mouth
Lysozyme present in saliva destroys bacteria.

Nose
Hairs in the nose help to prevent microorganisms from entering on dust particles. The process of expelling dust and microbes is assisted by the sneeze reflex.

Respiratory tract
Mucus secreted by cells lining the throat, windpipe, and bronchi traps microbes, which are then swept away by cilia (hairs on cells in the lining) or engulfed by phagocytes (types of white cells). The cough reflex also helps to expel microbes.

Stomach and intestines
Stomach acid destroys the vast majority of microbes. The intestines contain harmless types of bacteria (commensals) that compete with and control the harmful microorganisms.

Genito-urinary system
The vagina and urethra also contain commensals and are protected by mucus.

Skin
Intact skin provides an effective barrier against most microbes. The sebaceous glands secrete chemicals that are highly toxic to many bacteria.

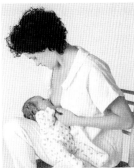

Breast-feeding
Antibodies (proteins with a protective role) formed by the mother against particular microbes are transferred to the baby in breast milk. Breast-feeding provides some extra immunity until the baby can form his or her own specific antibodies.

ACTION OF PHAGOCYTES

These white blood cells are attracted to sites of infection, where they adhere to, engulf, and digest microorganisms and debris.

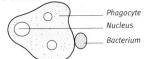

1 Adherence The phagocyte comes into contact with a microbe and recognizes it as foreign. This process is assisted by chemicals released during inflammation.

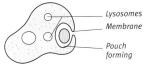

2 Ingestion The phagocyte engulfs the microbe in a pouch formed in its membrane. Fluid-filled particles, lysosomes, move towards the microbe.

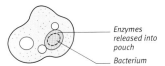

3 Digestion Enzymes within the lysosomes are released into the pouch to help digest the microbe. Debris from this process is later ejected.

THE **ADAPTIVE IMMUNE SYSTEM**

This system is based on white blood cells called lymphocytes. It has two parts. Humoral immunity relies on the action of B-lymphocytes; these cells produce antibodies, which circulate and attack specific microbes. In cellular immunity, cells called T-lymphocytes are activated and attack specific microbes or abnormal cells (such as virally infected cells or tumour cells).

HUMORAL IMMUNITY

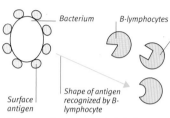

Bacterium
B-lymphocytes
Surface antigen
Shape of antigen recognized by B-lymphocyte

1 A humoral response is started when an antigen (foreign protein), here on the surface of a bacterium, is recognized by one type of B-lymphocyte and activates it.

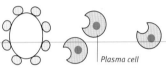

Plasma cell

2 This particular type of B-lymphocyte multiplies, forming cells called plasma cells, which make antibodies designed specifically to attack the bacterium.

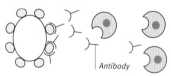

Antibody

3 After a few days, the antibodies are released. They attach themselves to the antigen. This triggers more reactions, which ultimately destroy the bacterium.

Second exposure

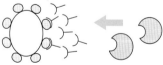

4 Some B-lymphocytes remain in the body as memory cells; if the bacterium enters the body again, they rapidly produce large amounts of antibodies to halt the infection.

CELLULAR IMMUNITY

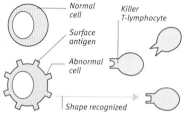

Normal cell
Killer T-lymphocyte
Surface antigen
Abnormal cell
Shape recognized

1 An antigen, here on the surface of an abnormal cell (such as a virus-infected cell or a tumour cell), is recognized by specific killer (cytotoxic) T-lymphocytes and activates them.

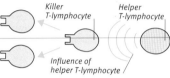

Killer T-lymphocyte
Helper T-lymphocyte
Influence of helper T-lymphocyte

2 With the assistance of helper T cells (another type of T-lymphocyte), the appropriate killer T-lymphocyte begins to multiply.

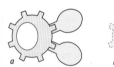

a *b*

3 The killer T-lymphocytes attach themselves to the abnormal cells (a), leading to the cells' destruction (b). The T-lymphocytes survive and may go on to kill more targets.

Second exposure

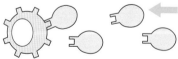

4 Some of the killer T-lymphocytes remain in the body as memory cells, and quickly attack abnormal cells if they reappear (for example, after reinfection with a virus).

EXAMPLES OF INFECTIOUS ORGANISMS COMBATED

Humoral immunity particularly important against:	• Some viruses (e.g. hepatitis) • Many bacteria (e.g. cholera) • Some parasites (e.g. malaria)
Cellular immunity particularly important against:	• Many viruses (e.g. herpes simplex) • Some bacteria (e.g. tuberculosis) • Some fungi (e.g. candidiasis)

group of blood proteins called the complement system, which act to destroy the invading organisms.

ACQUIRED IMMUNITY

The second part of the immune system, which is known as acquired (or adaptive) immunity, comes into play when the body encounters certain organisms that overcome the innate defences. The acquired, or adaptive, immune system responds specifically to each type of invading organism, and retains a memory of the invader so that defences can be rallied instantly in any future invasion.

The acquired immune system first must recognize part of an invading organism or tumour cell as an antigen (a protein that is foreign to the body). One of two types of response (humoral or cellular) is then mounted against the invading antigen.

HUMORAL IMMUNITY

Humoral immunity is important in the defence against bacteria. Following a complex recognition process, certain B-*lymphocytes* multiply and produce vast numbers of antibodies that bind to the antigens on the invading organism; the bacterium is then engulfed by phagocytes and destroyed. The binding of antibody and antigen may activate the complement system, which increases the efficiency of the phagocytes.

CELLULAR IMMUNITY

Cellular immunity is particularly important in the defence against viruses, some types of parasites that hide within cells, and, possibly, against cancer cells. Cellular immunity involves two types of

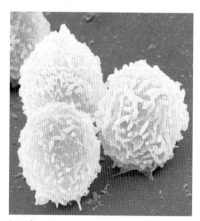

Lymphocytes
These types of white blood cells are found in the blood and the lymphoid organs (the lymph nodes, spleen, and thymus). The two main types (B- and T-lymphocytes) have different functions but look similar under the microscope.

TYPES OF **IMMUNIZATION**

Two main types of immunization exist. In passive immunization, antibodies (protective proteins) are injected into the body and provide immediate, but short-lived, protection against specific disease-causing bacteria, viruses, or toxins. Active immunization primes the body to make its own antibodies against such microorganisms and confers longer-lasting immunity.

PASSIVE IMMUNIZATION

1 Blood is taken from a person or, rarely, an animal previously exposed to a particular microorganism. The blood will contain antibodies against that microorganism.

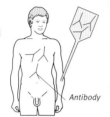

Antibody

2 An extract from the blood containing the antibodies (known as immune serum or antiserum) is injected into the person to be protected.

Serum

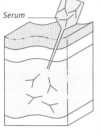

3 The antibodies help to destroy the microorganism if it is present in the blood or enters it over the following few weeks.

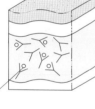

Disease-causing microorganism

ACTIVE IMMUNIZATION

1 The person to be protected is inoculated with a killed or modified microorganism (vaccine) that does not cause disease.

Vaccine

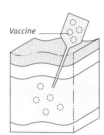

2 The immune system is provoked to make antibodies against the modified microorganism; it also retains a "memory" of the organism.

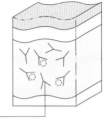

Antibody

3 If the real microorganism then enters the blood, antibodies can be produced quickly and in large numbers.

Disease-causing microorganism

T-lymphocyte: helper cells, which play a role in the recognition of antigens, and killer cells (the second type of T-lymphocyte), which are activated by helper cells and destroy cells that have been invaded.

immune system disorders

Disorders of the immune system include immunodeficiency disorders and *allergy*, in which the immune system has an inappropriate response to usually innocuous antigens such as pollen.

In certain circumstances, such as after tissue or organ transplants, *immunosuppressant drugs* are used to suppress the immune system and thus prevent the body from rejecting the donor tissue or organ as a foreign organism.

immunity

A state of protection against disease through the activities of the *immune system*. Natural (innate) immunity is present from birth and is passively acquired from the mother through the placenta. Acquired (adaptive) immunity develops either through exposure to invading microorganisms or through *immunization* and can be active or passive. Active immunity occurs through *vaccination* with killed or weakened microorganisms, which primes the body to produce antibodies as a defence against future invaders of this type; passive immunity involves the administration of specific antibodies to fight the infection, for example, following exposure to chickenpox.

immunization

The process of artificially inducing *immunity* as a preventive measure against *infectious diseases*.

TYPES AND BENEFITS

Immunization may be active or passive. In the passive form, *antibodies* are injected into the blood to provide immediate but short-lived protection against specific *bacteria*, *viruses*, or *toxins*. Active immunization, also called vaccination, primes the body to make its own antibodies and confers longer-lasting immunity. It also protects the more vulnerable members of a community, such as the very old or the very young (see *herd immunity*). The vaccines used in active immunization may consist of live, weakened forms of an infectious microorganism (such as a virus or bacterium); inactivated preparations of an infectious microorganism; or extracts or detoxified toxins from an infectious microorganism.

WHO SHOULD BE IMMUNIZED

Routine childhood immunization programmes exist for diseases such as *diphtheria*, *tetanus*, *pertussis*, *poliomyelitis*, HAEMOPHILUS INFLUENZAE type B (Hib), *measles*, *mumps*, *rubella*, *meningitis* C, and *pneumococcus* (see *DTaP/IPV or dTaP/IPV*; *DTaP/IPV/Hib*; *Hib vaccine*; *MMR vaccination*; *Td/IPV*). For injections and timings, see *Typical childhood immunization schedule*, overleaf.

Additional immunizations may also be recommended for certain groups; such immunizations include *influenza* immunization, *BCG vaccination* against *tuberculosis*, and immunization against *hepatitis B*. Immunization against strains of *human papillomavirus* associated with cervical cancer is being introduced for girls aged 12 to 13. Other immunizations may be necessary or recommended before foreign travel (see *travel immunization*).

POSSIBLE RISKS

Most immunizations are given by injection, and usually have no after-effects. However, some vaccines cause pain and swelling at the site of injection and may produce a slight fever or flulike symptoms. Others may produce a mild form of the disease. Very rarely, severe reactions occur as a result of, for example, an allergy to one of the vaccine's components.

In general, people with *immunodeficiency disorders*, widespread *cancer*, or those taking high-dose *corticosteroid drugs* should not receive live vaccines and should discuss their condition with their doctor before starting a vaccination

TYPICAL CHILDHOOD **IMMUNIZATION** SCHEDULE

Age	Disease
2 months	Diphtheria/tetanus/pertussis/poliomyelitis/Haemophilus influenzae b (Hib)*. Pneumococcal infection.
3 months	Diphtheria/tetanus/pertussis/poliomyelitis/Haemophilus influenzae b (Hib)*. Meningococcus C.
4 months	Diphtheria/tetanus/pertussis/poliomyelitis/Haemophilus influenzae b (Hib)*. Meningococcus C. Pneumococcal infection.
Around 12 months	Haemophilus influenzae b (Hib)/meningococcus C*.
Around 13 months	Measles/mumps/rubella (MMR)*. Pneumococcal infection.
3 years 4 months– 5 years	Diphtheria/tetanus/pertussis/poliomyelitis*†. Measles/mumps/rubella*†.
13–18 years	Diphtheria/tetanus/poliomyelitis*†.
Any age (at-risk infants and children)	Bacillus Calmette Guerin (BCG) against tuberculosis.

*1 combined injection †Booster

programme. Medical advice should also be sought if a person has had a severe reaction to a previous dose of a vaccine, or if a person has an acute illness when an immunization is due to be given. Some vaccines should not be given to young children or pregnant women.

immunoassay

A group of laboratory techniques, which include radioimmunoassay and ELISA (enzyme-linked immunosorbent assay), that are used in the diagnosis of infectious diseases, to confirm *immunity*, and also to investigate *allergies*. The tests are performed to determine the presence or absence of particular *antigens* (proteins that are present on the surface of microorganisms or allergens) or *antibodies* (proteins that are formed by the immune system to combat a particular microorganism or allergen). Immunoassay procedures may also be used to measure blood levels of *hormones* (which are also proteins).

immunocompromised

A term used to describe a person whose immune system activity has been reduced by disease (such as *AIDS* or *cancer*) or by certain medical treatments (such as treatment with *immunosuppressant drugs*). An immunocompromised person is at a greater than normal risk of contracting infections, particularly so-called *opportunistic infections* (diseases caused by organisms that rarely pose a threat to healthy people).

immunodeficiency disorders

Disorders in which the defences of the *immune system* fail to fight infection and tumours. Immunodeficiency disorders may be due to an inherited or a *congenital* defect or may be the result of acquired disease. The result is persistent or recurrent infection, including infections with organisms that would not ordinarily cause disease (see *opportunistic infections*), and an undue susceptibility to certain forms of *cancer*. Opportunistic infections include *pneumocystic pneumonia*, *fungal infections*, and widespread *herpes simplex* infections.

INHERITED IMMUNODEFICIENCY

Congenital or inherited deficiencies can occur in either of the two prongs of the adaptive immune system – humoral or cellular immunity – or in both.

Deficiencies of the humoral system include hypogammaglobulinaemia and agammaglobulinaemia. The former may cause few or no symptoms, depending on the severity of the deficiency, but agammaglobulinaemia can be fatal if not treated with *immunoglobulin*.

Congenital deficiencies of T-*lymphocytes* may lead to problems such as persistent and widespread *candidiasis* (thrush). A combined deficiency of both humoral and cellular components of the immune system, called severe combined immunodeficiency (SCID), is usually fatal in the first year of life unless treatment can be given by *stem cell* or *bone marrow transplant*.

ACQUIRED IMMUNODEFICIENCY

Acquired immunodeficiency may be due to disease processes (such as infection with *HIV*, which leads to *AIDS*). It may also be caused by damage to the immune system as a result of its suppression by drugs, either intentionally as in treatment for autoimmune diseases or after organ transplantation, or as a side effect of treatment for another condition. Severe malnutrition and many cancers can also cause immunodeficiency. Mild immunodeficiency arises through a natural decline in immune defences with age.

immunoglobulin

Also known as an *antibody*, a type of protein found in blood and tissue fluids. Such proteins are produced by B-lymphocytes (a type of white blood cell). Their function is to bind to substances in the body that are recognized as foreign *antigens*, such as proteins on the surfaces of bacteria and viruses. This binding is crucial for the destruction of antigen-bearing microorganisms. Immunoglobulins also play a key role in *allergies* and *hypersensitivity* reactions.

There are five main classes of immunoglobulin in the blood (IgA, IgD, IgE, IgG, and IgM). IgA is mainly found in secretions of the respiratory tract, intestine, and urinary tract. Only low levels of IgD are present in the body and its function is not known. IgE is involved in the immune response to worm infestations; high levels are also produced to fight atopic (allergic) conditions. IgG is the major class of immunoglobulin, with four subclasses; its molecule consists of two parts, one of which binds to an antigen and the other to other cells of the immune system, which then engulf the microorganisms bearing the antigen. The most important function of IgG is to mount a response to bacterial infections. IgM is produced promptly in response to infection and then levels fall; IgM present in an infant at birth is an indicator of intrauterine infection.

Immunoglobulins can be extracted from the blood of people who have recovered from certain infectious diseases and used for passive *immunization*.

immunoglobulin injection

The administration of *immunoglobulin* preparations (antibodies) to prevent or treat infectious diseases. Such preparations, also known as immune globulin or gamma-globulin injections, work by passing on antibodies obtained from the blood of people who have previously been exposed to these diseases. The main use of these injections is to prevent infectious diseases in people exposed to infection who are not already immune, or in those who are at special risk. They are also given intravenously for *immunodeficiency disorders*. Side effects of such injections include rash and fever, and pain and tenderness at the injection site if injected into a muscle.

immunology

The discipline that is concerned with the *immune system*. Immunologists study the immune system's functioning; investigate and treat immune system disorders, including *autoimmune disorders*, *allergies*, and *immunodeficiency disorders*; and investigate ways of stimulating the immune system. In addition, they play a role in *transplant surgery*, looking for a good match between donor and recipient and using *immunosuppressant drugs* to minimize the risk of organ rejection.

immunostimulant drugs

COMMON DRUGS
- Aldesleukin • BCG • Interferon alfa
- Interferon beta • Peginterferon alfa

A group of drugs that increase the efficiency of the body's *immune system*. They include *vaccines*, *interferon*, and aldesleukin (interleukin-2). Interferon alfa is used to treat persistent viral infections, such as hepatitis C. Interferon beta is used to treat some types of *multiple sclerosis*. Aldesleukin is used in the treatment of *kidney cancer*.

immunosuppressant drugs

COMMON DRUGS
| ANTICANCER DRUGS • Azathioprine |
| • Chlorambucil • Cyclophosphamide |
| • Methotrexate • Mycophenolate mofetil |
| CORTICOSTEROID DRUGS • Prednisolone |
| ANTIBODIES • Anti-lymphocyte globulin |
| • Basiliximab • Daclizumab |
| OTHER DRUGS • Ciclosporin • Tacrolimus |

A group of drugs used to reduce the activity of the *immune system*. Immunosuppressants are given to prevent rejection of donor tissue after *transplant surgery*. They are also given to slow the progress of *autoimmune disorders* such as *rheumatoid arthritis* and systemic *lupus erythematosus*. The drugs work by suppressing the production and activity of white blood cells called *lymphocytes*. Side effects vary, but all immunosuppressant drugs increase the risk of infection and of the development of certain *cancers*.

immunotherapy

Stimulation of the *immune system* as a treatment for *cancer*. The term is also used to describe *hyposensitization* treatment for *allergy*.

One type of immunotherapy used in the treatment of cancer uses *immunostimulant drugs*; for example, the treatment of bladder cancer may involve introducing BCG into the bladder. Another types uses monoclonal antibodies (see *antibody, monoclonal*) directed against tumours. *Interferon* or chemical poisons can be linked to these antibodies in order to increase their ability to destroy tumour cells without damaging normal cells.

Imodium

A brand name for *loperamide*, an *antidiarrhoeal drug*.

impaction, dental

Failure of a tooth to emerge completely from the gum. It may occur because of *overcrowding* or when a tooth grows in the wrong direction.

Impacted wisdom teeth are common when the teeth come through in early adulthood. If they cause no symptoms, they do not need to be removed. In some cases, however, impacted wisdom teeth partially penetrate the gum, leaving a flap of tissue over most of the crown. *Plaque*, bacteria, and food debris may then collect between the tooth and the gum, causing pain and inflammation in the gum tissues (see *gingivitis*). If the problem persists, the affected teeth need to be removed.

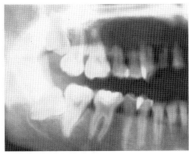

Impacted wisdom teeth
This X-ray shows impacted upper and lower wisdom teeth. The teeth are wedged against an adjacent molar and are unable to erupt normally; the tooth in the lower jaw is lying horizontally.

impaction, faecal

See *faecal impaction*.

impedance audiometry

A *hearing test* used to investigate the performance of the middle ear in cases of conductive *deafness*.

imperforate

A term meaning "without an opening". The term is used to describe a body structure, such as the *hymen* or the anus (see *anus, imperforate*), which should have an opening but does not.

impetigo

A highly contagious skin infection, common in children, that most commonly occurs around the nose and mouth, but can affect the skin anywhere on the body.

CAUSE AND SYMPTOMS
Impetigo is caused by bacteria (usually staphylococci) entering areas of broken

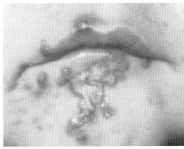

The appearance of impetigo
Fluid-filled blisters appear on the skin (in this case, on a young child's mouth and chin). The blisters often burst, releasing fluid that dries to leave pale brown crusts on the skin.

skin. The skin reddens and small, fluid-filled blisters appear. The blisters tend to burst, leaving moist, weeping areas that dry to leave honey-coloured or golden crusts. In severe cases, there may be swelling of the *lymph nodes* in the face or neck and fever.

TREATMENT AND PREVENTION
Treatment is with topical (locally administered) *antibiotic drugs* unless the condition is widespread, in which case oral antibiotics are usually given.

As the condition is highly contagious, to prevent the spread of the infection, towels, flannels, and pillowcases should not be shared. Children should not go to school or mix with others until they have been treated and the condition has cleared up.

implant

Any material, either natural or artificial, that is inserted into the body for medical or cosmetic purposes.

implantation, egg

Attachment of a fertilized *ovum* (egg) to the wall of the *uterus*. Implantation occurs about six days after *fertilization*, when the blastocyst (early embryo) comes into contact with the uterus wall.

As the cells of the developing *embryo* continue to divide, the outer cell layer penetrates the lining of the uterus to obtain oxygen and nutrients from the mother's blood; later, this layer develops into the *placenta*. The embryo usually implants in the upper part of the uterus; if it implants low down near the cervix, *placenta praevia* may develop. Rarely, implantation occurs outside the uterus, possibly in a fallopian tube, resulting in an *ectopic pregnancy*.

implant, dental

A post that is surgically embedded in the jaw for the attachment of a dental prosthesis (an artificial tooth). Titanium or synthetic materials may be used. A dental implant is fitted under a local anaesthetic (see *anaesthesia, dental*). A hole is drilled in the jaw and the post inserted. Several months later, an attachment that protrudes from the gum is screwed into the post; a few weeks after that, the prosthesis is fitted.

implosive therapy

A form of *behaviour therapy*, also known as *flooding*, used for desensitizing a person to the cause of a *phobia*.

impotence

The inability to achieve or maintain an *erection*, now more commonly known as *erectile dysfunction*.

impression, dental

A mould taken of the *teeth*, *gums*, and *palate*. A quick-setting material, such as alginate, is placed in a mould over the teeth. The mould is then removed, and plaster of Paris poured into it to obtain a model of the area. This model is then used as a base on which to build a *denture*, *bridge*, *crown*, or dental *inlay*. Dental impressions are also used in *orthodontics* to study the position of the teeth, and to make *orthodontic appliances* to correct irregularities.

impulse

A sudden, spontaneous force or action. In biology and medicine, the term "impulse" is usually used to refer to electrical activity that travels along a *nerve* which may result, for example, in a muscle contraction.

inattention, sensory

In *neurology* (the study of diseases of the nervous system), a term meaning the inability to recognize a tactile stimulus (such as a pinprick) on one side of the body, while reacting normally to a simultaneous stimulus on the other side. Visual inattention (failure to respond to local visual stimuli) may also be present. The condition is most commonly the result of a *stroke*.

inborn errors of metabolism

See *metabolism, inborn errors of*.

incest

Sexual intercourse between close relatives, such as with a parent, a son or daughter, a brother or sister, an uncle or aunt, a nephew or niece, or a grandparent or grandchild. Incest is illegal or taboo in most societies and is against the teaching of many religions.

incidence

One of the two principal measures (the other is prevalence) of how common a disease is in a defined population. The incidence of a disease is the number of new cases that occur during a given period (for example, 17 new cases per 100,000 people per year). The prevalance of a disease is the total number of cases of the disease in existence at any one time in a defined population. The prevalence figure is usually expressed as the number of cases per 100,000 people.

incision

A cut made into the tissues of the body by a scalpel (surgical knife). Most incisions are made to gain access to tissue inside the body, usually to repair or remove a diseased organ. An incision may also be made to allow pus to drain from an *abscess* or boil.

incisional hernia

A type of *hernia* in which the intestine bulges through a scarred area of the abdominal wall because the surrounding muscle has been weakened by a previous surgical *incision*.

incisor

One of the eight front *teeth* (four in the upper jaw and four in the lower) used for cutting through solid food.

incompatible blood transfusion

A blood transfusion in which the patient's immune system reacts against the donor blood as a foreign invader (see *blood transfusion, incompatible*).

incompetence

A medical term applied to a structure that should close tightly but does not. For example, valve incompetence (see *aortic incompetence*; *mitral incompetence*) causes leakage of blood; *cervical incompetence* may result in a miscarriage.

incomplete miscarriage

The retention in the uterus of placental or fetal tissue after a *miscarriage* or a medical abortion (see *abortion, induced*). If this tissue is not promptly removed, it may become infected, resulting in a dangerous condition called *septic abortion* and haemorrhage (bleeding).

incontinence, faecal

Inability to retain *faeces* in the *rectum*, leading to involuntary defaecation.
CAUSES
A common cause of faecal incontinence is *faecal impaction*, which often results from long-standing *constipation*. In this condition the rectum becomes overfull, causing faecal fluid and small pieces of faeces to be passed involuntarily around the impacted mass of faeces. Temporary loss of continence may also occur in severe *diarrhoea*. Other causes include injury to the anal muscles (as may occur during childbirth), *paraplegia* (damage to the nerves in the lower trunk, including those supplying the intestines), and *dementia* (loss of normal brain functions, such as control of the bowels).
TREATMENT
Faecal incontinence can usually be successfully treated. If the underlying cause of faecal impaction is constipation, recurrence may be prevented by eating a high-fibre diet. Suppositories containing *glycerol* or *laxative drugs* may be recommended. Pelvic floor and anal sphincter

damage can often be surgically repaired. Faecal incontinence in people with dementia or a nerve disorder may be avoided by regular use of *enemas* or *suppositories* to empty the rectum.

incontinence, urinary

Involuntary passing of *urine*, often due to injury or disease of the *urinary tract*. Damage to or disorders of the nervous system are also common causes.

TYPES AND SYMPTOMS

Stress incontinence refers to the involuntary escape of urine when a person coughs, laughs, picks up a heavy object, runs, or jumps. It develops when the urethral sphincter muscles (which normally keep the bladder outlet closed) have been stretched and weakened. Stress incontinence is common in women, particularly after childbirth or in patients with prolapse of the uterus or vagina. This condition results in the loss of small amounts of urine.

In urge incontinence, also known as irritable bladder, an urgent desire to pass urine (even though the bladder is not full) is accompanied by inability to control the bladder as it contracts. Once urination starts, it cannot be stopped, leading to the loss of large volumes of urine. Urge incontinence is often caused by irritability of the bladder lining. The problem may be caused by infection or inflammation (see *cystitis*). It may also result from the presence of stones (see *calculus, urinary tract*) or bladder tumours; disorders affecting the nerves that supply the bladder (such as *stroke* or *multiple sclerosis*); or *anxiety*. In some cases the bladder muscles are too sensitive to increasing pressure within the bladder, inappropriately triggering emptying.

Total incontinence is a complete lack of bladder control due to loss of function in the urethral sphincter. It may be associated with spinal cord damage, due to disease or injury, that affects the nerves supplying the bladder.

Overflow incontinence occurs in long-term *urinary retention*, often because of an obstruction such as an enlarged *prostate gland*. The bladder is always full, leading to constant dribbling of urine.

Incontinence due to lack of control by the brain commonly occurs in young children (see *enuresis*) or elderly people, and in those with *learning difficulties*.

TREATMENT

A wide range of treatments is available, and most affected people achieve significant improvement. If weak pelvic muscles are causing stress incontinence, *pelvic floor exercises* may help. Sometimes, surgery may be needed to tighten the pelvic muscles or correct a prolapse. *Anticholinergic drugs* may be used to relax the bladder muscle if irritable bladder is the cause. *Collagen* injections into the urethral wall, performed under anaesthetic, may also be effective.

If normal bladder function cannot be restored, incontinence pants can be worn; men can wear a penile sheath leading into a tube connected to a urine bag. Some people can avoid incontinence by means of self-catheterization (see *catheterization, urinary*). Permanent catheterization is necessary in some cases.

incoordination

Loss of the ability to produce smooth, muscular movements, leading to clumsiness and unsteady balance. The term "incoordination" can also mean the failure of a group of organs to work together successfully. (See also *ataxia*.)

incubation period

The time during which an *infectious disease* develops, from the point when the infectious organism enters the body until symptoms appear. Different infections have characteristic incubation periods; for example, 10–21 days for chickenpox and 7–14 days for measles. The incubation period for cholera may be as short as several hours.

incubator

A transparent plastic cot that provides premature or sick infants with ideal conditions for survival. In an incubator, oxygen, temperature, and humidity levels are controlled. Incubators have portholes to allow handling of the baby, and smaller ones through which monitoring cables and intravenous and respiratory tubing can pass.

incus

One of the three tiny, linked bones (*ossicles*) in the middle *ear* that convey sound vibrations. The incus (the Latin name for an anvil) is so called because it is said to resemble an anvil.

indapamide

A *diuretic drug* used in the treatment of *hypertension* (high blood pressure). Possible side effects of indapamide include headaches, fatigue, and muscle cramps. Less common adverse effects include dizziness, fainting, a pins-and-needles sensation, sore throat, rash, and *jaundice*; these problems need prompt medical attention.

Inderal

A brand name for *propranolol*, a *beta-blocker drug* used to treat heart and circulatory disorders as well as some cases of anxiety.

Indian medicine

Traditional Indian, or Ayurvedic, medicine was originally based largely on herbal treatment, although simple surgical techniques were also used. Indian medicine later developed into a scientifically based system with a wide range of surgical techniques (such as operations for cataracts and kidney stones) alongside other therapies such as diet, yoga, breathing exercises, and the herbal tradition.

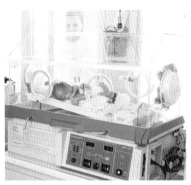

Premature infant in an incubator
Portholes make it possible for medical staff or parents to handle the infant without disturbing the special conditions in the incubator.

indigenous

Native to a particular place or country. In medicine, this concept is important when investigating the effect of environmental factors on disease patterns.

indigestion

A common term (known medically as dyspepsia) covering a variety of symptoms brought on by eating, including *heartburn*, *abdominal pain*, *nausea*, and *flatulence* (excessive wind in the stomach or intestine, that causes belching and discomfort).

Discomfort in the upper abdomen is often caused by eating too much, eating too quickly, or by eating very rich, spicy, or fatty foods. Persistent or recurrent indigestion may be due to a *peptic ulcer*, *gallstones*, *oesophagitis* (inflammation of the oesophagus), or, rarely, *stomach cancer*.

Antacid drugs help to relieve the symptoms, but they may mask an underlying cause that needs medical attention. They should not be taken for longer than two weeks without medical advice.

indole

A substance produced by the breakdown of the *amino acid* tryptophan in the intestine. Indole is excreted in urine. An indole compound (5-hydroxyindole acetic acid) is measured in the urine in the investigation of possible *carcinoid tumours*.

indolent ulcer

A term describing an *ulcer* that is slow to heal but usually causes little pain.

indometacin

A *nonsteroidal anti-inflammatory drug* (NSAID) used to relieve pain, stiffness, and inflammation caused by disorders such as *rheumatoid arthritis*, *osteoarthritis*, and *tendinitis*. Indometacin is also prescribed to relieve the pain caused by injury to soft tissues, such as muscles and ligaments.

Side effects may include abdominal pain, nausea, heartburn, headache, and dizziness. Indometacin should not be used by people who have had a previous reaction to it (for example, *asthma*, *rhinitis*, or rash) or to any other NSAID, including aspirin. Indometacin should also not be used by people who have, or have ever had, a peptic ulcer. Indometacin may be associated with a small increased of certain cardiovascular problems, such as *myocardial infarction* (heart attack) or stroke, particularly if taken in high doses and for prolonged periods. To minimize any risk of adverse effects, it is recommended that the lowest effective dose of indometacin should be taken for the shortest duration.

indoramin

An *alpha-blocker drug* used to treat *hypertension* (high blood pressure). It acts by relaxing the muscles in the blood vessel walls, thus allowing the vessels to widen and easing the flow of blood. In lower doses, indoramin is also prescribed to relieve the symptoms of an enlarged prostate gland (see *prostate, enlarged*); it relaxes the muscle of the prostate and thereby enables urine to be passed more easily.

When first taken, indoramin can cause a rapid fall in blood pressure. For this reason, the first dose is usually small and is taken lying down. Indoramin may also cause drowsiness at the start of treatment and whenever the dosage is increased.

induction of labour

The use of artificial means to begin *labour*. Labour is induced if the health of the mother or baby would be at risk if the pregnancy was allowed to continue for longer.

WHY IT IS DONE

The most common reason for inducing labour is that the pregnancy has continued past the estimated delivery date, which increases the chance of complications during childbirth. Other reasons for induction are *pre-eclampsia* (a serious condition involving high blood pressure and fluid accumulation), *rhesus incompatibility* (a difference between the blood groups of mother and fetus), or *intrauterine growth retardation* (poor growth of the developing fetus).

HOW IT IS DONE

Different methods of induction are used, depending on the stage of labour and cervical condition. A *prostaglandin* pessary may be inserted high into the vagina to encourage the cervix to soften and open. The hormone *oxytocin* may also be given as a continuous intravenous infusion in order to stimulate uterine contractions.

induration

A specific medical term meaning the hardening or thickening of areas of soft tissue (for example, the skin or blood vessel walls) or an organ (such as the lung or liver) due to inflammation or disease. (See also *sclerosis*.)

industrial diseases

See *occupational disease and injury*.

industrial psychology

A field of *psychology* in which human behaviour is studied in relation to the effects and influences of the workplace. The principles of industrial psychology are applied to such issues as leadership, communications, motivation, job analysis, and selection of employees.

indwelling catheter

A *catheter* (flexible tube) that remains in place for a prolonged period. The term usually refers to a urinary catheter that is used to drain the contents of the bladder via the *urethra*; it is held in place with a balloon (see *balloon catheter*).

in extremis

The Latin term for "at the point of death".

Infacol

A brand name for *dimeticone* (an antifoaming agent used to relieve *colic*).

infant

A term usually applied to a baby up to the age of 12 months.

infantile autism

An alternative term for *autism*, a disorder that usually develops in early childhood and causes severe impairment of language and communication skills.

infantile cataract

A *congenital* disorder (one present from birth) in which a baby's sight is seriously impaired by opacity of the lens of the eye (see *cataract*). Causes include infections, such as *rubella* (German measles) and *toxoplasmosis*, passed from mother to baby before birth. Surgical removal of the cataract may be beneficial.

infantile colic

See *colic, infantile*.

infantile eczema

An alternative term for atopic *eczema* that first develops in early childhood.

infantile spasms

A rare type of recurrent seizure, also called progressive myoclonic encephalopathy or salaam attacks, that affects babies. The condition is a form of *epilepsy* and first occurs around four to nine months of age.

Spasms may occur hundreds of times a day, each lasting a few seconds. During a seizure, the baby's head suddenly falls forwards, the body stiffens, and the limbs bend, then the arms and hands extend and move outwards. These seizures are usually a sign of brain damage; affected babies usually have severe *developmental delay*.

infant mortality

The number of infants who die during the first year of life per 1,000 live births (usually expressed as per year). The majority of infant deaths occur during the neonatal period (the first month of life). Most of those who die are very premature and of low birth weight, or have severe congenital abnormalities. *Sudden infant death syndrome* (SIDS) is another significant cause of infant mortality.

infarction

Death of an area of tissue due to isch-aemia (lack of blood supply). One common example is *myocardial infarction*, commonly called a heart attack, in which an area of heart muscle dies. Another is pulmonary infarction, which is lung damage caused by a *pulmonary embolism* (a blood clot that has moved into a vessel in the lung and is obstructing the flow of blood). (See also *necrosis*).

infection

The establishment in the body of dis-ease-causing microorganisms (such as pathogenic *bacteria*, *viruses*, or *fungi*). The organisms reproduce and cause dis-ease by direct damage to cells or by releasing toxins. This activity normally provokes the *immune system* into res-ponding, which accounts for many common symptoms.

Infection can be localized within a particular area or tissue, as in a boil, or be systemic (spread throughout the body), as in *influenza*. Localized infec-tion may result from the spread of organisms through wounds, or during surgery. This form of infection is gener-ally associated with pain, redness, swelling, and formation of a pus-filled abscess at the site of infection, and a rise in temperature. Weakness, aching joints, and fever are expressions of systemic infectious disease.

Many minor infections are dealt with by the immune system and need no specific treatment. A localized infection that has produced pus may be drained surgically. Severe systemic infections may need treatment with drugs such as *antibacterials*, *antivirals*, or *antifungals*. For further information about different infectious diseases, see the accompany-ing tables on the following pages.

infection, congenital

Infection that is acquired by a baby in the uterus or during birth.

INFECTIONS ACQUIRED IN THE UTERUS

Many infectious microorganisms can pass from the mother, by way of the placenta, into the circulation of the growing fetus. Particularly serious infections that may be acquired in the uterus are *rubella* (German measles), *syphilis*, *toxoplasmosis*, *cytomegalovirus*, and *HIV*. All these infections may cause *intrauterine growth retardation*. Rubella that occurs in early pregnancy may cause *deafness*, congenital *heart disease*, and eye disorders in the baby.

Some diseases in later pregnancy may also damage the fetus severely. One such condition is infection with a *herpes* virus. A woman who is infected with *HIV* risks passing it on to her baby dur-ing pregnancy, but the risk can be reduced by use of *antiretroviral drugs* during the pregnancy.

INFECTIONS ACQUIRED DURING BIRTH

Infections acquired during birth are almost always the result of microorgan-isms in the mother's vaginal secretions or uterine fluid. Premature rupture of the membranes is associated with increased risk of disease, particularly *streptococcal infections*. Conditions that may be acquired during delivery include *herpes simplex*, *chlamydial infec-tions*, and *gonorrhoea*.

TREATMENT

Treatment of the baby depends on the type of infection. Some birth defects caused by infection (such as certain types of heart defect) can be treated; others (such as congenital deafness) are usually not treatable.

infectious disease

Any illness that is caused by a specific microorganism. The most important disease-causing organisms are *viruses*, *bacteria* (including rickettsiae, chlamy-diae, and mycoplasmas), and *fungi*. Others are *protozoa* and *worms*.

INCIDENCE

In affluent countries, infectious diseases are generally less of a threat than in the past because of better methods to con-trol the spread of disease organisms (such as improved sanitation and water purification); effective drugs; *immuniza-tion*; and better general health and nutrition. In poorer countries, such dis-eases still pose a threat, both to people who live in these countries and to trav-ellers who visit them.

INCUBATION PERIOD

For most infectious diseases, there is a time gap between the entry of the microorganisms into the body and the first appearance of symptoms. This incubation period, during which an infected person is able to pass the microorganism to others, may vary from a few hours or days to, in some cases, several months.

TREATMENT

Antibiotic drugs and other antimicrobials are the mainstay of treatment for bacte-rial infection. However, for most viral infections drug treatment is restricted to severe infections and treatment often relies on supportive measures alone.

OUTLOOK

Progress has been made in the fight against infectious diseases, but many problems remain. The spread of diseas-es such as *sexually transmitted infections*

HOW **INFECTIOUS DISEASES** ARE TRANSMITTED

In affluent countries, infections are usually spread by sexual transmission, airborne transmission, blood-borne transmission, or direct skin contact. In poorer countries, insects, food, and water are other important mechanisms of transmission. Certain infectious diseases can also pass from a pregnant woman's blood across the placenta into the blood of the fetus.

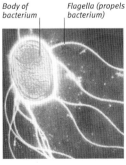

Body of bacterium   *Flagella (propels bacterium)*

Salmonella bacterium
This image shows the bacterium *Salmonella enteritidis*, which can cause food poisoning. These bacteria may be found in meat, eggs, and milk.

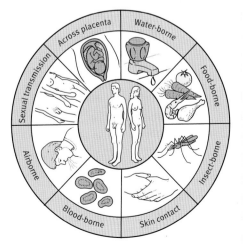

is difficult to control and, for many infections, no effective *vaccine* exists. In addition, some bacteria have developed *resistance* to the drugs available, and this could lead to a rise in potentially fatal bacterial infections similar to those that were common before the development of antibiotics.

The majority of viral infections cannot be combated with drugs. *HIV* is a notable exception but it still poses a major threat to world health because the *antiretroviral drugs* used to treat HIV do not cure the disease and are too expensive for many developing countries, which is where HIV incidence is highest.

infectious mononucleosis
See *mononucleosis, infectious*.

infective arthritis
An alternative term for septic *arthritis*.

infective endocarditis
See *endocarditis*.

INFECTIOUS DISEASES: VIRAL INFECTIONS

Disease	Infective agent	Transmission	Incubation period	Symptoms	Treatment
AIDS/HIV infection	Human immunodeficiency virus (HIV)	Sexual contact; sharing hypodermic needles; mother to fetus or to breast-fed baby; unscreened blood transfusions	6–8 weeks	Flulike illness; fever; fatigue; sore throat; muscle aches; swollen lymph nodes; skin disorders; fungal, viral, or bacterial infections	Treatment given for complicating infections; antiretroviral drugs can prolong life expectancy
Chickenpox	Varicella-zoster virus (herpes zoster virus)	Airborne droplets; direct contact	10–21 days	Slight fever; malaise; crops of itchy blisters	Relief of symptoms; aciclovir beneficial in some cases
Common cold	Numerous rhino- and adenoviruses; coronaviruses	Airborne droplets; hand-to-hand contact	1–3 days	Sneezing; chills; muscle aches; runny nose; cough	Relief of symptoms
Hepatitis, viral	Hepatitis virus types A, B, C, D, or E	A, E: infected food or water. B, C: sexual contact; infected blood; sharing needles; body piercing/tattooing; mother to fetus. D: sexual contact; infected blood; sharing needles	A, E: 3–6 weeks B, C, D: a few weeks to several months	Flulike illness; jaundice; many people are asymptomatic	Interferon, ribavirin, and lamivudine may be beneficial in some cases
Influenza	Influenza virus types A, B, or C	Airborne droplets	1–3 days	Fever; chills; aches; headache; sore throat; cough; runny nose	Relief of symptoms; fluids
Measles	Measles virus (a paramyxovirus)	Airborne droplets	7–14 days	Fever; coldlike symptoms; mottled red rash that fades to leave staining; conjunctivitis	Relief of symptoms
Meningitis, viral	Various viruses	Various methods, including via rodents	Variable	Fever; headache; drowsiness; confusion	Relief of symptoms
Mononucleosis, infectious (glandular fever)	Epstein–Barr virus	Possibly via saliva	1–6 weeks	Swollen glands; fever; sore throat; headache; malaise; lethargy	Relief of symptoms; rest; fluids
Poliomyelitis	3 polioviruses	From faeces to mouth via hands; airborne droplets	3–21 days	Minor illness: headache; sore throat; vomiting. Major illness: fever; stiff neck and back; muscle aches; paralysis	Relief of symptoms
Rabies	Rabies virus (a rhabdovirus)	Bite, or lick on broken skin, from infected animal	Usually 2–8 weeks, but may be over 1 year	Fever; malaise; irrationality; throat spasms; hydrophobia	Wound cleansing; prompt rabies vaccine and immunoglobulins for post-exposure treatment in the unimmunized
Rubella	Rubella virus	Airborne droplets; mother to fetus	14–21 days	Low fever; characteristic rash; congenital abnormalities in fetus, including ear, eye, and heart defects	Relief of symptoms

INFECTIOUS DISEASES: BACTERIAL INFECTIONS

Disease	Infective agent	Transmission	Incubation period	Symptoms	Treatment
Gonorrhoea	NEISSERIA GONORRHOEAE	Sexual contact; mother to baby at delivery	2–10 days	Pain on passing urine; discharge; pain in abdomen	Cephalosporin or quinolone antibiotics
Meningitis, bacterial	NEISSERIA MENINGITIDIS (meningococcus); STREPTOCOCCUS PNEUMONIAE; others	Airborne droplets	Less than 3 weeks; may be less than 48 hours	High fever; stiff neck; nausea; confusion; purple rash that does not fade (in meningococcus)	Immediate treatment with antibiotics
Pertussis (whooping cough)	BORDETELLA PERTUSSIS	Airborne droplets	7–10 days	Runny nose and moderate fever; slight cough leading to characteristic cough spasms and vomiting	Erythromycin to prevent spread of infection; small children may require hospital admission
Pneumonia	STREPTOCOCCUS PNEUMONIAE; MYCOPLASMA PNEUMONIAE; others	Airborne droplets	1–3 weeks	Cough; fever; chest pain; shortness of breath	Antibiotics
Tuberculosis	MYCOBACTERIUM TUBERCULOSIS	Airborne transmission; unpasteurized cows' milk	4–12 weeks for primary infection; disease may be reactivated later in life	Fever; malaise; weight loss; cough; shortness of breath; chest pain	Multiple antituberculous drugs for several months
Typhoid fever	SALMONELLA TYPHI	Food or water contaminated with infected faeces	1–2 weeks, sometimes longer	Headache; lethargy; constipation; very high, prolonged fever; dry cough	Antibiotics

INFECTIOUS DISEASES: CHLAMYDIAL INFECTIONS

Disease	Infective agent	Transmission	Incubation period	Symptoms	Treatment
Nongonococcal urethritis (in men) / Chlamydia (in women)	CHLAMYDIA TRACHOMATIS	Sexual contact	1–4 weeks	Nongonococcal urethritis: pain on passing urine; watery mucous discharge. Nonspecific genital infection: often no symptoms	Antibiotics
Psittacosis	CHLAMYDIA PSITTACI	Inhalation of dust containing faeces from infected birds	1–3 weeks	Flulike and feverish symptoms; shortness of breath	Antibiotics

INFECTIOUS DISEASES: RICKETTSIAL INFECTIONS

Disease	Infective agent	Transmission	Incubation period	Symptoms	Treatment
Q fever	COXIELLA BURNETII	Inhalation of infected dust	2–4 weeks	Sudden onset of fever and sweating; cough; chest pains; headache	Antibiotics
Epidemic typhus	RICKETTSIA PROWAZEKII	Bite from infected body louse	About 7 days	Severe headache; high fever; muscle aches; weakness; rash	Antibiotics

INFECTIOUS DISEASES: FUNGAL INFECTIONS

Disease	Infective agent	Transmission	Incubation period	Symptoms	Treatment
Tinea (ringworm)	TRICHOPHYTON RUBRUM; MICROSPORUM CANIS; others	Direct contact with infected humans or animals	Variable	Itchy skin patches; patchy hair loss; cracking skin between toes	Topical or systemic antifungal drugs
Meningitis, fungal	CRYPTOCOCCUS NEOFORMANS	Inhalation of fungus from pigeon droppings	Unknown	Headache; stiff neck; photophobia	Antifungal drugs

INFECTIOUS DISEASES: PROTOZOAL INFECTIONS

Disease	Infective agent	Transmission	Incubation period	Symptoms	Treatment
Amoebiasis	ENTAMOEBA HISTOLYTICA	Food or water contaminated by faeces	A few weeks to many years	Severe, sometimes bloody diarrhoea	Antiprotozoal drugs (such as metronidazole)
Giardiasis	GIARDIA LAMBLIA	Food or water contaminated by faeces; sexual contact	7–40 days	Diarrhoea; abdominal discomfort; bloating	Antiprotozoal drugs (such as metronidazole)
Malaria	PLASMODIUM FALCIPARUM; PLASMODIUM VIVAX; others	Bite from infected mosquito	10–40 days	Chills; high fever; sweating; headache; fatigue	Proguanil/atovaquone, artemether/lumefantrine, quinine (for falciparum); chloroquine, primaquine (for vivax and others).

inferior

An anatomical term that is used to describe the lower of two body structures, surfaces, or organs.

inferiority complex

A neurotic state of mind that develops because of repeated hurts or failures in the past. Inferiority complex arises from a conflict between the positive wish to be recognized as someone worthwhile and the fear of frustration and failure.

Attempts to compensate for the sense of worthlessness may take the form of aggression and violence, or an overzealous involvement in activities. (See also *superiority complex*.)

infertility

The inability to produce offspring, which may result from a problem in either the male or the female reproductive system, or, in many cases, from a combination of problems in both.

MALE INFERTILITY

The main cause of male infertility is a lack of healthy sperm. In *azoospermia*, no sperm are produced; in *oligospermia* only a few sperm are produced. In some cases, sperm are produced but are malformed or short-lived.

The underlying cause of these problems may be blockage of the spermatic tubes or damage to the spermatic ducts, usually due to a *sexually transmitted infection*. Abnormal development of the testes due to an endocrine disorder (see *hypogonadism*) or damage to the testes by *orchitis* may also cause defective sperm. Smoking, toxins, or various drugs can lower the sperm count (the number of sperm cells in a sample of semen). Other causes are disorders affecting ejaculation (see *ejaculation, disorders of*). Rarely, male infertility is due to a chromosomal abnormality, such as *Klinefelter's syndrome*, or a genetic disease, such as *cystic fibrosis*.

FEMALE INFERTILITY

The most common cause of female infertility is failure to ovulate. Other causes are blocked, damaged or absent *fallopian tubes*; disorders of the uterus, such as *fibroids* and *endometriosis*; problems with *fertilization*; or difficulties with implantation in the uterus (see *implantation, egg*). Infertility also occurs if the woman's cervical mucus contains antibodies that kill or immobilize her partner's sperm. Rarely, a chromosomal abnormality, such as *Turner's syndrome*, is the cause of a woman's infertility.

INVESTIGATION

The initial investigation performed for male infertility is *semen analysis*, which includes a sperm count. Investigations to discover the cause of a woman's infertility may include blood and urine tests to check that ovulation is occurring, ultrasound scanning or X-ray examinations to assess whether the fallopian tubes are blocked, and *laparoscopy* to determine if a condition, such as *endometriosis*, is present.

TREATMENT

There are various possible treatments for male infertility, depending on the cause. In azoospermia due to blockage of the spermatic ducts, it may be possible to take sperm directly from the testis or epididymis. The sperm sample may then be used for *intracytoplasmic sperm injection* (ICSI) in conjunction with *in vitro fertilization* (IVF). In some cases of male infertility due to a hormonal

INVESTIGATING **INFERTILITY**

First, a general check-up and/or a personal interview regarding sexual behaviour are carried out. If no cause for infertility is found at this stage, more specialized tests may be performed.

It is important that both partners are tested for infertility, because infertility can be attributed to one person, to both people, or to mutual incompatibility.

CAUSES OF INFERTILITY

Conception is a complicated process; the reproductive organs can be affected in numerous ways, resulting in infertility. Some of the principal underlying causes of infertility in men and in women are illustrated on the right.

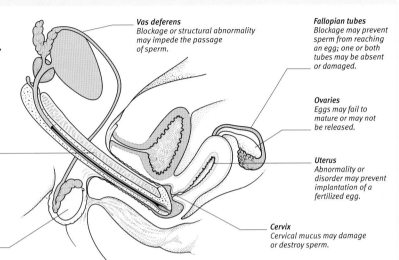

Penis
There may be failure to achieve or maintain an erection, or abnormality of ejaculation.

Testes
Too few sperm may be produced; sperm could be abnormally shaped, too short-lived, or have impaired motility.

Vas deferens
Blockage or structural abnormality may impede the passage of sperm.

Fallopian tubes
Blockage may prevent sperm from reaching an egg; one or both tubes may be absent or damaged.

Ovaries
Eggs may fail to mature or may not be released.

Uterus
Abnormality or disorder may prevent implantation of a fertilized egg.

Cervix
Cervical mucus may damage or destroy sperm.

FEMALE INFERTILITY

Investigations to discover the cause of a woman's infertility may include taking a menstrual history and a study of the woman's body temperature during her menstrual cycle (below). There may also be blood and urine tests to discover whether ovulation is normal, hysterosalpingography (right), and/or laparoscopy (below right).

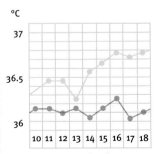

Body temperature and ovulation
Charting the changes in a woman's body temperature during her menstrual cycle can reveal abnormalities of ovulation. The chart above shows typical daily temperature fluctuations during a normal menstrual cycle (coloured line) and temperature changes associated with failure to ovulate (grey line).

Hysterosalpingography
This is an X-ray technique that is used to show the uterus and/or fallopian tubes. Here, the right-hand tube (on the left of the image) is totally blocked, and the left-hand tube appears enlarged.

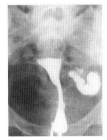

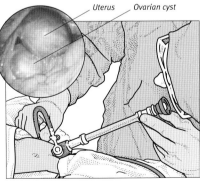

Uterus   Ovarian cyst

Laparoscopy
In this technique, a laparoscope (a type of viewing tube) is inserted through the abdominal wall to examine the woman's reproductive organs and determine whether an abnormality or disorder, such as blocked fallopian tubes or endometriosis, is present. The laparoscopic view above shows an ovarian cyst.

MALE INFERTILITY

The first test for investigating male infertility is semen analysis (below). If it reveals a low sperm count, more tests may be needed to investigate the underlying cause.

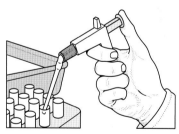

Semen analysis
Semen produced by masturbation is examined as soon as possible, and the number, shape, and degree of motility (movement) of the sperm are determined. A postcoital semen test may also be performed.

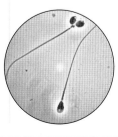

Abnormal sperm
If a man's semen contains large numbers of abnormally shaped sperm, such as the two-headed one at the top of this image, his fertility may be reduced.

imbalance, drugs such as *clomifene* or *gonadotrophin hormone* therapy may prove useful. If no sperm at all are produced by the testis, the only options are adoption of children or *artificial insemination* by a donor.

Failure of the woman to ovulate requires ovarian stimulation with a drug such as clomifene, given either with or without a gonadotrophin hormone. *Microsurgery* can sometimes repair damage to the fallopian tubes. If surgery is unsuccessful, IVF is an option. Uterine abnormalities or disorders, such as fibroids, may require treatment. In some cases, provided the woman has normal fallopian tubes, either *gamete intrafallopian transfer* (GIFT) or *zygote intrafallopian transfer* (ZIFT) may be carried out.

infestation

The presence of animal parasites (such as mites, ticks, or lice) in the skin or hair, or of worms (such as tapeworms) inside the body.

infibulation

A form of female circumcision in which the labia majora (the outer lips surrounding the vagina) are removed and the entrance to the vagina narrowed (see *circumcision, female*).

infiltrate

The term used for a build-up of substances or cells within a tissue that are either not normally found in it or are usually present only in smaller amounts.

The word "infiltrate" may also refer to a drug (such as a local anaesthetic) that has been injected into a tissue, or to the build-up of a substance within an organ (for example, fat in the liver caused by excessive alcohol consumption). In addition, radiologists use the term to refer to the presence of abnormalities, most commonly on a *chest X-ray*, due to conditions such as infection.

inflammation

Redness, swelling, heat, and pain in a tissue due to injury or infection. When body tissues are damaged, *mast cells* release the chemical *histamine* and other substances. Histamine increases the flow of blood to the damaged tissue and also makes the blood capillaries more leaky; fluid then oozes out and into the tissues, causing localized swelling. The inflammatory chemicals stimulate the nerve endings, causing pain. Inflammation is usually accompanied by a local increase in the number of white blood cells. These cells help to destroy invading microorganisms and are involved in repairing the damaged tissue.

Inflammation may be suppressed by *corticosteroid drugs* or by *nonsteroidal anti-inflammatory drugs*.

inflammatory bowel disease

A collective term for chronic disorders that affect the small and/or the large intestine and cause abdominal pain, bleeding, and diarrhoea. *Crohn's disease* and *ulcerative colitis* are the most common types of inflammatory bowel disease.

inflammatory oedema

A term sometimes used to describe the swelling associated with *inflammation*, such as the swelling that develops around a cut as it heals.

infliximab

A monoclonal antibody (see *antibody, monoclonal*) that inhibits the activity of tumour necrosis factor (TNF), a chemical released by *lymphocytes* causing tissue damage and pain. Such drugs are known as TNF blockers or anti-TNF drugs. Infliximab is used to treat severe *rheumatoid arthritis*, *Crohn's disease*, *ulcerative colitis*, and *psoriasis* that have not responded to other drug treatment.

influenza

Popularly known as "flu", a viral infection of the respiratory tract (air passages). Influenza is spread by infected droplets from coughs or sneezes. It usually occurs during the winter months, typically in small outbreaks but, every few years, in epidemics.

CAUSES

There are three main types of influenza virus: A, B, and C. A person who has had an attack caused by the type C virus acquires *antibodies* that provide immunity against type C for life. Infection with a strain of type A or B virus produces immunity only to that particular strain. Type A and B viruses, however, are capable of altering to produce new strains; type A has been the cause of pandemics (disease outbreaks affecting millions of people) in the last century. Occasionally, another strain of influenza virus that primarily affects birds may also affect humans, such as *avian influenza*.

SYMPTOMS AND COMPLICATIONS

Types A and B produce classic flu symptoms: fever, headache, muscle aches, and weakness. Type C causes a mild illness that is indistinguishable from a common cold.

Flu usually clears up within 7–10 days, although sufferers may not feel completely recovered for another week or two. Rarely, however, it takes a severe form, causing acute *pneumonia* that may be fatal within a day or two, even in healthy young adults.

Type B infections in children sometimes mimic *appendicitis*, and they have been implicated in *Reye's syndrome*. In elderly people and those with lung or heart disease, influenza may be followed by a bacterial infection such as *bronchitis* or pneumonia.

TREATMENT

Analgesics (painkillers) help to relieve aches and pains and reduce fever. The drugs *oseltamivir*, *zanamivir*, and *amantadine* may be used for the prevention and/or treatment of influenza in certain cases. *Antibiotic drugs* may be used to combat secondary bacterial infection.

PREVENTION

Flu vaccines containing killed strains of the types A and B virus currently in circulation are available but have only a 60–70 per cent success rate. The immunity they provide is only short-lived and vaccination must be repeated annually. Influenza vaccination is advised for those over 65 and for people with chronic respiratory disease, chronic heart disease, chronic kidney disease, chronic liver disease, immunosuppression (which may be due to disease or medication), or *diabetes mellitus*. Vaccination is also recommended for people in long-stay residential care and for healthcare workers who have regular contact with vulnerable groups. The human influenza vaccines do no protect against avian influenza.

informed consent

See *consent*.

infra-

A prefix meaning "below", commonly used in medical terminology.

infrapatellar bursitis

Inflammation of the *bursa* (fluid-filled sac) that lies below the *patella* (kneecap) and over the top of the *tibia* (shinbone) acting as a cushion against friction. The condition is usually the result of prolonged kneeling in an upright position (which it is why it is sometimes called "clergyman's knee"). Infrapatellar bursitis is similar to prepatellar bursitis, or *housemaid's knee*; however, this second condition often results from prolonged kneeling while leaning forwards, which puts excessive pressure on the bursa that lies in front of the kneecap.

Infrapatellar bursitis causes swelling and pain. Knee movement may also be restricted. The swelling usually reduces with rest; *nonsteroidal anti-inflammatory drugs* may help to relieve the discomfort. For persistent symptoms, a doctor may drain the fluid from the bursa and inject a *corticosteroid drug* into the sac. Frequent changes in position and use of foam padding is recommended.

infra-red

A term denoting the part of the electromagnetic spectrum that is immediately beyond the red end of the visible light spectrum (see *colour vision*).

Infra-red radiation is directed on to the skin and heats the skin and the tissues immediately below it. An infra-red lamp is one means of giving *heat treatment* to promote healing from injuries and inflammatory conditions.

infundibulum

The medical term for a funnel-shaped passage or structure. Specifically, infundibulum refers to the short stalk carrying nerve fibres connecting the *hypothalamus* in the brain to the *pituitary gland*.

infusion, intravenous

See *intravenous infusion*.

ingestion

The act of taking any substance (for example, food, drink, or medications) into the body through the mouth. The term "ingestion" also refers to the process by which certain cells (for example, some white blood cells) surround and then engulf small particles.

ingrowing toenail

See *toenail, ingrowing*.

inguinal

A word relating to the groin (the area between the abdomen and thigh), as in *inguinal hernia*.

inguinal hernia

A type of *hernia* in which part of the intestine protrudes through the abdominal wall in the groin. It can be either direct or indirect. In a direct inguinal hernia, there is a localized weakness in the abdominal wall through which the intestine pushes. In an indirect inguinal hernia the intestine protrudes through the inguinal canal (in males the passage through which the testes descend into the scrotum). An indirect inguinal hernia may also occur in females.

inhalation

The act of taking in breath (see *breathing*). An inhalation is also a medication designed to be breathed in and prepared in the form of a gas, vapour, powder, or aerosol.

inhaler

A device used for administering a drug in powder or vapour form. Inhalers are used mainly in the treatment of various respiratory disorders, including *asthma* and chronic *bronchitis*. Metered-dose inhalers deliver a precise dose when the inhaler is pressed. Drugs taken by inhalation include *bronchodilators* and *corticosteroids*. See the illustrated box for information on using an inhaler.

inheritance

The transmission of characteristics and disorders from parents to their children through the *genes*. Genes are units of *DNA* (deoxyribonucleic acid) contained in the cells; DNA controls all aspects of the body's growth and functioning. Half of a person's genes come from the mother and half from the father.

GENES AND CHROMOSOMES

Genes are organized into *chromosomes* (long, thread-like structures) in the cell nucleus. Genes controlling most characteristics come in pairs, one from each parent. Every individual has 22 pairs of chromosomes (called autosomes), with each chromosome in a pair bearing one of the paired genes. In addition, there are two sex chromosomes: females have two X chromosomes, and males have an X and a Y chromosome.

MECHANISMS OF INHERITANCE

Most physical characteristics, many disorders, and some mental abilities and aspects of personality are inherited. The inheritance of normal traits and disorders can be divided into three groups: those controlled by a single pair of genes on the autosomal chromosomes (unifactorial inheritance); those controlled by genes on the sex chromosomes (sex-linked inheritance, such as haemophilia); and those controlled by the combination of many genes (multifactorial inheritance, such as height).

UNIFACTORIAL INHERITANCE

Either of the pair of genes controlling a trait may take any of several forms, known as *alleles*.

HOW TO USE A METERED-DOSE **INHALER**

The user puts the mouthpiece of the inhaler in the mouth, presses the end, and simultaneously breathes in through the mouth. If the device is used correctly, the drug is dispersed to the bronchi. Young children, or people who find it difficult to use an inhaler, can use a spacer. A *nebulizer* is a device that delivers the drug directly as a fine mist, through a face-mask or mouthpiece, over several minutes.

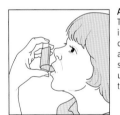

Aerosol inhaler
This type of inhaler delivers a dose of the drug as an aerosol spray when the user presses the top of the inhaler.

Top of inhaler is pressed

Canister of liquid drug

Spacer
The inhaler fits on to the spacer and the drug dose is released into it. The user inhales normally from the spacer's mouthpiece.

Mouthpiece

Spacer

Inhaler fits on to end of spacer

For example, the genes controlling eye colour exist as two main alleles, coding for blue and brown eye colour. The brown allele is dominant over blue in that it "masks" the blue allele, which is described as "recessive" to the brown allele. Only one of the pair of genes controlling a trait is passed to a child from each parent. For example, someone with the brown/blue combination for eye colour has a 50 per cent chance of passing on the blue gene, and a 50 per cent chance of passing on the brown gene, to any child. This factor is combined with the gene coming from the other parent, according to dominant or recessive relationships, to determine the child's eye colour. Certain genetic disorders are also inherited in a unifactorial manner (for example, *cystic fibrosis* and *achondroplasia*).

SEX-LINKED INHERITANCE
Sex-linked inheritance depends on the two sex chromosomes, X and Y. The most obvious example of this type of inheritance is gender of an individual. Male gender is determined by genes on the Y chromosome, which is present only in males.

Any faults in a male's genes on the X chromosome tend to be evident because there is no second, normal X chromosome that would mask the faults (as there is in females). Faults in the genes of the X chromosome include those responsible for colour vision deficiency, haemophilia, and other sex-linked inherited disorders, which almost exclusively affect males.

MULTIFACTORIAL INHERITANCE
Multifactorial inheritance, along with the effects of lifestyle (such as diet) and environment (such as exposure to diseases or toxins), may play a part in causing certain disorders, such as *diabetes mellitus* and *neural tube defects*.

inhibition
The process of preventing any mental or physical activity. Inhibition in the brain and spinal cord is carried out by certain *neurons* (nerve cells), which damp down the action of other nerve cells in order to keep the brain's activity in balance.

In *psychoanalysis*, the term "inhibition" refers to the unconscious restraint of instinctual impulses.

injection
Introduction of a substance into the body from a syringe via a needle. Injections may be intravenous (given into a vein); intramuscular (into a muscle); intradermal (into the skin); subcutaneous (into the tissue layer under the skin); or intra-articular (into a joint).

injury
Physical harm to any part of the body. Injury may have many possible causes, including environmental influences (for example, force, heat, cold, electricity, and radiation), chemical causes (such as poisons), bites, or oxygen deprivation.

ink-blot test
An outdated psychological test in which the subject was asked to interpret the appearance of several ink blots; the responses were thought to reveal aspects of mental function such as emotions and psychological conflicts. The most widely used example was the *Rorschach test*.

inlay, dental
A filling of porcelain or gold used to restore a badly decayed tooth where the cavity is too big to receive amalgam. An inlay may be needed for the back teeth or to protect a weakened tooth.

innate
A term to describe a condition or trait that is present from birth (see *congenital*).

inner ear
The deepest part of the *ear*, lying closest to the brain, that contains the organs of hearing and balance. The inner ear registers air vibrations and other sensory stimuli, such as head movement; cells convert the information into electrical impulses, which pass along nerves to the brain. The other parts of the ear are the outer and middle ear.

innervation
A term meaning the supply of nerves to an organ or other part of the body.

innocent murmur
A *murmur* (a sound made by blood flow through the heart, as heard through a stethoscope) that is not due to any disease of the heart or its valves. Innocent heart murmurs are commonly found in children and may be more noticeable after exercise or during a fever. If there is any doubt about the significance of a murmur, tests such as *echocardiography* or *ECG* may be requested.

inoculation
The act of introducing a small quantity of a foreign substance into the body, usually by injection, for the purpose of stimulating the *immune system* to produce *antibodies* (protective proteins) against the substance, a process known

INHERITANCE OF EYE COLOUR

Eye colour is determined by two main alleles (forms of a gene), one coding for brown eyes and the other for blue eyes. The brown allele is dominant to the blue one (which is therefore recessive).

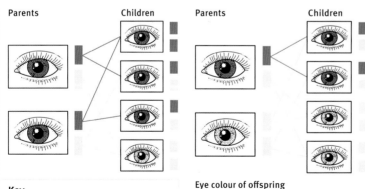

Key

Allele for brown eyes

Allele for blue eyes

Brown eyes

or

Blue eyes

Eye colour of offspring
Two brown-eyed parents, each with the brown/blue combination of alleles, have a one-in-four chance of producing a blue-eyed child (above left). However, when one parent is brown-eyed (with brown/blue alleles) and the other is blue-eyed (with blue alleles), there is a one-in-two chance that they will have a blue-eyed child (above).

as active *immunity*. Inoculation is usually done to protect individuals against future infection by particular bacteria or viruses (see *immunization*).

inoperable

A term applied to any condition that cannot be alleviated or cured by surgery, particularly cancers.

inorganic

A term used to refer to any of the large group of substances that do not contain carbon. Some examples of inorganic substances include table salt (sodium chloride) and bicarbonate of soda (sodium bicarbonate). The term "inorganic" is also applied to a few of the most simple carbon compounds, such as *carbon dioxide* and *carbon monoxide*.

inotropic

A term used to refer to anything that affects the force or energy of muscular contractions, either positively (strengthening the contractions) or negatively (weakening the contractions).

Inotropic drugs are drugs that stimulate, and increase the force of, heart muscle contractions. Inotropic drugs are sometimes needed immediately after a *myocardial infarction* (heart attack) to maintain blood pressure and tissue circulation. In such cases, drugs such as *dopamine* and dobutamine are given by intravenous infusion. In cases of chronic *heart failure*, *digitalis drugs*, and especially *digoxin*, may be used for the same purpose.

inpatient treatment

Care or therapy in hospital following patient admission.

inquest

An official inquiry by a *coroner* into a death that is of unknown cause or is suspected of being unnatural.

INR

The abbreviation for *International Normalized Ratio*.

insanity

A term commonly used for serious mental disorder. Although used legally, the term has no real medical meaning.

insect bites

Puncture wounds inflicted by bloodsucking insects such as gnats, mosquitoes, fleas, and lice. Most bites cause only temporary pain or itching, but some people have severe skin reactions. In the tropics and subtropics, insect bites are potentially more serious because certain biting species are capable of transmitting disease (see *insects and disease*).

All insect bites provoke a skin reaction to substances in the insect's saliva or faeces, which may be deposited at or near the site of the bite. Reactions vary from red pimples to painful swellings or an intensely itching rash. Some insects, such as bees and wasps, have stings (see *insect stings*) that can produce fatal allergic reactions. (See also *lice*; *spider bites*; *mites and disease*; *ticks and disease*.)

insecticides

See *pesticides*.

insects and disease

Relatively few insect species cause disease directly in humans. Some parasitize humans, living under the skin or on the body surface (see *lice*; *chigoe*; *myiasis*). The most troublesome insects are flies and biting insects. Flies can carry infectious microorganisms from human or animal excrement via their feet or legs and contaminate food or wounds.

A number of serious diseases are spread by biting insects. These disorders include *malaria* and *filariasis* (transmitted by mosquitoes), *sleeping sickness* (from tsetse flies), *leishmaniasis* (sandflies), epidemic *typhus* (lice), and *plague* (rat fleas). Mosquitoes, sandflies, and ticks can also spread illnesses such as *yellow fever*, *dengue*, *Lyme disease*, and some types of viral *encephalitis*. Organisms picked up when an insect ingests blood from an infected animal or person are able to survive or multiply in the insect. Later, the organisms are either injected into a new human host via the insect's saliva or deposited in the faeces at or near the site of the bite.

Most insect-borne diseases are confined to the tropics and subtropics, although tick-borne Lyme disease occurs in some parts of the UK.

PREVENTION

The avoidance of insect-borne disease is largely a matter of keeping flies off food, discouraging insect bites by the use of suitable clothing and insect repellents (such as *DEET*), and, in parts of the world where malaria is present, the use of mosquito nets and screens, *pesticides*, and antimalarial tablets.

insect stings

Reactions that are produced by the *stings* of insects such as bees and wasps. Venom injected by the insect contains inflammatory substances that cause local pain, redness, and swelling for about 48 hours.

A sting in the mouth or throat is dangerous because the swelling may obstruct breathing. A severe allergic reaction can occur in response to insect venom, leading to *anaphylactic shock*.

If the symptoms of anaphylactic shock develop, it is essential to seek emergency medical treatment immediately. Anyone who is known to be hypersensitive to bee or wasp venom should obtain and carry an emergency kit for the self-injection of *adrenaline* (epinephrine).

insecurity

Lack of self-confidence and uncertainty about one's abilities, aims, and relationships with others. A feeling of insecurity may be a feature of *anxiety* and other neurotic mental disorders.

INSECT-BORNE DISEASES

Malaria is by far the most prevalent of the insect-borne diseases, causing about 300 million acute illnesses and 1 million deaths each year.

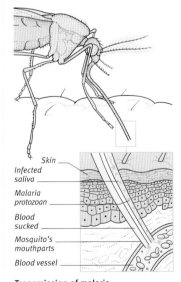

Skin
Infected saliva
Malaria protozoan
Blood sucked
Mosquito's mouthparts
Blood vessel

Transmission of malaria
When an infected *Anopheles* mosquito feeds on a person's blood, it injects saliva through its mouthparts to stop the blood from clotting; the protozoa that cause malaria enter the blood via the insect's saliva.

insemination

The term used for the introduction of a man's *semen* into a woman's *uterus*. Insemination may occur through *sexual intercourse* or by the use of instruments as part of *infertility* treatment (see *artificial insemination*).

insight

Being aware of one's own mental state. In a general sense, "insight" means knowing one's own strengths, weaknesses, and abilities. The term also has the specific psychiatric meaning of knowing that one's symptoms are an illness. Loss of insight may be a feature of psychotic disorders (see *psychosis*).

in situ

A Latin term meaning "in place". The phrase "carcinoma in situ" is used to describe tissue (particularly of the skin or cervix) that is cancerous only in its surface cells.

insomnia

A regular inability to fall asleep or stay asleep, leading to excessive tiredness.

CAUSES

The most common cause of insomnia is stress, but other causes include physical symptoms such as a cough, itching, or conditions such as *restless legs*. Environmental and lifestyle factors (such as jet lag, noise, and excessive caffeine or alcohol) or misuse of *sleeping drugs* are also common causes. Insomnia can be a symptom of a psychological problem, such as *anxiety* and/or *depression*. Withdrawal symptoms from *antidepressants*, *antianxiety drugs*, sleeping drugs, and some illicit drugs (see *drug abuse*) may also cause insomnia.

PREVENTION AND TREATMENT

People with insomnia should ensure that they get sufficient exercise during the day and moderate their alcohol and caffeine intake. They should also avoid eating late at night and should establish regular routines and times for going to bed and waking. If insomnia is severe or persistent, *cognitive-behavioural therapy* or *counselling* may be helpful, particularly if the underlying cause is a psychological problem.

Sleeping drugs should be used only for short-term treatment and only on medical advice. Possible complementary therapies for insomnia include *acupuncture* and *aromatherapy* using lavender oil. (See also *nightmares*; *night terrors*; *sleepwalking*.)

inspiratory capacity

The volume of air that can be drawn into the lungs in a maximum inhalation following a normal expiration.

inspiratory reserve volume

The volume of air that can be drawn into the lungs beyond the end of a normal inhalation.

inspiratory stridor

A harsh, high-pitched sound heard on inhaling. Inspiratory stridor is associated with damage to or a disorder of the respiratory tract, particularly in the area of the *larynx* (voicebox). (See also *expiratory stridor*; *stridor*.)

inspissation

Thickening or drying up of secretions as a result of dehydration or evaporation. Inspissated secretions in the airways, for example, can lead to blockage and collapse of areas of lung tissue.

instep

The arched area of the *foot* between the heel and ball of the foot.

instinct

An innate primitive urge, such as the need for warmth, food, and sex, and the instinct for survival. An instinct is different from a *reflex*, which is an involuntary response to a stimulus (such as withdrawing quickly from a source of pain).

institutionalization

Loss of personal independence that stems from living for long periods under a rigid regime, such as in a prison or other large institution. Apathy, obeying orders unquestioningly, accepting a standard routine, and loss of interests are the main features.

insufficiency

The inability of an organ or body part to perform its intended function. In hepatic insufficiency, for example, the liver cannot carry out its normal work (see *liver failure*). In another example, venous insufficiency, which usually affects the legs, the blood does not drain adequately through the veins, which may lead to swelling and leg *ulcers*.

insufflation

A technique in which air, another type of gas, or powder is blown into a body cavity. Insufflation may be used during medical investigations to make it easier to view organs or to identify blockages. In *laparoscopy*, for example, the abdomen is insufflated using carbon dioxide.

insulin

A hormone produced by clusters of cells in the *pancreas*, known as the *Islets of Langerhans*, that regulates the level of *glucose* in the blood. It is produced continuously, but the amount increases in response to a raised glucose level after a meal. Insulin is essential if glucose is to be absorbed into cells where it is converted into energy. Insulin thus prevents a buildup of glucose in the blood and ensures that tissues have sufficient amounts of glucose.

Failure of insulin production results in *diabetes mellitus*. An *insulinoma* is a rare tumour that causes excessive production of insulin and consequent attacks of *hypoglycaemia* (an abnormally low blood glucose level).

INSULIN THERAPY

Insulin replacement is used in the treatment of diabetes mellitus. Insulin is usually self-administered by subcutaneous injection or through an infusion pump (see *pump, insulin*). Insulin cannot be taken orally because it is destroyed by stomach acid. This treatment prevents *hyperglycaemia* (high blood glucose) and *ketosis* (a buildup of acids in the blood), which, in severe cases, may cause coma. Human insulin preparations are produced by *genetic engineering*, although older beef or pork insulins are still available.

Too high a dose of insulin will cause hypoglycaemia, which can be reversed by consuming food or a sugary drink. Severe hypoglycaemia may cause coma, for which emergency treatment with an intravenous injection of glucose, or *glucagon* (a hormone that opposes the effects of insulin) given into a muscle, vein, or subcutaneously is necessary.

insulinoma

A rare noncancerous tumour of the insulin-producing cells of the *pancreas*. The tumour causes abnormal quantities of insulin to be produced, with the result that the amount of glucose in the blood can fall to dangerously low levels (*hypoglycaemia*). Unless sugar is given immediately, this situation can cause *coma* and death. Once the condition has been diagnosed, a drug (diazoxide) is given to prevent hypoglycaemia from occurring until the tumour is removed.

insulin resistance

An impaired response of body cells to the effects of *insulin*, a hormone produced by the *pancreas* to regulate blood sugar levels. The most common cause of mild insulin resistance is obesity; and sensitivity is regained with weight loss. In type 2 *diabetes mellitus*, raised blood glucose levels are partly due to insulin resistance, but also to a reduced capacity to produce insulin.

Insulin resistance is also a feature of other conditions, such as *polycystic ovary syndrome* and *acanthosis nigricans*. People with unstable diabetes occasionally require massive doses of insulin to achieve a reduction in blood sugar. In such cases, the cause of the insulin resistance is often not known.

insulin shock

An uncommon term for *hypoglycaemia* (abnormally low blood glucose levels).

Intal

A brand name for inhaled *sodium cromoglicate*, an *antiallergy drug* commonly used to prevent *asthma*.

intelligence

The ability to understand concepts and to reason them out. Intelligence can be considered as having three separate forms: abstract (understanding ideas and symbols); practical (aptitude in dealing with practical problems such as repairing machinery); and social (coping reasonably and wisely with human relationships). Intelligence is partly inherited and partly influenced by external factors such as environment and physical health.

Intelligence is formally evaluated with *intelligence tests*, which test a range of mental abilities and express the result as an intelligence quotient (IQ). The tests are designed so that a person of average mental ability has an IQ of 100. Extremes of intelligence occur in *learning difficulties* (defined by a low IQ) and in the gifted (defined by a high IQ – generally over about 130).

intelligence quotient (IQ)

See *intelligence*; *intelligence tests*.

intelligence tests

Tests designed to provide an estimate of a person's mental abilities. Among the most widely used are Wechsler tests. There are two basic types: the Wechsler Adult Intelligence Scale (WAIS) and the Wechsler Intelligence Scale for Children (WISC). Each is divided into verbal (language skills) and performance sections including measures of visual–spatial and perceptual ability (interpretation of shapes) and constructional ability. Other tests include the Stanford–Binet test, used mainly as a measure of scholastic ability.

In most intelligence tests, scoring is based on mental age (MA) in relation to chronological age (CA). The intelligence quotient (IQ) is MA divided by CA, multiplied by 100. The tests are devised to ensure that 3 in 4 people have an IQ between 80 and 120. They are standardized so that the score indicates the same relative ability at different age levels.

Intelligence tests may be used to assess school or job aptitude. They have, however, been criticized for their alleged bias regarding gender, race, and culture.

intensive care unit

A medical facility in which critically ill patients are given intensive care (constant close monitoring and treatment).

Intensive care units (ICUs), sometimes called intensive treatment/ therapy units (ITUs), contain electronic equipment to monitor vital functions such as blood pressure and heart rate. Blood pressure is monitored by an automatic sphygmomanometer, and heart rate and rhythm by an ECG machine. Frequently, patients in ICUs require mechanical *ventilation*, in which a machine takes over or assists with breathing. Urine is collected via a catheter. Urine output, fluid balance, and blood chemistry are recorded regularly and fluids are given intravenously. If nutrients are needed, they may be supplied directly to the stomach through a tube or are administered intravenously. Body fluids and blood sugar levels are maintained by intravenous infusion of salts and glucose. Monitors are fitted with alarms to alert the staff to any dangerous fluctuations.

An ICU contains a high ratio of specially trained nursing and medical staff to patients, which enables treatment to be tailored to a patient's condition as it changes. (See also *coronary care unit*.)

intention tremor

A form of *tremor* (involuntary, rhythmic shaking of the muscles) occurring only when a person tries to carry out a conscious movement, such as touching or picking up an object. The tremor worsens as the object is approached. The condition is usually due to disease or

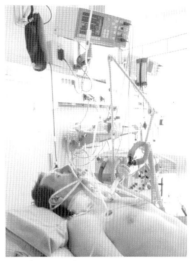

Intensive care unit
An intensive care unit has sophisticated equipment for constant monitoring of a seriously ill patient. He or she is usually sedated and connected to a ventilator to maintain breathing.

damage affecting the *cerebellum* (the area at the back of the brain responsible for coordinating movement).

inter-

A prefix that means between, as in *intercostal* (between the ribs). (See also *intra-*.)

intercostal

A term meaning "between the *ribs*", as in the intercostal muscles, thin sheets of muscle between each rib.

intercourse, painful

Pain during *sexual intercourse*, known medically as dyspareunia, which can affect both men and women. Pain may be superficial (around the external genitals) or deep (within the pelvis).

CAUSES

In men, superficial pain may be due to anatomical abnormalities such as *chordee* (bowed erection) or *phimosis* (tight foreskin). *Prostatitis* (inflammation of the prostate gland) may cause a widespread pelvic ache, a burning sensation in the penis, or pain on ejaculation.

In women, one possible cause of pain is scarring (after childbirth, for example) and lack of vaginal lubrication, especially after the *menopause*. *Psychosexual dysfunction* may also cause pain during intercourse. *Vaginismus*, a condition in which the muscles of the vagina go into spasm, is usually psychological in origin. Deep pain is frequently caused by pelvic disorders (such as *fibroids*, *endometriosis, ectopic pregnancy,* or *pelvic inflammatory disease* due to sexually transmitted infections), disorders of the ovary (such as *ovarian cysts*), and disorders of the *cervix.* Other causes of deep and superficial dyspareunia are *cystitis* and *urinary tract infections.*

TREATMENT

Treatment of painful intercourse is directed at the underlying cause of the pain. If the discomfort is psychological in origin, special counselling may be needed (see *sex therapy*).

intercurrent

A term used to describe a condition, usually an infection, that develops in a person who is already suffering from another disorder.

interdigital

A term meaning between two fingers or toes. Interdigital is used to refer to the skin in such an area.

interferon

One of a group of proteins produced naturally by body cells in response to viral infections and other stimuli. Interferon inhibits viral multiplication and increases the activity of *natural killer cells* (a type of lymphocyte that is part of the *immune system*). The substance may also be produced artificially for use as a drug in the treatment of various disorders. Interferon has to be given by injection.

There are three main types: interferon alfa, beta, and gamma. Interferon alfa is used in the treatment of certain *lymphomas* and *leukaemias*, malignant melanoma (see *melanomoa, malignant*), chronic *hepatitis B* and *C*, and AIDS-related *Kaposi's sarcoma.* Peginterferon, a modified form of interferon alfa, remains in the circulation longer and is used particularly in the treatment of hepatitis C. Interferon beta is used to treat some patients with relapsing *multiple sclerosis.* Interferon gamma is used in the treatment of a rare condition called chronic granulomatous disease.

Adverse reactions to interferons are common including fever, headaches, lethargy, depression, and dizziness.

interleukin

One of a group of proteins that occur naturally in the body. Interleukins are involved in the production of different types of *blood cells* and also help to regulate the *immune system.* At least 18 different interleukins have been identified. One form of interleukin, known as interleukin-2 or aldesleukin, is believed to slow the progress of advanced *kidney cancer.* However, it often has very severe side effects, including damage to the brain and bone marrow and leakage of fluid into the lungs.

intermenstrual bleeding

Bleeding from the vagina between menstrual periods (see *menstrual cycle*). The condition may be due to a disorder of the uterus, but is also a common side effect of oral contraception (see *breakthrough bleeding*).

intermenstrual pain

Pelvic pain occurring between menstrual periods, which may have a variety of causes. In one type, pain occurs in the middle of the *menstrual cycle*, around the time of ovulation (see *mittelschmerz*).

intermittent claudication

Cramping pain in the legs due to inadequate blood supply (see *claudication*).

intermittent positive pressure ventilation (IPPV)

A form of mechanical *ventilation* in which air is delivered into a person's lungs under pressure and in short bursts, to simulate intakes of breath. IPPV can be administered through a tube into a lung, which may be carried out in an *intensive care unit.* A similar procedure of continuous positive airway pressure (CPAP) can be delivered by mask to treat *sleep apnoea.*

internal cardiac massage

A procedure carried out during surgery on the chest to maintain circulation if the heart has stopped beating (see *cardiac massage*). In internal cardiac massage, the surgeon reaches into the open rib cage and squeezes the heart directly.

internal fixation

A procedure for treating fractured bones (see *fracture*) by surgically inserting metal plates, pins, rods, or wires to hold the broken bone ends together. The procedure is used to treat severe fractures that cannot be stabilized by other means. Once the bone has healed, the devices used for internal fixation are often left in place if they are not causing any problems. In some cases, however, it is necessary to remove them in another operation.

internal haemorrhoids

Swollen veins that develop within the rectum (see *haemorrhoids*).

International Normalized Ratio (INR)

A measure introduced by the World Health Organization to standardize the control of *anticoagulant drug* therapy internationally. The ratio is based on comparing the prothrombin time (see *blood-clotting tests*) of a patient's blood with a control time. It gives a standardized measure of a patient's anticoagulation status.

intersex

A group of abnormalities in which the affected person has ambiguous genitalia (abnormal external sex organs) or external genitalia that have the opposite appearance to the chromosomal sex of the individual (see *sex determination*).

interstitial

A word used medically to refer to gaps (interstices) between cells, tissues, or other body structures. For example, *tissue fluid* between the body cells is called interstitial fluid. (See also *interstitial radiotherapy.*)

interstitial cystitis

A chronic inflammation of the bladder lining that causes pain and a frequent urge to pass urine. An *ulcer* usually develops in the bladder wall and, eventually, the bladder muscles thicken and contract (shorten).

Interstitial cystitis is most likely to occur in women. Unlike most other bladder inflammation (see *cystitis*) the disorder is not due to bacterial infection and the cause is unknown.

The disorder is difficult to treat. In a procedure carried out under general anaesthesia, the bladder may be stretched by being filled with water or other liquids. *Anti-inflammatory drugs* may also be given as a treatment.

interstitial pulmonary fibrosis

Scarring of lung tissue mainly affecting the alveoli (the tiny air sacs in the lungs; see *alveolus, pulmonary*). Interstitial pulmonary fibrosis (IPF) may have various causes, including occupational exposure to mineral dusts; *fibrosing alveolitis* (an *autoimmune disorder* in which the immune system attacks the lung tissue); and an allergic reaction (see *allergy*) that causes inflammation of the alveoli.

HOW **INTERFERON** FIGHTS VIRAL INFECTIONS

Interferon is part of the body's immune system, providing a defence against many different types of virally infected cells or tumour cells. It is produced naturally in the body during viral infections, but can also be administered as a drug to enhance its natural actions.

VIRAL MULTIPLICATION

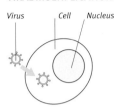

Virus   Cell   Nucleus

1 A virus can multiply only by first invading one of its host's cells.

2 The genetic material of the virus takes over the cell's chemical machinery to make copies of the virus.

3 The copies of the virus escape, killing the host cell, and invade more cells.

HOW INTERFERON WORKS

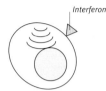

Interferon

1 Interferon attaches to the membrane of host cells and primes them against viral attack.

Antiviral enzymes

2 If a virus invades a cell primed by interferon, enzymes are produced that impair viral copying.

3 Being unable to copy itself, the virus is nullified, and the infection is either stopped altogether or shortened.

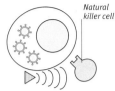

Natural killer cell

1 Interferon also causes natural killer cells to attack virally infected cells or tumour cells.

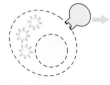

2 A natural killer cell attaches to the abnormal host cell and makes the cell disintegrate.

3 The effect of this process is to help limit a viral infection or to slow down the growth of a tumour.

SYMPTOMS AND DIAGNOSIS

Symptoms of interstitial pulmonary fibrosis include progressive shortness of breath, coughing, chest pain, and *clubbing* (abnormal thickening and broadening) of the fingertips. There may also be additional symptoms caused by any underlying disease.

The diagnosis of IPF is based on the symptoms and a physical examination; it is confirmed by *chest X-ray* and a *biopsy* (removal of a sample of lung tissue for microscopic examination).

TREATMENT AND OUTLOOK

Treatment for interstitial pulmonary fibrosis depends on the cause. Treatment for fibrosing alveolitis often includes use of immunosuppressant drugs and *corticosteroid drugs*, which suppress the the immune system. There is no known treatment for localized fibrosis due to radiotherapy. In other cases, treatment is directed at the underlying cause.

For people with fibrosing alveolitis, the outlook is poor: the lungs become progressively stiffer and *heart failure* and *bronchopneumonia* may develop. Transplantation of a single lung (see *transplant surgery*) may be considered. The outlook of occupational dust disease depends on the type of dust involved and the level of exposure. If IPF is due to an allergy, however, the condition can more easily be treated and the outlook is better.

interstitial radiotherapy

Treatment of a cancerous tumour by inserting radioactive material into the cancerous growth or into neighbouring tissue. Using this method, which is a type of brachytherapy, radiation can be targeted at the diseased area.

Radioactive material (usually artificial radioisotopes) contained in wires, small tubes, or seeds is implanted into or near to the diseased tissue under general anaesthesia. The material is left in place for variable amounts of time depending on the radioactive substance and the tumour that is being treated. In some cases, such as in prostate cancer, the material is left in place permanently as the radiation decays after a relatively short period of time. (See also *radiotherapy*.)

intertrigo

Inflammation of the skin due to two surfaces rubbing together. It is most common in obese people. The affected skin is red and moist and may have an unpleasant odour, and is often accompanied by a fungal infection, such as *candidiasis*; there may also be scales or blisters. The condition gets worse with sweating.

Treatment consists of weight reduction and keeping the affected areas clean and dry. A cream containing *antifungal drugs,* with or without a *corticosteroid,* is used if candidiasis is present.

intervertebral cartilage

The strong tissue, also called fibrocartilage, that makes up the platelike, shock-absorbing discs between the bones of the spine (see *cartilage; disc, intervertebral*).

intervertebral disc

See *disc, intervertebral*.

intervertebral foramen

A natural opening between adjacent *vertebrae* in the spine formed by the space between small notches in each side of the *vertebrae*. Such gaps are the exit points for the peripheral nerves branching from the *spinal cord*.

intestinal imaging

See *barium X-ray examinations*.

intestinal lipodystrophy

See *Whipple's disease*.

intestine

The major part of the digestive tract (see *digestive system*), extending from the exit of the stomach to the anus. It forms a long tube divided into two main sections: the small and large intestines.

SMALL INTESTINE

The small intestine is about 6.5 m in length and has three sections: the *duodenum*, the *jejunum* and the *ileum*. Partially digested food from the stomach is forced along the intestine by *peristalsis*.

The small intestine is concerned with the digestion and absorption of food. Digestive enzymes and *bile*, which break down food to release nutrients, are added to the partly digested food in the duodenum via the bile and pancreatic ducts (see *biliary system*). Glands within the walls of each section of the small intestine produce mucus and other enzymes, which also help to break down the food. Blood vessels in the intestinal walls absorb nutrients and carry them to the *liver* for distribution to the rest of the body.

LARGE INTESTINE

The large intestine is approximately 1.5 m long. The main section, the *colon*, is divided into an ascending, a transverse, a descending, and a pelvic portion (the sigmoid colon). The *appendix* hangs from a pouch (the *caecum*) between the small intestine and the colon. The final section before the *anus* is the *rectum*.

Unabsorbed material leaves the small intestine as liquid and fibre. As this material passes through the large intestine, water and mineral salts are absorbed into the bloodstream, leaving faeces that are made up of undigested food residue, fat, various secretions, and bacteria. The faeces are compressed and pass into the rectum for evacuation.

intestine, cancer of

A malignant tumour in the small or large intestine. Cancer of the small intestine is rare; cancer of the large intestine is one of the most common cancers (see *colon, cancer of*; *rectum, cancer of*). Both the small and large intestine may develop carcinoid tumours (causing *carcinoid syndrome*) and *lymphomas*.

intestine, obstruction of

A partial or complete blockage of the small or large intestine.

CAUSES

Possible causes include a strangulated *hernia* (protrusion of the intestines through the abdominal wall); stenosis (narrowing) of the intestine, often due to cancer in the intestine; intestinal *atresia* (congenital closure); *adhesions* (scar tissue); *volvulus* (twisting of loops of bowel); and *intussusception* (in which the intestine telescopes inside itself).

Intestinal obstruction can also occur in diseases that affect the intestinal wall, such as *Crohn's disease* or paralysis of the muscles in the intestinal wall (see *ileus, paralytic*).

Less commonly, an internal blockage of the intestine is caused by impacted food, *faecal impaction*, *gallstones*, or by an object of some kind that has been accidentally swallowed.

SYMPTOMS

A blockage in the small intestine usually causes intermittent cramplike pain in the centre of the abdomen with increasingly frequent bouts of vomiting and failure to pass wind or faeces. An obstruction in the large intestine causes pain, distension of the abdomen, and failure to pass wind or faeces.

TREATMENT

Treatments involve emptying the stomach via a *nasogastric tube* and replacing lost fluids through an intravenous drip; in some instances, these measures will be sufficient to correct the problem. In many cases, however, a surgical operation to deal with the cause of the blockage is necessary.

intestine, tumours of

Cancerous or noncancerous growths in the intestine. Cancerous tumours most commonly affect the large intestine (see *colon, cancer of*; *rectum, cancer of*); the small intestine is only rarely affected. *Lymphomas* and carcinoid tumours (leading to *carcinoid syndrome*) may sometimes develop in the intestine. Noncancerous tumours include *polyps* in the colon, and *adenomas*, *leiomyomas*, *lipomas*, and *angiomas* in the small intestine.

intoxication

A general term for a condition resulting from *poisoning*. It customarily refers to the effects of excessive drinking (see *alcohol intoxication*). The term may also be used of *drug poisoning*; poisoning from the accumulation of the by-products of *metabolism* in the body; or the effects of industrial poisons.

intra-

A prefix that means "within", as in the term "intramuscular" (within a muscle). (See also *inter-*.)

DISORDERS OF THE INTESTINE

The intestine is subject to the effects of many infective organisms and parasites. It may also be affected by tumours, structural defects, and other disorders.

Infection and inflammation

Generalized inflammation of the intestine may be caused by viral or bacterial infections such as *food poisoning*, *traveller's diarrhoea*, *cholera*, *typhoid fever*, *amoebiasis*, or *giardiasis*, or by infestation with *roundworms* or *tapeworms*. It may also have noninfectious causes, as in *ulcerative colitis* and *Crohn's disease*. *Gastroenteritis* is the term commonly applied to inflammation of the stomach and intestines. Sometimes, inflammation is localized, as in *appendicitis* and *diverticular disease*.

Tumours

Tumours of the small intestine are rare, but noncancerous growths, *lymphomas*, and carcinoid tumours (causing *carcinoid syndrome*) may occur. Tumours of the large intestine are common (see *colon, cancer of*; *rectum, cancer of*). Some forms of familial *polyposis*, a condition causing the development of noncancerous growths, may progress to cancer.

Structural abnormalities

Structural defects may be congenital (present from birth) or may develop later. They include *atresia* (congenital closure), *stenosis* (narrowing), and *volvulus* (twisting of loops of bowel). These abnormalities can cause blockage of the intestine (see *intestine, obstruction of*). In newborn babies with cystic fibrosis, meconium (fetal intestinal contents) is much thicker than normal and may block the intestine.

Obstruction

Impaired blood supply (*ischaemia*) to the intestine may result from partial or complete obstruction of the arteries in the abdominal wall (from diseases such as *atherosclerosis*) or from the blood vessels being compressed or trapped, as in *intussusception* or *hernias*. Loss of blood supply may cause *gangrene*.

Other disorders

Other disorders that affect the intestine include *peptic ulcers*, *diverticulosis*, *malabsorption*, *coeliac disease*, and *irritable bowel syndrome*.

LOCATION OF THE **INTESTINE**

Situated below the stomach and the liver, the intestine occupies a large proportion of the central and lower part of the abdomen.

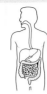

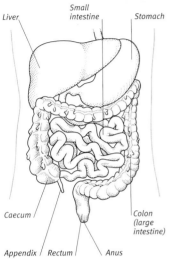

Liver · Small intestine · Stomach · Caecum · Colon (large intestine) · Appendix · Rectum · Anus

intra-articular cartilage

See *hyaline cartilage*.

intracavitary therapy

Treatment of a cancerous tumour in a hollow organ by placing a radioactive implant or *anticancer drugs* within the cavity of the organ.

Intracavitary *radiotherapy* is a type of brachytherapy (the practice of implanting radioactive wires or grains close to the tumour) that is mainly used to treat cancers of the uterus and cervix (see *uterus, cancer of*; *cervix, cancer of*). Implants of radioactive material (usually in the form of artificial radioisotopes in small tubes) are placed near the tumour and left there for a period of time. This varies from hours to days depending on the type of radioactive substance used and the type of tumour being treated.

Intracavitary therapy may be used to treat a malignant effusion (a collection of fluid that contains cancerous cells). A needle, sometimes with a *catheter* (flexible tube) attached, is passed through the wall of the abdomen into the abdominal cavity or through the wall of the chest into the pleural cavity (the space around the lungs). As much of the fluid as possible is withdrawn from the cavity before anticancer drugs are injected directly into it. (See also *interstitial radiotherapy*.)

intracerebral haemorrhage

Bleeding into the tissue of the brain from a ruptured blood vessel. Intracerebral haemorrhage is one of the three principal mechanisms by which a *stroke* can occur.

CAUSES

This disorder mainly affects middle-aged or elderly people and is usually due to *atherosclerosis* (accumulation of fatty deposits in the walls of the arteries). Untreated *hypertension* (high blood pressure) increases the risk of intracerebral haemorrhage.

SYMPTOMS

The ruptured artery is usually in the *cerebrum* (the main mass of the brain). The escaped blood seeps out, damaging brain tissue. The symptoms are sudden headache, weakness, and confusion, and often loss of consciousness. Speech loss, facial paralysis, or one-sided muscle weakness may develop, depending on the area affected.

TREATMENT AND OUTLOOK

Surgery is usually impossible; treatment is aimed at life-support and at the reduction of blood pressure. Large haemorrhages are usually fatal. For the survivor of an intracerebral haemorrhage, rehabilitation and outlook are the same as for any type of stroke.

intracranial aneurysm

The abnormal dilation of an artery occurring anywhere inside the area enclosed by the *cranium* (skull bones). Intracranial aneurysms may cause no symptoms. However, they can suddenly enlarge or rupture, causing *subarachnoid haemorrhage* or *stroke*, which are potentially fatal. (See also *aneurysm*; *berry aneurysm*.)

intracranial hypertension, benign

A condition in which *intracranial pressure* is substantially raised. The cause of the condition is unknown, but it often occurs in obese young women with menstrual irregularities. Rarely it is caused by drugs, including *corticosteroid drugs*. Symptoms may include headache, vomiting, and visual disturbance. The condition is not fatal but can damage the *optic nerves*, leading to permanent visual loss. Treatment is with *diuretic*

drugs; occasionally, excess *cerebrospinal fluid* may be diverted by way of a surgically inserted *shunt* (artificial passage).

intracranial pressure (ICP)

Pressure exerted by *cerebrospinal fluid* (fluid that cushions and nourishes the brain and spinal cord) around the brain. ICP can be assessed during a *lumbar puncture*. Following serious head injury or some types of *neurosurgery*, ICP may be monitored continuously using a transducer that is inserted through the skull.

Raised ICP may be due to a *brain tumour*, *head injury*, *meningitis*, or benign *intracranial hypertension*. Untreated, it can result in permanent neurological damage and may be serious and, in some cases, life-threatening.

intracranial tumour

Any tumour that develops within the *skull*.

intractable

A term used to describe any condition that does not respond to treatment.

intracytoplasmic sperm injection (ICSI)

A treatment for male *infertility* in which a single sperm, collected from a sample of semen or directly from the testis or epididymis, is injected into an *ovum* (see *in vitro fertilization*) to fertilize it. The fertilized ovum is then placed in the woman's uterus.

intradermal

A medical term meaning "into or within the skin". For example, an intradermal injection is made into the skin, whereas a *subcutaneous injection* is made into the layer of fat under the skin.

intradermal naevus

A type of pigmented *naevus* (skin blemish) formed by groups of *melanocytes* (pigment-producing cells) within the dermis (the thick inner layer of the skin). An intradermal naevus is usually raised and may range in colour from dark brown to pink. They are noncancerous and may disappear spontaneously. (See also *junctional naevus*.)

intramuscular

A medical term meaning "within a muscle", as in an intramuscular injection, in which a drug is injected deep within a muscle.

intraocular pressure

The pressure within the eye that helps to maintain the shape of the eyeball. Normal intraocular pressure is produced by a balance between the rate of production and removal of aqueous *humour*, the watery fluid that fills the front of the eyeball. Aqueous humour is continually produced from the *ciliary body* and exits from the drainage angle (a network of tissue between the iris and cornea). If drainage is impeded, intraocular pressure builds up; this condition is called *glaucoma*. If the ciliary body is damaged (as a result of prolonged inflammation), insufficient aqueous fluid may be produced and the eyeball may become soft.

intrauterine contraceptive device

Also known as an IUCD or coil, a mechanical plastic and copper device inserted into the uterus for *contraception*. See *IUD*.

intrauterine growth retardation

Poor growth in a *fetus* (an unborn baby within the uterus). Intrauterine growth retardation usually results from a failure of the *placenta* to provide adequate nutrients (which is often related to *pre-eclampsia*) or sometimes from a fetal defect. Severe maternal disease, such as chronic *kidney failure*, can reduce fetal growth. If the mother smokes during pregnancy, this may also reduce growth and birth weight. Problems in the fetus, such as an intrauterine infection or *genetic disorder*, can also impair growth.

Intrauterine growth retardation may be suspected on *antenatal* examination; *ultrasound scanning* may be performed to assess the problem.

The underlying cause is treated, if possible. If the baby's growth is slowing, *induction of labour* or a *caesarean section* may be necessary. Most babies whose growth was retarded in the uterus gain weight rapidly after delivery. If an intrauterine infection or genetic disorder was the cause, however, poor growth may continue after birth.

intrauterine system

A contraceptive device that fits inside the uterus and releases progestogen hormone (see *IUS*).

intravenous

A term meaning "within a vein", as in intravenous infusion (slow introduction of a substance into a vein) and intravenous injection (rapid introduction of a substance into a vein).

intravenous infusion

The slow introduction of fluid into the bloodstream through a cannula (thin plastic tube) inserted into a vein. An intravenous injection is given over several hours or days and is commonly known as a drip. The procedure is used to give blood (see *blood transfusion*) or, more commonly, fluids or essential salts. Other uses of intravenous infusion include providing nutrients to people who are unable to digest food (see *feeding, artificial*) as well as the administration of certain drugs. A machine known as an infusion pump may be used to control the amount of the drug or fluid being infused.

intravenous urography

An X-ray procedure, commonly abbreviated to IVU, that is used to give a clear image of the *urinary tract*.

The procedure involves intravenous injection of a *contrast medium* (a substance that is opaque to X-rays) into the arm. The medium is carried in the blood to the urinary system, where it passes through the kidneys, ureters, and bladder to be excreted in the urine. X-rays taken at intervals show outlines of the urinary system. IVU reveals abnormalities such as tumours and obstructions, and signs of kidney disease.

intraventricular haemorrhage

Bleeding into the ventricles (the fluid-filled cavities of the brain). Premature babies are at greater risk because the nearby blood vessels are underdeveloped and fragile, but the bleeding may occur in babies carried to full term.

There may be no obvious signs that a haemorrhage has occurred; alternatively, the baby may be pale and limp. *Seizures* may also occur.

Ultrasound scanning of the baby's brain through the fontanelle (a gap in the baby's skull) is used to check for bleeding. Intraventricular haemorrhage may cause no long-term problems. In some cases, however, it may lead to disability or *hydrocephalus* (a buildup of fluid around the brain). In the most severe cases, it may be life-threatening.

intrinsic asthma

The name sometimes given to a type of *asthma* that is not associated with an identifiable allergic trigger, such as pollen. (See also *allergy*; *hypersensitivity*.)

intrinsic factor

A chemical produced by the stomach lining that is necessary for the absorption of vitamin B_{12}. A lack of intrinsic factor leads to a deficiency in vitamin B_{12}; this problem, in turn, results in *pernicious anaemia*.

introitus

A general term for the entrance to a body cavity or space. The word is most commonly used to refer to the vagina.

introspection

The contemplation or analysis of one's own thoughts, feelings, and other mental processes. (See also *insight*.)

introvert

A person who is more concerned with his or her inner world than the external or social environment. Introverts prefer to work alone, are shy and quiet, and become withdrawn when under stress. (See also *extrovert*; *personality*.)

intubation

A term that is most commonly used to refer to the process of passing an *endotracheal* (breathing) *tube* into the trachea (windpipe). Endotracheal intubation is carried out if mechanical *ventilation* is needed to deliver oxygen into the lungs.

To carry out intubation, an anaesthetist first looks down the patient's throat with a laryngoscope (viewing instrument) to identify the vocal cords. The tube is then passed through the mouth or nose and down the throat between the vocal cords and trachea.

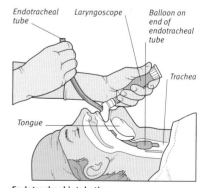

Endotracheal intubation
Guided by an anaesthetist, the endotracheal tube is passed through the patient's mouth and down the throat into the trachea.

The term "intubation" is also used to refer to the placement of a gastric or intestinal tube in the stomach for purposes of suction or the giving of nutrients (see *feeding, artificial*).

intussusception

A condition in which part of the intestine telescopes in on itself, forming a tube within a tube. Intussusception usually occurs at the junction of the ileum and caecum, where the last part of the small intestine joins the large intestine. The condition usually results in intestinal obstruction (see *intestine, obstruction of*).

CAUSES
In some cases intussusception is associated with a recent infection. In other cases, it may start at the site of a *polyp* or *Meckel's diverticulum* (a pouch-like projection from the ileum).

SYMPTOMS AND COMPLICATIONS
Intussusception occurs most commonly in children under the age of two. An affected child usually develops severe abdominal colic; vomiting is common, and blood and mucus are often found in the faeces.

In severe cases of intusseption, the blood supply to the intestine becomes blocked. If this occurs, *gangrene* (tissue death), followed by *peritonitis* (inflammation of the abdominal lining) or *perforation* (rupture), may result.

TREATMENT
In some cases, an *enema* can be used to force the abnormal area of intestine back into a normal position. In other cases, surgery may be necessary to reposition the intestine. Most affected children recover fully after treatment.

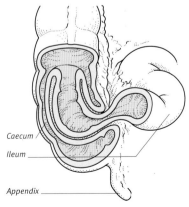

Caecum
Ileum
Appendix

Intussusception
This disorder is characterized by part of the intestine telescoping in on itself. The problem usually occurs at the junction between the ileum and the caecum.

invasive

A term used to describe anything that forcibly enters or spreads through the body. The term is usually applied to cancerous tumours or harmful microorganisms that tend to spread throughout body tissues. It can also be used to refer to surgery. In an "invasive" procedure, the body tissues are penetrated by an instrument during surgery. (See also *minimally invasive surgery*; *noninvasive*.)

inverted nipple

An indrawing of the *nipple*. The condition can be longstanding or may develop in later life as a result of changes in the breast tissue. Possible causes include normal changes associated with aging or, in some cases, an underlying cancer.

in vitro

The performance of biological processes in a laboratory rather than within the body. The term literally means "in glass".

in vitro fertilization (IVF)

A technique used to treat *infertility* when its cause cannot be determined or treated or if there is a blockage in a fallopian tube. IVF is also used to treat couples affected by a *genetic disorder* because the embryo can be tested for abnormalities before implantation. IVF involves surgical removal of an *ovum* from the ovary and its fertilization outside the body.

HOW IT IS DONE
The woman is given a course of *fertility drugs* to stimulate the release of mature ova, followed by *ultrasound scanning* to

PROCEDURE FOR **IN VITRO FERTILIZATION**

Fertilization of eggs outside a woman's body can be performed to treat some types of infertility. One such technique used is in vitro fertilization; the main stages involved in this procedure are illustrated below.

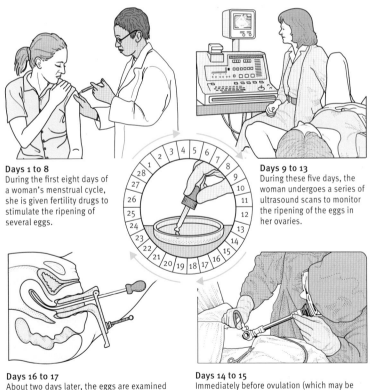

Days 1 to 8
During the first eight days of a woman's menstrual cycle, she is given fertility drugs to stimulate the ripening of several eggs.

Days 9 to 13
During these five days, the woman undergoes a series of ultrasound scans to monitor the ripening of the eggs in her ovaries.

Days 16 to 17
About two days later, the eggs are examined to see if they have been fertilized and have started to develop into embryos. If they have, one or two of the best embryos are introduced into the woman's uterus through the vagina. Further embryos may be frozen and stored.

Days 14 to 15
Immediately before ovulation (which may be induced with drugs), ripe eggs are removed by laparoscopy (above) or by ultrasound-guided needle aspiration through the vagina or the abdomen. The eggs are mixed with the man's sperm in a dish (above, centre), which is then put in an incubator.

check the ova. The ova are collected immediately before ovulation using the guidance of ultrasound, either by *laparoscopy* or via the vagina under sedation. They are then mixed with sperm – usually from the partner, but sometimes from a donor – in the laboratory and are incubated at body temperature for about 48 hours to allow fertilization to take place. One or two fertilized ova are introduced into the woman's uterus through a thin tube fed through the cervix. If they become safely implanted in the uterine wall, the pregnancy usually continues normally.

More than one in four couples who undergo IVF eventually achieve pregnancy, although several attempts may be necessary. Modifications of the technique, such as *intracytoplasmic sperm injection* (ICSI), *gamete intrafallopian transfer* (GIFT), and *zygote intrafallopian transfer* (ZIFT) are generally more effective than the original method.

ADVERSE EFFECTS AND RISKS
The procedures involved in IVF may be uncomfortable, particularly for the woman, who may suffer side effects from the fertility drugs and experience discomfort during egg collection.

IVF may result in multiple pregnancy (see *pregnancy, multiple*) and some techniques carry an increased risk of *ectopic pregnancy* (implantation of a fertilized egg outside the uterus, most commonly in the fallopian tubes). Rarely, the fertility drugs may overstimulate the ovaries (a condition known a ovarian hyperstimulation syndrome, or OHSS), which may cause pain and bloating and may jeopardize the IVF treatment. In severe cases of OHSS, hospitalization may be necessary.

in vivo

Literally "in the living organism"; biological processes occurring within the body. (See also *in vitro*.)

involuntary movements

Uncontrolled movements of the body. These movements occur spontaneously and may be slow and writhing (see *athetosis*); rapid, jerky, and random (see *chorea*); or predictable, stereotyped, and affecting one part of the body, usually the face (see *tic*).

involuntary muscle

An alternative name for smooth *muscle*, which lines the walls of internal body structures such as the blood vessels, airways, and digestive tract.

involution

A term meaning a return to normal size; it is most commonly used to refer to the shrinkage of the enlarged *uterus* following *childbirth*.

iodine

A *trace element* essential for formation of the *thyroid hormones*, triiodothyronine (T_3) and thyroxine (T_4), which control the rate of *metabolism* (internal chemistry) as well as growth and development of the body.

Iodine must be obtained from the diet; it is found in seafood and dairy products, as well as in vegetables grown in soil containing iodides. Dietary shortage may lead to enlargement of the thyroid gland known as goitre or *hypothyroidism*. A deficiency in newborn babies can, if left untreated, lead to mental deficiency and incomplete physical development. Shortages are very rare in developed countries due to bread and table salt being fortified with iodide or iodate.

Radioactive iodine is sometimes used to reduce thyroid gland activity in cases of thyrotoxicosis and in the treatment of thyroid cancer. Iodine compounds are used as antiseptics, in radiopaque contrast media in some X-ray procedures (see *imaging techniques*), and in some cough remedies.

ion

A particle that carries an electrical charge; positive ions are called cations and negative ions anions. Many vital body processes, such as the transmission of nerve impulses, depend on the movement of ions across cell membranes. Sodium is the principal cation in the fluid that bathes all cells (extracellular fluid), affecting the movement of water into and out of cells (see *osmosis*) and thereby influencing the concentration of body fluids.

The acidity of the blood and other body fluids is dependent on the level of hydrogen cations, which are produced by metabolic processes. To prevent the fluids from becoming too acidic, hydrogen cations are neutralized by bicarbonate anions in the extracellular fluid and the blood, and by phosphate anions inside cells (see *acid-base balance*).

IMPORTANT IONS AND THEIR ROLES

Types of ion	Name	Major roles in body
Cations (positively charged ions)	Ammonium (NH_4^+)	Acid–base balance; produced by protein metabolism
	Calcium (Ca^{2+})	Nerve conduction; muscle contraction; blood clotting; bone and tooth formation; heart muscle contraction
	Hydrogen (H^+)	Acid–base balance; component of stomach acid
	Magnesium (Mg^{2+})	Nerve conduction; muscle contraction; bone and tooth formation; enzyme activation; protein metabolism
	Potassium (K^+)	Nerve conduction; muscle contraction; water balance; acid–base balance; heart rhythm
	Sodium (Na^+)	Nerve conduction; muscle contraction; water balance; acid–base balance
Anions (negatively charged ions)	Bicarbonate (HCO_3^-)	Acid–base balance; neutralizes stomach acid
	Chloride (Cl^-)	Acid–base balance; water balance; component of stomach acid
	Phosphate (PO_4^{3-})	Acid–base balance; bone and tooth formation; protein metabolism; energy metabolism; structure of cell membranes

ionizer

A device that produces *ions*. Some people believe that use of an ionizer, which produces negative ions, reduces symptoms, such as headaches and fatigue, that may result from a buildup of the positive ions from electrical machines.

ionizing radiation

A type of *radiation*.

ipecacuanha

A drug (also called ipecac) previously used to induce vomiting in the treatment of types of *poisoning*.

ipratropium bromide

A *bronchodilator drug* used in the treatment of *breathing difficulties*.

IQ

The abbreviation for intelligence quotient (see *intelligence; intelligence tests*).

iridectomy

A procedure performed on the eye to remove part of the *iris*. The most common type of iridectomy, known as a "peripheral iridectomy", is usually performed to treat acute *glaucoma*. A small opening is made, surgically or with a laser, near the outer edge of the iris to form a channel through which *aqueous humour* can drain.

iridocyclitis

Inflammation of the *iris* and *ciliary body*. Iridocyclitis is more usually known as anterior *uveitis*. (See *eye, disorders of*).

iridotomy

A surgical procedure performed on the eye to treat acute *glaucoma*. In the procedure, a laser or knife is used to make one or more tiny holes in the iris (but without removing any iris tissue) to enable excess aqueous humour to drain away. (See also *iridectomy*).

iris

The coloured part of the eye. It is made up of a framework of transparent *collagen* and two sets of muscle fibres (one radial and one circular) that lies behind the *cornea* and in front of the *lens*. It is connected at its outer edge to the ciliary body and has a central aperture, the *pupil*, through which light enters the eye and falls on the *retina*. The iris constricts and dilates to alter the size of the pupil, thereby controlling the amount of light that passes through to reach the retina.

LOCATION OF THE IRIS

The iris lies behind the cornea and in front of the lens. The outer edge is connected to a ring of muscle called the ciliary body (not shown). At the centre is an aperture called the pupil.

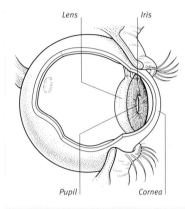

The colour of the iris is inherited from the parents (see *inheritance*) and is determined principally by the amount of *melanin* (dark pigment) in its tissues. Brown eyes contain a high level of melanin. Blue and grey eyes contain very little melanin, their colour comes instead from the collagen tissues themselves. Hazel and green eyes contain moderate levels of melanin; their colour comes partly from the pigment and partly from the collagen tissues. Flecks of colour in the iris are due to scattered light reflected off blood vessels and muscle tissue. It is possible for people to have eyes of different colours (a fairly rare condition called heterochromia iridium). People with *albinism* have no melanin in their bodies and therefore the colour is governed by the tissues. Such people have light blue or even pink eyes.

iritis

Inflammation of the *iris*, now often termed anterior *uveitis*.

iron

A mineral that is essential for the formation of certain *enzymes*, *haemoglobin* (the oxygen-carrying pigment in red blood cells), and *myoglobin* (the oxygen-carrying pigment in muscle cells). Iron is found in foods such as liver, cereals, fish, green leafy vegetables, nuts, and beans. During pregnancy, iron supplements may be required. Iron deficiency leading to anaemia (see *anaemia, iron*

deficiency) is usually caused by abnormal blood loss, such as from a *peptic ulcer* or particularly heavy periods but may also be due to diet.

Iron supplements may cause nausea, abdominal pain, constipation, or diarrhoea and may colour the faeces black. Excessive iron in the tissues is a feature of *haemochromatosis*, which commonly results in *cirrhosis* or other forms of organ damage.

iron-deficiency anaemia

See *anaemia, iron-deficiency*.

irradiation

See *radiation hazards*; *radiotherapy*.

irradiation of food

Treatment of food with ionizing *radiation* in order to kill bacteria, moulds, insects, and other parasites. Irradiation improves the keeping qualities of food and is a means of controlling some types of *food poisoning*. It does not, however, destroy bacterial toxins and may destroy *vitamins*. Irradiation does not render food radioactive, and there is no evidence that it poses a risk to human health.

irrigation, antral

See *antral irrigation*.

irrigation, wound

Cleansing of a dirty or contaminated wound by washing it out repeatedly with a medicated solution or sterile saline solution.

irritable bladder

Intermittent, uncontrolled contractions of the muscles in the *bladder* wall that may cause urge incontinence (see *incontinence, urinary*).

Irritable bladder can occur if there is a urinary tract infection (see *cystitis*); a catheter in the bladder; a bladder stone (see *calculus, urinary tract*); or an obstruction to the outflow of urine by an enlarged *prostate gland*; however often the cause of discomfort is not known. In some cases, symptoms may be relieved by *antispasmodic drugs*; other treatment is directed at any underlying cause. Bladder training may also be used.

irritable bowel syndrome (IBS)

A combination of intermittent abdominal pain and constipation, diarrhoea, or bouts of each, that occurs in the absence of other diagnosed disease.

CAUSE AND INCIDENCE

The precise cause of IBS is unknown, but *anxiety* and *stress* tend to exacerbate the condition. IBS affects up to one in five people at some time during their lives and accounts for more referrals to gastroenterologists than any other disorder. It is twice as common in women as in men and the disorder is generally found to begin in early or middle adulthood.

SYMPTOMS AND SIGNS

Symptoms of IBS include intermittent, cramplike pain in the abdomen; abdominal distension, often on the left side; transient relief of pain by bowel movement or passing wind; a sense of incomplete evacuation of the bowels; excessive wind; passage of mucus; diarrhoea; constipation; and nausea. Some people also have symptoms unrelated to the digestive tract, such as headache, back pain, and tiredness.

Symptoms are typically intermittent, and usually recur throughout life, though they may become less frequent and severe with time. The condition is unlikely to lead to complications.

DIAGNOSIS AND TREATMENT

There is no single test to diagnose IBS as opposed to another disorder of the digestive tract, and the disorder is usually diagnosed from the symptoms and a physical examination. However, tests may be needed if the patient is middle-aged or older, or if there is rectal bleeding, weight loss, infection, or a family history of bowel cancer (see *colon, cancer of; rectum, cancer of*) or *inflammatory bowel disease*. The tests may include endoscopy (examination using a viewing tube) such as *colonoscopy* (examination of the colon) or *gastroscopy* (examination of the stomach); *ultrasound scanning*; or a barium enema (see *barium X-ray examinations*).

IBS can sometimes be controlled through a change in diet and use of relaxation techniques. An individual may need to experiment to find the approach that works best.

If constipation is the main problem, a high-fibre diet or bulk-forming agents (see *laxative drugs*), such as *bran* or *methylcellulose*, may be helpful. Short courses of *antidiarrhoeal drugs* may be given for persistent diarrhoea. *Antispasmodic drugs* may be prescribed to relax the contractions of the digestive tract and relieve abdominal pain. *Hypnosis, cognitive-behavioural therapy*, and *counselling* have proved effective in some cases.

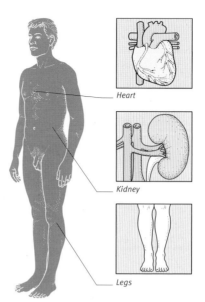

Symptoms of ischaemia
Ischaemia (insufficient blood supply) of the heart causes the chest pain of angina pectoris. Ischaemia of blood vessels in the legs may cause a cramplike pain during exercise. The condition may also affect the kidneys, causing kidney failure, or the brain (not shown), resulting in a stroke.

ischaemia

Insufficient blood supply to a specific organ or tissue. It is usually caused by a disease of the blood vessels, such as *atherosclerosis*, but may also result from injury, constriction of a blood vessel due to spasm of the muscles in the vessel wall, or an inadequate blood flow due to inefficient pumping of the heart. Symptoms depend on the area affected.

Treatment may include *vasodilator drugs* to widen the blood vessels or, in more severe cases, an *angioplasty* and insertion of a *stent* (rigid tube) or *bypass operation*.

ischaemic attack

See *transient ischaemic attack*.

ischaemic colitis

A form of *colitis* (inflammation of the colon) caused by an interruption of the blood supply to the colon. Ischaemic colitis most commonly affects people over 50 years old. People with diseases affecting blood vessels elsewhere in the body, such as *stroke* or *peripheral vascular disease*, are more likely to be affected. Other risk factors include a history of congestive *heart failure* or *diabetes mellitus*; surgery that has resulted in damage to the colon's blood supply; and treatment of the abdomen with *radiotherapy*.

SYMPTOMS AND COMPLICATIONS

Like other forms of colitis, ischaemic colitis may cause abdominal pain, diarrhoea (which may contain blood), fever, and vomiting. A longstanding reduction in the blood supply may lead to the formation of a stricture (narrowed area) in the affected part of the colon. Sudden total loss of blood supply, due to *thrombosis* or to an *embolism*, can cause *gangrene* (tissue death) of the colon.

DIAGNOSIS AND TREATMENT

The condition may be diagnosed by viewing the colon (see *colonoscopy; sigmoidoscopy*) and by taking a *biopsy* (sample of colon tissue). *Angiography* may also be performed to locate any blocked blood vessels.

In mild ischaemia, treatment with drugs used to treat *heart failure* and *hypertension* in combination with *lipid-lowering drugs* and, in some cases, antiplatelet or *anticoagulant drugs* is often sufficient, but acute ischaemia may require surgery in order to remove any blockages in the blood vessels. Areas of colon that have been irreparably damaged must be removed before *peritonitis* and *gangrene* (tissue death) develop (see *colectomy*).

ischaemic necrosis

The death of tissue as a result of an inadequate blood supply (see *necrosis*).

ischaemic optic atrophy

See *optic atrophy*.

ischium

One of the bones that form the lower part of the *pelvis*.

islets of Langerhans

Clusters of *endocrine* (hormone-producing) cells within the *pancreas*. The islets of Langerhans contain at least four different types of cells, which secrete hormones that control the level of *glucose* in the body. One type of cell secretes *insulin*, which lowers the blood glucose level; another type secretes *glucagon*, which raises the blood glucose level; a third type secretes a hormone called somatostatin, which inhibits the secretion of insulin; and a fourth type, about which relatively little is known, secretes a pancreatic polypepetide (a protein molecule).

One common disorder affecting the islets of Langerhans is type 1 *diabetes mellitus*, in which the insulin-secreting cells are destroyed. Other, less common disorders include the growth of tumours in particular groups of cells, leading to excessive hormone production by those cells (see *glucagonoma*; *insulinoma*).

Isogel

A brand name for ispaghula husk, a bulk-forming agent used as a *laxative drug*. Isogel is also used to control some types of *diarrhoea*.

isoimmunization, rhesus

See *rhesus isoimmunization*.

isolation

Nursing procedures (also called barrier nursing) designed to prevent a patient from infecting others or from being infected. The patient is usually isolated in a single room.

Complete isolation is used if a patient has a contagious disease, such as *Lassa fever*, that can be transmitted to others by direct contact and airborne germs. In this case, all bedding, equipment, and clothing are either sterilized or incinerated after use. Partial isolation is carried out if the disease is transmitted in a more limited way (by droplet spread, as in *tuberculosis*, for example).

Reverse isolation, also called reverse barrier nursing, is used to protect a patient whose resistance to infection is severely lowered by disease or treatment such as *chemotherapy*. The air supply to the room is filtered and staff and visitors must wear caps, gowns, masks, and gloves. Occasionally, long-term reverse isolation may be required for patients with severe combined immunodeficiency (see *immunodeficiency disorders*).

isometric

A system of *exercise* that involves no body movement, and in which muscles build up strength by working against resistance. The resistance is provided by either a fixed object or an opposing set of muscles. (See also *isotonic*.)

isoniazid

An *antibacterial drug* that is used in the treatment of *tuberculosis*. Isoniazid is given in combination with other anti-tuberculous drugs, usually for a minimum of six months.

isoprenaline

A drug used to stimulate the heart in cases of severe *shock*. It is used only in hospitals, mainly in intensive care units.

isosorbide

A *nitrate drug* that acts as a vasodilator drug (by widening blood vessels). Isosorbide is used to reduce the severity and frequency of *angina pectoris* (chest pain caused by impaired blood supply to the heart). It is also given to treat severe *heart failure*. There are two forms of isosorbide: mononitrate and dinitrate. Isosorbide dinitrate is converted by the body into isosorbide mononitrate, which is the active form of the drug.

Side effects include headache, hot flushes, and dizziness. In addition, tolerance to the drug may develop, especially in patients who are using a long-acting preparation; a change in the dosage, frequency, or timing, or changing to a different drug, may be required.

isotonic

Having the same tension. It is used to define a system of *exercise*, such as weight lifting, in which muscle tension is kept constant as the body works against its own, or an external, weight. The term "isotonic" also describes fluids, such as intravenous fluids or drinks, with the same osmotic pressure (see *osmosis*) as the blood. (See also *isometric*; *hypotonic solutions*.)

isotope

Any one of the different atoms of a chemical element. Different isotopes of an element have the same number of protons (positively charged particles) but different numbers of neutrons (neutral particles) in their nucleus, and therefore a different atomic weight.

Radioactive isotopes are unstable and break down into more stable forms, with the accompanying release of electromagnetic *radiation*. This radiation release means that such isotopes may be used in some medical procedures, such as *radiotherapy* for cancer and imaging tests such as *radionuclide scanning*.

isotope scanning

See *radionuclide scanning*.

isotretinoin

A drug derived from *vitamin A* used in the treatment of *acne*. Isotretinoin works by reducing the formation of sebum (natural skin oils) and keratin (a tough protein that is the major component of the outer layer of skin).

Isotretinoin can be used as a topical gel to treat mild to moderate cases of acne, or it may be taken orally in the treatment of severe, scarring acne that is unresponsive to other treatments. Side effects of topical treatment include inflammation and peeling of the skin; sunlight should be avoided. Isotretinoin should only be taken orally under medical supervision. In this form, it may cause drying of the skin and the mucous membranes, nosebleeds, sore eyes, and disorders of the blood.

Isotretinoin may damage a developing fetus and therefore before starting treatment a woman is given a pregnancy test to ensure she is not pregnant. She should then avoid getting pregnant while taking the drug and for at least one month after stopping it.

ispaghula

A bulk-forming *laxative drug* that is used to treat *constipation*, *diverticular disease*, and *irritable bowel syndrome*. As ispaghula travels through the intestine, it absorbs water, thereby softening and increasing the volume of the faeces. Ispaghula is also used in people who have chronic, watery *diarrhoea* and in those patients who have had a *colostomy* or an *ileostomy* to control the consistency of faeces.

Adverse effects include flatulence, abdominal distension, and discomfort.

isthmus

A narrow connecting structure or tissue between two larger body parts, such as the portion of tissue connecting the two lobes of the *thyroid gland*.

Istin

A brand name for *amlodipine*, a *calcium channel blocker drug* used in the treatment of disorders such as *angina pectoris* (chest pain due to insufficient blood supply to the heart muscle) and *hypertension* (high blood pressure).

itching

Known medically as pruritus, an intense irritation or tickling feeling in the skin.

TYPES AND CAUSES

Generalized itching may result from excessive bathing, which removes the natural oils from the skin and may leave the skin excessively dry. Some people experience general itching after taking certain drugs. Many elderly people suffer from dry, itchy skin, especially on their backs. Itching commonly occurs during pregnancy.

Conditions that produce a rash, such as *chickenpox*, *urticaria* (nettle rash), and

THE **IUD** (INTRAUTERINE CONTRACEPTIVE DEVICE)

The IUD, also known as the IUCD, is a small plastic and copper contraceptive device inserted into the uterus. IUDs work by preventing sperm from reaching the egg; they may also inhibit implantation of a fertilized egg in the uterus. All types of IUD can be fitted, by specially trained healthcare personnel, in family planning clinics, hospitals, or general practitioners' surgeries.

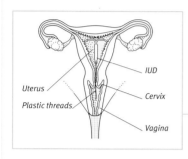

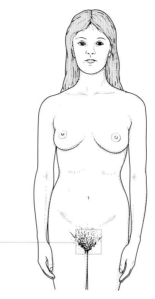

Uterus

Plastic threads

IUD

Cervix

Vagina

Site of an IUD
An IUD is inserted into the uterus. Most types have two arms that hold them in position. The base of the IUD has one or two plastic threads that extend through the cervix to the vagina. The threads enable the user to check that the device is in place.

WHO SHOULD NOT USE IUDS
IUDs can be used by most women who want to do so. However, they are not usually recommended for women with *fibroids* or an irregular uterine cavity, nor for women with an untreated pelvic or *sexually transmitted infection*. If menstrual flow is heavy, a progestogen IUD (IUS) may be recommended.

RISKS AND COMPLICATIONS
IUDs seldom cause problems and can be easily removed by a doctor or nurse. Rarely, pregnancy can occur while using an IUD and, if it does, there is a slightly increased risk that the pregnancy will be ectopic (see *ectopic pregnancy*). Nonprogestogen IUDs can increase the risk for *pelvic inflammatory disease* (PID) in certain groups of women, such as those with multiple partners. A rare complication of IUD use is perforation of the uterus, which most commonly occurs at the time of insertion.

IUS

An abbreviation for intrauterine system. An IUS is a mechanical contraceptive device that resembles an *IUD* but also contains the *progestogen hormone* levonorgestrel. Like the IUD, the device is fitted inside the uterus, where the hormone is released slowly and continuously for up to five years. The IUS prevents pregnancy by affecting the uterine lining and thickening the cervical mucus; it may also suppress ovulation in some women. Compared with the IUD, the IUS has a lower risk for *pelvic inflammatory disease* and *ectopic pregnancy*. The IUS is not suitable for emergency contraception.

In addition to its contraceptive effect, the IUS may make menstrual periods lighter and less painful and so may be used as treatment for heavy periods (see *menorrhagia*). It may also sometimes be used to deliver progestogen as part of *hormone replacement therapy* (HRT).

IVF

See *in vitro fertilization*.

IVU

The abbreviation for *intravenous urography* (an X-ray imaging technique for visualizing the urinary tract).

---

eczema, often produce itching at the site of the rash. Generalized skin itchiness can be a result of *diabetes mellitus*, *kidney failure*, *jaundice*, and *thyroid* disorders.

Pruritus ani (itching around the anal region) occurs with *haemorrhoids* and *anal fissure*. *Threadworm infestation* is the most likely cause of anal itching in children. Pruritus vulvae (itching of the external genitalia in women) may be due to the condition *candidiasis*, hormonal changes, or to use of spermicides or vaginal ointments and deodorants. *Insect bites, lice,* and *scabies* infestations cause intense itching.

TREATMENT
Specific treatment for itching depends on the underlying cause. Cooling and soothing lotions, such as *calamine*, may help to relieve irritation; emollients (substances that moisten and soften the skin) may reduce dryness.

-itis

A suffix meaning "inflammation of". Virtually every organ or tissue can suffer inflammation, so "itis" is a very common word-ending in medicine.

ITP

An abbreviation for *idiopathic thrombocytopenic purpura*.

itraconazole

A type of *antifungal drug*.

IUCD

An abbreviation for intrauterine contraceptive device (see *IUD*).

IUD

An abbreviation for intrauterine contraceptive device. An IUD, also known as an IUCD or coil, is a mechanical plastic and copper device inserted into the uterus for *contraception*. One type of IUD releases small amounts of *progestogen hormone* and is known as an intrauterine system (see *IUS*). IUDs act by preventing sperm from reaching the egg and may also inhibit the implantation of a fertilized egg in the wall of the uterus (see *implantation, egg*).

HOW IUDS ARE USED
An IUD is inserted through the vagina and cervix into the uterine cavity. Once in position, an IUD provides immediate and highly effective protection. IUDs have one or two threads attached to make removal easier and to indicate their presence when in place. IUDs may be left in place for up to ten years, depending on the type. Most IUDs can also be used as emergency contraception; the exception is the progestogen-releasing type (the IUS).

Jaccoud's arthropathy

Also called Jaccoud's arthritis or Jaccoud's syndrome, a rare form of chronic arthritis associated with systemic *lupus erythematosus*. The disorder causes fibrous changes in the *joint* capsules and tendons at the base of the fingers, leading to pain and swelling.

Jacksonian seizures

A temporary brain disturbance in which *seizures* begin in one part of the body, such as a limb or the face, and then spread to other areas or even the whole body (a progression called the march of the seizure). The person usually retains consciousness but may have *amnesia* (memory loss). (See also *epilepsy*.)

Jahnke's syndrome

A form of *Sturge–Weber syndrome* in which there is malformation of blood vessels in the face and brain but without the *glaucoma* (increased fluid pressure in the eye) that is usually associated with the syndrome.

Jakob–Creutzfeldt disease

See *Creutzfeldt–Jakob disease*.

Japanese B encephalitis

An epidemic, mosquito-borne form of *encephalitis* (brain inflammation) occurring in Japan, India, and parts of southeast Asia. In most cases the infection causes no symptoms; however, some people develop severe encephalitis leading to paralysis, seizures, coma, and death. Immunization is available for those travelling to high-risk areas.

jargon aphasia

A form of *aphasia* (loss of language skills) in which the affected person cannot form grammatical sentences but utters meaningless phrases composed of jumbled words or neologisms (made-up words). Jargon aphasia may be due to a lesion in the dominant temporal lobe of the *brain*, or, rarely, may be a sign of *schizophrenia*.

jaundice

Yellowing of the skin and whites of the eyes, caused by an accumulation of the yellow-brown pigment *bilirubin* in blood and tissues. Jaundice is the chief sign of many disorders of the *liver* and *biliary system*. Many otherwise healthy babies are affected briefly by jaundice soon after birth (see *jaundice, neonatal*).

TYPES AND CAUSES
Bilirubin is formed from *haemoglobin* (the oxygen-carrying pigment in red blood cells) when old red cells are broken down, mainly by the *spleen*. It is absorbed by the liver, where it is made soluble in water and excreted in *bile*.

There are three main types of jaundice: haemolytic, hepatocellular, and obstructive. In haemolytic jaundice, too much bilirubin is produced for the liver to process. This condition results from excessive *haemolysis* (breakdown of red blood cells), which can have many causes (see *anaemia, haemolytic*).

In hepatocellular jaundice, bilirubin accumulates because it is prevented from passing from liver cells into the bile. This form of jaundice is usually due to acute *hepatitis* (inflammation of the liver) caused by taking certain drugs or by *liver failure*.

In obstructive jaundice, also called cholestatic jaundice, bile cannot leave the liver because of *bile duct obstruction*, which may be caused by gallstones or due to a tumour anywhere in the duct. Obstructive jaundice can also occur if the bile ducts are underdeveloped (as in *biliary atresia*) or have been destroyed by disease. *Cholestasis* (stagnation of bile in the liver) then occurs and bilirubin overflows into the blood.

DIAGNOSIS AND TREATMENT
Blood tests, and possibly also a *liver biopsy* (removal of a sample of tissue for analysis), may be performed to identify the cause of the jaundice. Investigation of the bile duct may be carried out using such imaging techniques as *ERCP* and *MRI*. Treatment is for the underlying cause.

jaundice, neonatal

Yellowing of the skin and whites of the eyes in newborn babies, due to accumulation of the yellow-brown bile pigment *bilirubin* in the blood. Neonatal jaundice usually results from the *liver* being too immature to excrete bilirubin efficiently. The condition, which tends to be more common in breast-fed babies, is usually harmless and disappears within a week.

In rare cases, severe or persistent neonatal jaundice can be caused by the blood disorder *haemolytic disease of the newborn*; the genetic condition *G6PD deficiency*; *hepatitis* (inflammation of the liver); *hypothyroidism* (underactivity of the thyroid); *biliary atresia* (abnormal formation or absence of the bile ducts); or infection. such as a urinary tract infection.

Jaundiced babies usually require extra fluids and may be treated with *phototherapy* (light therapy) or, in severe cases, exchange transfusion (see *blood transfusion*). If severe neonatal jaundice is not treated promptly, *kernicterus* (a form of brain damage) may occur.

jaw

The mobile bone of the face, also called the mandible (or lower jaw). The term sometimes includes the *maxilla* (upper jaw), the bone that extends from the inner rims of the eyes to the mouth.

The mandible bears the lower teeth on its upper surface, and is connected to the base of the skull at the *temporomandibular joints*. Muscles attached to the jaw move the bone to enable chewing, biting, and side-to-side and downward motions.

ANATOMY OF THE **JAW**

The U-shaped jaw bone (mandible) joins the skull in front of the ears, at the temporomandibular joint. The jaw can move in several directions to enable biting and chewing.

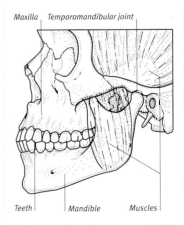

jaw, dislocated

Displacement of the lower *jaw* from one or both *temporomandibular joints* (which connect the jaw to the base of the skull), usually due either to a blow or to yawning. There is usually pain in front of the ear on the affected side, and the jaw projects forwards. The mouth cannot be fully closed, which makes eating and speaking difficult. Surgery may be performed to stabilize the joint, but dislocation tends to recur.

jaw, fractured

A fracture of the *jaw* bone, most often caused by a direct blow. A minor fracture may cause tenderness and pain on biting. In severe injuries, jaw movement may be limited, and there may be loss of feeling in the lower lip.

Minor fractures are normally left to heal on their own. Severe fractures with bone displacement, however, require surgery and immobilization of the jaw (see *wiring of the jaws*).

JC virus

A type of virus called a polyomavirus. JC virus does not usually cause symptoms in healthy adults but can be dangerous in people with a depressed immune system due to diseases such as *leukaemia*, *lymphoma*, or *AIDS*. In such cases, JC virus causes a brain disease called progressive multifocal leucoencephalopathy, which leads to dementia.

jealousy, morbid

Preoccupation with the potential sexual infidelity of one's partner. The sufferer, most often a man, becomes convinced that his partner is having an affair. Morbid jealousy is usually caused by a *personality disorder*, *depression*, or *paranoia*, but may also result from *alcohol dependence* or organic brain syndrome (see *brain syndrome, organic*).

jejunal biopsy

A diagnostic test in which a small piece of tissue is removed from the lining of the *jejunum* (middle section of the small intestine) for microscopic examination. It is especially useful in the diagnosis of *coeliac disease*, intestinal *lymphoma*, and other causes of *malabsorption*. The biopsy is taken through an *endoscope* introduced via the mouth, or with a device called a Crosby capsule, which is attached to a thread and swallowed.

jejunum

The middle, coiled section of the small *intestine*, joining the *duodenum* to the *ileum*. The main functions of the jejunum are to digest food and absorb nutrients. It may be affected by *coeliac disease*, *Crohn's disease*, and *lymphoma*.

ANATOMY OF THE JEJUNUM

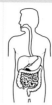

This section of the small intestine joins the duodenum (first section) to the ileum (final section). It is wider than the ileum and has a thicker wall.

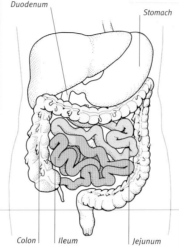

Duodenum

Stomach

Colon   Ileum   Jejunum

jellyfish stings

Injections of venom from the stinging cells of jellyfish. In most instances of jellyfish stings, there is only mild pain or itching, but some jellyfish venom causes vomiting, breathing difficulties, and collapse. Dangerous species live mainly in tropical waters. *Antivenoms* may be used to treat severe cases.

jerky nystagmus

A form of *nystagmus* (involuntary eye movement) in which the eyes move slowly in one direction, then dart back.

jet-lag

Fatigue and disruption of the sleep–wake cycle, caused by disturbance of normal body *biorhythms* as a result of flying across different time zones. Jet-lag causes daytime sleepiness and insomnia at night. Other symptoms include reduced physical and mental activity, and poor memory. Jet-lag tends to be worse after an eastward flight (which shortens the traveller's day) than after a westward one

jigger

An alternative name for a *chigoe*, which is also sometimes known as a sand flea.

jogger's nipple

Soreness of the nipple caused by friction from clothing, usually during sports such as jogging or long-distance running. Both men and women can be affected. Prevention is by applying petroleum jelly to the nipple before prolonged running.

joint

The junction between two or more bones. Many joints are highly mobile, while others are fixed or allow only a small amount of movement (see *Types of joint* box opposite).

STRUCTURE

In all types of joint, the bones are held together by soft tissues. In fixed joints, such as those in the skull, the bones are firmly secured by fibrous tissue. In semi-mobile joints (such as those in the spine), the bones are connected by cartilage, which allows limited movement. Mobile joints (such as those in the limbs) are supported by strong *ligaments*. They are moved by *muscles*, which are attached to the bones by *tendons*. Each mobile joint is also sealed within a tough, fibrous capsule.

TYPES

There are several types of mobile joint, each allowing a specific form of movement. Hinge joints, such as those in the fingers, knees, and elbows, principally allow bending and straightening. Pivot joints, such as the joint between the first and second vertebrae (see *vertebra*), allow rotation only. Ellipsoidal joints, such as the wrist, allow all types of movement except pivotal. Ball-and-socket joints, such as the shoulder and hip, allow movement in all directions.

DISORDERS

Common joint injuries include *sprains* (minor tears) or rupture of ligaments; damage to cartilage; and tearing of joint capsules. Such injuries may be caused by sudden twisting or wrenching movements, often during sport or vigorous exercise, or in a fall. Separation of the bone ends (see *dislocation, joint*), and partial displacement (see *subluxation*), are also usually caused by injury, but are occasionally present from birth. Rarely, the bone ends are fractured, which may cause bleeding into a joint (*haemarthrosis*). Joint *effusion* (buildup of fluid in a joint) is usually due to *synovitis* (inflammation of the joint lining).

One of the main diseases of the joints is *arthritis*, which causes pain, stiffness, inflammation, and degeneration of the joints. Other disorders include *bursitis*

TYPES OF **JOINT**

There are several types of joint. Some are fixed (such as the skull joints), some allow only a little movement (the vertebral joints, for example), and some are mobile. Of the mobile joints, ball-and-socket have the widest range of movement. Pivot joints allow rotation only. Ellipsoidal joints allow movement in most directions. Hinge joints mainly allow bending.

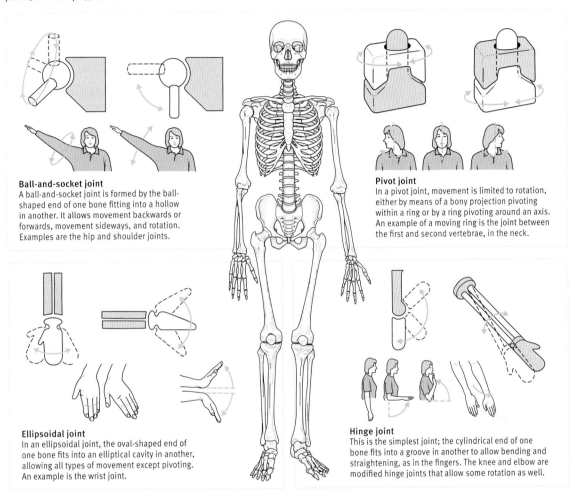

Ball-and-socket joint
A ball-and-socket joint is formed by the ball-shaped end of one bone fitting into a hollow in another. It allows movement backwards or forwards, movement sideways, and rotation. Examples are the hip and shoulder joints.

Pivot joint
In a pivot joint, movement is limited to rotation, either by means of a bony projection pivoting within a ring or by a ring pivoting around an axis. An example of a moving ring is the joint between the first and second vertebrae, in the neck.

Ellipsoidal joint
In an ellipsoidal joint, the oval-shaped end of one bone fits into an elliptical cavity in another, allowing all types of movement except pivoting. An example is the wrist joint.

Hinge joint
This is the simplest joint; the cylindrical end of one bone fits into a groove in another to allow bending and straightening, as in the fingers. The knee and elbow are modified hinge joints that allow some rotation as well.

STRUCTURE OF A FIXED JOINT

Fixed joints are firmly secured by fibrous tissue. The joints between the bones of the skull (known as sutures) are an example.

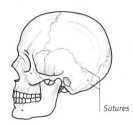

Sutures

STRUCTURE OF A MOBILE JOINT

The surfaces of the bone ends are coated with very smooth cartilage to reduce friction as they move against each other. The ends are sealed within a tough fibrous capsule; this is lined with synovial membrane, which produces a sticky lubricating fluid. The joint is surrounded by strong ligaments that support it and prevent excessive movement. Its movement is controlled by muscles that are attached to bone by tendons on either side of the joint. Most mobile joints have at least one bursa (fluid-filled sac) nearby, which cushions a pressure point.

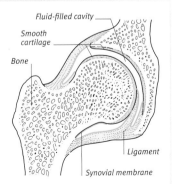

Fluid-filled cavity
Smooth cartilage
Bone
Ligament
Synovial membrane

J

(inflammation of a fluid-filled cushion around a joint); distortion or rupture of an intervertebral disc (see *disc, slipped*); *gout*; and *bunions*.

joint replacement

See *arthroplasty*.

Joubert's syndrome

An autosomal recessive *genetic disorder* in which part of the *cerebellum* fails to develop properly, causing impaired balance and coordination; abnormal breathing patterns; decreased muscle tone; and, sometimes, *seizures*.

joule

The international unit of *energy*, work, and heat. Approximately 4,200 joules (symbol J) or 4.2 kilojoules (kJ) equal 1 kilocalorie (kcal); 1 kJ is equal to about 0.24 kcal. (See also *calorie*.)

jugular vein

One of three veins on each side of the neck (the internal, external, and anterior jugular veins) that return deoxygenated blood from the head to the heart. The internal jugular vein, the largest of the three, arises at the base of the skull and travels down the neck alongside the *carotid arteries*, before passing behind

ANATOMY OF THE JUGULAR VEINS

There are three jugular veins on each side of the neck that return blood from the head to the heart.

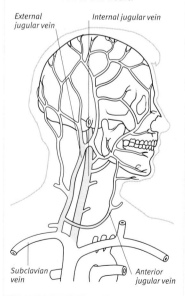

External jugular vein

Internal jugular vein

Subclavian vein

Anterior jugular vein

the *clavicle* (collarbone), where it joins the subclavian vein (the large vein that drains blood from the arms).

jugular venous pressure

An assessment of the pressure within the internal *jugular vein*. Raised jugular venous pressure may be an indication of *heart failure*.

junctional naevus

A pigmented *naevus* formed by a cluster of melanocytes (pigment-producing cells) in the skin, at the junction between the epidermis (outer layer) and the dermis (inner layer). The naevus looks like a flat, non-hairy, brown mole. (See also *intradermal naevus*.)

Jungian theory

Ideas put forward by the Swiss psychiatrist Carl Gustav Jung (1875–1961). He theorized that certain ideas (called archetypes) inherited from experiences in a person's distant past were present in his or her unconscious and controlled the way he or she viewed the world. Jung called these ideas the "collective unconscious". He believed that each individual also had a "personal unconscious" containing experiences from his or her life. Jungian therapy was aimed at putting people in touch with this source of ideas, particularly through dream interpretation. Jung's approach was also based on his theory of personality, which postulated two basic types: extrovert and introvert. One of these types dominates a person's consciousness and the other must be brought into consciousness and reconciled with its opposite for the person to become a whole individual.

juvenile arthritis

See *juvenile chronic arthritis*.

juvenile chronic arthritis

A rare form of *arthritis* affecting children. Juvenile chronic arthritis occurs more often in girls, and usually develops between two and four years of age or around puberty. The cause is not known but genetic factors may be involved.

TYPES
There are three main types, all of which cause joint pain, swelling, and stiffness. The most common form is pauciarticular juvenile arthritis, which affects four joints or fewer and usually occurs in very young girls. Polyarticular juvenile arthritis affects five or more joints, and is more common in girls. *Still's disease*

(systemic onset juvenile arthritis) affects both boys and girls. It starts with fever, rash, enlarged lymph nodes, abdominal pain, and weight loss. These symptoms last for several weeks. The joint problems may not develop for some months.

COMPLICATIONS
Possible complications include short stature, *anaemia*, *pleurisy* (inflammation of the membranes around the lungs), *pericarditis* (inflammation of the membrane around the heart), and enlargement of the *liver* and *spleen*. *Uveitis* (inflammation of parts of the eye) may develop. Rarely, *amyloidosis* (in which an abnormal protein is deposited in body organs) or *kidney failure* may develop.

DIAGNOSIS
Diagnosis is based on the symptoms, together with the results of *X-rays* and *blood tests*; it is made only if the condition lasts for longer than three months.

TREATMENT AND OUTLOOK
Treatment may include *disease-modifying antirheumatic drugs* such as gold, methotexate, and azathioprine, *corticosteroid drugs*, *nonsteroidal anti-inflammatory drugs*, or aspirin. Splints may be worn to rest inflamed joints and reduce the risk of deformities. *Physiotherapy* reduces the risk of muscle wasting and deformity. The arthritis usually clears up after several years, although it may sometimes persist into adult life.

juvenile muscular atrophy

A form of muscle atrophy (wasting and weakness) that occurs in children and adolescents, and is caused by an autosomal recessive *genetic disorder*. Muscle atrophy is most obvious in the legs, and later the arms. Respiratory muscles may also be involved. Most affected children eventually become wheelchair bound.

juvenile-onset diabetes

A form of type 1 (insulin-dependent) *diabetes mellitus* that develops suddenly in childhood or adolescence.

juvenile osteoporosis, idiopathic

A rare form of *osteoporosis* that occurs in children of eight to 14 years. Idiopathic juvenile osteoporosis causes leg and back pain; *kyphosis* (curvature of the upper spine); walking difficulty; and increased susceptibility to fractures. The disorder usually begins suddenly and often disappears spontaneously after two to four years. Treatment is aimed at preventing fractures and maintaining mobility.

J

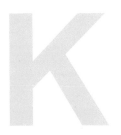

kala-azar

A form of the parasitic disease *leishmaniasis*, which is spread by sandflies. Kala-azar occurs in parts of Africa, India, the Mediterranean, and South America.

Kallmann's syndrome

An inherited condition in which there is a deficiency of gonadotrophin-releasing hormone (GnRH). This hormone, produced in the hypothalamus, regulates the release of other hormones in the pituitary gland that in turn stimulate the testes. The deficiency of GnRH delays or sometimes prevents normal sexual development at puberty. The condition is also associated with colour blindness and lack of a sense of smell. Treatment is with hormones that replace GnRH.

kaolin

An *aluminium* compound used as an ingredient in some *antidiarrhoeal drugs*. Kaolin is taken orally and increases the bulk of the faeces.

Kaposi's sarcoma

A cancerous tumour arising from blood vessels in the skin or, less commonly, in internal organs. Kaposi's sarcoma usually occurs in people who have a weakened immune system, such as those with *AIDS* or those taking *immunosuppressant drugs* (after a transplant, for example), and is associated with infection with a specific herpes virus. Several tumours are often present, appearing as pinkish-purple, raised areas of skin. The tumours can spread rapidly over the body; they usually develop first on the feet and the ankles, spread up the legs, then occur on the hands and the arms. Internal tumours, such as those affecting the gastrointestinal and respiratory tracts, may cause severe bleeding.

Skin tumours may be treated with *radiotherapy*. *Anticancer drugs* may be used if the skin is widely affected or for internal tumours. *Antiretroviral drugs* often control the cancerous growths and may shrink them.

Kaposi's varicelliform eruption

A generalized, serious skin eruption, consisting of pus-filled blisters, caused by a viral infection in areas of pre-existing atopic *dermatitis*. The disorder is also known as eczema herpeticum. The viruses usually responsible are herpes simplex virus (HSV1 and HSV2) and coxsackievirus.

Kartegener's syndrome

An inherited disorder in which the heart is situated on the right instead of the left side of the chest (a condition known as dextrocardia). This is associated with abnormal functioning of the cilia (hair-like projections) lining the airways, which impairs clearance of mucus and results in *bronchiectasis* and *sinusitis*.

karyotype

The characteristics of *chromosomes*, in terms of number, size, and structure, in an individual or a species. The term "karyotype" is also applied to a diagram of chromosome pairs arranged in their assigned numerical order.

Kawasaki disease

A rare, acute illness of unknown cause that most commonly affects children under two years of age. The disease is characterized by fever lasting one to two weeks; conjunctivitis; dryness and cracking of the lips; swollen *lymph nodes* in the neck; reddening of the palms and soles; and a generalized rash. By the end of the second week of illness, the skin at the tips of the fingers and toes peels and other symptoms subside. The heart muscle and *coronary arteries* are affected in some cases.

High doses of gamma-globulin (see *immunoglobulin injections*) and *aspirin* may be given in order to prevent associated heart complications. The majority of children recover completely.

Keller's operation

A type of surgery sometimes used to treat *hallux valgus* (a deformity of the big toe). The operation involves cutting away a piece of bone from the base of the first joint of the toe. Fibrous tissue forms in the gap, although the toe is left shorter. (See also *bunion*.)

keloid

A raised, hard, irregularly shaped, itchy scar on the skin due to a defective healing process in which too much *collagen* (a tough, fibrous protein) is produced, usu-

ally after a skin injury. Keloids can develop anywhere on the body, but the breastbone and shoulder are common sites. Black people are affected more commonly than white people. After several months, most keloids flatten and cease to itch.

Injection of *corticosteroid drugs* into the keloid may reduce itchiness more quickly and cause some shrinkage.

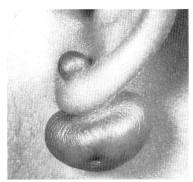

Keloid on the earlobe
This large overgrowth of scar tissue has formed on the earlobe after the ear was pierced. Black people are particularly susceptible to keloids.

keratin

A fibrous *protein* that is the main constituent of the tough outermost layer of the *skin*, *nails*, and *hair*.

keratitis

Inflammation of the *cornea* (the transparent front part of the eyeball). It often takes the form of a *corneal ulcer* and may result from injury, contact with chemicals, or an infection. Symptoms include pain and excessive watering of the eye, blurred vision, and *photophobia* (abnormal sensitivity to bright light).

Noninfective keratitis is treated by keeping the affected eye covered until is has healed. Drugs such as antibiotics may be given to treat infective keratitis. (See also *disciformis keratitis*.)

keratoacanthoma

A type of harmless skin nodule that commonly occurs in elderly people, most often on the face or arm. The cause is unknown, but many years of exposure to strong sunlight or long-term use of *immunosuppressant drugs* may be contributory factors. Initially, the nodule resembles a small wart, but it grows to 1–2 cm across in about eight weeks. Although the nodule usually disappears gradually after this time, surgical removal is often recommended to prevent scarring.

K

keratoconjunctivitis

Inflammation of the *cornea* (the transparent front part of the eyeball) that is associated with *conjunctivitis* (inflammation of the conjunctiva, the membrane covering the eyeball). The most common form of the disorder, epidemic keratoconjunctivitis, is caused by a virus and is highly infectious. The inflammation is often severe and in some cases may destroy the surface of the conjunctiva. Tiny, opaque spots develop in the cornea that may interfere with vision and persist for some months.

There is no specific treatment, but corneal spots may be minimized by using eye-drops containing *corticosteroid drugs*.

keratoconjunctivitis sicca

Persistent dryness of the *cornea* (the transparent front part of the eyeball) and the *conjunctiva* (the membrane covering the eyeball) caused by deficiency in tear production. The condition is associated with *autoimmune disorders* such as *rheumatoid arthritis*, *Sjögren's syndrome*, and systemic *lupus erythematosus*, all of which can damage the tear glands. Prolonged dryness may lead to blurred vision, itching, grittiness, and, in severe cases, the formation of a *corneal ulcer*. The most effective treatment is frequent use of artificial tears (see *tears, artificial*).

keratoconus

An inherited disorder of the *eye*, in which the cornea (the transparent front part of the eyeball) becomes gradually thinned and conical. The condition affects both eyes and usually develops around puberty, giving rise to increasing *myopia* (shortsightedness) and progressive distortion of vision that cannot be fully corrected by glasses. Hard *contact lenses* improve vision in the early stages, but later it is generally necessary to perform a *corneal graft* to restore normal vision permanently.

keratolytic drugs

Drugs that loosen and remove the tough outer layer of *skin*. Keratolytic drugs, which include *urea* and *salicylic acid* preparations, are used to treat skin and scalp disorders, such as *warts*, *acne*, *dandruff*, and *psoriasis*.

keratomalacia

A progressive disease of the *eye*, caused by severe *vitamin A* deficiency, in which the cornea (the transparent front part of the eyeball) becomes opaque and ulcerated. Perforation of the cornea is also common, often leading to loss of the eye through infection. The disorder usually occurs only in severely malnourished children and is a common cause of blindness in developing countries.

In the early stages, the damage can be reversed by treatment with large doses of vitamin A but, if the condition is left untreated, blindness is usually inevitable.

keratopathy

A general term used to describe a variety of disorders of the *cornea* (the transparent front part of the eyeball).

TYPES

Actinic keratopathy is a painful condition in which the outer layer of the cornea is damaged by *ultraviolet light* emitted from the sun, reflected from surfaces such as snow (in which case the problem is called snow-blindness), or given off by artificial sources such as sunbeds or arc-welding torches.

Exposure keratopathy is corneal damage due to loss of the protection afforded by the tear film and blink reflex. It may occur in conditions in which the eyelids inadequately cover the cornea, including severe *exophthalmos*, *facial palsy*, and *ectropion*.

keratoplasty

See *corneal graft*.

keratosis

A skin growth that is caused by an overproduction of the tough, fibrous protein *keratin*. Keratoses occur mainly in elderly people.

TYPES

Seborrhoeic keratoses are harmless growths that occur mainly on the trunk. They range in appearance from flat, dark-brown patches to small, wartlike protrusions. The growths do not need treating unless they are unsightly.

Solar keratoses are small, wartlike red or flesh-coloured growths that appear on exposed parts of the body as a result of overexposure to the sun over many years. Rarely, they may develop into skin cancer, usually *squamous cell carcinoma*.

TREATMENT

Seborrhoeic keratoses can be removed by curettage (scraping away). Surgery is required for solar keratoses that have become cancerous, however.

keratosis pilaris

A common condition, usually occurring in adolescents, in which patches of rough skin appear on the upper arms, thighs, and buttocks. The openings of the hair follicles become enlarged by plugs of *keratin* (a tough, fibrous protein), and hair growth may be distorted.

The condition is not serious and usually clears up on its own. In severe cases, applying a mixture of salicylic acid and soft paraffin and scrubbing with a loofah may help.

keratotomy, radial

An uncommon procedure in which radiating incisions are made in the *cornea* (the transparent front part of the eyeball) up to, but not through, its innermost layer, in order to reduce *myopia* (shortsightedness). Radial keratotomy has been largely replaced by laser procedures, such as *LASIK*, which carry less risk of permanent damage to the eye.

kerion

A red, painful swelling, oozing fluid, that appears on the scalp due to infection with scalp ringworm (see *tinea*). Treatment with oral *antifungal drugs* needs to be continued for several weeks before the scalp heals. The disorder may leave scarring and an area of permanent hair loss.

kernicterus

The abnormal accumulation of the pigment *bilirubin* in the brain of a newborn baby, as a result of severe *jaundice*. Kernicterus causes permanent brain damage, but the effective treatment of jaundice in newborn babies has made the condition rare.

ketamine

A general *anaesthetic* administered by injection. It is mainly given to children undergoing painful procedures, such as *bone marrow biopsy*. Ketamine may be abused for its stimulant effect.

ketoacidosis

A combination of *acidosis* and *ketosis*. (See also *diabetic ketoacidosis*.)

ketoconazole

An *antifungal drug* used to treat *fungal infections* of the gut, skin, and finger nails, and *candidiasis* (thrush) of the mouth or vagina. It is also used as a shampoo to treat dandruff. Adverse effects include nausea and rash.

ketone

Any of a group of chemicals related to acetone (which is found in solvents such as nail polish remover). Certain ketones are produced during the *metabolism* of fats; if excessive amounts build up in the body, they cause *ketosis*.

ketoprofen

A type of nonsteroidal *anti-inflammatory drug* (NSAID) that is prescribed as an *analgesic drug* (painkiller) for injuries to soft tissues, such as muscles and ligaments. Ketoprofen also reduces joint pain and stiffness in arthritic conditions. It may cause abdominal pain, nausea, indigestion, and an increased risk of *peptic ulcer*.

ketosis

A potentially serious condition in which excessive amounts of chemicals called *ketones* accumulate in the body. Ketones are normal products of fat *metabolism*, but are produced in excess when body cells cannot use *glucose* as an energy source. This occurs in starvation, in prolonged vomiting, and in untreated *diabetes mellitus* (see *diabetic ketoacidosis*) when a lack of insulin prevents glucose from entering cells. Symptoms include sweet, acetone-smelling breath, loss of appetite, nausea, and abdominal pain. Ketosis may eventually result in confusion, unconsciousness, and death. Treatment is of the underlying cause.

keyhole surgery

Another name for *minimally invasive surgery*.

kidney

Either of the two organs that filter the blood and excrete waste products and excess water as *urine*. The kidneys are situated at the back of the abdominal cavity, on either side of the spine.

STRUCTURE

Each kidney is surrounded by a fibrous capsule and is made up of an outer layer (cortex) and an inner layer (medulla). The cortex contains specialized capillaries (tiny blood vessels) called glomeruli; these vessels, together with a series of tubules, make up the *nephrons*, the filtering units of the kidney. Urine, the waste product from filtering, passes through tubules to the medulla, collects in an area called the renal pelvis, then travels through tubes called ureters to the bladder.

FUNCTIONS

The nephrons filter blood under pressure and then selectively reabsorb water and certain other substances into the blood. Urine is formed from substances that are not reabsorbed (see box: *The function of the kidneys*, p.449).

(see box: *The function of the kidneys*, p.449)

LOCATION OF THE **KIDNEYS**

The kidneys are situated at the back of the abdominal cavity, just above the waist, on either side of the spine. The right kidney lies below the liver (not shown), and the left kidney lies below the spleen. Each kidney is connected to the bladder by a ureter. The renal arteries, which supply the kidneys, arise directly from the aorta, and the renal veins join on to the inferior vena cava. The two adrenal glands sit on top of each kidney.

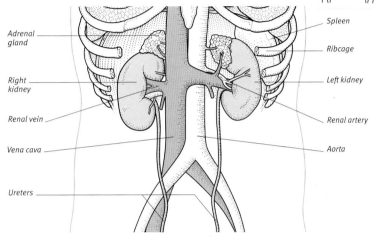
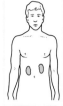

Adrenal gland

Right kidney

Renal vein

Vena cava

Ureters

Spleen

Ribcage

Left kidney

Renal artery

Aorta

The kidneys also regulate the body's fluid balance. To do this, they excrete excess water, and when water is lost from the body (for example, as a result of sweating), they conserve it (see *ADH*). In addition, they control the body's *acid–base balance* by adjusting urine acidity. Lastly, the kidneys produce hormones involved in the regulation of red *blood cell* production and *blood pressure*.

kidney biopsy

A procedure in which a small sample of *kidney* tissue is removed and examined under a microscope. Kidney biopsy is performed to investigate and diagnose serious disorders such as *glomerulonephritis*, *proteinuria*, *nephrotic syndrome*, and *acute kidney failure*, or to assess the kidneys' response to treatment.

There are two basic techniques: percutaneous needle biopsy, in which a hollow needle is passed through the skin into the kidney under local anaesthesia; and open surgery under general anaesthesia.

kidney cancer

A cancerous tumour of the *kidney*. Most kidney cancers originate in the kidney itself, but in rare cases cancer spreads to the kidney from another organ.

TYPES

There are three main types of cancer that affect the kidney: renal cell carcinoma, nephroblastoma, and transitional cell carcinoma.

Renal cell carcinoma

Also known as hypernephroma or adenocarcinoma, this is the most common type of kidney cancer. It usually occurs in people over the age of 40 and affects twice as many men as women. A common symptom is blood in the urine. There may also be pain in the back, a lump in the abdomen, fever, or weight loss. The cancer often spreads to the lungs, bones, liver, and brain.

Nephroblastoma

Nephroblastoma (also called Wilms' tumour) is a fast-growing tumour that mainly affects children under five years old. Nephroblastoma sometimes runs in families, but its cause is unknown. Symptoms may include swelling of the abdomen, abdominal pain or discomfort, and, occasionally, blood in the urine. Nephroblastoma may spread to the lungs, liver, and brain.

Transitional cell carcinoma

This type of kidney cancer arises from cells lining the renal pelvis (the urine-collecting system within the kidney); it is most common in smokers or in people

DISORDERS OF THE KIDNEY

The *kidneys* are susceptible to a wide range of disorders. Only one normal kidney is needed for good health, however, so disease is rarely life-threatening unless it affects both kidneys and is at an advanced stage. *Hypertension* (high blood pressure) can be both a cause and an effect of kidney damage. Other effects of serious damage include *nephrotic syndrome* and *kidney failure*.

Congenital and genetic disorders

Congenital abnormalities, such as *duplex kidney* (in which a kidney is partially duplicated) and *horseshoe kidney* (in which the two kidneys are joined at their base), are fairly common and usually harmless. Serious inherited disorders include polycystic kidney disease (see *kidney, polycystic*), in which multiple cysts develop on both kidneys; and *Fanconi's syndrome* and *renal tubular acidosis*, in which the kidney tubules function abnormally so that certain substances are inappropriately lost in the urine.

Impaired blood supply

Various conditions may cause damage to, or lead to blockage of, the blood vessels within the kidneys, impairing blood flow. Such conditions include *shock, haemolytic–uraemic syndrome, poly-arteritis nodosa, diabetes mellitus*, and systemic *lupus erythematosus*. Impaired blood flow through the kidneys can lead to tissue damage, hypertension, and kidney failure.

Autoimmune disorders

Glomerulonephritis includes a group of autoimmune disorders (in which the immune system attacks the body's own tissues) that cause the filtering units of the kidneys to become inflamed and unable to function normally.

Drugs

Allergic reactions to drugs, prolonged treatment with *analgesic drugs* (pain-killers), and some *antibiotics* can damage kidney tubules.

Tumours

Noncancerous *kidney tumours* are rare; *kidney cancer* is uncommon.

Metabolic disorders

Diabetes mellitus is the commonest cause of kidney failure in developed countries. Other metabolic disorders, such as *hyperuricaemia*, may cause kidney stones to form (see *calculus, urinary tract*).

Infection

Infection of the kidney is called *pyelonephritis* and can be a complication of *cystitis*. A predisposing factor to infection is obstruction of urine flow through the urinary tract due to a kidney or ureteral stone, tumour, or congenital defect.

Other disorders

Hydronephrosis (a kidney swollen with urine) is caused by obstruction of the urinary tract. *Crush syndrome* is a condition in which kidney function is disrupted by proteins released into the blood from damaged muscle.

INVESTIGATION

Kidney disorders are investigated by *kidney imaging* techniques such as *ultrasound scanning, urography, angiography, radionuclide scanning, CT scanning* and *MRI*; by *kidney biopsy* (removal of a small amount of tissue for analysis); by *blood tests*; and by *kidney function tests* such as *urinalysis*.

K

who have taken certain *analgesic drugs* for a long time. Blood in the urine is a common symptom; *hydronephrosis* (distension of the kidney with urine) may occur due to blockage of the ureter.

DIAGNOSIS, TREATMENT, AND OUTLOOK
The doctor will conduct a physical examination and test a urine sample for the presence of blood. Diagnosis can be confirmed by *ultrasound scanning*, *CT scanning*, *MRI*, or intravenous *urography*.

All types of kidney cancer require surgical removal of the affected kidney and sometimes also of the *ureter*. Any remaining cancerous cells are destroyed using *radiotherapy* and/or treatment with *anticancer drugs* (for example, *interleukin* or *medroxyprogesterone* are given to treat some cases of renal cell carcinoma).

Survival rates vary, depending on the type of cancer and how early treatment is commenced. In the case of nephroblastoma, about four in every five affected children survive; cure rates for this form of kidney cancer are relatively high even if it has spread by the time diagnosis is made.

kidney cyst

A fluid-filled sac in the *kidney*. Cysts commonly develop in people over 50, and can occur either singly or multiply in one or both kidneys. Most cysts occur for no known reason, are noncancerous, and do not usually produce symptoms unless they become large enough to cause lower back pain due to pressure on surrounding tissues. Large numbers of kidney cysts, however, may be associated with polycystic kidney disease (see *kidney, polycystic*), which often leads to *kidney failure*.

Simple cysts do not usually require treatment. For cases in which the cysts are painful or recurrent, however, aspiration (withdrawal of fluid) or surgical removal may be carried out.

kidney, duplex

See *duplex kidney*.

kidney failure

A reduction in the function of the kidneys. Kidney failure causes waste products such as urea and excess fluid to accumulate in the body, and also produces other chemical imbalances in the blood and body tissues.

TYPES
Kidney failure can be acute or chronic. In the acute form, kidney function often returns to normal once the underlying cause has been discovered and treated. In chronic kidney failure, however, kidney tissue is progressively damaged over several months or years. This condition may develop into end-stage kidney failure, a life-threatening condition in which kidney function is usually irreversibly lost.

CAUSES
Causes of acute kidney failure include a severe reduction in blood flow to the kidneys, as occurs in *shock*; an obstruction to urine flow, for example due to a bladder tumour; or certain rapidly developing types of kidney disease, such as *glomerulonephritis*.

Chronic kidney failure can be the result of a disease that causes progressive damage to the kidneys, such as polycystic kidney disease (see *kidney,*

THE FUNCTION OF THE **KIDNEYS**

The kidneys' main function is to filter the blood. This activity is essential in regulating the body's fluid balance and acid-base balance. Each kidney has about 1 million nephrons, where the filtering takes place. A nephron consists of a knot of capillaries, which is called a glomerulus, and a tubule, where urine is formed. Urine drains out of the kidney via the ureter; the normal daily output is 1 to 2 litres.

RENAL FUNCTION AND AGE

The efficiency of the kidneys diminishes with age as the number of functional nephrons is reduced.

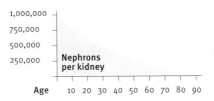

1,000,000	
750,000	
500,000	
250,000	**Nephrons per kidney**
Age	10 20 30 40 50 60 70 80 90

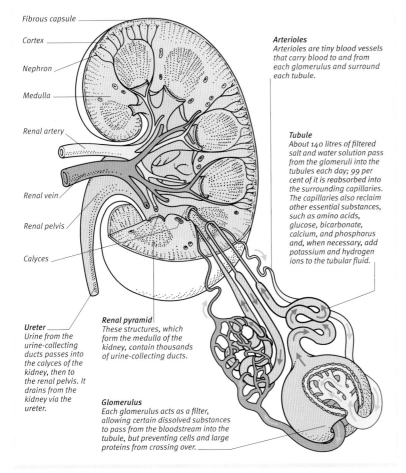

Fibrous capsule

Cortex

Nephron

Medulla

Renal artery

Renal vein

Renal pelvis

Calyces

Ureter
Urine from the urine-collecting ducts passes into the calyces of the kidney, then to the renal pelvis. It drains from the kidney via the ureter.

Renal pyramid
These structures, which form the medulla of the kidney, contain thousands of urine-collecting ducts.

Glomerulus
Each glomerulus acts as a filter, allowing certain dissolved substances to pass from the bloodstream into the tubule, but preventing cells and large proteins from crossing over.

Arterioles
Arterioles are tiny blood vessels that carry blood to and from each glomerulus and surround each tubule.

Tubule
About 140 litres of filtered salt and water solution pass from the glomeruli into the tubules each day; 99 per cent of it is reabsorbed into the surrounding capillaries. The capillaries also reclaim other essential substances, such as amino acids, glucose, bicarbonate, calcium, and phosphorus and, when necessary, add potassium and hydrogen ions to the tubular fluid.

polycystic), *diabetes mellitus*, and *hypertension* (high blood pressure), or from longstanding obstruction to urine flow.
SYMPTOMS
The most obvious symptom of acute kidney failure is oliguria (a reduced volume of urine). Urea and other waste products build up in the blood and tissues causing drowsiness, nausea, and breathlessness.

Symptoms of chronic kidney failure develop more gradually, and may include malaise, nausea, loss of appetite, and weakness. The kidney damage leads to conditions such as *anaemia* and *hyperparathyroidism*.
DIAGNOSIS AND TREATMENT
A person with suspected kidney failure will initially need blood and urine tests.

Other tests, such as *kidney biopsy* (examination of a tissue sample) and *intravenous urography* (taking X-rays of the urinary tract), may be carried out to identify the cause of the kidney failure if this is not already obvious.

If acute kidney failure is due to a sudden reduction in blood flow, blood volume and pressure can be normalized by saline *intravenous infusion* or *blood transfusion*. If there is an obstruction in the urinary tract, surgery may be needed. Acute kidney disease may be treated with *corticosteroid drugs*. Treatment may also involve *diuretic drugs* and temporary *dialysis* (artificial purification of the blood).

A high-carbohydrate, low-protein diet with controlled fluid and salt intake is important in the treatment of acute and chronic kidney failure, because this reduces the workload on the kidneys. Good control of hypertension and diabetes is also essential in both acute and chronic kidney failure.

For end-stage kidney failure, long-term dialysis or a *kidney transplant* is the only effective treatment.

kidney function tests

Tests that are performed to investigate *kidney disorders*. *Urinalysis* is a simple test in which a urine sample is examined under a microscope for blood cells, pus cells, and casts (cells and mucous material that accumulate in the tubules of the kidneys and pass into the urine). Urinalysis is used to test for substances, such as proteins, that leak into the urine when the kidneys are damaged. Kidney function can be assessed by measuring the concentration in the blood of substances that the kidneys normally excrete, such as *urea* and *creatinine*; by creatinine clearance, in which levels of creatinine in the blood are compared with creatinine excreted in urine over 24 hours; and by *kidney imaging* with radioisotopes.

kidney imaging

Techniques for visualizing the *kidneys*, usually performed for diagnosis.

Ultrasound scanning is often the first investigation and can be used to identify kidney enlargement, a cyst or tumour, and the site of any blockage. Conventional *X-rays* show the outline of the kidneys and most kidney stones. *Intravenous urography* shows the internal anatomy of the kidney and ureters. *Angiography* is used to image blood circulation through the kidneys. *CT scanning* and *MRI* provide

K

KIDNEY IMAGING

The various kidney imaging techniques can provide different types of information to help doctors investigate and diagnose kidney disorders.

MRI and CT scanning
These techniques produce cross-sectional images of body tissues, displayed as computer-generated pictures. They clearly show structural abnormalities such as tumours and cysts. This MRI scan of the abdomen shows a polycystic kidney (on the right of the image).

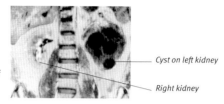

Cyst on left kidney

Right kidney

IVU (Intravenous urography)
This is a type of X-ray in which fluid containing a contrast medium (a substance opaque to X-rays) is introduced into the urinary system, then X-rays are taken. The images show how the fluid moves through the kidneys, ureters, and bladder, and can show up any obstructions, such as stones in the urinary tract.

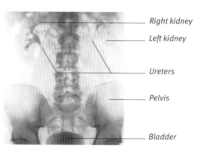

Right kidney

Left kidney

Ureters

Pelvis

Bladder

Ultrasound scanning
This is a quick technique, which provides clear images of the structure of the kidney. It can reveal fluid-filled structures such as cysts, which can be clearly differentiated from the kidney tissue surrounding them.

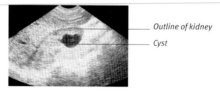

Outline of kidney

Cyst

Radionuclide scanning
This produces coloured images to show the functioning of the kidneys. (This scan is taken from the back.) Areas that are brighter than normal show overactive cells, as in a tumour; colours that are less intense than normal show underactivity, as in kidney failure.

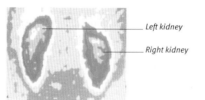

Left kidney

Right kidney

detailed cross-sectional images of kidney tissue and the urine-collecting system, and can show abscesses or tumours.

Two types of *radionuclide scanning* are used for the kidneys: DMSA and DTPA/MAG3 scanning. A DMSA scan gives information about the size, shape, and position of the kidneys. A DTPA/MAG3 scan provides information about blood flow to the kidneys and kidney function.

kidney, polycystic

An inherited disorder in which both *kidneys* develop numerous *cysts* that gradually enlarge until most of the normal tissue is destroyed. Polycystic kidney disease is distinguished from multiple simple *kidney cysts*, which occur commonly with increasing age.

TYPES
There are two types of polycystic disease. The most common type usually appears in middle age, producing abdominal swelling, pain, and blood in the urine. As the disease progresses, *hypertension* (high blood pressure) and *kidney failure* may result.

The second type of polycystic disease, which is rare, causes enlargement of the kidneys and kidney failure in infants and young children.

TREATMENT AND PREVENTION
There is no effective treatment for preserving kidney function in either type of the condition, but symptoms of kidney failure can be treated by *dialysis* (artificial purification of the blood) and *kidney transplant*.

People with a family history of this disease may need *genetic counselling* before starting a family. The adult form is an *autosomal dominant disorder* and an affected parent has a 50 per cent chance of passing on the defective gene. If both parents carry the gene for the juvenile form (*autosomal recessive disorder*), their fetus can be examined using *ultrasound scanning* to detect kidney enlargement.

kidney stone

See *calculus, urinary tract*.

kidney transplant

An operation in which a person with chronic *kidney failure* receives a healthy kidney from a living or, more commonly, a dead donor. One donor kidney can maintain the health of the recipient.

The new kidney is placed in the *pelvis* through an incision in the abdomen and carefully positioned so that it can be connected easily to a nearby vein and artery and to the *bladder*. The diseased kidneys may be left in place.

The transplant removes the need for *dialysis* (artificial purification of blood) and often allows a return to a normal lifestyle. The procedure is more straightforward than transplantation of other organs. Unless the donor is an identical twin, *immunosuppressant drugs* are given to avoid rejection of the kidney.

kidney tumours

Growths in the *kidney*. Kidney tumours may be cancerous (see *kidney cancer*) or noncancerous. The latter type, which include *fibromas, lipomas,* and *leiomyomas,* are often symptomless, although a *haemangioma* (composed of a collection of blood vessels) may grow very large and cause blood to appear in the urine.

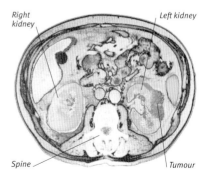

Right kidney

Left kidney

Spine

Tumour

CT scan of a kidney tumour
In this scan, the body is seen from below, with the spine at the base of the image. The kidneys are the round shapes on either side. A tumour (dark mass) can be seen on the left kidney (right of image).

PROCEDURE FOR A **KIDNEY TRANSPLANT**

A kidney transplant is performed when a person's kidneys have lost almost all of their normal function (so-called end-stage kidney failure). Just one healthy donor kidney can allow a patient to have a normal lifestyle. The donated kidney comes from a close relative of the patient, or from any person who consented to medical use of his or her organs after death. To prevent rejection of the kidney by the recipient's *immune system*, the tissue-type and blood group of recipient and donor must be a close match (see *transplant surgery*).

DIALYSIS AND TRANSPLANTATION

A significant proportion of patients with end-stage kidney failure are suitable for a kidney transplant, but many have to remain on dialysis for some time until a suitable donor kidney becomes available. A computer system is used to match donors with the most suitable recipients. The number of available donor kidneys is considerably less than the number of people waiting for a transplant.

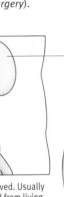

Donor kidney (from living donor)

The surgeon inserts the donated kidney in its new position in the pelvis.

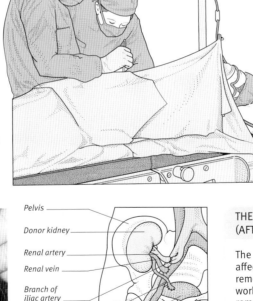

Site of incision
The donor kidney is inserted low in the patient's pelvis, close to the bladder and major blood vessels.

K

1 The donor kidney is removed. Usually the left kidney is removed from living donors, because it has a longer vein than the right and is easier to remove safely. With donation from people who have died (cadavers), both kidneys are used and each kidney usually goes to a separate recipient. Kidneys from a cadaver can be maintained for transplantation by a machine that passes a cooling saline solution through them. Donor organs may need to be transported over long distances, and occasionally to other countries, to reach the recipient.

2 After it has been removed, a donor kidney is flushed with chilled saline solution in order to preserve the tissues and internal structures. The donor kidney should then be transplanted as soon as possible in order to maximize the chance of the transplant being successful.

Pelvis
Donor kidney
Renal artery
Renal vein
Branch of iliac artery
Ureter
Bladder

3 The donor kidney is usually placed in the pelvis. The renal artery and vein of the donor kidney are joined to a convenient artery (usually a branch of the external iliac artery) and vein of the recipient. The lower end of the donor ureter is connected to the recipient's bladder. The donor kidney usually begins working immediately after transplantation into the recipient.

THE DONOR (AFTER THE OPERATION)

The health of the donor is not affected by having a kidney removed because the body can work efficiently with just one. The remaining kidney enlarges to increase its capacity and takes over full function.

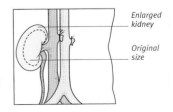

Enlarged kidney

Original size

A biopsy of the tumour may be needed to confirm that it is not cancerous. Treatment is usually not needed for noncancerous tumours unless they are large or painful.

Kiel classification

A system that is used for ranking non-Hodgkin's lymphoma (see *lymphoma, non-Hodgkin's*), any of several cancerous tumours of the lymphoid tissues in which the cells divide unchecked. The cancer is classified as high-grade or low-grade according to the type of cell and how rapidly the cells are dividing. Once widely used, Kiel classification has now been replaced by WHO classification.

Kienböck disease

Death of tissue cells (see *necrosis*) in the wristbone known as the lunate bone. The disorder, characterized by pain and stiffness in the wrist, is caused by an inadequate blood supply, often the result of an undiagnosed or unsuccessfully treated fracture. Treatment usually consists of resting the joint; in a few cases, surgery is needed.

killer T-cell

A type of white blood cell, also known as a cytotoxic T-lymphocyte or a CD8 *lymphocyte*, that has an important role in the *immune system*. Killer T-cells destroy an abnormal, cancerous, or virus-infected cell after a foreign *antigen* on its surface has been recognized by *helper T-cells*. (See also *natural killer cells*.)

kilocalorie

The unit of energy equal to 1,000 *calories*, abbreviated to kcal. In dietetics, a kilocalorie is sometimes referred to simply as a calorie (or C).

kilojoule

The unit of energy equal to 1,000 joules, abbreviated to kJ. One kcal (see *kilocalorie*) equals 4.2 kJ.

kinky-hair disease

A genetic disorder, also called Menkes' syndrome, in which body cells do not absorb sufficient copper. The condition is present from birth. It causes brittle, kinky hair; hypotonia (abnormal muscle slackness); feeding difficulties; seizures; and degeneration of brain tissue. Affected children die after a few years.

Kinky-hair disease is an *X-linked disorder*; it affects only male babies, but females may carry the gene. People

with a family history of the disorder may wish to consider genetic counselling before having children.

kiss of life

A common name for *rescue breathing*.

Klebsiella

A genus of rod-shaped bacteria that is commonly found in the human intestine. They may cause pneumonia, lung abscess, or *peritonitis* in people with *ascites* (excess fluid in the peritoneal cavity) due to liver disease. One type, KLEBSIELLA GRANULOMATIS, is the cause of the sexually transmitted infection granuloma inguinale or donovanosis, which is common in the tropics and produces a rash and ulceration of the genital area.

kleptomania

A recurring inability to resist impulses to steal, often without any desire for the stolen objects. The condition is usually a sign of an immature personality. It is sometimes associated with *depression*, and may also result from *dementia* or some forms of *brain damage*.

Klinefelter's syndrome

A *chromosomal abnormality* in which a male has one, or occasionally more, extra X chromosomes in his cells, giv-

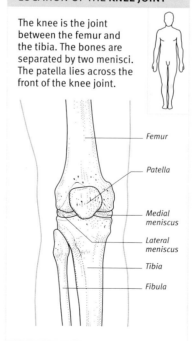

LOCATION OF THE **KNEE JOINT**

The knee is the joint between the femur and the tibia. The bones are separated by two menisci. The patella lies across the front of the knee joint.

Femur

Patella

Medial meniscus

Lateral meniscus

Tibia

Fibula

ing a complement of XXY instead of XY. The risk of a baby having the condition increases with maternal age.

SYMPTOMS AND SIGNS
Features of the syndrome vary in severity and may not become apparent until the child reaches puberty, when *gynaecomastia* (breast enlargement) occurs and the testes remain small. Affected males are usually infertile (see *infertility*). They tend to be tall and thin with a female body shape and absence of body hair. Incidence of learning difficulties is higher in people with Klinefelter's syndrome than in the general population.

TREATMENT
There is no cure, but hormonal treatment can induce signs of puberty (see *sexual characteristics, secondary*) such as the growth of facial hair, and surgery may be used to correct gynaecomastia.

Klippel–Fiel syndrome

A condition characterized by an abnormally short neck, due to fused cervical vertebrae. Affected people have restricted neck movement and a low hairline.

Klippel–Trenaunay–Weber syndrome

A rare condition, usually affecting a limb, in which massive malformation of blood vessels (including both arteries and veins) leads to overgrowth of the affected area.

Klumpke's paralysis

Paralysis of the lower arm, with wasting of the small muscles in the hand, and numbness of the fingers (but not the thumb) and the inner forearm.

Klumpke's paralysis is caused by injury to the eighth cervical and the first thoracic nerves (two of the *spinal nerves*) in the brachial plexus (the network of nerves located behind the shoulderblade), which usually results from injury to the shoulder.

knee

The hinge *joint* between the *femur* (thigh bone) and *tibia* (shin). The *patella* (kneecap) covers the front of the joint.

STRUCTURE
Two protective discs of cartilage called menisci (see *meniscus*) cover the surfaces of the femur and tibia to reduce friction. Bursas (fluid-filled sacs) located above and below the patella, and behind the knee, cushion the joint. External ligaments on either side of the knee provide support, and cruciate ligaments within

K

PROCEDURE FOR A **KNEE REPLACEMENT**

This procedure is carried out to replace a diseased or eroded knee joint. The surgeon usually makes a long, straight incision, cutting through the joint capsule and synovial membrane, then pushes aside the patella to reach the joint. Special instruments are used to make precise measurements and cut away areas of bone so that the artificial knee replacement components will fit and move correctly.

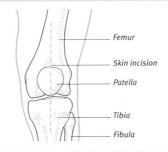
Femur
Skin incision
Patella
Tibia
Fibula

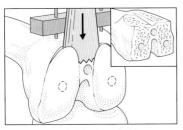

1 The lower end of the femur (thigh-bone) is shaped and holes are drilled into it to accept the femoral component of the prosthesis (see inset). Accuracy is achieved by using the surgical equivalent of a mitre box.

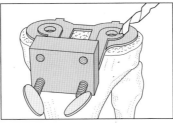

2 The upper end of the tibia (shin-bone) is shaped, and holes are drilled into it to accept the tibial component of the prosthesis. The cutting and drilling of the bone are again carried out using the special orthopaedic instruments.

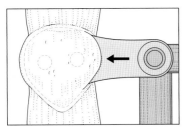

3 Often the patella is left undamaged, but repairs may be carried out to its surface. In this case, the back part of the patella is cut away to leave a flat surface. Small holes are then drilled into this surface to accept the patellar component of the artificial joint.

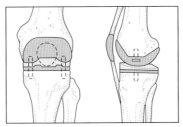

4 After achieving a satisfactory fit using trial components, the three parts of the final prosthesis are then cemented in place. Any excess cement is then removed from around the new joint and a final check is made of the joint movements.

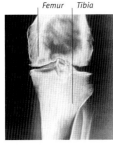
Femur   Tibia

X-ray of arthritic knee
Severe wear and tear of the bone and cartilage can easily be seen on this knee X-ray.

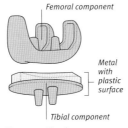
Femoral component
Metal with plastic surface
Tibial component

Knee prosthesis
The main artificial components fit over the femur and tibia (the patellar component is not shown). The prostheses come in different types and sizes.

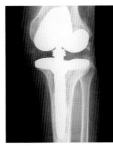

X-ray of artificial knee
This X-ray shows the three components of the prosthesis in position after surgery.

---

the joint prevent overstraightening and overbending. The quadriceps muscles, at the front of the thigh, straighten the knee, and the hamstring muscles at the back of the thigh bend it.

DISORDERS

Injuries of the knee are common, and include ligament sprains, torn meniscus, *dislocation* of the patella, and *fracture* of any of the bones. A painful inflammatory condition, *chondromalacia patellae*, is common in adolescents, and *knock-knee* and *bowleg* are common temporary defects in children.

kneecap

See *patella*.

knee-jerk reflex

An involuntary response, also known as a patellar reflex, that occurs when the tendon just below the kneecap (patella) is tapped. The tendon stretches and the thigh muscles contract, straightening the knee. (See also *reflex*.)

knee-joint replacement

Surgery to replace a diseased *knee* joint with an artificial one, usually made of metal or plastic. Knee-joint replacement is most commonly carried out on older people whose knees are severely affected by the inflammatory conditions *osteoarthritis* or *rheumatoid arthritis*.

Kniest syndrome

A very rare inherited disorder due to abnormal collagen (a protein in bone, cartilage, and connective tissue). It causes severe dwarfism (see *short stature*) with curvature of the spine (*kyphoscoliosis*).

knock-knee

Inward curving of the legs so that the knees touch, causing the feet to be positioned further apart than normal.

CAUSES

Knock-knee is common in children between the ages of three and five and may be part of normal development. In some children, knock-knee may be caused by *rickets*, a disease that softens the bones. In adults, causes include *osteoarthritis* and *rheumatoid arthritis* of the knee. A leg *fracture* that has not healed correctly may also cause knock-knee in children or adults.

TREATMENT

In children, the condition usually disappears by about seven years. Knock-knee that persists, or is due to a disorder, may require *osteotomy*, a surgical procedure

K

K

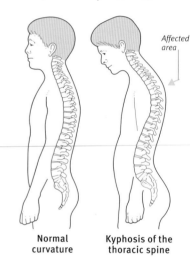

The appearance of knock-knee
This condition is common in young children but almost always disappears by the age of seven.

in which the *tibia* (shin) is cut and realigned to straighten the leg. In adults, *knee-joint replacement* may be needed.

knuckle
The name for a *finger* joint.

Koch's bacillus
Another name for MYCOBACTERIUM TUBERCULOSIS, the microorganism responsible for *tuberculosis*.

Koebner's phenomenon
A reaction in people with skin disorders such as *psoriasis* and *lichen planus*. New lesions develop, often due to scratching.

koilonychia
A condition in which the *nails* are brittle and thin, and become spoon-shaped. It may be congenital, and may be associated with iron-deficiency *anaemia* or the skin disease *lichen planus*.

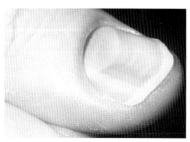

The appearance of koilonychia
In koilonychia, the nails look fragile and are flattened in the middle and elevated at the ends.

Konakion
A brand name for the *vitamin K* supplement *phytomenadione*, given routinely to newborn babies to prevent bleeding.

Koplik's spots
Tiny spots that appear in the mouth during the incubation period of *measles*.

Korsakoff's psychosis
See *Wernicke–Korsakoff syndrome*.

Krabbe's disease
A very rare inherited metabolic disorder (see *metabolism, inborn errors of*) that causes death in early childhood. Krabbe's disease is caused by deficiency of an *enzyme* (a substance that promotes a biochemical reaction) called galactocerebrosidase. The deficiency leads to the accumulation of toxic chemicals within cells of the nervous system. Symptoms, including *seizures*, deteriorating vision, deafness, and muscle weakness, usually begin to develop by nine months.

kraurosis vulvae
See *vulvitis*.

kuru
A rare, fatal form of *spongiform encephalopathy* (a disease in which the brain tissue shrinks and spaces develop in it) that affects some inhabitants of New Guinea. Kuru is caused by a *prion* that has a long incubation period and is spread by cannibalism. Symptoms of kuru include progressive difficulty in controlling movements and *dementia*. Typically, death occurs within about a year of symptoms appearing.

kwashiorkor
A severe form of *malnutrition* in young children that occurs principally in poor rural areas in the tropics.

SYMPTOMS AND COMPLICATIONS
Affected children have stunted growth and a puffy appearance due to oedema (accumulation of fluid in the tissues). The liver often enlarges, dehydration may develop, and the child loses resistance to infection, which may have fatal consequences. The advanced stages are marked by jaundice, drowsiness, and a fall in body temperature.

TREATMENT
Initially, the child is fed small, frequent amounts of milk, and vitamin and mineral tablets. A nutritious diet is then gradually introduced. Most treated children recover, but those under two years may have permanently stunted growth.

kyphoscoliosis
A combination of the two types of spinal curvature: *kyphosis* and *scoliosis*.

kyphosis
Excessive outward curvature of the *spine*. Kyphosis usually affects the spine at the top of the back, resulting in a hump or pronounced rounding of the back. When kyphosis is combined with a curvature of the spine to one side (*scoliosis*), the condition is known as kyphoscoliosis.

Kyphosis may be caused by various spine or muscle disorders, *osteoporosis*, or it may occur as a *congenital* abnormality. Treatment is of the underlying disorder, but is rarely successful.

Affected area

Normal curvature

Kyphosis of the thoracic spine

The appearance of kyphosis
In kyphosis, the thoracic part of the spine is excessively curved (as indicated by the arrow, above), producing a humped appearance.

L

Laband's syndrome

An autosomal dominant *genetic disorder* affecting tissues throughout the body. It causes bone deformities; overly flexible joints; clubbing of the fingers, and missing nails. Other features include a bulbous nose, overgrowth of the gums, thickened ears, and an enlarged liver and spleen. Some people may also have *learning difficulties*.

labetolol

A *beta-blocker drug* that is used to treat *hypertension* (high blood pressure) and *angina pectoris* (chest pain caused by an impaired blood supply to the heart). Possible adverse effects include indigestion, nausea and, in rare cases, *depression*, temporary *erectile dysfunction*, and liver damage.

labia

The folds of skin of the *vulva* that protect the vaginal and urethral openings. There are two pairs of labia. The outer pair, the labia majora, are fleshy folds that contain sweat glands and grow hair. They cover the smaller, hairless inner folds, the labia minora, which meet to form the hood of the *clitoris*.

LOCATION OF THE **LABIA**

The labia majora extend forwards from the perineum and fuse at the front at the mons pubis. The labia minora lie within.

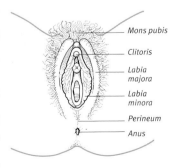

- Mons pubis
- Clitoris
- Labia majora
- Labia minora
- Perineum
- Anus

labile

A term meaning "unstable" or "likely to undergo change".

labour

See *childbirth*; *induction of labour*.

labour pains

Painful muscle contractions in the *uterus* during *childbirth*. The contractions dilate (widen) the *cervix* and then move the baby through the birth canal for delivery.

labyrinth

The collective term for the structures of the inner *ear*. The first part of the labyrinth is the *cochlea*, which contains the mechanisms that enable *hearing*. Situated behind the cochlea are two sacs (the saccule and the utricle) and three fluid-filled semicircular canals, all of which are concerned with *balance*.

labyrinthitis

Inflammation of the *labyrinth* in the inner ear. The disorder is almost always caused by a viral infection, which may develop during illnesses such as the common cold or influenza. Less commonly, labyrinthitis may be caused by a bacterial infection, as a complication of *otitis media* (middle-ear infection).

SYMPTOMS

The main symptom is *vertigo*. Nausea, vomiting, *nystagmus* (abnormal, jerky eye movements), *tinnitus* (ringing in the ears), and hearing loss may also occur.

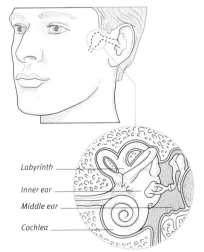

- Labyrinth
- Inner ear
- Middle ear
- Cochlea

Mechanism of labyrinthitis
In labyrinthitis, inflammation of the fluid-filled chambers (labyrinth) of the inner ear causes disruption of the individual's sense of balance. The inflammation is usually caused by viral or bacterial infection.

TREATMENT

Viral labyrinthitis clears up on its own, but symptoms may be relieved by *antiemetic drugs*. Bacterial labyrinthitis needs immediate treatment with *antibiotic drugs*, otherwise permanent *deafness* or *meningitis* (inflammation of the membranes covering the brain) may result.

laceration

A torn, irregular *wound*.

lacrimal apparatus

The system in the eye that produces and drains *tears*. The lacrimal apparatus includes the main and accessory lacrimal glands and nasolacrimal drainage duct (see *lacrimal apparatus* box, overleaf).

The main lacrimal glands lie just within the upper and outer margin of the eye orbit and drain onto the *conjunctiva* (the transparent membrane covering the white of the eye and the inside of the eyelids). They secrete tears during crying and when the eye is irritated.

The accessory glands lie within the conjunctiva, and maintain the normal tear film, secreting it directly onto the conjunctiva; the fluid is spread across the eye surfaces by blinking.

Tears drain from the eye through the lacrimal puncta, tiny openings towards the inner ends of the upper and lower eyelids. The puncta are connected by narrow tubes to the lacrimal sacs, which lie within the lacrimal bones on the sides of the nose. Leading from the sacs are the nasolacrimal ducts, which open inside the nose.

lactamase

An enzyme, also called penicillinase or beta-lactamase, that is produced by STA-PHYLOCOCCUS bacteria (see *staphylococcal infections*). Lactamase inactivates *antibiotic drugs* of the penicillin and cephalosporin groups, making them ineffective against the bacteria.

lactase deficiency

A condition in which there is an absence of *lactase*, an enzyme that breaks down *lactose* (milk sugar), in the cells of the small intestine. Lactase deficiency reduces ability to digest lactose. This is called *lactose intolerance* and usually appears in adolescence or adulthood; rarely, it is present at birth (especially in premature babies). Lactase deficiency may also occur temporarily after *gastroenteritis* or treatment with antibiotics, particularly in young children.

FUNCTIONS OF THE **LACRIMAL APPARATUS**

Tear production must be sufficient to compensate for evaporation and maintain the tear film. Accessory lacrimal glands in the conjunctiva perform this function. The main lacrimal glands secrete tears when excess fluid is required. Surplus tears drain into the nose through the lacrimal puncta, lacrimal sac, and lacrimal duct.

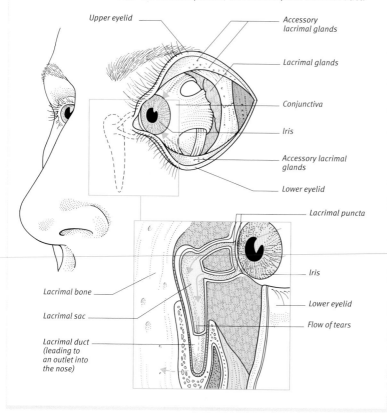

SYMPTOMS

The undigested lactose ferments in the intestines, causing symptoms such as abdominal cramps, bloating, *flatulence*, and *diarrhoea*.

DIAGNOSIS AND TREATMENT

The condition may be diagnosed by testing faeces for the presence of lactose. Alternatively, an *exclusion diet* may be used, in which consumption of dairy products is stopped for a few days and then resumed to see if this causes any changes in the symptoms.

Treatment is with a lactose-free diet. Some people are able to tolerate small amounts of dairy produce but others must avoid dairy products completely, including milk, yoghurt, cream, butter, and cheese. It is possible to obtain milk products in which lactose has already been broken down, and enzyme supplements containing lactase, which can be added to milk, or eaten with food.

lactation

The production and secretion of breast milk (see *breast-feeding*).

lactic acid

A weak acid that is produced when body cells break down *glucose* by *anaerobic* metabolism (chemical processes that do not require oxygen) to generate energy. Lactic acid is produced by muscles during vigorous exercise and is one of the factors that contribute to *cramp*.

Lactic acid is also produced in body tissues when they receive insufficient oxygen through impairment of their blood supply. This situation may be the result of a *myocardial infarction* (heart attack) or *shock*.

Normally, lactic acid is removed from the bloodstream by the liver. If this does not happen, the lactic acid accumulates in the body and causes a condition known as lactic *acidosis*.

lactobacillus

A type of rod-shaped *bacteria* found in fermented plant and dairy products. Some types of lactobacilli colonize the human intestine and the vagina, where they prevent the overmultiplication of harmful bacteria.

lactose

One of the sugars present in milk; a disaccharide *carbohydrate*.

lactose intolerance

The inability to digest *lactose* (see *lactase deficiency*).

lactulose

An osmotic *laxative drug* that is used to treat *constipation*.

Lafora-body disease

A degenerative disease of the nervous system that causes *epilepsy*. The disease is an autosomal recessive *genetic disorder* that first appears in childhood or adolescence, often with *seizures*. Subsequent signs include impaired movement and coordination, and *dementia*. There is no treatment. Death usually occurs within 10 years of onset.

Lambert–Eaton syndrome

A neuromuscular disorder in which nerve cells fail to release sufficient amounts of the *neurotransmitter* acetylcholine. It is often associated with the type of lung cancer known as *small cell carcinoma*. The main symptom is profound muscle weakness in the trunk and limbs.

lambliasis

Another name for *giardiasis*.

laminectomy

The partial surgical removal of one of the laminae (the bony arches on each *vertebra*). It is performed as the first stage of spinal canal decompression (see *decompression, spinal canal*) or in the treatment of a prolapsed disc (see *disc prolapse*).

Lamisil

A brand name for the antifungal drug *terbinafine*.

lamivudine

A nucleoside reverse transcriptase inhibitor *antiretroviral drug* used in the treatment of *HIV* infection to slow the progression of the illness. It is always prescribed in combination with another drug for HIV, to prevent the virus from

L

becoming resistant to it. Often, when treatment is started, three drugs are used: two nucleoside reverse transcriptase inhibitors and a third drug from another class, such as a non-nucleoside reverse transcriptase inhibitor or a *protease inhibitor*. Lamivudine may also be used to treat longstanding *hepatitis B* infections.

Nausea, vomiting, and diarrhoea are the most common side effects; others include a cough, headache, and pins and needles. Side effects such as fever, rash, hair loss, jaundice, or sore throat should be reported to a doctor. If severe abdominal pain develops, urgent medical help should be sought.

lamotrigine

An *anticonvulsant drug* used either alone or with other anticonvulsants in the treatment of *epilepsy*. Lamotrigine can cause various minor side effects such as rash, nausea, headache, and blurred vision. Rarely, serious skin reactions may occur, particularly in children. There may also be flulike symptoms, bruising, sore throat, and facial swelling, which should be reported to a doctor promptly.

lance

To incise (cut into) using a *lancet* or a surgical *scalpel*.

lancet

A small, pointed, double-edged knife used to open and drain lesions, such as boils and abscesses.

Landouzy–Dejerine dystrophy

See *facioscapulohumeral dystrophy*.

language disorders

Problems affecting a person's ability to communicate and/or comprehend the spoken and/or the written word (see *speech*; *speech disorders*).

lanolin

A mixture of purified water and a yellow, oily substance that is obtained from sheep's wool. Lanolin is used as an *emollient* in the treatment of dry skin and mild *dermatitis*. In occasional cases, lanolin may cause an allergic reaction.

Lanoxin

A brand name for the digitalis drug *digoxin*.

lansoprazole

A drug used to treat disorders that are caused by excess stomach acid, such as *peptic ulcer* and *gastro-oesophageal reflux disease*. Lansoprazole belongs to a group of drugs known as *proton pump inhibitors*. These drugs work by inhibiting the production of stomach acid.

Common side effects of lansoprazole include abdominal pain, constipation, diarrhoea, headache, fatigue, and dizziness. More serious side effects include muscle or joint pain, swollen hands and feet, and excessive bruising; all of these symptoms should be reported to a doctor. If a rash, itching, wheezing, or

breathing difficulties develop, the affected individual should stop using the drug immediately and seek urgent medical help.

lanugo hair

The fine, soft, downy hair that covers a *fetus*. Lanugo hair first appears in the fourth or fifth month of gestation and usually disappears by the ninth month. It can still be seen in some premature babies.

Lanugo hair sometimes reappears in adults who have cancer. It may also occur in those with the eating disorder *anorexia nervosa* or be a side effect of certain drugs, especially *ciclosporin*.

laparoscopy

Examination of the interior of the abdomen using a viewing instrument called a laparoscope, which is a type of *endoscope*. Laparoscopy is carried out in order to investigate the possible causes of abdominal pain, such as *appendicitis*. The procedure is also used in *gynaecology* for the diagnosis of disorders and investigation of infertility. Laparoscopy is also used to perform *minimally invasive surgery* such as *appendicectomy*, *cholecystectomy*, and female sterilization (see *sterilization, female*).

laparotomy

Any operation in which the abdomen is opened either for diagnostic purposes or for surgical treatment.

L

PRODECURE FOR **LAPAROSCOPY**

A hollow needle is inserted into the abdomen just below the navel (under anaesthesia), and carbon dioxide gas is pumped through to expand the abdominal cavity. The laparoscope is inserted through another incision to view the internal organs. The gas is removed afterwards but small amounts may remain for a day or two and cause some discomfort.

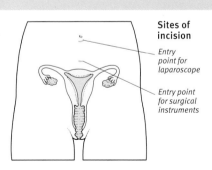

Sites of incision
Entry point for laparoscope
Entry point for surgical instruments

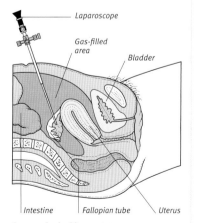

Laparoscope
Gas-filled area
Bladder
Intestine
Fallopian tube
Uterus

Gynaecological laparoscopy
Laparoscopy is used in diagnosis and is also sometimes used for removing ova for in vitro fertilization. Laparoscopy is commonly used to perform female sterilization.

LAPAROSCOPE

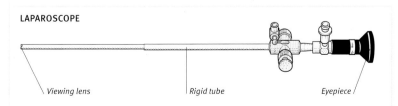

Viewing lens   *Rigid tube*   *Eyepiece*

Largactil

A brand name for the antipsychotic and anti-emetic drug *chlorpromazine*.

large intestine

The last section of the *gastrointestinal tract*. It begins at a pouch called the *caecum* (from which the *appendix* hangs). The main part, the *colon*, has four sections: the ascending, transverse, descending, and sigmoid colon. The intestine ends at the *rectum*, which is connected to the *anus*.

The large intestine processes the remains of food after nutrients have been extracted. It reabsorbs water, vitamins, and mineral salts into the bloodstream, and expels the waste material as *faeces*.

Lariam

The brand name for the antimalarial drug *mefloquine*.

larva migrans

Infections that are characterized by the presence of the larval (immature) forms of certain parasitic worms in the body. Visceral larva migrans (*toxocariasis*) is caused by a type of worm that normally parasitizes dogs. Cutaneous larva migrans (creeping eruption) is caused by a form of *hookworm infestation*; the larvae penetrate the skin and move around, leaving intensely itchy red lines that are sometimes accompanied by blistering. Both types of larva migrans can be treated with *anthelmintic drugs*.

LOCATION OF LARYNGEAL NERVES

Both nerves leave the brain at the base of the skull and pass down the neck. One hooks around an artery behind the right clavicle, the other hooks around the aorta; both return to the larynx.

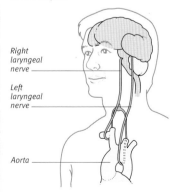

Right laryngeal nerve

Left laryngeal nerve

Aorta

PROCEDURE FOR **LARYNGOSCOPY**

There are two techniques for examination of the larynx. The patient's throat is examined with the use of a mirror in indirect laryngoscopy. In direct laryngoscopy, the patient's throat is viewed with an instrument called a laryngoscope. If a flexible laryngoscope is used, only local anaesthesia is needed; if a rigid laryngoscope is used, general anaesthesia is required.

INDIRECT LARYNGOSCOPY

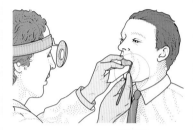

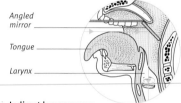

Angled mirror

Tongue

Larynx

Indirect laryngnocopy
The patient sticks out his or her tongue and the doctor rests an angled mirror on the soft palate. A lamp or mirror on the doctor's head illuminates the larynx, which is visible in the angled mirror.

DIRECT LARYNGOSCOPY

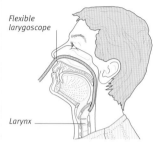

Flexible laryngoscope

Larynx

Flexible laryngoscope
A flexible laryngoscope is passed down the throat via the nostril; a rigid laryngoscope is passed via the mouth.

View of larynx
This view was obtained with a laryngoscope. The vocal cords are at the centre and the epiglottis forms the arc at the top.

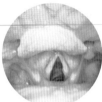

laryngeal nerve

One of a pair of *nerves* that carry instructions from the *brain* to the *larynx* (voicebox) and send sensations from the larynx to the brain.

laryngeal nerve palsy

Paralysis of one or both of the *laryngeal nerves*. Larangeal nerve palsy may be caused by disorders that cause pressure on the nerve, such as an *aneurysm* (localized swelling) in the aorta or a tumour in the thyroid gland, oesophagus, or lung. The condition may also result from infections or poisoning affecting the nerves, or damage during surgery on the thyroid gland, lung, or heart. Laryngeal nerve palsy causes complete or partial *vocal cord* paralysis, resulting in varying degrees of voice loss.

laryngeal stridor

A form of *stridor* (an abnormal, high-pitched sound during breathing) that emanates from the *larynx* (voicebox). It may occur if the larynx is inflamed, or partially blocked by an inhaled object. The condition may also appear at birth, or soon after, when it is known as congenital stridor; the cause is thought to be abnormal softness of the cartilage in the larynx (laryngomalacia).

Congenital laryngeal stridor rarely causes serious problems and usually corrects itself as the baby grows. However, medical or surgical treatment may be needed if the condition interferes with breathing.

laryngectomy

Surgical removal of all or part of the *larynx* (voicebox) to treat advanced cancer (see *larynx, cancer of*). If the entire larynx is removed, a stoma (opening) is then made in the trachea (windpipe), through which the patient will breathe. After the operation (called a tracheotomy) normal speech is no longer possible, but many patients learn to speak using *oesophageal speech*. There are also electronic devices available that help to generate speech.

laryngitis

Inflammation of the *larynx* (voicebox) that may be acute, lasting only a few days, or chronic, persisting for a long period.

CAUSES

Acute laryngitis is usually caused by a viral infection, such as a cold. It can also be due to an *allergy* or straining the laryngeal muscles. Chronic laryngitis may be caused by overusing the voice; violent coughing; irritation from tobacco smoke or fumes; or damage during surgery. Alcohol, particularly spirits, may aggravate laryngitis.

SYMPTOMS

Hoarseness is the most common symptom and may progress to loss of voice. Throat pain or discomfort and a dry, irritating cough may also occur. Laryngitis due to a viral infection is often accompanied by fever and a general feeling of illness.

TREATMENT

Treatment depends on the cause. Acute laryngitis due to a viral infection usually disappears by itself. There is no treatment for chronic laryngitis other than resting the voice, taking mild analgesic drugs (painkillers) if needed, using steam inhalation, and avoiding tobacco smoke and alcohol. If hoarseness persists for more than two weeks, medical advice should be sought in order to exclude the possibility of laryngeal cancer (see *larynx, cancer of*). In some cases, chronic laryngitis responds to speech therapy.

laryngoscopy

Examination of the *larynx* (voicebox) using a mirror held against the back of the palate (indirect laryngoscopy), or a rigid or flexible viewing tube known as a laryngoscope (direct laryngoscopy).

Laryngoscopy is performed to investigate pain in the throat; difficulty in swallowing; persistent hoarseness; and abnormal noises during breathing (such as *stridor*). Indirect laryngoscopy can show clear abnormalities, such as inflammation, paralysis of the vocal cords (see *laryngeal nerve palsy*), *singer's nodes*, or tumours. Direct rigid laryngoscopy is usually performed under general anaesthesia, and direct flexible laryngoscopy is usually carried out using local anaesthesia. These techniques enable doctors to examine the tissues of the larynx more closely, as well as to take a *biopsy* (sample of tissue) or remove foreign bodies or benign tumours.

laryngotracheobronchitis

Inflammation of the *larynx* (voicebox), *trachea* (windpipe), and *bronchi* (main airways to the lungs), caused by a viral or a bacterial infection. The disorder is usually mild but in some cases can be life-threatening. It is a common cause of *croup* in young children.

larynx

The organ in the throat responsible for voice production, commonly called the voicebox. It lies between the *pharynx* (throat) and the *trachea* (windpipe).

STRUCTURE AND FUNCTION

The larynx consists of areas of *cartilage*, the largest of which is the thyroid cartilage, which projects forwards to form the Adam's apple. Below the thyroid cartilage is the cricoid cartilage, which joins it to the trachea. Situated on the back of the cricoid cartilage are two pyramid-shaped structures called the arytenoid cartilages. The inside of the larynx is lined with mucous membrane.

LOCATION OF THE **LARYNX**

The larynx, commonly called the voicebox, is situated deep in the throat between the pharynx and the trachea (windpipe).

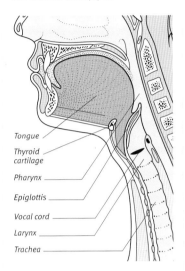

Tongue
Thyroid cartilage
Pharynx
Epiglottis
Vocal cord
Larynx
Trachea

Within the larynx, stretching between the thyroid and arytenoid cartilages, are two fibrous sheets of tissue called the *vocal cords*. The cords vibrate to produce vocal sounds when air from the lungs passes through them. These vibrations are modified by the tongue, mouth, and lips to produce *speech*.

Attached to the top of the thyroid cartilage is the *epiglottis*, which is a leaf-shaped flap of cartilage that closes

DISORDERS OF THE **LARYNX**

Disorders of the *larynx* (voicebox) usually cause *hoarseness*; other symptoms of a disorder include breathing difficulties, *stridor* (an abnormal sound during breathing), sore throat, and coughing.

Inflammation

Laryngitis (inflammation of the larynx) is the most common laryngeal disorder in adults. *Croup* (inflammation of the airways) is common in young children, up to the age of about four. Much rarer is *epiglottitis* (inflammation of the epiglottis, the flap of cartilage that covers the larynx).

Congenital defects

Rarely, a baby is born with a soft, limp larynx and epiglottis, a condition called laryngomalacia. This defect causes noisy breathing (see *laryngeal stridor*).

Tumours

Various kinds of noncancerous tumour may develop on the vocal cords. The most common is a *polyp* (a noncancerous swelling caused by smoking, an infection such as influenza, or straining the voice). Warts and small noncancerous growths called *singer's nodes* can also occur on the vocal cords. The larynx may also develop cancerous tumours

(see *larynx, cancer of*), which may cause persistent hoarseness.

Other disorders

Lesions, infection, or other disorders affecting the throat tissues, or surgery on the throat, may damage the nerves supplying the larynx. As a result, one or both of the vocal cords may become paralysed (see *laryngeal nerve palsy*).

INVESTIGATION

Disorders of the larynx are investigated by *laryngoscopy*. Sometimes a *biopsy* sample is taken.

over the larynx to prevent food and liquid from passing into the trachea during swallowing.

larynx, cancer of

A cancerous tumour of the *larynx* (voice-box). In more than half of the cases, the tumour develops on one of the *vocal cords*; in the remainder, tumours arise just above or below the cords.

CAUSES

The exact causes are not known, but smoking and high alcohol consumption are known risk factors.

SYMPTOMS

Hoarseness is the main symptom, particularly when the tumour originates on the *vocal cords*. At an advanced stage, symptoms may include difficulty in breathing and swallowing, and coughing up blood. The cancer may have spread to the *lymph nodes* in the neck; if so, the nodes will be enlarged.

DIAGNOSIS AND TREATMENT

If *laryngoscopy* reveals a tumour on the larynx, a *biopsy* (tissue sample) is taken. If the tumour is small, *radiotherapy* or *laser treatment* may be used to destroy it. For unresponsive or large tumours, partial or total *laryngectomy* (removal of the larynx) may be considered.

laser

A device that produces an intense beam of light. Lasers have many medical uses (see *laser treatment*).

laser treatment

Use of a *laser* beam in a variety of medical procedures. Lasers can cut through tissues, seal blood vessels, and destroy abnormal cells. They can be focused precisely so that tissues surrounding an operation site are not damaged.

TYPES

There are many different medical laser systems, and they can be operated in a variety of ways. Some emit light in brief bursts and are known as pulsed lasers; others emit a steady beam and are called continuous wave lasers.

One of the most commonly used devices is the carbon dioxide (CO_2) laser, which can be operated in either continuous or pulsed mode. Of all lasers, the CO_2 laser has an action most similar to that of a conventional scalpel. It is used both for internal surgery, including excision of brain tumours, and for skin treatments, such as the removal of noncancerous moles and scarring, and the reduction of wrinkles.

The argon continuous laser emits a light that is easily absorbed by the blood, causing it to clot. This laser has applications in ophthalmology (particularly in the treatment of abnormalities in the *retina* as a result of *diabetes mellitus*), surgery on the inner ear, and reduction of birthmarks such as port-wine stains. Another versatile laser is the yttrium-aluminium-garnet (YAG) system for treatments such as dentistry, hair and tattoo removal, and lithotripsy (breaking up of kidney stones). Tattoo removal and other dermatological treatments are also often carried out with a system known as the ruby laser, the light from which is strongly absorbed by the pigment melanin in hair and skin.

LASIK

The abbreviation for laser-assisted in-situ keratomileusis, a type of eye surgery in which a *laser* is used to reshape the *cornea* (transparent front part of the eye). LASIK is performed to correct refractive errors (see *refraction*) such as shortsightedness (see *myopia*) and *astigmatism*. A flap is cut partway through the cornea, some of the area beneath is removed by laser, and the flap is replaced. A newer procedure, known as LASEK (laser-assisted subepithelial keratomileusis), is similar to LASIK but cuts less deeply into the cornea.

Lasix

A brand name for the diuretic drug *furosemide* (frusemide).

Lassa fever

A serious infectious disease caused by a rodent-borne virus. Lassa fever, which is transmitted though contact with the urine, faeces, or saliva of rodents, is largely confined to West Africa. Symptoms appear after an incubation period of three to 21 days with fever, headache, muscular aches, and a sore throat. Later, severe diarrhoea and vomiting develop. In extreme cases, the condition leads to fatal heart or kidney failure. Treatment of Lassa fever is with the antiviral drug *ribavirin*, and *serum* containing *antibodies* to the virus.

Lassar's paste

A traditional skin preparation used in scaling conditions such as *psoriasis*. It contains *salicylic acid* and *zinc oxide*. Sometimes, *dithranol* is added.

USE OF A **LASER**

The concentrated beam of light produced by a laser has a variety of medical uses. Among its applications are removal of skin lesions, including birthmarks and tattoos, surgery on the eye and inner ear, treatment of tumours, and dentistry. Laser devices operate at varying wavelengths and energy levels for precise control; some are used to treat specific conditions only.

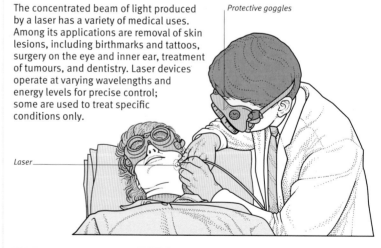

Protective goggles

Laser

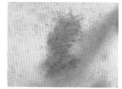

Before treatment

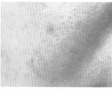

After treatment

Removing skin blemishes
These photographs, which were taken before and after laser treatment, show the removal of a port-wine stain (a type of haemangioma). In some cases, treatment is less successful, leaving scars.

lassitude

A term describing a feeling of *tiredness*, weakness, or exhaustion.

latanoprost

A *prostaglandin drug* used as eye-drops in the treatment of the eye condition *glaucoma* (increased pressure of fluid within the eyeball).

lateral

Relating to, or situated on, one side. "Bilateral" means "on both sides".

lateral cutaneous nerve entrapment

Compression of the thigh's lateral cutaneous nerve, which supplies the skin of the front and outer areas of the thigh. The nerve passes underneath the inguinal ligament (the fibrous band of tissue that extends across the crease of the groin); if, for any reason, the ligament puts pressure on the nerve the result is a burning, tingling sensation and sometimes a condition known as *meralgia paraesthetica* (numbness in the thigh).

In many cases, the problem is due to obesity. It may also result from overstretching of the hip joint, for example, when playing sport, or wearing constricting clothes around the hips.

There is no specific treatment for the condition. In obese people, weight loss may help to relieve the symptoms. Rarely, surgery is performed to try to reduce the pressure on the nerve.

latex fixation test

Also called the latex agglutination test, a procedure that is performed on body fluids, such as urine, blood, and saliva, in order to detect the presence of particular infections. Tiny beads of latex are coated with *antibodies* (proteins produced by the immune system) against a certain infectious organism and then added to a sample of body fluid. If the organism is present in the sample, it reacts with the antibodies on the beads, causing them to clump together.

latissimus dorsi

A large, flat, triangular-shaped *muscle* in the back. One end of the muscle is fixed to the lower chest vertebrae (spinal bones) and the back of the *pelvis*, while the other end of the muscle is joined to the top of the *humerus* (upper-arm bone). Contraction of the latissimus dorsi muscle moves the arm downwards and backwards.

laughing gas

The popular name for *nitrous oxide*, used with oxygen in general *anaesthesia*.

Laurence–Biedl–Moon syndrome

A rare inherited disorder characterized by obesity, *retinitis pigmentosa* (degeneration of the retina that may lead to blindness), *learning difficulties*, *polydactyly* (extra digits), and *hypogonadism* (underactivity of the ovaries or testes). (See also *genetic disorders*.)

lavage, gastric

Washing out the stomach with water, usually to remove toxins. The person is laid on one side, with the head lower than the stomach. One end of a lubricated, flexible tube is passed down the *oesophagus* (gullet) into the stomach. The other end is attached to a funnel. Water is poured into the tube until the stomach is full, then the funnel end is lowered, allowing the stomach contents to drain into a bucket. The procedure is repeated until the water runs clear.

Lavage is not used if a corrosive poison has been swallowed because of the risk that the tube may perforate tissues in the oesophagus or stomach.

laxative drugs

COMMON DRUGS		
BULK-FORMING ●Ispaghula ●Methylcellulose ●Sterculia		
STIMULANT ●Bisacodyl ●Co-danthramer ●Co-danthrusate, ●Docusate sodium ●Senna ●Sodium picosulfate		
LUBRICANT ●Arachis oil ●Liquid paraffin		
OSMOTIC ●Lactulose ●Magnesium hydroxide ●Magnesium sulphate ●Sodium acid phosphate		

A group of drugs used to treat *constipation* by making faeces pass through the intestines more quickly and easily. Laxatives are also given to people with *haemorrhoids* (piles), to prevent straining during defecation. In addition, they may be used to clear the intestine before investigative procedures such as *colonoscopy* or barium *enema*, or before abdominal surgery.

TYPES

There are various types of laxative, all of which work on the large intestine, either by increasing the speed with which faeces pass through the bowel, or by increasing their bulk and/or water content. Bulk-forming laxatives are not absorbed as they pass through the digestive tract. They contain particles that absorb many times their own volume of water, thereby increasing the volume and softness of the faeces and making them easier to pass. Stimulant laxatives prompt the intestinal wall to contract more strongly and speed up the elimination of faeces. Lubricant laxatives soften and facilitate the passage of the faeces. Osmotic laxatives cause water to be retained in the intestine, thus increasing the softness and volume of the faeces.

POSSIBLE ADVERSE EFFECTS

If they are used in excess, laxative drugs may cause abdominal cramps, diarrhoea, flatulence, and disturbances in body chemistry. Lubricants may prevent the fat-soluble vitamins (A, D, E, and K) from being absorbed in the intestine. Prolonged use of stimulant laxatives may lead to dependence on them for normal bowel function. For these reasons, laxatives should be used only if absolutely necessary, and for as little time as possible. When taken to relieve constipation, their use should be discontinued as soon as normal bowel movements have resumed. If constipation lasts for more than a week, a doctor should be consulted.

lazy eye

A term for the visual defect that commonly results from squint (see *amblyopia*).

LDL

See *low density lipoprotein*.

lead poisoning

Damage to the *brain*, *nerves*, red *blood cells*, and digestive system caused by inhaling lead fumes or swallowing lead salts. Acute poisoning, which occurs when a large amount of lead is taken into the body over a short period of time, is sometimes fatal but is rare. Chronic poisoning can be caused by exhaust fumes from vehicles running on leaded petrol, or by old paint or water pipes containing lead.

SYMPTOMS AND SIGNS

Symptoms of acute poisoning include severe, colicky abdominal pain, diarrhoea, and vomiting. There may also be *anaemia*, appetite loss, and, in chronic lead poisoning, a blue, grey, or black line along the gum margins.

Chronic poisoning can have especially severe effects on children: it can damage the brain and nervous system, leading to behavioural and learning

L

difficulties, and cause kidney problems and hearing difficulties. In adults, it can harm the kidneys, and the nervous and digestive systems.

DIAGNOSIS AND TREATMENT

Lead poisoning may be confirmed by blood and urine tests. *Chelating agents*, such as *penicillamine*, may be prescribed; they bind to the lead and enable the body to excrete it at a faster rate.

learning

The process by which knowledge or abilities are acquired, or by which behaviour is modified.

Various theories about learning have been proposed. Behavioural theories emphasize the role of *conditioning*, and cognitive theories are based on the concept that learning occurs through the building of abstract "cognitive" models, using mental capacities such as insight, *memory*, *intelligence*, and understanding. No one theory, however, can account for the complexities of learning.

learning difficulties

Problems with *learning*, which result from a range of mental and physical problems. Possible causes include *deafness*, *speech disorders*, and disorders of *vision*, as well as genetic and chromosomal problems. Learning difficulties may be either general or specific.

In general learning difficulties, all aspects of mental and physical functioning may be affected. Depending on the severity of the problem, a child with general learning difficulties may need to be educated in a special school.

Specific learning difficulties include *dyslexia* (difficulty in reading and/or writing), dyscalculia (inability to solve mathematical problems), and dysgraphia (a writing disorder). An affected child has problems in a particular area of learning but has normal intelligence. Treatment includes correction of any physical problems that interfere with learning, such as vision or hearing problems, and specialized teaching.

learning disability

A *learning difficulty*.

Leber's hereditary optic atrophy

See *optic atrophy*.

lecithin

A *phospholipid* (fatty substance) that is an important component of cell membranes. Lecithin is found in foods such as egg yolk, offal, and whole grains, and can be extracted from soya to be used as an emulsifier in processed foods. (See also *nutrition*.)

leech

A type of bloodsucking worm with a flattened body and a sucker at each end. Leeches of various types mainly inhabit tropical forests and waters. They bite painlessly, introducing their saliva into the wound before sucking blood. Leech saliva contains an anticlotting substance called hirudin, which may cause the wound to bleed for hours.

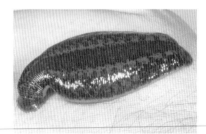

Use of leeches to drain blood
Leeches such as this are used in medicine (to drain a haematoma from the outer ear following injury, for example). The bites are painless, but the saliva contains an anticlotting agent, and the wound may bleed for several hours.

Leeches are sometimes used in medicine in order to drain a *haematoma* (collection of blood) from a wound. In addition, sometimes leeches are used in an effort to improve the circulation in tissues after surgery.

left atrium

The upper left chamber of the *heart*. In each heartbeat, the left atrium fills with oxygenated blood, which travels from the lungs via the pulmonary veins. The *mitral valve* then opens, allowing blood to be squeezed into the *left ventricle*, to be pumped around the body.

left bundle branch block

See *heart block*.

left ventricular failure

A disorder in which the left ventricle fails to empty normally, despite increased pressure from the blood within it. (See also *heart failure*.)

leg, broken

See *femur, fracture of*; *fibula*; *tibia*.

Legg-Calvé-Perthes' disease

See *Perthes' disease*.

legionnaires' disease

A form of *pneumonia* that is caused by LEGIONELLA PNEUMOPHILA, a bacterium that breeds in warm, moist conditions and stagnant water. Legionnaires' disease can occur in outbreaks. The source of infection is often an air-conditioning system in a large public building; the disease is contracted by the inhalation of droplets of contaminated water.

The first symptoms include headache, muscular and abdominal pain, diarrhoea, and a dry cough. Over the next few days, pneumonia develops, resulting in high fever, shaking chills, coughing up of thick *sputum* (phlegm), drowsiness, and sometimes *delirium*. Liver and kidney damage may occur.

Treatment is with antibiotic drugs such as *erythromycin*. The majority of people recover but mortality rates are higher among the elderly.

leg, shortening of

Shortening of the leg is usually caused by faulty healing of a fractured *femur* (thigh-bone) or *tibia* (shin). Other causes are an abnormality present from birth, surgery on the leg, or muscle weakness associated with *poliomyelitis* or another neurological disorder.

legs, restless

See *restless legs*.

leg ulcer

An open sore on the leg that is slow to heal, usually resulting from poor blood circulation in the area.

TYPES

There are two main types of leg ulcer: venous (also called gravitational or stasis) and arterial. Venous ulcers are by far

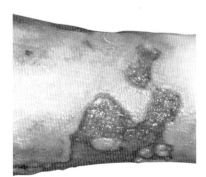

Venous ulcer on the leg
This type of ulcer, also known as a stasis ulcer, is caused by impaired drainage of blood from the leg by the veins. It is usually accompanied by oedema (fluid accumulation) in the lower leg.

L

the most common and occur mainly near the ankles and on the lower legs. They are caused by valve failure in veins and usually appear in conjunction with *varicose veins*.

Arterial ulcers, which form on the foot, are caused by poor blood flow through arteries. These ulcers are most likely to occur in people with *diabetes mellitus* and *sickle cell anaemia*.

TREATMENT
Treatment depends on the cause of the ulcer. The affected area should be bandaged in order to prevent infection, reduce swelling, and improve the circulation. If an ulcer is exuding pus, a dressing is applied under bandages and changed every few days. Measures such as exercising regularly, wearing support stockings, and keeping the leg raised when sitting may also help to improve circulation. A leg ulcer may take several months to heal, however, and the problem often recurs. In rare cases, a skin graft is necessary.

leiomyoma

A noncancerous tumour of smooth *muscle*. Leiomyomas, also called *fibroids*, usually occur in the *uterus*. More rarely, they develop in the walls of blood vessels in the skin, forming tender lumps. Leiomyomas may require surgical removal if they cause symptoms.

leiomyosarcoma

Also known as LMS, leiomyosarcoma is a cancerous tumour of the smooth *muscle*. Leiomyosarcomas most commonly occur in the stomach, small intestine, bladder, uterus, and prostate and are among the most common types of *sarcoma* (connective tissue cancer) of soft tissue. Leiomyosarcomas mainly affect adults; they are rare in children.

Treatment of a leiomyosarcoma is with surgery to remove the tumour and surrounding tissue, and chemotherapy and/or radiotherapy if the tumour cannot be removed completely.

leishmaniasis

Any of a variety of diseases caused by single-celled *parasites* called leishmania. These parasites are harboured by dogs and rodents and are transmitted by the bites of sandflies.

TYPES
The most serious form of leishmaniasis is called kala-azar or visceral leishmaniasis. This disease is prevalent in some parts of Asia, Africa, and South America,

and also occurs in some Mediterranean countries. In addition, there are several types of cutaneous leishmaniasis, some of which are prevalent in the Middle East, North Africa, and the Mediterranean.

SYMPTOMS
Kala-azar causes persistent fever, enlargement of the *spleen, anaemia*, and, later, darkening of the skin. The illness may develop any time up to two years after infection, and, if untreated, may be fatal. The cutaneous forms of the disease have the appearance of a persistent ulcer at the site of the sandfly bite.

TREATMENT
All varieties of leishmaniasis can be treated with drugs, such as sodium stibogluconate, given by intramuscular or intravenous *injection*.

People visiting areas in which leishmaniasis occurs should take measures to minimize the risk of *sandfly bites*.

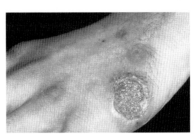

Leishmaniasis ulcer
This skin ulcer, which has developed at the site of a sandfly bite, is typical of the lesions found on the skin of people who are suffering from cutaneous leishmaniasis.

lens

The internal part of the *eye* that is responsible for focusing; also called the crystalline lens (to distinguish it from the *cornea*, which is also a form of lens). The lens is a disc of elastic, transparent tissue situated behind the *iris* and suspended on delicate fibres from the *ciliary body*. It is slightly less convex on the front surface than on the back.

The lens directs light precisely on to the retina (the layer of light-sensitive cells lining the eyeball). The muscles of the ciliary body act on it to change its curvature and thus alter its focus, so that near or distant objects can be seen sharply (see *accommodation*).

One common disorder that may affect the lens is *cataract* (a condition in which the lens tissue gradually turns opaque, restricting sight). Other possible problems are *lens dislocation* and *aphakia* (absence of the lens).

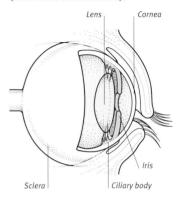
lens dislocation

Displacement of the crystalline *lens* from its normal position in the eye. Lens dislocation is almost always due to an injury that ruptures the fibres connecting the lens to the *ciliary body*. In people with the genetic disorder *Marfan syndrome*, these fibres are particularly weak; lens dislocation is common in such individuals.

A dislocated lens may produce severe visual distortion or double vision. If it slips forwards, it may cause a form of *glaucoma* (increased pressure within the eyeball) if drainage of fluid from the front of the eye is affected. If glaucoma is severe, the lens may need to be removed. (See also *aphakia*.)

lens implant

A plastic *prosthesis* (artificial substitute) used to replace the removed opaque *lens* in *cataract surgery*.

lentigo

A flat, brown area of skin that is also known as an age spot or liver spot. Lentigines (the plural of lentigo) are similar to freckles, except that they occur on both covered and exposed areas of skin and do not fade in winter. They are usually harmless and need no treatment. Any raised, darker brown areas within a lentigo need to be investigated, however, because they could develop into malignant melanomas (see *melanoma, malignant*).

leprosy

See *Hansen's disease*.

leptin

A *protein* that has a role in the regulation of fat storage by the body.

leptospirosis

A rare disease that is caused by a type of *spirochaete* bacterium harboured by rodents and excreted in their urine. It is usually transmitted to humans by contact with contaminated water or soil.

Symptoms of leptospirosis develop one to three weeks after infection. They include fever, chills, intense headache, severe muscle aches, and a skin rash. If the disease is left untreated, the nervous system may also be affected, often producing signs of *meningitis* (inflammation of the membranes covering the brain). The most severe form of leptospirosis is known as Weil's disease; it causes widespread internal bleeding, as well as kidney and liver damage. *Antibiotic drugs* are effective but the recovery of kidney and liver function may be slow.

lesion

An all-encompassing term for any abnormality of structure or function in any part of the body. The term may refer to a wound, infection, tumour, abscess, or chemical abnormality.

lethargy

A feeling of *tiredness*, drowsiness, or lack of energy.

leucocyte

An alternative spelling for leukocyte, a type of *blood cell*.

leukaemia

Any of several types of cancer in which there is a disorganized proliferation of abnormal white *blood cells* in the bone marrow. This increase in white cells interferes with production of normal blood cells in the marrow. A reduced number of red blood cells leads to *anaemia*, while a reduction in normal white cells increases the body's susceptibility to infection. Inadequate numbers of platelets may cause abnormal bleeding (see *thrombocytopenia*). Also, organs such as the liver, spleen, lymph nodes, or brain may cease to function properly if they become infiltrated by abnormal cells.

Leukaemias are classified as *acute* or *chronic* (acute types generally develop faster than chronic). They are also classified according to the type of white cell that is proliferating abnormally. If the abnormal cells are *lymphocytes* or lymphoblasts (precursors of lymphocytes), the leukaemia is called lymphocytic or lymphoblastic leukaemia. If the abnormal cells are derived from other types of white cell or their precursors, the disease is called myeloid, myeloblastic, hairy cell, or granulocytic leukaemia. (See also *leukaemia, acute*; *leukaemia, chronic lymphocytic*; *leukaemia, chronic myeloid*.)

leukaemia, acute

A type of *leukaemia* in which excessive numbers of immature white blood cells called blasts are produced in the bone marrow. If left untreated, acute leukaemia can cause death within a few weeks or months.

TYPES

The abnormal cells may be of two main types: lymphoblasts (immature *lymphocytes*) in acute lymphoblastic leukaemia, or ALL, and myeloblasts (immature forms of other types of white blood cell) in acute myeloblastic leukaemia, or AML.

CAUSES

In most cases, the cause of acute leukaemia is unknown. However, exposure to certain chemicals (such as benzene) or high levels of radiation may be a risk factor. Previous treatments for cancer may also increase the risk of leukaemia developing. Inherited factors are thought to play a part; there is increased incidence in individuals who have certain genetic disorders (such as *Fanconi's anaemia*) and chromosomal abnormalities (such as *Down's syndrome*). In addition, people who have blood disorders such as aplastic anaemia (see *anaemia, aplastic*) or primary *polycythaemia* are at increased risk because their bone marrow is already abnormal.

SYMPTOMS AND SIGNS

The symptoms and signs of acute leukaemia are due to the abnormal white cells crowding the bone marrow and infiltrating the bloodstream and body tissues (see *Leukaemia* box, opposite). They include bleeding gums, headache, easy bruising, bone pain, enlarged lymph nodes, and symptoms of *anaemia*, such as *tiredness*, pallor, and breathlessness on exertion. There may also be repeated chest or throat infections.

DIAGNOSIS AND TREATMENT

Blood tests (and, in some cases, tests on the cerebrospinal fluid, which surrounds the brain and spinal cord) may reveal the presence of abnormal white cells, but diagnosis is confirmed by a *bone marrow biopsy*.

Treatment is divided into two phases: remission induction to control the disease, and consolidation to prevent recurrence. Procedures include transfusions of blood and platelets; the use of *anticancer drugs* to kill abnormal cells in the bone marrow; and possibly *radiotherapy* to destroy any abnormal cells in the brain. A *bone marrow transplant* or *stem cell* transplant may also be required.

OUTLOOK

Chemotherapy has increased success rates, but the outlook depends on the type of leukaemia and the age of the patient. People with ALL generally respond better to treatment than those with AML, and many children with ALL can now make a full recovery. Treatment of AML is less likely to be successful in people over the age of 50.

leukaemia, chronic lymphocytic

A type of *leukaemia* caused by a proliferation of mature *lymphocytes* (white blood cells that are normally involved in fighting infection and harmful cells). There is no cure for the disease, but it is not always fatal. The cause is unknown.

SYMPTOMS

Symptoms develop slowly, often over many years. There may be enlargement of the *liver*, *spleen*, and *lymph nodes*, persistent raised temperature, and night sweats. Recurrent infections and anaemia also are common.

DIAGNOSIS AND TREATMENT

Diagnosis is by blood tests and a *bone marrow biopsy*. In many mild cases, treatment is not needed. To treat severe cases, *anticancer drugs* and monoclonal antibodies (see *antibody, monoclonal*) are given, sometimes with *radiotherapy*.

leukaemia, chronic myeloid

Also known as chronic granulocytic leukaemia, a type of *leukaemia* caused by overproduction of granulocytes (a type of white *blood cell*) or, in particular, neutrophils (a type of granulocyte). The cause of the condition is unknown but almost all affected people have a *chromosomal abnormality* called the Philadelphia chromosome, in which part of one chromosome is attached to another.

Chronic myeloid leukaemia usually has two phases: a chronic phase, which may last for several years, and an accelerated, or acute, phase that may last for several months.

LEUKAEMIA

In all forms of leukaemia, abnormal white cells proliferate in the bone marrow and spill into the blood. There are four main types: acute lymphoblastic leukaemia (ALL), acute myeloblastic leukaemia (AML), chronic lymphocytic leukaemia (CLL), and chronic myeloid leukaemia (CML). The acute types have a rapid onset. There is a risk of death from overwhelming infection or blood loss, but modern treatment has greatly improved survival rates, particularly in childhood leukaemias.

The chronic forms of leukaemia progress much more gradually than the acute types, but many of them are essentially incurable.

Symptoms of acute leukaemia
Symptoms are caused partly by the abnormal white cells crowding out the bone marrow (so that it fails to produce sufficient normal blood cells of all types) and partly by the invasion of other body organs by abnormal cells.

Gum bleeding
Gums may bleed as a result of insufficient production of platelet cells by the bone marrow; platelets are needed for the arrest of bleeding.

Bone tenderness
Tenderness of the bones may be felt as the bone marrow becomes packed with immature white cells.

Easy bruising and bleeding
Reduced numbers of platelets may lead to bleeding from nose and gums and bruising after mild trauma.

Headache
Headache may be caused by abnormal white cells affecting the nervous system.

Enlarged lymph nodes
The lymph nodes in the neck, armpits, and groin may be swollen with huge numbers of immature white cells. The liver, spleen, and testes may also be swollen.

Anaemia
Anaemia develops if there is insufficient production of red blood cells by the bone marrow. Anaemia causes tiredness, breathlessness on exertion, and pallor.

Infections
White blood cells play a major part in the defence against infection. However, in acute leukaemia, only immature, nonfunctioning white cells are made, so the patient may suffer from repeated chest or throat infections, herpes zoster, or skin and other infections.

HOW LEUKAEMIA ATTACKS THE BODY

Leukaemia is a form of cancer, but with the abnormally growing cells (mutated white blood cells) forming in the bone marrow rather than grouped into a tumour in a specific area. The abnormal cells may spill into the bloodstream and infiltrate and interfere with the function of other organs. But worse, these cells "take over" the marrow and prevent it from making enough normal blood cells (including normal white cells, red cells, and platelets). This leaves the sufferer highly susceptible to serious infections, anaemia, and bleeding episodes.

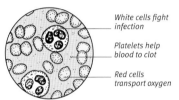

White cells fight infection

Platelets help blood to clot

Red cells transport oxygen

Normal appearance of blood
In a normal blood smear, there are large numbers of red cells, many platelets, and a few white cells.

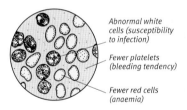

Abnormal white cells (susceptibility to infection)

Fewer platelets (bleeding tendency)

Fewer red cells (anaemia)

Appearance of blood in leukaemia
In leukaemia, the blood usually contains many abnormal white cells, and fewer red cells and platelets.

L

SYMPTOMS

During the chronic phase, symptoms are not always obvious, although they may include fever, night sweats, and weight loss. High numbers of white cells may cause the blood to become very thick and unable to flow through the smallest vessels, leaving tissues starved of oxygen. The results include visual disturbances, as blood vessels in the eye are affected, and abdominal pain due to the death of tissues in the spleen; *priapism* (persistent, painful erection of the penis) may also occur.

The symptoms of the accelerated phase are like those of acute leukaemia (see *leukaemia, acute*).

DIAGNOSIS AND TREATMENT

The diagnosis is made from blood tests and a *bone marrow biopsy*.

Treatment of the chronic phase includes *anticancer drugs* or alpha *interferons*. A *stem cell* or *bone marrow transplant* may also be possible. When the disease transforms into the acute phase, the treatment is similar to that given for acute leukaemia.

leukocyte

Any type of white *blood cell*.

leukodystrophies

A rare group of inherited childhood diseases in which the *myelin* sheaths that form a protective covering around many nerves, particularly in the brain and the spinal cord, are destroyed. The leukodystrophies cause severely disabling conditions, such as impaired speech, *blindness*, *deafness*, and *paralysis*, and are always fatal.

leukoplakia

Raised white patches on the *mucous membranes* of the *mouth* or *vulva* due to tissue thickening. It is most common in elderly people and in those with *AIDS*.

CAUSES

Leukoplakia in the mouth, which most commonly occurs on the tongue, is usually due to *smoking* or to rubbing by a rough tooth or denture. It is not known what causes the condition to develop on the vulva.

SYMPTOMS AND TREATMENT

The raised patches are usually harmless and painless, but they occasionally result in a cancerous change in the affected tissue. For this reason, leukoplakia should always be reported to a doctor.

If the condition persists, the patches are removed under either general or local *anaesthesia* and the tissue is examined microscopically for any signs of malignant change. (See also *mouth cancer*; *vulva, cancer of.*)

leukorrhoea

See *vaginal discharge*.

leukotriene receptor antagonists

A group of *antiallergy drugs* that are used to prevent the symptoms of mild to moderate *asthma*. Leukotriene receptor antagonists, which include *montelukast* and *zafirlukast*, work by blocking the effects of leukotrienes (naturally occurring substances that are released in the lungs during an allergic reaction).

Leukotriene receptor antagonists are not *bronchodilator drugs* and will not relieve an existing asthma attack. Instead, they are usually used with bronchodilators and inhaled *corticosteroids* to reduce the frequency of attacks.

Side effects of the drugs can include gastrointestinal disturbances and headache. In addition, hypersensitivity and skin reactions may occur.

levamisole

An *anthelmintic drug* given by mouth in a single dose to eliminate *roundworm* infestation. Side effects are rare but can include mild nausea or vomiting.

levodopa

A drug used to treat *Parkinson's disease*. Levodopa is usually combined with carbidopa or benserazide, substances that enhance levodopa's effects and help to reduce its side effects, including nausea, vomiting, nervousness, and agitation.

levonorgestrel

A *progestogen drug* used in some *oral contraceptives* and, in combination with an oestrogen drug, in *hormone replacement therapy (HRT)*. Norgestrel is a related drug with a similar action. Levonorgestrel is also used alone for emergency contraception (see *contraception, emergency*).

levothyroxine

A synthetic version of the *thyroid hormone* thyroxine, which is used to treat *hypothyroidism* (underactivity of the thyroid gland). Side effects, such as rapid heartbeat and tremor, may occur if the initial dose is too high.

Lewy-body dementia

A form of *dementia* in which spherical structures called Lewy bodies develop in the brain. There may be fluctuating episodes of confusion and visual hallucinations. Falls are also common.

Leyden–Mobius muscular dystrophy

A form of *muscular dystrophy*, also called limb-girdle muscular dystrophy, that affects the areas where the limbs join the body. Leyden–Mobius muscular dystrophy can occur in either sex, and it usually appears in childhood. It causes muscle weakness and wasting in the pelvic girdle (pelvifemoral muscular dystrophy) or the shoulder girdle (scapulohumeral muscular dystrophy).

LH

The abbreviation for *luteinizing hormone*.

LH-RH

The abbreviation for *luteinizing hormone-releasing hormone*.

libido

Sexual desire. Loss of libido may be a symptom of many physical illnesses; psychological difficulties such as *depression*; *drug abuse*; and *alcohol* abuse. (See also *sexual desire, inhibited*.)

lice

Small, wingless insects that feed on human blood. There are three species that infest humans: PEDICULUS HUMANUS CAPITIS (head louse), PEDICULUS HUMANUS CORPORIS (body louse), and PHTHIRUS PUBIS (crab, or pubic, louse). All have flattened bodies and may measure up to 3 mm across.

Head lice live on the scalp and are spread by direct contact. (The lice prefer clean hair, and their spread is not due to poor hygiene.) Their tiny eggs (nits) are attached to hairs close to the scalp. The bites from head lice cause intense itching.

Body lice live and lay eggs on clothing next to the skin. They can transmit epidemic *typhus* and *relapsing fever*.

Crab lice live in pubic hair or, more rarely, in armpits, beards, or eyelashes; they are usually transmitted during sexual contact (see *pubic lice*).

TREATMENT

Various preparations can be applied to kill lice and their eggs. In addition, lice on clothes, bedding, and items such as soft toys can be killed by washing the items in very hot water (60°C or above) then putting them in the hot cycle of a dryer for at least 20 minutes. Items that cannot be washed should be dry-cleaned or, if that is not possible, put in an airtight bag for two weeks. Carpets and upholstery should be vacuumed thoroughly.

lichenification

Thickening and hardening of areas of the *skin* caused by repeated scratching, often to relieve the intense itching of skin disorders such as *atopic eczema* or *lichen simplex*.

lichen planus

A common *skin* disease of unknown cause that usually affects middle-aged people. Small, shiny, intensely itchy, pink or purple raised spots appear on the skin of the inner wrists, forearms, or lower legs. There is often a lacy network of white spots covering the inside lining of the cheeks. The disease is treated with topical *corticosteroid drugs*.

lichen sclerosus et atrophicus

A chronic skin condition of the anogenital area. The skin is scarred and white, and the anatomy of areas such as the vaginal opening or foreskin may become distorted. Treatment is with potent topical *corticosteroid drugs*.

lichen simplex

Patches of thickened, itchy, and sometimes discoloured, skin that result from repeated scratching. Typical sites are the neck, wrist, elbow area, and ankles. Lichen simplex is most common in women and is often *stress*-related. Treatment is with oral *antihistamine drugs* and creams containing *corticosteroid drugs*, and may also involve addressing any underlying stress or anxiety.

L

lid lag

A momentary delay in the normal downward movement of the upper eyelids that occurs when the eye looks down. Lid lag is a characteristic feature of *thyrotoxicosis* (overactivity of the thyroid gland), and usually occurs in conjunction with *exophthalmos* (protrusion of the eyeball).

lidocaine

A local anaesthetic (see *anaesthesia, local*) that is used to numb tissues prior to minor surgical procedures. Lidocaine is also used as a *nerve block*. The drug is commonly given by injection, but it may also be applied to the surface of the skin as an anaesthetic cream; to mucous membranes as a spray or gel; or to the eyes as eye-drops.

In addition, lidocaine may be given by intravenous injection after a *myocardial infarction* (heart attack), to suppress *ventricular tachycardia* and reduce the risk of *ventricular fibrillation* (both of which are life-threatening abnormalities in the heart rhythm).

lie

In *pregnancy*, the position of the *fetus* relative to the mother's body. Normally, by the end of pregnancy, the long (head to tailbone) axis of the fetus is parallel to that of the mother. If the fetus is lying at an angle to the mother's body, or is horizontal (transverse lie), this may cause *malpresentation* in labour: the fetus's shoulder or body, rather than the head, is positioned over the cervix and delivery by *caesarean section* is needed.

life cycle

The series of stages through which an organism passes as it begins its life, reaches maturity, reproduces, and eventually dies. The term is most often used in the context of animals that assume various forms at different stages of life, such as insects and worms.

life expectancy

The number of years for which an individual at a specified age can expect to live. Life expectancy is often measured from birth. Assuming that patterns of health and illness in a community do not change, it is possible to estimate life expectancy. The proportion of a population that reaches its natural lifespan (the number of years for which people live in the absence of disease) depends on the general health of the population; for

this reason, life expectancy may be used to compare levels of general health within or between countries.

life support

The process of keeping a person alive by artificially inflating the lungs (see *ventilation*) and, if necessary, maintaining the heartbeat.

ligament

A band of tough, fibrous, partly elastic tissue that connects or supports certain body structures. Ligaments are most commonly found in *joints*; they bind the ends of the bones together and prevent excessive movement. Some ligaments are also involved in supporting various internal organs, such as the uterus, bladder, and liver.

Ligaments, especially those in the ankle or knee joints may sometimes be damaged by injury. Minor ligament injuries such as *sprains* are treated with ice, bandaging, and sometimes *physio-*

FUNCTION OF **LIGAMENTS**

These tough, fibrous bands of tissue bind bone ends together.

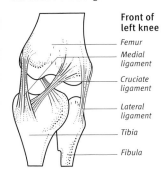

Front of left knee

- Femur
- Medial ligament
- Cruciate ligament
- Lateral ligament
- Tibia
- Fibula

Torn ligament
A common injury of football players, torn knee ligaments usually result from twisting stress when the knee is turned while weight is on that leg.

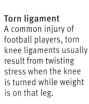

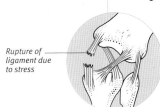

Rupture of ligament due to stress

therapy. If a ligament has been torn (ruptured), the joint is either immobilized by a *plaster cast*, which allows healing to occur, or is repaired surgically.

ligation

The surgical process of tying off a *duct* or a blood vessel with a *ligature* (a piece of thread or similar material). Ligation is carried out to stop bleeding from blood vessels, or to close a duct or other tubal body structure. The term is used in tubal ligation, a form of sterilization in which the fallopian tubes are tied off (see *sterilization, female*).

ligature

A length of thread or other material used for *ligation*.

lightening

A feeling that is experienced by many pregnant women at the time when the baby's head descends into the pelvic cavity. Lightening usually occurs in the final three weeks of pregnancy, and, because it leaves more space in the upper abdomen, it relieves pressure under the *diaphragm*.

lightheadedness

A general term for unsteadiness and a feeling of faintness. (See also *dizziness*; *fainting*.)

light reflex

A form of inborn *reflex* in which the pupil of the *eye* automatically responds to the amount of light falling on the eye. Normally, the pupil constricts in response to bright light, to restrict the amount of light entering the eye, and dilates (widens) in response to dim light. Abnormal light reflex can be a sign of disease in the eye or brain.

light treatment

See *phototherapy*.

lignocaine

The former name for *lidocaine*.

limb, artificial

An artificial leg or arm, known medically as a *prosthesis*, which is fitted to replace a limb that has been missing from birth (see *limb defects*) or lost as a result of *amputation*.

Prosthetic limbs enable the wearer to carry out many normal activities, such as walking. In addition, some prosthetic arms and hands contain electronic

L

circuitry that detects and responds to impulses from the wearer's nervous system. This enables the wearer to perform complex hand and finger actions, such as gripping objects.

limb defects

The incomplete development of one or more limbs at birth. Limb defects are rare and may be inherited or form part of a *syndrome*.

In a condition called *phocomelia*, hands, feet, or tiny finger- or toe-buds are attached to limb stumps or grow directly from the trunk. The sedative drug *thalidomide*, when taken by pregnant women, is known to have caused phocomelia in fetuses.

limbic system

A ring-shaped area in the centre of the *brain* consisting of a number of connected clusters of nerve cells. The limbic system plays a role in influencing the *autonomic nervous system*, which automatically regulates body functions; the emotions; and the sense of smell. The system is extensive, and contains various different substructures including the *hippocampus*, the cingulate gyrus, and the amygdala.

limb, phantom

See *phantom limb*.

limited cutaneous systemic sclerosis

See *systemic sclerosis*.

limp

An abnormal pattern of *walking* in which the movements of one leg (or of the *hip* on one side of the body) are different from those of the other. If a child is limping, a doctor should be consulted within 24 hours, because the problem may result from a hip disorder that requires prompt treatment.

linctus

A bland, usually sweetened mixture taken to soothe irritation caused by an inflamed *throat*. A simple linctus contains no active drug, but linctuses are commonly used as a basis for cough suppressants (see *cough remedies*).

linea alba

A vertical line of fibrous tissue running down the middle of the abdominal wall. The linea alba is the site of attachment of the rectus abdominis *muscles* and extends from the xiphoid process (the lowest part of the breastbone) to the pubic symphysis (the joint between the two pubic bones). The skin over the linea alba becomes pigmented during pregnancy (see *linea nigra*).

linea nigra

A pigmented, vertical line that appears down the front of the abdomen during *pregnancy*. The linea nigra is a visible form of the *linea alba* and often fades again after childbirth.

linear accelerator

A device for accelerating subatomic particles, such as electrons, to a speed approaching that of light so that they have extremely high energies. A linear accelerator can also be used to generate high-energy *X-rays*. High-energy electrons or X-rays are used in *radiotherapy* to treat certain cancers.

lingual

A term meaning "of the tongue", as in "sublingual drug" (a drug that is administered under the tongue).

liniment

A liquid that is rubbed on the skin to relieve aching muscles and stiff joints. Liniments may contain rubefacients (substances that increase blood flow beneath the skin), or certain drugs, such as *nonsteroidal anti-inflammatory drugs*.

linkage analysis

A type of *gene mapping*. Linkage analysis determines the presence or absence of an abnormal gene by detecting another gene located close to it on the same *chromosome*.

linkage, sex

The association of a particular *genetic disorder* with the sex chromosomes (see *sex-linked inheritance*).

linoleic acid

An essential *fatty acid* found principally in plant seed oils, such as maize oil and soya bean oil. Linoleic acid is used by the body in the synthesis of *prostaglandins* and cell membranes. Linoleic acid has to be obtained from the diet because the body cannot manufacture its own supplies.

linolenic acid

An essential *fatty acid*, found in fish oils and some plant seed oils, that is used by the body to form *prostaglandins*. Various forms of linolenic acid are nutritionally important, including alpha-linolenic acid (ALA), gamma-linolenic acid (GLA), and dihomo-gamma-linolenic acid (DGLA).

lint

A soft, absorbent fabric used in surgical dressings.

liothyronine

A *thyroid hormone* used as replacement therapy in *hypothyroidism* (underactivity of the thyroid gland). Liothyronine acts faster than *levothyroxine* and is cleared from the body more rapidly.

lip

One of two fleshy folds around the entrance to the mouth. The main substructure of the lips is a ring of muscle that helps to produce speech. Smaller muscles at the corners of the lips are responsible for facial expression.

Disorders of the lips include *chapped skin*, *cheilitis* (inflammation, cracking, and dryness), *cold sores*, and *lip cancer*.

lipaemia

An abnormally high level of fat in the blood. (See also *hyperlipidaemias*.)

lip cancer

A *malignant* tumour (usually a *squamous cell carcinoma*), commonly on the lower *lip*. Lip cancer is largely confined to older people, particularly those who have been exposed to a lot of sunlight and those who have smoked cigarettes or a pipe for many years.

The first symptom is a white patch that develops on the lip and soon becomes scaly and cracked with a yellow crust. The affected area grows and eventually becomes ulcerated. In some cases, the cancer spreads to the *lymph nodes* in the jaw and neck.

Lip cancer is diagnosed by *biopsy* (taking a sample of lip tissue for examination). Treatment is surgical removal, *radiotherapy*, or a combination of both.

lipectomy, suction

A type of *body contour surgery*, commonly known as liposuction, in which excess fat is sucked out through small skin incisions, using a cannula (thin tube) attached to a vacuum device.

lipid disorders

Metabolic disorders that result in abnormal amounts of *lipids* (fats) in the body. The most common lipid disorders are

L

the *hyperlipidaemias*, which are characterized by high levels of lipids in the blood. Hyperlipidaemia can cause *atherosclerosis* (narrowing of the arteries by deposits of fatty material) and *pancreatitis* (inflammation of the pancreas). There are also some very rare lipid disorders, such as *Tay–Sachs disease*, that are due solely to heredity.

lipid-lowering diet

A diet containing low levels of *cholesterol* and saturated fats (see *fats and oils*). By lowering the blood levels of lipids, such diets help to prevent *atherosclerosis* (accumulation of fatty deposits on the walls of arteries) and thereby lower the risk for cardiovascular disorders such as *coronary artery disease*, *myocardial infarction* (heart attack), and *stroke*. For the greatest cardiovascular risk reduction, lipid-lowering diets should be used in conjunction with other measures, such as stopping smoking, regular exercise, controlling raised blood pressure, and, if appropriate, *lipid-lowering drugs*.

lipid-lowering drugs

COMMON DRUGS

STATINS • Atorvastatin • Fluvastatin • Pravastatin • Rosuvastatin • Simvastatin	
FIBRATES • Bezafibrate • Ciprofibrate • Fenofibrate • Gemfibrozil	
NICOTINIC ACID AND DERIVATIVES • Acipimox • Nicotinic acid	
DRUGS THAT BIND TO BILE SALTS • Colestipol • Colestyramine	
OTHER DRUGS ACTING ON THE LIVER • Omega-3 marine triglycerides	

A group of drugs that are used to treat, or provide protection against, *hyperlipidaemia* (abnormally high levels of the fatty substances *cholesterol* and *triglycerides* in the blood). These drugs help to prevent, or slow the progression of, *atherosclerosis* (accumulation of fatty deposits on artery walls), which, in turn, reduces the risk for cardiovascular disorders such as *coronary artery disease*, *myocardial infarction* (heart attack), and *stroke*. To maximize cardiovascular risk reduction, lipid-lowering drugs should be used together with other measures, such as a stopping smoking, a *lipid-lowering diet*, regular exercise, and controlling raised blood pressure. In most cases, statins are the drugs of first choice for treating or preventing hyperlipidaemia.

HOW THEY WORK

Most groups of lipid-lowering drugs act on the liver to inhibit the processes by which fatty acids are converted into *lipids*. Statins cause the liver to produce less cholesterol, while fibrates and nicotinic acid reduce the formation of both cholesterol and triglycerides. Omega-3 marine triglycerides reduce the levels of triglycerides.

Drugs that bind to bile salts reduce the absorption of these salts (which contain high levels of cholesterol) from the small intestine into the bloodstream. The lowered blood levels of bile salts stimulate the liver into converting more cholesterol into bile salts.

POSSIBLE ADVERSE EFFECTS

Statins may cause muscle inflammation and may also affect liver function. Fibrates may cause an increased susceptibility to *gallstones*. Drugs that bind to bile salts may cause constipation, and sometimes nausea and diarrhoea, as a result of the increased amount of bile in the digestive tract. They may also reduce the absorption of fat-soluble vitamins. Rarely, combinations of drugs that act on the liver may cause a painful muscle condition called *rhabdomyolysis*.

lipidosis

Any disorder involving the *metabolism* (chemical transformation) of *lipids* in body cells. An example of a lipidosis is *Gaucher's disease*, which causes a build-up of fatty deposits in the liver, spleen, bone marrow, and sometimes the brain.

lipids

A general term for *fats and oils*. Lipids include triglycerides (simple fats), phospholipids (important constituents of cell membranes and nerve tissue), and sterols, such as *cholesterol*.

lipoatrophy

Wasting of the subcutaneous fat layer, which lies just beneath the skin. This condition may be associated with *lipodystrophy* and also sometimes occurs at sites of insulin injections in people with *diabetes mellitus*.

lipodystrophy

A type of disorder in which the metabolism (chemical transformation) of fat in the body is disturbed, leading to abnormalities in body fat distribution.

TYPES

One type of lipodystrophy occurs in people undergoing treatment with protease inhibitor drugs for *HIV*; it causes wasting of the limbs, buttocks, and face, but excessive fat deposits in the abdominal cavity, chest or breasts, back, and neck. Affected people also have raised levels of *lipids* in the blood.

Another form, total lipodystrophy, is due to an autosomal recessive genetic disorder. In this disorder, loss of fat over the whole body is associated with raised basal metabolic rate, hirsutism (excessive body hair), liver enlargement, and insulin-resistant *diabetes mellitus*.

lipoma

A common noncancerous tumour of fatty tissue. Lipomas are slow-growing, soft swellings that may occur anywhere on the body, most commonly on the thigh, trunk, or shoulder. They are painless and harmless, but may be surgically removed for cosmetic reasons.

lipoprotein

A small particle that is made up of a fatty core surrounded by a water-soluble form of fat (known chemically as a phospholipid) and a protein (apoprotein). Lipoproteins are the form in which fats are transported in the bloodstream.

liposarcoma

A rare cancer of fatty tissue that most commonly develops during late middle age. Liposarcomas produce firm swellings, usually in the abdomen or the thigh. The tumours can generally be removed by surgery but tend to recur.

Lipostat

The brand name for the lipid-lowering drug *pravastatin*.

liposuction

The popular term for suction lipectomy (see *lipectomy, suction*).

lip-reading

A way of understanding speech by interpreting movements of the mouth and tongue.

liquid paraffin

A lubricant *laxative drug* obtained from petroleum. It can cause anal irritation and prolonged use may impair the absorption of vitamins from the intestine into the blood.

liquor

A medical term for a liquid, particularly a water-based solution, that contains a medicinal substance. The term is also used to describe body fluids, such as *amniotic fluid*.

L

lisinopril

An *ACE inhibitor drug* commonly used to treat *hypertension* (high blood pressure) and *heart failure*. The first dose may cause a rapid fall in blood pressure, especially in someone who is also taking a *diuretic*; a person should lie down for a couple of hours after taking it. The drug may also produce various minor side effects, such as a persistent dry cough or a disturbance in taste sensation.

lisp

A common *speech disorder* caused by protrusion of the tongue between the teeth so that the "s" sound is replaced by "th". In most cases, there is no physical cause, but sometimes it is due to a cleft palate (see *cleft lip and palate*).

Unless there is an underlying cause, lisping usually disappears by the age of about four. If it persists beyond this time, speech therapy may be needed.

listeriosis

An infection that is common in animals and also affects humans.

CAUSE

Listeriosis is caused by the bacterium LISTERIA MONOCYTOGENES, which is widespread in the environment, especially in soil. Possible sources of human infection include soft cheese, ready-prepared coleslaw and salads, and improperly cooked meat.

SYMPTOMS

In most otherwise healthy adults, the only symptoms may be fever, aching muscles, diarrhoea, and abdominal pain. However, in elderly people, those with reduced immunity, and newborn babies, listeriosis can be life-threatening. *Pneumonia*, *septicaemia* (blood poisoning), and *meningitis* (inflammation of the membranes covering the brain) may develop. In pregnant women, infection may cause a miscarriage or stillbirth.

DIAGNOSIS AND TREATMENT

The condition is diagnosed by *blood tests* and analysis of other body fluids, such as cerebrospinal fluid. Treatment is with *antibiotic drugs*.

lithium

A mood-stabilizing drug used in the long-term treatment of *mania* and *bipolar disorder*, and to help prevent recurrence of severe depression. Side effects include nausea, vomiting, tremor, and excessive thirst. High levels of lithium may cause blurred vision, drowsiness, rash, and possibly *hypothyroidism*

and kidney damage. Regular tests are needed to monitor lithium levels in the blood, and any side effects should be reported promptly to a doctor.

lithotomy

Surgical removal of a *calculus* (stone) from the *urinary tract*. The procedure is performed only for large stones; smaller stones are usually crushed and removed using *cystoscopy*, or pulverized ultrasonically by *lithotripsy*.

lithotomy position

A position in which a patient lies on his or her back with the hips and knees bent and the legs wide apart; the feet

may be supported on firm surfaces or in stirrups. Once used for *lithotomy* (removal of bladder stones), the position is now widely used for *pelvic examinations* and some types of surgery.

lithotripsy

The use of highly concentrated shock waves or ultrasonic waves to break up *calculi* (stones) inside the kidneys, upper *ureters*, and *gallbladder* so that they can be comfortably excreted.

The most common type is extracorporeal shock-wave lithotripsy (ESWL), which is performed to break up small stones. ESWL uses a machine called a *lithotripter*, which produces shock waves

---

LITHOTRIPSY

Calculi (stones) can sometimes be broken up by lithotripsy, a procedure that uses ultrasonic or shock waves. In extracorporeal shock-wave lithotripsy (ESWL), the most common form of the treatment, no major surgery is needed. If the stones are in the kidney or ureter, fragments of the stones are passed in the urine.

EXTRACORPOREAL SHOCK-WAVE LITHOTRIPSY (ESWL)

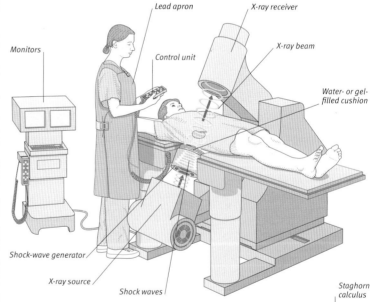

Patient receiving ESWL
The patient is given a general or epidural anaesthetic. The lithotripter produces shock waves that are focused on the stone. The image intensifier (X-ray equipment) allows the operator to locate the stones and adjust the lithotripter to ensure that the shock waves target the stones accurately. Nearly all the energy is dissipated in the stone, shattering it. The patient then drinks liberally to flush out stone fragments. There may be some blood in the urine and abdominal bruising, but serious complications are uncommon.

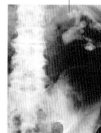

Kidney stone
This X-ray shows a staghorn calculus (stone) in the left kidney (on the right in the X-ray). With lithotripsy, stones such as these can be removed without the need for surgery.

that are transmitted into the body through a water- or gel-filled cushion placed over the organ being treated.

Ureteric colic (severe spasmodic pain in the side, occurring if the ureter is obstructed by small fragments of stone) may occur after ESWL. People treated for *gallstones* may need drug treatment to aid the elimination of stone residues.

lithotripter
The machine used in extracorporeal shock-wave *lithotripsy* (ESWL) to destroy small *calculi* (stones).

Little's area
An area near the front of the nasal septum (partition between the nostrils) that is richly supplied with blood vessels and is a common site of *nosebleeds*.

Little's disease
See *spastic diplegia*.

live birth
The delivery of a baby that breathes spontaneously and has a heartbeat. Statisticians may calculate the number of live births per year per 1000 women of childbearing age (usually 15 to 44), a measure called the fertility rate, to help them assess the health and growth of a population (see *statistics, vital*).

livedo reticularis
A netlike, purple or blue mottling of the skin, usually on the lower legs, caused by enlargement of blood vessels under the skin. It is more common in people with vasculitis (inflammation of the blood vessels) and those who suffer from excessive sensitivity to cold. The condition is harmless, and tends to be worse in cold weather.

liver
The largest organ within the body, this wedge-shaped, reddish-brown structure lies in the upper right abdominal cavity, directly below the *diaphragm*.

STRUCTURE
The liver is divided into two main lobes, each consisting of many lobules. The lobules are surrounded by branches of the hepatic artery, which supplies the liver with oxygenated blood, and the portal vein, which supplies nutrient-rich blood from the small intestine. Deoxygenated blood from the liver drains into the hepatic veins. A network of ducts carries the digestive juice *bile* from the liver to the *gallbladder* and the small intestine.

FUNCTION
The liver plays a vital role in the body because it produces and processes a wide range of chemical substances (see *Disorders of the liver* box and *Structure and function of the liver* box overleaf).

The chemicals produced by the liver include important proteins for blood *plasma*, such as *albumin* and *clotting factors*. The liver also produces *cholesterol* and proteins that help the blood to carry fats around the body. In addition, liver cells secrete bile, which removes waste products from the liver and aids the breakdown and absorption of fats in the small intestine (see *biliary system*).

Another major function is the processing of nutrients for use by cells. The liver also stores excess *glucose* as glycogen. In addition, it controls the blood level of *amino acids* (the building blocks of proteins). If the level of amino acids is too high, the liver converts the excess into glucose, proteins, other amino acids, or *urea* (for excretion).

Finally, the liver helps to clear the blood of drugs and poisons. These substances are broken down and excreted in the bile.

liver abscess
A localized collection of *pus* in the *liver*. The most common cause is an intestinal infection. Bacteria may spread from areas inflamed by *diverticulitis* or *appendicitis*, and *amoebae* may invade the liver as a result of *amoebiasis*. Symptoms are high fever, pain in the upper right abdomen, and (especially in the elderly) confusion.

Ultrasound scanning usually reveals the abscess, and the organism responsible may be identified by examination of a blood or tissue sample. The abscess can sometimes be treated by *aspiration* (sucking out the pus through a needle), but often surgery is needed.

liver biopsy
A diagnostic test in which a small sample of tissue is removed from the liver, usually under local *anaesthesia*. The main purpose of this test is to aid diagnosis of liver diseases. (See also *biopsy*.)

liver cancer
A cancerous tumour in the *liver*. The tumour may be primary (originating in the liver) or, far more commonly, secondary (having spread from elsewhere, often the stomach, pancreas, or large intestine). There are two main types of primary tumour: a *hepatocellular carcinoma*, also known as a hepatoma, which develops in the liver cells; and a *cholangiocarcinoma*, which arises from cells lining the bile ducts. Hepatocellular carcinomas are often linked to infection with *hepatitis B* or *hepatitis C* and to *cirrhosis*.

L

LOCATION OF THE **LIVER**
The liver is a large, red-brown organ, made up of two lobes, that occupies the upper right-hand portion of the abdominal cavity. It lies immediately beneath the diaphragm, to which its upper side is attached. Its base is in contact with the stomach, right kidney, and intestines. Tucked within a depression on the underside of the liver is the gallbladder.

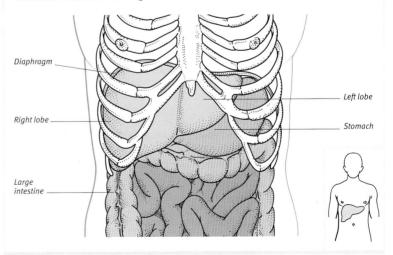

The most common cause of liver disease in developed countries is excessive alcohol consumption. Alcohol-related disorders (see *liver disease, alcoholic*) include *hepatitis* (liver inflammation) and *cirrhosis*. Many other types of liver disorder may occur, including infections, tumours, metabolic disorders, and congenital defects.

Liver failure (complete loss of liver function) may occur as a result of acute hepatitis, poisoning, or cirrhosis. *Jaundice* and hepatomegaly (enlargement of the liver) are common signs of liver disease.

Infection and inflammation
Hepatitis is a general term for inflammation of the liver. It can be caused by viruses (see *hepatitis, viral*) or bacteria, which may spread up the biliary system to the liver, causing *cholangitis* (inflammation of the bile duct) or *liver abscess*. Parasitic diseases, including *schistosomiasis*, *liver fluke*, *amoebiasis*, and *hydatid disease*, can also affect the liver.

Tumours
The liver is a common site for cancerous tumours that have spread from elsewhere in the body (in which case they are known as secondary tumours of the liver). Primary tumours of the liver (those that originate in the liver) are much rarer. (See *liver cancer*.)

Metabolic disorders
Two main *metabolic disorders* affect the liver: *haemochromatosis* (in which there is too much iron in the body) and *Wilson's disease* (in which there is an excess of copper in the liver).

Congenital defects
Occasionally, defects of liver structure are present from birth. Abnormalities such as these principally affect the bile ducts. A choledochal cyst is a malformation of a main bile duct. These cysts require surgery because, in infants, they may obstruct the flow of bile, causing jaundice. *Biliary atresia*, in which the bile ducts are missing, also causes jaundice.

Poisoning and drugs
Normally, the liver can break down drugs and toxins. However, drug overdose or allergy may damage liver cells in the process, and overdose of paracetamol can lead to severe liver damage. Poisoning by certain types of mushroom can cause acute liver failure.

Other disorders
In *Budd–Chiari syndrome*, the veins draining the liver become blocked by blood clots, which causes painful swelling of the liver. Obstruction of the portal vein is one cause of *portal hypertension* (high blood pressure in the portal vein), which can lead to *oesophageal varices* (swollen veins in the oesophagus) and *ascites* (collection of fluid in the abdomen).

Enlargement of the liver is a common symptom of *leukaemias* and *lymphomas*. *Liver failure* (complete loss of liver function) may be caused by acute hepatitis, poisoning, or cirrhosis.

INVESTIGATION
Disorders of the liver may be investigated by *liver biopsy* (removal of a tissue sample for examination), *liver-function tests*, and *liver imaging* (which includes *ultrasound scanning*, *CT scanning*, and *MRI*).

SYMPTOMS
The most common symptoms of any liver cancer are loss of appetite, weight loss, lethargy, and sometimes pain in the upper right abdomen. The later stages of the disease are marked by *jaundice* (yellowing of the skin and the whites of the eyes, due to accumulation of the bile pigment *bilirubin*) and *ascites* (excess fluid in the abdomen).

DIAGNOSIS AND TREATMENT
Blood tests (see *liver-function tests*) may be used to assess liver function, which can be disturbed by cancer. Tumours are often detected by *ultrasound scanning*, *CT scanning*, or *MRI*; diagnosis may be confirmed by *liver biopsy* (tissue sampling).

Primary liver cancer can sometimes be cured by total removal of the tumour and a surrounding area of normal tissue. Alternatively, if the tumour is small and localized, it may be possible to destroy it by injecting it with chemicals (a procedure called tumour ablation) or by subjecting it to intense laser light or radiofrequency waves (see *radiofrequency ablation*). In other cases, *anticancer drugs* can help to slow the the disease's progress. *Radiotherapy* may also be used to treat cholangiocarcinomas but is not usually used for hepatomas. Rarely, a liver transplant may be a possibility.

It is usually not possible to cure secondary liver cancer, but anticancer drugs or, in some cases, removal of a solitary *metastasis* (secondary cancerous tumour) may significantly improve the outlook.

liver, cirrhosis of
See *cirrhosis*.

liver disease, alcoholic
Damage to the *liver* resulting from excessive *alcohol* consumption. Alcohol-related liver disease increases the risk of developing *liver cancer*.

The longer that heavy alcohol consumption goes on, the more severe the damage. The initial effect is the formation of fat globules inside liver cells, a condition called fatty liver, which is then followed by alcoholic *hepatitis* (liver inflammation). Damage progresses to *cirrhosis* (scarring of liver tissue), resulting in severe structural damage to the liver that eventually leads to loss of liver function.

Liver-function tests show a characteristic pattern of abnormalities, and *liver biopsy* (tissue sampling) may be needed to assess the severity of damage. There is no particular treatment, but abstinence from alcohol prevents further damage. Treatment for *alcohol dependence* may be required in some cases.

liver failure
Severe impairment of *liver* function that develops suddenly (acute liver failure) or at the final stages of a chronic liver disease (chronic liver failure). Because the liver breaks down toxins in the blood, liver failure causes the levels of the toxins to rise, affecting the functioning of other organs, particularly the brain.

SYMPTOMS
Symptoms of acute liver failure develop rapidly; they may include impaired memory, agitation, and confusion, followed by drowsiness. The functioning

L

of other organs may also become impaired, and the condition may lead to *coma* and death.

Features of chronic liver failure develop much more gradually. They include *jaundice*; itching; easy bruising and bleeding; ascites (swollen abdomen due to accumulated fluid); red palms; and, in males, *gynaecomastia* (enlarged breasts) and shrunken testes. Chronic liver failure may suddenly deteriorate into acute liver failure.

TREATMENT
Acute liver failure requires urgent hospital care. Although no treatment can repair damage that has already occurred in acute or chronic liver failure, certain measures, such as prescribing *diuretic drugs* to reduce abdominal swelling, may be taken to reduce the severity of symptoms. Consumption of alcohol should cease in all cases.

OUTLOOK
The prognosis for sufferers of chronic liver failure varies depending on the cause, but some people survive for many years. For both chronic and acute liver failure, a *liver transplant* is necessary to increase the chances of survival.

liver fluke

Any of various species of flukes (flatworms) that infest the *bile ducts* in the *liver*. The only significant fluke in the UK is FASCIOLA HEPATICA, which causes the disease *fascioliasis*.

Fascioliasis has two stages. During the first stage, young flukes migrate through the liver, causing it to become tender and enlarged; other symptoms include fever and night sweats. In the second stage, adult worms occupy the bile ducts. Their presence may lead to *cholangitis* (inflammation of the bile duct) and bile duct obstruction, which can cause *jaundice*. Treatment with an *anthelmintic drug* may be effective.

liver-function tests

Tests of blood chemistry that can detect changes in the way the *liver* is making new substances and breaking down and/or excreting old ones. The tests can also show whether liver cells are healthy or damaged (see *Liver-function tests* table, overleaf).

liver imaging

Techniques that produce images of the *liver*, *gallbladder*, *bile ducts*, and blood vessels supplying the liver, to aid the detection of disease.

Ultrasound scanning is the most widely used technique for imaging the liver; *CT scanning* and *MRI* are also commonly used. *Radionuclide scanning* may reveal cysts and tumours and show bile excretion. *X-ray* imaging techniques include *cholangiography*, *cholecystography*, and *ERCP* (endoscopic retrograde cholangio-pancreatography). In these procedures, a *contrast medium* is used to outline the *biliary system*. *Angiography* reveals the blood vessels in the liver.

liver palms

Redness accompanied by warmth in the palms of the hands. This combination of symptoms is often associated with chronic liver disease. (See *liver failure*.)

STRUCTURE AND FUNCTION OF THE **LIVER**

The liver is a large organ with numerous functions. It absorbs nutrients from blood that has come from the intestines, and regulates the blood's glucose and amino-acid levels. It helps break down drugs and various toxins, and manufactures important proteins, such as albumin and blood coagulation factors. The liver also produces bile, which contains waste products and helps with the digestion of fats in the small intestine.

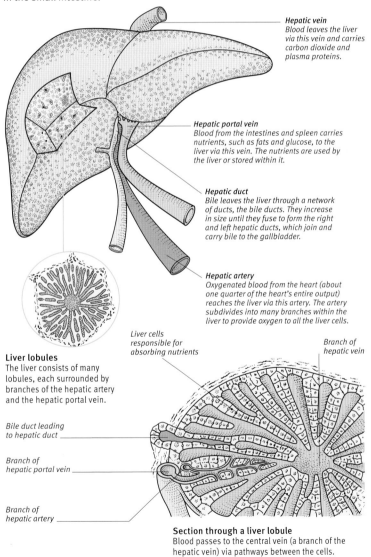

Hepatic vein
Blood leaves the liver via this vein and carries carbon dioxide and plasma proteins.

Hepatic portal vein
Blood from the intestines and spleen carries nutrients, such as fats and glucose, to the liver via this vein. The nutrients are used by the liver or stored within it.

Hepatic duct
Bile leaves the liver through a network of ducts, the bile ducts. They increase in size until they fuse to form the right and left hepatic ducts, which join and carry bile to the gallbladder.

Hepatic artery
Oxygenated blood from the heart (about one quarter of the heart's entire output) reaches the liver via this artery. The artery subdivides into many branches within the liver to provide oxygen to all the liver cells.

Liver lobules
The liver consists of many lobules, each surrounded by branches of the hepatic artery and the hepatic portal vein.

Bile duct leading to hepatic duct

Branch of hepatic portal vein

Branch of hepatic artery

Liver cells responsible for absorbing nutrients

Branch of hepatic vein

Section through a liver lobule
Blood passes to the central vein (a branch of the hepatic vein) via pathways between the cells.

L

LIVER-FUNCTION TESTS

Test	Significance
Serum bilirubin	Bilirubin is the yellow breakdown product of red blood cells that is passed to the liver and excreted in bile. It is this substance that gives the yellow colour to the skin in jaundice. High blood bilirubin levels may indicate excessive breakdown of red blood cells, obstruction to bile flow, defective processing of bile by the liver, or Gilbert's syndrome.
Serum albumin	Albumin is one of the main proteins in blood. Made by the liver, one of its actions is to hold fluid inside the blood vessels. A low level is found in many chronic liver disorders and is often associated with ascites and ankle oedema (fluid collection in the abdomen and around the ankles).
Serum alkaline phosphatase	Alkaline phosphatase is an enzyme found in the cells that line the bile ducts and also in other tissues such as bone. The blood level of this enzyme rises when there is obstruction to the flow of bile (cholestasis).
Gamma-glutamyl transpeptidase	An enzyme present in liver cells. When the flow of bile is obstructed, the blood level of this enzyme is raised, along with a raised level of alkaline phosphatase. A gamma-glutamyl transpeptidase level raised in isolation is related to alcohol intake. its measurement can also be used as a screening test for glutamyl transpeptidase deficiency.
Serum aminotransferases (transaminases)	The aminotransferases are enzymes released from liver cells into the blood when the liver cells are damaged. The levels will be raised in any condition that damages liver cells, including poisoning, and acute and chronic hepatitis.
Prothrombin time	A normal result in this test of blood clotting depends on the presence in the blood of a protein made by the liver from a fat-soluble vitamin, vitamin K. The test result can be abnormal in two types of disorder: when the protein is not made because of liver cell damage, and when there is a blockage to bile flow in the liver, causing a lack of bile in the intestines (which interferes with fat and vitamin K absorption).

liver spot

See *lentigo*.

liver transplant

Replacement of a diseased *liver* with a healthy liver removed from a donor. In most cases, the donor is a dead person, but sometimes (for example, when a liver transplant is performed on a child) part of the liver may be donated by a living relative of the patient.

WHY IT IS DONE
Liver transplants are most successful in treating advanced liver *cirrhosis* in people who have chronic *hepatitis* or primary *biliary cirrhosis*. People who have primary liver cancer may be considered for a transplant if the tumour is relatively small.

HOW IT IS DONE
During this procedure, the liver, the *gallbladder*, and portions of the connected blood and *bile* vessels are removed. The donor organs and blood vessels are then connected to the recipient's vessels.

RECOVERY PERIOD
After the transplant, the recipient is monitored in an *intensive care* unit for a few days and remains in hospital for up to four weeks. Immunosuppressant drugs to prevent rejection of the new organ must be taken for life.

live vaccine

A *vaccine* containing live but weakened forms of an infectious organism. Live vaccines include those given for *measles*, *mumps*, *rubella*, and *tuberculosis*.

living will

An advance directive, signed by an adult of sound mind, that gives instructions about what type of medical treatment the person does or does not want to receive if he or she becomes incapable of giving or refusing consent.

LLETZ

An abbreviation for large loop excision of the transformation zone, a procedure that may be used to treat *cervical intra-epithelial neoplasia*. It involves using a heated wire loop passed through the vagina to remove areas of abnormal tissue from the cervix.

Loa loa

The parasitic worm responsible for the disease *loiasis*.

lobar pneumonia

A form of *pneumonia* (inflammation of the lung) in which only one lobe of a lung is affected.

lobe

One of the clearly defined parts into which certain organs, such as the brain, liver, and lungs, are divided. The term may also be used to describe the earlobe, the soft, fleshy part of the external ear.

lobectomy

An operation performed to cut out a *lobe* in the liver (see *hepatectomy, partial*), the lung (see *lobectomy, lung*), or the thyroid gland (see *thyroidectomy*).

lobectomy, lung

An operation to cut out one of the *lobes* of a *lung*, usually to remove a cancerous tumour in the lung.

lobotomy, prefrontal

The cutting of some of the fibres that link the brain's frontal lobes to the rest of the brain. This operation was formerly used to treat severe psychiatric disorders. It often caused harmful personality changes, however, and is now very rarely performed.

lobular

A word meaning "relating to a lobule".

lobule

A smaller division of a lobe of an organ such as the *liver* or *lung*. Lobules are separated by boundaries such as septa (dividing walls).

local anaesthetic

See *anaesthesia, local*.

localized amnesia

Loss of memory for all events occurring within a particular period of time. See also *amnesia*.

localizing sign

A sign that is found during a physical examination that pinpoints the cause of a disorder.

lochia

The discharge, after childbirth, of blood and fragments of uterine lining from the area where the *placenta* was attached. The discharge is bright red for the first three or four days and then becomes paler. The amount of lochia decreases as the placental site heals, and the discharge usually ceases completely within six weeks.

locked knee

Temporary inability to move the *knee*. A locked knee may be the result of a torn cartilage or of small fragments of bone or cartilage in the joint (*loose bodies*).

lockjaw

A painful spasm of the jaw muscles that makes it difficult or impossible for a person to open the mouth. Lockjaw is the most common symptom of *tetanus*.

locomotor

Relating to movement from one place to another, as in locomotor *ataxia*.

locus

The medical term for a region or site in the body. In genetics, the word is used to describe the position of a gene on a chromosome.

lofepramine

A *tricyclic antidepressant* drug used in the long-term treatment of *depression*. It is particularly helpful if the depression is accompanied by lethargy. Possible side effects include dry mouth, sweating or flushed skin, drowsiness, or blurred vision. If the drug causes constipation, difficulty in passing urine, or dizziness, a doctor should be consulted.

Löffler's syndrome

A rare form of allergic reaction affecting the lungs. Possible causes include drug allergy and roundworm infestation of the lungs (see *ascariasis*). The symptoms include a dry cough, fever, wheezing, shortness of breath, and chest pain. The disease often disappears spontaneously.

log-roll technique

A method of turning a casualty on to his or her back without altering the position of the spine. The technique is used if a spinal injury is suspected and resuscitation is needed (see *cardiopulmonary resuscitation*). The aim is to prevent further injury by keeping the head, trunk, and toes in a straight line.

loiasis

A form of the tropical parasitic disease *filariasis*, which is caused by an infestation by the worm LOA LOA. The worms travel beneath the skin, producing itchy areas of inflammation known as Calabar swellings, and can sometimes be seen moving across the front of the eye. Loiasis is treated with a course of diethylcarbamazine to kill the worms.

loin

The part of the back on each side of the spine between the lowest pair of ribs and the top of the pelvis.

Lomotil

A brand-name *antidiarrhoeal drug* containing *atropine* and *diphenoxylate*.

longsightedness

See *hypermetropia*.

loop of Henlé

Part of the long renal tubule within each of the kidney's filtering units, or *nephrons*. The U-shaped loop of Henlé absorbs water and certain soluble substances back into the bloodstream.

loose bodies

Fragments of *bone*, *cartilage*, or capsule linings within a *joint*. Loose bodies may occur whenever there is damage to a joint, as in injury, *osteoarthritis*, or *osteochondritis dissecans*.

The fragments can cause a joint to lock, resulting in severe pain. *X-rays* or *arthroscopy* (viewing of the interior of a joint with an endoscope) may reveal their presence. Gentle manipulation of the joint may be required, in order to unlock it. If locking occurs frequently, the loose bodies may be removed during arthroscopy or by surgery.

loperamide

An *antidiarrhoeal drug* that slows intestinal activity and reduces the loss of water and salts from the body. It is usually used to treat sudden and recurrent bouts of diarrhoea.

Loperamide occasionally produces a rash; other rare adverse effects are abdominal cramps, and bloating. They require prompt attention from a doctor.

Lorain-Lévi syndrome

A form of *dwarfism* in which a child retains the appearance of an infant, due to insufficient secretion of growth hormone and a lack of gonadotrophin.

loratadine

An *antihistamine drug* used to relieve symptoms of allergic *rhinitis*, such as sneezing, runny nose, and itching eyes, and to treat allergic skin problems such as chronic *urticaria*. It is less likely to cause drowsiness than some other antihistamines. Side effects are uncommon; they include headache, fatigue, and nausea.

lorazepam

A *benzodiazepine drug* used in the treatment of *insomnia* and *anxiety*, or for premedication prior to an operation or other procedure.

lordosis

Inward curvature of the *spine*. This curvature is normally present to a minor degree in the lower back but can become exaggerated by poor posture or by *kyphosis* (excessive curvature of the upper spine). Pronounced lordosis is usually permanent and can lead to *disc prolapse* (slipped disc) or spinal *osteoarthritis*.

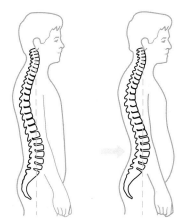

Normal and abnormal lordosis
The normal inward curvature of the spine (left) is exaggerated in abnormal lordosis (right).

losartan

An *angiotensin II antagonist* drug used to treat *hypertension* (high blood pressure). Side effects are rare and mild; they include dizziness, diarrhoea, and fatigue.

Losec

The brand name for the anti-ulcer drug *omeprazole*.

lotion

A liquid drug preparation applied to the skin. Some examples of drugs prepared as a lotion include *calamine* and *betamethasone*, both of which are used to treat skin inflammation.

L

Lou Gehrig's disease

The most common type of *motor neuron disease*; also known as amyotrophic lateral sclerosis (ALS).

low birthweight

See *birthweight*.

low-density lipoprotein

One of a group of proteins combined with *lipids* in the blood *plasma*. Low-density lipoproteins (LDLs) are involved in the transport of *cholesterol* in the bloodstream; they also deposit cholesterol around the body. An excess of LDLs (see *hyperlipidaemias*) is associated with *atherosclerosis* (narrowing of the arteries by deposits of fatty material). (See also *high-density lipoprotein*.)

lower back pain

See *back pain*.

Lowe's syndrome

A rare, X-linked *genetic disorder* affecting the eyes, kidneys, and brain. Lowe's syndrome is a metabolic disorder in which an *enzyme* found in cell membranes does not function. Only males are affected.

Eye problems include *glaucoma*; *cataracts*; and *nystagmus* (abnormal, jerky eye movements). The kidney dysfunction causes chemical imbalances such as *acidosis* and a form of *rickets* that is resistant to vitamin D treatment. The brain disorders include *learning difficulties*, behavioural problems, and sometimes *seizures*.

lozenge

A medicated sweet or tablet that dissolves in the mouth, usually taken to relieve a sore mouth or throat.

LSD

The abbreviation for lysergic acid diethylamide, a synthetic *hallucinogenic drug* that is derived from the fungus *ergot*. LSD is used illegally as a recreational drug. It causes visual and sometimes auditory hallucinations (perceptions that occur with no external stimulus); it may also produce unusual emotional states such as "mystical" experiences. The user may also have abnormal thoughts, such as believing that he or she can fly unaided.

LSD sometimes produces panic and physical side effects such as nausea and dizziness. In addition, individuals who have used it frequently may experience "flashbacks" (recurrences of the hallucinations) for months or even years after their last use of the drug. LSD is not addictive but regular users rapidly develop *tolerance*.

Ludwig's angina

A rare bacterial infection that affects the floor of the mouth, usually due to an infected tooth or area of gum. Ludwig's angina occurs most commonly in people who tend to have poor *oral hygiene* habits.

Symptoms include fever; pain and swelling in the mouth; and difficulty in opening the mouth and swallowing. If left untreated, the disorder may cause life-threatening swelling in the throat that obstructs breathing and needs immediate treatment with *antibiotic drugs*.

lumbago

A general term for lower *back pain*. Lumbago may be due to an intervertebral *disc prolapse* (slipped disc). It may also arise if *synovium* (joint membrane) is trapped between the surfaces of a small intervertebral joint, or if there is momentary subluxation (partial dislocation) of an intervertebral joint with *sprains* of the ligaments. In many cases, however, no cause is found.

Treatment is with *analgesic drugs* (painkillers) and gentle physical activity. (See also *lumbosacral spasm*.)

lumbar

A word referring to the part of the back between the lowest ribs and the top of the pelvis. The lumbar part of the *spine* is made up of the five lumbar *vertebrae*.

lumbar disc protrusion

See *disc prolapse*.

LOCATION AND STRUCTURE OF THE LUNGS

The lungs lie in the chest within the ribcage. Air entering the body through the nose and mouth travels down the trachea to the main bronchi, which divide into smaller bronchi and then into bronchioles. These in turn lead to alveoli, where the exchange of oxygen and carbon dioxide takes place. During expiration (breathing out), air leaves the body by the same routes.

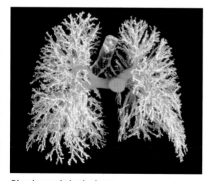

Blood vessels in the lungs
The tiniest "twigs" of this extensive blood vessel "tree" form into capillaries that surround the alveoli (air sacs) in the lung. Oxygen and carbon dioxide are exchanged between the alveoli and the capillaries.

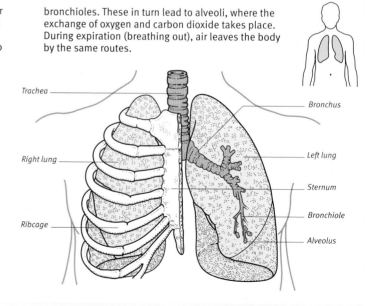

Trachea

Bronchus

Right lung

Left lung

Sternum

Bronchiole

Ribcage

Alveolus

lumbar puncture

A procedure in which a hollow needle is inserted into the lower part of the spinal canal, between two lumbar *vertebrae*, to withdraw *cerebrospinal fluid* or to inject drugs or other substances.

Lumbar puncture is usually carried out to collect a sample of cerebrospinal fluid in order to diagnose and investigate disorders of the brain and spinal cord (such as *meningitis* and *subarachnoid haemorrhage*). The procedure takes about 15 minutes and is carried out under local *anaesthesia*.

lumbosacral spasm

Excessive tightening of the muscles that surround and support the lower region of the *spine*, causing *back pain*. Treatment of lumbosacral spasm may include *analgesic drugs* (painkillers).

lumbosacral spine

The area of the lower *spine* consisting of the lumbar vertebrae and the *sacrum* (the fused vertebrae that form the back of the pelvis).

lumen

The space within a tubular organ or structure such as the intestine.

lumpectomy

A surgical treatment for *breast cancer* in which only the cancerous tissue is removed, rather than the entire breast. (See also *mastectomy*; *quadrantectomy*.)

lumpy jaw

A nonmedical name for *actinomycosis*.

lunacy

An outdated term for serious mental disorder.

lung

One of the two main organs of the *respiratory system*. The lungs supply the body with the oxygen needed for *aerobic* metabolism and eliminate the waste product carbon dioxide.

STRUCTURE AND FUNCTION

Air is delivered to the lungs through the *trachea* (windpipe); this air passage divides into two main bronchi, with one *bronchus* supplying each lung. The main bronchi divide again into smaller bronchi and then into bronchioles, which lead to air passages that open out into grapelike air sacs called alveoli (see *alveolus, pulmonary*). Oxygen and carbon dioxide diffuse into or out of the blood through the thin walls of the alveoli.

Each lung is enclosed in a double membrane called the *pleura*; the two layers of the pleura secrete a lubricating fluid that enables the lungs to move freely as they expand and contract during breathing. (See also *respiration*.)

lung cancer

The second most common form of *cancer* in the UK (after skin cancer).

CAUSES

Smoking of tobacco is the main cause of lung cancer in the UK, accounting for about 90 per cent of all cases. Other causes include exposure to certain air pollutants and industrial substances such as silica and asbestos. Passive smoking (inhalation of tobacco smoke by non-smokers) is also a risk factor.

TYPES

There are several types of lung cancer, each of which affects a different group of lung cells. The most common types are squamous cell carcinoma and small cell (or oat cell) carcinoma; the other main types are adenocarcinoma and large cell carcinoma. *Mesothelioma* is a type of lung cancer that affects the *pleura* (the membrane that covers the lungs and lines the chest cavity) associated with exposure to asbestos.

L

DISORDERS OF THE LUNG

The lungs are continuously exposed to airborne particles, such as bacteria, viruses, and allergens, all of which can cause disease. Disorders may also arise within the lung tissue or in associated structures such as blood vessels.

Infection

Lung infections are common. These include *pneumonia* (inflammation of the lung), *tracheitis* (inflammation of the lining of the windpipe), and *croup* (a viral infection in young children). *Bronchitis* and *bronchiolitis*, which are inflammatory disorders affecting the airways within the lungs, can be complications of colds or influenza. The disorder *bronchiectasis* (abnormal widening of the bronchi) may be a complication of bacterial pneumonia or *cystic fibrosis*.

Allergies

Inhalation of certain substances, such as pollen, *dander* (skin cells from animals), and house mite faeces, can provoke allergic disorders in susceptible people. The most significant of these disorders is *asthma*. Another such disorder is allergic *alveolitis*, which is usually a reaction to dust of plant or animal origin.

Tumours

Lung cancer is one of the most common of all cancers; cancerous tumours may also spread to the lungs from other areas. Noncancerous tumours of the lung are far less common.

Injury

Injury to the lung, usually by penetration of the chest wall, can allow air or blood to collect between the two layers of the pleura (the membrane around each lung), and the lung may collapse (see *pneumothorax; haemothorax*). Injury to the interior of the lungs can be due to inhalation of toxic substances (see *asbestosis; silicosis*).

Other disorders

The blood supply to the lungs may be reduced by *pulmonary embolism* (a condition in which a clot obstructs a blood vessel in the lung).

Oxygen intake may be severely impaired by diseases affecting the tiny air sacs in the lungs (see *alveolus, pulmonary*). in *emphysema*, the alveoli are destroyed, thereby reducing the area of lung tissue where oxygen is absorbed into the blood (see also *pulmonary disease, chronic obstructive*). *Respiratory distress syndrome* in adults occurs when fluid leaks into the alveoli from the tiny blood vessels surrounding them, thereby preventing the alveolar walls from absorbing sufficient oxygen.

INVESTIGATION

Lung disorders are investigated by *chest X-ray*, *CT scanning*, *bronchoscopy*, *pulmonary function tests*, *sputum analysis*, and *blood tests*. Sometimes, a lung *biopsy* (removal of a tissue sample) is performed.

Each form of lung cancer has a particular growth pattern and response to treatment. Small cell carcinoma is the most highly malignant form of lung cancer; it grows rapidly and spreads very quickly throughout the body. In contrast, squamous cell carcinoma grows more slowly than the other forms and does not spread outside the lung until late in the course of the disease.

SYMPTOMS

The first and most common symptom of lung cancer is a persistent cough. Other symptoms include coughing up blood, shortness of breath, and chest pain. The tumour may obstruct the airway, causing *pneumonia* (inflammation in the lung), or involve the pleura, causing an accumulation of fluid called *pleural effusion*. A tumour developing at the top of the lung may press on the nerves supplying the arm on that side, causing pain and weakness in the arm.

Lung cancer can spread to other parts of the body, especially the liver, brain, and bones, causing pain and other problems in these areas.

DIAGNOSIS AND TREATMENT

In most cases, the cancer is revealed in a *chest X-ray* or diagnosed from abnormal cells in a sputum sample. A *bronchoscopy* to view inside the airways and *CT scanning* may also be used to make an initial diagnosis. To confirm the diagnosis, a *biopsy* (tissue sample) is taken and examined microscopically for the presence of cancerous cells. Blood tests, and CT scanning or *MRI*, may be used in order to determine whether or not the cancer has spread to other areas.

If lung cancer is diagnosed at an early stage, *pneumonectomy* (removal of the whole lung) or *lobectomy* (removal of the diseased lobe of the lung) may be a possibility. Surgery is usually considered only in cases in which the tumour is still relatively small and has not spread beyond the lung. *Anticancer drugs* and *radiotherapy* may be used in order to contain the spread of the tumour and to treat any metastases (cancerous cells that have spread to other areas of the body). Small cell carcinoma is usually treated by means of radiotherapy and chemotherapy.

lung, collapse of

See *atelectasis*; *pneumothorax*.

lung disease, chronic obstructive

See *pulmonary disease, chronic obstructive*.

lung-function tests

See *pulmonary function tests*.

lung imaging

Techniques that are used to provide images of the lungs in order to facilitate the diagnosis of lung disease. Most *lung disorders* can be detected by means of *chest X-ray*. *CT scanning* and *MRI* play an important role in detecting the presence and the spread of *lung tumours*. *Ultrasound scanning* is sometimes used to reveal *pleural effusion* (buildup of fluid around a lung). *Radioisotope scanning* is used to detect evidence of *pulmonary embolism* (in which a clot obstructs a blood vessel in a lung); alternatively, a pulmonary *angiogram* contrast X-ray may be performed.

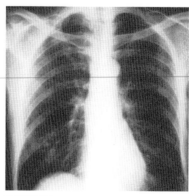

Chest X-ray
This is the most important lung imaging technique. It provides information about the lungs, their blood vessels and main airways.

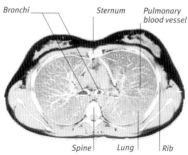

CT scan of the lungs
This scan shows a detailed horizontal slice through the lungs. CT scans are useful for showing the extent and spread of lung tumours.

lung lobectomy

See *lobectomy, lung*.

lung tumours

Growths in the lungs. These tumours may be either cancerous (see *lung cancer*) or noncancerous.

Noncancerous tumours occur less frequently than cancers. The most common of these tumours is a bronchial *adenoma*, which arises in the lining of a bronchus. Adenomas often cause bronchial obstruction; affected people may also cough up blood. Treatment of adenoma involves surgical removal of the tumour.

Other rare noncancerous tumours include *fibromas* (which consist of fibrous tissue) and *lipomas* (which consist of fatty tissue). No treatment is necessary for these, unless the tumours are causing problems.

lupus erythematosus

An *autoimmune disorder* that causes inflammation of *connective tissue*. The most common type of this disorder is discoid lupus erythematosus (DLE), which affects only exposed areas of skin. The more serious form, systemic lupus erythematosus (SLE), affects many of the body systems, including the skin.

SYMPTOMS

In both varieties of lupus erythematosus, the symptoms periodically subside and recur with varying severity.

In DLE, the rash starts as one or more red, circular, and thickened areas of skin. The rash may be triggered or worsened by exposure to sunlight. The affected areas of skin subsequently become scarred. The patches may occur on the face, behind the ears, and on the scalp.

SLE causes a variety of symptoms. A characteristic red, blotchy, butterfly-shaped rash may appear on the cheeks and the bridge of the nose; other symptoms include fatigue, fever, nausea, loss of appetite, joint pain, and weight loss. There may also be associated problems including *anaemia*, neurological or psychiatric problems, *kidney failure*, *pleurisy* (inflammation of the membrane that lines the lungs), arthritis, and *pericarditis* (inflammation of the membrane surrounding the heart).

DIAGNOSIS AND TREATMENT

Diagnosis of DLE is made by *blood tests* and sometimes a *skin biopsy*. SLE is usually diagnosed from the symptoms, medical history, and blood tests.

DLE is usually treated with topical *corticosteroid drugs*. Both DLE and SLE may be treated with the antimalarial drug hydroxychloroquine. Sufferers of mild forms of SLE may have near normal health for many years, and

L

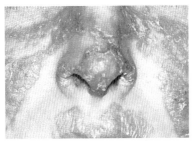

Systemic lupus erythematosus on face
The disease can cause a skin eruption across the nose and cheeks. The distinctive pattern this causes is known as a butterfly rash.

treatment with *corticosteroid drugs* and *immunosuppressant drugs* can improve life expectancy. Other treatments are available to treat specific features of the disease; however, SLE is still a potentially fatal disorder.

lupus pernio

A form of *sarcoidosis* affecting the skin, in which purple swellings resembling chilblains appear on the ears, nose, or cheeks.

lupus vulgaris

A rare form of *tuberculosis* affecting the skin, especially on the head and neck. Painless, clear, red-brown nodules appear and ulcerate; the ulcers eventually heal, leaving deep scars.

Lüscher colour test

Developed in the 1960s by Dr. Max Lüscher, the Lüscher colour test is based on the idea that psychological information about a person can be gained through that person's choices and rejections of eight colours: grey, blue, green, red, yellow, violet, brown, and black. The test is sometimes used in the workplace to test job applicants for suitability. It can also be a useful tool for psychologists when they are trying to determine the current state of mind of an individual.

luteinizing hormone

Also known as LH, a *gonadotrophin hormone* produced by the *pituitary gland*.

luteinizing hormone-releasing hormone

A naturally occurring *hormone*, also known as LH-RH or gonadotrophin-releasing hormone (GnRH), that is released by the *hypothalamus* in the brain. LH-RH stimulates the release of *gonadotrophin hormones* from the *pituitary*

gland. Gonadotrophin hormones control the production of *oestrogen hormones* and *androgen hormones*. There is a medicinal preparation of LH-RH known as *gonadorelin*.

Lyell's syndrome

Also known as toxic epidermal necrolysis, a life-threatening drug reaction in which the skin, mucous membranes, and lining of internal organs such as the bladder and intestine blister and slough off. Drugs that are known to have caused this condition include *penicillin*, *carbamazepine*, and *nonsteroidal anti-inflammatory drugs* (NSAIDS). Cases of Lyell's syndrome require treatment in an *intensive care* unit.

Lyme arthritis

Inflammation of the joints as a result of *Lyme disease* (a bacterial infection transmitted by the bite of a tick). *Arthritis* affects up to half of those infected with Lyme disease. It develops within a few weeks to two years of the original infection and causes joint pain and swelling. The knee is the most commonly affected joint.

Lyme disease

A disease caused by the bacterium Borrelia burgdorferi, which is transmitted by ticks. The ticks are found in forests (mainly deciduous forests), heathland, moorland, and also in suburban parks. Areas in which deer live are especially likely to harbour the ticks.

SYMPTOMS

At the site of a tick bite, a red dot may appear and gradually expand to form a circular rash (known as erythema migrans) that may be up to 15 cm across. Symptoms including fever, headache, and muscle pain usually develop; they are followed by joint inflammation, which typically affects the knees and other large joints. Symptoms of Lyme disease may vary in severity and occur in cycles lasting for about one to three weeks.

COMPLICATIONS

If Lyme disease is not treated promptly, complications may develop; these include *meningitis* (inflammation of the membranes covering the brain), *facial palsy*, and an abnormal heartbeat (see *arrhythmia, cardiac*). The most serious long-term complications of Lyme disease are *Lyme arthritis* and persistent neurological disorders that are similar to *multiple sclerosis*.

TREATMENT

Treatment of Lyme disease is with *antibiotic drugs*, such as amoxicillin or doxycycline, and is most effective when given soon after initial infection.

In areas that are known to be infested with the ticks, people should take measures to prevent tick bites. Such measures includes wearing clothes that cover the body and fit closely at the wrists and ankles, applying a *DEET* insect repellent on exposed areas of skin, and taking care not to walk through thick undergrowth.

lymph

A watery or milky body fluid containing *lymphocytes* (a type of white blood cell), proteins, and fats. It plays an important role in the *immune system* and in absorbing fats from the intestine.

Lymph accumulates outside the blood vessels in the intercellular spaces of body tissues, and is collected by the vessels of the *lymphatic system*. This system filters the fluid and eventually returns it to the bloodstream.

lymphadenitis

A medical term for inflammation of the *lymph nodes*, which is a common cause of *lymphadenopathy*.

lymphadenopathy

The medical term for swollen *lymph nodes* (see *glands, swollen*).

lymphangiography

A diagnostic procedure that involves injecting a *contrast medium* into lymph vessels (see *lymphatic system*) in order that the vessels and lymph nodes, and any abnormalities, can be seen on *X-rays*. Lymphangiography has been largely superseded by *CT scanning* and *MRI*.

lymphangioma

A rare, noncancerous tumour consisting of a mass of lymph vessels and often affecting the skin and the deeper tissues. It may be present from birth. Lymphangiomas are sometimes removed with *laser treatment*.

lymphangitis

Inflammation of the lymphatic vessels (see *lymphatic system*) due to the spread of *bacteria* (commonly streptococci) from an infected wound. The inflammation causes the appearance of tender red streaks on the skin overlying the lymphatic vessels. These red streaks extend

L

from the infection site towards the nearest *lymph nodes*. The affected nodes become swollen and tender, and the affected individual usually has a fever and a general feeling of illness.

Lymphangitis requires urgent treatment with *antibiotic drugs* to prevent *septicaemia* (a life-threatening disorder resulting from high levels of bacteria, and bacterial toxins, in the blood).

lymphatic system

A system of vessels (lymphatic vessels) that drains *lymph* from tissues all over the body back into the bloodstream. The lymphatic system is part of the *immune system* and has a major function in defending the body against infection and cancer. The lymphatic system also plays a part in the absorption of fats from the intestine.

STRUCTURE AND FUNCTION

All body tissues are bathed in lymph, a watery fluid that is derived from the bloodstream. Much of this fluid is returned to the bloodstream through the walls of the capillaries (see *circulatory system*), but the remainder of the fluid is transported to the heart through the lymphatic system.

Lymph is moved along the lymphatic vessels during physical activity, in which the contraction of muscles compresses the vessels; valves inside the vessels ensure that the lymph always flows in the correct direction.

Situated on the lymphatic vessels are *lymph nodes*, through which the lymph passes. These nodes filter the lymph and trap or destroy infectious microorganisms or other foreign bodies. Also included in the lymphatic system are the *spleen* and the *thymus*, which produce *lymphocytes* (white blood cells that fight infection or harmful cells).

DISORDERS

If infection or inflammation occurs in any part of the body, the lymph nodes in that area may become swollen and tender as the white blood cells within them try to combat the organisms or cells causing the problem. If an infection is particularly severe, the lymphatic vessels leading from the nodes may also become inflamed (see *lymphangitis*).

If a lymphatic vessel becomes obstructed (for example, by worms or cell debris), lymph will collect in the nearby tissues, leading to *lymphoedema*.

Cancer commonly spreads to other parts of the body through the lymphatic system. If a primary tumour invades

the lymphatic vessels, cells from the tumour may break off and enter the vessels (see *metastasis*). They may then become lodged in lymph nodes situated nearby, where they may then grow into secondary tumours. In *breast cancer*, for example, the cells from a breast tumour may spread to the lymph nodes in the armpit.

lymph gland

A popular name for a *lymph node*. (See also *lymphatic system*.)

lymph node

A small organ lying along the course of a lymphatic vessel (see *lymphatic system*). Lymph nodes are commonly, but incorrectly, called lymph glands. Lymph nodes vary in size; they can be microscopic or can be up to about 2.5 cm in diameter.

STRUCTURE

A lymph node is composed of a thin, fibrous outer capsule and an inner mass of lymphoid tissue. Penetrating the capsule are several small lymphatic vessels, which transport lymph into the node. Each lymph node contains sinuses (spaces) in which the lymph is filtered. A single, larger vessel carries lymph out of the node.

FUNCTION

Lymph nodes act as a barrier to the spread of infection by destroying or filtering out bacteria before they can pass into the bloodstream. As lymph passes through a node, narrow channels in the sinuses slow down its movement; this reduction in the flow of lymph allows macrophages (white blood cells that engulf and destroy foreign and dead material) to filter microorganisms from the lymph. In addition, germinal centres, which are located in the lymph node, release white blood cells known as *lymphocytes*. These cells also help to fight infection.

lymphocyte

Any one of a group of white *blood cells* that are of crucial importance to the *immune system* because they combat infectious organisms and cancer. There are two principal types of lymphocyte: B- and T-lymphocytes.

B-LYMPHOCYTES

B-lymphocytes produce *immunoglobulins* or *antibodies* (proteins that attach to *antigens* (proteins) on the surface of bacteria). This starts a process that leads to the destruction of the bacteria.

T-LYMPHOCYTES

The T-lymphocytes are classified in two main groups, according to the type of antigens found on their surfaces. One group (known as CD8) includes killer (cytotoxic) and suppressor cells; the other group (CD4) includes helper cells. The killer T-lymphocytes attach themselves to abnormal cells (such as tumour cells, cells that have been invaded by viruses, and those in transplanted tissue) and release chemicals that help to destroy the abnormal cells. Suppressor T-cells act to "damp down" the immune response. Helper T-cells enhance the activities of the killer T-cells and the B-cells, and also orchestrate the immune response.

MEMORY FUNCTION

Some B- and T-lymphocytes do not participate directly in immune responses but serve as a memory bank for antigens that have been encountered. These lymphocytes are created when the immune system cells respond to an infection, and they contain information on how to deal with that infection. Once the immune response is over, the memory cells are then stored in the body in order to aid subsequent immune responses to that infection.

lymphocytosis

An increase in the number of *lymphocytes*, a type of white blood cell that mounts the immune response, either by attacking foreign cells directly or by producing antibodies that cause their destruction. Lymphocytosis, which can be detected by blood test, most commonly occurs in viral infections. Rarely, a massive increase in lymphocytes may be due to *leukaemia*.

lymphoedema

An abnormal accumulation of *lymph* in the tissues, which occurs when the normal drainage of lymph is disrupted (see *lymphatic system*).

CAUSES

There are various possible causes for lymphoedema. Cancer can lead to the condition if the vessels become blocked by deposits of cancer cells. Surgical removal of *lymph nodes* under the arm (as in radical *mastectomy*) or in the groin, or *radiotherapy* to an area containing lymph nodes, may also result in lymphoedema. In the tropical disease *filariasis*, the lymphatic vessels may be blocked by parasitic worms. Rarely, the condition is due to a *congenital* abnormality of the

L

STRUCTURE AND FUNCTION OF THE **LYMPHATIC SYSTEM**

The lymphatic system is a collection of organs, ducts, and tissues that has the dual role of draining tissue fluid (lymph) back into the bloodstream and of fighting infection. Lymph is drained by a system of channels (the lymphatic vessels).

White cells that are produced by the bone marrow, thymus, and spleen are present in lymph nodes, or they circulate through the lymphatic system and the bloodstream, providing defences against infection.

The lymphatic network
The lymphatic system consists of a network of lymph nodes connected by lymphatic vessels. The nodes generally occur in clusters, mainly around the neck, armpits, and groin. The lymphatic system also includes organs such as the spleen and thymus.

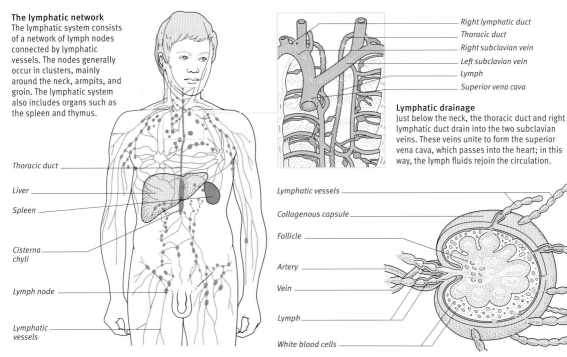

Thoracic duct

Liver

Spleen

Cisterna chyli

Lymph node

Lymphatic vessels

Right lymphatic duct
Thoracic duct
Right subclavian vein
Left subclavian vein
Lymph
Superior vena cava

Lymphatic drainage
Just below the neck, the thoracic duct and right lymphatic duct drain into the two subclavian veins. These veins unite to form the superior vena cava, which passes into the heart; in this way, the lymph fluids rejoin the circulation.

Lymphatic vessels

Collagenous capsule

Follicle

Artery

Vein

Lymph

White blood cells

Structure of a lymph node
Any fluid absorbed into the lymphatic system passes across at least one lymph node before it returns to the circulation. The fluid filters through a mesh of tightly packed white blood cells – some of which are grouped into follicles consisting of similar cells – which attack and destroy harmful organisms. Every lymph node is supplied by its own tiny artery and vein.

MOVEMENTS OF BODY FLUIDS

Lymph is constantly moving around the body, but the lymphatic system has no central pump equivalent to the heart. Lymph is circulated by the movement of the body's muscles; a system of one-way valves in the lymphatic vessels ensures that it moves in the right direction. Exertion also pushes fluid from body tissues into the bloodstream.

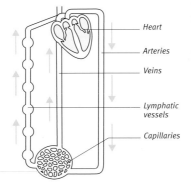

Heart

Arteries

Veins

Lymphatic vessels

Capillaries

Remaining fluid passes from tissues to lymphatic system

Cells

Lymphatic vessel

Tissue fluid

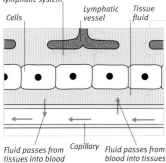

Fluid passes from tissues into blood

Capillary

Fluid passes from blood into tissues

Fluid exchange
During a 24-hour period, approximately 24 litres of serumlike fluid pass from the bloodstream to the body's tissues. This fluid bathes the cells and provides them with oxygen and nutrients. During the same period of time, approximately 20 litres of fluid pass back from the tissues to the bloodstream, carrying carbon dioxide and other waste products. The remaining 4 litres pass from the tissues to the lymphatic system and return eventually to the circulation from there.

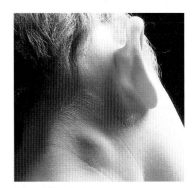

Enlarged lymph nodes
This photograph shows a child with an enlarged lymph node in the neck. One cause of such enlargement is infection. Enlarged nodes may also be a result of Hodgkin's disease, a rare cancer of the lymph nodes.

L

lymphatic vessels known as Milroy's disease. In addition, lymphoedema may occur for no known reason.

SYMPTOMS

Lymphoedema causes painless swelling in the tissues and thickening of the skin over the affected area. It usually develops in the legs; the swelling may start at the ankle and extend up the leg, and may occur to an incapacitating degree in some individuals. If a limb that is affected by lymphoedema is subsequently injured, infection can easily enter the site of injury and spread rapidly through the body tissues.

TREATMENT

There is no known cure for lymphoedema. Treatment consists of taking *diuretic drugs*, wearing an elastic bandage or compression sleeve, massage, and special exercises; these measures may bring about some improvement.

lymphogranuloma venereum

A sexually transmitted disease caused by a *chlamydial infection*; it is most common in tropical areas.

The first sign of lymphogranuloma venereum may be a small genital blister that heals in a few days. There may also be fever, headache, muscle and joint pains, and a rash. The *lymph nodes*, particularly in the groin, become painfully enlarged and inflamed. *Abscesses* may form, and persistent *ulcers* may develop, on the skin over the affected nodes. Treatment is with *antibiotic drugs*.

lymphoma

Any of a group of cancers in which the cells of lymphoid tissue (found principally in the *lymph nodes* and the *spleen*) multiply unchecked.

Lymphomas fall into two principal categories. If certain characteristic abnormal cells (Reed–Sternberg cells) are present, the condition is called *Hodgkin's disease*. All other forms are known as non-Hodgkin's lymphoma (see *lymphoma, non-Hodgkin's*).

lymphoma, non-Hodgkin's

Any cancer that affects the lymphoid tissue (found mainly in the *lymph nodes* and *spleen*) other than the condition *Hodgkin's disease*.

CAUSES

In most cases, non-Hodgkin's lymphoma has no known cause. Occasionally, however, the disease is associated with suppression of the *immune system*, particularly after an organ transplant. One

type of non-Hodgkin's lymphoma, called *Burkitt's lymphoma*, is associated with the *Epstein–Barr virus*.

SYMPTOMS

There is usually painless swelling of *lymph nodes* in the neck or groin. The *liver* and *spleen* may enlarge, and lymphoid tissue in the abdomen may be affected. Many other organs may become involved, leading to diverse symptoms ranging from headache to skin ulceration. In some cases, there may be fever, marked weight loss, and recurrent infections.

DIAGNOSIS

Diagnosis is based on a *biopsy*, usually taken from a lymph node. Further investigations, such as *chest X-ray*, *CT scanning*, *MRI*, *bone marrow biopsy*, and *lymphangiography*, may be needed to assess the extent of the disease.

TREATMENT

In cases where the lymphoma is confined to a single group of lymph nodes, treatment consists of *radiotherapy*, *anticancer drugs*, and *corticosteroid drugs*. More often, however, the disease is more extensive, and in such cases anticancer drugs and monoclonal antibodies (see *antibody, monoclonal*) are given. A *stem cell* or *bone marrow transplant*, with drug treatment and/or radiotherapy, may be considered for some people. Many people with non-Hodgkin's lymphoma can be cured or have a long period of remission.

lymphopenia

A decrease in the number of *lymphocytes*, a type of white blood cell that mounts the immune response, either by a direct attack on abnormal cells or invading organisms or by producing antibodies that cause their destruction. This condition may occur when the bone marrow fails to produce enough blood cells, as in aplastic anaemia (see *anaemia, aplastic*) or treatment with *radiotherapy* or *anticancer drugs*.

lymphosarcoma

The former name for a condition that is now classified as a type of non-Hodgkin's lymphoma (see *lymphoma, non-Hodgkin's*).

lysergide

see *LSD*.

lysis

A medical term for breaking down or destruction. The term lysis is usually

applied to the destruction of cells by disintegration of their outer membrane. A common example is *haemolysis*, the breakdown of red blood cells.

Lysis may be caused by chemical action, for example the action of an *enzyme*, or by physical action, for example the action of heat or cold. The term "lysis" is also occasionally used to refer to a sudden recovery from a fever.

lysosomal storage disease

One of several different conditions, also known as inborn errors of metabolism (see *metabolism, inborn errors of*) in most of which an enzyme is missing from the *lysosome* within cells. This absence leads to a buildup of abnormal substances within the cells that causes tissue damage.

lysosome

One of a variety of structures present within every cell that are responsible, when the cell dies, for breaking down the components of the cell for the purposes of recycling.

lysozyme

An *enzyme* found in tears, saliva, sweat, nasal secretions, breast milk, and many tissues. It destroys bacteria by disrupting their cell walls.

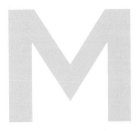

M

macro-

A prefix meaning "large", as in *macrophage* (a large type of cell found in the *immune system*) or *macroglossia* (enlargement of the tongue).

macrobiotics

A dietary system in which foods with a balance of *yin and yang* are eaten. Foods are classed as yin or yang depending on factors such as colour, texture, and taste.

macrocytosis

A condition in which the red *blood cells* are larger than normal. Macrocytosis has many possible causes, the most common of which are megaloblastic anaemia (see *anaemia, megaloblastic*) and the effects of alcohol.

macroglobulinaemia, Waldenström's

A type of *lymphoma* in which *lymphocytes* (a type of white *blood cell*) produce excessive amounts of a protein called immunoglobulin M (IgM), which is normally created to fight disease (see *immunoglobulins*). It tends to occur most commonly in men over 50 years old.

The excess IgM causes the blood to become overly viscous (thick), impairing its flow through the smallest blood vessels. Signs and symptoms include fatigue; headache; dizziness; visual disturbances; easy bruising and bleeding; and numbness and tingling in the hands and feet. The spleen, liver, and *lymph nodes* may become enlarged.

There is no cure, but treatment can relieve the symptoms. Blood viscosity can be lowered by *plasmapheresis*, in which a machine removes excess IgM from the blood plasma. *Anticancer drugs* and *corticosteroids* may also be given.

macroglossia

Abnormal enlargement of the tongue. Macroglossia is a feature of the chromosomal abnormality *Down's syndrome*; *hypothyroidism* (an underactive thyroid gland); and *acromegaly* (a hormonal disorder causing enlargement of several body parts). It is also caused by some tumours of the tongue, such as a *haemangioma* or a *lymphangioma*.

macrognathia

An abnormally large upper and/or lower *jaw*. Macrognathia can be a feature of the condition *acromegaly*. (See also *prognathism*).

macrolide drugs

A class of *antibiotic drugs* used to treat a wide range of infections, including those of the ear, nose, throat, respiratory and gastrointestinal tracts, and skin. Common macrolides include *azithromycin* and *erythromycin*.

macrophage

A cell in the *immune system*. Macrophages are large *phagocytes*, which can engulf and destroy microorganisms and other foreign particles. They are found in most body tissues.

macroscopic

Visible to the naked eye.

macula

The specific area of the *retina* (the light-sensitive layer at the back of the eye) that is responsible for seeing fine detail. The macula surrounds the *fovea*, the part of the retina that contains the highest density of visual cells.

macular degeneration

A progressive, painless deterioration of the *macula*. It is a common disorder in elderly people, and is the most common cause of people being registered as blind in the UK. The cause is unknown.

There are two forms of macular degeneration: dry and wet. In dry macular degeneration, cells within and just beneath the macula die. In wet macular degeneration, fragile new blood vessels grow beneath the macula; and these vessels may easily leak blood or other fluid, which damages the cells. Both forms of macular degeneration produce a roughly circular area of blindness that increases in size. It does not cause total blindness because the vision is retained around the edges of the visual fields.

Diagnosis is by *ophthalmoscopy* and *vision tests*. If wet macular degeneration is suspected, fluorescein *angiography* (imaging of the blood vessels in the retina) may be performed to detect abnormal blood vessels.

For wet macular degeneration, early treatment is essential to prevent further visual loss. Treatment may involve *laser treatment* or photodynamic therapy to destroy the abnormal blood vessels, although recurrence of the condition is common and repeat treatments may be needed. In some cases, it may be possible to slow progression of wet macular degeneration with periodic injections into the eye of drugs that prevent abnormal blood vessels from forming. There is no treatment for dry macular degeneration, although the affected individual may benefit from visual aids such as magnifying instruments.

macule

A spot that is level with the skin's surface and discernible only by difference in colour or texture.

maculopathy, diabetic

A complication of *diabetes mellitus* that is characterized by damage to the *macula*, at the back of the retina. Usually, the remainder of the retina is also affected (see *retinopathy*).

madarosis

Loss of the eyelashes or eyebrows.

mad cow disease

The commonly used name for *bovine spongiform encephalopathy* (BSE).

Madelung's disease

The development of multiple, symmetrical, fatty masses resembling *lipomas* under the skin of the head, neck, upper trunk, and upper arms. The disease, also called multiple symmetrical lipomatosis or Lanois–Bensaude syndrome, occurs primarily in adult men. The cause of the disease is unknown, but it has been associated with long-term, excessive alcohol use (see *alcohol-related disorders*).

Madopar

A brand-named drug, containing *levodopa* with benserazide (a drug that enhances the effect of levodopa), used in the treatment of *Parkinson's disease*.

Madura foot

A fungal and/or bacterial infection of the foot that occurs in tropical or subtropical regions such as Central and South America, Africa, India, and Southeast Asia. Madura foot usually affects men aged 20 to 40, often as a result of outdoor work.

The infection enters the foot through broken skin. A nodule or abscess forms, and grows into a mass of diseased tissue with sinuses (abnormal channels) that discharge bloody or pus-filled fluid. The fluid typically contains very small granules, which are fragments of infectious organisms. The infection may progress to involve the foot bones.

Treatment involves removal of diseased tissue (or, if necessary, *amputation*) and the use of *antibiotics* or *antifungal drugs* to destroy the infection.

Maffucci's syndrome

A syndrome characterized by enchondromas (benign tumours of *cartilage*) together with *haemangiomas* (benign tumours of the blood vessels) on the skin or internal organs. The condition develops during childhood, and is more common in males than in females.

Magnapen

A brand-named antibiotic drug containing *ampicillin* with *flucloxacillin*.

magnesium

A mineral that is essential for the formation of bones and teeth, muscle contraction, nerve impulse transmission, and activation of many *enzymes*. Dietary sources include cereals, milk, nuts, soya beans, and fish.

magnesium sulphate

A magnesium compound used as a *laxative drug* and an *anticonvulsant drug*.

magnesium trisilicate

A magnesium compound that is used in *antacid drugs*.

magnetic resonance imaging

See *MRI*.

malabsorption

Impaired absorption of nutrients by the lining of the small intestine.

CAUSES

Malabsorption may be caused by many conditions. One possible cause is an inflammatory disorder, such as chronic *pancreatitis* (long-term inflammation of the pancreas) or *Crohn's disease* (an inflammatory bowel condition). Another is infection, such as *giardiasis* (an infection of the small intestine).

Genetic disorders resulting in abnormal intestinal structure or function can also cause malabsorption, as in *lactase deficiency* (lack of an enzyme needed to digest milk sugar), *cystic fibrosis* (a disorder in which an excess of mucus is produced in the intestines), or *coeliac disease* (hypersensitivity to gluten, a substance in certain cereals).

Other causes of malabsorption include *amyloidosis* (a condition in which a starchy substance is deposited in vital organs), *Whipple's disease* (a rare bacterial disorder), and *lymphoma* (cancer of lymph tissue). In addition, the removal of some of the small intestine, and certain operations on the stomach, may also result in malabsorption.

SYMPTOMS

Common symptoms of malabsorption are diarrhoea and weight loss. In severe cases, there may also be malnutrition (see *nutritional disorders*), *vitamin* deficiency, *mineral* deficiency, or *anaemia*.

DIAGNOSIS AND TREATMENT

Diagnosis may be made by tests on faeces, *blood tests*, *barium X-ray examination* and *jejunal biopsy*. In most cases, dietary modifications or supplements are successful in treating the disorder. In severe cases, intravenous infusion of nutrients is needed (see *feeding, artificial*).

maladjustment

Failure to adapt to a change in one's environment, resulting in inability to cope with daily activities. Maladjustment can occur as a reaction to stressful situations such as divorce or moving house.

The person may have feelings of *depression* or *anxiety*; children and adolescents may show disturbed behaviour (see *behavioural problems in children*). Maladjustment often disappears when a person is removed from the stressful situation or if he or she manages to adapt to it.

malaise

A vague feeling of being unwell.

malalignment

Positioning of the *teeth* in the *jaw* so that they do not form a smooth arch shape when viewed from above or below (see *malocclusion*).

The term "malalignment" may also refer to a *fracture* in which the bone ends are not in a straight line.

malar flush

A high colour over the cheekbones, with a bluish tinge caused by reduced oxygen concentration in the blood. Malar flush is considered to be a sign of *mitral stenosis* (narrowing of one of the heart valves), which often follows *rheumatic fever*. However, malar flush is not always present in mitral stenosis, and many people with this colouring do not have heart disease.

malaria

A serious disease caused by *protozoa* called plasmodia. The infection is spread by the bite of ANOPHELES mosquitoes and is prevalent throughout the tropics. Malaria causes severe fever, and, in some cases, fatal complications affecting the kidneys, liver, brain, and blood.

CAUSES

There are four species of plasmodia that cause malaria: PLASMODIUM FALCIPARUM, PLASMODIUM VIVAX, PLASMODIUM OVALE, and PLASMODIUM MALARIAE. When a mosquito carrying the infection bites a human, the plasmodia enter the bloodstream. They invade the liver and red blood cells, where they multiply. The red cells then rupture, releasing the new parasites. Some of them infect new red cells, and the others develop into forms that can infect more mosquitoes. Falciparum malaria infects more red cells than the other species and thus causes a more serious infection. Most cases of this form occur in Africa.

SYMPTOMS

Symptoms of malaria include fever, shaking, and chills. There may also be severe headache, general malaise, and vomiting. The fever often develops in cycles, occurring every other day (in vivax and ovale infections) or every third day (in malariae infections).

Falciparum malaria can be fatal within days. Infected red cells become sticky and block blood vessels in vital organs. The *spleen* becomes enlarged and the *brain* may be affected, leading to *coma* and convulsions. Destruction of red blood cells causes haemolytic anaemia (see *anaemia, haemolytic*). Kidney failure and jaundice often occur.

DIAGNOSIS AND TREATMENT

A *blood film* examination is carried out to detect the parasites. There is also a specific blood test that can confirm the diagnosis. Falciparum malaria is treated with *quinine* or *proguanil* and atovaquone, or artemether with lumefantrine. *Chloroquine* is the usual treatment for species other than falciparum. People with vivax or ovale malaria must also take the drug *primaquine* to eradicate parasites in the liver. In severe cases, blood transfusions may be necessary.

THE LIFE-CYCLE OF **MALARIA**

Malaria parasites (plasmodia) are transmitted by the bites of infected *ANOPHELES* mosquitoes. The plasmodia invade the liver and then the red blood cells, where they multiply. When the red blood cells rupture, they release the parasites; some of the plasmodia invade more red cells, while others develop into forms that can infect mosquitoes.

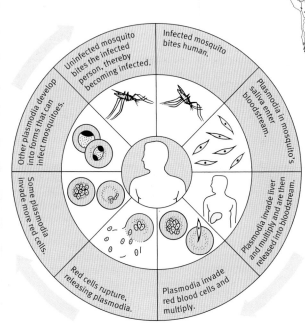

Prevalence of malaria
Malaria, although rare in the UK, is a major problem in the tropics. It affects about 300 million people worldwide, and kills more than one million people a year in Africa alone.

Key
Areas in which malaria is prevalent
Areas with limited risk
Areas with no malaria

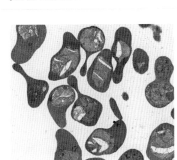

Malarial infection of blood cells
Some of the red blood cells on this TEM (transmission electron micrograph) contain the typical "signet ring" forms of one type of malarial parasite.

M

PREVENTION
Preventive antimalarial drugs should be taken by people visiting malarial areas. A doctor should be consulted for up-to-date advice about the choice and dosages of drugs to be taken. Avoiding mosquito bites by wearing suitable clothing and using insect repellents (such as *DEET*) and mosquito nets is also important in helping prevent infection.

Malarone
A brand-named *antimalarial drug* containing *proguanil* with atovaquone.

malathion
An *antiparasitic drug* for skin or hair infestations such as *lice* and *scabies*. The drug kills parasites by interfering with their nervous systems. Malathion is applied as a shampoo or a lotion. It should not be used on broken or infected skin. If they are used correctly, preparations that contain malathion should not produce adverse effects. However, some alcohol-based lotions may give off fumes that cause wheezing in people with asthma.

male
The term that is used for a man or a boy. Male sex is determined by the possession of a Y *sex chromosome*, and by the presence of a *penis* and *testes* (see *sexual characteristics, primary*).

male-pattern baldness
The most common type of *alopecia*.

malformation
A deformity, particularly one that results from the faulty development of a baby in the mother's uterus. (See *embryo* and *uterus*).

malignant
A term used to describe a condition that tends to become progressively worse and eventually result in death. The term "malignant" is primarily used with reference to a cancerous *tumour* whose cells spread from the original site to form secondary tumours in other parts of the body.

malignant hypertension
Severe *hypertension* in which the blood pressure rises suddenly to a very high level, usually for no obvious cause, resulting in damage to arterioles and capillaries (tiny blood vessels). The condition occurs in a small minority of people with existing hypertension, particularly if it is due to kidney disorders; it is more common in young adults.

Most of the symptoms are caused by increased pressure in blood vessels in the head; they include headache, blurred vision, confusion, drowsiness, nausea, and vomiting. There may also be chest pain and shortness of breath. In addition, the pressure may produce changes in internal organs; for example, it causes *papilloedema* (swelling of the optic nerve) and enlargement of the heart, and may also cause retinal bleeding and acute kidney failure. If not treated promptly, malignant hypertension may cause life-threatening complications.

Diagnosis is based on measurement of blood pressure and tests to detect damage to organs such as the kidneys. An affected person will need hospital treatment to lower blood pressure.

malignant hyperthermia
See *hyperthermia, malignant*.

malignant melanoma
See *melanoma, malignant*.

malingering
The deliberate simulation of symptoms for a particular purpose, such as taking time off work or obtaining compensation. Malingering is different from *factitious disorders* and *hypochondriasis*, in which the motivation for illness is not under the individual's voluntary control.

malleolus
The bony protuberance on each side of the *ankle*.

mallet finger
A common sports injury, mallet finger is injury to the tendon or bone in a fingertip that forces the tip into a bent position. Treatment is with a splint or by temporary insertion of wire through the bones to hold the finger straight. The injury heals in two to three months.

mallet toe
See *claw-toe*.

malleus
One of the three tiny bones (known collectively as the auditory ossicles) that are situated in the middle ear. The malleus, together with the *incus* and the *stapes*, transmits sound vibrations from the eardrum to the inner ear.

Mallory–Weiss syndrome
A tear at the lower end of the *oesophagus*, causing vomiting of blood. The syndrome is commonly caused by retching and vomiting after drinking excess alcohol, or

as a result of food poisoning. Less often, violent coughing, a severe asthma attack, or epileptic convulsions may be the cause.

An *endoscope* is passed down the oesophagus to confirm the diagnosis. The tear generally heals within about ten days, with no special treatment required; however, a *blood transfusion* may sometimes be necessary.

malnutrition
See *nutritional disorders*.

malocclusion
An abnormal relationship between the upper and lower sets of *teeth* when they are closed, affecting the bite or the appearance of the teeth.

CLASSES OF **MALOCCLUSION**

Unsatisfactory contact between the upper and lower teeth is known as malocclusion. There are three main classes, as shown below.

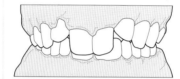

Class 1 malocclusion
In this (the most common) type, the jaw relationship is normal. However, because the teeth are poorly spaced, tilted, or rotated, the upper and lower set do not meet properly.

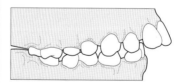

Class 2 malocclusion
In this type –called retrognathism – the lower jaw is lying too far back; the normally small overbite of the upper incisors is greatly increased, and the molar bite is displaced backwards.

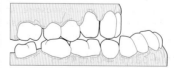

Class 3 malocclusion
In this (the least common) type – called prognathism – the lower jaw is lying too far forward; the lower incisors meet, or lie in front of, the upper ones, and the molar bite is displaced forwards.

Malocclusion usually develops during childhood. In some cases, it may be inherited. Alternatively, it may be due to thumb-sucking or to a mismatch between the teeth and jaws – for example, the combination of large teeth and a small mouth (see *overcrowding, dental*).
TREATMENT
Orthodontic appliances (braces) may be used to reposition the teeth; if there is dental overcrowding, some of the teeth may be extracted. *Orthognathic surgery* is used to treat severe recession or protrusion of the lower jaw. Treatment is best carried out in childhood or adolescence.

malpresentation
A condition in which a baby is not in the usual head-first position for *childbirth*. Malpresentation includes breech presentation (in which the baby's bottom appears first), face presentation, and shoulder presentation (in which the baby is lying across the uterus). Breech presentations are the most common. A breech baby may be born by *breech delivery* or *caesarean section*. A shoulder presentation baby usually has to be delivered by caesarean section.

MALT
The abbreviation for mucosa-associated lymphoid tissue. This tissue is part of the *lymphatic system*, which helps to defend the body against infection. It is found in the digestive tract, particularly in the *tonsils* and in areas called *Peyer's patches* in the small intestine.

maltose
A sugar composed of two *glucose* molecules (see *disaccharide*). Maltose is found in germinating cereal seeds.

mammary dysplasia
Normal variations in *breast* tissue that cause thickening and general lumpiness of the breasts. It may develop just before menstruation and subside afterwards. The condition is common in women between 30 and 50 years of age but is lower in those taking *oral contraceptives*.

The condition is not a disorder and does not lead to breast cancer. In many cases, no treatment is needed; in more severe cases, oral contraceptives may be prescribed. In contrast, any distinct *breast lump* should be assessed by a doctor.

mammary gland
See *breast*.

mammography

An X-ray procedure for examining the *breast*. The breast is flattened between an X-ray plate and a plastic cover so that as much tissue as possible can be imaged. Mammography is used to investigate *breast lumps* and to screen for *breast cancer*. In the UK, all women aged 50 to 70 are offered routine mammography every three years. Such screening has improved the detection of early breast cancer and has led to a reduction in the number of deaths from the disease.

mammoplasty

An operation that is performed in order to make large breasts smaller, to enlarge small breasts, or to reconstruct a breast following surgery for *breast cancer*. In many cases, mammoplasty is performed

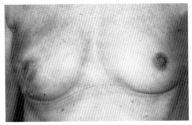

Reconstruction of a breast
The right breast (left in the image) was removed in an earlier mastectomy operation. The breast has been reconstructed using a silicone implant.

for cosmetic reasons. However, the reduction of excessively large breasts may have the physical benefit of reducing back pain.

PROCEDURES

In breast reduction, excess tissue and skin is removed and the tissue is raised and reshaped to correct drooping. Breast enlargement or augmentation involves the insertion of a soft, fluid-filled *breast implant* behind the breast tissue or behind the muscles of the chest wall. In women undergoing a *mastectomy* (removal of a breast) for cancer, breast reconstruction may be carried out either at the same time or as a separate procedure. The normal contours of the breast are restored by the insertion of an implant.

RISKS

Breast reduction carries few risks, but enlargement may cause complications. These problems include leakage from the implant, hardening of the surrounding breast tissue, scarring, and infection. Complications may necessitate further surgery.

PROCEDURE FOR **MAMMOGRAPHY**

Mammography is a simple, safe procedure and causes only slight discomfort. Only low-dose X-rays are used. The breast may be X-rayed from above, the side, or both; and sometimes an oblique (angled) view is taken.

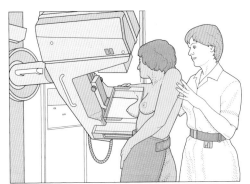

How mammography is done
In the method shown here, the breast is place on the machine and gently compressed between the X-ray plate below and a plastic cover above. This flattens the breast so that as much tissue as possible can be imaged. Several views may be taken. In another method, the breast hangs freely and is X-rayed from the side.

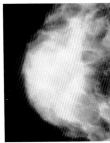

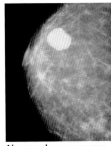

Mammograms
The mammogram on the far left shows a side view of the healthy, relatively dense, breast tissue of a younger woman. In the mammogram on the left, a fibroadenoma (noncancerous tumour made up of fibrous tissue) is present on the upper part of the breast. A biopsy (removal of a tissue sample for analysis) can confirm whether or not a tumour is cancerous.

Normal mammogram   **Abnormal mammogram**

PROCEDURES FOR **MAMMOPLASTY**

One of the most common cosmetic operations, mammoplasty is carried out to improve the appearance of the breasts by removal of excess fat and skin or by using an implant to increase their size.

BREAST REDUCTION   **BREAST ENLARGEMENT**

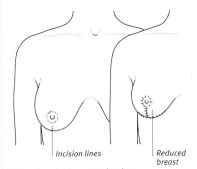

Incision lines   *Reduced breast*

Procedure for breast reduction
Incisions are made around the edge of the nipple, in the crease under the breast, and from the nipple to the crease. Excess tissue and skin are removed, and the nipple is repositioned, then the incisions are closed.

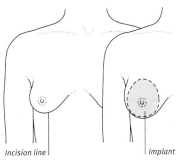

Incision line   *Implant*

Procedure for breast enlargement
An incision is made in the armpit or along the crease under the breast, and a pocket is created behind the breast or the chest muscles to receive the implant. After the implant has been inserted, the incision is stitched.

M

mandible

The lower *jaw*. The mandible consists of two fused pieces of bone forming a U shape. The upper surface bears the lower set of teeth. The mandible is joined to the rest of the skull at the *temporomandibular joint*. It is the only skull bone capable of movement; it is moved by the cheek muscles for chewing and speech.

mania

A mental disorder characterized by episodes of overactivity, elation, or irritability. Mania usually occurs as part of *bipolar disorder*.

SYMPTOMS

Manic behaviour may include extravagant spending; repeatedly starting new tasks; sleeping less than normal; an increased appetite for food, alcohol, sex, and exercise; outbursts of inappropriate anger or laughter; a sudden increase in socializing; and delusions of grandeur. Milder forms are called hypomania.

TREATMENT

Severe mania is usually treated in hospital with *antipsychotic drugs*. Taking *lithium* or *carbamazepine* may prevent relapses.

manic–depressive illness

An alternative term for *bipolar disorder*.

manipulation

A therapeutic technique involving the use of the hands to move parts of a patient's body in order to treat certain disorders. Manipulation is important in *orthopaedics*, *physiotherapy*, *osteopathy*, and *chiropractic*. It may be used to treat deformity and stiffness caused by bone and joint disorders, to realign bones in a displaced *fracture*, to reposition a joint after a *dislocation*, or to stretch a *contracture*. Occasionally, manipulation is used to help treat *frozen shoulder*.

mannitol

An osmotic *diuretic drug* used to treat *oedema* (accumulation of fluid) in the brain and to relieve *glaucoma* (a buildup of fluid, and pressure, in the eyeball).

manometry

The measurement of pressure (of either a liquid or a gas) using an instrument called a manometer. Manometry is used to measure the blood pressure by means of an instrument called a *sphygmomanometer*.

Manson's disease

See *schistosomiasis*.

mantoux test

A skin test that is performed to detect tuberculosis (see *tuberculin tests*).

manubrium

The top part of the *sternum* (breastbone).

MAOI

An abbreviation for *monoamine oxidase inhibitor* drugs.

maple syrup urine disease (MSUD)

An inherited defect in body chemistry (see *metabolism, inborn errors of*) that interferes with the normal breakdown of amino acids. Abnormal acids accumulate in the blood and urine, giving the urine a characteristic smell of maple syrup, and causing severe *ketoacidosis*, *seizures*, and *coma*.

If left untreated, MSUD leads to learning difficulties and eventually to death during infancy. The condition can, however, be controlled with a low-protein diet.

marasmus

A severe form of protein and calorie malnutrition that usually occurs in famine or semi-starvation conditions. Marasmus is common in young children in developing countries. It causes stunted growth, emaciation, and loose folds of skin on the limbs and buttocks due to loss of muscle and fat. Other signs include sparse, brittle hair; diarrhoea; and dehydration.

Treatment includes keeping the child warm and giving a high-energy, protein-rich diet. Persistent marasmus can lead to learning difficulties and can also cause impaired growth. (See also *kwashiorkor*.)

marble bone disease

See *osteopetrosis*.

Marburg virus disease

A rare form of *haemorrhagic fever*, also known as green monkey disease, that is transmitted to humans by African vervet monkeys.

The onset of the disease is sudden, with fever; severe headache; chest and abdominal pain; vomiting; diarrhoea; and a rash on the trunk. The symptoms become increasingly severe; they may include weight loss, delirium, *jaundice*, massive haemorrhaging (internal bleeding), failure of the liver and other organs, and *shock*.

There is no specific treatment for the disease; affected people must be admitted to hospital, where their blood and fluid levels will be maintained and any further infections treated.

march fracture

A break in one of the *metatarsal bones* (the long bones in the foot) that is caused by running or walking for long distances on a hard surface. The fracture results in pain, tenderness, and swelling; however, it may not show on *X-rays* until callus (new bone) has started to form. Treatment for a march fracture involves rest and, occasionally, immobilization of the foot in a plaster *cast*. (See also *stress fracture*.)

Marfan syndrome

A *genetic disorder* of *connective tissue* (material that holds body structures together) that results in skeletal, heart, and eye abnormalities. It is inherited in an autosomal dominant manner. Marfan syndrome is one of the most common disorders of connective tissue.

The features of the syndrome usually appear after the age of 10. Affected people are very tall and thin. They have long, thin limbs, fingers, and toes, and weak ligaments and tendons. The chest and spine are often deformed and the lens of the eye may be dislocated. The heart is often abnormal and the *aorta* weakened.

There is no cure for Marfan syndrome, but children are monitored and any complications are treated as they arise. Many affected children need glasses. Children may also be given *beta-blockers* to help prevent weakening of the aorta, and those with defects of the heart valve or aorta may undergo corrective surgery.

If a family has a member with Marfan syndrome, tests may be used (see *genetic counselling*) to find out whether or not relatives will pass on the gene.

marijuana

The flowering tops and dried leaves of the Indian hemp plant CANNABIS SATIVA, containing the active ingredient THC (tetrahydrocannabinol). The leaves are usually smoked but can also be drunk as tea or eaten in food.

Physical effects of marijuana include dry mouth, mild reddening of the eyes, slight clumsiness, and an increased appetite. The main subjective feelings are usually of calmness and wellbeing, but depression occurs occasionally.

M

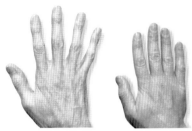

Features of Marfan syndrome
One of the characteristic features of Marfan syndrome is long, thin, "spider" fingers (arachnodactyly). The condition is apparent when the hand of a person with Marfan syndrome (left) is compared to that of a normal person.

Large doses may cause panic, fear of death, and delusions. In rare cases, *drug psychosis* occurs, with symptoms such as paranoid delusions and confusion, which usually disappear in a few days.

There is increasing evidence that regular use of marijuana can aggravate or trigger mental health problems, particularly *depression* and *schizophrenia*; adolescents are most at risk. Regular marijuana use may also reduce fertility in both men and women and, if used in pregnancy, may contribute to premature birth. In addition, regular smoking of marijuana may cause worse lung damage than that caused by tobacco alone.

Maroteaux–Lamy syndrome

A form of *mucopolysaccharidosis* caused by a deficiency in levels of the *enzyme* arylsulphatase B. The condition causes features similar to those of *Hurler's syndrome*, such as coarsening of the facial features, skeletal deformities, cardiac abnormalities, and enlargement of the liver and spleen; however, the affected child's level of intelligence is normal. The condition often appears early in childhood. There is no specific treatment, and death from *heart failure* often occurs between 20 and 30 years of age.

marriage guidance

See *relationship counselling*.

marrow, bone

See *bone marrow*.

marsupialization

A surgical procedure that is carried out to drain some types of *abscess* or *cyst* and to prevent further abscesses. It is used to treat certain types of cyst affecting the *pancreas* and *liver*, and cysts affecting the *Bartholin's glands* at the entrance to the vagina.

In marsupialization, the cyst is first cut open and drained, then its edges are stitched to the surrounding skin or tissue (to form a pouch) so that it is kept open until it has healed.

Marvelon

A brand-named *oral contraceptive* containing the synthetic female hormones *ethinylestradiol* (an oestrogen drug) and *desogestrel* (a progestogen).

masculinization

See *virilization*.

masking

A technique used in a *hearing test* that involves applying a noise to one ear while testing the hearing of the other.

The term "masking" may also be used in connection with pairs of *genes* in which the effects of an abnormal gene are concealed by its normal equivalent. (See *genetic disorders*; *inheritance*.)

masochism

A desire to be physically, mentally, or emotionally abused. The term "masochism" is primarily used to refer to obtaining sexual excitement through one's own suffering in activities such as bondage, flagellation, and verbal abuse. (See also *sadism*; *sadomasochism*.)

massage

Rubbing and kneading areas of the body, usually with the hands. Massage increases the blood flow and relaxes muscles; it may be used to relieve muscle spasm, treat muscle injury, and reduce *oedema* (accumulation of fluid in body tissues). Although massage is most effective when carried out by someone else, self-massage can alleviate pain caused by muscle tension.

masseter

The large muscle in the cheek that stretches between the cheekbone and the angle of the lower jaw. The muscle lifts the lower jaw during chewing.

mass hysteria

Intense emotion and irrational behaviour that spreads through a group of people in response to a highly exciting or upsetting event. The term may also be used to describe the occurrence of identical physical or emotional symptoms simultaneously in a particular group of people, such as children in the same class or school.

mastalgia

The medical term for pain in the *breast*.

mast cell

A type of cell that plays an important part in *allergy*. In an allergic response, antibodies (proteins produced by the immune system to neutralize an allergen) attach themselves to mast cells. The cells burst and release a chemical called *histamine*, which produces an inflammatory response in surrounding tissues, thereby causing many of the symptoms of allergic conditions.

mastectomy

The surgical removal of all of the *breast*, usually performed to treat *breast cancer*. Mastectomy may be used if the cancer cannot be removed by *lumpectomy* (removal of the tumour and a small area of surrounding tissue) or *quadrantectomy* (removal of part of the breast) because of its size or position. Occasionally, a prophylactic mastectomy may be recommended for women who have a high risk of developing breast cancer because they carry an abnormal gene that is associated with the disease.

HOW IT IS DONE

Formerly, a procedure called radical mastectomy was used; this involved removal of the breast together with an extensive area of muscle down to the chest wall. Today, however, the usual procedure is a total mastectomy. This operation involves removal of all of the breast tissue and usually some or all of the *lymph nodes* in the armpit. Cells from the nodes are examined to determine whether cancerous cells have spread. The operation is performed under a general *anaesthesia* and usually requires a stay in hospital of a few days. *Plastic surgery* to reconstruct the breast may be carried out at the same time as the mastectomy or at a later date (see *mammoplasty*).

RISKS

After the operation, the scar may be tender. If the lymph nodes have been removed, there is a risk of *lymphoedema* developing in the arm.

mastication

The process of chewing food. The canines and incisors (front teeth) shear the food. The tongue then pushes it between the upper and lower premolars and molars (back teeth) to be ground by movements of the lower jaw. *Saliva* is mixed with the food to help break it down for swallowing.

TYPES OF **MASTECTOMY**

The type of operation depends on many factors, including the size and site of the tumour and the woman's wishes. A small tumour may be treated by lumpectomy; other cases may require more extensive surgery.

LUMPECTOMY

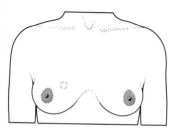

Site of incision for a lumpectomy
Only the cancerous tissue (shown here by a dotted line) and some of the surrounding normal tissue is removed. Lumpectomy leaves the breast looking relatively normal.

TOTAL MASTECTOMY

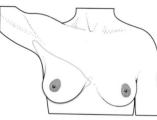

1 A large, elliptical incision that encompasses the nipple and sometimes the entire breast, is made. Part of the incision is extended into the armpit. All of the breast tissue, including the skin and some of the fat, is dissected (separated by cutting) down to the chest muscles. The dissection is continued under the skin into the armpit, to free the upper and outer "tail" of breast tissue with its lymph nodes.

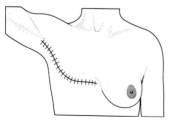

2 All of the bleeding vessels are tied off, then a drainage tube is inserted and the skin is closed with stitches or clips. The scar runs diagonally across the chest. The woman may wear a prosthesis or may have an implant inserted later.

mastitis

Inflammation of *breast* tissue. Mastitis is usually caused by bacterial infection and sometimes by hormonal changes.

CAUSES

Mastitis usually occurs when bacteria enter the nipple during *breast-feeding*. It can also be caused by changes in levels of *sex hormones* in the body – for example, at the onset of *puberty*.

SYMPTOMS

The condition causes pain, tenderness, and swelling in one or both breasts. Bacterial mastitis during breast-feeding also causes redness and *engorgement* and may result in a *breast abscess*.

TREATMENT

Mastitis due to infection is treated with *antibiotic drugs* and *analgesic drugs*, and by *expressing milk* to relieve engorgement. Mastitis caused by hormonal changes usually clears up in a few weeks without treatment.

mastocytosis

An unusual condition in which itchy, irregular, yellow or orange-brown swellings occur on the skin, most commonly on the trunk. Mastocytosis may also affect body organs, including the liver, spleen, and intestine, and may cause symptoms such as diarrhoea, vomiting, and fainting. Very rarely, it leads to *anaphylactic shock* (a severe form of allergic reaction), which can be fatal.

Mastocytosis usually begins in the first year of life and clears up by adolescence. *Antihistamine drugs* may be helpful in relieving the symptoms.

mastoid

The lower part of the temporal bone in the *skull*. The mastoid has a projection, called the mastoid process, which can be felt behind the ear. The bone is honeycombed with cavities called air cells; these spaces are connected to a larger cavity called the mastoid antrum, which leads into the middle ear.

In some cases, infections of the middle ear (see *otitis media*) spread through the mastoid bone to cause acute *mastoiditis*.

mastoiditis

Inflammation of the *mastoid* (lower part of the temporal bone in the skull).

CAUSE

Mastoiditis is due to infection spreading from the middle ear (see *otitis media*) to the air cells in the mastoid through a cavity called the mastoid antrum.

SYMPTOMS

The condition causes earache and severe pain, swelling, and tenderness behind the ear. There is usually also fever, a creamy discharge from the ear, progressive hearing loss, and displacement of the outer ear.

If the infection spreads, it may lead to complications such as *meningitis*, a *brain abscess*, blood clotting in veins within the brain, or *facial palsy*.

TREATMENT

Mastoiditis is treated with *antibiotic drugs*. However, if the infection persists, an operation called a mastoidectomy may be carried out; in this procedure, the mastoid is opened and the infected air cells are removed.

LOCATION OF **MASTOID**

The mastoid is the lower part of the temporal bone. The mastoid process can be felt as a hard prominence just behind the ear.

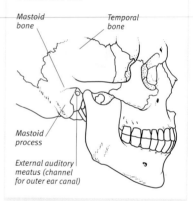

masturbation

Sexual self-stimulation, usually to produce *orgasm*. Massaging the *penis* or the *clitoris* with the hand is the usual method of masturbation.

maternal mortality

The death of a woman during *pregnancy*, or within 42 days of *childbirth, miscarriage*, or an *induced abortion*, from any pregnancy-related cause. Maternal mortality rate is the number of such deaths per 100,000 live births as measured over a given year.

Maternal deaths may be a direct result of complications of pregnancy or they may be caused indirectly by a medical condition that is worsened by pregnancy. The major direct causes of death include *pulmonary embolism* (blood clots in the lungs), *antepartum haemorrhage*, *postpartum haemorrhage*, *hypertension* (high blood pressure), *eclampsia* (a condition causing seizures in late pregnancy), and *puerperal sepsis* (infection following childbirth). Indirect causes of maternal mortality include heart disease, *epilepsy*, and some cancers.

Maternal mortality is lowest for second pregnancies. After the age of 20, it rises with age, being greatest for women over the age of 40.

maturation

The process by which full development is reached. The term "maturation" is used with reference to cells (particularly *ova* and *sperm*) and some microorganisms; it may also be used of physical and emotional development in people.

maxilla

Each of a pair of bones that together form the centre of the face, the upper jaw, and the roof of the mouth. In addition, the top of the maxilla forms the base of the orbit (eye socket). Each bone contains a large, air-filled cavity called the maxillary sinus (see *sinus, facial*), which is connected to the nasal cavity.

MCADD

A rare inherited metabolic disorder in which there is lack of an enzyme needed to convert fats into energy. As a result, affected children cannot go without food for long before their blood glucose falls to potentially dangerous levels.

SYMPTOMS

Typically, symptoms do not appear until between about three months and two years after birth and are often triggered by an illness or a period of feeding poorly. Initially there may be irritability, extreme sleepiness, and sometimes fever, diarrhoea, and vomiting. Without prompt treatment, breathing problems, seizures, and unconsciousness may develop. In some cases, there may brain damage, heart failure, or even death.

TREATMENT AND OUTLOOK

Treatment primarily consists of ensuring that an affected child feeds regularly. A dietitian will be able to advise about a suitable diet. With early detection, a suitable dietary regimen, and careful monitoring, an affected child should be able to live a normal life.

PREVENTION

MCADD cannot be prevented but it can be detected shortly after birth by *blood spot screening tests*.

McArdle's disease

A rare *genetic disorder* characterized by muscle stiffness and painful cramps that increase during exertion and afterwards. The cause is a deficiency of an *enzyme* in muscle cells that stimulates breakdown of the carbohydrate *glycogen* into glucose. The result is a buildup of glycogen and low levels of glucose in the muscles. Damage to the muscles occurs, causing myoglobinuria (the presence of pigment from muscle cells in the urine); this, in turn, may lead to *kidney failure*.

There is no treatment, but symptoms may be relieved by eating glucose or fructose before exercise.

MDMA

The hallucinogenic substance methylenedioxymethamfetamine, which has the street name *Ecstasy*.

ME

The abbreviation for myalgic encephalomyelitis (see *chronic fatigue syndrome*).

measles

A potentially dangerous viral illness that causes fever and a rash. Measles mainly affects children, but can occur at any age. It is spread primarily by airborne droplets of nasal secretions. There is an *incubation period* of about 12 to 14 days after infection before the rash appears. Measles is highly contagious from the time symptoms first appear until four days after the appearance of the rash.

LOCATION OF THE **MAXILLA**

The maxillae are a pair of bones that form the base of the eye sockets, the centre of the face, the upper jaw, and the roof of the mouth.

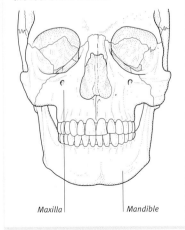

Maxilla   Mandible

SYMPTOMS AND SIGNS

The illness starts with a fever, runny nose, sore eyes, cough, and a general feeling of being unwell. After three to four days, a red rash appears, usually starting on the head and neck and spreading to cover the body. The spots sometimes join to produce large red blotches, and the *lymph nodes* may be enlarged. After three days, the rash starts to fade and the symptoms subside.

COMPLICATIONS

The most common complications are ear and chest infections, which usually develop two to three days after the rash has appeared. Diarrhoea, vomiting, and abdominal pain may occur. Febrile convulsions (see *convulsion, febrile*) are also common, but are not usually serious.

In a tiny minority of cases, *encephalitis* (inflammation of the brain) occurs, causing headache, drowsiness, and vomiting. Seizures and *coma* may follow, sometimes leading to *brain damage* or even death. In very rare cases, a progressive brain disorder called *subacute sclerosing panencephalitis* develops several years after infection.

If a woman has measles during pregnancy, the infection may be fatal to the fetus; however, there is no evidence that measles causes birth defects.

TREATMENT

There is no specific treatment. Plenty of fluids and *paracetamol* are given for fever. In addition, *antibiotic drugs* may be given to treat bacterial infections that occur as complications.

PREVENTION

Immunization with the *MMR vaccination* is recommended at around 13 months of age, with a booster at between three years four months and five years of age. This measure produces immunity in over 90 per cent of cases.

meatus

A canal or passageway through part of the body. The term usually refers to the external auditory meatus, the canal in the outer *ear* that leads from the outside of the ear to the eardrum.

mebendazole

An *anthelmintic drug* that is used to treat various *worm infestations* of the intestine. Possible adverse effects include abdominal pain and diarrhoea.

mebeverine

An *antispasmodic drug* that is used to treat *irritable bowel syndrome*.

M

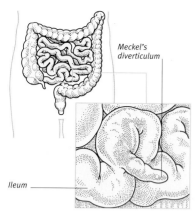

Anatomy of Meckel's diverticulum
In this common birth defect, an appendix-type sac protrudes from the ileum (the last section of the small intestine).

Meckel's diverticulum

A common abnormality, present at birth in about 1 in 40 people, in which a small, hollow, wide-mouthed sac protrudes from the *ileum*. Symptoms only occur if the diverticulum becomes infected, obstructed, or ulcerated. The most common symptom is painless bleeding from the rectum; this bleeding may be sudden and severe, making immediate *blood transfusion* necessary. Inflammation may cause symptoms very similar to those of *appendicitis*, such as lower abdominal pain. Meckel's diverticulum occasionally causes *intussusception* (telescoping) or *volvulus* (twisting) of the small intestine.

Diagnosis of the abnormality may be made by using technetium *radionuclide scanning*. If any complications develop, they will be treated by surgical removal of the diverticulum.

meconium

The thick, sticky, greenish-black faeces that is passed by infants in the first day or two after birth. Meconium consists of *bile*, mucus, and intestinal cells that have been shed.

Occasionally, the fetus passes meconium into the *amniotic fluid* while still in the uterus. This problem is more common in those babies who experience *fetal distress* during labour or who are over 40 weeks' gestation. Meconium in the amniotic fluid may be inhaled when the baby starts to breathe, sometimes blocking the airways and damaging the lungs. In some babies with *cystic fibrosis*, the meconium is so thick and sticky that it blocks the intestine (see *intestine, obstruction of*).

medial

A medical term that means "situated towards the midline of the body". Less commonly, the term refers to the middle layer of a body structure.

median nerve

One of the main nerves of the arm. The median nerve is a branch of the *brachial plexus* and runs down the arm from the shoulder into the hand. It controls the muscles that carry out bending movements of the wrist, fingers, and thumb, and the muscles that rotate the forearm palm-inwards. The nerve also conveys sensations from the thumb and first three fingers, and from the region of the palm at their base.

DISORDERS
Damage to the nerve may result from injury to the shoulder, a *Colles' fracture* just above the wrist, or pressure on the nerve where it passes through the wrist (*carpal tunnel syndrome*). Symptoms of damage include numbness and weakness in areas controlled by the nerve.

mediastinoscopy

Viewing of the *mediastinum* using an *endoscope* inserted through an incision just above the sternum (breastbone). The procedure is performed under general anaesthesia.

Mediastinoscopy is used mainly to perform a *biopsy* of a *lymph node*, often in diagnosing *lymphoma*. The tissue sample is removed by tiny blades attached to the endoscope.

mediastinum

The membranous partition between the lungs and the other structures within the chest cavity. These other structures include the *heart* and associated blood vessels; the *trachea* (windpipe); the *oesophagus*; the *thymus* gland; *lymph nodes*; lymphatic vessels; and nerves.

MedicAlert bracelet

An item, available from a charitable organization called the MedicAlert foundation, that provides vital information about a person's identity and medical status in case he or she needs urgent medical help. The items are designed to be worn by individuals with a hidden medical condition (such as *epilepsy* or *diabetes mellitus*) or a serious allergy (such as *penicillin allergy*).

MedicAlert bracelets, and necklaces, are engraved with an emblem that is instantly recognizable to medical workers. The bracelets and necklaces carry details of important medical conditions that affect the wearer, a personal identification number, and a 24-hour telephone number so that any further medical details can be accessed anywhere in the world.

medical ethics

The professional values and guidelines that govern medical decisions, particularly medical practitioners' treatment of patients and their relatives and of colleagues. Ethical requirements also play a part in medical research; for example, when new drugs or other treatments are tested on patients, the trials must be designed so that they will not cause any harm to the patients involved.

medical history

See *history-taking*.

medical tests

See *tests, medical*.

medication

Any substance prescribed to treat disease. (See also *drug; medicine*.)

medicine

The study of human diseases and their causes, frequency, treatment, and prevention. The term "medicine" is also used of a substance that is prescribed to treat an illness. In some circumstances, it is used to refer to treatments that do not involve surgery.

medicolegal

A term used of matters in which medicine and the law overlap. Among the issues on which medicolegal experts advise people are laws concerning damages for injuries that are due to medical negligence or malpractice; evidence concerning the extent of injury in a civil action; the use of paternity tests; the mental competence of people who have drawn up wills; and restrictions placed on mentally ill people.

Medicolegal issues also include an individual's right to die (see *brain death*; *euthanasia*; *living will*); the necessity for informed *consent* to any surgical procedure; the legal aspects of *artificial insemination*, *in vitro fertilization*, *sterilization*, and *surrogacy*; and a patient's right to *confidentiality* concerning his or her illness or other medical informaation. (For the medical aspects of criminal law, see *forensic medicine*.)

LANDMARKS IN **MEDICINE**: DIAGNOSIS

Date	Development
c.400 BC	**Disease concept** Introduced by the Greek physician Hippocrates.
1612	**Medical thermometer** Devised by the Italian physician Sanctorius.
c.1660	**Light microscope** Single-lens microscope developed by the Dutch naturalist Antonj van Leeuwenhoek, who discovered microorganisms with it. A practicable compound microscope was not developed until the 19th century.
1810	**Stethoscope** Invented by the French physician René Laennec.
1850–1900	**Germ theory of disease** Proposed by the French scientist Louis Pasteur and developed by the German bacteriologist Robert Koch.
1851	**Ophthalmoscope** Invented by the German scientist Herman von Helmholtz.
1895	**X-rays** Discovered by the German physicist Wilhelm Roentgen. He also produced the first X-ray picture of the body.
1906	**Electrocardiograph (ECG)** Invented by the Dutch physiologist Willem Einthoven.
c.1932	**Transmission electron microscope (TEM)** Constructed by the German scientists Max Knoll and Ernst Ruska.
1938	**Cardiac catheterization** First performed by George Peter Robb and Israel Steinberg in New York.
1957	**Fibre-optic endoscopy** Pioneered by the South African-born doctor Basil Hirschowitz at the University of Michigan.
1972	**CT scanner** Invented by the British engineer Godfrey Hounsfield of EMI Laboratories, England, and the South African-born physicist Alan Cormack of Tufts University, Massachusetts.
1975	**Monoclonal antibodies** Large-scale production method for monoclonal antibodies developed by the Argentinian-born scientist César Milstein at the Medical Research Council Laboratories, England.
1976	**Chorionic villus sampling** Developed by Chinese gynaecologists as an aid to the early diagnosis of genetic disorders.
1981	**MRI scanner** Developed by scientists at Thorn-EMI Laboratories and Nottingham University, England.
1985	**Polymerase chain reaction** Rapid copying of DNA sequences developed by Kary Mullis of the Cetus Corporation, California.
1995	**Genetics** Chromosome sequence of first nonviral organism, *Haemophilus influenzae*, identified.
2003	**Human Genome** Completion of the Human Genome Project by the International Human Genome International Consortium, following first draft produced in 2001.

meditation

Concentration on an object, a word, or an idea with the aim of inducing an altered state of consciousness. At its deepest level, meditation can resemble a trance. More commonly, it is a calming therapy and can be a way to reduce stress levels and treat stress-related disorders. A common form of meditation practised in Europe and North America is transcendental meditation (TM).

Mediterranean diet

A diet based on the traditional foods eaten in Mediterranean countries, where people have a lower risk of cardiovascular disease and *cancer* than people in northern European countries. The bulk of the diet consists of fruit, vegetables, and grain-based foods such as pasta and couscous. The major source of fat is olive oil, a *monounsaturated* fat (see *fats and oils*). The diet also includes fish, but only small amounts of meat, poultry, eggs, and dairy products.

Mediterranean fever

See *brucellosis*.

Mediterranean fever, familial

See *familial Mediterranean fever*.

medroxyprogesterone

A *progestogen drug* used to treat *endometriosis* (a condition in which fragments of uterine lining are found in the pelvic cavity), as well as uterine cancer (see *uterus, cancer of*). In addition, medroxyprogesterone is sometimes used to treat menstrual disorders such as *amenorrhoea* (absence of menstruation). The drug can also be used as a contraceptive, given by injection at three-month intervals (see *contraception, hormonal methods of*) and, with oestrogen, as *hormone replacement therapy*. Possible adverse effects of medroxyprogesterone include weight gain, swollen ankles, and breast tenderness.

medulla

The innermost part of a body structure; for example, the adrenal medulla is the central area of an *adrenal gland*. In addition, the word "medulla" is sometimes used to refer to the *medulla oblongata*.

medulla oblongata

Also called the *medulla*, the lowest part of the *brainstem*. The medulla oblongata lies at the base of the skull. It connects the brain to the *spinal cord*.

M

LANDMARKS IN **MEDICINE:** SURGERY

Date	Development
1545	**Basic surgical** principles Established by the French surgeon Ambroise Paré.
1842	**General anaesthesia** First operation using general anaesthesia performed by the American surgeon Crawford Long, who used ether. In 1845, the American dentist Horace Wells used nitrous oxide (laughing gas) as an anaesthetic. In 1847, the British obstetrician James Simpson introduced chloroform anaesthesia.
1870	**Antiseptic surgery** Pioneered by the British surgeon Joseph Lister, who used a carbolic acid (phenol) spray during surgery to help prevent infection.
1901	**Blood groups** ABO blood groups discovered by the Austrian pathologist Karl Landsteiner, so establishing the basis for safe transfusions.
1951	**Coronary artery bypass graft** First attempted by the Canadian surgeon Arthur Vineberg at the Royal Victoria Hospital, Montreal.
1955	**Kidney transplant** First successful kidney transplant (between identical twins) performed by a team of American surgeons, led by Joseph Murray, of the Harvard Medical School, Massachusetts.
1967	**Heart transplant** First human heart transplant performed by the South African surgeon Christian Barnaard at the Groote Schur Hospital, Cape Town.
1976	**Coronary angioplasty** Introduced by the Swiss surgeon Andreas Grüntzig at the University Hospital, Zurich.
1987	**Minimally invasive surgery** The first cholecystectomy (gallbladder removal) using laparoscopic techniques under video control performed by the French doctor P. Mouret, in Lyon.
1998	**Robotic surgery** First coronary artery bypass surgery using a robot performed by a team under Professor Friedrich-Wilhelm Mohr, at Leipzig Heart Centre, Germany.

LANDMARKS IN **MEDICINE:** OTHER TREATMENTS

Date	Development
c.1270	**Glasses** Thought to have been invented in Italy. Contact lenses were invented in 1887 by the Swiss optician Eugen Frick.
1817	**Dental plate** Introduced by the American dentist Anthony Plantson.
1891	**Baby incubator** Introduced by the French doctor Alexandre Lion.
1901	**Hearing-aid (electric)** Developed by the American inventor Miller Reese Hutchinson. The first truly miniature hearing-aid was introduced in 1952 by the Sonotone Corporation.
1545	**Kidney dialysis machine** Developed by the Dutch surgeon Willem Kolff.
1978	**"Test-tube baby"** Louise Brown, the first baby resulting from in vitro fertilization, was born in the UK. The IVF techniques were developed by the British gynaecologist Patrick Steptoe and the embryologist Robert Edwards.
1979	**Shock-wave lithotripsy** Pioneered by researchers at the University Hospital, Munich, Germany.
1990	**Gene therapy** First attempted at the US National Institute of Health, by doctors W. French Anderson, Michael Blaese, and Kenneth W. Culver, to treat a four-year-old girl with a form of severe combined immunodeficiency (SCID). Gene therapy has since had some success, but to date it is still at an experimental stage.

medulloblastoma

A type of cancerous *brain tumour* that occurs mainly in children. It usually arises from the *cerebellum*, the region of the brain concerned with posture, balance, and coordination. The tumour grows rapidly and may spread to other parts of the brain and to the *spinal cord*. A morning headache, repeated vomiting, and a clumsy gait develop. There are also frequent falls.

The tumour is diagnosed by *CT scanning* or *MRI* and is treated with surgery, *radiotherapy*, and *anticancer drugs*.

mefenamic acid

An NSAID (see *nonsteroidal anti-inflammatory drugs*) used to relieve pain and inflammation. Mefenamic acid may be given for conditions such as headache, toothache, and *dysmenorrhoea* (painful menstrual periods), and to reduce *menorrhagia* (excessive menstrual bleeding). It may also be prescribed for relief of joint pain and stiffness in *osteoarthritis* and *rheumatoid arthritis*.

Possible adverse effects are typical for NSAIDs; they include abdominal pain, indigestion, nausea, and vomiting.

mefloquine

A drug used to prevent *malaria* in parts of the world where the parasite that causes it is resistant to *chloroquine*.

Side effects include nausea, vomiting, and diarrhoea. Rarely, there may be *panic attacks*, *hallucinations*, and *psychosis*. Mefloquine is not recommended for people who have a history of disorders such as *depression* or seizures.

mega-

A prefix meaning "very large", as in *megacolon*. The prefix "megalo-" has the same meaning.

megacolon

A gross distension (enlargement) of the *colon*, usually accompanied by severe, chronic *constipation*.

CAUSES
In children, the main causes of megacolon are *anal fissures*, *Hirschsprung's disease*, and psychological factors that may have arisen during toilet-training. In elderly people, causes include long-term use of strong *laxative drugs*. People suffering from chronic *depression* or *schizophrenia* often have megacolon. Other, rarer causes include *hypothyroidism*, *spinal injury*, and the use of drugs such as *morphine* and *codeine*.

LANDMARKS IN **MEDICINE**: DRUGS

Date	Development
1666	**Quinine** The British physician Thomas Sydenham popularized the use of Jesuits' bark (containing quinine) for treating malaria.
1785	**Digitalis** The use of digitalis to treat heart failure described by the British physician William Withering.
1796	**Smallpox vaccination** The first vaccination to be performed, by the British physician Edward Jenner. The first true vaccine (consisting of weakened microorganisms), against chicken cholera, was developed in 1880 by the French scientist Louis Pasteur.
1805	**Morphine** Extracted from opium and used to relieve pain, by the German pharmacist Friedrich Sertürner.
1911	**Salvarsan** Introduced by the German bacteriologist Paul Ehrlich to treat syphilis.
1928	**Penicillin** Antibacterial action first recognized by the British bacteriologist Alexander Fleming. Produced as a drug in 1940, by the Australian-born British pathologist Howard Florey and the German-born British biochemist Ernst Chain.
1935	**Sulphonamides** Antibacterial action discovered by the German pharmacologist Gerhard Domagk.
1951	**Oral contraceptive** Developed by the American doctors Gregory Pincus and John Rock, and the Austrian-born American chemist Carl Djerassi.
1959	**Librium (chlordiazepoxide)** The first benzodiazepine minor tranquillizer, introduced by the Swiss pharmaceutical company Hoffmann-LaRoche.
1962	**Nethalide (pronethalol)** The first beta-blocker heart drug, developed by scientists at Imperial Chemical Industries, England.
1984	**Genetically engineered human insulin** Developed by scientists at Genentech, California.
1986	**Zidovudine (originally called AZT)** Introduced to treat AIDS after development by scientists at Burroughs Wellcome Research Laboratories, North Carolina.
1998	**Viagra (sildenafil)** Introduced as a treatment for erectile dysfunction after development by the Pfizer Corporation, US.

SYMPTOMS

Megacolon causes constipation and abdominal bloating. Some affected individuals experience loss of appetite, which may lead to weight loss. Diarrhoea may occur if semi-liquid faeces leak around the obstructing hard faeces.

DIAGNOSIS AND TREATMENT

The diagnosis is made by *proctoscopy*, *barium X-ray examination*, and tests to assess the functioning of the intestinal muscles. If Hirschsprung's disease is suspected, *biopsy* of the large intestine may be performed.

Impacted faeces are often removed using *enemas*. In severe cases, the faeces must be removed manually.

megaloblastic anaemia

See *anaemia, megaloblastic*.

megalomania

An exaggerated sense of one's importance or ability that often occurs in *mania*. Megalomania may take the form of a *delusion* of grandeur, or may manifest itself as a desire to organize large-scale activities that are expensive and involve many people.

-megaly

A suffix that means "enlargement", as in *acromegaly*, a rare disorder in which the jaw, skull, hands, feet, and internal organs are enlarged.

megaureter

Gross distension (widening) of a *ureter*, the tube that carries urine from each kidney to the bladder. One possible cause of megaureter is a long-standing blockage in the ureter that stops the flow of urine. Another is backward flow of urine from the bladder into the ureters while the bladder is being emptied (see *vesicoureteric reflux*). In some cases, the condition is congenital (present at birth) and has no known cause.

Megaureter is treated by surgery to remove blockages or to relieve reflux.

megestrol

A *progestogen drug* that is used to treat uterine cancer (see *uterus, cancer of*) and certain types of *breast cancer*. Megestrol may be prescribed when a tumour is inoperable, if a tumour has recurred after surgery, or when other *anticancer drugs* or *radiotherapy* prove ineffective.

Possible adverse effects of the drug include swollen ankles, weight gain, nausea, dizziness, headache, rash, and, rarely, raised blood calcium levels.

meibomian cyst

See *chalazion*.

meibomian gland

A small sebaceous (oil-secreting) gland situated under the *conjunctiva* (membranous lining) of each eyelid. If one of the glands becomes blocked, it enlarges to create a swelling known as a *chalazion*.

meibomianitis

Inflammation of the *meibomian glands*, the sebaceous (oil-secreting) glands within the eyelids. The condition is caused by excessive or unusually thick glandular secretions, which result in an overgrowth of bacteria on the eyelids. Conditions that can increase the secretions include skin disorders affecting the face (such as *acne* or *rosacea*), allergic reactions, and the hormonal changes that occur in adolescence.

Symptoms of meibomianitis include swelling of the eyelid edges, brief blurring of the vision due to oily tears, and frequent *styes*. Careful cleansing of the eyelids may relieve the symptoms. Antibiotic eye ointment may be prescribed to clear up infection.

Meig's syndrome

A rare condition in which a tumour of an *ovary* is accompanied by *ascites* (an accumulation of fluid in the abdomen)

M

and a *pleural effusion* (fluid around one of the lungs). The fluid usually disappears when the tumour is removed.

meiosis

A type of cell division that occurs in the *ovaries* and *testes* during the production of egg and sperm cells. During meiosis in humans, a cell containing 23 pairs of *chromosomes* (46 in total) divides to form four sperm or egg cells, each with 23 single chromosomes.

First, each chromosome is duplicated (making a total of 92); the doubled chromosomes are joined at a point called the centromere. Matching pairs of doubled chromosomes line up and exchange genetic material. The cell then divides twice to form four daughter cells, with each taking one copy of each chromosome.

Egg and sperm cells therefore have 23 single chromosomes, which is only half the usual chromosome content of a body cell, so each parent contributes half of the offspring's genetic material. The exchange between chromosomes means that each daughter cell has a unique genetic make-up. (See also *mitosis*).

melaena

Black, tarry *faeces* caused by bleeding, usually in the upper gastrointestinal tract. The blood is blackened by the action of secretions during digestion. Melaena is usually caused by a *peptic ulcer* but may indicate cancer.

melancholia

Former term for *depression*.

melanin

The brown or black pigment that gives skin, hair, and the iris of the eyes their colouring. Melanin is produced by cells called *melanocytes*.

Exposure to sunlight increases the production of melanin, which protects the skin from the harmful effects of ultraviolet rays and causes the skin to darken. Localized overproduction of melanin in the skin can result in a pigmented spot, most commonly a *freckle* or mole (see *naevus*).

melanocyte

A specialized type of skin cell that produces the pigment *melanin*. Melanocytes can be damaged by overexposure to sunlight; this damage may result in a form of skin cancer known as malignant melanoma (see *melanoma, malignant*).

MECHANISM OF **MEIOSIS**

In meiosis, a cell in the *testis* or *ovary* containing 46 chromosomes undergoes chromosome duplication then divides to form four germ cells (sperm or eggs), each with 23 chromosomes. Germ cells have only half the usual chromosome content because a child can receive only half the genes of each parent.

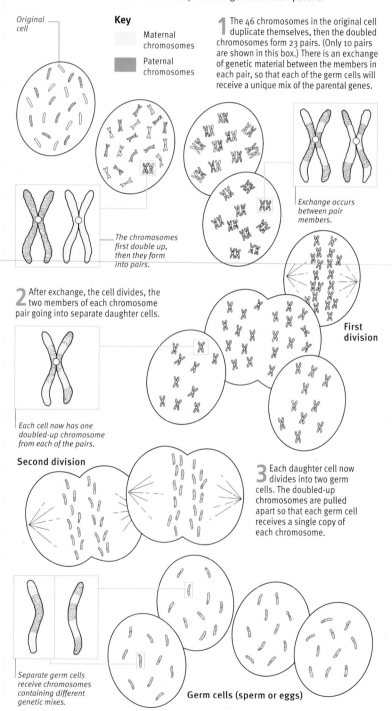

1 The 46 chromosomes in the original cell duplicate themselves, then the doubled chromosomes form 23 pairs. (Only 10 pairs are shown in this box.) There is an exchange of genetic material between the members in each pair, so that each of the germ cells will receive a unique mix of the parental genes.

Original cell

Key
Maternal chromosomes
Paternal chromosomes

The chromosomes first double up, then they form into pairs.

Exchange occurs between pair members.

2 After exchange, the cell divides, the two members of each chromosome pair going into separate daughter cells.

Each cell now has one doubled-up chromosome from each of the pairs.

First division

Second division

3 Each daughter cell now divides into two germ cells. The doubled-up chromosomes are pulled apart so that each germ cell receives a single copy of each chromosome.

Separate germ cells receive chromosomes containing different genetic mixes.

Germ cells (sperm or eggs)

melanoma, juvenile

A raised, reddish-brown skin blemish, also called a Spitz naevus, which sometimes appears on the face or legs in early childhood (see *naevus*). Despite the name, it is noncancerous. Although it is harmless, an unsightly growth, or one that is suspected of being skin cancer, may be removed surgically.

melanoma, malignant

The most serious of the three types of skin cancer. (The other two forms of the disorder are *basal cell carcinoma* and *squamous cell carcinoma*.) If left untreated, the cancer may be fatal.

CAUSE AND INCIDENCE

Malignant melanoma is a tumour of melanocytes (cells that produce the pigment *melanin*) and is due to long-term exposure to strong sunlight. It is most common in middle-aged and elderly people with pale skin and fair hair who have spent many years in sunny climates.

There are increasing numbers of new cases and deaths in the UK each year from this skin cancer, probably due to people sunbathing and taking holidays in sunny countries. Severe sunburn during childhood doubles the risk of developing melanoma in later life. The use of sunbeds is also associated with an increased risk of developing melanoma.

SYMPTOMS

Tumours usually develop on areas of exposed skin but may occur anywhere on the body, including in the eye. In many cases, a melanoma grows from an existing mole. An affected mole may change colour, increase in size, or develop an irregular edge. Other signs include a mole becoming lumpy, bleeding or crusting, forming a scab, or becoming itchy or inflamed. Such changes should be reported to a doctor immediately. A melanoma may also develop in normal skin, and sometimes a melanoma does

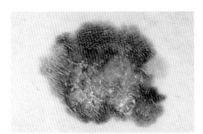

Development of malignant melanoma
Only one mole in a million becomes malignant. However, change of shape, darkening, tenderness, pain, itching, or ulceration are warning signs of a malignant melanoma.

not have any pigment (known as amelanotic melanoma). If left untreated, the cancer can grow down through the layers of skin and rapidly spread to other parts of the body.

DIAGNOSIS AND TREATMENT

Early diagnosis is vital to help prevent life-threatening spread of the cancer. Diagnosis is by a *skin biopsy*, in which tissue from the growth, together with some of the surrounding skin, is removed for microscopic examination. Samples from nearby *lymph nodes* may also be examined; the presence of any cancerous cells in these samples would indicate that the cancer has spread.

The melanoma, together with a wide area of surrounding skin, will be removed surgically. Treatment may also include *radiotherapy, anticancer drugs*, and *immunotherapy*.

melanonychia

Black or dark coloration of a fingernail or toenail, due to an excess of the pigment *melanin*. The colour often forms a vertical streak down the nail.

Melanonychia is normal in some black and Asian people. In white people, it may be caused by a *naevus* (pigmented blemish) beneath the nail; melanoma (see *melanoma, malignant*); a reaction to a drug; or *HIV* infection.

melanosis coli

Black or brown discoloration of the colon lining. Melanosis coli is associated with chronic *constipation* and prolonged use of certain *laxative drugs*, such as senna, rhubarb, and cascara.

The discoloration is most common in elderly people and is usually symptomless. It clears up when the laxatives are no longer used. Rarely, it is associated with colon cancer (see *colon, cancer of*).

melasma

See *chloasma*.

melatonin

A *hormone* secreted by the *pineal gland* in the brain that is thought to play a part in controlling daily body rhythms and regulating the sleep-wake cycle. Levels of melatonin rise in response to decreasing light, preparing the body for sleep.

melphalan

An *anticancer drug* used to treat *multiple myeloma* as well as certain types of *breast cancer* and ovarian cancer (see *ovary, cancer of*). Possible adverse effects

include nausea, vomiting, sore throat, loss of appetite, reduced numbers of red and other blood cells (see *anaemia, aplastic*), abnormal bleeding, and increased susceptibility to infection.

membrane

A layer of tissue that covers or lines a body surface or forms a barrier.

memory

The ability to remember. Memory is usually regarded as comprising three stages: registration, retention, and recall. In registration, information is perceived, is understood, and is then held in the short-term memory. In retention, more important information is transferred into the long-term memory and then stored. Recall involves bringing information into the conscious mind at will. There are a number of factors that determine how well information is remembered, including its familiarity and how much attention has been paid to it.

Where in the brain the memory process takes place is not known. However, the temporal lobe and *limbic system* may be involved. The mechanisms for storing memory are also unknown.

THE STAGES OF MEMORY

Stage 1: Registration
Information is perceived and understood, then held in a short-term memory system. This system seems to be very limited in the amount of material that it can store at one time. Unless refreshed by constant repetition, the contents of short-term memory are lost within minutes, to be replaced by other material.

Stage 2: Retention
If information is sufficiently important, it is transferred into long-term memory for storage. The process of storage involves association of the information with certain words or meanings, with visual imagery evoked by it, or with other experiences, such as smell or sound.

Stage 3: Recall
Information that has been stored at an unconscious level, in long-term memory, is brought into the conscious mind by an act of will. The reliability of the recall process depends on how well the information was encoded in stage 2.

DISORDERS

Most memory disturbances are due to failure at the retention or recall stage (see *amnesia*). In some cases, the problem occurs at the registration stage. Some people with *temporal lobe epilepsy* have uncontrollable flashbacks of distant past events. The most common memory disorder is the normal difficulty in recall that develops with age. More severe loss of memory may be an early symptom of *dementia*.

memory B-cell

A type of white blood cell, also known as a memory B-lymphocyte (see *lymphocyte*), that is involved in the *immune system* response to invading *bacteria*. Memory B-cells recognize bacteria that the body has previously encountered. They promptly produce huge quantities of *antibodies* that inactivate the bacteria, thus preventing or shortening the organisms' effects. (See also *memory T-cell*.)

memory, loss of

See *amnesia*.

memory T-cell

A type of white blood cell, also known as a memory T-lymphocyte (see *lymphocyte*), that is involved in the *immune system* response to viruses, parasites, and cancer cells. Memory T-cells recognize viruses, parasites, or cancer cells that the body has previously encountered. Some belong to the class of *killer T-cells*, which attach themselves to infected cells and then release toxic proteins to destroy the cells. (See also *memory B-cell*.)

menarche

The onset of *menstruation*. Menarche usually occurs around the age of 12 or 13, two years after *puberty* starts.

Mendelian inheritance

A form of *inheritance* first described by the Austrian monk Gregor Mendel. He discovered that certain distinct, unchanging physical characteristics are controlled by factors that are now called *genes*, which are transmitted through many generations. He also revealed the existence of *dominant* and *recessive* genetic characteristics.

Mendel formulated two laws concerning inheritance. Mendel's first law, or the law of segregation, states that the characteristics of an organism are determined by pairs of genes, and that

during reproduction the genes in each pair separate, with only one *allele* (gene from a pair) being carried in a *gamete* (egg or sperm cell) and passed on to an offspring (see *meiosis*). Mendel's second law, or the law of independent assortment, states that each gene in a pair can be combined with either of the genes from any other pair, so that gametes can show all possible combinations of nonpaired genes.

Mendelson's syndrome

Inhalation of regurgitated stomach contents by someone who is under general *anaesthesia*; also called pulmonary acid aspiration syndrome. Stomach acid can damage the mucous membranes lining the airways; it can also cause bronchospasm (sudden constriction of the airways leading to each lung), and pulmonary oedema (a buildup of fluid in the lungs). Breathing may be severely impaired and the person may die.

The problem is particularly associated with general anaesthesia for emergency obstetric procedures during labour. It can be prevented by giving drugs to inhibit stomach acid secretion before operating.

Ménière's disease

An inner *ear* disorder characterized by recurrent *vertigo* (a spinning sensation), *deafness*, and *tinnitus* (ringing in the ears). It is uncommon before the age of 40.

CAUSE

The cause of the disorder is an accumulation of fluid in the *labyrinth*. The buildup may damage the labyrinth and sometimes the adjacent *cochlea*.

SYMPTOMS

There is a sudden attack of vertigo, lasting from a few minutes to several hours. This is usually accompanied by nausea, vomiting, *nystagmus* (abnormal jerky eye movements), and deafness, tinnitus, and a feeling of pressure or pain in the affected ear.

DIAGNOSIS AND TREATMENT

Diagnosis is usually made with audiometry (see *hearing tests*) or other hearing tests, and a *caloric test*.

Treatment with certain *antihistamine drugs*, such as *cinnarizine*, or with *betahistine* usually relieves the symptoms. *Prochlorperazine* may be given, either rectally or by injection, for severe attacks. Severe Ménière's disease that cannot be controlled by drugs can be treated by surgery to the inner ear. If deafness eventually becomes total, the other symptoms usually disappear.

meninges

The three membranes that cover and protect the *brain* and the *spinal cord*. The outermost membrane, the dura mater, is tough and fibrous; it lines the inside of the skull and forms a loose sheath around the spinal cord. The middle membrane, the arachnoid mater, is elastic and weblike. The innermost membrane, the pia mater, lies next to the surface of the brain.

The pia mater is separated from the arachnoid mater by the subarachnoid space, which contains *cerebrospinal fluid*. Another space, called the subdural space, separates the arachnoid mater from the dura mater.

meningioma

A rare, noncancerous tumour of the *meninges* (the membranes surrounding the brain). A meningioma arises from the arachnoid mater (the middle membrane) and, in most cases, it then becomes attached to the dura mater (the outer membrane).

The meningioma slowly expands and may become very large before any symptoms appear. The symptoms may include headache, vomiting, and impaired mental function. There may also be speech loss or visual disturbance. If the tumour invades the overlying skull bone, there may be thickening and bulging of the skull.

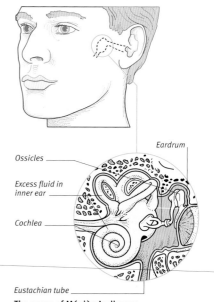

Ossicles

Eardrum

Excess fluid in inner ear

Cochlea

Eustachian tube

The cause of Ménière's disease
This condition is caused by excessive fluid in the labyrinth and cochlea, in the inner ear. These structures may become damaged as a result.

M

ANATOMY OF THE **MENINGES**

The pia mater lies on the brain. It is separated from the arachnoid mater by the subarachnoid space. The outermost membrane, the dura mater, lines the inside of the skull.

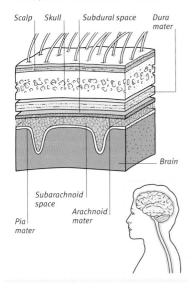

Meningiomas can be detected by *X-ray*, *CT scanning*, *MRI*, or *angiography*. The tumours can often be completely removed by surgery. Otherwise, treatment is by *radiotherapy*.

meningitis

Inflammation of the *meninges* (membranes covering the *brain* and *spinal cord*), usually due to infection.

CAUSES

Viral meningitis tends to occur in epidemics in winter; it is usually relatively mild. Bacterial meningitis, however, is life-threatening. It is mainly caused by HAEMOPHILUS INFLUENZAE, STREPTOCOCCUS PNEUMONIAE (also known as pneumococcus), or MENINGOCOCCUS types B and C.

The infection usually reaches the meninges via the bloodstream from an infection elsewhere in the body, often in the nose or throat. Less commonly, it passes through skull cavities from an infected ear or *sinus*, or from the air following a *skull fracture*.

SYMPTOMS

The main symptoms are fever, severe headache, nausea, vomiting, dislike of light, and a stiff neck. In viral meningitis, the symptoms are mild and may resemble influenza. In bacterial meningitis, the main symptoms may develop over only a few hours, followed by drowsiness and, occasionally, loss of consciousness. In about half the cases of meningococcal meningitis, there is also *meningococcaemia* (a potentially life-threatening condition in which bacteria multiply rapidly in the blood). This causes a reddish-purple rash under the skin, which does not fade with pressure (see *glass test*). The rash starts as pinprick spots that can expand to give a bruiselike appearance.

DIAGNOSIS AND TREATMENT

To make a diagnosis, a *lumbar puncture* is performed to remove a small sample of cerebrospinal fluid.

Viral meningitis needs no treatment and usually clears up in a week or two. Bacterial meningitis is a medical emergency treated with intravenous *antibiotic drugs*. With prompt treatment, a full recovery is usually made. The earlier treatment is given, the better the outlook, but in some cases, *deafness* or *brain damage* may occur, or an area of skin, or fingers or toes may be lost.

PREVENTION

Vaccines are now given to protect children and teenagers against three of the major types of bacterial meningitis: those caused by HAEMOPHILUS INFLUENZAE, by MENINGOCOCCUS type C, and by pneumococcus (see *immunization*). Antibiotic drugs may be given as a protective measure to people who have come into contact with these infections.

Immunization against some forms of meningitis is recommended for those travelling to Saudi Arabia for the Hajj and Umrah pilgrimages, and for people travelling to some parts of sub-Saharan Africa and certain other destinations.

meningocele

A protrusion of the spinal cord's *meninges* (protective coverings) under the skin. It is caused by a congenital defect in the spine (see *spina bifida*).

meningococcaemia

Also called meningococcal septicaemia, an acute, life-threatening infection of the bloodstream caused by MENINGOCOCCUS bacteria. It may occur with uncontrolled *meningococcal meningitis* and produces the characteristic, reddish-purple rash often seen in this condition.

Meningococcaemia can cause *shock*; *kidney failure*; and the loss of areas of skin, or fingers and toes. It can be fatal. Affected people need to be admitted to hospital immediately. Treatment is with *antibiotic drugs* followed by *intensive care*.

meningococcal meningitis

One of the most common forms of bacterial *meningitis*. Most cases occur in children or young adults. The disease is transmitted by exhaled droplets; it can spread rapidly through groups of people who are in close contact with each other, such as children in boarding schools. If not treated promptly, it may progress to the life-threatening disorder *meningococcaemia*.

meningococcal rash

A rash that occurs in about half of all cases of *meningococcal meningitis* and meningococcal *septicaemia*. The rash arises as pin-prick spots beneath the skin that join together to give the appearance of a bruise (see *purpura*). The rash associated with meningococcal infection does not fade when pressure is applied (see *glass test*).

meningoencephalitis

Inflammation of the *brain* and the *meninges* (the membranes surrounding the brain), usually as a result of a viral infection. See *encephalitis*.

meningomyelocele

Another name for *myelomeningocele*.

meniscectomy

A surgical procedure in which all or part of a damaged *meniscus* (cartilage disc) is removed from a joint, almost always from the knee.

WHY IT IS DONE

Meniscectomy may be performed when damage to the meniscus causes the knee to lock or to give way repeatedly. It cures these symptoms and reduces the risk of premature *osteoarthritis* in the joint.

HOW IT IS DONE

Arthroscopy (in which a viewing instrument is inserted into the joint through a small incision) may be carried out to confirm and locate the damage. The damaged area may then be removed by instruments passed through the arthroscope. Alternatively, the meniscus may be removed through an incision at the side of the *patella* (kneecap).

OUTLOOK

There is an increased risk of osteoarthritis in later life, but this is less than if the damaged meniscus had been left in place.

meniscus

A crescent-shaped disc of cartilaginous tissue found in several joints. The *knee* joint has two menisci, and the *wrist* joints, and the *temporomandibular joints*

M

MENISCI

The diagram (right) shows the sites of the menisci. The menisci of the knee are shown in detail below.

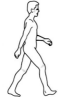

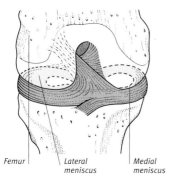

Femur | Lateral meniscus | Medial meniscus

M

of the jaw, have one meniscus each. The menisci are held in position by *ligaments* and help to reduce friction during joint movement.

menopause

The cessation of *ovulation* (egg production) and of *menstruation* (discharge of blood and tissue from the uterus). This process usually occurs between the ages of 45 and 55, the average age being 52 years. The term "menopause" usually refers to a period of physical and psychological changes that occur as a result of reduced *oestrogen* production.

The menopause usually occurs gradually; it is signalled by a change in menstrual patterns (see *perimenopause*) followed by *amenorrhoea* (the cessation of menstrual periods). It can also be brought on by medical procedures that halt the activity of the ovaries, such as *oophorectomy* (surgical removal of the ovaries), *radiotherapy*, or *chemotherapy*. In a few women, the menopause may occur abnormally early, usually before age 40 (see *premature menopause*).

SYMPTOMS

Some women have few difficulties with the menopause. Other women may have symptoms including *hot flushes* and night sweats; vaginal dryness caused by thinning of the vaginal lining; and a decrease in vaginal secretions. The tissues in the neck of the bladder and the urethra also become thinner, which can cause a feeling of needing to urinate frequently. In addition, the breasts tend to decrease in size. Some women experience psychological symptoms, such as poor concentration, tearfulness, loss of interest in sex, and *depression*.

Changes in *metabolism* occur during the menopause but they may not cause symptoms until later. In all women, the bones become thinner; this process happens most rapidly in the years immediately after the menopause. The loss of bone density may result in *osteoporosis*. The risk of heart disease also increases, gradually approaching that for men of a similar age, due to the drastic reduction in oestrogen hormones (which protect premenopausal women against heart disease).

TREATMENT

Women going through the menopause can protect themselves from losing bone density by regularly taking weight-bearing exercise, such as walking, and by eating foods that are rich in *calcium*, such as dairy products and green, leafy vegetables. Measures such as avoiding fatty foods, stopping smoking, and limiting alcohol intake can help to protect women against heart disease.

Hormone replacement therapy (HRT) may relieve menopausal symptoms but is usually given only for short-term use around the menopause because of the risks associated with long-term use, such as the increased risk of *breast cancer*, *stroke*, and *thromboembolism*. In the long term, HRT may protect against osteoporosis but it is not usually recommended for this purpose because of the associated risks. However, whether or not HRT is appropriate depends on the woman concerned, and women considering HRT should consult their doctor for specific individual advice.

menorrhagia

Excessive loss of blood during *menstruation*. Menorrhagia may be caused by an imbalance of *oestrogen hormones* and *progesterone hormone*, which control menstruation. The imbalance leads to an excessive buildup of *endometrium* (the uterine lining). Disorders affecting the uterus, such as *fibroids*, *polyps*, a *pelvic infection*, or, very rarely, uterine cancer (see *uterus, cancer of*), can also cause menorrhagia.

Treatment of menorrhagia depends on the cause. It may include *nonsteroidal anti-inflammatory drugs*, drugs that affect blood clotting, hormones, or the fitting of an *IUS* (intrauterine system), which releases small amounts of *progestogen*. Menorrhagia may also be treated by *endometrial ablation*, or, rarely, by *hysterectomy*.

menotrophin

A *gonadotrophin hormone* given as a drug to stimulate cell activity in the *ovaries* and *testes*. It is used as a treatment for certain types of male and female *infertility*, as it prepares the ovary for ovulation and may help stimulate sperm production. It is used along with human chorionic gonadotrophin (see *gonadotrophin, human chorionic*).

In women, menotrophin may cause multiple pregnancy, abdominal pain, bloating, and weight gain. In men, it may cause enlargement of the breasts.

menses

Another name for a menstrual period. The word "menses" may also mean the blood, tissue, and fluid that is discharged from the uterus during a menstrual period (see *menstruation*).

menstruation

The periodic shedding of *endometrium* (the lining of the uterus), accompanied by bleeding, that takes place in women who are not pregnant. Menstruation usually begins at *puberty* and continues until the *menopause*.

The loss of the endometrium occurs at the end of the menstrual cycle, which usually lasts for 28 days (with the normal range being between 21 and 35 days). At the beginning of the cycle, a hormone from the *pituitary gland*, known as follicle-stimulating hormone (FSH), prompts several follicles (collections of cells containing eggs) within the *ovaries* to mature. The egg follicles secrete *oestrogen hormones*, which cause the endometrium to thicken.

Ovulation (the release of a mature egg from a follicle) usually occurs in the middle of the cycle. The empty follicle (called the corpus luteum) produces *progesterone hormone*. This hormone causes the endometrium to retain fluid and grow thicker, so that a fertilized egg can implant in the tissue. If pregnancy does not occur, production of oestrogens and progesterone diminishes. The endometrium is shed about 14 days after ovulation. Uterine contractions force the tissue, together with fluid and blood, to be expelled via the vagina; this process lasts for one to eight days.

THE **MENSTRUAL CYCLE**

During menstruation, the endometrium (the lining of the uterus) is shed. Following menstruation, a pituitary hormone called follicle-stimulating hormone (FSH) triggers the growth of follicles containing eggs. The follicles secrete oestrogen. Another hormone, luteinizing hormone (LH), causes one of them to release a mature egg. The empty follicle produces progesterone, which, along with oestrogen, prepares the endometrium to receive the egg. If the egg is unfertilized, then levels of oestrogen and progesterone fall and a new menstrual cycle begins.

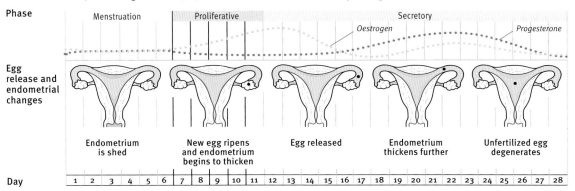

menstruation, anovular

The occurrence of a menstrual period when *ovulation* (the release of an egg from an ovary) has not occurred (see *menstruation*). Anovular menstruation is common in girls who have just started to menstruate, and in women who are approaching the menopause. It may produce irregular menstrual cycles.

menstruation, disorders of

Abnormalities in menstrual bleeding. Menstrual disorders may indicate a problem in the pelvic area, such as *fibroids*, *endometriosis*, or *pelvic inflammatory disease*, but the cause is often unknown.

Dysmenorrhoea (painful periods) is the most common type of menstrual disorder. Other types are *amenorrhoea* (absence of menstruation), polymenorrhoea (overly frequent menstruation), oligomenorrhoea (infrequent periods or scanty blood loss), and *menorrhagia* (excessive bleeding).

Some women have extreme variations in the length of menstrual cycles or periods, or in the amount of blood lost (see *menstruation, irregular*).

menstruation, irregular

A variation in the normal pattern of *menstruation*. Irregular menstruation includes variations in the interval between periods, the duration of bleeding, or the amount of blood that is lost.

The most common cause is a disturbance in the balance between *oestrogen hormones* and *progesterone hormone*. Other causes include *stress*, travel, a change in *contraception*, unsuspected pregnancy, or early *miscarriage*. Menstruation is often irregular for the first few years, and for several years before the *menopause*.

menstruation, retrograde

The backward flow of tiny amounts of menstrual discharge (see *menstruation)* from the *uterus* through the *fallopian tubes* instead of the *vagina*. Retrograde menstruation is thought to be a possible cause of *endometriosis*.

menstruation, suppressed

The failure of menstrual (monthly) bleeding (see *menstruation*) to occur. (See also *amenorrhoea*).

mental age

A measurement of the intellectual development of a person, with regard to the normal age at which that level of achievement is attained. For example, a 13 year-old child with *learning difficulties* may have a mental age of five years.

mental handicap

Impaired intellectual development. This condition is also known as general *learning difficulties* or disability.

Mental Health Act

The Mental Health Act (1983) details the rights of people with *mental illness* and the grounds for admitting people to psychiatric hospitals against their will. It also outlines forms of legal guardianship for such patients. The Act, which applies in England and Wales, is divided into several sections for different situations. (These divisions have given rise to the term "being sectioned" to describe compulsory admission to a mental hospital.) When individuals are endangering their own or other people's health or safety because of a recognized mental illness, they may be compulsorily taken into hospital to be given treatment. If people break the law because of a mental disorder, the courts may remand them to hospital.

mental illness

A general term that describes any form of disorder affecting mental functions such as thought, emotion, perception, or memory. Such illnesses are distinct from *learning difficulties*.

Mental illnesses include forms of *psychosis*, in which a person loses contact with reality, and disorders such as *anxiety, obsessive-compulsive disorder*, and *post-traumatic stress disorder*, in which mental processes are abnormal but the affected person is fully aware of his or her condition.

mental retardation

See *learning difficulties*.

menthol

An alcohol prepared from mint oils. Menthol is an ingredient of several over-the-counter inhalation preparations used to treat a blocked or stuffy nose.

M

mentum

The medical term for the *chin*.

meprobamate

An *antianxiety drug* occasionally used in the short-term treatment of *anxiety* and *stress*. It also acts as a muscle relaxant. Meprobamate can, however, induce dependence (see *drug dependence*).

meptazinol

An opioid *analgesic drug* used for the short-term relief of moderate to severe pain, such as after surgery and during childbirth. Possible side effects include nausea, vomiting, and dizziness.

meralgia paraesthetica

Abnormal sensations such as burning pain, numbness, and tingling, in the outer surface of the thigh. The condition occurs in the area supplied by the lateral femoral cutaneous nerve, and is due to the nerve being trapped at the point where it passes under the inguinal ligament, in the groin. (See also *lateral cutaneous nerve entrapment*).

mercaptopurine

An *anticancer drug* used to treat certain types of *leukaemia*. Adverse effects include nausea, mouth ulcers, and loss of appetite. Rarely, it may cause liver damage, *anaemia*, and abnormal bleeding.

Mercilon

A brand-named *oral contraceptive* containing the synthetic female hormones ethinylestradiol (an *oestrogen drug*) and desogestrel (a *progestogen*).

mercury

The only metal that is liquid at room temperature. It is used in amalgam fillings for teeth (see *amalgam, dental*).

mercury poisoning

Toxic effects of mercury on the body.
CAUSES
The most common cause of mercury poisoning is breathing in vapour given off by liquid mercury, usually as a result of industrial exposure. Also, mercury compounds may be absorbed through the intestines (producing symptoms such as nausea, vomiting, diarrhoea, and abdominal pain) or through the skin (causing severe inflammation).
SYMPTOMS
After entering the body, mercury accumulates in organs, principally the brain and kidneys. Mercury deposits in the

brain cause tiredness, incoordination, excitability, tremors, and numbness in the limbs. In severe cases, there may be impaired vision and *dementia*. Deposits of mercury in the kidneys may lead to *kidney failure*.
TREATMENT
Treatment of mercury poisoning may involve the use of *chelating agents*, which help the body to excrete the mercury quickly; haemodialysis (see *dialysis*); and induced vomiting or pumping out the stomach, if mercury has been swallowed within the previous few hours.

Merkel cell tumour

A rare form of cancerous skin tumour that occurs in people over 60 years old, on areas of skin that have been exposed to the sun. The tumour arises from Merkel cells, which are found deep in the skin, close to nerve endings; these cells are thought to be part of the neuroendocrine system, which produces hormones that trigger nerve signals.

The cancer is initially treated by surgery, but metastasis (migration of cancer cells to other parts of the body) may occur. In this case, *radiotherapy* or *chemotherapy* may be given, but these treatments rarely produce a cure.

mesalazine

A drug that is used in the treatment of *ulcerative colitis* and *Crohn's disease*. For ulcerative colitis, it is used to reduce intestinal inflammation and may be prescribed to relieve symptoms in acute attacks or given as a preventive measure. For Crohn's disease, mesalazine is used to maintain remission of the symptoms. Adverse effects of the drug include nausea, diarrhoea, abdominal pain, and headache.

mescaline

A *hallucinogenic drug* obtained from the crowns of the Mexican peyote cactus (LOPHOPHORA WILLIAMSII).

mesenteric lymphadenitis

An acute abdominal disorder, mainly affecting children, in which *lymph nodes* in the *mesentery* (a membrane that anchors organs to the abdominal wall) become inflamed.

The main symptoms are pain and tenderness in the abdomen, which may mimic appendicitis. There may also be mild fever. Mesenteric lymphadenitis usually clears up rapidly, needing only *analgesic drugs* to reduce pain and fever.

mesentery

A membrane that attaches organs to the abdominal wall. The term particularly refers to the membranous fold that encloses the small intestine, attaching it to the back of the abdominal wall. The mesentery contains the blood vessels, nerves, and lymphatic vessels for the intestines.

mesial

A word meaning the same as "medial" (relating to, or situated at, the centre of an organ, tissue, or the body). The term "mesial" is often used in dentistry, to refer to a tooth surface or position.

mesomorph

A term used for an individual whose body is characterized by a square head; a large heart; broad and muscular chest and shoulders; powerful arms and legs; and little body fat. The term has no clinical significance, however. (See also *ectomorph*; *endomorph*.)

mesothelioma

A cancerous tumour of the *pleura* (the membrane that lines the chest cavity and covers the lungs). Exposure to asbestos dust is a risk factor (see *asbestos-related diseases*). Symptoms may appear 20 to 40 years after exposure to asbestos and may include cough, chest pain, and breathing difficulty, especially if a *pleural effusion* (a collection of fluid around the lung) develops.

Diagnosis is made with a *chest X-ray* or *CT scan*, followed by pleural *biopsy* or examination of a sample of fluid from any effusion. If the tumour is small, surgery may be successful. Otherwise, there is no effective treatment, although *anticancer drugs* and *radiotherapy* may alleviate symptoms.

mesothelium

A type of *epithelium* (surface cell layer) covering the *peritoneum* (the membrane lining the abdominal cavity), the *pleura* (the membrane lining the chest cavity and surrounding the lungs), and the *pericardium* (the covering of the heart).

messenger RNA

An RNA chain (see *nucleic acids*), also called mRNA, involved in *protein synthesis* within cells. The mRNA is made from free nucleotide bases (of which three types are the same as those of DNA, and one is unique to mRNA); these nucleotide bases attach themselves to corresponding bases on a single strand of DNA. By following the sequence of bases in a length of DNA, the mRNA copies instructions for making a protein. The mRNA then passes from the cell's nucleus to its cytoplasm, where the sequence of bases is decoded to form the protein.

mesterolone

An *androgen hormone* (male sex hormone) used as replacement therapy in *hypogonadism*. Adverse effects of mesterolone can include prostate problems, headache, and *depression*.

mestranol

An *oestrogen drug* that is used in some *oral contraceptives*.

metabolic acidosis

Increased acidity of the blood and tissues due to chemical processes in the body. It may result from uncontrolled or abnormal processes, as in *diabetic keto-acidosis* and *lactic acidosis*, or from a failure to remove waste from normal processes, as in kidney disease (see *renal tubular acidosis*). Alternatively, it may be due to loss of alkali in conditions such as diarrhoea. Acidosis may also be due to poisoning with antifreeze (ethylene glycol) or aspirin. If untreated, it can be fatal. Treatment involves giving sodium bicarbonate to correct the acidosis, together with measures to relieve the underlying cause. (See also *acidosis; acid–base balance*.)

metabolic alkalosis

Increased alkalinity of the blood and body tissues, due to chemical processes in the body. One possible cause is loss of stomach acids through prolonged vomiting. Metabolic alkalosis can also result from excessive consumption of alkaline substances, such as sodium bicarbonate in *antacid drugs*.

Treatment is for the underlying cause. (See also *alkalosis; acid–base balance*.)

metabolic disorders

A group of disorders in which some aspect of body chemistry is disturbed. Some metabolic disorders result from an inherited malfunction or deficiency of an *enzyme* involved in a particular chemical reaction (see *metabolism, inborn errors of*). Others result from under- or overproduction of a hormone that controls metabolic activity, as occurs in *diabetes mellitus* and *hypothyroidism*.

metabolism

A collective term for all of the chemical processes that take place in the body. It is divided into catabolism (in which complex substances are broken down into simpler ones) and anabolism (in which complex substances are built up from simpler ones). Usually, catabolism releases energy, while anabolism uses it. These chemical processes are regulated by proteins called *enzymes*.

METABOLIC RATE

The energy needed to keep the body functioning at rest is called the basal metabolic rate (BMR). It is measured in kilojoules (or kilocalories) per square metre of body surface per hour. The BMR increases in response to factors such as stress, fear, exertion, and illness. It is chiefly controlled by hormones such as *thyroxine, adrenaline (epinephrine)*, and *insulin*. (See also *metabolism, inborn errors of; metabolic disorders*.)

metabolism, inborn errors of

Inherited defects of body chemistry.

CAUSE AND TYPES

Inborn errors of metabolism are caused by single *gene* defects, which lead to the abnormal functioning of an *enzyme*. Some defects are harmless, but others are severe enough to cause death or physical or mental disability. Examples are *Tay–Sachs disease, phenylketonuria, Hurler's syndrome*, and Lesch–Nyhan syndrome.

SYMPTOMS

Symptoms of these inborn metabolic disorders are usually present at or soon after birth. They may include unex-

plained illness or failure to thrive, developmental delay, floppiness, persistent vomiting, or *seizures*.

DIAGNOSIS AND TREATMENT

Routine tests are performed on newborn babies for some genetic disorders, such as phenylketonuria.

For some inborn errors of metabolism, no treatment is needed. For others, avoidance of a specific environmental factor, such as certain foods, may be sufficient. In some cases, the missing enzyme or the protein that it produces can be manufactured with the use of *genetic engineering* techniques, or a vitamin supplement can help to compensate for the defective enzyme. If the enzyme is made in blood cells, a *stem cell* or *bone marrow transplant* may provide a cure.

PREVENTION

People with a child or a close relative who is affected may wish to consider having *genetic counselling* before planning a new pregnancy.

metabolite

Any substance involved in a metabolic reaction (a chemical reaction in the body). The term "metabolite" is sometimes used only for the products of such a reaction. (See also *metabolism*.)

metacarpal bone

One of five long, cylindrical bones in the hand. The bones run from the wrist to the base of each digit, with the heads of the bones forming the knuckles.

metaphysis

The part of a long *bone* that forms new tissue to lengthen the bone during normal childhood growth. The metaphysis is situated between the *diaphysis* (bone shaft) and *epiphysis* (bone end). In children the area consists of spongy bone, but in adults it has become hard and fused with the epiphysis.

metaplasia

A change in tissue that results from the transformation of one type of cell into another. Metaplasia is usually harmless but is occasionally precancerous. It can affect the lining of various organs in the body, such as the bronchi (airways), bladder, and oesophagus.

metastasis

A secondary cancerous tumour (one formed from cells that have spread from a primary *cancer* to another part of the body). The term metastasis also applies

---

LOCATION OF THE METACARPAL BONES

The five metacarpals lie between the carpal (wrist) bones and the phalanges of the fingers.

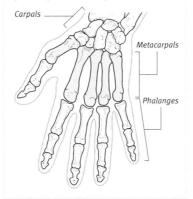

Carpals

Metacarpals

Phalanges

M

to the process by which such migration occurs. Metastases can spread through the *lymphatic system*, in the bloodstream, or across a body cavity.

metastatic abscess

An *abscess* (localized collection of pus) formed by bacteria that have spread from another site via the blood or *lymph*. The bacteria may come from an existing (primary) abscess or from an infected wound. One example of this process is the spread of bacteria from the heart valves (see *endocarditis*) to form an abscess in the brain.

metatarsal bone

One of five long, cylindrical bones in the foot. The metatarsal bones make up the central skeleton of the foot, connecting the *phalanges* (the bones of each toe) to the *tarsal bones* (which form the ankle). The bones are held together in an arch by the *ligaments* that surround them.

metatarsalgia

Pain in the foot. Causes include fracture of a *metatarsal bone*, *flat-feet*, or *neuroma* of a nerve in the foot.

LOCATION OF THE METATARSAL BONES

The five metatarsals lie between the tarsal bones (which form the ankle and the back of the foot) and the phalanges of the toes.

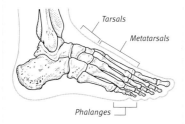

Tarsals

Metatarsals

Phalanges

metatarsophalangeal joint

The joint between each *metatarsal bone* and its adjoining toe bone (see *phalanges*). The metatarsophalangeal joint at the base of the big toe is commonly affected by *gout* and by *hallux rigidus* (immobility due to osteoarthritis).

metformin

An oral hypoglycaemic drug (see *hypoglycaemics, oral*) that lowers blood glucose levels and is used either alone

or with other hypogycaemic drugs to treat type 2 *diabetes mellitus*. Possible adverse effects include loss of appetite, a metallic taste in the mouth, nausea, vomiting, and diarrhoea.

methadone

A synthetic opioid *analgesic drug* that resembles *morphine*. Methadone is administered, under supervision, in gradually decreasing doses, to people who are undergoing a *heroin* or morphine withdrawal programme. It may also be used to treat severe pain in people who cannot tolerate morphine. Side effects may include nausea, vomiting, constipation, dizziness, and dry mouth.

methaemoglobin

An abnormal substance formed by oxidation of the iron in *haemoglobin* (the pigment in red blood cells). Unlike *oxyhaemoglobin*, this compound cannot take up and transport oxygen.

Normal blood usually carries a small amount of methaemoglobin. Excessive blood levels (methaemoglobinaemia) may result from poisoning with substances such as nitrates and chlorates. In some cases, the excess is due to a *congenital* defect in haemoglobin. The resulting symptoms include *cyanosis* (blue-grey colouring of the extremities and lips), headache; drowsiness; and shortness of breath. Very high levels of methaemoglobin lead to coma and death. Treatment is with a substance called methylene blue.

methane

A colourless, odourless, highly inflammable gas that occurs naturally in oil wells and coal mines. Methane is also produced by the decomposition of organic matter; it is one of the gases present in intestinal gas (see *flatus*).

methanol

A poisonous type of *alcohol* used as a solvent or paint remover and in some types of antifreeze. Methanol poisoning usually occurs from drinking it as a substitute for ordinary alcohol. Symptoms of poisoning include headache, dizziness, nausea, vomiting, and unconsciousness. Damage may also occur to the *retina* and *optic nerve*, causing blurred vision. Repeated or large doses of methanol may result in permanent blindness.

methicillin-resistant staphylococcus aureus

See *MRSA*.

methotrexate

An *anticancer drug* and *disease-modifying antirheumatic drug*. It is used to treat *lymphoma* (cancer of the lymph nodes), some forms of *leukaemia*, and cancers of the uterus, breast, ovary, lung, bladder, and testis. Methotrexate slows the progression of disease in some inflammatory conditions and may be used to treat some cases of *rheumatoid arthritis* and severe *psoriasis*. Possible adverse effects include nausea, vomiting, diarrhoea, mouth ulcers, anaemia, increased susceptibility to infection, liver damage, and abnormal bleeding.

methyl alcohol

An alternative name for *methanol*.

methylcellulose

A bulk-forming *laxative drug* that is used in the treatment of *constipation*, *irritable bowel syndrome (IBS)*, and *diverticular disease*. It increases the firmness of faeces in chronic watery *diarrhoea* and regulates their consistency in people who have a *colostomy* or *ileostomy*. The drug causes a feeling of fullness, so it is sometimes used to help treat *obesity*.

methyldopa

An *antihypertensive drug* that controls high blood pressure by acting on the part of the brain that regulates the diameter of blood vessels.

Methyldopa is not known to affect unborn babies, so may be prescribed for women who have high blood pressure during pregnancy. It may also be used for people with kidney disorders, because it does not impair blood flow to the kidneys. Side effects include drowsiness, depression, and nasal congestion. The drug may also cause premature destruction of red blood cells (see *anaemia, haemolytic*).

methylenedioxy-methamfetamine

See *Ecstasy*.

methylphenidate

A central nervous system *stimulant drug* used, under specialist supervision, to treat *attention deficit hyperactivity disorder (ADHD)* in children. Possible adverse effects include loss of appetite, tremors, sleeplessness, and rashes.

methylprednisolone

A *corticosteroid drug* used to treat severe *asthma*, skin inflammation, *inflammatory*

M

bowel disease, and certain types of *arthritis*. Adverse effects are the same as for other *corticosteroid drugs*; they are more likely to occur if the drug is taken over long periods of time.

methysergide

A drug that is used to prevent *migraine* and *cluster headaches*. Methysergide is usually administered only under hospital supervision, when other treatments have been ineffective.

Adverse effects of the drug can include dizziness, drowsiness, and nausea. Long-term treatment may cause chest pain, *kidney failure*, or leg cramps.

metoclopramide

An *antiemetic drug* that is used to prevent and treat nausea and vomiting, including that which is associated with *migraine* or caused by *anticancer drugs*, *radiotherapy*, or *anaesthetic drugs*. Metoclopramide may be given with a premedication to reduce the risk of a person inhaling vomit when he or she is under general anaesthesia (see *anaesthesia, general*).

Adverse effects of the drug include dry mouth, sedation, or diarrhoea. Large doses may cause uncontrollable movements of the face, mouth, and tongue.

metolazone

A *diuretic drug* used to treat *hypertension* (high blood pressure). Metolazone is also given to reduce *oedema* in people who have *heart failure*, kidney disorders, or *cirrhosis* of the liver. Adverse effects can include weakness, lethargy, and dizziness.

metoprolol

A cardioselective *beta-blocker drug* that acts mainly on nerve endings in the heart and blood vessels. It is used to prevent the heart from beating too fast, in *angina pectoris* (chest pain due to insufficient blood supply to the heart), and for *hypertension* (high blood pressure). It is also given after a *myocardial infarction* (heart attack) to reduce the risk of further damage to the heart. In addition, metoprolol is used to relieve symptoms of *hyperthyroidism* (overactivity of the thyroid gland) and to prevent *migraine* attacks. Adverse effects include lethargy, cold hands and feet, nightmares, and rash.

metronidazole

An *antibiotic drug* used to treat infections caused by *anaerobic* bacteria, such as dental *abscess* and *peritonitis*. Metronidazole is also used to treat protozoan infections such as *trichomoniasis* and *amoebiasis*. In addition, it may be applied topically as a gel to treat skin conditions such as *acne* and *rosacea*, and it is used to treat gum disease.

Adverse effects include nausea and vomiting, loss of appetite, abdominal pain, and dark-coloured urine. Alcohol should be avoided during treatment.

metropathia haemorrhagica

Abnormal, excessive, sometimes continuous menstrual bleeding (see *menstrual cycle*) due to excessive production of *oestrogen hormones*. The high oestrogen levels cause hyperplasia (overgrowth) of the endometrium (uterus lining).

mexiletine

An *antiarrhythmic drug* used to treat certain serious heart-rhythm disorders, usually after a *myocardial infarction* (heart attack). Possible adverse effects include nausea, vomiting, dizziness, and tremor.

mianserin

An *antidepressant drug* that is used to treat severe *depression*, especially if the illness is accompanied by *anxiety* or *insomnia*. Mianserin usually takes several weeks to become fully effective. Possible adverse effects include dry mouth, blurred vision, constipation, dizziness, and drowsiness. Rarely, the drug may cause reduced blood cell production; regular *blood counts* are therefore carried out during treatment.

miconazole

An *antifungal drug* that is used topically (applied directly to the skin), in the form of creams, ointments, or powder, to treat *tinea* skin infections such as *athlete's foot*, or as vaginal suppositories for vaginal *candidiasis* (thrush). Miconazole in the form of a cream or vaginal suppository may, in rare cases, cause a burning sensation or a rash. Preparations used in the vagina may damage *diaphragms* or latex *condoms*.

micro-

A prefix meaning "small", as in *microorganisms* (tiny organisms).

microalbuminuria

A slight increase in the level of the protein *albumin* in the urine, usually due to early kidney damage. Microalbuminuria is a very early sign of kidney disease in people with *diabetes mellitus*. (See also *albuminuria*.) If left untreated, it may lead to diabetic kidney disease (see *diabetic nephropathy*) in people with type 1 diabetes, or may increase the risk of cardiovascular disorders in those who have type 2 diabetes.

Microalbuminuria may be detected by dipstick tests on the urine and can be confirmed by testing urine collected over 24. Treatment with *ACE inhibitor drugs* is usually advised, even if the affected person's blood pressure is normal.

microaneurysm

A tiny, localized swelling in a *capillary* (the smallest form of blood vessel). Microaneurysms in the vessels of the *retina* are a characteristic sign of *diabetic retinopathy* in *diabetes mellitus*; they may also be due to blockage of a retinal vessel. The swellings can be seen as small red dots when the retina is examined with an *ophthalmoscope*.

microangiopathy

Any disease or disorder of the smallest blood vessels. It may be a feature of conditions such as *diabetes mellitus*, *septicaemia*, *eclampsia*, *glomerulonephritis*, and advanced *cancer*. When microangiopathy occurs with these conditions, the small blood vessels become distorted and the red *blood cells* are damaged, leading to microangiopathic haemolytic anaemia (see *anaemia, haemolytic*).

microbe

A popular term for a microorganism, particularly a type that causes disease.

microbiology

The study of microorganisms, particularly of pathogenic types (organisms that cause disease).

microcephaly

An abnormally small head. Microcephaly is associated with *learning difficulties*. It may be the result of certain *chromosomal abnormalities*; in addition, it may occur if the brain is damaged before or during birth, or if it is injured or diseased in early infancy.

microcytic anaemia

Any form of *anaemia* in which there is a defect in the production of *haemoglobin* (the oxygen-carrying pigment in the blood), causing a reduction in size of the *red blood cells*. An example of microcytic anaemia is *iron-deficiency anaemia*. (See also *normocytic anaemia*.)

M

microdiscectomy

Surgery to relieve pressure on the spinal cord, or on a nerve root emerging from it, due to protrusion of the core of an intervertebral disc (see *disc prolapse*). The procedure is performed under general anaesthesia (see *anaesthesia, general*) and involves removing the protruding tissue via a small incision in the outer coat of the intervertebral disc.

microfilaria

The immature forms of certain types of worm. Microfilaria are produced by adult worms that have infected a human being or an animal (see *filariasis*), and circulate in the blood or *lymph*. They complete their life cycle when they are ingested by mosquitoes or other insects that bite infected people or animals; they turn into larvae within the insect, and are then passed on when it bites another victim.

The presence of microfilaria in the body can be determined by microscopic examination of blood samples.

microglioma

An obsolete term for a *primary central nervous system lymphoma* (PCNSL).

microglossia

An abnormally small tongue. The condition is often due to a *genetic disorder* and associated with *micrognathia* (an abnormally small jaw).

micrognathia

An abnormally small jaw (usually the lower jaw). Micrognathia is *congenital* (present at birth), and may stop a baby from feeding properly. It is a feature of various *chromosomal abnormalities*. In many cases, the problem disappears as the child's skull grows.

micrograph

A photographic image of a tiny object seen through a *microscope*.

Microgynon 30

A brand-named *oral contraceptive* that contains the female hormones *ethinylestradiol* (an *oestrogen drug*) and *levonorgestrel* (a *progestogen*).

microinvasion

The spread of cancerous cells into normal tissue adjacent to the tumour. It is detectable only by microscopic examination of a tissue sample. This is a transitional stage between *carcinoma in situ* and invasion (see *staging*).

Micronor

A brand-named *oral contraceptive* that contains the female hormone *norethisterone* (a *progestogen*).

microorganism

A single-celled living organism. Most microorganisms are too small to be seen by the naked eye. The main groups of disease-causing microorganisms are *bacteria*, *viruses*, *protozoa*, and *fungi*.

microphthalmos

A rare congenital eye disorder. Affected children are born with an abnormally small eye on one or both sides.

microscope

An instrument for producing a magnified image of a very small object. Microscopes are used to examine the structure and chemical composition of cells and tissues, and to investigate microorganisms and diseased tissues. In the operating theatre, microscopes are used in *microsurgery*.

LIGHT MICROSCOPES

Compound microscopes are the most widely used type. They have two lens systems (the objective and the eyepiece), mounted at opposite ends of a tube called the body tube. There is a stage to hold the specimen, a light source, and an optical condenser which concentrates the light. The maximum magnification is about 1,500 times.

Phase-contrast and interference microscopes are modified light microscopes that allow unstained transparent specimens to be seen. They are used for examining living cells and tissues.

Fluorescence microscopes use ultraviolet light to study specimens stained with fluorescent dyes.

ELECTRON MICROSCOPES

Electron microscopes give much higher magnifications than light microscopes by using a beam of electrons instead of light. There are two types: transmission electron microscopes (TEMs) and scanning electron microscopes (SEMs). TEMs can magnify objects up to about 5,000,000 times, enabling tiny viruses and molecules to be seen. SEMs have a lower maximum magnification (100,000 times), but produce three-dimensional images, so are useful for studying surface structures of cells and tissues.

microsurgery

Surgery on minute, delicate, or not easily accessible tissues in the body. In procedures involving microsurgery, the surgeon views the operation site using a special binocular microscope with pedal-operated magnification, focusing, and movement. He or she carries out the procedure using tiny, specially adapted surgical instruments, such as forceps, clamps, and very fine suturing needles and thread.

The techniques of microsurgery are applied to a variety of procedures. They are used for eye operations such as repairing a detached *retina* or replacing a diseased *lens*. Microsurgery may be carried out to fit a prosthesis to replace a diseased bone in the inner ear (see *stapedectomy*). After serious injuries, microsurgery may be performed to rejoin the severed ends of blood vessels or nerves. Microsurgery may also be used to reverse female or male sterilization (see *sterilization, female*; *vasectomy*), by rejoining structures that had been surgically severed in the original sterilization operation.

microvillus

One of the many microscopically small, hairlike structures covering the surface of a *villus* (a tiny projection from the wall of the small intestine).

microwave therapy

A form of *diathermy* that uses microwaves (electromagnetic waves of very short wavelength). It is used to treat *benign prostatic hypertrophy* (noncancerous enlargement of the prostate gland) and is also being investigated as a possible treatment for *breast cancer* and *prostate cancer*.

micturition

A medical term for passing *urine*.

micturition syncope

A brief loss of consciousness (see *syncope*) that occurs during or just after *micturition* (passing urine), usually when a person has got out of bed to urinate at night. The condition is more common in older men. It is thought to result from a drop in blood pressure as the person gets up (see *orthostatic hypotension*), combined with changes in blood flow as the bladder empties.

midazolam

A *benzodiazepine drug* that is used as *premedication*. Adverse effects of midazolam include confusion, drowsiness, and dizziness.

M

TECHNIQUES OF **MICROSURGERY**

Microsurgery started with ophthalmic surgeons, whose demands for more delicate operating instruments led to the adoption of the operating microscope. The results were so favourable that surgeons working in other specialties began to use the technique for intricate operations.

The operating microscope
This surgeon is performing microsurgery with the aid of an operating microscope. The photograph below shows a blood vessel as seen through the microscope.

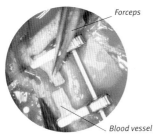

Forceps

Blood vessel

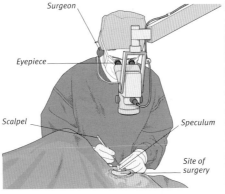

Surgeon

Eyepiece

Scalpel

Speculum

Site of surgery

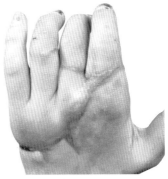

Replantation microsurgery
A major application of microsurgery is the replantation of severed fingers, toes, hands, feet, or even entire limbs. This is successful only if the severed blood vessels and nerves are accurately rejoined so that regeneration occurs.

midbrain

The top part of the *brainstem*, situated above the pons. The midbrain is also called the mesencephalon.

middle ear

See *ear*.

middle-ear effusion, persistent

See *glue ear*.

middle-ear infection

See *otitis media*.

mid-life crisis

A popular term for the feelings of distress that affect some people in early middle age when they realize that they are no longer young. Counselling and support are usually effective in helping people to come to terms with aging.

midwifery

The profession concerned with assisting women in pregnancy and childbirth, and in the weeks just after a birth.

mifepristone

A *sex hormone* drug that is used together with a *prostaglandin* drug to induce medical termination of a pregnancy (see *abortion, induced*). Possible adverse effects include malaise, faintness, nausea, rash, and uterine bleeding.

migraine

A severe headache, typically lasting from four to 72 hours, accompanied by light and noise sensitivity and/or nausea and vomiting. Migraine attacks are due to spasm, followed by excessive dilation, of blood vessels in the brain.

CAUSES

There is no single cause of migraine, although it tends to run in families. Stress-related, food-related, or sensory-related factors (such as eating cheese or chocolate, or drinking red wine) may trigger migraine attacks. In women, *menstruation*, *oral contraceptives*, and *hormone replacement therapy (HRT)* may also be triggers.

TYPES AND SYMPTOMS

There are two types: migraine with aura (an impression of flashing lights and/or other neurological symptoms such as numbness and tingling) and migraine without aura. In migraine without aura, there is a slowly worsening headache, often on one side of the head, with nausea and sometimes vomiting and/or light and noise sensitivity.

In migraine with aura, there may be visual disturbances for up to an hour, followed by a severe, one-sided headache, nausea, vomiting, and sensitivity to light and noise. Other temporary neurological symptoms, such as weakness in one half of the body, may occur.

DIAGNOSIS AND TREATMENT

Diagnosis is usually made from the history and a normal outcome from any physical examinations between attacks. Treatment for an attack is an *analgesic drug* such as *aspirin*, *paracetamol*, or a *nonsteroidal anti-inflammatory*

drug, together with an *antiemetic drug*, if needed. If this is not effective, drugs called 5HT₁ agonists (see *serotonin agonists*), such as *sumatriptan*, may be prescribed. These drugs are taken as early as possible at the start of an attack, and may prevent the development of a full-blown attack. Sleeping in a darkened room may hasten recovery.

For people who suffer frequent migraine attacks, preventive treatment may be required. Keeping a diary can help sufferers to identify trigger factors, and prophylactic drugs may be prescribed. Drugs that contain *ergotamine* may prevent an attack if they are taken before the headache begins, but are now rarely used; they have largely been replaced by *serotonin antagonists* such as *pizotifen*. *Beta-blocker drugs*, or low doses of tricyclic *antidepressant drugs*, may also be used to prevent attacks. (See also *cluster headaches*.)

migrainous neuralgia

See *cluster headaches*.

Migraleve

A brand-named drug for migraine relief that contains the *analgesic drugs* (painkillers) *paracetamol* and *codeine* and the *antiemetic drug* buclizine.

Migril

A brand-named drug for migraine relief containing *caffeine*, *ergotamine* (to relieve migraine symptoms), and the *antihistamine drug* cyclizine (to relieve nausea).

M

milia

Tiny, harmless, hard, white spots that usually occur in clusters around the nose and on the upper cheeks in newborn babies and also in young adults.

miliary tuberculosis

A potentially life-threatening form of *tuberculosis* in which bacteria from the original site of infection enter the bloodstream and then spread throughout the body to form millions of tiny tubercles (nodular masses) in other organs and tissues. The condition occurs in only a small minority of people with tuberculosis; it is most common in *immunocompromised* people, such as those with *AIDS* or those taking *corticosteroid drugs*.

milk

A *nutrient* fluid produced by the mammary glands of female mammals. Milk contains fat, carbohydrate, protein, vitamins, and minerals. The composition of milk varies between different species; for example, human breast milk contains more sugar (lactose) and less protein than cows' milk.

milk–alkali syndrome

A rare type of *hypercalcaemia* (abnormally high level of calcium in the blood) together with *alkalosis* (reduced acidity of the blood) and *kidney failure*. The syndrome is caused by excessive, long-term intake of *antacid drugs* containing calcium and of milk. It is most common in people with a *peptic ulcer*. Symptoms include weakness, muscle pains, irritability, and apathy. Treatment is to reduce the intake of milk and antacids.

Milk of Magnesia

A magnesium preparation used as an *antacid* and *laxative drug*.

milk teeth

See *primary teeth*.

Milroy's disease

An inherited form of *lymphoedema* (the accumulation of *lymph* in tissues) caused by a malformation of the lymphatic vessels that prevents the free flow of lymph. The disease is a *genetic disorder* inherited in an autosomal dominant manner and is *congenital* (present from birth). The condition usually affects the legs.

Minamata disease

A severe form of *mercury poisoning* that occurred in the mid-1950s in people who had eaten polluted fish from Minamata Bay, Japan. Many affected people suffered severe nerve damage, and some died.

mineral

A chemical element that is defined in *nutrition* as being essential in the diet for maintaining health. At least 20 minerals are vital for health, including calcium, iron, potassium, and sodium. Some, such as zinc, are needed in only tiny amounts (see *trace elements*). A well-balanced diet should provide all the minerals the body needs. (See also *Minerals and main food sources*, opposite; *Reference nutrient intake (RNI)*, below.)

mineralization, dental

The deposition of calcium crystals and other mineral salts in developing teeth. (See *calcification, dental*.)

mineralocorticoid

The term used for a *corticosteroid hormone* that controls the amount of salts that are excreted in urine.

REFERENCE NUTRIENT INTAKE (RNI) FOR SELECTED **MINERALS**

The table below gives the reference nutrient intake (RNI) of selected minerals for which amounts have been established; when different, the RNI for males and females is denoted by the letters M and F. The figures given are for healthy children (aged over one year) and adults. The figures are not applicable for babies or for individuals who have medical conditions or special nutritional requirements, such professional sports players.

	1–3 years	4–6 years	7–10 years	11–14 years	15–18 years	19–50 years	51+ years	Extra needed: Pregnancy	Breast-feeding
Calcium (mg/day)	350	450	550	M 1000 F 800	M 1000 F 800	700	700	0	+550
Iodine (mcg/day)	70	100	110	130	140	140	140	0	0
Iron (mg/day)	6.9	6.1	8.7	M 11.3 F 14.8*	M 11.3 F 14.8*	M 8.7 F 14.8*	8.7	0	0
Magnesium (mg/day)	85	120	200	280	300	M 300 F 270	M 300 F 270	0	+50
Phosphorus (mg/day)	270	350	450	M 775 F 625	M 775 F 625	550	550	0	+440
Selenium (mcg/day)	15	20	30	45	M 70 F 60	M 75 F 60	M 75 F 60	0	+15
Sodium (mg/day)	500	700	1200	1600	1600	1600	1600	0	0
Zinc (mg/day)	5	6.5	7	9	M 9.5 F 7	M 9.5 F 7	M 9.5 F 7	0	+6

* Insufficient for women with heavy menstrual periods, who should take iron supplements.

Units: mg = milligrams (thousandths of a gram)
mcg = micrograms (millionths of a gram)

mineral supplements

Dietary supplements containing one or more *minerals* in tablet or liquid form. Most people obtain sufficient amounts from their diet; supplements are only necessary for those with a recognized deficiency. Some mineral supplements may even be harmful if taken in excess. (See also entries for individual minerals.)

Iron, the most commonly taken mineral supplement, is used to treat people with *iron-deficiency anaemia*, which may occur in women who have heavy menstrual periods or are pregnant or breast-feeding, and vegans.

miner's lung

See *pneumoconiosis*.

minilaparotomy

A procedure for female sterilization (see *sterilization, female*).

minimal access surgery

See *minimally invasive surgery*.

minimal brain dysfunction

A hypothetical condition that is thought to account for behavioural and other problems in children for which no physical cause is found. It may be a possible cause of some *learning difficulties*, difficulty in concentrating, impulsiveness, and *hyperactivity*.

minimally invasive surgery

Surgery using a rigid *endoscope* passed into the body through a small incision. Further small openings are made for instruments so that the operation can be performed without a long incision.

Minimally invasive surgery may be used for a range of operations on the abdomen (see *laparoscopy*), including *appendicectomy*, *cholecystectomy*, *hernia repair*, and many *gynaecological* procedures. Operations on the knee (see *arthroscopy*) are also often performed by minimally invasive surgery.

minipill

Also known as the progestogen-only pill (POP), an *oral contraceptive* that contains only a *progestogen drug*. The minipill makes the cervical mucus thick and impenetrable by sperm and causes thickening of the uterine lining, thereby reducing the chance of a fertilized egg implanting successfully. A newer type of minipill that contains the progestogen desogestrel also inhibits ovulation. Possible adverse effects may include menstrual irregularities, bleeding between periods, headaches, and breast discomfort.

minocycline

A tetracycline *antibiotic drug* used to treat *acne*, respiratory tract infections such as *pneumonia*, and some genitourinary infections, such as *gonorrhoea* and *nongonococcal urethritis*.

The most common side effects are nausea, dizziness, and diarrhoea. The drug may also interfere with the balance mechanism within the inner ear, causing dizziness or *vertigo*, but these problems usually disappear once the drug is no longer being used. Very rarely, minocycline can cause systemic *lupus erythematosus*.

minoxidil

A *vasodilator drug* used to treat severe *hypertension* (high blood pressure) when other drugs have been ineffective.

Prolonged use can stimulate hair growth, especially on the face. This effect may be a problem for people using the drug to control high blood pressure. It can, however, be beneficial for male-pattern baldness (see *alopecia*) and topical preparations containing minoxidil are available to stimulate hair regrowth.

miosis

Constriction of the pupil of the *eye*. Miosis may be caused by drugs such as *pilocarpine* or *opium*, by a disease affecting the *autonomic nervous system*, or by bright light. A degree of miosis is normal in older people.

miotic drugs

Drugs used in the treatment of *glaucoma* to reduce pressure in the eye. When applied to the eye, miotic drugs cause

MINERALS AND MAIN FOOD SOURCES

Mineral	Sources
Calcium	Milk, cheese, calcium-fortified bread, butter and margarine, green vegetables, pulses, nuts, soya bean products, hard water
Chromium	Red meat, cheese, butter and margarine, whole-grain cereals and breads, green vegetables
Copper	Red meat, poultry, liver, fish, seafood, whole-grain cereals and breads, green vegetables, pulses, nuts, raisins, mushrooms
Fluorine	Fish, fluoridated water, tea
Iodine	Milk, cheese, butter and margarine, fish, whole-grain cereals and breads, iodized table salt
Iron	Red meat, poultry, liver, eggs, fish, whole-grain cereals and breads, dried fruit
Magnesium	Milk, fish, whole-grain cereals and breads, green vegetables, pulses, nuts, hard water
Phosphorus	Red meat, poultry, liver, milk, cheese, butter and margarine, eggs, fish, whole-grain cereals and breads, green vegetables, root vegetables, pulses, nuts, fruit
Potassium	Whole-grain cereals and breads, green vegetables, pulses, fruit
Selenium	Red meat, liver, milk, fish, seafood, whole-grain cereals and breads
Sodium	Red meat, poultry, liver, milk, cheese, butter and margarine, eggs, fish, whole-grain cereals and breads, green vegetables, root vegetables, pulses, nuts, fruit, table salt, processed foods
Zinc	Red meat, fish, seafood, eggs, milk, whole-grain cereals and breads, pulses

M

the pupil to contract, which opens up the drainage channels and drains fluid from the front of the eye. Side effects include headache, particularly over the eye, and blurred vision. Common miotics include carbachol and *pilocarpine*. (See also *mydriatic drugs*.)

Mirena

A brand-name intrauterine progestogen-only system (a type of contraceptive device, also known as an intrauterine system, see *IUS*) containing the progestogen hormone *levonorgestrel*. The Mirena device is fitted inside the uterus, then releases a low dose of the drug continually for up to five years.

miscarriage

Loss of the fetus before the 24th week of pregnancy or loss of fetal viability (the ability to survive outside the uterus without artificial support). The majority of miscarriages occur in the first 12 weeks of pregnancy, and may be mistaken for a late menstrual period.

TYPES

Miscarriages are classified into three types. In a threatened miscarriage the fetus remains alive in the uterus. In an inevitable miscarriage the fetus dies and is expelled from the uterus. In a missed miscarriage the fetus dies but remains in the uterus.

CAUSES

Miscarriages may occur because of *chromosomal abnormalities*, *genetic disorders*, or developmental defects in the fetus. Problems in the mother that may cause miscarriage include severe illness, placental failure, an *autoimmune disorder*, *cervical incompetence*, a defect in the uterus, or large uterine *fibroids* (noncancerous growths). However, in many cases no cause is found.

SYMPTOMS

The symptoms of miscarriage are heavy bleeding with cramping. Slight blood loss with severe pain may be a symptom of either a threatened miscarriage or *ectopic pregnancy* (development of the fetus outside the uterus).

INVESTIGATION AND TREATMENT

A *pelvic examination*, urine test, and *ultrasound scanning* may be performed to assess the pregnancy. If all of the contents of the uterus have been expelled, no further treatment may be necessary. Otherwise, medication or a *D and C* may be required. A missed miscarriage requires medication to induce a miscarriage, a D and C, or *induction of labour*,

depending on the duration of the pregnancy. Rhesus-negative women are given *anti-D(Rh$_o$) immunoglobulin* to prevent complications related to *rhesus incompatibility* in future pregnancies.

misoprostol

A synthetic *prostaglandin drug* that may be used to induce a medical abortion (see *abortion, induced*). Misoprostol is also used to prevent and treat peptic ulcers associated with the use of *nonsteroidal anti-inflammatory drugs* (NSAIDs) because it inhibits gastric secretion; for this reason it is combined with an NSAID in some preparations.

mites and disease

Mites are very small animals, usually less than about 1 mm long, with eight legs. Many species of mites have piercing and bloodsucking mouthparts.

Species that may cause disorders include the *scabies* mite, which burrows in human skin causing intense itching; the house-dust mite, which can cause *asthma* when inhaled; and chiggers (American harvest mites), which are found in grass and cause an itchy rash when they bite. Mites in grain or fruit may cause skin irritation – sometimes called grocers' or bakers' itch. Certain mites transmit diseases, particularly scrub *typhus* and rickettsial *pox*.

mitochondria

Small *organelles* found inside *cells* in which cell *respiration* occurs. The mitochondrial wall has two membranes. The inner one is highly folded to provide a surface for respiration reactions. Cells that use a lot of energy, such as muscle cells, contain many mitochondria.

mitochondrial DNA

A particular form of *DNA* existing in *mitochondria*. In human mitochondria, the DNA is a double-helical circle that codes for 13 proteins. Mitochondria have a distinctive genetic code, and their genomes are not changed by *meiosis* during reproduction; these features make the DNA useful in genetic studies.

The significance of mitochondria having their own DNA is that diseases can be inherited via abnormalities of mitochondrial DNA, and inheritance of the DNA is maternal, directly from the egg.

mitosis

A type of cell division in which the *chromosomes* in a cell nucleus are dupli-

cated into each of two daughter cells. Before cell division, the chromosomes duplicate themselves and coil up with the two copies joined together. The doubled chromosomes line up in the centre of the cell and are pulled apart to opposite ends of the cell, which then divides. Each daughter cell therefore has the same chromosome content as the original cell. (Egg and sperm cells, in contrast, divide by means of a process called *meiosis*.)

mitral incompetence

Failure of the *mitral valve* of the *heart* to close properly, allowing blood to leak back into the left atrium (upper chamber) when it has been pumped out of the left ventricle (lower chamber). The disorder, also known as mitral regurgitation, may occur in conjunction with *mitral stenosis* (narrowing of the valve).

SYMPTOMS

Symptoms include increasing breathlessness and fatigue, sometimes with *palpitations*. Later, as *heart failure* develops, the ankles may swell.

DIAGNOSIS AND TREATMENT

Diagnosis may be made by hearing a characteristic heart *murmur*; from *X-rays*; *ECG*; and *echocardiography*. The heart's interior may also be investigated with a catheter (see *catheterization, cardiac*).

Treatment may include *diuretic drugs*, *ACE inhibitor drugs*, and *anticoagulant drugs*. If symptoms are disabling, *heart-valve surgery* may be considered.

Before dental or other surgery, people with mitral incompetence are given *antibiotic drugs* to prevent *endocarditis*.

mitral stenosis

Narrowing of the opening of the *mitral valve* in the *heart*. The left atrium (upper chamber) has to work harder to force blood through the narrowed valve. Mitral stenosis is more common in women and may be accompanied by *mitral incompetence* (failure of the mitral valve to close properly). It is usually due to damage caused by *rheumatic fever*.

SYMPTOMS

The main symptom is breathlessness on exertion. As mitral stenosis worsens, breathing difficulty eventually occurs when the person is at rest. Other signs include *palpitations*, *atrial fibrillation* (a rapid, uncoordinated, irregular heartbeat), and flushed cheeks. The person may also cough up blood and feel fatigued. The possible complications of mitral stenosis are the same as those for mitral incompetence.

THE MECHANISM OF **MITOSIS**

Mitosis is the simplest type of cell division. It provides new body cells to replace those that have died. Each of the new cells receives an identical copy of the chromosomes from the original cell.

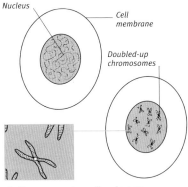

Nucleus

Cell membrane

Doubled-up chromosomes

1 Chromosomes in a cell nucleus are invisible, long threads. Before cell division, the threads replicate, coil up, and shorten, appearing as dark rods. The two copies of each chromosome are joined at a point called the centromere, so they appear X-shaped.

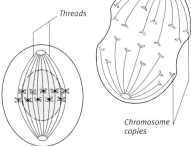

Threads

2 The doubled chromosomes line up in the centre of the cell. The cell nucleus breaks down, and threads appear in the cell. The two copies of each chromosome then move apart along the threads.

Chromosome copies

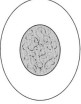

3 The two identical groups of single chromosomes now gather at opposite ends of the cell, and a nuclear membrane forms around each group. The rest of the cell then divides.

Nuclear membrane

4 When division has finished and new nuclei have fully formed in the two daughter cells, the chromosomes uncoil to resume their invisible, threadlike form. Mitosis is now complete.

DIAGNOSIS AND TREATMENT

A diagnosis is made from the patient's history, listening to heart sounds, and by various investigations such as an *ECG*, *chest X-rays*, *echocardiography*, and cardiac *catheterization*. Drug treatment is broadly the same as for mitral incompetence. Similarly, people with mitral stenosis are given prophylactic *antibiotic drugs* before dental or orther surgery.

If symptoms persist, balloon *valvuloplasty* may be carried out to stretch the valve. Alternatively, *heart-valve surgery* may be performed to replace the valve.

mitral valve

A valve in the left side of the *heart*. The mitral (or bicuspid) valve is made up of two flaps, allowing one-way blood flow from the left *atrium* (upper chamber) into the left *ventricle* (lower chamber).

mitral valve prolapse

A common, slight deformity of the *mitral valve*, in the left side of the *heart*, that can produce a degree of *mitral incompetence* (failure of the valve to close properly). The prolapse is most common in women and causes a heart *murmur*. It may be inherited, but the cause is often unknown.

Usually, there are no symptoms. Occasionally, however, the condition may produce chest pain, *arrhythmia* (irregular heartbeat), or, rarely, *heart failure*.

Often, no treatment is required, but some people may be treated with *beta-blocker drugs*, *diuretic drugs*, *antiarrhythmic drugs*, or, rarely, *heart-valve surgery*.

mittelschmerz

Lower abdominal pain experienced by some women at the time of *ovulation*. The pain usually occurs on one side of the abdomen and lasts for only a few hours. It may be accompanied by slight vaginal blood loss. In cases of severe mittelschmerz, *oral contraceptives* may be prescribed to suppress ovulation.

mixed connective tissue disorder

An *autoimmune disease* that affects the *connective tissue* (which supports body structures) throughout the body. It combines features of *systemic sclerosis*, systemic *lupus erythematosus*, *polymyositis*, and *rheumatoid arthritis*.

Mixed connective tissue disorder is diagnosed by blood tests that reveal antibodies to a cellular protein called ribonucleic protein (RNP). Treatment is similar to that for systemic lupus erythematosus, with *corticosteroid drugs* and *immunosuppressant drugs*.

MMR vaccination

Administration of a combined *vaccine* that gives protection against *measles*,

mumps, and *rubella*. The MMR vaccination is offered to all children at around 13 months of age, with a booster shot at three years four months to five years of age. Vaccination is postponed if a child is feverish, and is not given to children whose immune systems are suppressed or who have had a severe reaction to a previous dose of the vaccine.

Mild fever, rash, and malaise may occur after vaccination. In a minority of cases, mild, noninfectious swelling of the *parotid glands* develops three to four weeks after vaccination. There is no evidence for a link between MMR and *Crohn's disease* or autism.

mobilization

The process of making a part of the body capable of movement. Mobilization is treatment that is designed to increase mobility in a part of the body that is recovering from injury or affected by disease.

Surgeons use the term to refer to the freeing of an organ or structure from surrounding *connective tissue* or fibrous adhesions (bands of tissue joining normally unconnected parts of the body).

Möbius' syndrome

A rare *genetic disorder* that is characterized by *paralysis* of both sides of the face, due to the absence or underdevel-

M

opment of the sixth and seventh *cranial nerves* (the abducent nerve and the facial nerve, respectively). The condition is *congenital* (present from birth).

An affected child has a masklike facial expression and cannot move the eyes fully from side to side. Newborn babies are unable to feed properly. In some cases, the syndrome is associated with abnormalities of the limbs or with *learning difficulties*. There is no specific treatment, but surgery may restore some facial expression.

moclobemide

An *antidepressant drug* that is used to treat resistant depression and social phobia. Moclobemide is a reversible *monoamine oxidase inhibitor* and is less likely than other MAOIs to interact with certain foods and drugs to cause a dangerous rise in blood pressure. However, the same dietary and medication restrictions still apply for people taking moclobemide; for example, they should not consume foods such as cheese, meat, or yeast extracts, or drink red wine or beer.

Mogadon

A brand name for the benzodiazepine drug *nitrazepam*.

molar

See *teeth*.

molar pregnancy

A pregnancy in which a tumour develops from the placental tissue and the embryo does not develop normally. A molar pregnancy may be noncancerous (a *hydatidiform mole*) or may invade the wall of the uterus (an invasive mole). A molar pregnancy that becomes cancerous is called a *choriocarcinoma*.

If the dead embryo and placenta are not expelled from the uterus after a *miscarriage*, the dead tissue forms a mass called a carneous mole.

mole

A type of pigmented *naevus*. (See also *molar pregnancy*.)

molecule

The smallest complete unit of a substance that can exist independently and still retain the characteristic properties of that substance. Almost all molecules consist of two or more atoms bonded together. Those that consist of only one atom are called monatomic molecules.

molluscum contagiosum

A harmless viral infection characterized by shiny, pearly white papules (tiny lumps) on the skin surface. Each papule has a central depression, and releases a cheesy fluid when it is squeezed. A crust forms before healing occurs.

The papules often appear on the genitals, the insides of the thighs, or the face. Children are more commonly affected than adults. The infection is transmitted by direct skin contact or during sexual intercourse; it usually clears up within a few months, but may last for up to 18 months.

Mongolian blue spot

Blue-black pigmented spots found on the lower back and buttocks at birth. The spots are a type of *naevus*, caused by a concentration of melanocytes (cells that produce pigment). Mongolian blue spots are commonly found in black or Asian children. They usually disappear by the age of three to four years.

Mongolism

An outdated name for *Down's syndrome*.

moniliasis

See *candidiasis*.

monitor

To maintain a constant watch on the condition of a patient. The word "monitor" is also used to refer to any device used to carry out monitoring.

monoamine oxidase inhibitors

Also known as MAOIs, one of the three main types of *antidepressant drug*. They work by preventing the breakdown of certain *neurotransmitters* by the *enzyme* monoamine oxidase. The increased levels of neurotransmitters that result are associated with improved mood.

Common drugs include *phenelzine* and isocarboxazid. All MAOIs interact with certain other drugs and foods such as cheese and red wine, which can lead to a dangerous rise in blood pressure. *Moclobemide*, however, is a type called a reversible MAOI, or RIMA, and adverse interactions are less likely; nevertheless, the same foods and drugs should still be avoided by people taking moclobemide.

monoarthritis

Inflammation that affects a single joint, causing pain and stiffness. Common causes of monoarthritis include *osteoarthritis*, *gout*, and *infection*.

monoclonal antibody

See *antibody, monoclonal*.

monocyte

One of the three main types of leukocyte (white *blood cell*), with a large, kidney-shaped nucleus. (The other main types of white blood cell are granulocytes and lymphocytes.) Monocytes are *phagocytes* (cells that surround and engulf invading microorganisms and tissue debris) and play an important role in the *immune system*.

mononucleosis, infectious

An acute viral infection, commonly called glandular fever, that is characterized by a high temperature, sore throat, and swollen *lymph nodes*.

CAUSE

The infection is caused by the *Epstein–Barr virus*. It is transmitted via saliva, through close personal contact (including kissing), or possibly on cups or cutlery.

SYMPTOMS

In the body, the virus multiplies in the *lymphocytes* (also called mononuclear cells). If the infection occurs in early childhood, it may cause no symptoms. However, symptoms are common in adolescence or early adulthood; and the first to appear are a fever and headache, followed by swollen lymph nodes (particularly in the neck) and a severe sore throat. In rare cases, enlargement of the tonsils may obstruct breathing. The spleen may become enlarged. In addition, the liver may become inflamed, sometimes causing *jaundice*.

DIAGNOSIS AND TREATMENT

Diagnosis of the condition is often made from the symptoms and from a blood test (see *monospot test*); affected lymphocytes have an atypical appearance. Recovery usually takes four to six weeks, with rest the only treatment needed. Contact sports should be avoided until the spleen has returned to its normal size. For two to three months after recovery, people often feel depressed, lacking in energy, and sleepy during the day.

monorchism

The presence of only one *testis*. The most probable causes of monorchism are surgery (see *orchidectomy*) and *congenital* absence of the testis.

monosaccharide

An alternative term for a simple sugar (see *carbohydrates*).

M

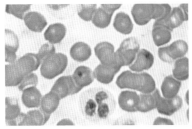

Blood smear in mononucleosis
The large cell with a three-lobed nucleus, surrounded by many red blood cells, is an atypical lymphocyte (it is bigger than normal). Such cells are a feature of mononucleosis.

monosodium glutamate

A *food additive* used as a flavour enhancer and seasoning in food. Monosodium glutamate (MSG) is the sodium salt of an *amino acid*. Some people who eat foods that contain MSG develop a short-lived illness, with pain in the neck and chest, *palpitations*, feeling hot, and a headache.

monospot test

A blood test used in the diagnosis of infectious mononucleosis (see *mononucleosis, infectious*). It is designed to detect certain antibodies (proteins produced by the immune system to fight infection) that are associated with this disorder.

monounsaturated

A term that is used to describe a form of unsaturated fatty acid that is found in certain oils that are used for food, such as olive oil and groundnut oil. (See *fats and oils*.)

monozygotic twins

The medical term for identical twins. (See *twins*.)

mons pubis

The rounded area over the front of the *pubic bone*. The mons pubis is formed by a pad of fatty tissue underneath the skin. It becomes covered with pubic hair at *puberty*.

Monteggia's fracture

Fracture of the *ulna* (the bone on the inner side of the forearm) just below the elbow, together with dislocation of the *radius* (the outer forearm bone) from the elbow joint.

montelukast

A specific *leukotriene receptor antagonist drug* that is used in the management of asthma. It is not, however, used to treat acute attacks.

Montgomery's tubercles

Raised sebaceous glands on the *areola* (the pigmented area around the nipple). The glands tend to become more obvious during pregnancy.

mood

See *affect*; *affective disorders*.

mood swings

Rapid changes in mood. Milder forms of mood swings, such as changes from a calm state to a state of anxiety, irritability, or tearfulness, may occur in women suffering from *premenstrual syndrome* or those who are going through the *menopause*. Extreme mood swings, from *mania* (abnormal overactivity and elation) to *depression*, are associated with *bipolar disorder*.

moon face

Rounding of the face that is due to abnormally high levels of natural corticosteroid hormones in the body, as in *Cushing's syndrome*, or to prolonged courses of *corticosteroid drugs*.

Moraxella

A group of bacteria that exist in a variety of mammals, including humans. The bacteria can cause a wide range of disorders; for example, MORAXELLA LACUNATA may cause *conjunctivitis* and infections of the *cornea* (the transparent covering over the front of the eye), and MORAXELLA CATARRHALIS occasionally causes *otitis media* (infection of the middle ear) and certain infections of the upper respiratory tract, such as *sinusitis* and *bronchitis*.

morbid anatomy

Also called pathological anatomy, the study of the structural changes that occur in body tissues as a result of disease, especially the changes that are visible to the naked eye.

morbidity

The state of being diseased. In medical statistics, the morbidity ratio is the proportion of diseased people to healthy people in a particular community.

morbilli

Another name for *measles*.

morning-after pill

See *contraception, emergency*.

morning sickness

See *vomiting in pregnancy*.

Moro reflex

An automatic movement in infants (see *reflex, primitive*) in which the arms are flung outwards before coming together in an embracing movement, the head jerks backwards, and the legs extend. The Moro reflex occurs in response to a stimulus such as the head being allowed to fall back momentarily.

morphine

An opioid *analgesic drug* derived from the opium poppy. Morphine is given to relieve severe pain caused by *myocardial infarction* (heart attack), major surgery, serious injury, and *cancer*. It blocks the transmission of pain signals at sites called opiate receptors in the *brain* and *spinal cord*. The drug also induces a sense of wellbeing or euphoria.

Side effects include drowsiness, dizziness, constipation, nausea, vomiting, and confusion. Long-term use of morphine may lead to *drug dependence*, with severe flulike symptoms when the drug is withdrawn (see *withdrawal syndrome*).

morphoea

A condition in which one or more hard, flat patches develop on the skin. It is a type of *scleroderma* but is confined to the skin. Although harmless, the condition can be disfiguring.

mortality

The death rate – the number of deaths per 100,000 (or 10,000 or 1,000) of the population per year. Mortality is often calculated for specific groups. For example, *infant mortality* measures the deaths of liveborn infants during the first year of life.

Standardized mortality is a measure that allows comparison of the death rate in, for example, a particular occupational or socioeconomic group with that for the entire population. (See also *life expectancy*; *maternal mortality*.)

morula

A stage in the development of an *embryo* following *fertilization*. The fertilized egg divides repeatedly as it travels down the *fallopian tube* towards the *uterus*. Once it has developed into a ball of cells, it is called a morula.

mosaicism

The presence of two or more groups of cells containing different genetic material within one person. Some people who have syndromes that are caused by *chromosomal abnormalities* (such as

M

Down's syndrome and *Turner's syndrome*) also have mosaicism. Depending on the proportion of the abnormal cells and the type of abnormality, such people range from appearing physically normal to having features that are typical of the syndrome.

mosquito bites

Mosquitoes are flying insects found throughout the world. The females bite humans or animals to obtain blood, which they need to produce eggs. The males do not bite. A doctor should be consulted if there is a severe skin reaction to a mosquito bite.

DISEASE TRANSMISSION

In addition to causing skin irritation, mosquito bites are also capable of transmitting diseases. The main types of disease-transmitting mosquitoes belong to three different groups: ANOPHELES (which transmits *malaria*), AEDES (which carries *yellow fever*), and CULEX (which transmits *filariasis*).

PREVENTION

Preventive measures should be taken in any area where mosquitoes are rampant. The most effective measures are wearing long-sleeved shirts and socks, fitting mosquito screens over windows, and using insect-repellents, such as *DEET*, or slow-burning impregnated coils that release insecticidal smoke. In addition, mosquito nets should be placed over beds. (See also *insect bites*; *insects and disease*.)

motility stimulant drugs

Drugs that stimulate movement through the gastrointestinal tract. There are two main types of motility stimulant: those that work as *antiemetic drugs* and affect the upper gastrointestinal tract (*metoclopramide* and *domperidone*, for example); and intestinal stimulant *laxative drugs*, such as *dantron* and *senna*, which are used to treat constipation.

motion sickness

A problem that some people experience during road, sea, or air travel. Symptoms range from uneasiness and headache to distress, excessive sweating and salivation, pallor, nausea, and vomiting.

Motion sickness is caused by the effect of repetitive movement on the organ of balance in the inner *ear*. Factors such as anxiety, a fume-laden atmosphere, or the sight of food may make the condition worse. So, too, can focusing on nearby objects; sufferers

DANGEROUS MOSQUITOES

Mosquito	Appearance	Habits	Diseases transmitted
ANOPHELES species	Head and body in straight line and at an angle to surface.	Mainly rural; bite at night.	Malaria; filariasis.
CULEX species	Body parallel to surface; head bent down; whining sound in flight; brown colour.	Urban or rural; bite in evening or at night.	Viral encephalitis; filariasis.
AEDES species	Body shape as for CULEX, but tropical species are black and white.	Urban or rural; bite during day.	Dengue; yellow fever; viral encephalitis.

should look at a point on the horizon. The sickness may be prevented or controlled by *antiemetic drugs*.

motor

A term used to describe any body structure that brings about movement, such as a *muscle* or a *nerve*.

motor nerve

A bundle of *nerve* fibres that carry electrical impulses from the *central nervous system* (the brain and spinal cord) to a muscle to bring about activity. (See also *sensory nerve*.) A group of muscle fibres that are activated by a single motor nerve fibre is called a motor unit.

motor neuron disease

A group of disorders in which there is degeneration of the *nerves* in the *central nervous system* that control muscular activity. This nerve degeneration causes weakness and wasting of the muscles. The cause is unknown.

TYPES AND SYMPTOMS

The most common type of the disease is amyotrophic lateral sclerosis (also called ALS, or Lou Gehrig's disease). It usually affects people over the age of 50 and is more common in men. Some cases run in families. Usually, symptoms start with weakness in the hands and arms or legs, and muscle wasting. There may be irregular muscle contractions, and muscle cramps or stiffness. Soon, all four extremities are affected.

Progressive muscular atrophy and progressive bulbar palsy are conditions that both start with patterns of muscle weakness different from ALS but usually develop into ALS.

There are two types of motor neuron disease that first appear in childhood or adolescence. In most cases, these disorders are inherited. *Werdnig–Hoffman disease* affects infants at birth or soon afterwards. In almost all cases, progressive muscle weakness leads to death within only a few years. Chronic spinal muscular atrophy begins in childhood or adolescence, causing progressive weakness but not always serious disability.

DIAGNOSIS

There are no specific tests for motor neuron disease. Diagnosis is based on careful clinical examination by a neurologist. Tests including *EMG*, muscle *biopsy*, *blood tests*, *myelography*, *CT scanning*, or *MRI* may be performed.

TREATMENT AND OUTLOOK

The disease typically progresses to affect the muscles involved in breathing and swallowing, leading to death within two to four years.

The nerve degeneration cannot be slowed down, but *physiotherapy* and the use of various aids may help to reduce disability. The drug riluzole is used to extend life (or extend the time until mechanical *ventilation* is required) in people who have ALS.

mould

Any of a large group of *fungi* that exist as many-celled, filamentous colonies. Some moulds are the source of *antibiotic drugs*. Others, however, can cause diseases such as *aspergillosis*.

mountain sickness

An illness that can affect people who have ascended rapidly to heights above 2,400–3,000 m. Mountain sickness, also

M

called altitude sickness, is caused by the reduced atmospheric pressure and oxygen levels that exist at high altitude.

SYMPTOMS AND SIGNS

Affected people breathe abnormally fast and deeply (see *hyperventilation*) to compensate for the lack of oxygen; as a result, the level of carbon dioxide in the blood falls abnormally low. Other symptoms include nausea, headache, anxiety, and exhaustion. In severe cases, *pulmonary oedema* (the accumulation of fluid in the lungs) may occur, leading to acute shortness of breath (see *respiratory distress syndrome*). Fluid may also accumulate in the brain (see *cerebral oedema*), causing confusion, loss of consciousness, or *coma*.

TREATMENT

An affected person should be returned to a lower altitude as rapidly and safely as possible. He or she may need extra oxygen. Pulmonary or cerebral oedema will need treatment in hospital.

PREVENTION

Mountain sickness can be prevented or minimized by ascending gradually, stopping for one or two days of rest for every 600 m above 2,400 m. It is also helpful to drink plenty of fluids, have regular high-carbohydrate meals, and avoid drinking alcohol. *Acetazolamide* may be used to help prevent or treat symptoms of mountain sickness but is not a substitute for proper acclimatization. Those with existing heart or lung disorders should avoid ascending to high altitudes.

mouth

The oral cavity. The mouth breaks down food for swallowing (see *mastication*) and is used in breathing. In addition, it helps to convert sound vibrations from the *larynx* into speech.

mouth breathing

Breathing through the open mouth, rather than through the nose. It may be due to obstruction of the nasal passages by thick secretions (as in a heavy *cold* or *sinusitis*) or by enlarged *tonsils* or *adenoids*. (See also *snoring*.)

mouth cancer

Forms of cancerous tumour that develop in the lips, tongue, and oral cavity. Lip cancer and tongue cancer are the most common types.

CAUSES AND INCIDENCE

Predisposing causes of mouth cancer are *smoking*, poor *oral hygiene*, drinking alcoholic spirits, chewing tobacco, and inhaling snuff. Irritation from ill-fitting dentures or jagged teeth are other risk factors. Men are affected twice as commonly as women; most cases occur in men over the age of 40.

SYMPTOMS

In most cases, the cancer begins with a whitish patch, called *leukoplakia*, or a small lump. These lesions may cause a burning sensation, but are usually painless. As a tumour grows, it may develop into an *ulcer* or a deep fissure, which may bleed and erode surrounding tissue.

DIAGNOSIS AND TREATMENT

Diagnosis is based on a *biopsy*. Treatment consists of surgery, *radiotherapy*, or both. Surgical treatment may cause facial disfigurement and problems with eating and speaking, which may then necessitate *plastic surgery* to restore appearance and function. Radiotherapy may be given either externally or with implants in the area (brachytherapy); however, it sometimes damages the salivary glands (see *mouth, dry*).

When mouth cancer is detected and treated early, the outlook is good. Any nonhealing ulcer or lump in the mouth should be assessed by a doctor or dentist within two weeks, to maximize the chance of effective treatment.

mouth, dry

A condition caused by the inadequate production of saliva. A dry mouth is usually a temporary problem resulting from fear, infection of a *salivary gland*, or the action of *anticholinergic drugs*. Rarely, permanent dry mouth may result from *Sjögren's syndrome* or radiotherapy for mouth cancer. The dryness causes swallowing and speaking difficulty, impaired taste, and tooth decay (see *caries, dental*). Spraying the inside of the mouth with artificial saliva or taking *pilocarpine* tablets may help.

mouth-to-mouth resuscitation

See *rescue breathing*.

mouth ulcer

An open sore that is caused by a break in the *mucous membrane* that lines the mouth. Mouth ulcers are white, grey, or yellow spots with an inflamed border. The most common types are aphthous ulcers (see *ulcer, aphthous*) and ulcers caused by the *herpes simplex* virus.

A mouth ulcer may be an early stage of *mouth cancer*. Those that fail to heal within a month may need to be investigated with a *biopsy*.

mouthwash

A solution for rinsing the mouth. Many only leave the mouth feeling fresh and remove loose food debris from the teeth. Some, such as those containing *hydrogen peroxide*, can help to clean the teeth if the gums are too tender for proper toothbrushing, as may occur in some types of *gingivitis*. Mouthwashes that

M

ANATOMY OF THE MOUTH

The mouth has a complex structure, which reflects its various functions. For example, the tongue, lips, teeth, and palate play an essential role in speech production. The same parts of the mouth, with the salivary glands, also begin the process of digestion by taking in and swallowing food and drink.

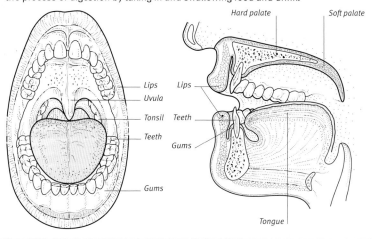

M

contain *chlorhexidine* are effective against plaque when routine dental hygiene is impossible. *Fluoride* mouthwashes help to prevent tooth decay (see *caries, dental*), and a mouthwash of warm salt water can help to ease painful inflammation caused by tooth disorders. Antiseptic mouthwashes intended to combat *halitosis* are usually ineffective because they do not treat the cause of the problem.

movement

Any motion of limbs or other areas of the body, or any motion within soft tissues and body organs. All movements are caused by the actions of muscles. They may be either voluntary (willed) or involuntary (automatic). Certain movements occur as *reflex* actions.

SKELETAL MOVEMENTS

These movements involve the bones, the joints, and the skeletal muscles. Most of them are voluntary. They are initiated in a part of the cerebrum (the main mass of the *brain*) called the motor cortex. Nerve signals are sent down the *spinal cord* along some nerve fibres, and, from there, along separate nerve fibres to the appropriate muscles. Control relies on information supplied by sensory nerve *receptors*, in the muscles and elsewhere, which detect the position of different body parts and the degree of contraction in each muscle. This information is integrated in the specific regions of the brain (including the *cerebellum* and *basal ganglia*) that control the coordination, initiation, and cessation of movement.

Skeletal movements can also occur as simple reflexes in response to certain sensory warning signals. These movements are automatic and less controlled, involving far fewer nerve connections.

OTHER MOVEMENTS

Some body movements do not involve the skeleton. For example, eye and tongue movements result from the contractions of muscles attached to other soft tissues. These movements may be voluntary or reflex.

The movements of the internal organs are involuntary; they include the *heartbeat* and *peristalsis*.

movement, loss of

See *akinesia*.

moxibustion

A form of alternative therapy, often used in conjunction with *acupuncture*, in which a cone of wormwood leaves

MOVEMENT

Various movements occur constantly throughout the body. All movement is either voluntary (willed) or involuntary (automatic). Visible movements are caused by the contraction of skeletal muscles or eye muscles, usually for only brief periods at a time.

SKELETAL MOVEMENT

This action involves the movement of bones relative to one another, often at the joints. Many muscles are involved. Some act to brace certain bones, while others move adjacent bones.

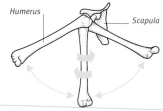

Arm movements
A ball-and-socket joint, the shoulder allows combined rotation and displacement movements in all directions.

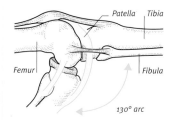

Knee movement
A hinge joint, the knee allows movement (through an arc of about 130°) in only one plane: forwards or backwards.

INVOLUNTARY MOVEMENT

Many movements in the body are involuntary (automatic), and are regulated by the autonomic nervous system. One example of involuntary movement is the beating of the heart, which automatically speeds up in response to increased demands for oxygenated blood by body tissues and slows down again when these demands decrease. Another example is peristalsis (see right).

EYE MOVEMENT

A group of six muscles act together on each eyeball to give a range of smooth, precise movements. The eyeball can move through an arc of about 100° horizontally and about 80° vertically.

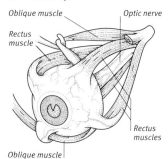

Eye muscles
The four rectus eye muscles run directly from the eyeball to a tendon at the back of the eye socket. The oblique muscles are attached to the eyeball at an angle.

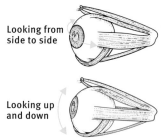

Actions of the eye muscles
Two rectus muscles control side-to-side movements. The other rectus muscles, with the oblique muscles, control up-and-down and rotational movements.

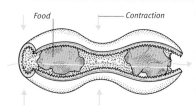

Peristalsis
This is an example of movement caused by involuntary muscle action. Waves of contraction pass along muscles in the intestinal wall, forcing the contents forwards and preventing obstruction.

(moxa) or certain other plant materials is burned just above the skin for the purpose of relieving internal pain.

moxisylyte

A *vasodilator drug* that is used to treat *Raynaud's disease*. Side effects include nausea, diarrhoea, hot flushes, head-ache, and dizziness.

MRI

The abbreviation for magnetic reso-nance imaging. MRI is a diagnostic technique that produces cross-sectional or three-dimensional images of organs and other body structures.

HOW IT IS DONE

The patient lies inside a scanner sur-rounded by a large, powerful magnet. A receiving magnet is placed around the part of the body to be investigated. If large areas, such as the abdomen, are to be imaged, the receiving magnet is fit-ted inside the scanner; for a smaller area, such as a joint, a magnet may be placed around the part to be scanned.

The scanner generates a strong mag-netic field, which causes the atoms in the body to line up parallel to each other. Short pulses of radio waves from a radiofrequency source briefly knock the atoms out of alignment. As the atoms realign they emit tiny signals, which are detected by the receiving magnet. Information about these signals is passed to a computer, which builds up an image based on the signals' strength and location.

MRI images can be enhanced by use of a *contrast medium* to highlight partic-ular body structures, such as tumours and blood vessels.

WHY IT IS DONE

Images from MRI are similar to those produced by *CT scanning*, but they give greater contrast between normal and abnormal tissues. MRI is useful for studying the brain and spinal cord, the internal structure of the eye and ear, the internal organs, and blood flow. A type of MRI called functional MRI (fMRI) can reveal areas of neural activi-ty in the brain.

RISKS

There are no known risks or side effects of MRI scanning. The scans do not use ionizing radiation and can be performed repeatedly. However, because the scan-ner uses powerful magnetic fields, it may interfere with the functioning of pacemakers, hearing aids, and other electrical devices.

MAGNETIC RESONANCE IMAGING (MRI)

A valuable diagnostic technique, MRI has been in use since the early 1980s. The patient lies down and is surrounded by a massive electromagnet and is exposed to short bursts of powerful magnetic fields and radio waves. The bursts stimulate protons (hydrogen nuclei) in the patient's tissues to emit radio signals, which are detected and analysed by computer to create an image of a "slice" of the patient's body.

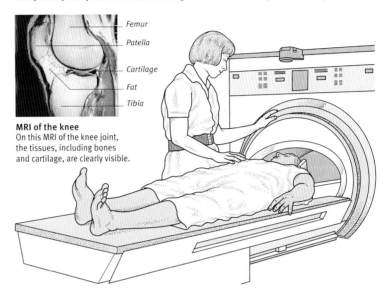

MRI of the knee
On this MRI of the knee joint, the tissues, including bones and cartilage, are clearly visible.

THE SCANNING PROCESS

An MRI scanner consists of a powerful electromagnet, a radio-wave emitter, and a radio-wave detector. A plane of the body is selected for imaging and the electromagnet is turned on.

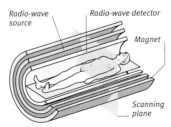

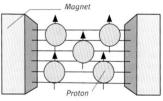

1 Normally, the protons (nuclei) of the body's hydrogen atoms point randomly in different directions, but under the influence of the scanner's powerful magnetic field they align themselves in the same direction.

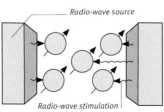

2 Next, the radio-wave source emits a powerful pulse of radio waves, which knocks the protons out of alignment.

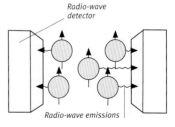

3 However, milliseconds later, the protons realign themselves. As they do so, they emit faint radio signals, which are picked up by the scanner's radio-wave detector.

MRSA

The abbreviation for methicillin-resistant STAPHYLOCOCCUS AUREUS, a bacterium that is resistant to methicillin and many other *antibiotic drugs*. MRSA is commonly known as the "hospital superbug" because most cases are contracted in hospital and infection is difficult to treat and can sometimes be fatal.

MS

The abbreviation for *multiple sclerosis*.

MSG

The abbreviation for the food additive *monosodium glutamate*.

MST Continus

A brand name for a modified-release preparation of the opioid analgesic (painkilling) drug *morphine*.

MSU

The abbreviation for midstream specimen of urine: a sample to be examined for microorganisms in the urinary tract. Allowing the first part of the stream to flow into the toilet helps clear contaminants from the skin or urethral lining.

mucocele

A sac or cavity in the body that is filled with *mucus* secreted by its inner lining.

mucolipidoses

A group of rare metabolic disorders (see *metabolism, inborn errors of*) in which a particular *enzyme* deficiency causes an abnormal accumulation of *lipids* and substances called mucopolysaccharides in cells. The disorders appear in childhood; they may cause *learning difficulties* and a variety of physical abnormalities.

mucolytic drugs

Drugs that make sputum (phlegm) less sticky and easier to cough up. An example is *carbocisteine*.

mucopolysaccharidosis

A group of rare inherited metabolic disorders (see *metabolism, inborn errors of*) of which *Hurler's syndrome* is the most well known. Mucopolysaccharidoses are *genetic disorders* in which there is an abnormality of a specific *enzyme*, causing the accumulation of substances called mucopolysaccharides in body cells.

SYMPTOMS

Features may include abnormalities of the skeleton and/or the central nervous system, with *learning difficulties* and, in some cases, a characteristic facial appearance. There may also be clouding of the *cornea*, enlargement of the liver, and stiffness in the joints.

TREATMENT AND OUTLOOK

No specific treatment is available; however, a *stem cell* or *bone marrow transplant* may be used to treat Hurler's syndrome.

Mild forms of mucopolysaccharidoses allow a child to have a relatively normal life. More severe types usually cause death in childhood or adolescence.

mucosa

A term for *mucous membrane*.

mucous membrane

The soft, pink, skinlike layer that lines many of the cavities and tubes in the body, including the *respiratory tract* and the *digestive tract*. Mucous membranes contain cells called goblet cells, which secrete a fluid containing *mucus*.

mucus

The thick, slimy fluid that is secreted by *mucous membranes*. Mucus moistens, lubricates, and protects parts of the body lined by mucous membranes.

mucus method of contraception

See *contraception, natural methods of*.

MUGA scan

A method of investigating how much blood the *heart* can pump with each heartbeat and whether different parts of the heart wall are contracting properly. The patient's *red blood cells* are injected with a radioactive *isotope* to enable an image to be formed of the blood pool within the heart at different times during the heart cycle. A MUGA scan, or multiple-gated acquisition scan, uses *ECG*, a *gamma camera*, and a computer.

multi-infarct dementia

A deterioration in brain function (see *dementia*) resulting from the death of small areas of brain tissue. It is the third most common cause of dementia after *Alzheimer's disease* and *Lewy-body dementia*. The disorder occurs when clots block small blood vessels within the brain, preventing the flow of blood to particular areas and thereby starving the tissue of oxygen. The risk of developing multi-infarct dementia is increased in people with *hypertension* (high blood pressure) and *atherosclerosis* (narrowing of the arteries by fatty deposits on the artery walls).

Symptoms vary depending on the part of the brain that is affected, but they become progressively worse, in distinct steps, after each attack. Symptoms include disruption of memory, so that the person cannot recall recent events or gets lost in familiar surroundings; difficulty in making decisions or carrying out simple tasks; and changes in mood, such as depression or agitation. Affected people often experience repeated *transient ischaemic attacks* or *strokes*.

Diagnosis is based on the symptoms and, if necessary, confirmed by *MRI* or *CT scanning* of the brain. *Antihypertensive drugs* may be prescribed to control blood pressure, and *aspirin* is often prescribed to reduce the risk of the condition progressing. People can also help to protect themselves from any further infarcts by following a low-fat diet and exercising regularly.

multiparous

A term for a woman who has had two or more pregnancies resulting in birth (whether or not the fetuses were alive at the time of birth).

multiple endocrine neoplasia (MEN)

The name for a group of rare, autosomal dominant *genetic disorders* that cause tumours to develop in several of the *endocrine glands*. Each disorder is caused by a different abnormal gene. One form of MEN causes tumours in the *pancreas*, *parathyroid glands*, and *pituitary gland*, and sometimes also in the *adrenal gland* and the *thyroid gland*. Another, less common form produces tumours in the adrenal, thyroid, and parathyroid glands. Tumours may arise simultaneously or at different times over several years. The affected glands may produce excess hormones. One type of thyroid tumour, which secretes the hormone calcitonin, is usually cancerous, but most tumours in other endocrine glands are not.

Tumours are usually removed by surgery, and the person will be monitored afterwards so that any further endocrine abnormalities can be detected. The person's relatives may be offered screening for the abnormal gene or the effects of the disorder (see *familial screening*).

multiple myeloma

A rare, cancerous disorder, also known as myelomatosis, in which the plasma cells in the *bone marrow* proliferate uncontrollably and function incorrectly. Multiple myeloma is more common in elderly people.

CAUSE

Plasma cells are a type of B-*lymphocyte* that produce *immunoglobulins*, which help protect against infection. In multiple myeloma, the proliferating plasma cells produce excessive amounts of one type of immunoglobulin while the production of other types is impaired. This makes infection more likely.

SYMPTOMS

Early in the disease there may be no symptoms but, as the disease progresses, proliferation of the abnormal cells in the bone marrow causes pain and destroys the bone tissue. Affected *vertebrae* may collapse and compress the *spinal cord* or spinal nerves, causing numbness or *paralysis*. As bone is destroyed, levels of calcium in the blood increase, as may the levels of one or more immunoglobulins. These changes in the blood may lead to damage of the kidneys, resulting in *kidney failure*. There may also be *anaemia* and a tendency for abnormal bleeding.

DIAGNOSIS AND TREATMENT

Multiple myeloma is diagnosed by *bone marrow biopsy*, *blood tests* or *urinalysis*, and *X-rays*.

People with no symptoms generally do not need treatment, although monitoring is necessary to check the progress of the disease. When treatment is necessary, it may include *chemotherapy* to slow the course of the disease; *radiotherapy* for localized bone deposits, to relieve pain and reduce the risk of fractures; and *stem cell* transplantation (sometimes together with chemotherapy) to replace diseased or damaged bone marrow. In addition, treatment may involve correction of associated problems, such as kidney failure, and supportive measures, including *blood transfusions*, *antibiotic drugs*, and *analgesic drugs* (painkillers). No treatment provides a cure, however.

The outlook for multiple myeloma varies depending on the severity of the illness. Some people remain well for months or years, and then the progression of the disease accelerates.

multiple organ failure

Loss of function in several organs at once. This life-threatening condition affects the lungs (see *respiratory distress syndrome*), kidneys and other organs, and the circulation. It is most often triggered by overwhelming infection, but may also be due to *shock* after severe injury.

multiple personality disorder

A rare disorder in which a person has two or more distinct personalities, each of which dominates at different times. Each personality may be unaware that the others exist. The transition from one personality to another is often sudden, and may be triggered by *stress*. The condition is thought to result from severe emotional trauma, such as violent *sexual abuse*, during childhood.

multiple pregnancy

See *pregnancy, multiple*.

multiple sclerosis (MS)

A progressive disease of the central *nervous system*, in which patches of *myelin* (the protective covering of nerve fibres) in the brain and the spinal cord are damaged. The damaged patches are called plaques. The nerves cannot conduct electrical impulses, so functions such as movement and sensation may be lost. Any part of the central nervous system may be affected.

CAUSES AND INCIDENCE

MS is an *autoimmune disorder* in which the body's immune system attacks the myelin sheath that covers some nerves in the brain and spinal cord. Women are more likely to develop MS than men, and there may be a genetic factor involved because MS sometimes runs in families. There may also be an environmental factor, as MS is more common in temperate zones than in the tropics.

SYMPTOMS

MS usually develops between the ages of 20 and 45, and the symptoms depend on the area of the brain or spinal cord affected. Spinal cord damage may cause tingling, numbness, weakness in the extremities, *spasticity*, *paralysis*, and *incontinence*. Damage to white matter (myelinated nerves) in the brain may cause fatigue, *vertigo*, clumsiness, muscle weakness, slurred speech, blurred vision, facial numbness, or facial pain. People with MS may also have difficulty concentrating, impaired memory, and have feelings of depression or anxiety. For further information see *Features of multiple sclerosis* box, overleaf.

An attack may last for several weeks or months. It is followed by a variable period of remission, in which dramatic improvements may be made. After a remission period, a further attack or a relapse occurs, which may be precipitated by injury, illness, or stress. Some people have mild relapses and long periods of remission (relapsing–remitting MS), with few permanent effects. Others have a form called chronic–progressive MS, becoming gradually more disabled from the first attack. A few have a form called fulminant MS, which progresses rapidly to gross disability in the first year of illness.

DIAGNOSIS

There is no single diagnostic test, but *MRI* may show damage to white matter in the brain, and a *lumbar puncture* may show abnormal proteins in the fluid around the spinal cord. *Evoked response* tests on the eyes may also provide confirmatory evidence.

TREATMENT

There is no specific treatment. A short course of *corticosteroid drugs* may reduce the severity of relapses, and beta *interferon* can lengthen the time between attacks in relapsing-remitting MS and reduce the rate of decline. The use of *rehabilitation*, *physiotherapy*, and *occupational therapy* is essential so that people can carry out daily activities more easily.

Many complementary therapies claim to be able to alleviate the symptoms of MS but there is little evidence that they are effective. However, there is some evidence that general wellbeing may be improved by certain therapies, such as reflexology, massage, and t'ai chi.

multivitamins

Over-the-counter preparations, containing a combination of vitamins, that are used as a dietary supplement. (See *vitamin supplements*.)

mumps

An acute viral illness usually occurring in childhood. The main symptom is inflammation and swelling of one or both

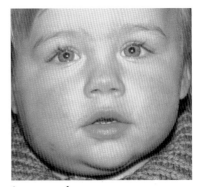

Appearance of mumps
The swelling may be present on either or both sides and can give the affected child's face a bloated appearance.

FEATURES OF **MULTIPLE SCLEROSIS**

The disease can affect any area of the white matter of the brain and spinal cord. The plaques of demyelination are areas in which the fatty myelin sheaths of the nerve fibres have been destroyed. The affected fibres cannot conduct nerve impulses, so functions such as movement and sensation may be lost. The patchy distribution of plaques causes very varied effects.

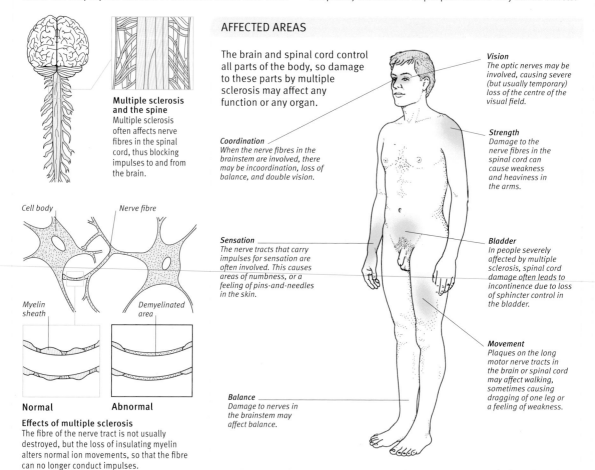

Multiple sclerosis and the spine
Multiple sclerosis often affects nerve fibres in the spinal cord, thus blocking impulses to and from the brain.

AFFECTED AREAS

The brain and spinal cord control all parts of the body, so damage to these parts by multiple sclerosis may affect any function or any organ.

Coordination
When the nerve fibres in the brainstem are involved, there may be incoordination, loss of balance, and double vision.

Sensation
The nerve tracts that carry impulses for sensation are often involved. This causes areas of numbness, or a feeling of pins-and-needles in the skin.

Balance
Damage to nerves in the brainstem may affect balance.

Vision
The optic nerves may be involved, causing severe (but usually temporary) loss of the centre of the visual field.

Strength
Damage to the nerve fibres in the spinal cord can cause weakness and heaviness in the arms.

Bladder
In people severely affected by multiple sclerosis, spinal cord damage often leads to incontinence due to loss of sphincter control in the bladder.

Movement
Plaques on the long motor nerve tracts in the brain or spinal cord may affect walking, sometimes causing dragging of one leg or a feeling of weakness.

Cell body

Nerve fibre

Myelin sheath

Demyelinated area

Normal   **Abnormal**

Effects of multiple sclerosis
The fibre of the nerve tract is not usually destroyed, but the loss of insulating myelin alters normal ion movements, so that the fibre can no longer conduct impulses.

M

parotid glands, which are situated inside the angle of the jaw. One attack of mumps confers lifelong immunity. Since routine *MMR vaccination*, epidemics of mumps no longer occur.

CAUSE
The mumps virus is spread in airborne droplets. The *incubation period* is two to three weeks; an affected person is infectious from 12 to 25 days after exposure to the virus.

SYMPTOMS
Infected children often have no symptoms, or they may feel slightly unwell and have some discomfort around the parotid glands. In more serious cases, there is pain around the glands and chewing becomes difficult; one or both glands then become swollen and tender. A fever and headache may develop. The swelling subsides within a week to ten days. When only one gland is affected, the second gland often swells as the swelling in the first subsides.

COMPLICATIONS
Mumps may lead to a number of other conditions including viral *meningitis* (inflammation of the membranes covering the brain and spinal cord), *pancreatitis* (inflammation of the pancreas), or, in adolescent or adult males, *epididymoorchitis* (inflammation of the testes).

DIAGNOSIS AND TREATMENT
Diagnosis is usually made from the symptoms. There is usually no treatment; rest and painkillers may ease symptoms.

Munchausen's syndrome

A chronic *factitious disorder* in which a person complains of physical symptoms that are pretended or self-induced in order to play the role of patient.

The usual complaints are abdominal pain, bleeding, neurological symptoms, rashes, and fever. People typically invent dramatic histories. Most sufferers are repeatedly admitted to hospital, and many have detailed medical knowledge and scars from self-injury or previous treatment. In Munchausen's syndrome by proxy, parents simulate disorders in children.

Treatment consists of protecting the sufferers from unnecessary operations and drug treatments.

mupirocin

An *antibacterial* cream or ointment used to treat skin infections such as *impetigo*. It is also sometimes used to eliminate staphylococcal bacteria from the skin.

mural aneurysm

A dilated, weakened area in the wall of the left *ventricle* in the heart; also called a *ventricular aneurysm*.

mural thrombus

A *thrombus* (blood clot) on the inner wall of a heart chamber, usually on the wall of a ventricle (lower chamber). The clot develops on an area of tissue that has been damaged by a *myocardial infarction* (heart attack).

murmur

A sound caused by turbulent blood flow through the *heart*, as heard through a *stethoscope*. Heart murmurs are regarded as an indication of possible abnormalities in the blood flow. Apart from *innocent murmurs*, the most common cause of extra blood turbulence is a disorder of the *heart valves*. Murmurs can also be caused by some types of congenital heart disease (see *heart disease, congenital*) or by rarer conditions such as a *myxoma* in a heart chamber. (See also *systolic murmur*.)

muscle

A structure composed of bundles of specialized cells, which are capable of contraction and relaxation to create movement. There are three types of muscle: skeletal, smooth, and cardiac.

SKELETAL MUSCLE

The skeletal muscles are the most prominent muscle group in the body (see *muscular system*). They are called voluntary muscles because they are under conscious control (see *The body's muscles* box, overleaf).

Skeletal muscles comprise groups of muscle fibres arranged in bundles called fascicles. A fibre is made up of longitudinal units called myofibrils, the working units of which are filaments of actin and myosin (two proteins that control contraction). Impulses from the brain cause the myosin filaments to slide over the actin, making the muscle fibres contract and move the body. Conversely, nerve fibres in the muscle register the force of contraction (while nerves in the tendon register how much it has stretched) and transmit this information back to the brain, which limits the strength of the contraction. The muscle activity is affected by changes in the chemical composition of the fluid that surrounds the muscle cells. A fall in the level of potassium ions causes muscle weakness; a decrease in calcium ions causes muscle *spasm*.

A state of partial contraction is constantly maintained, even when the muscles are not moving; this is called muscle tone (see *tone, muscle*). Some disorders may cause abnormalities in muscle tone, such as excessive rigidity (*spasticity*) or floppiness (*hypotonia*).

SMOOTH MUSCLE

This type of muscle exists in the walls of internal organs. It produces movements such as *peristalsis* in the intestine and contractions of the uterus in childbirth. Smooth muscle also forms part of the lining of hollow structures such as the blood vessels, airways, and bladder. It is also called involuntary muscle, because it is not under conscious control.

The muscle is made of long, spindle-shaped cells, and contracts by the same action of actin and myosin as skeletal muscle. It is stimulated by the *autonomic nervous system*; it also responds to *hormones* and to levels of chemicals in the fluid around the muscle.

CARDIAC MUSCLE

Cardiac muscle (also called myocardium) is found only in the *heart*. It is able to contract continually and rhythmically, about 100,000 times a day. Contraction is stimulated by the automatic nervous system, by hormones, and by the stretching of muscle fibres. The initial electrical stimulus comes from the *sinoatrial node*; it spreads through specialized conduction cells that form a network throughout the muscle fibres. The fibres are joined end to end by areas of extensive folds that enable contractions to be transmitted rapidly from onr fibre to another.

DISORDERS

The most common disorders are injury and lack of blood supply to a muscle. (See also *Disorders of muscle*, p.523.)

muscle enzymes

Proteins that regulate the rate of chemical reactions in muscle cells. Measuring the blood levels of muscle enzymes (see *blood tests*) can help in the diagnosis of certain disorders, such as *myocardial infarction* (heart attack), in which damaged

MUSCLE TYPES

In each main muscle type, the fibres form a distinctive structure that enables the muscle to fulfil a specific function.

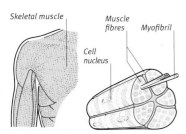

Skeletal muscle
Long bundles of muscle fibres, each containing myofibrils (contractile elements), allow skeletal muscle to contract briefly but powerfully.

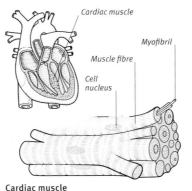

Cardiac muscle
This muscle comprises short, branching cells that interconnect, so that nerve signals can spread instantly throughout the heart.

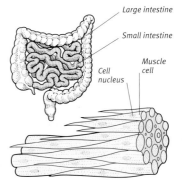

Smooth muscle
In smooth muscle, loosely woven, tapering cells form flat sheets of tissue. Contraction is slower than in other muscle types.

THE BODY'S **MUSCLES**

The most prominent muscles in the body are the skeletal muscles, which account for 40 to 45 per cent of body weight. These muscles are defined as voluntary because they are under conscious control; some important voluntary muscles are indicated on the illustration below. In contrast, many of the internal organs, such as the heart and the intestines, consist partly or entirely of involuntary muscle, which is not under conscious control.

M

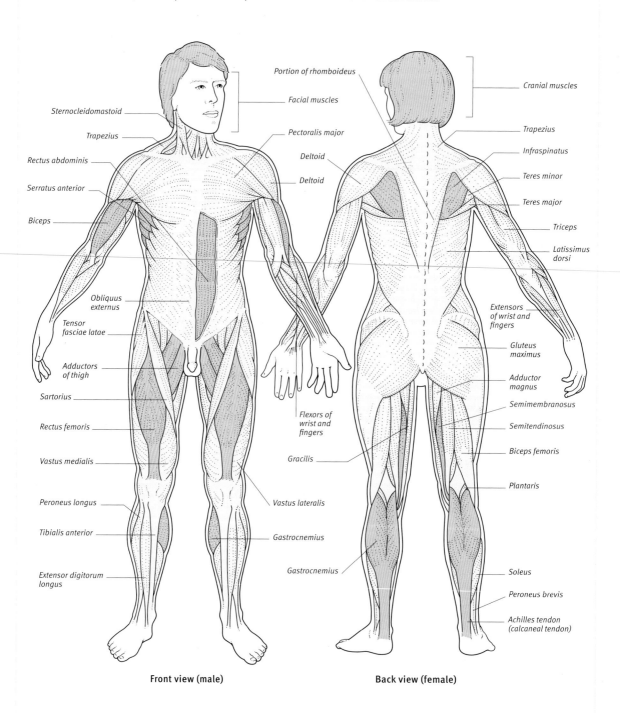

Front view (male)

Back view (female)

heart muscle leaks higher than normal levels of enzymes into the blood, and *muscular dystrophy*, in which the raised levels of muscle enzyme are due to death of muscle cells. Enzymes leaked from the heart muscle differ from those from skeletal muscle; this distinction helps to pinpoint the site of muscle damage.

muscle-relaxant drugs

A group of drugs used to relieve muscle spasm and *spasticity*, mainly in the treatment of nervous system disorders such as *multiple sclerosis* and painful muscular conditions such as *torticollis*. They are occasionally used to relieve muscle rigidity due to injury. Some types of muscle-relaxant drugs are used to produce temporary paralysis during surgery under general *anaesthesia*.

Most muscle-relaxants partially block nerve signals that stimulate muscle contraction. *Dantrolene*, in contrast, interferes with the chemical activity in muscle cells themselves. The drugs may cause muscle weakness and drowsiness. In rare cases, dantrolene causes liver damage.

muscle spasm

Sudden and involuntary contraction of a muscle. Spasm is a reaction to pain and inflammation around a joint. Common causes are *strain*, *disc prolapse* (slipped disc), and stress. Usually, the underlying cause is treated. *Muscle-relaxant drugs* may also be needed. (See also *spasticity*.)

DISORDERS OF MUSCLE

The most common muscle disorder is injury, followed by symptoms caused by a lack of blood supply to a muscle (including the heart muscle). There are also various other, rare disorders that can affect the muscles.

Injury

Muscle injuries, such as tears and *strains*, are very common. They cause bleeding into the muscle tissue. Healing may lead to the formation of a scar in the muscle, which shortens its natural length. Blunt injury may result in the formation of a *haematoma* (a localized collection of blood) from bleeding into the muscle. Rarely, bone may form in a blood clot, causing *myositis ossificans*.

Impaired blood supply

Muscles depend on a good blood supply in order to function normally. A temporary lack of blood flow, which is sometimes associated with severe exertion, may cause *cramp*. *Peripheral vascular disease*, in which blood vessels in the legs (and sometimes the arms) are narrowed, restricts the blood supply, causing *claudication* (muscle pain on exercise). *Angina pectoris* (chest pain caused by lack of blood supply to heart muscle) may occur in people with *coronary artery disease*.

The *compartment syndrome* is pain in muscles as a result of pressure that limits their blood supply. It may be brought on by injury or exercise, and occurs most often in athletes who have well-developed muscles.

Infection

The most serious infection of muscle is *gangrene*, which may complicate deep wounds (especially those contaminated by soil). *Tetanus* is acquired in a similar way; it causes widespread muscle spasm through the release of a powerful toxin.

Viruses (especially influenza B) may also infect muscles (causing *myalgia*), as may the organism causing *toxoplasmosis*. Lastly, a parasitic disease called *trichinosis* can occur in muscle tissue. This disease results from infestation with the worm TRICHINELLA SPIRALIS, which is acquired by eating undercooked meat (usually pork).

Tumours

Various forms of tumour may originate in the muscles. Such tumours, called primary muscle tumours, may or may not be cancerous. Noncancerous tumours are called *myomas;* those affecting smooth muscle are called *leiomyomas*, and those developing in skeletal muscle are called *rhabdomyomas*. Myomas of the uterus (see *fibroids*) are among the most common of all tumours. Cancerous tumours, called myosarcomas, are very rare; they include *rhabdomyosarcomas*, which are cancers of the skeletal muscle.

Secondary tumours, which spread from a primary site of cancer elsewhere in the body, very rarely involve muscle.

Hormonal and metabolic disorders

Muscle contraction depends on the maintenance of proper levels of sodium, potassium, and calcium in and around muscle cells. Any alteration in the concentration of these substances affects muscle function. For example, a severe drop in the level of potassium (*hypokalaemia*) causes profound muscle weakness and may stop the heart. A drop in blood calcium (*hypocalcaemia*) causes increased excitability of muscles and, occasionally, *muscle spasms*.

Thyroid disease is often associated with muscle disorders, the most common of which is swelling of the small muscles that move the eyes, causing a bulging eyeball (see *exophthalmos*). Adrenal failure (see *Addison's disease*) causes general muscle weakness.

Poisons and drugs

Several toxic substances can damage muscle tissue. Alcohol can cause damage following a prolonged drinking bout. Other substances that may cause muscle damage include the drugs *chloroquine* and *vincristine*.

Genetic disorders

These disorders include the various forms of *muscular dystrophy*, which cause progressive weakness and disability. Some types appear at birth, some in infancy, and some develop as late as the fifth or sixth decade. *Cardiomyopathy* (disease of the heart muscle) is also inherited in some cases.

Autoimmune disorders

Myasthenia gravis is a disorder involving the transmission of nerve impulses to muscles; it usually begins with drooping of the eyelids and double vision. Other autoimmune diseases that may affect the muscles are *lupus erythematosus, rheumatoid arthritis, systemic sclerosis, sarcoidosis,* and *dermatomyositis*.

INVESTIGATION

Muscle disorders are investigated by EMG (electromyography), which measures the response of muscles to electrical impulses, and by biopsy (removal of a sample of tissue for analysis). In addition, blood tests may be used to detect abnormal levels of muscle enzymes.

M

muscle wasting

See *muscular atrophy*.

muscular atrophy

Weakness and shrinking of muscle tissue. Muscular atrophy may have many possible causes, including injury, starvation, loss of function in a body part, degeneration of muscle cells, and disorders of the nerves supplying muscles.

Muscles can atrophy rapidly if a body part is not used and if no measures are taken to prevent the problem. In a broken leg, for example, muscle loss may be visible after only a week. The muscle fibres are not lost, however; they can return to normal if the muscle is stimulated and used.

muscular dystrophy

A group of rare inherited muscle disorders that cause slow, progressive wasting of muscle fibres. This degeneration may lead to disability and death.

TYPES AND SYMPTOMS

The most common and severe form of muscular dystrophy is Duchenne muscular dystrophy. This is caused by a recessive gene carried on the X chromosome (see *sex-linked inheritance*). Boys only have one X chromosome, so if they inherit a copy of the defective gene from their mother they develop the disorder. Girls (with two X chromosomes) are not affected but become carriers of the defective gene.

Affected boys walk with a waddle, find climbing difficult, and may have curvature of the spine. The disorder progresses rapidly: the ability to walk is lost by the age of 12, and few boys survive beyond the teenage years.

Becker's muscular dystrophy starts later in childhood and progresses at a slower rate. Myotonic dystrophy affects the muscles of the hands, face, neck, and feet, and causes *learning difficulties*. Limb-girdle muscular dystrophy mainly affects muscles in the hips and shoulders, and facioscapulohumeral muscular dystrophy affects muscles in the upper arms, shoulder girdle, and face. In this last form, severe disability is rare.

DIAGNOSIS

A diagnosis for Duchenne muscular dystrophy can be made with gene testing before symptoms develop. Once muscle weakness has developed, other tests may be used, including measurement of muscle *enzymes* and an *EMG*.

TREATMENT

There is no cure, and *physiotherapy* is the main treatment. Remaining as active

M

DUCHENNE MUSCULAR DYSTROPHY: A TYPICAL FAMILY TREE

Affected males always inherit the gene for the disorder from their mothers, who are carriers of the gene but are themselves unaffected. About half the sons of carriers are affected; the other sons are neither affected nor carriers. The daughters of carriers have a 50 per cent chance of being carriers themselves. Complex blood tests provide the only means of knowing whether or not a certain daughter (or granddaughter) is a muscular dystrophy carrier.

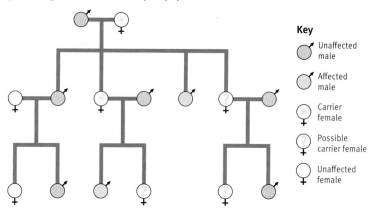

Key
Unaffected male
Affected male
Carrier female
Possible carrier female
Unaffected female

TYPES OF **MUSCULAR DYSTROPHY**

Duchenne muscular dystrophy	In this type, the child is slow in learning to sit up and walk, and does so much later than normal. The condition is rarely diagnosed before the age of three, but progresses rapidly. Affected children tend to walk with a waddle and have difficulty climbing stairs. In getting up from the floor, the child "climbs up his legs", pushing his hands against his ankles, knees, and thighs.	Sometimes there is curvature of the spine. Despite their weakness, the muscles (especially those in the calves) appear bulky; this is because wasted muscle is replaced by fat. By about the age of 12, affected children are no longer able to walk, few survive beyond their teenage years, usually dying from a chest infection or heart failure. Affected boys often have below-average intelligence.
Becker's muscular dystrophy	This type produces the same symptoms as the Duchenne type, but starts later in childhood and progresses much	more slowly. Patients often reach the age of 50. Both types of dystrophy have sex-linked inheritance.
Myotonic dystrophy	This form affects muscles of the face, hands, and feet. Infants are floppy and slow to develop. The main feature is that the muscles contract strongly but do not relax easily. Myotonic	dystrophy is associated with cataracts in middle age, baldness, mental retardation, and endocrine problems. The condition has an autosomal dominant pattern of inheritance.
Limb-girdle muscular dystrophy	This type takes different forms. It starts in late childhood or early adult life, and progression is slow. The muscles of the hips and shoulders are mainly	affected. Other nerve and muscle conditions must be eliminated before this form of dystrophy can be diagnosed confidently.
Facioscapulohumeral muscular dystrophy	This form usually appears first between the ages of 10 and 40; it affects only the muscles of the upper arms, shoulder girdle, and face. It is inherited in an	autosomal dominant pattern. In this form of muscular dystrophy, progression of the weakness is slow, and severe disability is rare.

as possible keeps healthy muscles in good condition. Surgery to the heel *tendons* may aid walking in some cases.

OUTLOOK

The long-term outlook depends on the particular form. Families in which a child or adult has developed any form of muscular dystrophy may wish to consider *genetic counselling*.

muscular system

The muscles of the body that are attached to the *skeleton*. These muscles are responsible for voluntary movement, and also support and stabilize the skeleton. In most cases, a muscle attaches to a bone (usually by means of a *tendon*) and crosses over a *joint* to attach to another bone.

FUNCTION

Muscles produce movement by contracting and shortening to pull on the bone to which they are attached. They can only pull, not push, and are therefore arranged so that the pull of one muscle or group of muscles is opposed to another, enabling a movement to be reversed. Although most actions of the skeletal muscles are under conscious control, *reflex* movements can occur in response to certain stimuli.

TYPES OF MUSCLE

There are more than 600 muscles in the body, classified according to the type of movement they produce. An extensor opens out a joint, a flexor closes it; an adductor draws a part of the body inwards, an abductor moves it outwards; a levator raises it, a depressor lowers it; and constrictor or sphincter muscles surround and close orifices.

musculoskeletal

Relating to muscle and/or bone. The musculoskeletal system is the skeleton and the muscles attached to it.

musculoskeletal pain

Pain in the bones, joints, muscles, or other parts of the musculoskeletal system. Such pain may have a wide variety of causes, from fever and temporary injuries to soft tissues (such as muscle or tendon *strains* and ligament *sprains*) to severe diseases such as *arthritis*.

mushroom poisoning

There are numerous species of poisonous mushrooms and toadstools in the UK, but many have an unpleasant taste and are therefore unlikely to be eaten in sufficient amounts to cause problems.

MUSCLE MOVEMENT

To move a particular part of the body, a skeletal muscle contracts. It shortens and draws together the bones to which it is attached.

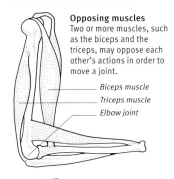

Opposing muscles
Two or more muscles, such as the biceps and the triceps, may oppose each other's actions in order to move a joint.

Biceps muscle
Triceps muscle
Elbow joint

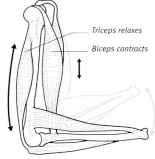

Triceps relaxes
Biceps contracts

Moving the elbow
Elbow movement relies on relaxation and contraction of the biceps, which bends the elbow, and the triceps, which straightens it.

DEATH CAP

Most fatal cases of mushroom poisoning in the UK are caused by AMANITA PHALLOIDES (death cap). This mushroom can be confused with the edible field mushroom, although it has white gills instead of pinkish-brown ones.

The death cap and some related species, such as AMANITA VIROSA (destroying angel), contain poisons called amanitins, which attack cells in the liver, kidneys, and small intestine. Symptoms such as severe abdominal pain, vomiting, and diarrhoea usually develop 8 to 14 hours after eating the mushrooms. Later, there may be liver enlargement and *jaundice*, which may lead to death from *liver failure*. There is no antidote; treatment consists of supportive measures only. For people who survive, recovery usually occurs after about a week.

FLY AGARIC

AMANITA MUSCARIA (fly agaric) has a red cap flecked with white. Symptoms of poisoning appear within 20 minutes to two hours and may include drowsiness, visual disturbances, *delirium*, muscle tremors, nausea, and vomiting. This type of poisoning (and other types that have rapidly developing symptoms) is treated with gastric lavage (see *lavage, gastric*) and activated charcoal. Recovery usually occurs within 24 hours.

MAGIC MUSHROOMS

"Magic" mushrooms contain the hallucinogen *psilocybin*. They may also cause high fever in children. The effects usually last for four to six hours.

mutagen

Any agent that increases the rate of *mutation* (genetic changes) in cells. The main mutagens are ionizing *radiation* (see *radiation hazards*), some chemicals, and certain illnesses.

mutation

A change in a cell's DNA. Many mutations are harmless; however, some are harmful, giving rise to *cancers*, *birth defects*, and hereditary diseases. Very rarely, a mutation may be beneficial.

CAUSES

A mutation results from a fault in the replication of DNA when a cell divides. A daughter cell inherits some faulty DNA, and the fault is copied each time the new cell divides, creating a cell population containing the altered DNA.

Some mutations occur by chance. Any agent that makes mutations more likely is called a *mutagen*.

TYPES

There are several types of mutation. Point mutations affect only one *gene* and may lead to the production of defective *enzymes* or other proteins. In other mutations, *chromosomes* (or parts of them) are deleted, added, or rearranged. This type may produce greater disruptive effects than point mutations.

EFFECTS

If a mutated cell is a somatic (body) cell, it can, at worst, multiply to form a group of abnormal cells. These cells often die out, are destroyed by the body's *immune system*, or have only a minor effect. Sometimes, however, they may become a *tumour*.

A mutation in a *germ cell* (immature egg or sperm) may be passed on to a child, who then has the mutation in all of his or her cells. This may cause an obvious birth defect or an abnormality in body chemistry. The mutation may also be passed down to the child's

M

descendants. *Genetic disorders* (such as *haemophilia* and *achondroplasia*) stem from point mutations that occurred in the germ cell of a parent, grandparent, or more distant ancestor. *Chromosomal abnormalities* (such as *Down's syndrome*) are generally due to mutations in the formation of parental eggs or sperm.

mutism

Refusal or inability to speak. It may be a symptom of profound congenital *deafness*, severe *bipolar disorder*, catatonic *schizophrenia*, or a rare form of *conversion disorder*.

Elective mutism is a rare childhood disorder (usually starting before age five) in which a child can speak properly but refuses to do so most of the time.

Akinetic mutism is a state of passivity caused by some brain tumours or by *hydrocephalus* (fluid surrounding the brain). Affected people are incontinent, require feeding, and respond at most with a whispered "yes" or "no".

myalgia

Medical term for *muscle* pain.

myalgic encephalomyelitis

Also known as ME, an alternative name for *chronic fatigue syndrome*.

myasthenia gravis

A rare disorder in which the muscles become weak and tire easily. The muscles of the eyes, face, throat, and limbs are most commonly affected.

CAUSE

Myasthenia gravis is an *autoimmune disorder*. In many cases, abnormalities in the thymus gland are present, and in some cases a *thymoma* (tumour of the thymus gland) is found.

SYMPTOMS

The disease is extremely variable in its effects. In most cases, it causes drooping eyelids, double vision, a blank facial expression, and a weak, hoarse, nasal voice that is hesitant and becomes slurred during extended conversation. The arm and leg muscles may also be affected. In severe cases, the respiratory muscles may become weakened, causing breathing difficulty.

DIAGNOSIS

One common test is injection of the drug edrophonium into a vein, which temporarily restores power to the weak muscles. *Blood tests* and *EMG* are also sometimes used. In some cases, *CT scanning* or *MRI* may be performed to detect a thymoma.

TREATMENT AND OUTLOOK

There is no guaranteed cure for myasthenia gravis, although there are treatments that can give good control of the symptoms. *Cholinesterase inhibitors* such as neostigmine facilitate the transmission of nerve impulses and can often restore a person's condition to near normal. In some people, the condition may improve, and is sometimes cured, with thymectomy (removal of the thymus gland). In more severe cases, regular *plasmapheresis* may be carried out. *Corticosteroid drugs* may also be given to suppress immune system activity. In a few people, however, *paralysis* of the throat and respiratory muscles may lead to death.

mycetoma

An uncommon tropical infection affecting skin and bone. Mycetoma is caused by *fungi* or by bacteria called actinomycetes. It usually occurs on one limb, causing a hard swelling and a discharge of pus. Infections caused by actinomycetes are treated with *antibiotic drugs*. Surgical removal of diseased tissue may be necessary for a fungal infection.

mycobacterial infections

Diseases caused by bacteria from the MYCOBACTERIUM group (see *tuberculosis*; *Hansen's disease*). An increasing range of mycobacterial infections is recognized in *immunocompromised* people, such as those with *AIDS*.

mycology

The study of *fungi*.

mycophenolate mofetil

An *immunosuppressant drug* used after organ transplants to reduce the risk of the body rejecting the organ.

mycoplasma

Any of a group of *bacteria* that are the smallest type capable of free existence. Mycoplasmas are about the same size as *viruses* but, unlike viruses, are capable of reproducing outside living cells. One species, MYCOPLASMA PNEUMONIAE, causes primary atypical *pneumonia*.

mycosis

Any disease caused by a fungus. (See *fungal infection*; *fungi*.)

mycosis fungoides

A rare type of *lymphoma* that primarily affects the skin of the buttocks, back, or shoulders. The cause is unknown. In its mildest form, mycosis fungoides produces a non-itchy, red, scaly rash, which may spread slowly or remain unaltered for many years. In more severe forms, thickened patches of skin, *ulcers*, and enlarged *lymph nodes* may develop.

Diagnosis is confirmed with a *skin biopsy*. Treatment may include *PUVA*, *radiotherapy*, nitrogen mustard, *anticancer drugs*, and *corticosteroid drugs*.

mydriasis

Dilation (widening) of the pupil. It occurs in the dark; with emotional arousal; after the use of certain eye-drops (for example those containing *atropine*); and also after drinking alcohol.

mydriatic drugs

A group of drugs used to treat *uveitis* and to dilate the pupil during examination of the inside of the eye and for surgery. Mydriatics work by relaxing the circular muscles of the *iris*, causing the pupil to dilate. Common mydriatic drugs include *tropicamide*, cyclopentolate, homatropine, and *phenylephrine*. (See also *cycloplegia*; *miotic drugs*.)

myectomy

Surgical removal of part or all of a muscle. Myectomy may be performed to treat severely injured and infected muscles or to remove a *fibroid* (an operation called a *myomectomy*) from the muscular wall of the uterus.

myel-

A prefix denoting a relationship to bone marrow (as in *multiple myeloma*) or to the spinal cord (as in *myelitis*). The prefix "myelo-" has the same meaning.

myelin

The fatty material made of *lipid* (fat) and protein that forms a protective sheath around some nerve fibres and increases the efficiency of nerve impulse transmission. (See also *demyelination*).

myelitis

Inflammation of the *spinal cord*. It is often caused by a viral infection. In transverse myelitis, the spinal cord becomes inflamed around the middle of the back. Common symptoms are back pain and gradual *paralysis* of the legs; in some cases, the paralysis becomes permanent. (See also *poliomyelitis*.)

myelocele

Another name for *myelomeningocele*.

M

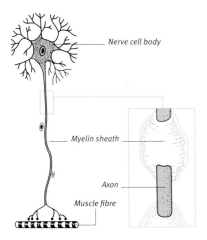

The myelin nerve sheath
The axon is the conducting fibre of a nerve. To transmit impulses more efficiently, some nerve axons have a myelin sheath.

Nerve cell body

Myelin sheath

Axon

Muscle fibre

myelofibrosis

An alternative term for *myelosclerosis*.

myelography

X-ray examination of the spinal cord, nerves, and other tissues within the spinal canal after injection of a contrast medium (a substance that is opaque to X-rays). The procedure has now been replaced by *CT scanning* and *MRI*.

myeloid leukaemia

See *leukaemia, chronic myeloid*.

myeloma, multiple

See *multiple myeloma*.

myelomatosis

See *multiple myeloma*.

myelomeningocele

A congenital abnormality seen in *spina bifida*. An affected baby has a raw swelling over the spine, containing an exposed, malformed section of the *spinal cord* and its *meninges* (protective membranes).

myelopathy

A disease or disorder of the *spinal cord*.

myeloproliferative disorders

Conditions characterized by the abnormal proliferation of one or more blood cell groups within the *bone marrow*. (See *leukaemia*; *polycythaemia*.)

myelosclerosis

An increase of fibrous tissue within the *bone marrow* (also called myelofibrosis), which interferes with the ability of the marrow to produce blood cells. Myelosclerosis may be primary (with no obvious cause) or secondary (resulting from another bone marrow disease).

The main symptoms of myelosclerosis are those of *anaemia*. In addition, enlargement of the *spleen*, night sweats, loss of appetite, and weight loss commonly occur. In secondary myelosclerosis, the underlying disease may cause other symptoms.

Treatment of primary myelosclerosis includes *blood transfusions* to relieve the symptoms. A few people, however, may develop acute *leukaemia*. Treatment of secondary myelosclerosis depends on the underlying cause.

myiasis

Infestation by fly larvae; the condition is primarily restricted to tropical areas. In Africa, the tumbu fly lays eggs on wet clothing left outside; the larvae hatch and penetrate the skin to cause swellings like boils. Other flies lay eggs in open wounds, on the skin, or in the ears or nose. Sometimes, larvae penetrate deeply into the tissues. Intestinal infestation can occur after eating food that has been contaminated.

Myiasis of the skin is treated by applying drops of oil to the swelling. The larva comes to the surface, where it can be carefully removed. In deeper tissues, surgery may be required. Intestinal myiasis is treated with a *laxative*. Preventive measures include keeping flies away from food, keeping open wounds covered, and ironing clothes that have been dried outdoors.

myo-

A prefix denoting a relationship to muscle (as in *myocarditis*).

myocardial infarction

Sudden death of part of the *heart* muscle due to a blockage in the blood supply to that area of the heart. The disorder is popularly known as a heart attack. Myocardial infarction is fatal in about 25 per cent of cases.

CAUSES

The usual cause is *atherosclerosis* of the coronary arteries. In this condition, plaques (fatty deposits) develop on the artery walls; a clot may then form over a plaque and block an artery (see *Features of myocardial infarction* box, overleaf).

Men are more likely to have a heart attack than women, and smokers are at greater risk than nonsmokers. Other risk factors include increased age, an unhealthy diet, obesity, lack of exercise, disorders such as *hypertension* (high blood pressure) and *diabetes mellitus*, and a family history of myocardial infarction at a young age.

SYMPTOMS

There is a sudden, crushing pain that starts in the centre of the chest and may spread into the arms or up to the jaw. Breathlessness, restlessness, clammy skin, and nausea and/or vomiting may also occur. In some cases, the first symptom is sudden collapse and loss of consciousness. A few people have only mild symptoms or have none at all; this type of heart attack is known as a silent myocardial infarct.

The damage to the heart tissue may cause immediate *heart failure* (reduced pumping efficiency) or *arrhythmias* (irregular heartbeat). *Ventricular fibrillation* is the most dangerous form of arrhythmia; it prevents the heart from pumping effectively and, if untreated, is fatal within a few minutes.

DIAGNOSIS

Diagnosis is made from the patient's history, together with an *ECG*. Tests are also carried out to measure levels of certain *enzymes*, and of a protein called troponin, which are released into the blood from damaged heart muscle.

TREATMENT

A myocardial infarction is a medical emergency and the sooner treatment is given, the greater the chance of survival. If a person is having a heart attack, he or she will normally be given an *aspirin* tablet to chew immediately to stop the clot in the artery from becoming larger and will be taken to hospital as soon as possible.

Initially, *oxygen* and *diamorphine* are given in order to relieve the pain and intravenous *thrombolytic drugs* ("clot busters") may be given to dissolve the blood clot (unless there is a risk that the drugs will cause excessive bleeding). If thrombolytic drugs fail to restore blood flow in the affected artery, an emergency angioplasty (see *angioplasty, balloon*) may be carried out, usually with insertion of a *stent* (rigid tube) in the artery to keep it open. Alternatively, a *coronary artery bypass graft* may be performed

Afterwards, patients are monitored in an intensive care or coronary care unit so that any complications, such as *heart failure*, arrhythmias (see *arrhythmia, cardiac*), or rupture of a heart valve can be detected and treated as early as possible.

M

FEATURES OF **MYOCARDIAL INFARCTION**

Myocardial infarction (heart attack), in which an area of heart muscle is deprived of blood and suffers tissue death as a result, causes severe pain and can be fatal. most cases result from atherosclerosis of the coronary arteries, a condition in which plaques (patches of fatty deposits) collect inside the arteries.

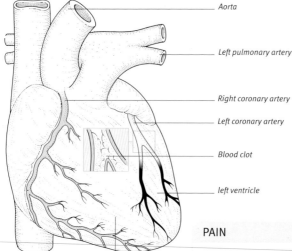

Aorta

Left pulmonary artery

Right coronary artery

Left coronary artery

Blood clot

left ventricle

Heart muscle

RISK FACTORS

- Uncontrollable factors include family history of heart disease, increasing age, and being male.

- Cigarette smokers have a substantially increased risk of dying of myocardial infarction.

- High blood pressure is a major risk factor, and the risk increases the higher the pressure.

- The risk of atherosclerosis and coronary artery disease increases in those who are obese and drink excessive amounts of alcohol.

- A raised level of cholesterol in the blood, a high-fat diet, and diabetes mellitus are significant risk factors.

- Physical inactivity is also a major risk factor.

Outer layer

Blood clot

Fatty deposit (atheroma)

Inner lining

Atherosclerosis
Plaques of atheroma develop on the inner lining of the arteries, restricting the blood flow. The plaques develop a fibrous covering, which may rupture or become roughened. Platelets (tiny blood cells) may then stick to the plaque and trigger the formation of a blood clot. The clot may completely block the artery, causing a sudden stoppage of blood flow to the heart.

PAIN

Some people who suffer myocardial infarction have a history of angina pectoris, in which blood flow through the coronary arteries is impaired but the resulting chest pain is relieved by rest. The pain of infarction usually comes on suddenly, and ranges from a tight ache to intense, crushing agony. It lasts for longer than 10 minutes, and is not relieved by rest.

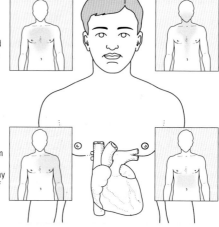

Central chest
A feeling of pressure in the central chest, ranging from mild to severe, occurs in almost every myocardial infarction that is due to coronary obstruction.

Jaw to back
In some cases, pain radiates up into the jaw and through to the back. Sometimes, it occurs only in these places.

Chest to arm
In many cases, pain radiates from the chest down the left arm; it may cause a feeling of weakness in the arm muscles.

Upper abdomen
More rarely, pain may be felt in the upper abdomen. If it occurs only here, it may be mistaken for another disorder.

After recovery from a heart attack, patients may be given *beta-blocker drugs* or *ACE inhibitors* to improve the function of the heart and to protect the heart muscle. *Statin* drugs may also be prescribed to lower blood *cholesterol*. In addition, patients will undergo a *rehabilitation* programme to help them return to full activity and to increase awareness of risk factors.

myocardial ischaemia

Insufficient blood supply to the *heart* muscle. It is usually caused by narrowing or blockage of the coronary blood vessels (which supply the heart muscle), due to *atherosclerosis* (fatty deposits on artery walls). Myocardial ischaemia causes the heart muscle to be deprived of oxygen, and may give rise to problems such as *angina pectoris* and *myocardial infarction*.

myocarditis

Inflammation of *heart* muscle. It may be caused by infection (usually a coxsackie-virus infection), drugs, or excessive alcohol use. Myocarditis is also a characteristic feature of *rheumatic fever*.

SYMPTOMS
Myocarditis often produces no symptoms. Rarely, there may be a serious disturbance of the heartbeat, breathless-

M

ness, chest pain, and *heart failure*. In severe cases of myocarditis, death may result from *cardiac arrest*.

DIAGNOSIS AND TREATMENT
Myocarditis may be suspected from the patient's history and from a physical examination. An *ECG* will show characteristic abnormalities of the heartbeat. Diagnosis also involves *echocardiography* and *blood tests*.

There is no specific treatment. Bed rest is usually recommended and *corticosteroid drugs* may be prescribed.

myocardium

The middle of the three layers of muscle that make up the wall of the heart. The myocardium is composed of cardiac muscle. (See also *cardiomyopathy*; *myocardial infarction*; *myocardial ischaemia*; *myocarditis*.)

myoclonus

Rapid, uncontrollable jerking or spasm of one or more muscles, either at rest or during movement. Myoclonus may be associated with a muscular or nervous disorder, but it also occurs in healthy people; for example, when the limbs twitch before sleep.

myofascial pain syndrome

See *temporomandibular joint syndrome*.

myoglobin

An oxygen-carrying pigment found in muscles. Myoglobin consists of a combination of iron and protein. It stores oxygen, releasing it when it is needed by the muscles.

Myoglobin may be released into the urine, causing myoglobinuria. Slight myoglobinuria may result from prolonged exercise. Severe myoglobinuria is usually due to the release of myoglobin from a large area of damaged muscle, and may cause *kidney failure*.

myoma

A noncancerous muscle *tumour*. (See also *fibroid*.)

myomectomy

Surgical removal of a *myoma*. The term is also used to describe the surgical removal of *fibroids* from the uterus.

myometrium

The muscular wall of the *uterus*. It is composed of smooth *muscle* and lined with *endometrium*. The myometrium contracts strongly during *childbirth* in order to dilate the cervix and push the fetus (and the *placenta*) out of the uterus. It also undergoes much smaller contractions during menstrual periods, which help to expel blood and tissue (see *menstruation*).

myopathy

A disease of *muscle* that is not caused by disease of the nervous system. A myopathy may be an inherited disorder, such as *muscular dystrophy*; it may also be caused by chemical poisoning, a chronic disorder of the *immune system*, or a *metabolic disorder*.

myopia

An error of *refraction*, commonly called shortsightedness, in which distant objects appear blurred. It is caused by the eye being too long from front to back. As a result, images of distant objects are focused in front of the retina.

Myopia, which tends to be inherited, usually appears around puberty, increasing until the early 20s. If it starts in early childhood it may become severe. The condition is detected during a *vision test*. Treatment is with concave *glasses* (or *contact lenses*) or by *photorefractive keratectomy* or *LASIK*.

myosin

A major protein component of *muscle* fibres. Together with *actin*, it provides the mechanism for muscles to contract. The myosin molecules slide along the actin filaments in order to make the muscle fibres shorten.

myositis

Inflammation of *muscle* tissue, causing pain, tenderness, and weakness. Types include *myositis ossificans*, *polymyositis*, and *dermatomyositis*.

myositis ossificans

A *congenital* (present from birth) or acquired condition in which bone is deposited in muscles. The congenital form is rare. The first symptoms are painful swellings in the muscles, which gradually harden and extend until the affected child is encased in a rigid sheet. There is no treatment, and the condition is eventually fatal.

The acquired form may develop after a bone injury, especially around the elbow; it causes severe pain and a swelling that hardens. Treatment with *diathermy*, and gentle, active movements, may be helpful.

myotomy

A surgical procedure that involves cutting into a *muscle*.

myotonia

Inability of a *muscle* to relax after the need for contraction has passed. It is a feature of myotonic dystrophy, a form of *muscular dystrophy*.

myringitis

Inflammation of the eardrum. Myringitis occurs in *otitis media*.

myringoplasty

Surgical closure of a perforation (hole) in the eardrum (see *eardrum, perforated*) by means of a tissue graft (see *grafting*).

myringotomy

A surgical opening made through the eardrum to allow drainage of the middle-ear cavity. It is usually performed to treat persistent *glue ear* in children. A *grommet* may be inserted into the eardrum at the same time.

myxoedema

A condition in which the skin and other body tissues (most noticeably in the face) thicken and coarsen. Myxoedema is usually due to *hypothyroidism*. The term "myxoedema" is sometimes used of adult hypothyroidism.

myxoma

A noncancerous, jellylike tumour composed of soft mucous material and loose fibrous strands. Myxomas usually occur singly, and may sometimes grow very large. They may develop under the skin, in the abdomen, or, very rarely, in the heart chambers. In this last case, thrombi (blood clots) may form, and the blood flow through the heart may be obstructed. Myxomas can usually be successfully removed by surgery.

myxovirus

One of a group of *RNA*-containing viruses that are responsible for various human and animal diseases. There are two families of myxovirus: *paramyxovirus* and *orthomyxovirus*.

M

N

nabilone

An *antiemetic drug* derived from *marijuana*. Nabilone is used to treat patients suffering from the nausea and vomiting caused by *anticancer drugs* that have not responded to other treatments.

nabothian cyst

A *cyst* (a small fluid-filled swelling or lump) that develops on the cervix (the neck) of the uterus when the ducts of a mucous gland become obstructed. A nabothian cyst, which is also known as a nabothian follicle, is harmless and requires no treatment.

NAD

The abbreviation for nicotinamide adenine dinucleotide, which is a coenzyme (an organic compound that plays an essential role in a reaction catalyzed by an *enzyme*) derived from *nicotinic acid*. NAD acts as a hydrogen acceptor (forming NADH) in the chemical process that produces energy within cells.

nadolol

A *beta-blocker* drug used to treat *hypertension* (high blood pressure), *angina pectoris* (chest pain due to impaired blood supply to the heart muscle), and certain types of *arrhythmia* (irregularity of the heartbeat). Nadolol is also used for controlling symptoms of *hyperthyroidism* (overactivity of the thyroid gland) and preventing *migraine* attacks.

Possible side effects are typical of other beta-blocker drugs; they include a reduction in the patient's capacity for strenuous exercise and aggravation of any existing symptoms of lung disease and *peripheral vascular disease*.

Naegeli syndrome

A rare inherited condition that has its onset in the first few years of life. Symptoms include weblike skin *pigmentation*, diminished function of the sweat glands, hypodontia (fewer teeth than normal), *hyperkeratosis* (thickening of the outer layer of skin) affecting the palms and soles, and blistering. Naegeli syndrome has an autosomal dominant pattern of inheritance (see *genetic disorders*) and affects both males and females.

naevus

A type of blemish on the skin. There are two main groups of naevus: pigmented naevi, which are caused by an abnormality in or overactivity of melanocytes (skin cells that produce the brown pigment *melanin*); and vascular naevi, which result from an abnormal collection of blood vessels near the surface of the skin.

PIGMENTED NAEVI

The most common type of pigmented naevus is a freckle, which is a small, flat, light-brown to dark-brown area that may occur on any part of the body exposed to the sun. The tendency to develop freckles on exposure to the sun is inherited; they are more common in people with fair skin and red hair. A *lentigo*, sometimes called an age spot or liver spot, is a light-brown spot similar to a freckle. These spots most commonly affect people over the age of 40 and appear both on covered and on sun-exposed areas of the body. *Café au lait spots* are another type of light-brown pigmented naevus.

Another common type of pigmented naevus is a mole, which is sometimes called a melanocytic naevus. Moles are brown to dark-brown in colour and usually measure less than 1 cm in diameter. Moles can form anywhere on the body and a tendency to develop them sometimes runs in families. Moles may appear soon after birth (see *birthmark*) or during childhood and early adolescence; almost all adults have between ten and 20 moles by the time they are 30. Most moles are noncancerous, but, rarely, a mole may undergo changes that make it cancerous (see *melanoma, malignant*). Red-brown naevi that occur in childhood are juvenile melanomas (see *melanoma, juvenile*).

Some naevi have a bluish coloration. Many black and Asian infants are born with blue-black spots on their lower backs (see *Mongolian blue spot*).

VASCULAR NAEVI

Port-wine stains and strawberry marks (see *haemangioma*) are vascular naevi. These types of naevi are usually present at birth. A port-wine stain is visible as an irregularly shaped red patch and may be distressing, especially if it affects the individual's face. The mark is usually permanent. Strawberry marks are common birthmarks and appear as raised, red swellings; they usually disappear by the time a child is about five years old. A *spider naevus* is another example of a vascular naevus. These are common in children and pregnant women.

TREATMENT

Most naevi are harmless. If, however, a naevus suddenly appears, grows, bleeds, or changes colour, medical advice should be sought immediately to exclude *skin cancer*. Permanent birthmarks can be treated with *laser treatment*.

nail

A hard, curved plate, found on each of the fingers and toes, composed of *keratin* (a tough protein that is also the main constituent of skin and hair). Nails grow from an area called the nail bed. At the base of each nail, a half-moon shape (the lunula) is crossed by a flap of skin known as the cuticle. The surrounding skin is the nail fold. A fingernail takes about six months to grow from its base to its tip, although there are seasonal growth variations; and toenails take twice as long.

DISORDERS

The nails are susceptible to damage through injury, usually as a result of crushing or pressure on the nail. Nails may also be damaged by bacterial or fungal infections, especially *tinea* and *candidiasis* (thrush). In *paronychia*, it is the nail folds that are infected. Some-

---

ANATOMY OF A **NAIL**

The nail bed is the area from which the nail grows. At the base of each nail, a half-moon shape, the lunula, is crossed by a flap of skin, the cuticle. The skin that surrounds the nail is the nail fold. The nail is composed of keratin, a tough protein also found in skin and hair.

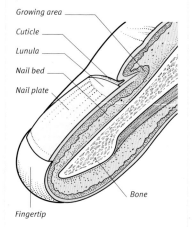

Growing area
Cuticle
Lunula
Nail bed
Nail plate
Bone
Fingertip

times the nails can become abnormally thick and curved, a condition known as *onychogryphosis*. This mainly affects the big toes of elderly people.

The nails may also be affected by skin diseases. Examples of the effects of skin disease on the nails include pitting of the nails in *alopecia* areata; pitting and separation of the nail from its bed in *psoriasis*; and scarring of the nails in *lichen planus*. Certain nail abnormalities may be signs of more generalized illness. Brittle, ridged, concave nails are a sign of iron-deficiency anaemia (see *anaemia, iron-deficiency*) and fibrous growths on the nail are a sign of *tuberous sclerosis*. Splinterlike black marks develop beneath the nails in particular *bleeding disorders*, indicating bleeding into the nail bed.

Abnormal nail colour may also indicate disease. A greenish discoloration may be caused by bacterial infection under the nail; blue nails may be a sign of respiratory or heart disease; and yellow nails that are hard and curved develop in the lung disorder *bronchiectasis* and in *lymphoedema* (an accumulation of lymph in the tissues). Nails may also become discoloured by smoking (due to nicotine) and by the use of nail polish.

Treatment of nail disorders can be difficult. Creams and lotions may not penetrate sufficiently; oral medication may take months to be effective.

nail-biting

A common habit in children during their early years at school. Most children grow out of it, although nail-biting sometimes continues as a nervous habit in adolescents and adults. Persistent nail-biting may make the nails unsightly and cause pain and, sometimes, bleeding.

Various preparations with an unpleasant taste can be painted on the nails as a preventive measure.

nalidixic acid

An *antibiotic drug* used in the prevention and/or treatment of *urinary tract infections*. Possible side effects of nalidixic acid include nausea, vomiting, increased sensitivity to sunlight, blurred vision, drowsiness, and dizziness.

naloxone

An opioid antagonist (a drug that counteracts the effects of opioid *analgesic drugs*). Naloxone reverses the breathing difficulty caused by high doses of opioid drugs given during surgery. It may also be given to people who have taken an overdose of an opioid drug. Naloxone may be given to newborn babies who are affected by opioid drugs used to relieve the mother's pain during childbirth.

Possible side effects of naloxone include nausea, vomiting, abdominal cramps, diarrhoea, and tremors.

naltrexone

An opioid antagonist (a drug that counteracts the effects of opioid *analgesic drugs*) that is used in the treatment of opioid addiction. Naltrexone works by blocking the action of opioid drugs and precipitating withdrawal symptoms in opioid-dependent people. The drug may be given to former addicts to help to prevent relapse. (See also *drug abuse*; *drug dependence*.)

nandrolone

An anabolic steroid (see *steroids, anabolic*) sometimes used in the treatment of certain types of aplastic anaemia (see *anaemia, aplastic*). Nandrolone is also used illegally by some body builders and athletes to increase their protein production and, therefore, muscle bulk.

Possible side effects of nandrolone include swollen ankles, nausea and vomiting, and *jaundice* (yellowing of the skin and the whites of the eyes). Nandrolone may cause irregular menstruation and abnormal hair growth in women.

nappy rash

An inflammatory skin condition common in babies, causing soreness and a red rash in the skin covered by a nappy.

CAUSES AND SYMPTOMS

Nappy rash is most commonly caused by urine or faeces irritating the skin. It usually occurs only where the skin and the soiled nappy have been in direct contact; it does not spread to creases in the baby's skin. Nappy rash becomes worse if the baby's nappy is not changed frequently or if the nappy area is not cleaned thoroughly. Perfumed skin products and some washing powders used to clean fabric nappies can also result in a rash.

Nappy rash may also be caused by a fungal infection of the skin, such as *candidiasis* (thrush), or, less commonly, by a bacterial infection, such as *impetigo*. A rash caused by infection affects the whole nappy area, including the creases in the baby's skin.

Discomfort from the rash may make a baby irritable. A severe rash may progress to blistering.

TREATMENT

If nappies are changed frequently and the affected area is regularly cleaned and covered in a barrier cream (such as zinc and castor oil cream), nappy rash generally clears up within a few days. In more severe cases, an ointment containing a mild *corticosteroid drug* may be prescribed to suppress the inflammation. If the area has become infected, *antibiotic drugs* or *antifungal drugs* may also be prescribed.

naproxen

A *nonsteroidal anti-inflammatory drug* (NSAID) that is used to relieve pain in the joints and stiffness in *arthritis* (including juvenile arthritis). Naproxen is also prescribed to speed recovery following injury to soft tissues, such as muscles or ligaments.

Side effects of naproxen may include nausea, abdominal pain, and *peptic ulcer*.

naratriptan

A *serotonin agonist* drug used in the treatment of acute attacks of *migraine*.

narcissism

Intense self-love. A narcissistic personality disorder is characterized by an exaggerated sense of self-importance, constant need for attention or praise, inability to cope with criticism or defeat, and poor relationships with other people. People with a narcissistic personality believe themselves to be unique, special, and superior to others; in addition, they may lack concern for the wellbeing or problems of others.

narcolepsy

A *sleep* disorder characterized by chronic daytime drowsiness with recurrent episodes of sleep occurring throughout the day. The exact cause of narcolepsy is unknown, although it can run in families. The condition usually develops before the age of 20.

SYMPTOMS

People who suffer from narcolepsy tend to fall asleep at any time of the day, often when they are carrying out a monotonous task. Sleep may occur at inappropriate times, such as while eating. Narcoleptic attacks may last from a few seconds to more than an hour. In narcolepsy, the REM (rapid eye movement) state of sleep is entered abnormally rapidly. Affected people can be awakened easily but may fall asleep again a short time afterwards.

N

Some people with narcolepsy have vivid hallucinations just before falling asleep. Others find that they are unable to move while they are falling asleep or waking up (see *sleep paralysis*). About three in four people with narcolepsy also have cataplexy, in which there is a temporary loss of strength in the limbs that causes the person to fall to the ground. Cataplexy is sometimes triggered by an emotional response, such as fear or laughter.

TREATMENT AND OUTLOOK
Treatment of narcolepsy usually involves regular naps, together with *stimulant drugs* such as dexamfetamine to control drowsiness and *antidepressant drugs* to suppress cataplexy.

Although narcolepsy is usually a lifelong condition, in some cases there is spontaneous improvement over time.

narcosis
A state of stupor, usually caused by an opioid *analgesic drug* or other chemical. Narcosis resembles sleep, being marked by reduced awareness and diminished ability to respond to external stimulation. However, unlike someone who is sleeping, a person in narcosis cannot be roused completely.

narcotic drugs
The former name for *opioid* drugs. (See also *analgesic drugs*.)

nasal congestion
Partial blockage of the nasal passage by swelling of the *mucous membrane* that lines the *nose*. It is sometimes accompanied by accumulation of thick nasal mucus, which further impedes breathing. Nasal congestion produces the feeling of a stuffy, "full" nose. There is a frequent desire to blow the nose, but this usually has little effect on the congestion.

CAUSES
Nasal congestion is a symptom of the common cold (see *cold, common*) and hay fever (see *rhinitis, allergic*). In these conditions, the swelling is due to inflammation of the membrane lining the inside of the nose. The swelling may become persistent in disorders such as chronic *sinusitis* or *nasal polyps*. The congestion may also be caused by certain drugs, such as *methyldopa* (an *antihypertensive drug*).

TREATMENT
Placing the head over a basin of hot water, possibly containing aromatic oils such as menthol or eucalyptus, and inhaling the steam for several minutes can help loosen the mucus.

Decongestant drugs in the form of drops and sprays should be used for only a few days. Longer term, nasal *corticosteroid drugs*, *sodium cromoglicate*, and topical *antihistamine drugs* may control symptoms. Persistent nasal congestion should be investigated by a doctor.

nasal discharge
The emission of fluid from the *nose*. Nasal discharge is commonly caused by inflammation of the *mucous membrane* lining the nose and is often accompanied by *nasal congestion*.

A discharge of mucus may indicate hay fever (see *rhinitis, allergic*), a cold (see *cold, common*), or an infection that has spread from the nearby sinuses (see *sinusitis*). A persistent runny discharge may be an early indication of a tumour (see *nasopharynx, cancer of*).

Bleeding from the nose (see *nosebleed*) is usually caused by injury or by a foreign body in the nose. In rare cases, bleeding from the nose may be a sign of an underlying *bleeding disorder* or a tumour. A discharge of cerebrospinal fluid from the nose may follow a fracture at the base of the skull (see *skull, fracture of*).

nasal obstruction
Blockage of the nasal passage on one or both sides of the *nose*, which interferes with breathing. The most common cause is inflammation of the *mucous membrane* lining the passage (see *nasal congestion*). Other causes include deviation of the *nasal septum*; *nasal polyps*; a *haematoma* (a collection of clotted blood), which is usually caused by injury; and, rarely, a cancerous tumour. In children, enlargement of the *adenoids* is a common cause of nasal obstruction.

nasal polyp
A growth in the lining of the *nose*, usually attached by a small stalk. Large or numerous nasal polyps may cause *nasal obstruction*, a runny nose, and an impaired sense of smell.

CAUSES
The exact cause of nasal polyps is not known. However, they are more common in people with *asthma* or *rhinitis* (a condition in which the membrane that lines the nose and throat becomes inflamed). Although nasal polyps are rare in children, they do sometimes develop in children with *cystic fibrosis*.

DIAGNOSIS
Nasal polyps are diagnosed by physical examination and sometimes also by

endoscopy (inspection and examination of the nasal cavity using a viewing instrument). Most nasal polyps are noncancerous; however, a *biopsy* (removal of a small sample of tissue for microscopic analysis) may be performed to exclude the rare possibility of cancer.

TREATMENT
Nasal polyps do not need treatment unless they are interfering with breathing, are cancerous, or are causing other symptoms. Small nasal polyps may be treated by using a corticosteroid nasal spray (see *corticosteroid drugs*), which shrinks the polyps over a few weeks. Larger or cancerous polyps may be removed during an endoscopic procedure or by surgery. In certain people, polyps may recur after treatment.

nasal septum
The dividing partition in the *nose*. The nasal septum consists of cartilage (connective tissue formed of collagen) at the front and bone at the rear, both of which are covered by *mucous membrane*.

DISORDERS
A deviated septum (twisting of the septum to one side) may be present from birth or caused by injury. The condition is rarely troublesome, but surgery may be needed if breathing is obstructed.

Injury may also lead to formation of a *haematoma* (a collection of clotted blood) between the cartilage of the septum and the wall of one of the nasal cavities. A haematoma may obstruct breathing and may become infected, causing an *abscess* (collection of pus) that may require surgical drainage. Occasionally, an abscess develops on a child's septum without prior injury.

Rarely, a hole may be eroded in the nasal septum by *tuberculosis*, *syphilis*, *Wegener's granulomatosis*, or as a result of snorting *cocaine*.

Naseptin
A brand name for a combination of chlorhexidine (an *antiseptic* for the skin) with *neomycin* (an *antibiotic drug*). Naseptin cream is used to eliminate organisms, such as staphylococci, from the inside of the nostrils.

nasogastric tube
A narrow plastic tube that is passed through the nose, down the oesophagus (gullet), and into the stomach.

WHY IT IS USED
Nasogastric tubes are commonly used to suck or drain digestive juices from

N

the stomach when there is a blockage in the intestine (such as in *pyloric stenosis*) or it is not working properly (as may occur after an abdominal operation). A nasogastric tube is also used to give liquid nourishment to patients who cannot eat (see *feeding, artificial*), to obtain specimens of stomach secretions for examination, and to wash out the stomach after a drug overdose or after swallowing poison (see *lavage, gastric*).

HOW IT IS USED

Inserting the tube is a quick, simple procedure that causes little discomfort and does not require an anaesthetic. After it has been lubricated, the tube is passed into one nostril and then, while the patient is swallowing, slid down the throat and into the stomach. To ensure that the tube is in the stomach, a sample of fluid is withdrawn through a syringe and may be tested for acidity. The stomach contents are then either allowed to drain or sucked out through a syringe or a suction device. Fluids for lavage or feeding may be introduced through a funnel. If the tube is to be left in place for some time, the protruding end is taped to the patient's face.

nasolacrimal duct

A channel that drains *tears* into the nose. The nasolacrimal duct forms part of the *lacrimal apparatus*.

nasopharynx

The passage that connects the nasal cavity behind the *nose* to the top of the throat behind the soft *palate*. The nasopharynx is part of the respiratory tract and forms the upper section of the *pharynx*. During swallowing, the nasopharynx is sealed off by the soft palate pressing against the back of the throat, thereby preventing food from entering.

The nasopharynx contains the lower openings of the *eustachian tubes* (passages connecting the back of the nose to the middle ear). In children, it also contains the *adenoids*, which can enlarge to block the nasopharynx, forcing the child to breathe through the mouth.

nasopharynx, cancer of

A cancerous tumour that originates in the *nasopharynx* (the uppermost part of the throat, behind the nose) and usually spreads to the nasal cavity, nasal sinuses, base of the skull, and neck *lymph nodes*.

CAUSES AND INCIDENCE

Cancer of the nasopharynx is rare in the West but relatively common in the Far East; the reasons for this are not clear. It occurs most often in people between the ages of 30 and 60.

Factors that increase the risk of this cancer include diet (a high intake of salt-cured fish); smoking; and viral infections, especially infection with the *Epstein–Barr virus*. People who inhale hardwood dust or nickel dust at work over a long period are also at increased risk and should take precautions.

SYMPTOMS

Initially, cancer of the nasopharynx may not cause any symptoms. It may remain unnoticed until the tumour spreads to a lymph node, causing a painless swelling in the neck.

If symptoms do develop, they may include facial swelling, recurrent nosebleeds, a runny nose, and discomfort on swallowing. Loss of the sense of smell, double vision, deafness, paralysis of one side of the face, voice change, and severe facial pain may also develop if nearby nerves are affected.

DIAGNOSIS AND TREATMENT

Diagnosis is through *endoscopy* (internal examination and inspection using a viewing tube), during which a *biopsy* (removal of a small sample of tissue for microscopic analysis) can also be taken. An *MRI* scan (a technique that produces cross-sectional or three-dimensional images of internal body structures) and *X-rays* are required to assess the extent of the tumour and the involvement of nearby structures.

Treatment is usually with *radiotherapy*, but, in some cases, the tumour may be surgically removed. If the tumour is treated early, the outlook can be good.

LOCATION OF THE NASOPHARYNX

The nasopharynx forms the upper part of the pharynx and connects the nasal cavity to the top of the throat.

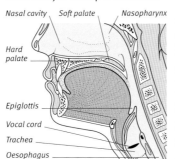

Nasal cavity   Soft palate   Nasopharynx
Hard palate
Epiglottis
Vocal cord
Trachea
Oesophagus

natriuretic peptide

See *atrial natriuretic peptide*.

natural childbirth

See *childbirth, natural*.

natural immunity

A type of *immunity* (protection against disease) that is manifested by a species not previously sensitized to the disease in question either through infection or through *vaccination*.

The mechanisms that are involved in natural immunity are still poorly understood. However, it is not believed to be stimulated by specific *antigens* (substances that trigger an immune response), as is the case with acquired immunity. Natural immunity (also known as innate immunity) is inherited and present at birth.

natural killer cells

A specific type of *lymphocyte* (a type of white blood cell) that is able to destroy cells infected with viruses as well as some types of *cancer* cell. Natural killer cells, also known as NK cells, constitute the *immune system*'s first line of defence against cancerous or infected cells. NK cells are neither T- nor B-lymphocytes (unlike *killer T-cells*, for example).

naturopathy

A form of *complementary medicine* based on the principle that disease occurs as a result of the accumulation of waste products and toxins in the body; symptoms are thought to reflect the attempts of the body to rid itself of these substances. Practitioners of naturopathy believe that health is maintained by avoiding anything artificial or unnatural in the diet or in the environment.

nausea

The sensation of needing to vomit. Although nausea may occur without *vomiting*, the causes are the same.

navel

A popular term for the *umbilicus*, the depression in the abdomen that marks the point at which the umbilical cord was attached to the fetus.

navicular bone

A foot bone that articulates with the head of the talus (one of the bones in the *ankle joint*) and with three of the bones in the tarsus (which makes up the back of the foot and the ankle).

N

nebulizer

An aerosol device used to administer drugs, such as *bronchodilators*, especially in the emergency treatment of *asthma*. Usually an electric pump sends a stream of air or oxygen across a chamber that contains the drug. This stream of air disperses the drug into a fine mist, which is then conveyed to the face mask and inhaled by the user.

neck

The part of the body that supports the head and serves as a passageway between the head (and brain) and the rest of the body. The neck contains many important structures: the *spinal cord* (which carries nerve impulses to and from the brain); the *trachea* (windpipe); the *larynx* (voicebox); the *oesophagus* (gullet); the *thyroid* and *parathyroid glands*; *lymph nodes*; and several major blood vessels. Seven spinal vertebrae are located in the neck; they are surrounded by a complex system of muscles.

DISORDERS

Torticollis (wry neck), in which the head is twisted to one side, may result from injury to a neck muscle or from skin *contracture* (shrinkage) after burns or other injuries. *Fractures* and *dislocations* of vertebrae in the neck, as well as *whiplash injury*, can cause injury to the spinal cord, causing paralysis or even death (see *spinal injury*).

Degeneration of the joints between the neck vertebrae may occur as a result of *cervical osteoarthritis*, resulting in neck pain, stiffness, and sometimes tingling and weakness in the arm and hand. Similar symptoms may also be caused by a *disc prolapse*. In *ankylosing spondylitis*, fusion of the vertebrae may result in permanent neck rigidity.

Cervical rib is a rare congenital defect in which there is a small extra rib in the neck. This condition often causes no symptoms until middle age, when it may result in pain, numbness, and a pins-and-needles sensation in the forearm and hand.

Neck pain of unknown origin is very common. However, as long as there are no neurological symptoms (such as loss of sensation or a decrease in muscle power), the condition is unlikely to be serious and usually disappears over the course of a few weeks. However, any condition causing a large swelling in the neck (such as enlargement of the thyroid gland) may interfere with breathing or swallowing.

ANATOMY OF THE NECK

The neck contains many important structures, including the larynx, thyroid and parathyroid glands (embedded in the back of the thyroid), many lymph nodes, and carotid arteries. The upper seven vertebrae of the spine are in the neck; a complex system of muscles is connected to these vertebrae, the clavicles, the upper ribs, and the lower jaw. Contraction of these muscles allows the head to turn and the jaw to open and close.

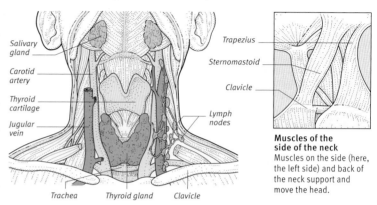

Muscles of the side of the neck
Muscles on the side (here, the left side) and back of the neck support and move the head.

neck dissection, radical

A surgical procedure for the removal of cancerous *lymph nodes* in the neck. The operation is often part of the treatment for cancer of the tongue, the tonsils, or other structures in the mouth and throat.

Under general anaesthetic (see *anaesthesia, general*), a flap of skin on the affected side of the neck is raised to expose the underlying sternomastoid muscle. The muscle is cut just above the clavicle (collarbone) and lifted up. All the components of the lymphatic system in the neck (the lymph vessels as well as the lymph nodes) are then removed, together with the internal jugular vein, the lower salivary gland, and other surrounding tissue.

neck rigidity

Marked stiffness of the neck caused by *spasm* of the muscles in the neck and spine. Neck rigidity is an important clinical sign of *meningitis* (inflammation of the membranes that envelop the brain and spinal cord). Severe neck rigidity may cause the head to arch backwards, especially in babies.

necrobiosis lipoidica

A skin condition, usually associated with *diabetes mellitus*, in which reddened patches with yellowish centres develop, most commonly on the shins. The skin in the centre of the patches becomes thin and may ulcerate.

necrolysis, toxic epidermal

A severe, blistering rash in which the surface layers of the skin peel off, exposing large areas of red, raw skin. The condition carries a risk of widespread infection and loss of body fluids and salts.

The most common cause of toxic epidermal necrolysis is an adverse reaction to a drug, particularly a *barbiturate*, *sulphonamide*, or *penicillin*. The condition usually clears up when the causative drug is discontinued. Intravenous fluid replacement is sometimes necessary.

In newborn babies, the condition may be due to a *staphylococcal infection* and is called scalded skin syndrome. Treatment is with *antibiotic drugs* and fluid replacement.

necrophilia

A rare sexual perversion in which orgasm is achieved by means of sexual acts with dead bodies.

necropsy

A little-used medical term for an *autopsy* (postmortem examination of a body).

necrosis

The death of tissue cells. Necrosis can occur as a result of *ischaemia* (inadequate blood supply), which may lead to *gangrene* (tissue death); infection; or damage by extreme heat or cold, noxious chemicals, or excessive exposure to X-rays or other forms of *radiation*.

N

The appearance of the dead tissue depends on the cause of the necrosis and on the type of tissue affected. In necrosis due to *tuberculosis*, the dead tissue is soft, dry, and cheeselike. Fatty tissue beneath the skin that has died as a result of damage or infection develops into tough scar tissue that may form a firm nodule.

necrotizing fasciitis

A rare but serious infection of tissues beneath the skin by a type of streptococcal bacterium (see *streptococcal infections*) and other bacteria. Necrotizing fasciitis is most likely to occur as a complication of surgery. Initial symptoms of the infection are inflammation and blistering of the skin. The infection spreads very rapidly and the bacteria release enzymes and toxins (poisons) that can cause extensive destruction of deeper tissues and damage to internal organs. Urgent treatment with *antibiotic drugs* and surgical removal of all infected tissue are essential. The infection is life-threatening.

nedocromil

A drug similar to *sodium cromoglicate* that is used to prevent *asthma* attacks and allergic *conjunctivitis*.

needle aspiration

See *biopsy*.

needle exchange

A health scheme that enables intravenous drug abusers to exchange used hypodermic needles for new, sterile ones. The scheme is aimed at reducing the risks of infections, such as *HIV* and *hepatitis*, that are transmitted by the sharing of contaminated needles.

needlestick injury

Accidental puncture of the skin by a contaminated hypodermic needle. Hospital staff are most likely to be at risk. Needlestick injuries carry the risk of serious infections, such as *HIV* and *hepatitis*, and need immediate medical attention. The wound should be cleaned thoroughly. If there is a risk of infection, preventive medication will be given. *Blood tests* will be carried out to determine whether infection has actually been transmitted.

nefopam

An *analgesic drug* that is used to relieve moderate pain caused, for example, by injury, surgery, or cancer. Possible adverse effects include nausea, nervousness, dry mouth, and difficulty sleeping.

negativism

The tendency to resist or oppose advice, suggestions, or commands. There are two principal types of negativism: active negativism and passive negativism. In active negativism, the individual does the opposite of what he or she is requested to do; such behaviour is seen in toddlers and is uncommon in adult life, although it may be a feature of *catatonia*. In passive negativism, the person does not cooperate simply by failing to do something that has been suggested. This often occurs in *depression* and may also be a feature of *schizophrenia*.

neisserial infections

Infections caused by *bacteria* belonging to the NEISSERIA genus. NEISSERIA GONORRHOEAE (gonococcus) causes *gonorrhoea* (a common *sexually transmitted infection*) in humans. NEISSERIA MENINGITIDIS (meningococcus), is the causative agent of the condition *meningococcal meningitis* (inflammation of the membranes covering the brain and spinal cord).

Nelson's syndrome

A rare disorder of the *endocrine system* that causes increased skin pigmentation. Nelson's syndrome results from enlargement of the *pituitary gland*, which can follow removal of the *adrenal glands* (to treat *Cushing's disease*).

Nelson's syndrome is treated by *hypophysectomy* (removal or destruction of the pituitary gland).

nematodes

The scientific name for a group of cylindrically shaped worms (see *roundworms*); some are human parasites.

neologism

The act of making up new words that have a special meaning for the inventor. The term neologism also refers to the invented word itself. Persistent neologism can be a feature of speech in people with *schizophrenia*.

neomycin

An *antibiotic drug* that is used to treat ear, eye, nose, and skin infections, often in combination with other drugs. Neomycin is also given to prevent infection of the intestine prior to surgery. Possible adverse effects include a rash and itching.

neonatal death

The *death* of a live-born infant in the first four weeks of life. Neonatal death is classified as early or late: early neonatal deaths are deaths that occur less than seven completed days from the time of birth; late neonatal deaths are those that occur after seven completed days and before 28 completed days after birth.

About half of all neonatal deaths in the UK are attributed to *prematurity*; about a quarter to congenital malformations; and the remainder to various causes, including infection and difficulties with delivery. (See also *infant mortality*; *stillbirth*.)

neonatal hypoglycaemia

An abnormally low blood glucose level (see *hypoglycaemia*) in an infant that is under four weeks of age. Neonatal hypoglycaemia commonly causes problems in the first 24 hours of life. Persistent low glucose levels may result in permanent damage to the brain (see *cerebral palsy*).

CAUSES AND INCIDENCE

Neonatal hypoglycaemia is uncommon in healthy babies who are carried to full term. The condition is likely to occur in premature infants and those of low birth weight, due to their reduced reserves of *glycogen* (main form of the body's stored carbohydrate). It is also more common in babies whose mothers had *diabetes mellitus* during pregnancy. These babies produce the extra insulin they require before delivery, but their glucose levels fall after birth. Also at risk of neonatal hypoglycaemia are infants with inborn errors of metabolism (see *metabolism, inborn errors of*) and those who are unwell at birth. Difficulties with *breast-feeding* during the first days of life may also cause the condition to develop.

SYMPTOMS AND SIGNS

Neonatal hypoglycaemia is usually characterized by jitteriness, *seizures*, irritability, floppiness, *apnoea* (interruption in breathing), and poor feeding.

DIAGNOSIS AND TREATMENT

A diagnosis of neonatal hypoglycaemia is confirmed using *blood tests* to check blood glucose levels.

In babies at increased risk of the condition, preventive treatment involves the immediate establishment of regular feeding, ideally breast-feeding. Hypoglycaemia that is severe enough to cause symptoms requires an intravenous infusion of glucose along with, if possible, treatment of the underlying cause.

N

neonatal jaundice

See *jaundice, neonatal*.

neonatal urticaria

See *urticaria, neonatal*.

neonate

A newly born infant, specifically up to the age of 27 days. (See also *newborn*.)

neonatology

The branch of *paediatrics* concerned with the care of *newborn* infants and the treatment of disorders that occur during the first few weeks of life. Such problems may be short-term (such as those associated with *prematurity* or low birth weight) or lifelong (such as *spina bifida*).

neoplasia

A medical term for the process of *tumour* formation, characterized by progressive, abnormal cell multiplication. The term neoplasia does not necessarily imply that the new growth is cancerous; neoplasia also results in noncancerous tumours.

neoplasm

A medical term for a *tumour* (any new abnormal growth). Neoplasms may be cancerous or noncancerous.

neostigmine

A drug used in the treatment of *myasthenia gravis* (an autoimmune disorder that causes muscle weakness). It increases the activity of *acetylcholine*, a *neurotransmitter* (a chemical released from nerve endings) that stimulates muscle contraction.

Possible side effects include nausea and vomiting, increased salivation, diarrhoea, abdominal cramps, blurred vision, muscle cramps, sweating, and twitching.

nephrectomy

The surgical removal of one or both of the *kidneys*.

WHY IT IS DONE
One of the most common reasons for nephrectomy is to remove a cancerous tumour (see *kidney cancer*). A kidney may also be removed if it is not functioning properly because of injury, infection, or the presence of stones (see *calculus, urinary tract*) or if it is causing severe *hypertension* (high blood pressure). Nephrectomy may also be necessary if a kidney is so badly injured that bleeding cannot be stopped.

HOW IT IS DONE
Nephrectomy is performed under general anaesthetic (see *anaesthesia, general*).

An incision is made along the lower edge of the ribs, from the spine to the front of the abdomen, in order to expose the kidney. The ureter (the tube that carries urine from the kidney to the bladder) and the renal blood vessels are tied off, then the kidney is removed. The incision is stitched up after insertion of a drainage tube, which is left in place for between 24 and 48 hours.

OUTLOOK
On removal of a single kidney, the remaining kidney takes over the workload. If both kidneys are removed, the patient requires regular *dialysis* (artificial purification of blood) or a *kidney transplant*.

nephritis

Inflammation of one or both of the *kidneys*. Nephritis may be caused by an infection (see *pyelonephritis*), by abnormal responses of the *immune system* (see *glomerulonephritis*), or by drugs – for example, penicillin. (See also *Disorders of the kidney* box.)

nephroblastoma

A type of *kidney cancer* that mainly affects children.

nephrocalcinosis

Deposits of *calcium* within the tissue of one or both of the *kidneys*. Nephrocalcinosis is not the same as kidney stones (see *calculus, urinary tract*), in which particles of calcium develop inside the drainage channels of the kidney.

Nephrocalcinosis may occur in any condition in which the level of calcium in the blood is raised – for example, in *hyperparathyroidism* (overactivity of the parathyroid gland) and *renal tubular acidosis* (in which the kidney produces urine of lower-than-normal acidity). Nephrocalcinosis may also occur as a result of taking excessive amounts of certain *antacid drugs* or *vitamin D*.

Treatment is of the underlying cause in order to prevent further calcification.

nephrolithotomy

The surgical removal of a kidney stone (see *calculus, urinary tract*) by cutting into the main part of the *kidney*.

Nephrolithotomy may be performed through an abdominal incision, an incision in the back, or using *pyelolithotomy* (a procedure in which a kidney stone is removed through an incision at the renal pelvis). Instruments are used to grasp and remove the calculus; large calculi may need to be broken up before removal.

It is now often possible to avoid surgery by using *lithotripsy* (a procedure that uses ultrasonic waves to break up calculi for excretion in the urine).

nephrology

The medical speciality concerned with the normal functioning of the *kidneys* and with the causes, diagnosis, and treatment of kidney disease.

Methods of investigating the kidneys include kidney *biopsy* (removal of a small sample of tissue for microscopic analysis), *kidney function tests*, and *kidney imaging* techniques, such as *ultrasound scanning* and *intravenous urography*.

Treatment of kidney disorders may involve drugs (for example, to control high blood pressure, inflammation, or infection) and surgery (for the treatment of stones or tumours). In advanced cases, regular *dialysis* (artificial purification of the blood) or a *kidney transplant* may be required. (See also *Disorders of the kidney* box.)

nephron

The functional microscopic unit of the *kidney* that consists of a glomerulus (a filtering unit made up of a cluster of capillaries) and a tubule. Each kidney contains about one million nephrons.

The nephrons filter waste products from the blood and modify the amount of salt and water excreted in the urine, according to the body's needs. This process involves blood filtration in the glomerulus followed by further processing of the filtrate as it flows through the various parts of the tubule: the proximal convoluted tubule, the *loop of Henlé*, and the distal convoluted tubule.

nephropathy

A term for any disease of, or damage to, the *kidneys*. The term is usually combined with a word that indicates the cause of the damage, for example diabetic nephropathy, toxic nephropathy, hypertensive nephropathy, and obstructive nephropathy. The treatment and outlook are dependent on the cause. (See also *Disorders of the kidney* box.)

nephrosclerosis

Hardening of the arterioles and arteries within the *kidney*, usually as a result of *atherosclerosis* (the deposition of fatty material within blood vessels).

nephrosis

See *nephrotic syndrome*.

N

nephrostomy

The introduction of a small tube into the *kidney* to drain urine to the abdominal surface, thereby bypassing the ureter and bladder. Nephrostomy is sometimes performed after an operation (typically removal of a kidney stone) on the ureter or the kidney–ureter junction.

nephrotic syndrome

A collection of symptoms and signs resulting from damage to the glomeruli (the filtering units of the *kidney*), which causes severe *proteinuria* (leakage of protein from the blood into the urine), low blood levels of protein, and swelling.

CAUSES

Nephrotic syndrome may occur as a result of *diabetes mellitus*, *amyloidosis* (accumulation of amyloid, an abnormal protein, in the tissues), or any type of *glomerulonephritis* (inflammation of the glomeruli). The conditions may also be due to severe *hypertension* (high blood pressure), reactions to poisons (such as *mercury* or *cadmium*), or adverse reactions to drugs, such as *gold* or *penicillamine*.

Nephrotic syndrome may also be a complication of an infection elsewhere in the body, such as *hepatitis B* or *malaria*. In children, the syndrome is most commonly due to a condition known as minimal change glomerulonephritis.

SYMPTOMS

The symptoms of nephrotic syndrome appear gradually over days or weeks and worsen as more and more protein is lost in the urine. Early signs include frothy urine and decreased urine production. The main symptom is swelling of the legs and face as a result of *oedema* (accumulation of fluid in the tissues). Fluid may also collect in the chest cavity, resulting in *pleural effusion* and shortness of breath, or in the abdomen, causing *ascites*. Lethargy and loss of appetite (leading to weight loss) may also occur.

DIAGNOSIS AND TREATMENT

Diagnosis involves *blood tests*; the urine must also be examined under a microscope and the amount and type of protein lost assessed over a 24-hour period (see *urinalysis*). In most cases, a kidney *biopsy* (removal of a small sample of tissue for microscopic analysis) is also required to establish the exact cause and help with treatment decisions.

Treatment is aimed at the underlying condition. A low-sodium diet may be recommended and *diuretic drugs* may be given to reduce oedema. Protein may need to be given intravenously, but the effects are short lived. *Corticosteroid drugs* may also be prescribed and are often effective in cases of nephrotic syndrome in childhood.

OUTLOOK

The outlook for someone with nephrotic syndrome depends on the extent of the kidney damage. Recurrent episodes may occur even after treatment. Problems with excessive blood clotting are common and may require treatment with *anticoagulant drugs*. Infections may occur as a result of *immunoglobulin* loss into the urine. Nephrotic syndrome is usually associated with raised cholesterol, which increases the risk of *myocardial infarction* (heart attack) due to *atherosclerosis* (fatty deposits on the artery walls). In the most severe cases, chronic *kidney failure*, and eventually an irreversible loss of kidney function, may develop.

nephrotoxic

A term meaning toxic (poisonous) to *kidney* cells, resulting in damage to or destruction of the cells.

nerve

A bundle of nerve fibres travelling to a common location. Nerve fibres, which are also known as axons, are the filamentous projections of many individual *neurons* (nerve cells).

STRUCTURE

The most obvious nerves in the body are the peripheral nerves, which extend from the *central nervous system* (consisting of the *brain* and the *spinal cord*) to other parts of the body. Of these, 12 pairs of *cranial nerves* link directly to the brain and 31 pairs of *spinal nerves* join the spinal cord. In the shoulder and hip regions, the spinal nerves join to form plexuses, from which branch the main nerves to the limbs, such as the median nerve in the arm and the sciatic nerve in the leg. Most nerves divide at numerous points to send branches to all parts of the body, particularly to the sense organs, the skin, the skeletal muscles, the internal organs, and the glands.

FUNCTION

Nerve fibres may have a sensory function, carrying information from a receptor or sense organ towards the central nervous system (CNS), or they may have a motor function, carrying instructions from the CNS to a muscle or a gland. The messages are carried by electrical impulses propagated along the fibres. Some nerves carry only sensory or motor fibres, but most carry both.

DISORDERS

Nerve function is sensitive to cold, pressure, and injury (see *nerve injury*). The peripheral nerves can be damaged by a variety of disorders, including infection, inflammation, poisoning, nutritional deficiencies, and metabolic disorders (see *neuropathy*). (See also *radiculopathy*.)

nerve block

The injection of a local anaesthetic (see *anaesthesia, local*) around a nerve in order to produce loss of sensation in a part of the body supplied by that nerve. For example, the palm of the hand may be anaesthetized by giving injections at sites up the arm, thereby blocking the ulnar and median nerves.

WHY IT IS DONE

A nerve block is performed when it is not possible to inject anaesthetic directly into the tissues being treated because the area is painfully inflamed or because there is a risk of spreading infection.

The technique may also be used to anaesthetize a large area or an area not suitable for injection because it is deep within the body or is covered with bone.

TYPES

Spinal nerve block A nerve may be blocked as it leaves the cord. This happens both in *epidural anaesthesia*, which is used mainly in childbirth, and in *spinal anaesthesia*, which is used for surgery on the lower abdomen and limbs.

Caudal block In a caudal block, an anaesthetic is injected around the nerves leaving the lowest part of the spinal cord. It produces a loss of sensation in the buttock and genital areas and is occasionally used in childbirth.

Pudendal block A pudendal nerve block involves the injection of an anaesthetic into nerves passing under the pelvis into the floor of the vagina. This type of nerve block is sometimes used during childbirth in a *forceps delivery*.

nerve conduction studies

Electrical tests carried out to assess the extent of nerve damage caused by disorders of the peripheral nervous system (see *neuropathy*). In the test, an electrical stimulus is applied to a nerve; the speed at which the nerve responds to the stimulus and transmits its signal is recorded by specialized equipment.

nerve injury

Damage or severance of conducting fibres within a *nerve* as a result of trauma, resulting in the loss of skin

N

sensation and muscle power. (See *neuropathy* for nerve damage from causes other than injury.)

Nerves may be damaged in many different injuries, including knife wounds, bullet wounds, penetrating injuries (such as from flying glass), or from accidental contact with powered devices (such as rotary saws and propellers).

PERIPHERAL NERVE INJURY
If injury to a peripheral nerve (a nerve outside the brain or spinal cord) results in severance of some, but not all, of the individual fibres within the nerve, the cut fibres degenerate on both sides of the injury. This leads to loss of power in the muscles and loss of sensation in the skin area supplied by the fibres.

In cases of partial severance in which the ends of the severed fibres are still aligned, new fibres can regenerate along channels left by the degenerated ones. These new fibres begin to grow within a few days of injury, but they grow slowly (at a rate of about 1 mm per day).

If there is total severance of a nerve, the individual fibres try to regenerate but, with no directing channels, simply bunch up to form a lump of tissue. In such cases, function does not recover.

Regenerating nerve fibres sometimes pass down the wrong channels. So, when function is restored, actions may differ from what was intended (for example, an attempt to move the index finger may move the middle finger as well). Movement skills and the interpretation of sensations may need to be relearned.

BRAIN AND SPINAL CORD INJURY
Nerve tracts within the brain and spinal cord are structurally different from the peripheral nerves, and severed fibres in these tracts do not regenerate. Vision cannot be restored if, for example, the *optic nerves* are cut.

TREATMENT
Surgery can sometimes repair a severed nerve, but such treatment is possible only for peripheral nerves. In *microsurgery*, the neurosurgeon ensures that the severed fibres are meticulously brought together and stitched into place using delicate needles and sutures. Careful realignment of the nerve ends gives the fibres the best chance of regenerating along the correct channels. However, even with the best surgical repair, recovery is rarely complete.

A programme of *physiotherapy* is needed to keep paralysed muscles healthy and free from *contracture* (abnormal shortening) during the recovery period.

nerve, trapped
Compression or stretching of a *nerve*, causing numbness, tingling, weakness, and, sometimes, pain in the area supplied by the nerve. Common examples of a trapped nerve include *carpal tunnel syndrome*, in which pressure on the median nerve as it passes through the wrist causes symptoms in the thumb, index, and middle fingers; a *disc prolapse*, in which pressure on the nerve root leading from the spinal cord produces symptoms in the back and legs; and *crutch palsy*, in which the radial nerve presses against the humerus (upper arm bone), producing symptoms in the wrist and hand.

A damaged nerve may take some time to heal. In severe cases, surgical decompression to relieve pressure on the nerve may be necessary.

nervous breakdown
A nontechnical term used to describe unusual behaviour (such as episodes of tearfulness or shouting and screaming) that may be part of a crisis of severe *anxiety*, *depression*, or other psychiatric illness. The condition affects the sufferer's ability to cope with everyday life.

nervous energy
A nontechnical term for the increased drive and activity of individuals who are always restless, anxious, and on the go.

nervous habit
A nontechnical term for a minor repetitive movement or activity. A nervous habit can consist of involuntary twitches and facial tics, such as in *Gilles de la Tourette's syndrome* and some forms of *dyskinesia*. Voluntary nervous habits, such as *nail-biting* and *thumb-sucking*, are common in young children, but usually disappear naturally with time. All nervous habits increase during periods of tension or anxiety and may be severe in some forms of *depression*, *anxiety disorder*, or drug withdrawal.

nervous system
The body system that gathers and stores information. It is in control of the body. (See *Nervous system* box, opposite.)
STRUCTURE
The *brain* and *spinal cord* form the *central nervous system* (CNS), which consists of billions of interconnected *neurons* (nerve cells). The input of information to the CNS comes from the sense organs. Motor instructions are sent out to skeletal muscles, the muscles controlling speech, internal organs and glands, and the sweat glands in the skin. This information is carried along *nerves* that fan out from the CNS to the entire body, together making up what is known as the peripheral nervous system (PNS).

Each nerve is a bundle consisting of the axons (filamentous projections) of many individual neurons.
FUNCTION
There are also functional divisions. Two of the most important are the *autonomic nervous system*, which is concerned with the automatic regulation of internal body functions, and the somatic nervous system, controlling the muscles responsible for voluntary movement.

The overall function of the nervous system is to gather and analyse information about the external environment and the body's internal state and to initiate appropriate responses aimed at satisfying certain drives.

The most powerful drive is for survival. Many survival responses, which range from avoiding physical pain and danger to shivering in response to the cold, are initiated unconsciously and automatically by the nervous system. Other drives are more complex, revolving around a need to experience positive emotions (such as pleasure and excitement) and to avoid negative emotions (such as pain, anxiety, and frustration).

The nervous system functions largely through automatic responses to stimuli (see *reflex*), but it can also improve its performance through *learning*, which relies on *memory*. Voluntary actions can be initiated via activity in conscious areas of the brain. Certain functions (such as visual perception, memory, thought, and speech production) are extremely complex and still not fully understood.
DISORDERS
Disorders of the nervous system may be caused by damage to or dysfunction of any of its parts (see *disorders of the brain* box; *spinal cord*; *neuropathy*; *nerve injury*). They may also be due to impaired sensory, analytical, or memory functions (see *vision, disorders of*; *deafness*; *numbness*; *anosmia*; *agnosia*; *amnesia*), or motor functions (see *aphasia*; *dysarthria*; *ataxia*).

netilmicin
An *antibiotic drug* usually prescribed only to treat serious infection in hospital, when other antibiotic drugs have proved ineffective. In rare cases, netilmicin can damage the inner ear or the kidneys.

N

NERVOUS SYSTEM

The nervous system detects and interprets changes in conditions inside and outside the body and responds to them. The central nervous system analyses information and initiates responses; the peripheral nervous system gathers information and carries the response signals. Some responses are involuntary; others are dictated by conscious thought. All nervous system activity consists of signals passed through pathways of interconnected neurons (nerve cells).

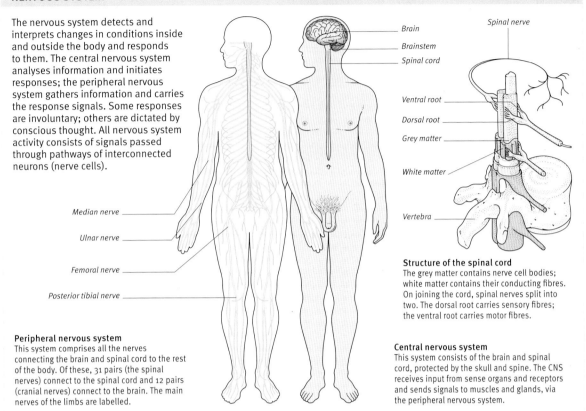

Median nerve
Ulnar nerve
Femoral nerve
Posterior tibial nerve

Brain
Brainstem
Spinal cord

Spinal nerve

Ventral root
Dorsal root
Grey matter

White matter

Vertebra

Structure of the spinal cord
The grey matter contains nerve cell bodies; white matter contains their conducting fibres. On joining the cord, spinal nerves split into two. The dorsal root carries sensory fibres; the ventral root carries motor fibres.

Peripheral nervous system
This system comprises all the nerves connecting the brain and spinal cord to the rest of the body. Of these, 31 pairs (the spinal nerves) connect to the spinal cord and 12 pairs (cranial nerves) connect to the brain. The main nerves of the limbs are labelled.

Central nervous system
This system consists of the brain and spinal cord, protected by the skull and spine. The CNS receives input from sense organs and receptors and sends signals to muscles and glands, via the peripheral nervous system.

N

HOW IT WORKS

Some possible events in response to a finger touching a hot object are shown. A receptor sends a message, via a sensory fibre, to the spinal cord. This triggers a signal that travels, via a motor fibre, back to a muscle, which contracts to move the finger away from the heat. This action is called a reflex arc. Other signals pass to the brain.

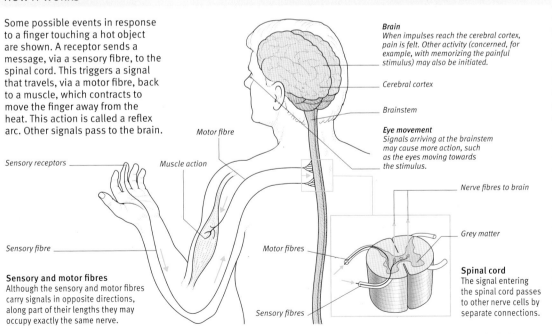

Brain
When impulses reach the cerebral cortex, pain is felt. Other activity (concerned, for example, with memorizing the painful stimulus) may also be initiated.

Cerebral cortex

Brainstem

Eye movement
Signals arriving at the brainstem may cause more action, such as the eyes moving towards the stimulus.

Nerve fibres to brain

Grey matter

Spinal cord
The signal entering the spinal cord passes to other nerve cells by separate connections.

Motor fibre
Muscle action
Sensory receptors
Sensory fibre
Motor fibres
Sensory fibres

Sensory and motor fibres
Although the sensory and motor fibres carry signals in opposite directions, along part of their lengths they may occupy exactly the same nerve.

nettle rash

A common name for *urticaria*.

neuralgia

Pain caused by irritation of, or damage to, a *nerve*. The pain usually occurs in brief bouts, may be severe, and can often be felt shooting along the affected nerve.

TYPES AND CAUSES

Some types of neuralgia are features of a disorder. *Migraine* sufferers commonly experience a form of neuralgia comprising attacks of intense, radiating pain around the eye. Postherpetic neuralgia is a burning pain that may recur at the site of an attack of *herpes zoster* (shingles) for months or even years after the illness.

Other types of neuralgia result from disturbance of a particular nerve. In glossopharyngeal neuralgia, intense pain is felt at the back of the tongue and in the throat and ear, all of which are areas supplied by the glossopharyngeal nerve. The cause is unknown. The same is true of *trigeminal neuralgia*, a severe paroxysm of pain affecting one side of the face supplied by the trigeminal nerve.

TREATMENT

Neuralgia may be relieved by *analgesic drugs* (painkillers), such as *paracetamol*. Glossopharyngeal, trigeminal, and postherpetic neuralgia may respond to treatment with *carbamazepine* or other *anticonvulsant drugs* (such as gabapentin), or to *tricyclic antidepressant drugs*.

neural tube defect

A developmental failure affecting the *spinal cord* or *brain* of the *embryo*. The neural plate, which develops along the back of the embryo by about the third week of pregnancy, then folds to form the neural tube that later becomes the brain, the spinal cord, and their coverings (the *meninges*). If the neural tube does not form properly, defects in any of these parts can result.

TYPES AND SYMPTOMS

The most serious neural tube defect is *anencephaly* (failure of the skull and brain to develop), which is fatal before birth or soon afterwards. More common is *spina bifida*, in which the vertebrae do not form a complete ring around the spinal cord. Spina bifida can occur anywhere on the spine, but it is most common in the lower back.

There are different forms of spina bifida. In spina bifida occulta, the only defect is a failure of the bony arches behind the spinal cord to fuse, which is sometimes associated with a tuft of hair over the area or a dimple in the skin. This may cause no problems, although there may be tethering of the spinal column, which may need releasing surgically.

If the bone defect is more extensive, there may be a meningocele (a protrusion of the meningeal membranes) or a myelomeningocele (a malformation in which part of the spinal cord and the meninges overlying it are completely exposed). Myelomeningocele is likely to cause severe handicap, with paralysis of the legs, loss of sensation in the lower body, and paralysis of the anus and bladder, causing incontinence (see *incontinence, faecal*; *incontinence, urinary*). The higher up the spine the malformation is, the more severe the handicap.

Associated problems include *hydrocephalus*, in which extra fluid forms in the brain; insertion of a shunt to relieve the pressure is often needed in the first few weeks of life. However, some children will also have *cerebral palsy*, *epilepsy*, or *learning difficulties*. Children with neural tube defects are at particular risk of developing *meningitis*, a serious infection of the membranes covering the brain and spinal cord.

CAUSES

The cause of neural tube defects is not fully understood, but they tend to run in families, which suggests that genetic factors are involved. Certain types of *anticonvulsant drug* are associated with neural tube defects if they are taken by women during pregnancy.

TREATMENT AND OUTLOOK

Surgery is usually performed a few days after birth. In mild cases, the defect can usually be corrected completely, but in myelomeningocele, some handicap will remain; affected children usually need lifelong care. *Physiotherapy* and mobility aids may be useful to maintain activity and allow as great a degree of independence as possible. Children with extensive damage to the brain and/or spinal cord usually have a reduced life expectancy.

PREVENTION

The risk of a neural tube defect can be substantially reduced if the mother takes the recommended dose of *folic acid* supplements before conception and during the first 12 weeks of pregnancy. If one of the parents has spina bifida or has previously had a child with a neural tube defect, a higher dose of folic acid is recommended.

Blood tests and *ultrasound scanning* in pregnancy can help to detect neural tube defects before birth. Over the last 25 years, there has been a substantial decline in the numbers of babies born with these defects.

neurapraxia

A type of *nerve injury* in which the outward structure of a nerve appears intact, but some conducting fibres have been damaged and thus do not transmit signals normally.

neurasthenia

An outdated term that literally means "nervous exhaustion". The term neurasthenia was once used to describe a number of physical and mental symptoms, such as insomnia, loss of energy, aches and pains, *depression*, irritability, and reduced concentration.

neuritis

A term that literally means inflammation of a *nerve*. True nerve inflammation may be caused by infection (for example, by a virus in *herpes zoster* or by a bacterium in *Hansen's disease*). The term neuritis is also often applied to nerve damage or disease from causes other than inflammation. It has become virtually synonymous with *neuropathy*.

neuroblastoma

A cancerous tumour that develops from nervous tissue in the *adrenal glands* or in part of the sympathetic nervous system (see *autonomic nervous system*). Neuroblastomas from the sympathetic nervous system usually develop in the sympathetic nerves along the back wall of the abdomen. Less commonly, tumours originate in the sympathetic nerves of the chest or neck. The tumours often spread to other sites in the body.

INCIDENCE AND CAUSE

Neuroblastomas are the most common extracranial (outside the skull), solid tumour of childhood. Most cases develop during the first ten years of life, especially in the first five. The disorder is slightly more common in boys than in girls.

The cause of these tumours is not known, although a genetic factor is thought to be involved.

SYMPTOMS

Symptoms may be present from birth or may develop gradually during childhood. Typical symptoms include a lump in the abdomen, tiredness, weight loss, aches and pains, pallor, and irritability. In some cases, there is also diarrhoea, *hypertension* (high blood pressure), and flushing of the skin.

N

If a tumour spreads through the body, other symptoms, such as bone pain or, if the lymph nodes are affected, swellings in the neck or armpits, may occur. *Anaemia* (a reduced level of the oxygen-carrying pigment *haemoglobin* in the blood) may result if the cancer spreads to the bone marrow.

DIAGNOSIS
The diagnosis of a neuroblastoma is made from *MRI* and *CT scanning* (techniques that produce cross-sectional or three-dimensional images of internal body structures), blood tests, urine tests, and *biopsy* (removal of a small sample of tissue for analysis) of the bone marrow and any accessible tumours.

TREATMENT AND OUTLOOK
If possible, the tumour is surgically removed; this is not possible if it has grown around the large blood vessels in the abdomen, however. Treatment is primarily with *anticancer drugs* (*chemotherapy*). *Radiotherapy* and a *stem cell* or *bone marrow transplant* are other treatments that may also be considered.

Neuroblastomas vary widely, from being relatively harmless to aggressively cancerous, and the outlook is therefore also highly variable.

neurocutaneous disorders
A group of conditions characterized by abnormalities of the skin and of the nerves and/or the *central nervous system*.

The best known of the neurocutaneous disorders is *neurofibromatosis*, in which there are brown patches on the skin and numerous fibrous nodules on the skin and nerves. Another example is *tuberous sclerosis*, which is characterized by small skin-coloured swellings over the cheeks and the nose, mental deficiency, and epilepsy.

neurodermatitis
An itchy, *eczema*-like skin condition caused by repeated scratching. (See also *lichen simplex*.)

neuroendocrinology
The study of the interactions between the *nervous system* and the *endocrine system* that control internal body functions and the body's response to the external environment.

neurofibromatosis
A *genetic disorder* that causes numerous soft, noncancerous growths, known as neurofibromas, to appear throughout the body. These tumours grow from nerve tissue and develop along nerve pathways. If the condition is severe, it can be very disfiguring.

TYPES AND CAUSES
There are two types of neurofibromatosis. The more common of the two, known as neurofibromatosis 1 or von Recklinghausen's disease, is usually apparent in early childhood. The other type, neurofibromatosis 2, is extremely rare and the symptoms do not usually appear until adulthood.

Both types are caused by an abnormal gene that shows an autosomal dominant pattern of inheritance.

SYMPTOMS
In neurofibromatosis 1, numerous pale-brown, flat patches with irregular edges, which are known as café au lait spots, develop on the skin. The growths under the skin feel soft to the touch and range in size from hardly noticeable to large bumps. In addition there may be numerous freckles in the armpit and the groin areas.

Adults with neurofibromatosis 2 tend to develop tumours in the inner ear, which can affect hearing, but they rarely have tumours under the skin.

COMPLICATIONS
Complications may occur when the growing tumours press on surrounding organs or nerves. For example, vision may be affected if a tumour develops on the optic nerve, which connects the eye to the brain. Tumours can also cause curvature of the spine. Some children with neurofibromatosis may develop epilepsy or have learning problems. In rare cases, tumours become cancerous.

TREATMENT
There is no cure for neurofibromatosis, and its progression cannot be slowed. However, surgical removal of neurofibromas may be carried out if there are complications or if large, disfiguring tumours are causing distress. Anyone with this disorder, and parents of an affected child, may wish to seek *genetic counselling* when planning a pregnancy.

OUTLOOK
In mild cases, life expectancy is normal, but if the tumours are extensive and become cancerous, lifespan is reduced.

neuroleptic drugs
An alternative name for *antipsychotic drugs*.

neurology
The medical discipline concerned with the study of the *nervous system* and its disorders. Neurologists are trained to examine the nerves, reflexes, motor and sensory functions, and muscles to determine a disorder's cause and extent. They are specialists in the treatment of conditions, such as *migraine* and *Parkinson's disease*, that have a neurological basis, and in the care and support of patients with progressive disorders such as *multiple sclerosis* and *muscular dystrophy*. (See also *neuropathology*; *neurosurgery*.)

neuroma
A noncancerous tumour of *nerve* tissue. In most cases, the cause is unknown; rarely, a neuroma develops as a result of damage to a nerve.

A neuroma may affect any nerve in the body. Symptoms vary according to the nerve involved. In most cases, there is intermittent pain in the areas of the body supplied by the affected nerve. The same areas may also become numb and weak if the neuroma develops in a confined space and presses on the nerve.

If symptoms are troublesome, the tumour may be surgically removed. (See also *acoustic neuroma*.)

neuron
The medical term for a *nerve* cell.

STRUCTURE
A typical neuron consists of a cell body, several branching projections called dendrites, and a filamentous projection called an axon (also known as a nerve fibre). An axon branches at its end to form terminals through which nerve signals are transmitted to target cells.

Most axons are coated with a layered insulating *myelin* sheath, which speeds the transmission of nerve signals. The myelin sheath is punctuated along its length by gaps called nodes of Ranvier, which help this process. Because the myelin sheath is nonconductive, ion exchange (depolarization) only occurs at a node; signals leap from node to node along the length of the axon.

FUNCTION
The nervous system contains billions of neurons, of which there are three main types: sensory neurons, which carry signals from sense receptors into the *central nervous system* (CNS); motor neurons, which carry signals from the CNS to muscles or glands; and interneurons, which form all the complex electrical circuitry within the CNS itself.

When a neuron transmits ("fires") a nerve impulse, a chemical called a *neurotransmitter* is released from the axon

N

STRUCTURE OF A **NEURON**

A neuron (nerve cell) consists of a cell body and several branching projections, which are called dendrites. Every neuron has a filamentous projection called an axon (nerve fibre). Axons vary greatly in length – from a fraction of a centimetre to about a metre. An axon branches at its end to form terminals, via which signals are transmitted to target cells, such as the dendrites of other neurons, muscle cells, or glands. Bundles of the axons of many neurons are known as nerves or, when they are located within the brain or spinal cord, as nerve tracts or pathways.

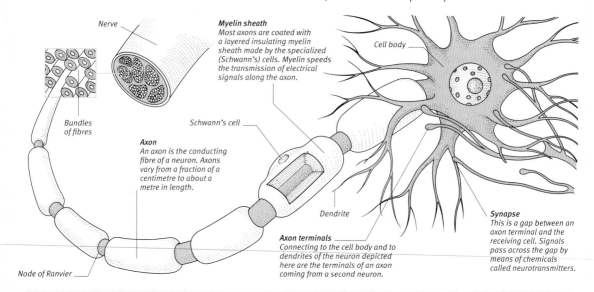

Nerve

Myelin sheath
Most axons are coated with a layered insulating myelin sheath made by the specialized (Schwann's) cells. Myelin speeds the transmission of electrical signals along the axon.

Cell body

Bundles of fibres

Schwann's cell

Axon
An axon is the conducting fibre of a neuron. Axons vary from a fraction of a centimetre to about a metre in length.

Dendrite

Synapse
This is a gap between an axon terminal and the receiving cell. Signals pass across the gap by means of chemicals called neurotransmitters.

Node of Ranvier

Axon terminals
Connecting to the cell body and to dendrites of the neuron depicted here are the terminals of an axon coming from a second neuron.

BASIC TYPES OF **NEURON**

Sensory neurons carry signals from sense receptors along their axons into the central nervous system (CNS). Motor neurons carry signals from the CNS to muscles or glands; the axon terminals form a motor endplate. Interneurons form all the complex interconnecting electrical circuitry within the CNS itself. For each sensory neuron in the body, there are about 10 motor neurons and 99 interneurons.

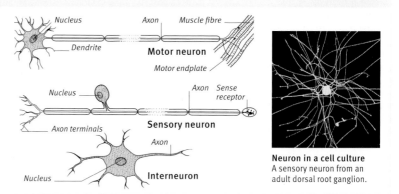

Nucleus   *Axon*   *Muscle fibre*

Dendrite   **Motor neuron**

Motor endplate

Nucleus   *Axon*   *Sense receptor*

Axon terminals   **Sensory neuron**

Nucleus   *Axon*

Interneuron

Neuron in a cell culture
A sensory neuron from an adult dorsal root ganglion.

terminals at *synapses* (junctions with other neurons). This neurotransmitter may make a muscle cell contract, cause an endocrine gland to release a hormone, or affect an adjacent neuron.

Different stimuli excite different types of neurons to fire. For example, physical stimuli such as cold, pressure, or light of a certain wavelength may excite sensory neurons. Most neurons' activity is controlled by the effects of neurotransmitters released from adjacent neurons. Certain neurotransmitters generate a sudden change in the balance of electrical poten-tial inside and outside the cell (an "action potential"), which occurs at one point on the cell's membrane and flows at high speed along it. Others stabilize neuronal membranes, preventing an action potential. Thus, a neuron's firing pattern depends on the balance of excitatory and inhibitory influences acting on it.

LIFESPAN
If the cell body of a neuron is damaged or degenerates, the cell dies and is never replaced. A baby is born with the maximum number of neurons, and this number decreases continuously through-out life. However, because people are born with a very large number of neurons, problems normally only arise when disease, injury, or persistent alcohol abuse affects the CNS and dramatically increases the rate at which neurons are lost.

If a peripheral nerve is damaged, its individual nerve fibres can regenerate themselves (see *nerve injury*; *neuropathy*).

neuropathic joint

A joint that has been damaged by inflammation and a series of injuries, which pass unnoticed due to a loss of sensation in the joint resulting from *neuropathy* (nerve damage caused by disease). Neuropathic joints develop in a number of conditions, including *diabetes mellitus* and untreated *syphilis*.

SYMPTOMS

When sensation to pain is lost, abnormal stress and strain on a joint do not stimulate the protective reflex spasm of the surrounding muscles; this failure of the protective reflex allows exaggerated movement that can lead to damage within and around the joint. *Osteoarthritis*, swelling, and deformity are features of a neuropathic joint.

TREATMENT AND OUTLOOK

An orthopaedic *brace* or *caliper splint* may be necessary to restrict any abnormal movement of the joint. Occasionally, *arthrodesis* (a surgical operation to fuse a joint) is performed. The nerve damage is irreversible.

neuropathology

The branch of *pathology* that is concerned with the causes and effects of disorders of the *nervous system*. (See also *neurology*.)

neuropathy

Disease or inflammation of, or damage to, the peripheral *nerves*, which connect the *central nervous system* (the brain and the spinal cord), to the muscles, glands, sense organs, and internal organs. The term neuritis is now used more or less interchangeably with neuropathy.

TYPES

Most nerve cell axons (the conducting fibres that make up nerves) are insulated by a sheath of the fatty substance *myelin*. Most neuropathies arise from damage to, or irritation of, either the axons or their myelin sheaths. This may cause the passage of nerve signals to be slowed or blocked completely.

Various types of neuropathy are described according to the site and the distribution of the damage. For example, a distal neuropathy starts with damage at the far end of a nerve (the end farthest from the brain or spinal cord). A symmetrical neuropathy affects nerves at the same places on each side of the body. Some neuropathies are described according to the underlying cause of the condition, for example *diabetic neuropathy*, *entrapment neuropathy*, or alcoholic neuropathy.

Polyneuropathy (also known as polyneuritis) refers to damage to several nerves; mononeuropathy (or mononeuritis) indicates damage to a single nerve. The term "neuralgia" describes pain caused by irritation or inflammation of a particular nerve.

CAUSES

There are some cases of neuropathy that have no obvious cause. Among the many specific causes are *diabetes mellitus*, dietary deficiencies (particularly of the B vitamins), excessive alcohol consumption, and metabolic upsets such as *uraemia*. Other causes include *Hansen's disease* (leprosy), *lead poisoning*, or poisoning by drug overdose.

Nerves may become acutely inflamed after a viral infection, such as occurs in *Guillain-Barré syndrome*. Neuropathies may also result from *autoimmune disorders* (disorders in which the immune system attacks the body's own healthy tissues) such as *rheumatoid arthritis*, systemic *lupus erythematosus*, or *polyarteritis nodosa*. In these disorders, there is often damage to the blood vessels supplying the nerves. Neuropathies may occur secondarily to cancerous tumours, such as lung cancer, or with *lymphomas* and *leukaemias*. There is also a group of inherited neuropathies, the most common being *peroneal muscular atrophy*.

SYMPTOMS

The symptoms of neuropathy depend on whether it affects mainly sensory nerve fibres or mainly motor nerve fibres. Damage to sensory nerve fibres may cause numbness, tingling, sensations of cold, and pain, which often starts in the hands and feet and spreads towards the centre of the body. Damage to motor fibres may cause muscle weakness and muscle wasting. Damage to nerves of the *autonomic nervous system* may lead to blurred vision, impaired or absent sweating, faintness, and disturbance of gastric, intestinal, bladder, and sexual functioning, including incontinence and *erectile dysfunction*.

Some neuropathies are linked with particular symptoms; for example, diabetic neuropathy can cause severe pain.

DIAGNOSIS

In order to determine the extent of the nerve damage, *nerve conduction studies* are carried out together with electromyography tests (see *EMG*), which record the electrical activity in muscles. Diagnostic tests such as *blood tests*, *MRI* scans (a technique that produces cross-sectional or three-dimensional images of body structures), and nerve or muscle *biopsy* (removal of a small sample of tissue for microscopic analysis) may also be required.

TREATMENT AND OUTLOOK

Treatment is aimed at the underlying cause. For example, vitamin injections may be given to correct a nutritional deficiency; blood sugar levels are carefully controlled to reduce the risk of further nerve damage and promote recovery in people with diabetes mellitus.

If the cell bodies of the damaged nerve cells have not been destroyed, full recovery from the neuropathy is possible. (See also *radiculopathy*.)

neuropsychiatry

The branch of medicine that deals with the relationship between psychiatric symptoms and neurological disorder (see *neurology*). This may include the effects of head injury and alcohol on the brain or specific disorders such as brain tumours, infections, inherited illnesses, and disorders causing brain damage in childhood. *Brain imaging* techniques are often used to demonstrate abnormalities of structure and function in disorders with psychiatric symptoms.

neurosis

An old term for a range of psychiatric disorders in which there was no loss of contact with reality (unlike *psychosis*). Disorders classed as neurotic included mild forms of *depression*, *anxiety*, *hypochondriasis*, and *dissociative disorders*.

neurosurgery

The specialty concerned with the surgical treatment of disorders of the *brain*, *spinal cord*, or other parts of the *nervous system*. Many generalized nervous system disorders do not respond to surgical treatment, but neurosurgery can deal with most conditions in which a localized structural change interferes with nerve function. Improvements in monitoring techniques and control of post-operative complications, such as swelling of the brain, have reduced the risk of serious problems developing.

Conditions treated by neurosurgery include *tumours* of the brain, spinal cord, or meninges (the membranes surrounding the brain and spinal cord); *brain abscesses*; trauma to part of the nervous system, such as that caused by a penetrating wound; abnormalities of the blood vessels supplying the brain, such as an *aneurysm* (a balloonlike swelling in an artery); bleeding inside the skull (see *extradural haemorrhage*; *intracerebral haemorrhage*; *subdural haemorrhage*); a number of birth defects (such as *neural*

N

tube defects and hydrocephalus); certain types of epilepsy; and nerve damage caused by illness or accidents. Neurosurgery may also be performed to relieve pain that is otherwise untreatable.

neurosyphilis

Infection of the brain or spinal cord that occurs in untreated syphilis many years after initial infection.

Damage to the spinal cord due to neurosyphilis may cause tabes dorsalis, a condition characterized by poor coordination of leg movements when walking, urinary incontinence, and intermittent pains in the abdomen and limbs. Damage to the brain may cause dementia, muscle weakness, and, in rare cases, total paralysis of the limbs.

neurotic

Suffering from neurosis (any of a range of psychiatric disorders in which there is no loss of contact with reality).

neurotoxin

A chemical that damages nervous tissue. The principal effects of neurotoxic nerve damage are numbness, weakness, or paralysis of the part of the body supplied by the affected nerve.

Neurotoxins occur in the venom of certain snakes (see snake bites) and are released by some bacteria (such as those that cause tetanus and diphtheria). Some chemical poisons, such as arsenic and lead, are neurotoxic; and certain drugs, such as nitrofurantoin, may cause neurological damage in high doses or in susceptible people.

neurotransmitter

A chemical released from a nerve ending that transmits impulses from one neuron (nerve cell) to another neuron or to a muscle cell.

ACTION

When a nerve impulse reaches a nerve ending, neurotransmitters are released from synaptic vesicles and cross a tiny gap (a synapse) to reach the target cell. Here, they cause channels in the target cell to open, letting through charged particles that stimulate an impulse in the cell. Alternatively, neurotransmitters may inhibit nerve impulses.

Scores of different chemicals fulfil this function in different parts of the nervous system. Many neurotransmitters also function as hormones, being released into the bloodstream to act on distant target cells.

TYPES AND FUNCTIONS

One of the most important neurotransmitters is acetylcholine, which causes skeletal muscles to contract when it is released by neurons connected to the muscles. Acetylcholine is also released by neurons that control the sweat glands and the heartbeat, and transmits messages between neurons in the brain and neurons in the spinal cord. Interference with the action of acetylcholine on skeletal muscles is the cause of myasthenia gravis. It is thought that depletion of the nerve cells that release acetylcholine in the brain may be a factor in Alzheimer's disease.

Another chemical, noradrenaline (norepinephrine), aids the nervous control of heartbeat, blood flow, and the body's response to stress. This substance is made by the adrenal glands as well as being produced by neurons.

The neurotransmitter dopamine plays an important role in parts of the brain that control movement. A malfunction of the neurons that respond to dopamine is thought to underlie Parkinson's disease.

Serotonin is one of the main neurotransmitters found in the parts of the brain concerned with conscious processes.

Another group of neurotransmitters are called neuropeptides. This group includes the endorphins, which are used by the brain to control sensitivity to pain.

neutropenia

An abnormally low number of neutrophils (a type of white blood cell) in the blood, which results in an increased susceptibility to infection. Symptoms may include a sore throat and fever. Neutropenia can be due to aplastic anaemia (see anaemia, aplastic), agranulocytosis, acute leukaemia (see leukaemia, acute), or drugs such as anticancer drugs.

neutrophil

A type of phagocyte (a cell in the immune system). Neutrophils are a very important part in the immune system, and their role is to engulf and destroy invading bacteria.

newborn

A general term for an infant at birth and during the first few weeks of life.

APPEARANCE OF A NEWBORN BABY

A full-term newborn baby weighs, on average, 3.5 kg, measures 51 cm long, and is well prepared for survival. The newborn baby may have an oddly shaped skull or a swollen skull as a result of the transition from the uterus to the outside world. Such differences are normal, and they usually disappear relatively quickly.

In a newborn baby, other structures, such as the long bones in the legs, are not yet fully formed. The eyelids are puffy and vision is poor even when the eyes are wide open. The umbilical cord, which is cut at delivery, shrivels and falls off within about ten days to form the navel. The skin is often covered with vernix, a greasy substance that protects the skin in the uterus. Premature babies may have downy hair, called lanugo hair, all over the body; this hair disappears after about a month. Blisters, or small white bumps, can sometimes be seen on the lips of a newborn baby; these are due to vigorous sucking. The genitals may appear large in relation to the rest of the body.

At birth, there are changes in the structure of the heart that result in all the blood circulating through the lungs (see fetal circulation).

The baby has primitive reflexes, such as a grasp reflex, which were important to survival, although these disappear with increasing age.

MEDICAL EXAMINATION

Immediately after birth, the newborn baby is usually given straight to the mother unless there is concern about its condition. Later, it is checked by the nurse, midwife, or doctor in attendance. This usually includes checking the heart rate with a stethoscope and establishing that breathing is normal.

The Apgar score and other tests are performed to confirm that the baby is in good health. The baby's sex, weight, length, and head circumference are noted and a check is made for any obvious birth defect. The vernix is wiped off and the baby is then usually given back to the mother to hold. If very small or sick, the baby may need to be monitored in a neonatal unit.

Within 72 hours of birth, the baby is given a complete medical examination. The skull, eyes, face, abdomen, heart, lungs, spine, hips, genitals, and limbs are checked, and the baby's posture, movements, behaviour, cry, reflexes, and responsiveness are noted. The doctor or midwife will confirm that the baby has passed urine and meconium (faeces). During the first week of life, blood spot screening tests are carried out to check for several rare but potentially serious disorders, including phenylketonuria (an

N

HOW **NEUROTRANSMITTERS** WORK

When an electrical impulse travels down a nerve cell axon, it causes the release of a chemical neurotransmitter at the axon terminals. The chemical released is not the same in every case; acetylcholine, noradrenaline (norepinephrine), dopamine, and serotonin are all important examples.

Example of neurotransmitter activity
Neurotransmitters enable the pupil to change size in different light conditions.

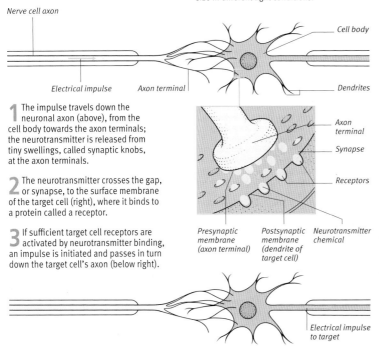

Nerve cell axon

Electrical impulse *Axon terminal*

Cell body

Dendrites

1 The impulse travels down the neuronal axon (above), from the cell body towards the axon terminals; the neurotransmitter is released from tiny swellings, called synaptic knobs, at the axon terminals.

2 The neurotransmitter crosses the gap, or synapse, to the surface membrane of the target cell (right), where it binds to a protein called a receptor.

3 If sufficient target cell receptors are activated by neurotransmitter binding, an impulse is initiated and passes in turn down the target cell's axon (below right).

Axon terminal

Synapse

Receptors

Presynaptic membrane (axon terminal) *Postsynaptic membrane (dendrite of target cell)* *Neurotransmitter chemical*

Electrical impulse to target

inherited enzyme defect), congenital *hypothyroidism* (underactivity of the thyroid gland), and sickle cell anaemia (an inherited disorder of red blod cells); in some areas, babies are also screened for *cystic fibrosis* (an inherited disorder that can affect the lungs and digestive system) and *MCADD* (an inherited metabolic disorder). A hearing test is also performed during the first few weeks of life. Other tests may also be performed, depending on family history and the baby's health.

CONDITIONS IN THE NEWBORN

Some babies suffer injury during birth (see *birth injury*), such as *cephalhaematoma* (a swelling of part of the head caused by bleeding between the scalp and the skull).

Jaundice (a yellowing of the skin and of the whites of the eyes; see *jaundice, neonatal*) is an extremely common con-dition that occurs in newborn babies, especially if the baby is breast-fed. Usually appearing on the second or third day of life, the jaundice usually disappears over the next few days. In most cases, neonatal jaundice is harmless; however, the condition may be serious if it occurs during the first 24 hours, if it is severe (see *kernicterus*), or if it affects a premature infant.

Some newborn baby girls have slight vaginal bleeding or discharge, and babies of either sex may have enlarged breasts. These conditions are harmless and are the result of the mother's circulating sex hormones that reach the fetus through the placenta. Any extra hormones leave the baby's bloodstream and their effects soon disappear.

Infections of the umbilical cord stump sometimes occur and need to be seen by a doctor. A blotchy, red rash (see *urticaria, neonatal*) affecting the face, chest, arms, and thighs of the baby may occur around the second day after birth; this condition is harmless, of no known cause, and disappears without treatment. (See also *prematurity; postmaturity*.)

newborn screening tests

A series of tests carried out on newborn babies to detect disorders of abnormalities so that, if necessary, treatment can be given as soon as possible. The tests include a complete physical examination; measurement of weight, head circumference, and length; *blood spot screening tests* for certain rare disorders; and hearing tests.

new variant CJD

One form of *Creutzfeldt–Jakob disease*.

NGU

An abbreviation for the condition *non-gonococcal urethritis*.

niacin

See *vitamin B complex*.

nickel

A metallic element that is present in the body in minute amounts. It is thought to activate certain *enzymes* (substances that promote biochemical reactions) and may also play a part in stabilizing chromosomal material in cell nuclei.

Disease due to a deficiency of nickel is unknown. Exposure to nickel may cause *dermatitis* (inflammation of the skin). *Lung cancer* has been reported in workers in nickel refineries.

niclosamide

An *anthelmintic drug* used to treat *tapeworm infestation*. Niclosamide causes the tapeworm to loosen its grip on the inner wall of the intestine. The worm is then passed out of the body in the faeces. Side effects of niclosamide include abdominal pain, lightheadedness, and itching.

nicorandil

A *potassium channel activator* drug used in the prevention and long-term treatment of *angina pectoris* (chest pain due to inadequate blood supply to the heart). Side effects, which include headache, flushing, nausea, vomiting, and dizziness, are mainly due to nicorandil's *vasodilation* (widening of the blood vessels) effects and usually wear off with continued treatment. Rarely, mouth ulcers and muscle pain can occur.

N

nicotinamide

See *vitamin B complex*.

nicotinamide adenine dinucleotide

See *NAD*.

nicotine

A stimulant drug found in tobacco that is responsible for tobacco dependence. After inhalation, nicotine in tobacco smoke passes rapidly into the bloodstream. Nicotine in chewing tobacco is absorbed more slowly via the lining of the mouth. The drug stimulates the nervous system until it is broken down by the liver and excreted in the urine.

EFFECTS

Nicotine acts primarily on the *autonomic nervous system*, which controls involuntary body activities such as heart rate. The effects of the drug vary from one person to another and also depend on dosage and past usage. In someone who is not used to smoking, even a small amount of nicotine may slow the heart rate and cause nausea and vomiting. However, in habitual smokers, the drug increases the heart rate and narrows the blood vessels, the combined effect of which is to raise blood pressure. Nicotine also stimulates the *central nervous system*, thereby reducing fatigue, increasing alertness, and improving concentration.

Regular use of tobacco results in tolerance to nicotine, so that a higher intake is needed for the same effects.

WITHDRAWAL

Because most regular smokers are physically dependent on nicotine, the act of stopping smoking often causes withdrawal symptoms such as headaches, fatigue, drowsiness, and difficulty in concentrating. *Nicotine replacement therapy*, such as the use of nicotine skin patches and chewing gum, can be effective in aiding withdrawal from nicotine. Drugs such as *amfebutamone* (bupropion) and *varenicline* may sometimes be prescribed for people who want to stop smoking but for whom other methods have failed. (See also *smoking*.)

nicotine replacement therapy

Preparations containing *nicotine* that are used in place of cigarettes as an aid to stopping *smoking*. Nicotine products are available in the form of *sublingual* tablets (placed under the tongue), chewing gum, skin patches, nasal spray, or inhalers.

Side effects of such preparations may include nausea, headache, palpitations,

cold- or flulike symptoms, hiccups, dry mouth, and vivid dreaming. Ideally, smoking should be stopped completely before staring nicotine replacement therapy, and it should be used as part of a complete package of measures, including the determination to succeed.

nicotinic acid

A form of niacin (see *vitamin B complex*). Nicotinic acid is prescribed as a *lipid-lowering drug* and is used together with a *statin* to treat certain types of *hyperlipidaemia* (a metabolic disorder in which there are high levels of fats in the blood). Possible adverse effects of nicotinic acid include flushing, dizziness, nausea, palpitations, and itching.

nifedipine

A *calcium channel blocker* drug used mainly to prevent and treat *angina pectoris* (chest pain due to inadequate blood supply to the heart). Nifedipine is also frequently used to treat *hypertension* (high blood pressure) and disorders affecting the circulation, such as *Raynaud's disease*.

Possible side effects of nifedipine include swelling of the hands and feet as a result of *oedema* (accumulation of fluid in tissues), flushing of the skin, headache, and dizziness.

night blindness

The inability to see well in dim light. Many people with night blindness have no discernible eye disease. The condition may be an inherited functional defect of the *retina* (the light-sensitive inner layer at the back of the eye), an early sign of *retinitis pigmentosa* (degeneration of the light-sensitive cells of the retina), or a result of *vitamin A* deficiency.

nightmare

An unpleasant, vivid dream, sometimes accompanied by a sense of suffocation. Nightmares occur during REM (rapid eye movement) *sleep* and they may be clearly remembered if the dreamer awakens completely during the course of the nightmare.

Nightmares are especially common in children aged between eight and ten and are particularly likely to occur when the child is unwell or anxious. In adults, nightmares may be a side effect of certain drugs, including *beta-blocker drugs* and *benzodiazepine drugs*. Repeated nightmares may be associated with traumatic experiences. However, there is no specific relationship with psychiatric illness.

Nightmares should not be confused with hypnagogic *hallucinations*, which occur while falling asleep, nor with *night terror*, which occurs in NREM (nonrapid eye movement) sleep and is not remembered on waking.

night terror

A disorder, occurring mainly in children, that consists of abrupt arousals from *sleep* in a terrified state. Night terror (or sleep terror) usually starts between the ages of four and seven, gradually disappearing in early adolescence.

Episodes of night terror occur during NREM (nonrapid eye movement) sleep, usually half an hour to three and a half hours after falling asleep. Sufferers wake up screaming, in a semiconscious state, and remain frightened for some minutes. They do not recognize familiar faces or surroundings and usually cannot be comforted. Physical signs of agitation, such as sweating or an increased heart rate, are common. The sufferer gradually falls back to sleep and has no memory of the event the following day.

Though distressing to parents, night terror in children has no serious significance. However, in adults, it is likely to be associated with an *anxiety disorder*.

nipple

The small prominence at the tip of each *breast*. Women's nipples contain tiny openings through which milk can pass. The nipple and the areola, the surrounding dark area, both increase in size during pregnancy. Involuntary muscle in the nipple allows it to become erect.

DISORDERS

Structural defects of the nipple are rare. One or both nipples may be absent or there may be additional nipples along a line extending from the armpit to the groin. An inverted nipple is usually a harmless abnormality of development, which can be corrected by drawing out the nipple between finger and thumb daily for several weeks. Nipple inversion that develops in older women is mostly due to aging, but *mammography* may be advisable to rule out the possibility of *breast cancer*.

Cracked nipples, which are common during *breast-feeding*, may lead to infective *mastitis* (inflammation of the breast tissue). Ensuring that the baby is correctly positioned while breast-feeding helps to prevent cracking.

Papilloma of the nipple is a noncancerous swelling attached to the skin by a stalk. *Paget's disease of the nipple* appears initially as persistent *eczema* of the nipple and is due to a slow-growing cancer arising in a milk duct. Surgical treatment is required.

Discharge from the nipple occurs for various reasons. A clear, straw-coloured discharge may develop in early pregnancy; a milky discharge may occur after breast-feeding is over. *Galactorrhoea* (milk discharge in someone who is not pregnant or breast-feeding) may be due to a hormone imbalance or, rarely, a *galactocele* (cyst under the areola). A discharge containing pus indicates a *breast abscess*. A bloodstained discharge may be due to a noncancerous breast disorder such as *fibroadenosis* (general lumpiness of the breast) or a cancerous tumour.

nitrate drugs

COMMON DRUGS
- Glyceryl trinitrate • Isosorbide dinitrate
- Isosorbide mononitrate

A group of *vasodilator drugs* used to treat or prevent attacks of *angina pectoris* (chest pain due to impaired blood supply to the heart) and to treat severe *heart failure* (reduced pumping efficiency).

Possible side effects of nitrate drugs include headaches, flushing of the skin, and dizziness. *Tolerance* (the need for greater amounts of a drug for it to have the same effect) may develop when some nitrate drugs are taken regularly. To avoid this, a change in dosage, frequency, or timing of the drug, or prescription of a different nitrate drug, may be required.

nitrazepam

A *benzodiazepine drug* used in the short-term treatment of *insomnia*. Nitrazepam is long-acting and may cause a hangover effect, with drowsiness and lightheadedness, the following day. Regular use over several weeks can lead to reduced effectiveness as *tolerance* develops.

Nitrazepam can lead to drug dependence and to withdrawal symptoms, such as nervousness and restlessness.

nitric oxide (NO)

A gas that is produced both outside the body as a pollutant (for example, in car exhaust fumes) and inside the body, where it takes the form of a molecule that acts as a messenger between cells.

Nitric oxide causes blood vessels to dilate, affecting the flow of oxygenated blood and regulating blood pressure. Overproduction of nitric oxide is associated with various disorders, including *toxic shock syndrome*, and *rheumatoid arthritis*; underproduction may cause *erectile dysfunction* and *angina*. The control of nitric oxide is an important element of many drug treatments.

nitrites

Salts of nitrous acid (a nitrogen-containing acid). To preserve meat, sodium nitrite is added in small amounts, together with potassium nitrate and salt, to inhibit the growth of potentially harmful bacteria. In large amounts, nitrites can cause dizziness, nausea, and vomiting.

nitrofurantoin

An *antibiotic drug* that is used in the treatment of *urinary tract infection*. Nitrofurantoin should be taken with food to reduce the risk of stomach irritation, which can cause abdominal pain and nausea. More serious side effects, such as breathing difficulty, numbness, and jaundice (yellowing of the skin and the whites of the eyes), occur rarely.

nitrogen

A colourless, odourless gas that makes up 78 per cent of the Earth's atmosphere. Atmospheric nitrogen has no biological action.

Nitrogen gas cannot be utilized by the body, but nitrogen compounds are essential to life. The most important of such compounds are *amino acids*, the building blocks of *proteins*. Humans cannot make certain amino acids (called essential amino acids), which must be obtained from the diet. The proteins are then broken down by digestion into their constituent amino acids to be absorbed and reconstituted into the specific proteins needed by the body. The processes of breakdown and reconstitution produce nitrogen-containing wastes, mainly *urea*, which are excreted in the urine. (See also *nitrate drugs*; *nitrites*.)

nitroglycerine

A former name for *glyceryl trinitrate*, a *nitrate drug*.

nitroprusside

An *antihypertensive drug* given as an infusion in the emergency treatment of *hypertension* (high blood pressure).

nitrous oxide

A colourless gas, also called laughing gas, that has a sweet smell and the chemical formula N_2O. Nitrous oxide is used with

The protrusion at the tip of the breast, surrounded by the areola. Milk ducts emerge at the nipple.

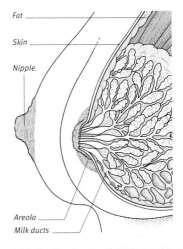

Fat
Skin
Nipple
Areola
Milk ducts

oxygen to provide *analgesia* (pain relief) and light anaesthesia (see *anaesthesia, general*) at the site of a serious accident or during childbirth, dental procedures, and minor surgery. For major surgery, which requires deeper anaesthesia, a nitrous oxide and oxygen mixture needs to be combined with other drugs.

The advantages of the combination of nitrous oxide and oxygen over other agents are its rapid action and nonflammability. Adverse effects of nitrous oxide may include nausea and vomiting during the recovery period.

nits

The eggs of *lice*. Both head lice and *pubic lice* produce eggs, which they stick to the base of hairs growing from their host's head or pubic area. Nits are tiny, measuring only about 0.5 mm in diameter. They are light brown when newly laid and white when hatched. Hatching takes place within about eight days of being laid. Louse infestations are frequently identified by the presence of nits.

nocardiosis

An infection caused by a funguslike bacterium present in soil. The infection, which is acquired through inhalation, usually starts in the lung and spreads to the brain and tissues under the skin. Nocardiosis is rare, except in people with *immunodeficiency disorders* or those already suffering from a serious disease.

N

The resulting illness, similar to pneumonia with fever and cough, fails to respond to short-term *antibiotic drug* treatment, and progressive lung damage occurs. Brain abscesses may follow.

Nocardiosis is diagnosed by microscopic examination of a sputum sample. Treatment, which may have to be continued over several months, is with drugs such as *co-trimoxazole*.

nocturia

The disturbance of sleep at night by the need to pass *urine*. In most people, a moderately full bladder does not usually disturb sleep, although light sleepers are more likely to wake with an urge to empty their bladders. Drinking alcohol in the evening stimulates urine production and may result in nocturia.

A common cause of nocturia in men is enlargement of the prostate gland (see *prostate, enlarged*), which obstructs the normal outflow of urine and causes the *bladder* to empty incompletely. In women, a common cause is *cystitis*, in which irritation of the bladder wall increases its sensitivity so that smaller volumes of urine trigger a desire to urinate. A common cause of nocturia in both sexes is *heart failure* (reduced pumping efficiency of the heart), leading to the retention of excess fluid in the legs during the day, which is absorbed into the bloodstream while lying down at night and is carried to the kidneys to make more urine.

Less common causes of nocturia include *diabetes mellitus*, in which greater volumes of urine are produced both during the day and night; chronic *kidney failure*, in which the normal ability of the kidney to produce a reduced quantity of more concentrated urine at night is lost; and *diabetes insipidus*, in which the kidneys fail to concentrate the urine due to the lack of a pituitary hormone.

nocturnal emission

Ejaculation that occurs during sleep, commonly called a "wet dream". Nocturnal emission is normal in male adolescents and may also occur in adult men.

nocturnal enuresis

See *enuresis, nocturnal*.

node

A small, rounded mass of tissue. The term commonly refers to a *lymph node* (a normal structure in the lymphatic system) or to the *sinoatrial node* or the *atrioventricular node*, which form part of the conducting system of the heart. (See also *Bouchard's node*; *Heberden's node*; *nodule*; *singer's nodes*.)

nodule

A small lump of tissue. A nodule may protrude from the skin's surface or form deep under the skin. Nodules may be hard or soft. (See also *rheumatoid nodules*; *surfer's nodules*.)

noise-induced hearing loss

Loss of *hearing* caused by prolonged or repeated exposure to excessive noise or by brief exposure to intensely loud noise.

LOUDNESS

The loudness of sounds is usually measured in units called decibels. On the decibel scale, an increase of three decibels is equivalent to doubling the loudness of a sound. Normal conversation is about 60 decibels, and the loudness of a jet aircraft from 30 metres away is about 130 decibels.

HEARING LOSS

Different individuals have different tolerances to noise and it is therefore impossible to establish absolute safe noise limits that apply to everybody. The noise levels given below should therefore be regarded as general guidelines.

Exposure to a sudden, extremely loud noise (above about 130 decibels) can cause immediate and permanent hearing loss. Normally, muscles in the middle ear respond to loud noise by repositioning the *ossicles* (bones that pass vibrations to the inner ear) to damp down the noise. If these reflexes have no time to respond, the full force of the vibrations is carried to the inner ear, severely damaging delicate hair cells in the cochlea. Loud noises can even rupture the *eardrum*.

More commonly, noise damage occurs by prolonged or repeated exposure to lower levels of noise. Prolonged or repeated exposure to noise above about 85 decibels may cause gradual destruction of the cochlea's hair cells, leading to permanent hearing loss.

Sounds at 85 to 90 decibels or above may initially cause pain and temporary deafness. Prolonged *tinnitus* (ringing or buzzing in the ears) after a noise has ceased is an indication of damage. The initial indication of permanent damage is loss of the ability to hear certain high tones. Later, deafness extends to all high frequencies, and speech perception is impaired. Eventually, lower tones are also affected.

PREVENTION

Avoiding exposure to excessive noise is the only way of preventing noise-induced hearing loss. As a general guide, if it is necessary to shout to make yourself heard by a person about two metres away, the noise level is potentially damaging. People who cannot avoid exposure to loud noise (for example, workers using pneumatic drills) should wear ear protection and have their hearing monitored regularly (see *hearing tests*).

noma

Also called cancrum oris, noma is the death of tissue in the lips and cheeks due to bacterial infection. The condition is largely confined to young, severely malnourished children in developing countries. Noma can also occur in the last stages of *leukaemia* (cancer of the blood).

The first symptom is inflammation of the gums and the inner surface of the cheeks. Without treatment, this leads to severe ulceration (with a foul-smelling discharge), eventual destruction of the bones around the mouth, and loss of teeth. Healing occurs naturally after a time, but scarring may be severe.

Antibiotic drugs and improved nutrition halt the disease's progress. Plastic surgery may be used to reconstruct damaged bones or improve facial appearance.

nonaccidental injury

See *child abuse*.

nongonococcal urethritis

Previously known as nonspecific urethritis (NSU), inflammation of the *urethra* (the tube that carries urine from the bladder to be excreted) due to a cause other than *gonorrhoea*. Worldwide, the condition is a very common type of *sexually transmitted infection*.

CAUSES

Almost half of all cases of nongonococcal urethritis are known to be caused by CHLAMYDIA TRACHOMATIS (see *chlamydial infections*); others may be caused by the virus that causes *herpes simplex*, the protozoan trichomonas (see *trichomoniasis*), or other microorganisms. In some cases, the cause remains unknown.

SYMPTOMS

Symptoms generally appear one to three weeks after infection. In men, the infection may cause a urethral discharge, which may be accompanied by stinging on passing urine. There may be redness, crusting, and soreness at the urethral opening. However, often no symptoms

N

are present. In women, infection often causes no symptoms, although in some cases there may be a stinging sensation on passing urine and vaginal discharge. Even if there are no symptoms, men and women who have the infection can pass it on to their sexual partners.

DIAGNOSIS AND TREATMENT

Diagnosis is made from a swab taken from the urethra and a urine sample; both enable identification of the causative organism. *Antibiotic drugs*, such as doxycycline and azithromycin, are the usual treatment. With treatment, the infection usually clears up in about a week. Follow-up visits may be advised after treatment because the infection can recur. Sexual partners must be tested and treated if necessary in oder to prevent reinfection.

COMPLICATIONS

In men, *epididymitis*, *prostatitis*, and *urethral stricture* can occur as complications of nongonococcal urethritis. *Reiter's syndrome* (in which there is arthritis and conjunctivitis as well as the urethritis) occurs as a complication in some men who develop nongonococcal urethritis.

In women, *pelvic inflammatory disease* and infection in the *Bartholin's glands* may occur. *Ophthalmia neonatorum*, a type of conjunctivitis, sometimes develops in babies born to women who have chlamydial cervicitis at delivery.

non-Hodgkin's lymphoma

See *lymphoma, non-Hodgkin's*.

noninvasive

A term used to describe any medical procedure that does not involve penetration of the skin or entry into the body through any natural opening. Examples of noninvasive procedures include *CT scanning* and *echocardiography*.

The term is sometimes also applied to noncancerous tumours that do not spread throughout body tissues.

non-nucleoside reverse transcriptase inhibitors

A type of *antiretroviral drug* that is used to delay the progression of *HIV* infection. (See also *AIDS*.)

nonoxinol 9

A *spermicide* used in contraceptive preparations such as gels, foams, and creams.

nonspecific urethritis

The former term for the condition *nongonococcal urethritis*.

nonsteroidal anti-inflammatory drugs

COMMON DRUGS

- Acemetacin • Aspirin • Benzydamine
- Diclofenac • Diflunisal • Felbinac • Fenbufen
- Fenoprofen • Flurbiprofen • Ibuprofen
- Indometacin • Ketoprofen • Mefenamic acid
- Meloxicam • Nabumetone • Naproxen
- Piroxicam • Sulindac • Tenoxicam
- Tiaprofenic acid

COX-2 INHIBITORS • Celecoxib • Etoricoxib
- Lumiracoxib

A group of drugs, also known as NSAIDs, that produce *analgesia* (pain relief) and reduce inflammation in joints and soft tissues such as muscles and ligaments. COX-2 inhibitors are classed as NSAIDS but the analgesic *paracetamol* is not classed as an NSAID because it has no anti-inflammatory effect

WHY THEY ARE USED

Nonsteroidal anti-inflammatory drugs (NSAIDs) are widely used to relieve symptoms caused by types of arthritis, such as *rheumatoid arthritis*, *osteoarthritis*, and *gout*. They do not cure or halt the progress of disease but they do help to improve mobility of the affected joints and relieve pain and stiffness. NSAIDs are also used in the treatment of back pain, menstrual pain, headaches, pain following minor surgery, and injuries to soft tissue.

HOW THEY WORK

NSAIDs reduce pain and inflammation by blocking the action of the enzyme cyclo-oxygenase (COX), which is involved in the body's production of *prostaglandins* (chemicals that cause inflammation and trigger transmission of pain signals to the brain, but that also protect the stomach lining). Most NSAIDs block both COX-2 (providing the anti-inflammatory effect) and COX-1 (leading to stomach irritation). COX-2 inhibitors were developed to block COX-2 alone, thereby reducing the risk of stomach irritation.

POSSIBLE ADVERSE EFFECTS

NSAIDs may cause a range of side effects, including nausea, indigestion, bleeding from the stomach, *fluid retention*, and, occasionally, *peptic ulcer*. They may also worsen *heart failure* or *kidney failure*. COX-2 inhibitors cause less gastrointestinal irritation than other NSAIDs, but, because they are associated with an increased risk of heart disease or stroke, they are not generally recommended for people who have had, or are at risk of having, these conditions. To minimize the risk of adverse effects,

the lowest effective dose of an NSAID should be taken for the shortest period. For other precautions about specific drugs, see the individual drug entries.

Noonan's syndrome

An inherited condition that shares many features with *Turner's syndrome*, but in which there is a full complement of chromosomes. Noonan's syndrome can affect both males and females. Features include congenital heart disease (see *heart disease, congenital*), *webbing* of the neck, *ptosis* (drooping eyelids), *myopia* (shortsightedness), feeding problems in infants, *short stature*, *hypotonia* (poor muscle tone), hearing difficulties, delayed speech development, delayed *puberty*, and undescended testes (see *testis, undescended*) in males.

Noonan's syndrome has an autosomal dominant pattern of inheritance (see *genetic disorders*). There is a family history of the condition in around half of all cases; the remainder are due to new *mutations*. There is no treatment for the condition, but many of its features (such as undescended testes and heart problems) may be treated successfully.

noradrenaline

Also known as norepinephrine, a *hormone* secreted by certain nerve endings (principally those of the *sympathetic nervous system*) and by the medulla (the central region) of the *adrenal glands*. Noradrenaline's primary function is to help maintain a constant blood pressure by stimulating certain blood vessels to constrict (narrow) when blood pressure falls. For this reason, it may sometimes be administered by injection in the emergency treatment of *shock* or severe bleeding. (See also *adrenaline*.)

norepinephrine

An alternative term for *noradrenaline*.

norethisterone

A *progestogen drug* that is used as an ingredient of some *oral contraceptives* and HRT preparations. Norethisterone alone is sometimes prescribed to postpone menstruation. It is also used to treat *premenstrual syndrome*, menstrual disorders such as *menorrhagia* (heavy periods), *endometriosis*, and certain types of *breast cancer*.

Possible side effects include swollen ankles, weight gain, depression and, rarely, *jaundice* (yellowing of the skin and the whites of the eyes).

N

norfloxacin

An *antibiotic drug* used in the treatment of *urinary tract infections*.

norgestrel

See *levonorgestrel*.

normocytic anaemia

Any form of *anaemia* in which the amount of *haemoglobin* (oxygen-carrying pigment) in the blood is reduced due to a reduction in the total number of *red blood cells*; the size and haemoglobin content of the individual red blood cells is normal. Normocytic anaemia can develop as a result of chronic diseases (such as *renal failure* or chronic inflammatory joint diseases such as *rheumatoid arthritis*), or as a result of a problem in the bone marrow itself. (See also *microcytic anaemia*.)

nose

The uppermost part of the respiratory tract and the organ of *smell*.

STRUCTURE

The nose is an air passage that connects the nostrils at its front to the *nasopharynx* (the upper part of the throat) at its rear. The *nasal septum*, which is made of cartilage at the front and bone at the rear, divides the nasal passage into two chambers.

The bridge of the nose is formed from two small nasal bones and from cartilage. The roof of the nasal passage is formed by bones at the base of the skull; the walls by the maxilla (upper *jaw*); and the floor by the hard palate. Three conchae (thin, downward-curving plates of bone) covered with *mucous membrane* project from each wall.

Air-filled, mucous membrane-lined cavities (called paranasal sinuses) open into the nasal passage. There is an opening in each wall to the nasolacrimal duct, which drains away tears. Projecting into the roof of the nasal passage are the hairlike endings of the *olfactory nerves*, responsible for the sense of smell.

FUNCTION

One important function of the nose is to filter, warm, and moisten inhaled air before it passes into the rest of the respiratory tract. Just inside the nostrils, small hairs trap large dust particles and foreign bodies. Smaller dust particles are filtered from the inhaled air by the microscopic hairlike projections of the conchae. The mucus on the conchae flows inwards, carrying microorganisms and other foreign bodies back towards the

ANATOMY OF THE **NOSE**

The nose is involved in breathing and the sense of smell. It is a hollow passage that connects the nostrils and the top of the throat. It warms and moistens air and traps particles to prevent them from being inhaled. The upper part contains the receptors that transmit sensations of smell.

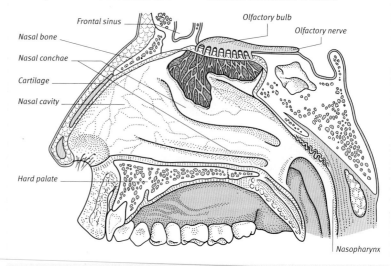

nasopharynx to be swallowed and destroyed in the stomach by gastric acid.

The nose also detects smells via the olfactory nerve endings, which, when stimulated by inhaled vapours, transmit this information to the olfactory bulb in the brain. (See also *nose* disorders box.)

nosebleed

Loss of blood from the *mucous membrane* that lines the nose. Nosebleeds are common in children, but the bleeding is usually minor and stops by itself. Nosebleeds are also common, but in some cases serious, in people over the age of 50. In this age group, bleeding may come from the back of the nose and be hard to stop. If the blood is swallowed, bleeding may not be seen.

CAUSES

Nosebleeds often occur spontaneously. In hot, dry environments or during the winter months, the membranes lining the nose may become dry and cracked, causing bleeding to occur. Nosebleeds may also occur if the lining of the nose is injured by a blow to the nose or by nose-picking or forceful nose-blowing. In children, nosebleeds often occur as a result of rough play.

A foreign body in the nose or infection in the upper respiratory tract may also cause a nosebleed. In people over the age of 50, the small blood vessels in

the nose may be more fragile and are therefore more likely to rupture. Rarely, recurrent nosebleeds are a sign of an underlying disorder, such as *hypertension* (high blood pressure), a bleeding disorder such as *thrombocytopenia*, or a tumour of the nose or paranasal sinuses. Nosebleeds may also be caused by drugs that prevent blood clotting (see *anticoagulant drugs*).

TREATMENT

The vast majority of nosebleeds are short-lived and do not require specific treatment. A nosebleed can usually be stopped by pressing on the soft part of the nose (pressing both sides together) for about 10 to 15 minutes. If membranes in the nose are dry or cracked, rubbing water-based ointment on the area may help to prevent nosebleeds.

A nosebleed that persists for more than about an hour requires medical attention. Treatment for a serious nosebleed may involve nasal sponges placed into the nostrils to absorb the blood or the insertion and inflation of a balloon catheter to stop the bleeding. If the cause is not obvious, the nasal passages may be examined with a viewing instrument to look for ruptured blood vessels or a tumour (see *endoscopy*). Alternatively, imaging techniques such as *X-rays* or *MRI* (a technique that produces cross-sectional or three-dimensional images

DISORDERS OF THE **NOSE**

The nose is susceptible to a wide range of disorders. Infections and allergic conditions, leading to stuffiness or sneezing, are common. Due to its prominent position, the nose is also prone to injury.

Infection

The common cold (see *cold, common*), a viral infection, causes inflammation of the lining of the nasal passages and excessive production of mucus, leading to nasal congestion. Small *boils* (infected hair follicles) sometimes occur just within the nostril, where they may cause pain. Backward spread of infection from the nose may cause *cavernous sinus thrombosis*, a serious condition that, without antibiotic drugs, can be fatal.

Tumours

Noncancerous tumours of blood vessels, known as *haemangiomas*, may affect the nasal cavity in babies. Many disappear spontaneously before puberty. *Basal cell carcinoma* and *squamous cell carcinoma* (types of skin cancer) may occur in or around the nostril. The nose may also be invaded by cancers originating in the sinuses.

Injury

Because of its prominent position, the nose is also particularly prone to injury. Fracture of the nasal bones (see *nose, broken*) is a common sports injury that can lead to deformity and may require corrective surgery. *Nosebleeds* are also common, particularly in children; they may be caused by fragile blood vessels, infection of the lining of the nose, or a blow to the nose.

Drugs

Repeated sniffing of cocaine interferes with the blood supply to the mucous membrane lining the nose and can cause perforation of the nasal septum. Persistent taking of snuff can irritate or damage the nasal lining.

Allergies

Hay fever (see *rhinitis, allergic*) is one of the most common allergies and may be brought on by a reaction to various allergens, such as pollens, animal dander, house mites, or fungal spores.

Obstruction

A *nasal polyp* (a projection of swollen mucous membrane) may block a nostril, causing a feeling of congestion. Young children frequently insert foreign bodies, such as beads, peas, or pebbles, into their nostrils. Objects can become stuck, leading to obstruction and discharge.

INVESTIGATION

To inspect the inside of the nose, the doctor uses a speculum to open up the nostrils. If a fracture is suspected, X-rays are taken. If cancer is suspected, MRI or CT scanning, nasal endoscopy, and a biopsy are performed.

---

of body structures) may be used. Treatment will then be of the underlying cause. Occasionally, surgery is required to tie off leaking blood vessels.

nose, broken

Fracture of the nasal bones or dislocation of the cartilage that forms the bridge of the *nose*. A blow from the side may knock the bones or cartilage out of position or cause displacement of the *nasal septum* (the dividing partition inside the nose). A frontal blow tends to splay the bones of the nose outwards, depressing the bridge. The fracture is

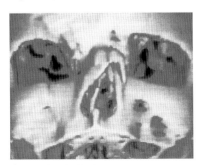

CT scan showing broken nose
In this three-dimensional image of the skull, a fracture of the nasal bone is clearly visible. The damaged bone is asymmetrical and has a V-shaped notch on the right-hand side.

usually accompanied by severe swelling of overlying soft tissue. A fractured nose is painful and remains tender for about three weeks after the injury.

TREATMENT
Resetting is usually carried out immediately following the injury, before the swelling has started, or after the swelling has subsided, usually about ten days after the injury. Occasionally, a displaced bridge can be carefully manipulated into position under a local anaesthetic (see *anaesthesia, local*). However, a general anaesthetic (see *anaesthesia, general*) is usually needed. A plaster splint is sometimes required during healing.

nosocomial

A term that means associated with hospitals. A nosocomial infection, for example, is an infection acquired by a patient during a stay in hospital.

notifiable diseases

Medical conditions that must be reported to the local health authority. The notification of certain potentially harmful infectious diseases enables public health physicians to monitor and control the spread of infection and records to be kept of disease patterns. Examples of notifiable infectious diseases are *food poisoning*, viral *hepatitis*, *measles*, *malaria*, *pertussis* (whooping cough), *tetanus*, *tuberculosis*, *meningitis*, *mumps*, and *rubella* (German measles). Similar information is also collected on cancers, occupational diseases, birth defects, and other noninfectious health problems. (See also *prescribed diseases*.)

NREM sleep

The abbreviation for nonrapid eye movement *sleep*, the period of sleep during which the brain is less active. NREM sleep occurs alternately with REM sleep throughout the night. An average cycle of sleep is made up of three-quarters NREM sleep and one-quarter REM sleep.

NSAID

The abbreviation for *nonsteroidal anti-inflammatory drugs*.

NSU

The abbreviation for nonspecific urethritis, the term formerly used for *nongonococcal urethritis*.

nuchal translucency scan

Ultrasound scanning performed in early pregnancy in order to identify fetuses at high risk of *chromosomal abnormalities*,

N

such as *Down's syndrome*. The scan investigates the nuchal fold, an area of skin at the back of the neck. The amount of fluid under the fold is measured as it is an indicator of a possible chromosomal abnormality.

nuclear energy

The energy that is released as a result of changes in the nuclei (see *nucleus*) of atoms. Nuclear energy is also known as atomic energy and it is principally released in the form of heat, light, and ionizing *radiation*, such as gamma rays. Nuclear energy may be released naturally, as in radioactive decay, or in devices such as nuclear reactors.

nuclear medicine

Techniques that use radioactive substances (see *radioactivity*) in the detection and treatment of disease.

Radioactive materials, which may be injected, inhaled, or swallowed, are taken up by body tissues or organs in different concentrations, and an instrument called a *gamma camera* is used to detect and map the distribution of radiation within the body (see *radionuclide scanning*). The technique uses only minuscule quantities of radiation.

In techniques for treatment, higher doses of radiation are used. Diseased tissues are destroyed by exposure to an external radioactive source or by insertion of a radioactive substance into a body cavity (see *radiotherapy*; *interstitial radiotherapy*; *intracavitary therapy*).

nucleic acid

A substance found in all living matter that has a fundamental role in the propagation of life. Nucleic acids provide the inherited coded instructions (or "blueprint") for an organism's development; they also provide the apparatus by which these instructions are carried out.

TYPES

There are two types of nucleic acid: deoxyribonucleic acid (DNA) and ribonucleic acid (RNA). In all animal and plant cells, including human cells, DNA permanently holds the coded instructions, which are first translated and then implemented by RNA. DNA is the main constituent of *chromosomes*, which are carried in the nucleus of the cell.

STRUCTURE

DNA and RNA are similar in structure: both of them consist of long, chainlike molecules. However, DNA usually consists of two intertwined chains, whereas RNA is generally single-stranded.

The basic structure of DNA is like a rope ladder; the chains form the two sides, and interlinking structures in between form the rungs. The ladder twists into a spiral shape called a double helix. Each DNA chain has a "backbone" consisting of a string of sugar and phosphate chemical groups. Attached to each sugar is a chemical called a base, which can be any of four types (adenine, thymine, guanine, and cytosine) and forms half a rung of the DNA ladder. The four bases can occur in any sequence along the chain. The sequence, often many millions of individual bases long, provides the code for the activities of the cell (see *genetic code*). Because the two bases that form each rung of the ladder conform to certain pairings, known as base pairs (adenine pairs with thymine; and guanine with cytosine) the sequence of bases on one chain determines the sequence on the other. This is of fundamental importance for the copying of DNA molecules when a cell divides.

RNA is like a single strand of DNA; the main difference is that the base thymine is replaced by another base, uracil, and the sugar and phosphate chain is chemically slightly different.

FUNCTION

DNA controls a cell's activities by specifying and regulating the synthesis of *enzymes* (substances that promote biochemical reactions) and other proteins in the cell. Different *genes* (sections of DNA) regulate the production of different proteins. For a particular protein to be made, an appropriate section of DNA acts as a template for an RNA chain. This "messenger" RNA then passes out of the nucleus into the cell cytoplasm (a thick fluid that forms the bulk of the cell), where it is decoded to form proteins (see *protein synthesis*).

When a cell undergoes mitotic (see *mitosis*) division, identical copies of its DNA must go to each of the two daughter cells. The structure of DNA makes this process possible. Starting at one end of the molecule, the two chains "unzip". As they do so, two more chains are formed (side by side with the original chains) by the linking of free, unlinked nucleotides that are present in cells. Because only certain base pairings are possible, the new double chains are identical to the original DNA molecule. Thus a dividing cell provides an exact copy of its DNA to its daughter cells. Each of a person's cells carries the same DNA replica that was present in the fertilized ovum, thus the DNA message passes from one generation of cells to the next.

nucleoside reverse transcriptase inhibitors

A group of *antiretroviral drugs* that are used to delay the progression of *HIV* infection. (See also *AIDS*.)

NUCLEIC ACIDS

Two types of nucleic acid are found in body cells: DNA and RNA, both of which are long, chainlike molecules (strands). DNA consists of two intertwined strands (a double helix), and RNA is usually just a single strand.

Nucleic acids are made up of units called nucleotides, each consisting of a sugar, a phosphate group, and a base.

There are four different bases in DNA: adenine (A), cytosine (C), guanine (G), and thymine (T). These bases pair up, adenine with thymine and cytosine with guanine, to form the characteristic double helix structure of DNA. RNA is like a single strand of DNA but has a base called uracil (U), instead of thymine, which pairs with adenine.

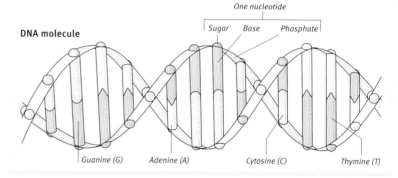

DNA molecule

One nucleotide

Sugar   Base   Phosphate

Guanine (G)   Adenine (A)   Cytosine (C)   Thymine (T)

N

nucleotide

A compound that consists of a base, linked to a sugar and a phosphate group. The *nucleic acids* DNA and RNA are chains of linked nucleotides. There are four different bases in DNA, adenine, cytosine, guanine, and thymine, which always pair up, adenine with thymine and cytosine with guanine, to form the characteristic double helix of DNA. RNA is like a single strand of DNA but has uracil as a base instead of thymine. The sugar molecule in DNA is deoxyribose; in RNA it is ribose.

nucleus

The central core, structure, or focus of any of a variety of objects or structures.

CELL NUCLEUS
The nucleus of a living *cell* is a roughly spherical unit at the centre of the cell. It contains *chromosomes* (composed mainly of *nucleic acid*), which direct cell activities, and is surrounded by a membrane. The membrane has small pores through which substances can pass between the nucleus and the cytoplasm, a thick fluid that forms the bulk of the cell. Usually, the nucleus has one nucleolus, a smaller dense region with no membrane concerned with protein manufacture.

NERVE NUCLEUS
A nerve nucleus is a group of *neurons* (nerve cells) within the brain and the spinal cord that work together to perform a particular function.

ATOMIC NUCLEUS
The nucleus of an atom is composed of protons and neutrons and accounts for almost the total mass of the atom, but only a tiny proportion of its volume. *Nuclear energy* is produced through changes in atomic nuclei.

nulliparous

A term that refers to a woman who has never given birth to a live infant, including a woman who has never conceived. (See also *grand multipara*; *multiparous*.)

numbness

Loss of sensation in part of the body caused by interference with the passage of impulses along sensory *nerves*.

CAUSES
Numbness can occur naturally (such as when blood supply to a nerve in the leg is cut off temporarily by sitting cross-legged); it can be induced artificially (for example by a local anaesthetic); or it may be the result of a disorder of the *nervous system* or its blood supply.

Multiple sclerosis can cause loss of sensation in any part of the body through damage to nerve pathways in the central nervous system (CNS). In a *neuropathy*, the peripheral nerves (nerves outside the CNS) are damaged. In a *stroke*, pressure on, or reduced blood supply to, nerve pathways in the brain often causes loss of feeling on one side of the body.

Severe cold, as in *frostbite*, causes numbness by direct action on the nerves. Numbness is a symptom of *Raynaud's disease*, a disorder of the blood vessels in which exposure to cold causes the small arteries supplying nerves in the fingers and toes to contract suddenly.

Numbness may indicate psychological disorders, such as *anxiety, panic attack*, or a hysterical *conversion disorder*.

DIAGNOSIS AND TREATMENT
Examination usually reveals an area of sensory loss or impairment corresponding to the skin distribution of a single peripheral nerve, several nerves, or a sensory area in the CNS. The distribution of the affected area may suggest the site and mechanism of the nerve damage. Treatment depends on the cause.

nummular

Round, flat, and disc-shaped. The term may also be used to describe a structure or condition that features round, flat, disc-shaped abnormalities. For example, nummular eczema is a skin disorder defined by the appearance of characteristic coin-shaped patches of itchy skin.

nurse

A person trained and experienced in the scientific basis of nursing. Nurses must meet certain standards of education and clinical competence. They must generally undergo a period of training in a hospital and pass a final examination in order to qualify in the profession.

The term nursing may also be used interchangeably with *breast-feeding*. (See also *doctor*; *midwifery*.)

nutrient

An essential dietary factor. (See *Essential nutrients* boxes, overleaf.)

nutrition

The scientific study of food and the processes of digestion and assimilation. Nutritionists look at the ways in which various types of food are used by the body, the chemical components of different foods, and the effects of eating certain foods on health. The knowledge

gained by nutritionists has led to the development of guidelines to ensure a healthy, balanced diet that can reduce the risk of ill health.

A BALANCED DIET
A good diet supplies adequate quantities of the main nutrients: *proteins, carbohydrates, fats and oils, vitamins, minerals*, dietary fibre (see *fibre, dietary*), and water. Each one of these elements makes an important contribution to health, but it is important that they are consumed in the correct proportions, with carbohydrates forming the bulk of the diet and fats only a relatively small proportion.

The daily diet should include foods from each of the five main food groups. Bread, potatoes, pasta, and other complex carbohydrates provide energy, plenty of dietary fibre, some minerals, and vitamins in the B group (see *vitamin B complex*). Milk and dairy foods provide protein and are a good source of *calcium* and certain vitamins, such as B_{12}, A, and D; low-fat versions are useful for reducing the overall fat intake in the diet. Meat, fish, and pulses provide protein, *iron*, B vitamins, and some minerals. A variety of fruit and vegetables should be eaten, ideally five portions each day. Fruit and vegetables provide fibre and carbohydrate and are rich in vitamins and minerals. Fatty and sugary foods (such as sweets, cakes, and chips), although providing *energy*, have little other nutritional value and should be limited in the diet. Consumption of saturated fats should be kept to an absolute minimum.

In addition to foods from the main groups, the diet should contain plenty of water, as much as eight glasses a day. The need for water is increased by diarrhoea, vomiting, and taking *diuretic drugs*. Drinks that contain sugar, caffeine, or alcohol should be consumed in moderation. Sugar contributes to tooth decay; carbonated drinks, even those low in sugar, can damage the teeth because they are acidic. Excessive intake of caffeine can cause palpitations and insomnia.

DIETARY SUPPLEMENTS
For an average healthy person eating a balanced diet, supplements are not necessary. Vitamin and mineral supplements are of unproven value in most healthy people and may be harmful if excessive amounts are taken. However, specific supplements may be recommended for certain groups, such as infants, women who have heavy menstrual periods, and women who are planning a pregnancy or are pregnant.

N

ESSENTIAL **NUTRIENTS**

Proteins	The main structural component of tissues and organs. We need proteins for growth and repair of cells. Each protein contains hundreds and sometimes thousands of units called amino acids in specific combinations. In the body there are 20 different amino acids; 12 of these can be manufactured by the body itself	and the remaining eight can only be obtained by eating a balanced diet. A vegetarian diet that contains eggs, milk, and cheese provides sufficient amounts of all the essential amino acids. A vegan diet, which also excludes dairy products, needs careful planning in order to prevent a deficient intake of protein (see *Veganism*).
Carbohydrates	The two carbohydrate food groups, sugars (simple carbohydrates) and starches (complex carbohydrates), are the main energy sources that are required for metabolism (chemical processes that take place in cells).	Complex carbohydrates should make up at least half of the diet. Complex carbohydrates found in cereals and fruit are rich in fibre and nutrients. Refined carbohydrates such as sugar and white flour should be kept to a minimum.
Fats	Fats provide energy for metabolism and are a structural component of cells. Most people in developed countries eat too much fat; fats should constitute no more than 30 per cent of total calorie intake. There are three types of dietary fats: saturated fats (found mostly in meat and dairy products), monounsaturated fats (found in olive oil and avocados), and polyunsaturated fats (found in fish and vegetable oils). Saturated fats	tend to increase the amounts of unwanted types of cholesterol in the blood whereas polyunsaturated fats and monounsaturated fats have the opposite effect. Studies have indicated that a high level of low-density lipoprotein cholesterol in the blood is associated with coronary artery disease. Our bodies naturally produce enough cholesterol for our needs; eating too much saturated fat contributes to excess cholesterol in the body.
Fibre	This is the indigestible structural material that is found in plants. Although fibre passes through the intestine unchanged, it is an essential part of a healthy diet. A diet low in fibre may lead to constipation, diverticular disease, and other disorders.	High-fibre diets (including plenty of fruit, raw vegetables, grains and cereals) provide bulk without excess calories. Low-fibre diets tend to be high in refined carbohydrates and fats, and thus increase the risk of developing obesity, heart disease, and some cancers.
Water	Our bodies are composed of about 60 per cent water. Water constitutes a high proportion of many foods, particularly fruit and vegetables, and is essential to maintain	metabolism (chemical processes in cells) and normal kidney and bowel function. Water is also the major component of the volume of blood in the circulation.
Vitamins	Regulators of metabolism. Vitamins ensure the healthy functioning of the brain, nerves, muscles, skin, and bones. Although vitamins do not supply energy, some enable energy to be released from the food. A healthy, balanced diet contains enough vitamins for most people's needs, and supplements are not	usually necessary. Indeed, some vitamins that are stored in fats (A, D, E, and K) are dangerous if taken in excess. The body can store only relatively small amounts of water-soluble vitamins (B and C), but even on a very restricted diet, vitamin deficiency is rare until several months have elapsed.
Minerals	A balanced diet provides enough minerals for most people. Calcium is necessary for the maintenance of healthy teeth and bones. Other minerals, such as zinc and magnesium, are needed in minute amounts to control cell metabolism.	The only mineral commonly required as a supplement is iron, which is used to prevent anaemia in women who have heavy periods. Sodium chloride (salt) is needed to maintain fluid balance; excess may cause high blood pressure.

N

ENERGY REQUIREMENTS

The body needs a constant reserve of energy to function properly. Energy from food is measured in units called kilojoules (kJ) or kilocalories (kcal), which are usually referred to simply as calories.

The number of calories needed by an individual depends on how much energy their body uses. This depends partly on how efficiently the body's cells use energy, which is genetically determined, and on the level of physical activity. The rate at which the body uses energy simply to maintain basic processes such as breathing and digestion is called the basal metabolic rate (BMR). Extra calories are needed for all other activities; energetic sports increase calorie requirement. Energy requirements also depend on gender (for example, an average woman requires about 2,000 kcal daily, compared with about 2,500 kcal for an average man) and age (a growing teenager requires more calories than an adult and the BMR declines with increasing age). A pregnant woman needs more calories than a nonpregnant woman.

If more calories are consumed than are needed, the excess energy is stored as fat and weight is gained. Weight loss occurs if demands for energy exceed calorie intake. (See also *energy requirements*; *metabolism*.)

nutritional disorders

Nutritional disorders may be caused by a deficiency or excess of one or more *nutrients*, or by the presence of a *toxin* (poisonous element) in the diet.

NUTRITIONAL DEFICIENCY

A diet deficient in *carbohydrates* is usually also deficient in *protein*, leading to protein–calorie malnutrition, which most often occurs as a result of severe poverty and famine (see *kwashiorkor*; *marasmus*).

Inadequate intake of protein and calories may also occur in people who restrict their diet excessively to lose weight (see *anorexia nervosa*), hold mistaken beliefs about diet and health (see *food fad*), or lose interest in food due to *alcohol dependence* or *drug dependence*.

Deficiency of specific nutrients is commonly associated with a disorder of the digestive system, such as *coeliac disease*, *Crohn's disease*, or pernicious anaemia (see *anaemia, megaloblastic*).

NUTRITIONAL EXCESS

Obesity results from taking in more *energy* (calories) from the diet than is used up by the body. It is a major threat to health and is associated with disorders such as *coronary artery disease*,

FOOD SOURCES OF ESSENTIAL **NUTRIENTS**

The tables list a selection of foods that are good sources of carbohydrate, protein, fat or fibre, together with the amount of the nutrient concerned in 100 g of each food. The figures given here are averages, because the exact nutrient content of many foods depends on variable factors such as the method of preparation. (See also *vitamins*; *minerals*.)

PROTEIN

Food	Protein content (g of protein per 100g of food)
Yeast extract	40
Beef, lean, roast	31
Tuna, canned	28
Wheatgerm	27
Cheese, cheddar	26
Chicken, lean, roast	26
Peanuts, shelled, roasted	24
Cod, grilled	17
Soya beans	14
Cottage cheese, low-fat	13
Eggs, boiled	12
Brazil nuts	12
Tofu (soft)	9
Chick peas	9

CARBOHYDRATE

Food	Carbohydrate content (g of carbohydrate per 100g of food)
Sugar, white	100
Sugar, brown	100
Rice, white, uncooked	87
Cornflakes	87
Pasta, uncooked	84
Brown rice	81
Honey	81
Flour, white	80
Apricots, dried, stoned	67
Chocolate, milk	57
Beans, haricot, uncooked	45
Bread, white	45
Bread, wholemeal	37
Prunes	34

FAT

Food	Fat content (g of fat per 100g of food)
Coconut oil (saturated fat)	92
Butter and margarine	81
Brazil nuts, shelled	67
Peanuts, shelled, roasted	49
Sausage, pork, cooked	42
Beef, lean with fat, roast	40
Low-fat spread	39
Cream, whipping	38
Cheese, cheddar	32
Chocolate, milk	30
Egg yolk	30
Olive oil (saturated fat)	14
Corn oil (saturated fat)	13
Sunflower oil (saturated fat)	9

FIBRE

Food	Fibre content (g of fibre per 100g of food)
Bran	44
Apricots, dried, stoned	24
Prunes	14
Peas, boiled	12
Blackcurrants	9
Brazil nuts	9
Bread, wholemeal	9
Peanuts, shelled, roasted	8
Sweetcorn	6
Celery	5
Tofu	4
Broccoli	4
Lentils	2
Bread, white	2

hypertension (high blood pressure), and *stroke* (damage to part of the brain due to interruption to its blood supply). An excessive intake of saturated fat is thought to be a factor in cardiovascular disease and in certain *cancers*. Nutritional disorders may also result from excessive intake of *minerals* and *vitamins*.

TOXINS
Naturally occurring toxins can interfere with the digestion, absorption, and/or utilization of nutrients or cause specific disorders due to their toxic effects. For example, the *ergot* fungus on rye can cause ergotism, symptoms of which include *gangrene* (tissue death) of the toes and fingers, *seizures*, and mental disorders. Industrial pollutants, pesticides, fertilizers, and various other chemicals may also contaminate food.

nystagmus

A condition in which there is involuntary movement of the *eyes*. This movement is usually horizontal, but can be vertical or rotatory. In almost all cases, both eyes move together.

TYPES
In the most common type, jerky nystagmus, the eyes repeatedly move slowly in one direction and then rapidly in the other. This may also occur as a normal effect of attempting to follow a sequence of objects rapidly passing the eyes, such as when looking out of the window of a moving vehicle. This phenomenon is known as "optokinetic nystagmus". Less commonly, nystagmus is "pendular", with the eyes moving evenly up and down or from side to side.

CAUSES
Nystagmus may be congenital (present at birth), in which case the cause is unknown. Because a steady gaze is impossible, there is almost always a moderate to severe defect of visual acuity. The condition also occurs in *albinism* and as a result of any very severe defect of vision present at birth, such as congenital *cataract*.

Persistent nystagmus appearing later in life usually indicates a nervous system disorder (such as *multiple sclerosis*, a *brain tumour*, or an *alcohol-related disorder*), or a disorder of the balancing mechanism in the inner ear. Adult-onset nystagmus is occasionally seen as an occupational disorder in people who work in poor light, such as coal miners.

INVESTIGATION AND TREATMENT
Electronystagmography, which is a method of recording eye movements, may be used to differentiate between the different types of nystagmus. Treatment is of the underlying cause, if possible.

nystatin

An *antifungal drug* used in the treatment of *candidiasis* (thrush). Nystatin may be taken as a tablet, liquid, pessary, cream, or ointment. High doses taken orally may cause diarrhoea, nausea, vomiting, and abdominal pain.

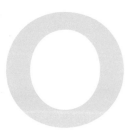

oat cell carcinoma

A form of *lung cancer*, also known as *small cell carcinoma*.

obesity

An increasingly common condition in which a large amount of excess fat has accumulated in the body. An adult with a *body mass index (BMI)* between 30 and 39.9 is classed as obese, and an adult with a BMI over 40 is classed as very obese (a BMI between 25 and 24.9 is classed as overweight). In the UK, about one in four adults are obese or very obese, and about one in five children.

CAUSES

Obesity is almost always caused by regularly consuming more calories than are expended. A person's calorie (energy) requirements are determined partly by metabolic rate (see *metabolism*) and partly by the level of physical activity. Genetic factors are occasionally a factor in becoming obese, and in a small minority of cases obesity is due to an underlying disorder, such as *hypothyroidism* (underactivity of the thyroid gland), *Cushing's syndrome*, damage to the *hypothalamus* (the area of the brain responsible for controlling the appetite), or the effects of drug treatment (such as with *corticosteroid drugs*).

EFFECTS ON HEALTH

Obesity has numerous adverse effects on health. The most immediately obvious are the low level of physical fitness and the difficulty and breathlessness experienced when undertaking physical tasks. Extra weight also puts additional strain on joints, which may aggravate existing conditions such as *osteoarthritis*.

Obesity substantially increases the risk of serious illness. *Hypertension* (high blood pressure), *stroke*, and type 2 *diabetes mellitus* are much more likely to occur in obese people. *Coronary artery disease* is also more common in obese people, particularly in obese men under 40. Obesity is also associated with an increased risk of cancer of the colon and rectum, venous *thrombosis* (blood clots in the veins), and *pulmonary embolism* (obstruction of the pulmonary artery, usually by a blood clot). In men, obesity increases the risk of prostate cancer, and in women of breast and uterine cancer.

TREATMENT

The first line of treatment is education in healthy eating habits and a weight-reducing diet (see *weight reduction*) plus regular exercise. Fad diets may cause a dramatic weight loss within a short period of time but, in almost all cases, the weight is quickly regained when normal eating habits are resumed. Drugs that reduce fat absorption, such as *orlistat*, or *appetite suppressants*, such as sibutramine, may be used as part of treatment in suitable patients.

Radical procedures are sometimes considered for severely obese people who have failed to lose weight using routine methods. *Wiring of the jaws* may be carried out to restrict food intake. An operation in which part of the stomach is stapled to reduce its capacity may be performed. Intestinal bypass operations are occasionally performed to reduce the length of the digestive tract and allow less food to be absorbed. However, due to the risk of adverse effects, such procedures are only considered if obesity is seriously endangering a person's health.

obsessive–compulsive disorder

A psychiatric condition, often known as OCD, in which an individual is dogged by persistent ideas (obsessions) that lead to repetitive, ritualized acts (compulsions). The disorder, which usually starts in adolescence, is rare. However, minor obsessional symptoms probably occur in about one sixth of the population, particularly at times of stress.

CAUSES

OCD may have a genetic element, but environmental factors also play a part. Personality traits of orderliness and cleanliness are thought to be related, as is a tendency to neurotic symptoms. Certain brain damage, especially that of *encephalitis*, can cause obsessional symptoms. Tests on people with OCD show overactivity in frontal areas of the brain.

SYMPTOMS

Obsessions are recurrent thoughts or feelings that come into the mind seemingly involuntarily. Although people who are affected regard such thoughts as senseless, they are unable to ignore or resist them. Thoughts of violence, fears of being infected by germs or dirt, and constant doubts (for example, whether the front door is shut or the oven turned off) are the most common obsessions. In obsessional rumination, there is constant brooding over a word, phrase, or unanswerable problem.

Compulsions are repetitive, apparently purposeful acts that are carried out in a ritualized fashion. They are performed for the purpose of warding off fears or relieving anxiety. Handwashing, counting, and checking are the most common. Compulsive acts may have to be performed so many times that they seriously disrupt work and social life.

The disorder is often accompanied by *depression* and *anxiety*. If severe, a person may become housebound.

TREATMENT

Many sufferers respond well to *cognitive-behavioural therapy* or to treatment with *selective serotonin reuptake inhibitors* (a group of antidepressants). Most recover within a year, but symptoms may recur under stress. For the most severely affected, OCD can be a lifelong problem.

obstetrics

The branch of medicine concerned with *pregnancy* and *antenatal care*, *childbirth*, and *postnatal care*. Obstetrics also involves the study of the structure and function of the female *reproductive system*. (See also *gynaecology*.)

obstructive airways disease

See *pulmonary disease, chronic obstructive*.

obstructive jaundice

A type of *jaundice* (yellowing of the skin and the whites of the eyes) resulting from an obstruction to the flow of *bile* (an alkaline liquid that carries waste products away from the *liver*) between the liver and the small intestine. Causes include *gallstones* and cancer of the pancreas (see *pancreas, cancer of*).

obstructive sleep apnoea

A type of *sleep apnoea* due to obstruction of breathing by repeated blockage of the upper airway during sleep.

occipital lobe

One of the two areas of *brain* tissue that lie beneath the occipital bone at the back of the brain. The occipital lobe is primarily concerned with vision.

occiput

The lower back part of the head, where it merges with the neck.

occlusion

Blockage of a passage, canal, opening, or vessel in the body. Occlusion may be caused by disease (for example, a *pulmonary embolism*) or may be medically induced. The term also describes eye-patching for the treatment of *amblyopia* (a defect of visual acuity) in children.

In dentistry, occlusion is the relationship between the upper and lower teeth when the jaw is shut. In an ideal occlusion the upper incisors and canines (front teeth) slightly overlap the lower ones; the front two upper incisors are aligned centrally with the front two lower incisors; the remaining upper teeth are positioned in an alternating pattern relative to the equivalent lower teeth; and the outer ridges of the lower premolars and molars (back teeth) fit into the hollows in the corresponding upper teeth. Few people have an ideal occlusion, but in most the arrangement of the teeth allows efficient biting and chewing. (See also *malocclusion*; *retinal artery occlusion*; *retinal vein occlusion*.)

occult

Hidden or obscure. For example, occult faecal blood is blood in faeces that is invisible to the naked eye but detectable by chemical tests.

occult blood, faecal

The presence in the *faeces* of blood that cannot be seen by the naked eye, but can be detected by chemical tests (see *faecal occult blood test*).

Faecal occult blood tests are widely used in screening for cancer of the colon (see *colon, cancer of*). Finding faecal occult blood may also be a sign of various gastrointestinal disorders including *oesophagitis* (inflammation of the gullet); *gastritis* (inflammation of the stomach lining); *stomach cancer*; cancer of the intestine (see *intestine, cancer of*); rectal cancer (see *rectum, cancer of*); *diverticular disease* (in which pouches form in the intestinal wall); *polyps* in the colon; *ulcerative colitis* (inflammation and ulceration of the lining of the colon and rectum); or irritation of the stomach or intestine by drugs such as aspirin. (See also *rectal bleeding*.)

occupational disease and injury

Illnesses, disorders, or injuries that are the result of exposure to chemicals or dust, or are caused by physical, psychological, or biological factors that occur in the workplace. Serious occupational diseases are far less common than formerly, but still make up an important group of conditions. They include the following main categories.

DUST DISEASES

The term *pneumoconiosis* is used to refer to *fibrosis* (formation of scar tissue) in the lung due to inhalation of industrial dusts, such as coal. *Asbestosis* is a lung condition associated with asbestos in industry. Allergic *alveolitis* (inflammation of the tiny air sacs in the lungs) is caused by inhalation of organic dusts (often containing fungal spores) (see *farmer's lung*).

CHEMICAL POISONING

Industrial chemicals can damage the lungs if they are inhaled, or other major organs if they enter the bloodstream through the lungs or skin. Examples of harmful chemicals include fumes of cadmium, beryllium, lead, and benzene. Carbon tetrachloride and vinyl chloride are causes of liver disease. Many of these compounds can cause kidney damage.

OCCUPATIONAL SKIN DISEASE

Work-related skin disorders include contact *dermatitis* (skin inflammation), which results from allergy or direct irritation by chemicals in contact with the skin, and *squamous cell carcinoma*, which may be caused by exposure to tar.

INFECTIOUS DISEASES

Rare infectious diseases that are more common in certain jobs include *brucellosis* and *Q fever* (acquired from livestock), *psittacosis* (acquired from birds), and *leptospirosis* (caused by a bacterium excreted in rats' urine). People who work with blood or blood products are at increased risk of viral hepatitis (see *hepatitis, viral*) and *AIDS*, as are healthcare professionals.

RADIATION HAZARDS

The nuclear industry and some healthcare professions use measures to reduce the danger from *radiation hazards*. Exposure to certain types of radiation increases the risk of cancer.

OTHER DISORDERS

Other occupational disorders include *writer's cramp*, *carpal tunnel syndrome*, and *singer's nodes*. *Raynaud's phenomenon* is associated with the handling of vibrating tools. Deafness may be caused by exposure to excessive noise.

occupational medicine

A branch of medicine that deals with the effects of various occupations on health and with an individual's capacity for particular types of work. It includes prevention of *occupational disease and injury* and the promotion of health in the working population.

Epidemiology is used to analyse patterns of sickness absence, injury, illness, and death. Clinical techniques are used to monitor the health of a particular workforce. Assessment of psychological stress and hazards of new technology are part of the remit.

occupational mortality

Death due to work-related disease or injuries. Annual death rates (deaths per million at risk) vary widely between occupations, ranging from very low levels in clothing and footwear manufacture to very high levels in industries such as the offshore oil and gas industries. The pattern of deaths varies over time as industrial standards change. Certain diseases that take many years to develop may reflect occupational practices that have since been improved.

occupational therapy

Treatment comprising individually tailored programmes of activities to help people who are disabled to improve their function and ability to carry out everyday tasks. Occupational therapy also involves recommending aids and changes to the home that help to increase an individual's independence.

octreotide

A *somatostatin analogue*, a hormone that acts on the *pituitary gland*. Given by injection, octreotide is used mainly in the treatment of *acromegaly* (a rare disorder that causes abnormal enlargement of certain body parts) and hormone-secreting intestinal tumours. Octreotide is also used to prevent complications following pancreatic surgery.

Side effects of octreotide may include various gastrointestinal disturbances such as nausea, vomiting, abdominal pain and bloating, flatulence, and diarrhoea.

ocular

Relating to or affecting the *eye* and its structures; also the eyepiece of an optical intrument, such as a *microscope*.

oculogyric crisis

A state in which the eyes are fixed, usually upwards, for minutes or hours. The crisis may occur with muscle spasm of the tongue, mouth, and neck, and is often triggered by stress. It may occur

O

following *encephalitis* (inflammation of the brain) and in *parkinsonism* (a movement disorder), or may be induced by drugs such as *phenothiazine* derivatives.

oculomotor nerve

The third *cranial nerve*, controlling most of the muscles that move the eye. The oculomotor nerve also supplies the muscle that constricts the pupil, that which raises the upper eyelid, and the ciliary muscle, which focuses the eye.

The oculomotor nerve may be damaged due to a fracture to the base of the skull or a tumour. Symptoms of damage include *ptosis* (drooping of the upper eyelid), *squint*, dilation of the pupil, inability to focus the eye, double vision, and a slight protrusion of the eyeball. (See also *trochlear nerve*; *abducent nerve*.)

LOCATION OF THE OCULOMOTOR NERVE

The oculomotor nerve originates high in the brainstem and passes forward through a slit in the bony eye socket to reach the muscles that move the eye and eyelids.

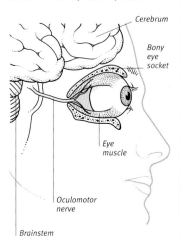

Cerebrum

Bony eye socket

Eye muscle

Oculomotor nerve

Brainstem

OD

The abbreviation for an overdose (see *drug overdose*).

odontoid

The peglike process on the second cervical *vertebra* (one of the vertebral bones in the neck) on which the first cervical vertebra rests. The odontoid is dislocated during judicial hanging, and the resultant pressure on the *spinal cord* is the cause of death.

oedema

Abnormal fluid accumulation in body tissues that may be localized (as in swelling from an injury) or generalized (as in *heart failure*).

WATER BALANCE IN THE BODY

Water accounts for roughly three-fifths of body weight and is constantly exchanged between blood and tissues. The pressure of blood being pumped around the body forces water out of the capillaries (tiny blood vessels) and into the tissues. By a reverse process, which depends on the water-drawing power of the proteins in the blood (see *osmosis*), water is reabsorbed into the capillaries and lymphatic vessels from the tissues. Normally, these two mechanisms are in balance, keeping the distribution of water between the blood and tissues more or less constant.

The action of the kidneys and hormones, including *ADH*, regulate the total amount of fluid in the body. Any excess is excreted from the body as urine.

CAUSES OF OEDEMA

Various disorders can disrupt these processes. Heart failure leads to congestion in the veins, which creates backward pressure in the capillaries. This overcomes osmotic pressure in the capillaries and causes more fluid than normal to be forced into the tissues. Backward pressure can also be created by a tumour pressing on veins, causing oedema in the area drained by the obstructed vein.

In *nephrotic syndrome*, an abnormal loss of protein from the blood reduces osmotic pressure and prevents enough fluid being drawn from the tissues into the blood. *Kidney failure* prevents salt being excreted from the body, allowing it to accumulate in the tissues and attract water to it.

Other disorders that can cause oedema include *cirrhosis* of the liver, which leads to blood congestion in the veins

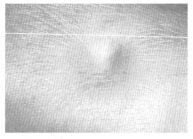

Appearance of oedema
This photograph shows the characteristic swelling that occurs with oedema and the dimpling of the skin when it is pressed.

of the liver, lowers blood protein (and therefore osmotic pressure), and causes salt retention. A deficiency of protein in the diet, as may occur in alcoholics, can also reduce osmotic pressure.

Injury or inflammation may lead to oedema by causing capillaries to leak. The blockage of lymphatic vessels may result in *lymphoedema*.

Oedema may also be caused by certain drugs, such as *corticosteroid drugs*, that have an action on the kidneys, resulting in salt retention.

SYMPTOMS

Symptoms of generalized oedema, such as swelling around the base of the spine (in bedridden people) or in the ankles, occur when excess body fluid increases by more than 15 per cent. In severe cases, fluid accumulates in large body cavities, such as the peritoneal cavity of the abdomen in *ascites* or the pleural cavity of the lungs in *pleural effusion*. In *pulmonary oedema*, the air sacs of the lungs become waterlogged, causing breathlessness.

TREATMENT

The underlying cause of the oedema should be remedied. If this is not possible, symptoms can be relieved by excretion of the excess fluid. Output of urine by the kidneys is increased by restricting dietary salt and by the use of *diuretic drugs*.

Oedipus complex

A psychoanalytic term defined as the unconscious sexual attachment of a child for the parent of the opposite sex, which is manifested by the consequent jealousy of, and desire to eliminate, the parent of the same sex.

oesophageal atresia

A rare *birth defect* in which the oesophagus forms into two separate sections during embryonic development. A short section of the *oesophagus* is absent, the part of the oesophagus above the gap terminates in a pouch, and the lower part of the oesophagus, projecting upwards from the stomach, may also be blind-ended. In most cases, however, the upper or lower section of oesophagus connects with the trachea (windpipe) to form an abnormal channel, called a *tracheoesophageal fistula*.

The condition may be suspected before birth if the mother has *polyhydramnios* (excess amniotic fluid); this indicates that the fetus is unable to swallow the amniotic fluid as normal.

SYMPTOMS

The infant cannot swallow saliva or milk, and drools and regurgitates milk continually. If there is an upper tracheo-esophageal fistula, milk may be sucked into the lungs, provoking coughing fits and *cyanosis* (a bluish skin coloration).

TREATMENT AND OUTLOOK

Immediate surgery is needed in order to join the blind ends of the oesophagus and close the fistula. In some cases, more than one operation may be necessary. If surgery is successful, the baby should develop normally.

oesophageal dilatation

A procedure to stretch the *oesophagus* when it has been narrowed by disease (see *oesophageal stricture*) and swallowing is difficult.

Endoscopy is used to locate the obstruction. The narrowed area is then stretched by passing bougies (cylindrical rods with olive-shaped tips) down the oesophagus, or by using a *balloon catheter* (a fine tube with an inflatable balloon at the end).

oesophageal diverticulum

A saclike protrusion of part of the wall of the *oesophagus*. There are two types: a pharyngeal pouch (also known as a Zenker's or pulsion diverticulum), and a mid-oesophageal diverticulum (also known as a traction diverticulum).

PHARYNGEAL POUCH

This type is located at the top of the oesophagus, at its entrance from the pharynx (throat). The pouch usually projects backwards. The cause is a failure of the sphincter (circular muscle) at the entrance to the oesophagus to relax during the act of swallowing, due to muscular incoordination. Instead, the sphincter resists the passage of food. As the powerful throat muscles used for swallowing work against this resistance, part of the lining of the oesophagus is forced through the oesophageal wall, forming the diverticulum.

Once the diverticulum is formed, it gradually enlarges. Food and fluids become trapped in it and may spill into the trachea (windpipe), causing coughing and recurrent chest infections. The condition is usually treated surgically.

MID-OESOPHAGEAL DIVERTICULUM

This disorder consists of a pouch that is formed further down the oesophagus. It rarely causes symptoms and may only be discovered accidentally. It does not usually require treatment.

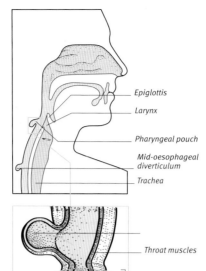

Labels: Epiglottis, Larynx, Pharyngeal pouch, Mid-oesophageal diverticulum, Trachea, Throat muscles, Sphincter

Location of oesophageal diverticula
A pharyngeal pouch forms at the top of the oesophagus as a reaction to the sphincter's failure to relax during swallowing. A mid-oesophageal diverticulum is a pouch further down the oesophagus. It is usually symptomless.

oesophageal spasm

Uncoordinated muscle contractions in the *oesophagus*, which cause intermittent swallowing difficulties and chest or upper abdominal pain. The spasm may be due to reflux *oesophagitis* but often occurs for no apparent reason. It is more common in women and in the elderly.

A barium swallow (see *barium X-ray examinations*) and *endoscopy* may be used to rule out a more serious condition, such as cancer. Treatment is of any underlying cause.

oesophageal speech

A technique for producing speech after surgical removal of the *larynx* (voice-box) (see *laryngectomy*). Air is trapped in the *oesophagus* and is gradually expelled while the tongue, palate, and lips form distinguishable sounds.

oesophageal stricture

Narrowing of the *oesophagus* that may cause pain, swallowing difficulties, regurgitation of food, and weight loss.

CAUSES

Oesophageal stricture may be due to cancer of the oesophagus (see *oesophagus, cancer of*) or to any of numerous noncancerous causes. These include

persistent reflux *oesophagitis*, in which constant irritation from gastric acid causes inflammation and swelling followed by the formation of fibrous scar tissue and narrowing. In *Plummer–Vinson syndrome*, a web of tissue forms in the upper oesophagus in association with iron deficiency anaemia (see *anaemia, iron deficiency*). A Schatzki ring (a noncancerous fibrous ring found in the lower oesophagus) can also cause difficulty swallowing. Prolonged use of a *nasogastric tube* may inflame the oesophagus, leading to a stricture, as may swallowing a corrosive liquid.

DIAGNOSIS AND TREATMENT

A barium swallow (see *barium X-ray examinations*) may help to confirm the diagnosis. *Endoscopy* (passage of a viewing instrument down the oesophagus) is used to look at the narrowed area, and a *biopsy* (removal of a sample of tissue for microscopic analysis) is carried out to exclude the possibility of cancer.

In some cases, the narrowed area can be stretched by *oesophageal dilatation*. In cases where the narrowing is caused by cancer, or in very rare cases where there is severe narrowing over a long segment of oesophagus (usually due to the swallowing of corrosives), the affected area may have to be removed surgically. The stomach can then be drawn up into the chest or the missing oesophagus replaced with a section of colon. In cases where such surgery cannot be performed, a stent (rigid tube) may be inserted as a palliative measure.

oesophageal varices

Widened veins in the walls of the lower *oesophagus* and, sometimes, the upper part of the stomach.

CAUSE

Oesophageal varices develop as a consequence of *portal hypertension* (an increase in blood pressure in the portal vein that is usually caused by liver disease). Blood in the portal vein, passing from the intestines to the liver, meets resistance due to liver disease, and is diverted into small veins in the walls of the oesophagus and stomach. The increased blood pressure causes the veins to balloon outwards.

SYMPTOMS

There are generally no symptoms until an episode of bleeding, which results in repeated episodes of haematemesis (vomiting of blood) and the passage of black faeces. There are usually other symptoms of chronic liver disease.

O

TREATMENT

To control acute bleeding, urgent endoscopic injection of a sclerosant to seal off the affected veins is required. Alternatively, banding (in which tight rubber bands are placed over the base of each enlarged vein) may be used. Replacement of lost blood and intravenous injection of drugs to constrict the blood vessels, such as octreotide and terlipressin, are also carried out. Creation of a shunt (a surgically created passage) to direct blood away from the varices may also be considered. However, despite treatment, an episode of bleeding may still prove fatal.

oesophagitis

Inflammation of the *oesophagus*. There are two main types: corrosive oesophagitis, caused by accidental or intentional swallowing of caustic chemicals, and reflux oesophagitis, caused by regurgitation of the stomach's contents.

CORROSIVE OESOPHAGITIS

Chemicals that are likely to cause severe corrosive oesophagitis include many cleaning and disinfecting products. The oesophagus may rupture, with fatal consequences; alternatively it may heal but may result in an *oesophageal stricture* (narrowing of the oesophagus).

REFLUX OESOPHAGITIS

Reflux oesophagitis is due to poor function of the muscles in the lower oesophagus, which permits the stomach's acidic contents to rise back into the oesophagus (see *gastro-oesophageal reflux disease*). The main symptom, heartburn, may be worsened by alcohol, smoking, obesity, and some foods and drinks (such as spicy foods and coffee). Poor function of the lower oesophagus may be linked with a *hiatus hernia*, in which the top part of the stomach slides back and forth through the muscular diaphragm between the chest and the abdomen.

COMPLICATIONS

Barrett's oesophagus is a complication of reflux oesophagitis in which cells that normally line the stomach extend up into the oesophagus. It may lead to cancer. Severe, chronic oesophagitis can cause an *oesophageal stricture*.

TREATMENT

The treatment for mild cases of reflux oesophagitis is a change of diet and lifestyle: weight loss, avoiding heavy meals, limiting alcohol intake, and stopping smoking; *antacid drugs* may also help to reduce acidity. In moderate or severe cases, *H2-receptor antagonists* or *proton pump inhibitors*, which greatly reduce gastric acid, may be used. Surgical treatment (such as *minimally invasive surgery*) may be necessary for a hiatus hernia.

oesophagogastroduodenoscopy

Examination of the upper digestive tract using an endoscope (see *gastroscopy*).

oesophagogastroscopy

Examination of the *oesophagus* and also the stomach with the use of an endoscope (see *gastroscopy*).

oesophagoscopy

Examination of the *oesophagus* using an endoscope (see *gastroscopy*).

oesophagus

The muscular tube that carries food from the throat to the stomach. The oesophagus is part of the digestive tract (see *digestive system*).

ANATOMY OF THE OESOPHAGUS

A muscular tube that propels food to the stomach from the throat. The upper and lower ends are bounded by sphincters – muscular valves that open to allow food to pass through.

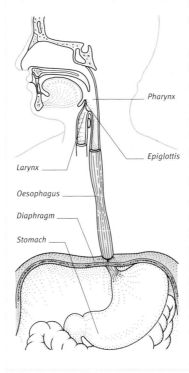

Pharynx

Epiglottis

Larynx

Oesophagus

Diaphragm

Stomach

STRUCTURE

The top end of the oesophagus is the narrowest section of the entire digestive tract. It is encircled by a sphincter (circular muscle) that is normally closed but can open to allow the passage of food. A similar sphincter operates where the oesophagus joins the stomach. The oesophageal walls consist of strong muscle fibres arranged in bundles: some circular, and others longitudinal. The inner lining of the oesophagus consists of smooth, squamous epithelium that is made up of flattened cells.

FUNCTION

Powerful waves of contractions (*peristalsis*) pass through the muscles in the oesophageal wall, propelling food and liquids down towards the stomach and intestines for digestion. Gravity plays little part in getting food into the stomach, making it possible to drink while upside down. (See also *swallowing*.)

oesophagus, cancer of

A malignant tumour of the *oesophagus*, most common in people over the age of 50, that leads to swallowing difficulties. Smoking and heavy alcohol intake are risk factors; people with certain disorders of the oesophagus (such as *Barrett's oesophagus*) are also at increased risk.

SYMPTOMS

The tumour is often present for some time before it begins to cause symptoms. Early symptoms may include pain on, and difficulty in, swallowing foods and/or liquids. The patient's condition progressively worsens to a point where food is immediately regurgitated and there is rapid weight loss. Regurgitated fluid spilling into the *trachea* (windpipe) often causes respiratory infections.

DIAGNOSIS AND TREATMENT

Diagnosis usually involves a barium swallow (see *barium X-ray examinations*) to detect obstruction in the oesophagus and a *biopsy* (removal of a tissue sample for analysis) taken during *endoscopy*.

Treatment depends on whether or not the cancer has spread to surrounding structures. Removal of the oesophagus may be possible in some localized, and early diagnosed, cancer. *Radiotherapy* may cause regression of the cancer, relieve symptoms, and occasionally cure older patients who might not be suitable for major surgery. Permanent insertion of a rigid tube (a stent) through the tumour, or laser treatment to burn through it, can help temporarily to relieve symptoms and improve nutrition.

DISORDERS OF THE **OESOPHAGUS**

Several disorders affect the oesophagus, many of which cause *swallowing difficulties* and/or chest pain.

Infection and inflammation

Infections of the oesophagus are rare but may occur in immunosuppressed patients whose defences are weakened. The most common are *herpes simplex* and *candidiasis* (thrush) spreading downwards from the mouth. Both cause pain on swallowing. *Oesophagitis* (inflammation of the oesophagus) is usually due to reflux of stomach contents, causing heartburn. A more severe form, corrosive oesophagitis, can occur as a result of swallowing caustic chemicals. Both types may cause an *oesophageal stricture* (narrowing of the oesophagus) with difficulty in swallowing. *Barrett's oesophagus* is a complication of long-term reflux oesophagitis; it may lead to cancer.

Congenital defects

Oesophageal atresia (the congenital absence of a section of the oesophagus, with the remaining sections ending in dead ends) requires urgent surgical treatment. Babies are occasionally also born with weblike constrictions of the oesophagus. These are rarely serious enough to require treatment, but they can be broken down with a dilator.

Tumours

Tumours of the oesophagus are relatively common. The initial symptom is usually difficulty in swallowing. The majority of oesophageal tumours are cancerous (see *oesophagus, cancer of*).

Injury

Severe vomiting and retching can tear the oesophageal lining and, in extreme cases, lead to rupture. A swallowed *foreign body* can also cause injury, even perforation, if it penetrates the oesophageal wall.

Other disorders

Oesophageal varices (dilated blood vessels) at the junction of the stomach and oesophagus may be associated with *cirrhosis*. An *oesophageal diverticulum* is a protruding sac in which food may collect, causing difficulty in swallowing. In *oesophageal spasm*, the oesophageal muscles contract uncontrollably. In *achalasia*, the sphincter at the junction between the oesophagus and stomach fails to relax to allow the passage of food, causing pain on swallowing and sometimes regurgitation of food.

INVESTIGATION

Disorders of the oesophagus are investigated by barium swallow (see *barium X-ray examinations*) and by endoscopy during which a biopsy (tissue sample) can be taken for microscopic examination.

oestradiol

See *estradiol*.

oestriol

See *estriol*.

oestrogen drugs

COMMON DRUGS

- Conjugated oestrogens • Diethylstilbestrol
- Estradiol • Estriol • Estrone • Estropipate
- Ethinylestradiol • Mestranol

A group of synthetically produced drugs that are used in *oral contraceptives* and additionally to supplement or re-place the body's own *oestrogen hormones* in *hormone replacement therapy (HRT)*. Oestrogen drugs are often used with *progestogen drugs*.

WHY THEY ARE USED

Oestrogens suppress the production of *gonadotrophin hormones*, which stimulate cell activity in the *ovaries*. They are used in HRT to treat, or sometimes to prevent, menopausal symptoms and disorders. Oestrogens may also be used to treat female *hypogonadism* (underactivity of the ovaries), abnormal menstrual bleed-ing, and *breast cancer*.

POSSIBLE ADVERSE EFFECTS

Oestrogens may cause breast tenderness and enlargement, bloating, weight gain, nausea, reduced sex drive, depression, migraine, and bleeding between peri-ods. Most of the side effects subside after two or three months. Oestrogens can also increase the risk of abnormal blood clotting (see *thrombosis, deep vein*), *breast cancer*, uterine cancer (see *uterus, cancer of*), and susceptibility to *hypertension* (high blood pressure).

Oestrogen drugs should not be taken during pregnancy because they may adversely affect the fetus.

oestrogen hormones

A group of *hormones* that are essential for normal female sexual development and healthy functioning of the reproductive system. In women, they are produced mainly in the *ovaries* and also in the *pla-centa* in pregnancy. Small amounts are produced in the *adrenal glands* in both men and women, but oestrogens have no specific function in men. When levels are low, oestrogen hormones can be replaced with *oestrogen drugs*.

oestrogen–progestogen pill

An alternative name for the combined pill (see *oral contraceptives*).

oestrone

See *estrone*.

ofloxacin

A *quinolone* antibiotic used to treat skin, soft tissue, and lower *respiratory tract* and *urinary tract infections*; *gonorrhoea*; *chlamydial infections*; and *pelvic inflam-matory disease*. It is usually taken in tablet form to treat infections that have not responded to other drugs but is also given by intravenous infusion for severe *systemic* infections. Side effects may include nausea, vomiting, diarrhoea, and abdominal pain.

oils

See *fats and oils*.

ointment

A greasy preparation that is used as a vehicle to apply drugs in dry skin con-ditions such as *eczema* or to protect or lubricate the skin.

olanzapine

An *antipsychotic drug* used for the treat-ment of *schizophrenia* and *mania*.

olecranon

The bony projection at the upper end of the *ulna* (the inner bone of the fore-arm) that forms the point of the elbow.

olecranon bursitis

Inflammation of the small, fluid-filled pad that cushions the *olecranon* at the tip of the elbow. The condition causes

O

LOCATION OF THE OLECRANON

This is the curved projection at the upper end of the ulna. It acts to prevent elbow overextension.

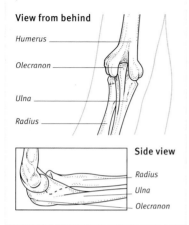

View from behind

Humerus

Olecranon

Ulna

Radius

Side view

Radius

Ulna

Olecranon

pain and swelling but usually clears up after a few days of rest and avoiding pressure on the joint. (See also *bursitis*.)

olfactory bulb

The swelling at the end of each *olfactory nerve* that deals with the sense of smell. These bulbs lie on the brain's lower surface, just above the roof of the nose.

olfactory nerve

The first *cranial nerve*, which conveys sensations of smell as nerve impulses from the nose to the brain. Each of the two olfactory nerves has receptors in the mucous membrane lining the nasal cavity. These receptors detect smells and send signals along nerve fibres, which pass through tiny holes in the roof of the nasal cavity and combine to form the olfactory bulbs. From here, nerve fibres come together to form the olfactory nerve, which leads to the olfactory centre in the brain. Sense of smell may be lost or impaired due to damage to the olfactory nerves, usually as a result of head injury.

oligo-

A prefix meaning few, scanty, or little, as in *oligospermia* (the presence of too few *sperm* in the *semen*).

oligodendroglioma

A rare and slow-growing type of primary *brain tumour* that originates in the oligodendroglial cells that support brain

cells. Oligodendroglioma mainly affect young or middle-aged adults. Surgical removal of the tumour can, in some cases, lead to a total cure.

oligohydramnios

A condition in which an insufficient amount of *amniotic fluid* surrounds a fetus in the uterus.

CAUSES

Amniotic fluid is produced partly by the *placenta*, but mainly from the urine produced by the fetus. Oligohydramnios may occur if the placenta is not functioning properly, which can occur in severe *pre-eclampsia*, or if there is an abnormality of the kidneys or bladder of the fetus. Reduced quantities of amniotic fluid may also result from leakage due to a premature rupture of the amniotic membranes.

TREATMENT AND OUTLOOK

Oligohydramnios may be suspected if the woman's uterus is smaller than expected; diagnosis is confirmed using *ultrasound scanning*.

In some cases, the underlying disorder can be treated, but this may not be possible (particularly if the fetus is not developing normally). If oligohydramnios occurs early in pregnancy, it usually results in *miscarriage*. In later pregnancy, the pressure of the uterus on the fetus may cause a deformity such as *talipes* (club-foot).

LOCATION OF THE OLFACTORY NERVE

Each olfactory bulb lies on top of a thin bony plate in the roof of the nose and connects to the brain via an olfactory nerve. Nerve twigs pass through the bony plate to enter the nasal lining.

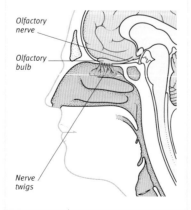

Olfactory nerve

Olfactory bulb

Nerve twigs

oligospermia

A temporary or permanent deficiency in the number of *sperm* in the *semen*. This condition is also known as oligozoospermia. It may be a cause of *infertility*, especially when other disorders of the sperm are also present.

CAUSES

Normally, there are more than 20 million sperm per millilitre of semen. A low sperm count can be due to various disorders, including hormonal disorders, *orchitis* (inflammation of a testis), undescended testis (see *testis, undescended*), and, infrequently, a *varicocele* (varicose vein in the scrotum). Smoking, alcohol abuse, and some drugs may also reduce the sperm count.

TREATMENT

Treatment of oligospermia is for the underlying cause. If the cause is a hormone deficiency, *gonadotrophin hormones* may be prescribed. If infertility is a problem, *artificial insemination* within the uterus or *in vitro fertilization* (IVF) with *intracytoplasmic sperm injection* may be successful. (See also *azoospermia*.)

oliguria

The production of low quantities of *urine* in proportion to the volume of fluid taken in. The condition may be caused by excessive sweating; in some cases, it is a sign of *kidney failure*.

olive oil

An oil, obtained from the fruit of the olive tree OLEA EUROPAEA, that may be used to soften earwax or to treat *cradle cap* in babies. Olive oil is high in monounsaturated fat (see *fats and oils*); it is an important part of a *Mediterranean diet*.

Ollier's disease

See *dyschondroplasia*.

-oma

A suffix denoting a tumour, which may be cancerous or noncancerous, as in *lipoma* and *carcinoma*.

omega-3 fatty acids

A group of *fatty acids* (constituents of fats and oils) that are vital for many body functions, including nerve function, immune system function, and fat transport. They cannot be made by the body and must be obtained from the diet. Good sources of omega-3 fatty acids include fish such as sardines, herring, mackerel, trout, and salmon, soya bean oil, and rapeseed oil.

Omega-3 fatty acids are thought to help reduce blood lipid levels, blood pressure, and the risk of cardiovascular disease. They may also help brain development in children. Pregnant and breast-feeding women may be advised to have an adequate intake of omega-3 fatty acids to support development of the baby's brain. Omega-3 fatty acids are sometimes prescribed as part of treatment to lower blood lipid levels.

omentum

A double fold of fatty membrane in the abdomen (peritoneum) hanging in front of the intestines that acts as a fat store.

omeprazole

A *proton pump inhibitor* used to treat *peptic ulcer*, *gastro-oesophageal reflux disease*, and *Zollinger–Ellison syndrome*. Possible adverse effects include rashes, headache, nausea, diarrhoea, and constipation.

onchocerciasis

A tropical disease, also called river blindness, caused by infestation with the worm ONCHOCERCA VOLVULUS. The disease, a type of *filariasis*, affects millions of people in some regions of Africa and Central and South America.

CAUSES AND SYMPTOMS

Onchocerciasis is transmitted from person to person by small, fiercely biting, black simulium flies. These flies, which breed in, and always remain near, fast-running streams, ingest microfilariae (tiny worms) and inject their larvae into human skin, where they multiply and spread around the body under the skin (see the illustrated box, below).

The dead larvae can cause an allergic reaction resulting in inflammation and the formation of fibrous tissue. When this occurs in the eye, the damage is permanent and leads to blindness. Symptoms of the condition include itchy, swollen patches; they usually arise about a year after infestation.

TREATMENT AND PREVENTION

Treatment involves taking *anthelmintic drugs*, which quickly kill the microfilariae. Such treatment needs to be repeated annually because the adult worms are not affected. Travellers to areas where the disease is prevalent should take measures to discourage *insect bites*, for example, by using an insect repellent such as *DEET*.

oncogenes

Genes found in every cell of the body that control growth, repair, and replacement. Activation of an oncogene is a factor in the development of cancerous cells. *Mutations* (structural changes) in oncogenes, resulting from damage by *carcinogens*, can cause a cell to grow uncontrollably and infiltrate and destroy normal tissues (see *cancer*). Factors known to encourage oncogene mutation include ultraviolet light, radioactivity, tobacco smoke, alcohol, asbestos, and some chemicals. In addition, some viruses can activate oncogenes.

oncology

The study of the causes, development, characteristics, and treatment of *tumours*, particularly *cancers* (malignant tumours). Because there are many different types of tumours and they may develop in virtually any tissue in the body, oncology is a wide-ranging discipline that includes surveying the frequency and distribution of tumours, investigating processes involved in tumour formation, studying genes associated with tumours, and developing new treatments.

ondansetron

A *serotonin antagonist* drug used to control the nausea and vomiting that occur following an operation or that are induced by *radiotherapy* or *anticancer drugs*. Ondansetron is taken in the form of tablets or suppositories or is given by injection. Side effects may include constipation, headache, and hiccups.

onychogryphosis

Abnormal thickening, hardening, and curving of the nails that occurs mainly in elderly people. It may be associated with *fungal infection* or poor circulation, or it may occur for no apparent reason.

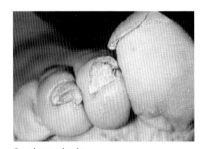

Onychogryphosis
This thickening, hardening, and overgrowth of the toenails occurs mainly in elderly people. It can also affect the fingernails.

onycholysis

Separation of the nail from its bed: a feature of many skin conditions, including *psoriasis* and *dermatitis*.

oocyte

One of the cells that are found in the *ovary* that, after undergoing *meiosis* (a type of cell division), form ova (egg cells; see *ovum*).

oogenesis

The process by which mature ova (egg cells; see *ovum*) are produced in the female's ovary. At birth, a female has her entire lifetime's complement of

LIFE-CYCLE OF **ONCHOCERCIASIS**

The infestation is spread by a fly that ingests microfilariae (tiny worms) from an infested person. The worms grow into larvae inside the fly and are deposited in the skin of a new human host when the fly bites. In the new host, the larvae develop into adults, which produce micro-filariae that migrate around the body.

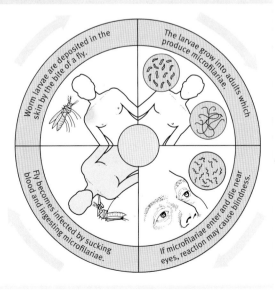

Worm larvae are deposited in the skin by the bite of a fly.

The larvae grow into adults which produce microfilariae.

If microfilariae enter and die near eyes, reaction may cause blindness.

Fly becomes infected by sucking blood and ingesting microfilariae.

oogonia (cells that divide by *meiosis* to develop firstly into *oocytes* and eventually into mature ova).

oophorectomy

Removal of the *ovaries*, usually done to treat *ovarian cysts* or cancer (see *ovary, cancer of*). A partial oophorectomy may be performed to preserve ovarian function in premenopausal women. In a *hysterectomy*, both ovaries may be removed if disease has spread from the uterus, or as a preventive measure. The ovaries may be removed as part of the treatment for *breast cancer* if growth of the tumour depends on hormones produced by the ovary. If both ovaries are removed before the onset of the menopause, *hormone replacement therapy (HRT)* may be needed.

-opathy

A suffix denoting disease or disorder, as in *neuropathy* (a disorder of the nerves).

open-angle glaucoma

An alternative name for chronic simple *glaucoma*, a gradual buildup of excessive fluid pressure in the eye.

open chest cardiac massage

Rhythmic compression that is applied directly to the heart through an incision in the chest wall in order to restart arrested heart action (see *cardiac arrest*). Open chest massage, which is also known as internal *cardiac massage*, is an emergency measure for the purpose of maintaining the circulation. It is not commonly performed.

open fracture

A type of *fracture*, also known as a compound fracture, in which the broken bone penetrates the overlying skin. An open fracture carries a greater risk of infection than a closed fracture because the skin has been punctured.

open heart surgery

Any operation on the *heart* in which it is stopped temporarily and its function taken over by a mechanical pump (a *heart–lung machine*). The main forms of open heart surgery include the correction of congenital heart defects (see *heart disease, congenital*), surgery for the repair of narrowed or leaky heart valves (see *heart-valve surgery*), and *coronary artery bypass* surgery.

OPERATING THEATRE

The operating table can be raised, lowered, and titled in any direction to allow optimum access to the patient. For some operations, it is best for the surgeon to stand but, during delicate procedures, such as microsurgery, the surgeon usually sits. The operating lamp is designed to give brilliant focal illumination without causing any shadow. The anaesthetic apparatus can maintain breathing in patients who have been given a muscle-relaxant drug.

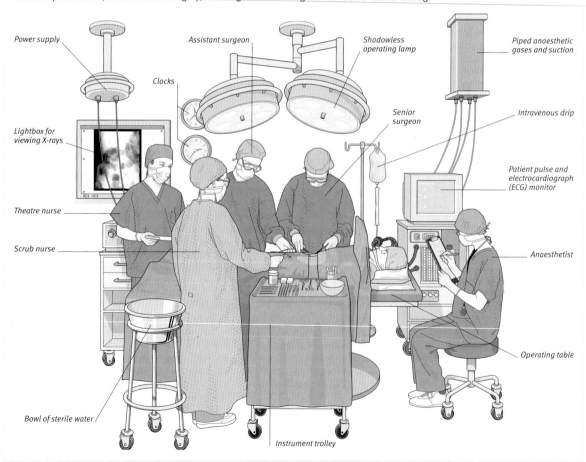

Power supply
Assistant surgeon
Shadowless operating lamp
Piped anaesthetic gases and suction
Clocks
Senior surgeon
Intravenous drip
Lightbox for viewing X-rays
Patient pulse and electrocardiograph (ECG) monitor
Theatre nurse
Scrub nurse
Anaesthetist
Operating table
Bowl of sterile water
Instrument trolley

Once the heart–lung machine has been connected, the heart is isolated, and the defects repaired. Surgical hypothermia is used to keep the heart cool and help prevent damage to the heart muscle from lack of oxygen (see *hypothermia, surgical*). Various techniques that enable procedures to be performed on a beating heart without the need to use a heart–lung machine are now becoming available.

operable

A term applied to a condition that is suitable for surgical treatment, such as an accessible noncancerous tumour. (See also *inoperable*.)

operating theatre

A specialized room in which surgical procedures are performed. An operating theatre is one of a suite of rooms, attached to an anaesthetic room and a recovery area. The risk of infection of open wounds during surgery is reduced by a ventilation system that continually provides clean, filtered air, and surfaces that are easily washable. Surgeons, assistants, and nurses use sterile brushes and bactericidal soaps to scrub their hands and forearms before putting on sterile gowns and gloves.

The operating theatre has a range of equipment, including shadowless operating lights; lightboxes for viewing *X-ray* images or scans; anaesthetic machines (see *anaesthesia, general*); and a *diathermy* machine, which is used for the control of bleeding. A *heart–lung machine* may also be used.

operation

A surgical procedure usually carried out with specialized instruments; but sometimes only the hands are used (as in the manipulation of a simple fracture).

ophryosis

Spasm (involuntary contraction) of the muscles of the eyebrow.

ophthalmia

An old term for *ophthalmitis*.

ophthalmia neonatorum

A type of eye inflammation and a discharge (*ophthalmitis*) that occur in newborn infants, usually as a result of being infected with the sexually transmitted diseases *gonorrhoea* or *chlamydia* at birth. Treatment of ophthalmia neonatorum is with *antibiotic drugs*.

ophthalmitis

A term that is used to describe any inflammatory eye disorder. Types of ophthalmitis include *ophthalmia neonatorum* and sympathetic ophthalmitis, a rare condition in which a penetrating injury to one eye is followed by severe *uveitis* (inflammation of the iris and choroid) that can lead to blindness in the other eye. Sympathetic ophthalmitis can be treated with *corticosteroid drugs*, but it is sometimes necessary to remove the injured eye in order to preserve the sight of the other.

ophthalmology

The study of the *eye* and the diagnosis and treatment of the disorders that affect it. Ophthalmology covers assessment of vision, prescription of glasses or contact lenses, and surgery for eye disorders, such as *cataracts* and *glaucoma*. (See also *eye, examination of*; *optician*; *optometry*; *orthoptics*.)

ophthalmoplegia

Partial or total paralysis of the muscles that move the eyes. Ophthalmoplegia may be caused by a disease that affects the eye muscles themselves, such as *Graves' disease*, or by a condition that affects the brain or the nerves supplying the eye muscles, such as *stroke*, a *brain tumour*, *encephalitis* (inflammation of the brain), or *multiple sclerosis*.

ophthalmoplegic migraine

A type of *migraine* (a severe headache that is often accompanied by visual disturbances) in which movement of an eye is affected. Movement of the pupil may or may not also be affected.

ophthalmoscope

An instrument that is used to examine the inside of the *eye*. The ophthalmoscope contains a deflecting prism or a perforated angled mirror, which allows illumination and viewing of the entire area of the back of the eye, including the light-sensitive *retina*.

ophthalmoscopy

A noninvasive procedure in which a doctor uses an *ophthalmoscope* to examine the inside of the *eye*. The ophthalmoscope is used first to direct a beam of light into the eye and then to examine various structures, such as the light-sensitive *retina*; the retinal blood vessels; the head of the *optic nerve*; and the jelly-like *vitreous humour*.

opiate

Any drug derived from, or chemically similar to, *opium*.

opioid

A type of *analgesic drug* (painkiller) used in the treatment of moderate to severe pain. Opioids, also known as narcotic drugs, may be abused for their euphoric effects; abuse may cause *tolerance* (the need for greater amounts of a drug to get the same effect), and physical and psychological *drug dependence*. Opioids in common use include *codeine*, *diamorphine*, *morphine*, and *pethidine*.

opisthotonus

A form of *spasm* in which the head is bent backwards and the back is arched. Opisthotonus may occur in people with *tetanus* or *meningitis* or as a result of a severe brain injury.

opium

A substance obtained from the unripe seed pods of the poppy plant PAPAVER SOMNIFERUM. Opium has an analgesic (pain-relieving) effect and may also cause sleepiness and euphoria. Opium and its derivatives, such as *codeine* and *diamorphine*, are known as *opiates* or *opioids*.

opportunistic infection

Infection by organisms that rarely have serious or widespread effects in people of normal health, but which can cause serious illness or widespread infection

O

OPHTHALMOSCOPE

An ophthalmoscope allows viewing of the entire area of the back of the eye, including the retina.

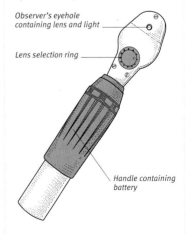

Observer's eyehole containing lens and light

Lens selection ring

Handle containing battery

in a person whose *immune system* is impaired. Malfunction of the immune system can be caused by diseases such as *AIDS* and *leukaemia* or by *chemotherapy*.

Opportunistic infections include a variety of viral, bacterial, protozoal, and fungal infections, including *tuberculosis*, *herpes simplex*, *pneumonia*, *cryptococcosis*, and *candidiasis* (thrush). Treatment of the infection is with the appropriate antimicrobial drugs.

oppositional defiant disorder

A type of behavioural disorder that usually appears in childhood or early adolescence. Typically, an affected child shows hostile, argumentative behaviour. While to some extent such behaviour is a common feature of adolescence, when law-breaking or violence occur the condition is considered pathological.

optic atrophy

A shrinkage or wasting of the *optic nerve* fibres due to disease of or injury to the optic nerve. The optic nerve is responsible for carrying electrical impulses from the light-sensitive layer of the eye, the *retina*, to the brain, where the information is processed to produce *vision*.

Damage to the fibres of the optic nerve leads to blurring of vision and may result in total visual loss. Damage to the optic nerve cannot be reversed. Optic atrophy may occur without prior signs of nerve disease.

The most common cause of optic atrophy is chronic *glaucoma* (raised pressure in the eyeball). Other causes include injury to the optic nerve; pressure on the nerve, from a tumour for example; and impaired blood supply to the nerve (ischaemic optic atrophy). It may also occur as a complication of certain nervous system disorders, such as *multiple sclerosis*. Rarely, optic atrophy has a familial cause, as in Leber's optic atrophy, a *genetic disorder*, most common in males, that causes degeneration of the optic nerve. The nerve degeneration first becomes apparent between 15 and 45 years of age.

Optic atrophy may be diagnosed by viewing the eye using an *ophthalmoscope*. The optic disc (the point where the optic nerve leaves the back of the eye) appears pale or white. *Vision tests* may also be performed.

If the underlying cause of the atrophy is identified and treated successfully, any further damage to the optic nerve can be prevented.

optic disc

The area on the *retina* (the light-sensitive layer at the back of the eye) where nerve fibres from the eyeball join the *optic nerve*. The optic disc is also known as the blind spot because of its lack of light-sensitive cells.

optician

A person who fits and sells *glasses* and *contact lenses*. An ophthalmic optician, or optometrist, examines the eyes for *myopia* (shortsightedness), *hypermetropia* (longsightedness), *presbyopia* (loss of focusing power with age), or *astigmatism* (uneven curvature of the cornea). Opticians also screen for eye disorders, such as *glaucoma*, and refer patients to ophthalmologists. (See also *ophthalmology*; *optometry*).

optic nerve

The second *cranial nerve*; the nerve of *vision*. The two optic nerves each consist of about one million nerve fibres that transmit impulses from the *retina* (the light-sensitive layer at the back of the eye) to the *brain*. The optic nerves converge behind the eyes, where fibres from the inner halves of the retina cross over. Nerve fibres from the right halves of both retinas go to the right side of the occipital lobes in the brain; and those from the left halves of the retinas go to the left side.

Disorders of the optic nerve include *optic atrophy* (shrinkage or wasting of the optic nerve), *optic neuritis* (nerve inflammation) and *papilloedema* (caused by pressure on the nerve from disease in the eye socket or by a *brain tumour*). Disease or injury occurring at a particular point on an optic nerve leads to loss of a specific part of the visual field.

optic neuritis

Inflammation of the *optic nerve*, often causing sudden loss of part of the visual field. Attacks are sometimes accompanied by pain on moving the eyes. Vision usually improves within six weeks, but some optic nerve fibres will be damaged. Recurrent attacks usually lead to permanent loss of visual acuity.

Most cases are thought to be due to demyelination of the optic nerve fibres in *multiple sclerosis*. The condition may also result from inflammation or infection of tissues around the optic nerve.

Corticosteroid drugs may help to restore vision, but have little effect on long-term outcome. (See also *optic atrophy*.)

THE FUNCTION OF THE **OPTIC NERVE**

Each optic nerve is a bundle of long fibres that relays electrical signals from the nerve cells in one of the retinas towards the brain. The optic nerves meet at the optic chiasma, where the information transmitted by both optic nerves is routed to the appropriate parts of the brain via the optic tracts. The brain coordinates this information into a complete visual picture.

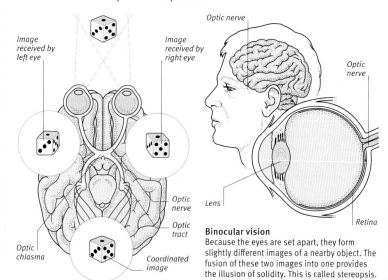

Image received by left eye

Image received by right eye

Optic nerve

Optic nerve

Optic chiasma

Optic nerve

Optic tract

Coordinated image

Lens

Retina

Binocular vision
Because the eyes are set apart, they form slightly different images of a nearby object. The fusion of these two images into one provides the illusion of solidity. This is called stereopsis.

optimum dose

The amount of an agent, such as a drug, that will produce a desired effect without causing unwanted side effects.

optometry

The practice of assessing *vision* to establish whether glasses or contact lenses are needed to correct a visual defect, as carried out by an optometrist. Disorders of the eye may require treatment by an ophthalmologist. (See also *ophthalmology*; *optician*.)

oral contraceptives

COMMON DRUGS

OESTROGENS • Ethinylestradiol • Mestranol
PROGESTOGENS • Desogestrel • Drospirenone
• Gestodene • Levonorgestrel
• Norethisterone • Norgestimate

A group of oral drug preparations containing one or more synthetic female *sex hormones* that are taken by women in a monthly cycle to prevent pregnancy. Oral contraceptives do not protect against sexually transmitted infections; if such protection is required, other measures, such as using a condom, are necessary (see *safer sex*).

TYPES

"The pill" commonly refers to the combined or the phased pill, which both contain an *oestrogen drug* and a *progestogen drug*, and the progestogen-only pill (POP), also sometimes known as the *minipill*. The combined pill is taken for three weeks out of every four. The POP is taken continuously.

EFFECTIVENESS

When oral contraceptives are used correctly, the number of pregnancies among women using them for one year is less than 1 per cent. However, actual failure rates may be higher, particularly for the minipill, which has to be taken at the same time each day.

If vomiting and/or diarrhoea occur after a pill has been taken, the woman should follow the manufacturer's advice for a missed pill. Certain drugs, such as some antibiotics, may make the contraceptive pill less effective. A woman who is taking other medications (including over-the-counter ones) as well as the pill should consult a doctor as additional contraceptive measures may be needed.

HOW THEY WORK

Combined and phased pills increase oestrogen and progesterone levels. This interferes with the production of two hormones, *luteinizing hormone* (LH) and

HOW **ORAL CONTRACEPTIVES** WORK

Combined pills (including phased pills) increase the levels of oestrogen and progesterone in the body, which interferes with the production by the pituitary gland of two *gonadotrophin hormones* called follicle-stimulating hormone (FSH) and luteinizing hormone (LH). This action in turn prevents ovulation. The progesterone-only pill (POP or minipill) works partly by making the mucus lining the inside of the cervix thick and impenetrable to sperm and partly by thickening the uterine lining itself. One type of POP also inhibits ovulation.

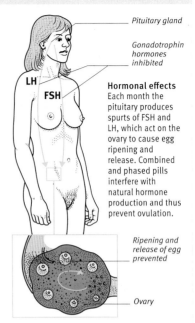

Pituitary gland

Gonadotrophin hormones inhibited

Hormonal effects
Each month the pituitary produces spurts of FSH and LH, which act on the ovary to cause egg ripening and release. Combined and phased pills interfere with natural hormone production and thus prevent ovulation.

Ripening and release of egg prevented

Ovary

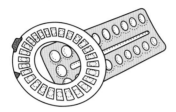

Pill packaging
Most oral contraceptives come in packs, called calendar packs, that clearly indicate which day of the week each pill should be taken.

Effects on eggs
FSH normally brings about egg ripening and LH causes the egg's release from the ovary; combined pills prevent this.

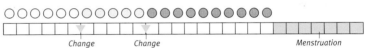

Menstruation

Combined pill
These pills contain an oestrogen and a progestogen drug in fixed doses. A course usually consists of one pill per day for 21 days, followed by seven pill-free days, during which bleeding may occur. A new course is then started, whether or not bleeding has occurred.

Change   Change   Menstruation

Phased pill
These are combined pills, containing both an oestrogen and a progestogen drug. Unlike other combined pills, the doses change from phase to phase (different times during the month). A course lasts for 21 days followed either by seven pill-free days or by seven inactive pills.

Menstruation

POP (minipill)
These pills contain only a progestogen drug in a fixed dose. The pills are taken continuously: one every day with no pill-free days in between. Bleeding usually occurs during the last few days of each cycle. The minipill has a slightly higher failure rate than combined pills.

follicle-stimulating hormone (FSH), which in turn prevents ovulation. Most POPs work by making the lining of the cervix too thick for sperm to penetrate and the uterine lining thinner so that implantation of a fertilized ovum is less likely. A type of POP containing *desogestrel* also works by inhibiting ovulation.

ADVANTAGES

Oestrogen-containing pills offer some protection against uterine, ovarian, and colon cancer, *ovarian cysts*, and *endometriosis* (fragments of uterine lining situated in other parts of the body). They also tend to make menstrual periods regular, lighter, and relatively pain-free.

POSSIBLE ADVERSE EFFECTS

Possible side effects of oestrogen-containing pills include raised blood pressure (see *hypertension*), weight changes, nausea, depression, swollen breasts, reduced sex drive, increased appetite, leg and abdominal cramps, headaches, and dizziness. There is also a risk of *thrombosis* (an abnormal blood clot) causing a *stroke* or a *pulmonary embolism*. These pills may also aggravate heart disease or cause *gallstones, jaundice*, and, very rarely, liver cancer. There may be a slightly increased long-term risk of *breast cancer* for women taking the combined pill.

All oral contraceptives can cause bleeding between periods, especially the POP. Other possible adverse effects of the POP include irregular periods, *ectopic pregnancy*, and ovarian cysts.

CONTRAINDICATIONS

Oestrogen-based pills should not be used by women who are or might be pregnant; women who are breast-feeding; women who have *liver disease* or certain types of *migraine*; women who have had or are at increased risk of thrombosis; women with breast cancer; or women with unexplained vaginal bleeding. They may be prescribed with caution to women with a family history of heart or circulatory disorders; to women with sickle cell disease; and to women with several risk factors for arterial disease, including *diabetes mellitus* (especially if there are complications), hypertension, smoking, obesity, *hyperlipidaemia*, and being 35 years old or over. In some cases, the POP or a low-oestrogen pill may be used by women who should avoid oestrogens. (See also *contraception; contraception, emergency*.)

oral hygiene

Measures to keep the mouth and teeth clean and to reduce the risk of tooth decay (see *caries, dental*), *gingivitis* and other gum disorders, and *halitosis* (bad breath). Oral hygiene includes regular, thorough *toothbrushing* and flossing (see *floss, dental*) to remove *plaque*. *Disclosing agents* can be used to help to reveal areas of plaque buildup. Dentures are brushed on all surfaces and soaked in cleansing solution.

Professional removal of *calculus* (a mineral deposit on teeth) and plaque by scaling and polishing is usually carried out by a dentist or hygienist during a routine check-up. In *periodontal disease*, treatment may be needed more often.

oral phase

A term used in *psychoanalytic theory* to refer to the earliest stage of a person's psychosexual development. It is thought to last from birth to about 18 months of age. (See also *anal phase; genital phase*.)

oral rehydration therapy

See *rehydration therapy*.

oral surgery

The branch of surgery concerned with the treatment of deformity, injury, or disease of the teeth, the jaws, and other parts of the mouth. Procedures include the extraction of impacted wisdom teeth (see *impaction, dental*) and *alveolectomy* (removal of tooth-bearing bone from the jaw).

More complicated oral surgery includes repair of a broken jaw; *orthognathic surgery*, (which is carried out to correct deformities of the jaw); plastic surgery in order to correct *cleft lip and palate*; and the removal of some noncancerous tumours from the mouth.

orange peel effect

See *peau d'orange*.

orbit

The socket in the *skull* containing the eyeball, protective fat, blood vessels, muscles, and nerves. The *optic nerve* passes from the eye to the *brain* through an opening in the back of the orbit.

LOCATION OF **ORBIT**

The orbits are the deep cavities in the skull that enclose and protect the eyeballs and the muscles that move the eyes.

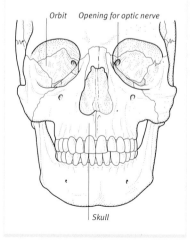

Orbit *Opening for optic nerve*

Skull

DISORDERS

A severe blow to the face may fracture the orbit, but the eyeball is often undamaged because it is squeezed backwards by protective muscles during reflex blinking. Fractures can often heal without treatment, but some may cause deformity and therefore require corrective surgery. In rare cases, bacterial infection spreads from a *sinus* or the face to cause *orbital cellulitis*.

orbital cellulitis

Bacterial infection of the tissues in the *orbit* (eye socket). Usually, the infection originates in a nearby sinus, but sometimes it spreads in the blood from a facial infection. The affected eye protrudes and is extremely painful and red. There is also severe swelling of the lids and conjunctiva (the membrane that lines the inside of the eyelids and covers the white of the eye).

Orbital cellulitis is a serious disorder and need urgent medical assessment. The eye may be damaged; there is also a slight risk that the infection may spread inwards to involve the brain. Treatment is with high doses of *antibiotic drugs*.

orchidectomy

The surgical removal of one or both of the *testes*. It may be performed for testicular cancer (see *testis, cancer of*), gangrene caused by torsion (see *testis, torsion of*), or to reduce production of the male hormone *testosterone* in the treatment of cancer of the prostate gland (see *prostate, cancer of*). Removal of only one testis does not affect sex drive, potency, or the ability to have children.

orchidopexy

An operation to bring down an undescended testis (see *testis, undescended*) into the scrotum. Orchidopexy is usually performed in early childhood to reduce the risk of later *infertility* or testicular cancer (see *testis, cancer of*).

orchitis

Inflammation of a *testis*. Orchitis may be caused by the *mumps* virus, particularly if infection occurs after puberty. Swelling and severe pain in the affected testis are accompanied by high fever. In *epididymo-orchitis*, the tube that carries sperm from the testis is also inflamed.

Treatment is with *analgesic drugs* (painkillers), bed rest, and *ice-packs* to reduce swelling; *antibiotic drugs* may be given, but not for mumps orchitis. The condition usually begins to subside within seven days but is followed in about half of cases by shrinking and loss of function of the testis.

orf

A skin infection occasionally transmitted to humans from sheep. Caused by a *pox* virus, orf usually produces a single persistent, fluid-filled blister on the arm or hand. Usually, no specific treatment is necessary as most cases clear up spontaneously in three to six weeks. However, large lesions may be removed surgically.

organ

A collection of various *tissues* integrated into a distinct structural unit to perform specific functions.

organ donation

The agreement of a person (or his or her family) to the surgical removal of one or more organs for use in *transplant surgery*. Most donor organs are removed immediately after death. Heart and lung function is sometimes maintained by machine after *brain death* has been certified until the organs have been removed. Living donors may be able to donate a kidney, but usually only to a close relative (see *tissue-typing*).

Although it is not legal in the UK, in some countries organ donors are paid for their organs. People can facilitate use of their organs after death by informing relatives and carrying a donor card. (See also *corneal graft*; *heart–lung transplant*; *heart transplant*; *heart-valve surgery*; *kidney transplant*; *liver transplant*.)

organelle

One of various specialized structures contained within a body *cell*.

organic

Related to a body *organ*; having organs or an organized structure; or related to *organisms* or substances from them. In medicine, the term indicates the presence of disease in the body. In chemistry, the term refers to certain compounds that contain carbon. (See also *inorganic*.)

organic brain syndrome

See *brain syndrome, organic.*

organic disease

A term used to refer to any disorder that is associated with changes in the structure of an organ or tissues. (See also *functional disorder*.)

organism

A general term for an individual animal or plant. Microscopically small organisms, such as *bacteria* and *viruses*, are termed *microorganisms*.

organ of Corti

A structure involved in hearing that is situated in the *cochlea* of the inner ear. Sensory hair cells in the organ of Corti vibrate in response to sounds and translate them into electrical impulses that travel via the cochlear nerve to the brain.

organomegaly

Abnormal enlargement of the body's internal organs, such as *hepatomegaly* (enlargement of the liver).

organophosphates

Highly poisonous agricultural insecticides that are harmful when absorbed through the skin, by inhalation, or by swallowing. Among the many possible symptoms are nausea, vomiting, abdominal cramps, diarrhoea, blurred vision, excessive sweating, headache, confusion, and twitching. In cases of severe poisoning, breathing difficulty, palpitations, seizures, and unconsciousness may occur. If left untreated, death may result.

Treatment of organophosphate poisoning may include washing out the stomach (see *lavage, gastric*) or removing soiled clothing and washing contaminated skin. Injections of *atropine* may be given, and *oxygen therapy* and/or artificial *ventilation* may be needed. With rapid treatment, people may survive doses that would otherwise have been fatal. Long-term effects of organophosphates in sheep dips are thought to be responsible for debilitating illness with neural, muscular, and mental symptoms.

orgasm

Intense sensations produced by a series of muscular contractions at the peak of sexual excitement. Orgasm usually lasts for about three to ten seconds but can last up to a minute in women.

In men, contractions of the muscles of the inner pelvis massage semen into the *urethra*; the semen is then forcefully propelled through the urethral orifice (see *ejaculation*).

Orgasm in women is associated with irregular contractions of the voluntary muscles of the walls of the *vagina* and, in some women, of the *uterus*, followed by relief of congestion in the pelvic area. Some women experience multiple

orgasms if stimulation is continued. Orgasm is usually followed by a refractory phase during which there is no physical response to further sexual stimulation. Both men and women may experience problems with orgasm (see *ejaculation, disorders of*; *orgasm, lack of*).

orgasm, lack of

Inability to achieve orgasm during sexual activity. The problem is more common in women than men. In either sex, failure to achieve orgasm may be due to inhibited sexual desire (see *sexual desire, inhibited*) or inability to become aroused or maintain arousal (see *frigidity*; *erectile dysfunction*). In men, there may be a problem achieving orgasm despite normal arousal (see *ejaculation, disorders of*). In women, lack of orgasm is the most common sexual problem, affecting up to 50 per cent of women at some time in their lives. Some are unable to achieve orgasm under any circumstances, others experience orgasm only occasionally.

For both sexes, contributory factors include problems with sexual technique or a relationship, lack of familiarity with sexual responses, psychological problems (such as anxiety, previous sexual trauma, or inhibitions), and fear of becoming pregnant.

Sex therapy, *relationship counselling*, and *psychotherapy* may be helpful.

orifice

A term used in anatomy to refer to any opening in the body, especially an entrance or outlet of a body cavity. An example of an orifice is the mouth.

orlistat

An anti-obesity drug used with a slimming diet to treat severe obesity. Unlike *appetite suppressants*, orlistat acts on the gastrointestinal tract, preventing the digestion of fats by lipases (pancreatic *enzymes*). Instead of being absorbed, the fats pass out of the body in faeces. Side effects are gastrointestinal in nature and can be minimized by reducing fat intake. Flatulence and faecal urgency are common. Deficiencies of fat-soluble vitamins may develop with prolonged use.

ornithosis

A disease of birds, caused by the microorganism CHLAMYDIA PSITTACI, that can cause *psittacosis* in humans.

oro-

A prefix pertaining to the *mouth*.

O

orphan drugs

Drugs that have been developed to treat rare conditions but are not manufactured generally.

orphenadrine

A *muscle-relaxant drug* used to treat the movement disorder *Parkinson's disease*. Side effects of orphenadrine include a dry mouth and blurred vision.

ORT

The abbreviation for *oral rehydration therapy*. (See also *rehydration therapy*.)

ortho-

A prefix meaning normal, correct, or straight, as in *orthopaedics*, a branch of surgery concerned with correcting disorders of the bones and joints.

orthodontic appliances

Fixed or removable devices, commonly known as braces, worn to correct *malocclusion* (an abnormal relationship between the upper and lower teeth) or to reposition overcrowded or *buck teeth*. Usually fitted during childhood and adolescence, a brace moves teeth using sustained gentle pressure.

A fixed appliance has brackets attached to the teeth through which an arch wire is threaded and tightened to exert pressure. These are usually kept in place for about a year, after which time a retainer plate may be needed to hold the teeth in place until tooth and jaw growth has finished.

Removable appliances, which consist of a plastic plate with attachments that anchor over the back teeth, are used when only one or a few teeth need correcting. They apply force by means of springs, wire bows, screws, or rubber bands fitted to the plate.

orthodontics

A branch of *dentistry* concerned with prevention and treatment of *malocclusion* (an abnormal relationship between the upper and lower teeth). The procedures are usually performed while teeth are developing and relatively manoeuvrable but can also be of benefit in adulthood.

An orthodontist may first make models of the teeth (see *impression, dental*) and take *X-rays* of the head and jaws. Certain teeth, often premolars, may be extracted to make room for the remaining teeth. Poorly positioned teeth are then moved by gentle pressure exerted by *orthodontic appliances*.

HOW **ORTHODONTIC APPLIANCES** WORK

The tooth sockets are remarkably responsive to sustained pressure against the teeth. Orthodontic appliances, which may be fixed or removable, provide such pressure. Even gentle pressure applied in a particular direction will move teeth. As they move, bone is remodelled so that the new position is stable.

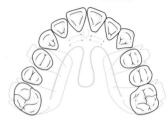

Overcrowding
This is frequently associated with malocclusion (poor alignment between upper and lower teeth). Some teeth have to be extracted to make room for others to be straightened.

FIXED APPLIANCES

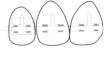

Appearance of brackets and wires
Brackets are fixed appliances cemented to the outer surface of the teeth; they have slots into which arch wires can be fitted.

Repositioning a tooth
By careful design of the arrangement of wires and spring, force can be exerted in any direction to move a tooth into the desired position.

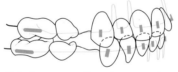

1 Teeth are removed to create space and an appliance made to correct the alignment of the remaining teeth and to close gaps between them.

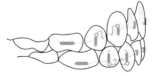

2 Once the teeth in the upper and lower jaws are completely aligned, the appliance is adjusted to tip or rotate the teeth in order to achieve a good appearance and bite.

REMOVABLE APPLIANCES

Arrangement of wires over teeth
These are easier to keep clean than fixed appliances and are less obtrusive, but they may interfere with speech; their efficiency relies on patients using them as directed. This type exerts pressure to push the teeth at the sides outwards.

Bow device
This simple wire spring acts by exerting force to straighten the tooth. Many bow devices are more complicated.

Direction of pull

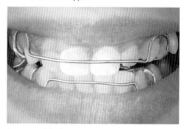

A removable bow
One of the many forms of orthodontic wire appliance, this bow device exerts pressure on the teeth at the sides, which straightens and moves them outwards.

---

orthognathic surgery

Operations to correct deformities of the jaw and the severe *malocclusion* (abnormal relationship between the upper and lower teeth) that is associated with them.

Orthognathic surgery is performed under general anaesthesia. A jaw that projects too far can be shortened by removing a block of bone from each side and manoeuvring the front of the jaw backwards. A jaw that is too short can be reshaped by dividing the bone on each side, sliding the front of the jaw forwards, and inserting bone grafts (taken from elsewhere in the body) into the gaps. After repositioning, the jaw bones often require wiring together (see *wiring of the jaws*) until they have healed.

orthomyxovirus

One of a family of *viruses* that includes the microorganisms responsible for respiratory tract diseases, especially *influenza*.

orthopaedics

The branch of surgery concerned with disorders of the *bones* and the *joints* and with their associated *muscles*, *tendons*, and *ligaments*.

orthopnoea

Difficulty in breathing when lying flat. Orthopnoea is a symptom of *heart failure* (the heart is no longer pumping blood efficiently) and *pulmonary oedema* (an accumulation of fluid in the lungs), and also occurs with *asthma* and chronic obstructive pulmonary disease (see *pulmonary disease, chronic obstructive*).

orthoptics

Techniques used mainly in children to measure and evaluate *squint*, including eye exercises, assessment of monocular and binocular vision, and measures to combat *amblyopia* (lazy eye).

orthostatic hypotension

Also called postural hypotension, low blood pressure that occurs on standing. Orthostatic hypotension may be caused by treatment with *antihypertensive drugs* or the failure of nerves that control the diameter of the blood vessels, often as a result of *diabetes mellitus*.

orthotics

Use of appliances to support or correct weakened or deformed limbs, joints, or other parts of the body.

os

An anatomical term for a bone. Os also refers to an opening in the body, as in the cervical os (entrance to the *uterus*).

oseltamivir

An *antiviral drug* used to prevent or treat *influenza* A and B virus infections. To be effective, the drug should be taken within 48 hours of the onset of symptoms. Oseltamivir is not a substitute for routine influenza vaccination, and it can be taken even by those who have been vaccinated. The drug may also help protect against the most serious effects of *avian influenza*. Possible side effects of oseltamivir include nausea, vomiting, and abdominal pain.

Osgood–Schlatter disease

Painful enlargement and tenderness of the tibial tuberosity, the bony prominence of the *tibia* (shin) just below the knee. The condition occurs most commonly in boys aged between 10 and 14 years of age. It may be the result of excessive, repetitive pulling of the *quadriceps muscle* at the front of the thigh due to repeated exercise. There is usually pain above and below the knee, which is worse during strenuous activity, and the tibial tuberosity is tender when touched. The disorder often clears up without treatment as long as sporting activity is restricted; severe pain may require *physiotherapy* or immobilization in a plaster *cast*.

Osler's disease

A rare inherited condition in which capillaries (tiny blood vessels) in the skin and mucous membranes, such as those lining the mouth and nose, become dilated, forming red spots. The condition, which is also known as hereditary haemorrhagic telangiectasia, is an autosomal dominant *genetic disorder*.

The lesions may bleed easily. Nosebleeds are a common symptom and may begin in childhood. Lesions may also develop in the digestive tract, causing recurrent bleeding leading to *anaemia*; in the lungs, causing blood to be coughed up; or in the brain, causing tissue damage and seizures.

Anaemia can be counteracted with iron supplements. In some cases, laser treatment is used to seal the lesions.

osmosis

The passage of a solvent from a weaker solution to a more concentrated one through a semipermeable membrane. All body cells are surrounded by such

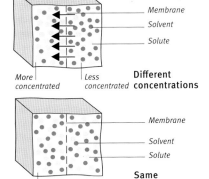

More concentrated — Less concentrated — **Different concentrations**

Membrane
Solvent
Solute

Same concentration — **Same concentration**

Membrane
Solvent
Solute

Osmosis
If two solutions, each consisting of different concentrations of a solute (e.g. salt) in a solvent (e.g. water), are separated by a semipermeable membrane, solvent moves from the weaker to the stronger solution until the two solutions attain equal concentration.

membranes, which allow water, salts, simple sugars (such as *glucose*), and *amino acids* (but not proteins) to pass through. Therefore, osmosis plays an important part in regulating the distribution of water and other substances that are present in body tissues.

osmotic diuresis

An increased output of *urine* by the *kidneys* due to the presence of one or more substances in the urine that draw water from the blood into the urine. Excessive amounts of *glucose* in the urine, as a result of *diabetes mellitus*, can produce this effect; another possible cause is treatment with one of the osmotic *diuretic drugs*, such as *mannitol*.

osseous

Bony or bonelike. The term "osseous" is sometimes used to refer to the bony parts of the inner *ear*. (See also *bone*.)

ossicle

A small bone, especially any of the three tiny bones in the middle *ear* (malleus, incus, and stapes) that are involved in conducting sound from the eardrum to the inner ear.

ossification

The process by which *bone* is formed, renewed, and repaired, which starts in the embryo and continues throughout a person's life. There are three main situations in which ossification occurs: bone growth, during which new bone forms at the *epiphyses* (ends) of bones; bone renewal as part of normal regeneration; and bone repair, which occurs following a *fracture*.

In newborn babies, the *diaphysis* (bone shaft) has begun to ossify and is composed mainly of bone tissue, while the epiphyses are made of cartilage that gradually hardens. In children, growth plates produce new cartilage to lengthen the bones and further bone forms at secondary ossification centres in the epiphyses. By the age of 18, the shafts, growth plates, and epiphyses have all ossified and fused into continuous bone, allowing no further growth.

osteitis

Inflammation of *bone*. The most common cause is infection, usually by bacteria (see *osteomyelitis*). Other causes of osteitis include *Paget's disease* and *hyperparathyroidism* (overactivity of the parathyroid glands).

O

osteitis deformans

An alternative term for *Paget's disease*.

osteo-

A prefix that is used to denote a relationship to bone, as in *osteoporosis*, which is a condition that causes the bones to become thin and weaken.

osteoarthritis

A common *joint* disease, osteoarthritis is characterized by degeneration of the cartilage that lines the joints or by formation of *osteophytes* (bony outgrowths), leading to pain, stiffness, and occasionally loss of function. Osteoarthritis is the most common form of *arthritis*. *Cervical osteoarthritis* is a particular form of osteoarthritis that affects mainly the joints between the cervical *vertebrae* (the bones in the neck).

CAUSES AND SYMPTOMS

Osteoarthritis is due to inflammation and destruction of the cartilage that occurs at joint surfaces and changes to the bone beneath. This condition is most likely to occur in the weight-bearing joints as well as in any joints that have previously suffered damage. However, these are not the only causes: genetic factors may also be involved.

Evidence of osteoarthritis can be seen on *X-rays* of almost everyone over the age of 60; however, not all of these people have symptoms. Factors that lead to the development of osteoarthritis at an earlier age include excessive wear of, or injury to, a joint; congenital deformity or misalignment of the bones in a joint; *obesity*; or inflammation from another disease such as *gout*. Severe osteoarthritis is more common in women than men.

Affected joints become enlarged and distorted by osteophytes, which are responsible for the gnarled appearance of arthritic hands. Weakness and shrinkage of surrounding muscles may occur if pain prevents regular use of the joint.

TREATMENT

There is no cure for osteoarthritis. Pain can be relieved by *analgesics* and *nonsteroidal anti-inflammatory drugs*; injection of *corticosteroid drugs* into an affected joint or of hyaluronic acid into an affected knee may temporarily relieve symptoms; *physiotherapy* to improve muscle strength around the affected joints can help limit the deterioration that otherwise results from joint instability. *Glucosamine* may also relieve symptoms in some people. In overweight people, weight loss often alleviates symptoms of osteoarthritis. If the condition is severe, various aids are available that can make everyday tasks easier. Surgery, including *arthroplasty* and *arthrodesis*, is only undertaken if the pain and disability are too severe to cope with.

osteoarthropathy, hypertrophic pulmonary

A *bone* disorder almost always associated with *lung cancer*. Symptoms include pain and swelling of the wrists and ankles, accompanied by clubbing of the fingers. The condition will disappear if the underlying cancer is treated successfully. Symptoms can be partially relieved with *nonsteroidal anti-inflammatory drugs*.

osteoblastoma

A painful, noncancerous *bone tumour* that is characterized by the formation of osteoid tissue and primitive bone. Osteoblastomas most commonly occur in the spine of a young person.

osteochondritis dissecans

Degeneration of a *bone* just under a joint surface, causing fragments of bone and cartilage to become separated; this may cause the joint to lock. The condition commonly affects the knee and usually starts in adolescence. Symptoms include aching discomfort and intermittent swelling of the affected joint.

If a fragment has not completely separated from the bone, the joint may be immobilized in a plaster *cast* to allow reattachment to occur. Loose bone or cartilage fragments in the knee are removed during *arthroscopy*. Disruption to the smoothness of the joint surface increases the risk of *osteoarthritis*.

OSTEOARTHRITIS

Osteoarthritis differs from rheumatoid arthritis and has a better outlook. It is characterized by degeneration of cartilage or by formation of bony outgrowths (osteophytes). It results from excessive wear on joints or to slight deformity or misalignment of bones in a joint. Inflammation from a disease, such as gout, may also lead to osteoarthritis. Weight-bearing joints, such as those in the neck, the lower back, the knees, and hips, are the areas most commonly affected.

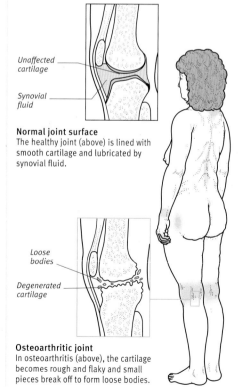

Unaffected cartilage
Synovial fluid

Normal joint surface
The healthy joint (above) is lined with smooth cartilage and lubricated by synovial fluid.

Loose bodies
Degenerated cartilage

Osteoarthritic joint
In osteoarthritis (above), the cartilage becomes rough and flaky and small pieces break off to form loose bodies.

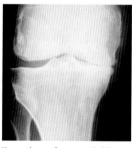

X-ray signs of osteoarthritis
In this X-ray of a knee joint, there is narrowing of the joint space with osteophyte production and an increase in density of the bone ends.

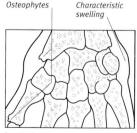

Osteophytes   *Characteristic swelling*

Osteophytes
These are outgrowths of new bone that tend to occur at the margins of the joint surfaces in osteoarthritis.

orthopaedics

The branch of surgery concerned with disorders of the *bones* and the *joints* and with their associated *muscles*, *tendons*, and *ligaments*.

orthopnoea

Difficulty in breathing when lying flat. Orthopnoea is a symptom of *heart failure* (the heart is no longer pumping blood efficiently) and *pulmonary oedema* (an accumulation of fluid in the lungs), and also occurs with *asthma* and chronic obstructive pulmonary disease (see *pulmonary disease, chronic obstructive*).

orthoptics

Techniques used mainly in children to measure and evaluate *squint*, including eye exercises, assessment of monocular and binocular vision, and measures to combat *amblyopia* (lazy eye).

orthostatic hypotension

Also called postural hypotension, low blood pressure that occurs on standing. Orthostatic hypotension may be caused by treatment with *antihypertensive drugs* or the failure of nerves that control the diameter of the blood vessels, often as a result of *diabetes mellitus*.

orthotics

Use of appliances to support or correct weakened or deformed limbs, joints, or other parts of the body.

os

An anatomical term for a bone. Os also refers to an opening in the body, as in the cervical os (entrance to the *uterus*).

oseltamivir

An *antiviral drug* used to prevent or treat *influenza* A and B virus infections. To be effective, the drug should be taken within 48 hours of the onset of symptoms. Oseltamivir is not a substitute for routine influenza vaccination, and it can be taken even by those who have been vaccinated. The drug may also help protect against the most serious effects of *avian influenza*. Possible side effects of oseltamivir include nausea, vomiting, and abdominal pain.

Osgood–Schlatter disease

Painful enlargement and tenderness of the tibial tuberosity, the bony prominence of the *tibia* (shin) just below the knee. The condition occurs most commonly in boys aged between 10 and 14 years of age. It may be the result of excessive, repetitive pulling of the *quadriceps muscle* at the front of the thigh due to repeated exercise. There is usually pain above and below the knee, which is worse during strenuous activity, and the tibial tuberosity is tender when touched. The disorder often clears up without treatment as long as sporting activity is restricted; severe pain may require *physiotherapy* or immobilization in a plaster *cast*.

Osler's disease

A rare inherited condition in which capillaries (tiny blood vessels) in the skin and mucous membranes, such as those lining the mouth and nose, become dilated, forming red spots. The condition, which is also known as hereditary haemorrhagic telangiectasia, is an autosomal dominant *genetic disorder*.

The lesions may bleed easily. Nosebleeds are a common symptom and may begin in childhood. Lesions may also develop in the digestive tract, causing recurrent bleeding leading to *anaemia*; in the lungs, causing blood to be coughed up; or in the brain, causing tissue damage and seizures.

Anaemia can be counteracted with iron supplements. In some cases, laser treatment is used to seal the lesions.

osmosis

The passage of a solvent from a weaker solution to a more concentrated one through a semipermeable membrane. All body cells are surrounded by such

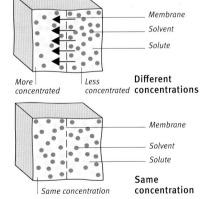

More concentrated | Less concentrated | **Different concentrations**

Membrane
Solvent
Solute

Same concentration | **Same concentration**

Membrane
Solvent
Solute

Osmosis
If two solutions, each consisting of different concentrations of a solute (e.g. salt) in a solvent (e.g. water), are separated by a semipermeable membrane, solvent moves from the weaker to the stronger solution until the two solutions attain equal concentration.

membranes, which allow water, salts, simple sugars (such as *glucose*), and *amino acids* (but not proteins) to pass through. Therefore, osmosis plays an important part in regulating the distribution of water and other substances that are present in body tissues.

osmotic diuresis

An increased output of *urine* by the *kidneys* due to the presence of one or more substances in the urine that draw water from the blood into the urine. Excessive amounts of *glucose* in the urine, as a result of *diabetes mellitus*, can produce this effect; another possible cause is treatment with one of the osmotic *diuretic drugs*, such as *mannitol*.

osseous

Bony or bonelike. The term "osseous" is sometimes used to refer to the bony parts of the inner *ear*. (See also *bone*.)

ossicle

A small bone, especially any of the three tiny bones in the middle *ear* (malleus, incus, and stapes) that are involved in conducting sound from the eardrum to the inner ear.

ossification

The process by which *bone* is formed, renewed, and repaired, which starts in the embryo and continues throughout a person's life. There are three main situations in which ossification occurs: bone growth, during which new bone forms at the *epiphyses* (ends) of bones; bone renewal as part of normal regeneration; and bone repair, which occurs following a *fracture*.

In newborn babies, the *diaphysis* (bone shaft) has begun to ossify and is composed mainly of bone tissue, while the epiphyses are made of cartilage that gradually hardens. In children, growth plates produce new cartilage to lengthen the bones and further bone forms at secondary ossification centres in the epiphyses. By the age of 18, the shafts, growth plates, and epiphyses have all ossified and fused into continuous bone, allowing no further growth.

osteitis

Inflammation of *bone*. The most common cause is infection, usually by bacteria (see *osteomyelitis*). Other causes of osteitis include *Paget's disease* and *hyperparathyroidism* (overactivity of the parathyroid glands).

osteitis deformans

An alternative term for *Paget's disease*.

osteo-

A prefix that is used to denote a relationship to bone, as in *osteoporosis*, which is a condition that causes the bones to become thin and weaken.

osteoarthritis

A common *joint* disease, osteoarthritis is characterized by degeneration of the cartilage that lines the joints or by formation of *osteophytes* (bony outgrowths), leading to pain, stiffness, and occasionally loss of function. Osteoarthritis is the most common form of *arthritis*. *Cervical osteoarthritis* is a particular form of osteoarthritis that affects mainly the joints between the cervical *vertebrae* (the bones in the neck).

CAUSES AND SYMPTOMS

Osteoarthritis is due to inflammation and destruction of the cartilage that occurs at joint surfaces and changes to the bone beneath. This condition is most likely to occur in the weight-bearing joints as well as in any joints that have previously suffered damage. However, these are not the only causes: genetic factors may also be involved.

Evidence of osteoarthritis can be seen on *X-rays* of almost everyone over the age of 60; however, not all of these people have symptoms. Factors that lead to the development of osteoarthritis at an earlier age include excessive wear of, or injury to, a joint; congenital deformity or misalignment of the bones in a joint; *obesity*; or inflammation from another disease such as *gout*. Severe osteoarthritis is more common in women than men.

Affected joints become enlarged and distorted by osteophytes, which are responsible for the gnarled appearance of arthritic hands. Weakness and shrinkage of surrounding muscles may occur if pain prevents regular use of the joint.

TREATMENT

There is no cure for osteoarthritis. Pain can be relieved by *analgesics* and *nonsteroidal anti-inflammatory drugs*; injection of *corticosteroid drugs* into an affected joint or of hyaluronic acid into an affected knee may temporarily relieve symptoms; *physiotherapy* to improve muscle strength around the affected joints can help limit the deterioration that otherwise results from joint instability. *Glucosamine* may also relieve symptoms in some people. In overweight people, weight loss often alleviates symptoms of osteoarthritis. If the condition is severe, various aids are available that can make everyday tasks easier. Surgery, including *arthroplasty* and *arthrodesis*, is only undertaken if the pain and disability are too severe to cope with.

osteoarthropathy, hypertrophic pulmonary

A *bone* disorder almost always associated with *lung cancer*. Symptoms include pain and swelling of the wrists and ankles, accompanied by clubbing of the fingers. The condition will disappear if the underlying cancer is treated successfully. Symptoms can be partially relieved with *nonsteroidal anti-inflammatory drugs*.

osteoblastoma

A painful, noncancerous *bone tumour* that is characterized by the formation of osteoid tissue and primitive bone. Osteoblastomas most commonly occur in the spine of a young person.

osteochondritis dissecans

Degeneration of a *bone* just under a joint surface, causing fragments of bone and cartilage to become separated; this may cause the joint to lock. The condition commonly affects the knee and usually starts in adolescence. Symptoms include aching discomfort and intermittent swelling of the affected joint.

If a fragment has not completely separated from the bone, the joint may be immobilized in a plaster *cast* to allow reattachment to occur. Loose bone or cartilage fragments in the knee are removed during *arthroscopy*. Disruption to the smoothness of the joint surface increases the risk of *osteoarthritis*.

OSTEOARTHRITIS

Osteoarthritis differs from rheumatoid arthritis and has a better outlook. It is characterized by degeneration of cartilage or by formation of bony outgrowths (osteophytes). It results from excessive wear on joints or to slight deformity or misalignment of bones in a joint. Inflammation from a disease, such as gout, may also lead to osteoarthritis. Weight-bearing joints, such as those in the neck, the lower back, the knees, and hips, are the areas most commonly affected.

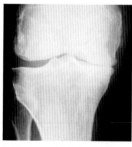

Normal joint surface
The healthy joint (above) is lined with smooth cartilage and lubricated by synovial fluid.

Unaffected cartilage
Synovial fluid

Loose bodies
Degenerated cartilage

Osteoarthritic joint
In osteoarthritis (above), the cartilage becomes rough and flaky and small pieces break off to form loose bodies.

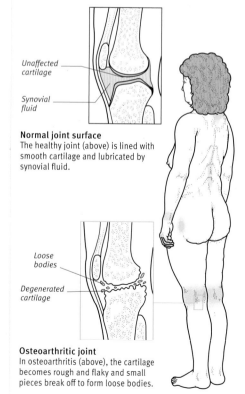

X-ray signs of osteoarthritis
In this X-ray of a knee joint, there is narrowing of the joint space with osteophyte production and an increase in density of the bone ends.

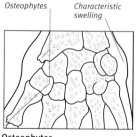

Osteophytes   *Characteristic swelling*

Osteophytes
These are outgrowths of new bone that tend to occur at the margins of the joint surfaces in osteoarthritis.

osteochondritis juvenilis

Inflammation of an *epiphysis* (growing end of bone) occurring in children and adolescents. Osteochondritis juvenilis causes pain, tenderness, and restricted movement if the epiphysis forms part of a joint. The inflammation leads to softening of the bone, which may result in deformity. The condition may be due to disruption of the bone's blood supply. There are several types of osteochondritis juvenilis: *Perthes' disease*; Scheuermann's disease, which affects several adjoining vertebrae; and other types that affect certain bones in the foot and wrist.

The affected bone may need to be immobilized in an orthopaedic *brace* or *plaster cast*. In Perthes' disease, surgery may be required to prevent more deformity. The bone usually regenerates within three years and rehardens, but deformity may be permanent and increases the risk of *osteoarthritis* in later life.

osteochondroma

A noncancerous *bone* tumour, which is formed from a stalk of bone capped with cartilage, and appears as a hard round swelling near a joint. An osteochondroma develops in late childhood and early adolescence, usually from the side of a long bone near the knee or shoulder. The tumour causes problems only if it interferes with the movement of tendons or the surrounding joint, in which case surgical removal may be necessary. Large osteochondromas can interfere with skeletal growth, and may cause deformity.

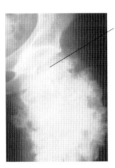

Head of femur

X-ray of osteochondroma
The X-ray shows the fluffy outline of an osteochondroma that is surrounding the head of the femur. These benign tumours are composed of cartilage-forming cells.

osteochondrosis

See *osteochondritis juvenilis*.

osteodystrophy

Any generalized bone defect caused by *metabolic disorders*. Types of osteodystrophy include *rickets*; *osteomalacia*; and bone cysts and bone mass reduction associated with chronic *kidney failure* or *hyperparathyroidism* (overactivity of the parathyroid glands). In adults, an osteodystrophy is usually reversible if the underlying cause is treated before bone deformity occurs.

osteogenesis imperfecta

A *congenital* condition characterized by abnormally brittle *bones* that are unusually susceptible to *fractures*.

CAUSE AND SYMPTOMS

The condition is caused by an inherited defect in the *connective tissue* that forms the basic material of bone. Severely affected infants are born with multiple fractures and a soft skull and they do not usually survive. Other sufferers have many fractures during infancy and childhood, often as a result of normal handling and activities, and it may be difficult to distinguish the condition from *child abuse*.

A common sign of osteogenesis imperfecta is that the whites of the eyes are abnormally thin, making them appear blue. Sufferers may also be deaf as a result of *otosclerosis*. In very mild cases, osteogenesis imperfecta may not be detected until adolescence or later.

TREATMENT AND OUTLOOK

There is no specific treatment for the condition. Fractures are immobilized and usually heal quickly, but they may cause shortening and deformity of the limbs, resulting in abnormal, stunted growth. Skull fractures may cause brain damage or death. Parents may have *genetic counselling* to estimate the risk of the condition occurring in future children. Severe cases can be diagnosed prenatally by *ultrasound scanning*.

osteogenic sarcoma

See *osteosarcoma*.

osteoid osteoma

A *bone* disorder in which a tiny abnormal area of bone, usually in a long bone, causes deep pain, which is typically worse at night. The condition is cured by removing the area of bone. (See also *osteoma*.)

osteoma

A hard, noncancerous, usually small tumour that may occur on any bone in the body. Surgical removal of the osteoma may be necessary if it causes symptoms through pressing on surrounding structures.

osteomalacia

The softening, weakening, and demineralization of an adult's *bones* as a result of a deficiency of *vitamin D*. Rickets is the equivalent disease in children.

The development and maintenance of healthy bone requires an adequate intake of calcium and phosphorus from the diet, but these minerals cannot be absorbed by the body without a sufficient amount of vitamin D. This vitamin is obtained from certain foods (such as butter, fish, eggs, and fish-liver oils) and from the action of sunlight on the skin.

CAUSES

Osteomalacia can be caused by various factors, including insufficient vitamin D in the diet; insufficient exposure to sunlight; or inadequate intestinal absorption of vitamin D (see *malabsorption*), caused by a disorder such as *coeliac disease*, or following intestinal surgery. Rare causes include *kidney failure, acidosis* (increased acidity of body fluids), and certain inherited *metabolic disorders*.

Osteomalacia is uncommon in developed countries, but it may affect people who have poor diets (especially dark-skinned people who have little exposure to sunlight).

SYMPTOMS

Osteomalacia causes bone pain, especially in the neck, legs, hips, and ribs. In addition, muscle weakness, particularly at the hips, can make it very difficult to stand up and to climb stairs. If the blood calcium level is very low, there may be *tetany* (muscle spasms) in the hands, feet, and throat. Weakened bones are vulnerable to distortion and fractures, which are often painless.

TREATMENT

Treatment is with a diet rich in vitamin D and increased exposure to sunlight; vitamin D supplements may be given in some cases. Calcium supplements may also be given if osteomalacia is due to malabsorption.

osteomyelitis

Infection, usually by bacteria, of *bone* and *bone marrow*. It is relatively rare in developed countries but is more common in children, most often affecting the long arm and leg bones and vertebrae; in adults, it usually affects the *vertebrae*. The condition may be either acute or chronic.

ACUTE OSTEOMYELITIS

In acute osteomyelitis, the infection (which is usually caused by the bacterium *STAPHYLOCOCCUS AUREUS*) enters the

O

bloodstream via a skin wound or as a result of infection elsewhere in the body. The infected bone and marrow become inflamed; pus forms, causing fever, severe pain and tenderness in the bone, and inflammation and swelling of the skin over the affected area.

Prompt treatment with high doses of *antibiotic drugs*, initially given intravenously and continued over several weeks or months, usually cures acute osteomyelitis. If the condition fails to respond, surgery has to be performed to remove infected and dead bone and drain away any pus.

CHRONIC OSTEOMYELITIS

Chronic osteomyelitis may develop if acute osteomyelitis is neglected or fails to respond to treatment; after a compound *fracture*; or due to infection of the bone with MYCOBACTERIUM TUBERCULOSIS, which causes *tuberculosis*.

The condition causes constant pain in the affected bone. Complications include persistent deformity and, in children, arrest of growth in the affected bone. Involvement of the spine can result in damage to the spinal cord if the condition is not treated. In the later stages of the disease, *amyloidosis* (abnormal deposits of a starchy substance in vital organs) may develop.

Chronic osteomyelitis requires surgical removal of all affected bone, sometimes followed by a *bone graft*; antibiotic drugs are also prescribed.

osteopathy

A system of diagnosis and treatment that recognizes the role of the musculoskeletal system in the healthy functioning of the body. The basic principle of osteopathy is that all body systems operate in unison, and disturbances in one system can alter the functions of others. An osteopath uses manipulation, rhythmic stretching, and pressure to restore mobility to the joints. He or she also uses traditional diagnostic and therapeutic methods to diagnose and treat dysfunction.

osteopenia

Any decrease in *bone* mass below the normal level. The term is used particularly to refer to a decrease in mass that occurs when the body makes too little new bone to compensate for normal bone lysis (breakdown or destruction). Osteopenia can occur throughout the skeleton or may be confined to a specific area, such as the bones adjacent to a diseased or damaged joint.

osteopetrosis

A very rare inherited disorder in which *bones* harden and become denser. Deficiency of one of the two types of bone cell responsible for healthy bone growth results in a disruption of normal bone structure. In its mildest form, there may be no symptoms. More severe forms result in abnormally high susceptibility to *fractures*; stunted growth; deformity; and *anaemia*. Pressure on nerves may cause blindness, deafness, and facial paralysis.

Most treatments aim to relieve symptoms. Bone marrow transplants of cells from which healthy bone cells might develop are done in some cases.

osteophyte

An outgrowth of *bone* at the boundary of a joint. The formation of osteophytes is a characteristic feature of *osteoarthritis* that contributes to the deformity and restricted movement of affected joints.

osteoporosis

A disease in which there is loss of bone tissue (and so loss of bone density), causing bones to become brittle and fracture easily.

CAUSES

Thinning of the bones is a natural part of the aging process. However, women are especially vulnerable to loss of bone density after the *menopause*, because their *ovaries* no longer produce *oestrogen hormones*, which help maintain bone mass.

Other causes of osteoporosis include premature removal of the ovaries; a diet that is deficient in calcium; certain hormonal disorders, such as an overactive thyroid gland (see *hyperthyroidism*); long-term treatment with *corticosteroid drugs*; and prolonged immobility. Osteoporosis is most common in heavy smokers and drinkers, and in very thin people.

SYMPTOMS

Osteoporosis may go undiagnosed for many years. The first sign is often a fracture, typically at the wrist or the top of the *femur* (thigh bone), after what may have been a trivial injury. One or several *vertebrae* may fracture spontaneously and cause the bones to crumble, leading to progressive height loss and/or pain due to compression of spinal nerve roots.

DIAGNOSIS AND TREATMENT

Osteoporosis is confirmed using *densitometry*, such as a *DEXA scan*.

Bone loss can be minimized with adequate dietary calcium and vitamin D, and regular, sustained exercise to build up the bones and maintain their strength. *Bisphosphonate drugs* may be prescribed to help prevent bone loss. If these drugs are not suitable, *raloxifene*, strontium ranalate (see *strontium*), or calcitonin may be given. *Hormone replacement therapy (HRT)* may be considered for postmenopausal women when other treatments have been ineffective or are unsuitable. Women who have gone through a premature menopause (before the age of 45) may be advised to have HRT until the age of 50 to protect against their higher risk of osteoporosis.

osteosarcoma

A cancerous tumour of the bone that can spread to the lungs and, less commonly, to other areas. An osteosarcoma usually develops in people between the ages of ten and 25, generally in a long bone of the arm or leg, often around the knee. Osteosarcomas may also be seen in elderly people as a rare complication of *Paget's disease* or of previous treatment with *radiotherapy*. The tumour causes pain and swelling of the affected bone if it occurs near the surface.

In the past, amputation of the affected limb was inevitable. However, the outlook has improved due to a combination of *chemotherapy* and surgery in which the diseased bone is replaced with a custom-made *prosthesis*.

osteosclerosis

Increased *bone density*, which is visible on *X-rays* as an area of extreme whiteness. Localized osteosclerosis may be caused by a severe injury that compresses the bone, the joint disorder *osteoarthritis*, chronic *osteomyelitis* (bone infection), or an *osteoma* (noncancerous bone tumour). Osteosclerosis occurs throughout the body in the inherited bone disorder *osteopetrosis*.

osteotomy

Surgery to alter the alignment or length of a *bone*, by cutting it. Osteotomy is used to correct *hallux valgus* (a deformity of the big toe) that has caused a *bunion*; *coxa vara* (a deformity of the hip); or deformity caused by congenital hip dislocation (see *developmental dysplasia of the hip*). Osteotomy is also used to straighten a long bone that has healed crookedly after a *fracture*, or to shorten the uninjured leg if a fractured leg has shortened during healing (see *leg, shortening of*).

ostium

An anatomical term for an opening.

OSTEOPOROSIS

In osteoporosis, the density of bones decreases, and their brittleness increases, although there is no change in size or composition. Women past the menopause are the most commonly affected because their ovaries no longer produce oestrogen, which helps to maintain bone mass. The risk of the condition is greater in a woman who undergoes the menopause early, or whose mother had osteoporosis.

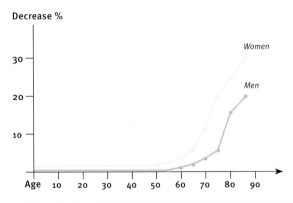

Normal bone cross-section
Bone consists of fibres of collagen (a protein), which give elasticity, and calcium, which gives hardness.

Bone marrow

Soft, spongy bone

Hard, dense bone

Less dense bone

Osteoporotic bone
Thinning is mainly due to loss of collagen, which takes calcium with it. Both hard and spongy bone tissues are affected.

Bone loss with age
The graph on the right shows how the percentage of bone lost increases in both sexes from age 50 onwards, with the losses particularly marked in women after the menopause. By age 80, up to half of all women have sustained at least one fracture due to osteoporosis, a much higher proportion than in men.

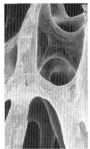

Decrease %

Women

Men

30

20

10

Age   10   20   30   40   50   60   70   80   90

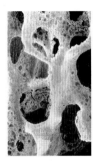

Bone tissue affected by osteoporosis
When compared with normal bone tissue (left), the osteoporotic bone (right) is far less dense and appears thin and brittle.

-ostomy

A term that is used to describe a surgical opening (for example, *colostomy*) or a junction of two hollow organs.

otalgia

The medical term for *earache*.

OTC drug

See *over-the-counter drug*.

otitis externa

Inflammation of the outer-ear canal, commonly due to infection (see *Ear infections* box, overleaf). It usually causes swelling, a discharge, and, in some people, *eczema* around the opening of the ear canal. The ear may be itchy and painful and blocked with pus, causing deafness.

CAUSES

Generalized infection of the canal, and sometimes of the pinna (external ear), may be due to a fungal or bacterial infection. The ear may also sometimes become inflamed as part of a generalized skin disorder such as atopic eczema or seborrhoeic *dermatitis*.

TREATMENT

Often, the only treatment required is to keep the ear clean and dry until the infection has cleared. Locally acting preparations that contain *antibiotic drugs*, *antifungal drugs*, and/or *corticosteroid drugs* may be used. Oral antibiotics may be given to treat bacterial infections if they are severe.

otitis media

Inflammation of the middle *ear*, the cavity between the eardrum and the inner ear, (see *Ear infections* box, overleaf).

CAUSES

This condition is due to a viral or bacterial infection that has usually travelled up the *eustachian tube*, the passage that runs from the back of the nose to the middle ear. The tube may become blocked by inflammation or enlarged *adenoids*, causing fluid and/or pus to accumulate in the middle ear rather than draining away through the tube. Children, particularly those under seven years, are especially susceptible to otitis media because of the shortness of their eustachian tubes; some children have recurrent attacks.

SYMPTOMS

Acute otitis media can cause sudden severe earache, a feeling of fullness in the ear, deafness, *tinnitus* (ringing or buzzing in the ear) and fever. The eardrum may burst, discharging pus and relieving pain, in which case healing usually occurs within a few weeks.

DIAGNOSIS AND TREATMENT

The condition is diagnosed by examination of the middle ear with an *otoscope*; the eardrum appears red and may bulge outwards. Treatment is with *analgesic drugs* (painkillers) and many cases clear up in a few days without further treatment. If the infection is severe or does not clear up quickly, *antibiotic drugs* may be prescribed, although such drugs are not effective against viral infections.

COMPLICATIONS

A complication of otitis media is *glue ear*, in which a thick fluid builds up in the ear and affects hearing. Glue ear may follow severe or recurrent otitis media, which occurs mainly in children.

In rare cases, the infection spreads inwards to cause *mastoiditis* (inflammation of the mastoid bone in the skull).

otoacoustic emission

An echo emitted by the inner *ear* in response to sound. The emission is produced only by a normally functioning ear and is recorded in a test to detect impaired hearing.

O

EAR INFECTIONS: **OTITIS MEDIA AND OTITIS EXTERNA**

Inflammation of the middle ear (otitis media) or ear canal (otitis externa) usually results from infection and may cause earache. Otitis media is more common in children and may be acute (with sudden onset of pain) or chronic (continuing over a long period).

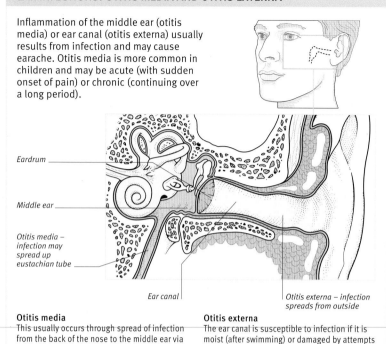

Eardrum

Middle ear

Otitis media – infection may spread up eustachian tube

Ear canal

Otitis externa – infection spreads from outside

Otitis media
This usually occurs through spread of infection from the back of the nose to the middle ear via the eustachian tube.

Otitis externa
The ear canal is susceptible to infection if it is moist (after swimming) or damaged by attempts to remove earwax.

otomycosis

A fungal *ear* infection that causes inflammation of the ear canal and the external ear (see *otitis externa*).

otoplasty

Cosmetic surgery on the external *ear* usually carried out to make protruding ears lie closer to the head. Otoplasty may also be performed to construct a missing ear in a child born with part or all of one missing, or to reconstruct a damaged ear.

otorhinolaryngology

A surgical speciality, also known as ENT surgery, concerned with diseases of the *ear*, *nose*, and *throat*. ENT specialists treat *sinus* problems, *otitis media*, *tonsillitis*, minor hearing loss, *otosclerosis*, *Ménière's disease*, airway problems in children, uncontrollable nosebleeds, and cancer of the *larynx* (voicebox) and *sinuses*.

otorrhoea

A discharge of pus or other fluid from the ear (see *ear, discharge from*).

otosclerosis

A disorder of the middle *ear* that causes progressive *deafness*. The condition usually develops in both ears.

CAUSES AND INCIDENCE

Otosclerosis occurs when overgrowth of bone immobilizes the *stapes* (the innermost one of the three tiny bones in the middle ear). As a result, sound vibrations are prevented from passing along the bone to the inner ear.

Otosclerosis frequently runs in families, and symptoms usually start to appear in early adulthood. The condition affects more women than men, and often develops during pregnancy.

SYMPTOMS AND SIGNS

To an affected person, sounds are muffled but can be distinguished more easily if there is background noise.

Hearing loss progresses slowly over 10 to 15 years and is often accompanied by *tinnitus* (ringing in the ears) and, more rarely, *vertigo* (a spinning sensation). A degree of sensorineural deafness may develop, making high tones difficult to hear and causing the sufferer to speak loudly.

DIAGNOSIS AND TREATMENT

The condition is diagnosed by *hearing tests*. It can be cured by *stapedectomy*, a surgical procedure in which the stapes is replaced by a tiny piston, which moves through a hole created in the inner ear. Because the piston can move

freely, it can transmit sound vibrations to the inner ear. Alternatively, a *hearing-aid* can markedly improve hearing.

otoscope

An instrument, also called an auroscope, for examining the outer-ear canal and the eardrum. An otoscope illuminates and magnifies the inside of the ear. Otoscopy (examination using an otoscope) is performed in order to detect physical abnormalities such as inflammation or pus in the outer-ear canal (see *otitis externa*) and distortion or rupture of the eardrum.

OTOSCOPE

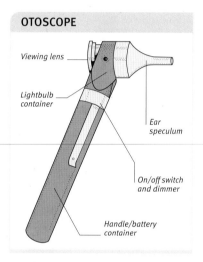

Viewing lens

Lightbulb container

Ear speculum

On/off switch and dimmer

Handle/battery container

ototoxicity

Toxic damage to the structures of the inner *ear*. High doses of certain drugs, such as *aminoglycoside* antibiotics, may cause this type of ear damage.

out-of-body experience

A feeling of leaving one's body and observing oneself from another dimension. The experience, thought to be due to disturbance of brain function, is reported by some patients after a general anaesthetic or a medical emergency.

outpatient treatment

Medical care on a same-day basis in a hospital or clinic.

ovarian cyst

An abnormal, fluid-filled swelling in an *ovary*. Ovarian cysts are common and, in most cases, noncancerous; however, the likelihood of a cyst being cancerous increases with age. In some cases, both of the ovaries have multiple cysts (see *ovary, polycystic*).

TYPES

The most common type of ovarian cyst, called a follicular cyst, is one in which the egg-producing ovarian follicle enlarges and fills with fluid. Cysts may also occur in the corpus luteum, a mass of tissue that forms from the follicle after *ovulation*.

Other types of ovarian cysts include *dermoid cysts* and mucous or serous cystadenomas (see *adenoma*), which can grow to a very large size. In some cases, an ovarian cyst may be due to *ovarian cancer*, particularly in postmenopausal women.

SYMPTOMS

Ovarian cysts often produce no symptoms, but some may cause abdominal swelling or discomfort, pain during sexual intercourse, or irregularities of menstruation, including *amenorrhoea*, *menorrhagia*, and *dysmenorrhoea*. Severe abdominal pain, nausea, and fever may develop if twisting or rupture of an ovarian cyst occurs. Surgery is required to treat these conditions.

DIAGNOSIS AND TREATMENT

An ovarian cyst may be discovered during the course of a routine *pelvic examination*. If a cyst is detected, *ultrasound scanning* will then be carried out to confirm its and its position and size.

In many cases, simple ovarian cysts (thin-walled or fluid-filled cysts) disappear without treatment. Complex cysts (such as dermoid cysts) usually require surgical removal. In some cases, aspiration (withdrawal by suction) of fluid under the guidance of ultrasound, or during *laparoscopy*, may be possible. If an ovarian cyst is particularly large, the ovary may need to be removed by surgery (see *oophorectomy*).

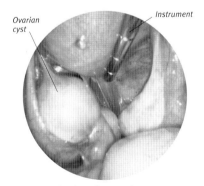

Laparoscopic view of an ovarian cyst
This photograph shows an ovarian cyst (centre left) that has formed at the ovary as a result of endometriosis, a condition in which fragments of uterine tissue locate in other parts of the body.

ovary

One of a pair of almond-shaped glands situated on either side of the *uterus* immediately below the opening of the *fallopian tubes*. Each ovary contains numerous cavities called *follicles*, in which egg cells (see *ovum*) develop. The ovaries also produce the female sex hormones *oestrogen* and *progesterone*.

ovary, cancer of

A malignant growth of the *ovary*. The cancer may be either primary (arising in the ovary) or secondary (resulting from the spread of cancer from another part of the body).

INCIDENCE AND CAUSES

Ovarian cancer can occur at any age but is most common in women after the *menopause* and in those who have never had children. A family history of cancer of the ovary, breast, or colon, especially in close relatives under 50, is an important risk factor. In particular, women who have inherited certain mutations on the *BRCA1 and BRCA2* genes (which are associated with breast cancer) have an increased risk of developing ovarian cancer. Having taken *oral contraceptives* in the past reduces the risk.

SYMPTOMS

In most cases, ovarian cancer causes no symptoms until it is widespread. The first symptoms may include vague discomfort and swelling in the abdomen; nausea and vomiting; and abnormal vaginal bleeding. The swelling may be due to the tumour itself or to *ascites* (excess fluid in the abdominal cavity).

DIAGNOSIS AND TREATMENT

Diagnosis of ovarian cancer involves a physical examination, *ultrasound scanning*, and *blood tests* to measure levels of a substance produced by the tumour. The tumour is usually surgically removed, along with the uterus (see *hysterectomy*) and the unaffected ovary. In younger women whose cancer is found early, it is sometimes possible to perform less radical surgery and preserve fertility. The extent of spread within the abdomen is assessed during surgery.

Surgery is followed by *chemotherapy*, unless the cancer was detected at a very early stage. Platinum-based drugs, which are combined with *paclitaxel*, are usually given. Survival rates depend on the type of tumour and how far advanced it is at the time of diagnosis. As the disease is often quite advanced, less than one in four women survive for more than five years.

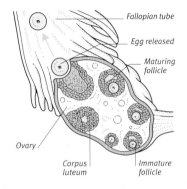

Each ovary consists of glandular cells and egg-producing follicles. After ovulation, each follicle forms a corpus luteum.

Fallopian tube

Egg released

Maturing follicle

Ovary

Corpus luteum

Immature follicle

ovary, disorders of

Disorders of the ovaries can occur for various reasons. The absence of ovaries, or their failure to develop normally, is rare and is due to a chromosomal abnormality (see *Turner's syndrome*). Oophoritis (inflammation of an ovary) may result from infections such as *gonorrhoea* or *pelvic inflammatory disease*. Ovarian cysts are common and usually noncancerous; multiple ovarian cysts, together with other characteristic features, occur in *polycystic ovary syndrome*. Ovarian cancer (see *ovary, cancer of*) occurs mainly in women after the menopause. Ovarian failure causes premature *menopause* in about 5 per cent of women.

ovary, polycystic

An ovary with multiple *ovarian cysts*. Symptomless ovarian cysts are present in about a quarter of the female population. In some women, however, ovarian cysts are associated with menstrual disorders and/or other symptoms; in these cases the condition is known as *polycystic ovary syndrome*.

overbite

Overlapping of the lower front *teeth* by the upper ones. A slight degree of overbite is normal as the upper jaw is larger than the lower jaw. In *malocclusion*, overbite may be greater than normal or the lower teeth may project in front of the upper teeth (prognathism).

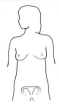

overbreathing

A common name for *hyperventilation*.

overcrowding, dental

Excessive crowding of the *teeth* so that they are unable to assume their normal positions in the jaw.

CAUSES

Dental overcrowding is commonly inherited and may occur because the teeth are too large for the jaw or the jaw is too small to accommodate the teeth. Overcrowding may also be caused, or aggravated, by premature loss of primary molar (back) teeth; this can cause the permanent teeth replacing them to move out of position and crowd the teeth further forward.

SYMPTOMS

Overcrowded teeth may lead to *malocclusion* (abnormal relationship between the upper and lower teeth) or may prevent certain teeth from erupting through the gum (see *impaction, dental*). The teeth can be difficult to clean, increasing the risk of dental decay (see *caries, dental*) and *periodontal disease*.

TREATMENT

Teeth may need to be extracted to allow room for others or for cosmetic reasons. Usually, an *orthodontic appliance* is fitted to the remaining teeth until they are positioned correctly.

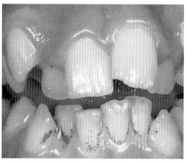

Overcrowded teeth
The top and bottom front teeth are crowded together because the molars, just behind them, have grown too far forward.

overdose

See *drug poisoning*.

overflow incontinence

A type of incontinence (see *incontinence, urinary*) in which urine leaks from the bladder, or a type of faecal incontinence in which semi-liquid faeces leak out around impacted faeces in constipation (see *incontinence, faecal*). Overflow urinary incontinence most commonly occurs in cases of long-term *urinary retention*, which is caused by an obstruction at the outlet of the bladder. Treatment is generally of the underlying problem.

over-the-counter (OTC) drug

A drug that can be bought without a prescription at a pharmacy or other shop, such as a supermarket.

overuse injury

Also called *repetitive strain injury*, a term for any injury caused by repetitive movement of part of the body. Symptoms include pain and stiffness in the affected joints and muscles.

Examples include *epicondylitis*: painful inflammation of one of the bony prominences at the elbow, caused by the pull of the attached forearm muscles during strenuous activities (see *golfer's elbow; tennis elbow*). Overuse injuries of the fingers, thumb, and wrist joints may affect assembly-line and keyboard workers, and musicians; injuries of the neck may affect violinists.

Rest usually relieves the symptoms. A change in the technique used during the activity may prevent recurrence.

overweight

Weighing more than the recommended *weight* for a particular height. (See also *obesity*.)

ovulation

The development and release of an *ovum* (egg; the female reproductive cell) from a follicle within an *ovary*. During the first half of the menstrual cycle (see *menstruation*), *follicle-stimulating hormone* (FSH) causes several ova to mature in the ovary. At mid-cycle, *luteinizing hormone* (LH) causes one ripe ovum to be released for potential fertilization.

Signs of ovulation include a rise in body temperature, changes in the consistency of the cervical mucus, and sometimes mild abdominal pain (see *mittelschmerz*). A yellow mass of tissue known as the corpus luteum develops from the follicle after *ovulation* and releases progesterone during the second half of the cycle.

After the release of the ovum, it travels along the *fallopian tube* and, if *fertilization* does not occur, it soon degenerates. Regular menstruation usually means that ovulation is occurring; exceptions to this occur around *puberty* and approaching the *menopause*.

ovum

The egg cell (the female cell of reproduction). An ovum contains a nucleus suspended in cytoplasm (a gel-like substance) and it is surrounded by a protective layer that is known as the *zona pellucida*.

About one million immature ova are present in each *ovary* at birth, but only about 200 per ovary mature to be released at *ovulation*. A *fertilized* ovum develops into an *embryo*.

ovum, blighted

A *zygote* (a fertilized egg cell) in which development has stopped at an early stage. This condition results in the appearance of an empty sac in the uterus, with no fetus visible on *ultrasound scanning*; blighted ovum is a common cause of *miscarriage*.

Ovysmen

A brand-name *oral contraceptive* containing *ethinylestradiol* (a synthetic form of the female sex hormone estradiol) and *levonorgestrel* (a progestogen drug).

oxalate

A substance that is synthesized by the body as well as being derived from certain foods, such as spinach, rhubarb, and tea. When blood oxalate levels are raised, kidney stones (see *calculus, urinary tract*) may develop.

oxazepam

A *benzodiazepine drug* used as a short-term treatment for *anxiety*. Oxazepam may cause dependence if it is taken regularly for more than two weeks (see *drug dependence*).

oximeter

An instrument that measures the amount of oxygenated haemoglobin (see *oxyhaemoglobin*) in the blood. A pulse oximeter is a photoelectric sensor attached either to a finger or to an ear to measure oxygen saturation continuously. Oximetry is used to monitor a patient during certain procedures, and always during *general anaesthesia*; it is also used to help diagnose and monitor many lung diseases.

oxprenolol

A *beta-blocker drug* used in the treatment of *hypertension* (high blood pressure), *angina* (chest pain due to insufficient blood supply to the heart), and cardiac *arrhythmias* (irregular heartbeat).

Oxprenolol may also be used to relieve symptoms of *anxiety* and control those of *hyperthyroidism* (overactivity of the thyroid gland).

oxybutynin

A drug used to treat frequent urination (see *urination, frequent*) and urge incontinence (see *incontinence, urinary*) by relaxing bladder muscle and increasing bladder capacity. Common side effects include dry mouth and blurred vision.

oxygen

A colourless and odourless gas that makes up 21 per cent of the Earth's atmosphere. Oxygen is essential for almost all forms of life, including humans, because it is necessary for the metabolic "burning" of foods to produce energy. This is a process that takes place in body cells and is known as *aerobic* metabolism.

Oxygen is absorbed through the lungs and into the blood, where it binds to the *haemoglobin* in red blood cells. As oxygen-rich blood circulates around the body, the oxygen is released from the red blood cells into the body tissues.

Additional supplies of oxygen are used to treat conditions such as severe *hypoxia* (inadequate oxygen in the body tissues) or *bronchitis*. High-pressure oxygen (see *hyperbaric oxygen treatment*) is sometimes used to treat *decompression sickness* or *carbon monoxide* poisoning. (See also *ozone*.)

oxygen concentrator

A device used in *oxygen therapy* that separates oxygen from the air and mixes it back in at a greater concentration. The oxygen-enriched air is delivered through a tube for prolonged inhalation. The device is used by people who have persistent *hypoxia* (inadequate oxygen in body tissues) due to severe chronic obstructive pulmonary disease (see *pulmonary disease, chronic obstructive*). (See also *hyperbaric oxygen treatment*.)

oxygen therapy

The process of supplying a person with oxygen-enriched air to relieve severe *hypoxia* (inadequate oxygen in body tissues). The oxygen is usually delivered through a face-mask or a nasal cannula (a length of narrow plastic tubing with two prongs that are inserted into the nostrils). The oxygen concentration of the air may be varied in accordance with the patient's needs. Piped oxygen is used in hospitals; oxygen in cylinders can be used when the patient is moving from place to place. Long-term therapy for people with persistent hypoxia, which results from diseases such as chronic obstructive pulmonary disease (see *pulmonary disease, chronic obstructive*) or *pulmonary fibrosis*, may involve the use of an *oxygen concentrator*. (See also *hyperbaric oxygen treatment*.)

oxyhaemoglobin

The substance formed when the *iron* in haem, the pigment in the *haemoglobin* of red blood cells, combines chemically with oxygen. Oxyhaemoglobin gives the blood in the arteries its bright red colour. This compound is the form in which oxygen is transported from the lungs to the tissues, where the oxygen is released (see *respiration*).

oxymetazoline

A *decongestant drug* used in the treatment of *allergic rhinitis* (hay fever), *sinusitis*, and the common *cold*.

oxytetracycline

A tetracycline *antibiotic drug* that is used to treat *chlamydial infections* such as *nongonococcal urethritis*. It is also used for a variety of other infective conditions, including *bronchitis* and *pneumonia*; the drug may also be used to treat severe *acne*.

Side effects may include nausea, vomiting, diarrhoea, skin rash, and increased sensitivity of the skin to sunlight. Oxytetracycline may discolour developing teeth and is not given to children under 12 or women who are pregnant or breast-feeding.

oxytocin

A *hormone* produced by the *pituitary gland*. Oxytocin causes uterine *contractions* during labour and stimulates milk-flow in *breast-feeding* women.

Synthetic oxytocin is used for *induction of labour*. It is given by intravenous infusion to produce uterine contractions. It is also often given with ergometrine as a single dose after delivery to prompt placental separation and expulsion, to reduce blood flow, or to empty the uterus after an incomplete *miscarriage* or a fetal death.

A possible adverse effect of synthetic oxytocin is abnormally strong, painful contractions. Rare side effects may include nausea, vomiting, palpitations, and allergic reactions.

oxyuriasis

An alternative name for enterobiasis or *threadworm infestation*.

ozena

A severe and rare form of *rhinitis*, in which the mucus membrane in the nose wastes away and a thick nasal discharge dries to form crusts. Ozena often causes severe *halitosis* (bad breath).

ozone

A form of oxygen, ozone (O_3) is a poisonous, faintly blue gas that is produced by the action of electrical discharges (such as lightning) on oxygen molecules (O_2) and by interactions between hydrocarbon pollutants and sunlight.

Ozone occurs naturally in the upper atmosphere, where it screens the Earth from most of the sun's harmful ultraviolet radiation. The ozone layer is being depleted by atmospheric pollutants, allowing increasing amounts of ultraviolet radiation to reach the Earth's surface. This increases the risk of affected populations developing higher rates of certain diseases and conditions, such as *skin cancer* and *cataracts* (see *sunlight, adverse effects of*).

Increased levels of ozone near the ground are an indicator of poor air quality. In these circumstances, the raised levels make the breathing problems of people with allergic lung diseases increasingly likely to worsen, particularly if they exercise.

O

P

pacemaker

A small device that supplies electrical impulses to the *heart* in order to maintain a regular *heartbeat*.

WHY IT IS USED

A pacemaker is needed when the heart's *sinoatrial node* malfunctions (see *sick sinus syndrome*), when the passage of the electrical impulses that stimulate heart contractions is impaired (see *heart block*), or when the heart rate is intermittently slow and fast or the rhythm is irregular.

TYPES

Pacemakers may be fitted externally, as a temporary measure until a permanent pacemaker can be fitted. They can also be internal (surgically implanted in the chest). Internal pacemakers can either discharge impulses at a steady (fixed) rate or discharge only at times when the heart rate slows or a beat is missed (demand pacemakers); some types can increase the heart rate during exercise or change an abnormal rhythm into a normal one. Internal pacemakers are also either single-chambered or dual-chambered. Single-chamber pacemakers work by passing a single wire into the right atrium or right ventricle; dual-chamber pacemakers have two wires, one that passes into the right atrium, and the other into the right ventricle.

pachyderma

Abnormal thickening of the skin. (See also *elephantiasis*.)

Pacinian corpuscle

A specialized form of sensory nerve ending (see *receptor*) found in the dermis (the lower layer of the skin). Pacinian corpuscles detect deep pressure and vibration.

packed red blood cells

A *blood product* comprising blood from which 70 per cent of the *plasma* (the fluid that carries blood cells and other substances) has been removed to leave a high concentration of *red blood cells*. In blood transfusions, packed red blood cells are used much more commonly than "whole" blood (blood that has had nothing removed), especially to treat *anaemia* and *haemolytic disease of the newborn*; if a smaller volume of blood is transfused, there is less risk of overloading the circulation.

paclitaxel

An *anticancer drug* that is used to treat certain types of cancer, such as ovarian cancer (see *ovary, cancer of*) and *breast cancer*.

The possible side effects of paclitaxel include nausea, vomiting, *anaemia*, and increased susceptibility to infection.

paediatrics

The branch of medicine that concentrates on the development of children and with the diagnosis, treatment, and prevention of childhood diseases and other conditions.

paedophilia

Persistent sexual attraction to, often leading to abuse of, children. Paedophilia is most often seen in men. It is thought to result from a combination of psychological and social factors that affect sexuality. Paedophiles often show *personality disorders* such as antisocial personality disorder, and have little concern for the effect of their behaviour on the child.

Paedophilic activity is illegal; many affected people are only identified once they have been arrested. Treatments are designed to reduce the urge to have sexual relations with children; they include *cognitive–behavioural therapy* and drug treatment to reduce sexual urges. (See also *child abuse*; *incest*.)

Paget's disease

A common disorder that occurs in middle-aged and elderly people that is characterized by the disruption of *bone* formation. The affected bones become weak, enlarged and thickened, and deformed. Paget's disease is sometimes called osteitis deformans,

Paget's disease usually affects the pelvis, skull, collarbone, vertebrae, and long bones of the leg. Normally, the maintenance of healthy bones involves a balance between the actions of cells that break down bone tissue and the activity of cells that create new tissue. In Paget's disease this balance is disturbed. The disorder may run in families and in some cases is thought to be caused by a viral infection.

SYMPTOMS

There are often no symptoms. If symptoms do occur, the most common ones are bone pain and deformity, especially bowing of the legs. Affected bones are susceptible to *fracture*.

INTERNAL **PACEMAKER**

An internal pacemaker is inserted just beneath the skin in the chest wall, usually under local anaesthetic. The device weighs only 20–50g, and most are powered by a lithium battery that lasts on average between six and 10 years before needing to be replaced. Each electrical impulse that the pacemaker discharges stimulates the heart into contracting and producing a heartbeat. Some pacemakers deliver continuous impulses: others deliver an impulse only when the heart rate falls too low or in order to override an excessively fast rate.

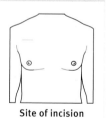

Site of incision

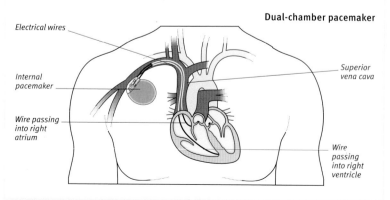

Dual-chamber pacemaker

Electrical wires

Internal pacemaker

Wire passing into right atrium

Superior vena cava

Wire passing into right ventricle

Skull changes may lead to leontiasis ossea (distortion of the facial bones producing a lionlike appearance) and cause damage to the inner-ear bones, sometimes resulting in deafness, *tinnitus* (ringing in the ears), *vertigo* (a spinning sensation), or headaches.

In the spine, enlarged vertebrae may press on the spinal cord, causing pain and sometimes paralysis of the legs. If the disease affects the pelvis, it may cause severe *arthritis* of the hip joints.

Occasionally, *bone cancer* may develop. In rare cases, when many bones are involved, increased blood flow through affected bones may cause *heart failure*.

DIAGNOSIS AND TREATMENT

Paget's disease is diagnosed by *X-rays*, which show areas of porous and thickened bone, and *blood tests*, which reveal abnormal levels of the substances involved in bone formation and breakdown.

Most people do not need treatment, or need only *analgesic drugs* (painkillers). In more severe cases, treatment with drugs such as *bisphosphonates* or *calcitonin* may be prescribed to control the rates of bone breakdown and renewal. The drugs will not reverse any existing deformity, but will slow the progression of the disease. Surgery may be needed to correct deformities or treat arthritis.

Paget's disease of the nipple

A rare type of *breast cancer* in which a tumour develops in the *nipple*. The disease resembles *eczema* and can cause itching and a burning feeling. A non-healing sore may develop. Without treatment, the tumour may spread into the breast. Diagnosis is made with a *biopsy* (sample of tissue).

pain

A localized, unpleasant sensation that can range from a feeling of mild discomfort to an excruciating experience. Pain serves the function of alerting the body to possible causes of injury, or making an affected person (or animal) withdraw from a source of harm. It may be acute (in which it appears and disappears suddenly) or chronic (in which it persists for days, weeks, or even longer).

MECHANISM OF PAIN

Pain results from the stimulation of sensory nerve endings called nociceptors in the skin. Pain receptors are also present in other structures, such as the blood vessels and tendons. Some nociceptors respond only to severe stimulation, such as cutting, pricking, or extreme heat; others respond to warning stimuli such as firm pressure or stretching. Signals that arise from the nociceptors are transmitted via nerves to the brain. In addition, chemicals called *prostaglandins* trigger inflammation and swelling, and further stimulate the nerve endings.

Pain that may be felt at a point some distance from the cause is known as referred pain (see *pain, referred*).

PSYCHOLOGICAL ASPECTS OF PAIN

Pain is usually associated with distress and anxiety, and sometimes with fear. People vary tremendously in their pain thresholds (the level at which the pain is felt and the person feels compelled to act). The cause and circumstances of the pain may also affect the way it is perceived by the sufferer. The pain of cancer, because of fear of the disease, may seem much greater and cause more suffering than similar pain that results from persistent indigestion. Unexplained pain is often worse because of the anxiety it can cause; once a diagnosis is made and reassurance given, the pain may be perceived as less severe. In some cases, pain may be felt due to emotional reasons rather than any obvious physical cause (see *pain, psychogenic*).

The experience of pain may be reduced or blocked by arousal or strong emotion; for example, an injury sustained during competitive sport or on the battlefield may go unnoticed in the heat of the moment. Some people believe that mental preparation for pain, in advance of situations such as childbirth or in experiments to test pain, can greatly reduce the response.

A person's response to pain is also greatly modified by past experience; the outcome of previous episodes of pain may affect the way in which the individual copes with subsequent pain. Factors such as *insomnia*, *anxiety*, and *depression*, which often accompany incapacitating chronic illness, lower tolerance to pain. Many hospitals now have specialist pain clinics, in which people with severe pain that has proved difficult to control may be assessed and treated. Such patients include those with advanced *cancer* and poorly understood conditions such as facial pain and various types of *neuralgia*.

TREATMENT

Treatment is for the underlying cause of the pain. It may involve *analgesic drugs*, electrical stimulation (*TENS*), surgery, or therapies such as *acupuncture*. (See also *pain relief*; *endorphins*.)

painful arc syndrome

A condition in which pain occurs when the arm is raised between 45 and 160 degrees from the side. The usual cause is an inflamed *tendon* or *bursa* in the *shoulder* joint that is being squeezed between the *scapula* (shoulderblade) and *humerus* (the upper-arm bone). Treatment includes *physiotherapy* and injections of *corticosteroid drugs*. (See also *subacromial bursitis*.)

painful heel

See *heel, painful*.

painkillers

See *analgesic drugs*.

painless haematuria

A form of *haematuria* (blood in the urine) that is not associated with pain when urine is passed (see *urination, painful*). Common causes of painless haematuria include *kidney tumours*; tumours in the ureters; *bladder tumours*; or *glomerulonephritis* (inflammation in the tiny filtering units of the kidneys).

pain, psychogenic

Pain that occurs in response to a mental or emotional stimulus rather than having a physical cause. Persistent pain that has no obvious physical cause may be due to a psychological disorder (see *somatization disorder*).

pain, referred

Pain that is felt in a site other than the affected part of the body. This form of pain occurs when the brain cannot distinguish the correct source of the pain signals (see the illustrated box overleaf). Examples of referred pain are pain in the left shoulder or the arm, related to *angina pectoris* (chest pain due to insufficient blood supply to the heart muscle) and *sciatica* (pain that radiates along the sciatic nerve in the leg).

pain relief

The treatment of pain, usually with *analgesic drugs*. *Paracetamol*, *aspirin* and *codeine* are among the most widely used drugs in this group. Pain accompanied by *inflammation* is often alleviated by *nonsteroidal anti-inflammatory drugs (NSAIDs)*. Severe pain may require treatment with *opioids*, such as *morphine*. Other types of drug may be used to treat nerve pain, such as *trigeminal neuralgia* or the burning sensation in the feet that may be a feature of *diabetes mellitus*. Examples are

P

PAIN

Pain mechanisms exist to provide a useful warning of possible injury or to caution against repeating an action that has led to injury. Certain diseases, such as arthritis and extensive cancer, may set off these same mechanisms, causing chronic pain that has no apparent function.

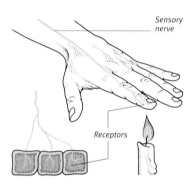

Sensory nerve

Receptors

Reflex action
The nerve pathways that warn of noxious stimuli (through the sensation of pain) may also initiate automatic, reflex actions that help prevent harm.

1 Receptors in the fingertip detect heat. Signals are sent along a sensory nerve to the spinal cord.

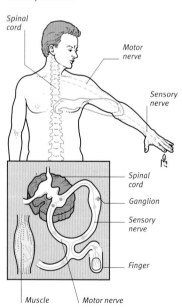

Spinal cord

Motor nerve

Sensory nerve

Spinal cord

Ganglion

Sensory nerve

Finger

Muscle   *Motor nerve*

2 The signals arriving in the spinal cord pass instantaneously to a motor nerve that connects to a muscle in the arm. The signals received via the motor nerve cause the muscle in the arm to contract, moving the arm away from the source of danger (the flame).

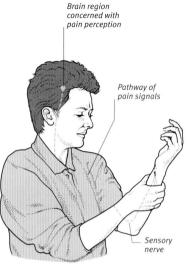

Brain region concerned with pain perception

Pathway of pain signals

Sensory nerve

Perception of pain
When an injury occurs, signals pass along nerve pathways concerned with pain, first to the spinal cord and then to the thalamus in the brain; there the pain is perceived.

REFERRED PAIN

A referred pain is one felt in a site other than an injured or diseased part. Sensory nerves from certain body areas converge before they enter the brain, causing confusion about the source of pain signals.

Tooth to ear region
A toothache may be felt in the ear, because the same sensory nerve supplies both parts.

Diaphragm to right shoulder
Inflammation of the diaphragm, often due to pneumonia, may be felt as a pain in the right shoulder.

Heart to left arm
Angina, a pain caused by reduced blood supply to the heart muscle, is often felt in the left shoulder or arm.

Hip to knee
Disorders that affect the hip, such as arthritis, may be felt as pain in the knee rather than in the hip.

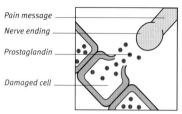

Pain message
Nerve ending
Prostaglandin
Damaged cell

Initiation of pain signals
Pain signals are set off by stimulation of special nerve endings – by pressure, heat, or the release of chemicals, including prostaglandins, by cells that have been damaged.

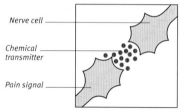

Nerve cell
Chemical transmitter
Pain signal

Signal transmission to brain
Within the brain and spinal cord, pain signals pass between nerve cells by means of chemicals that cross the gaps between the cells.

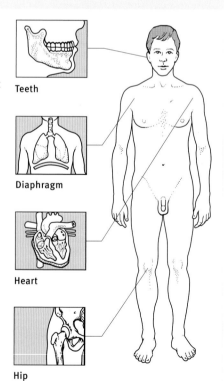

Teeth

Diaphragm

Heart

Hip

tricyclic antidepressants (such as amitriptyline) and *anticonvulsant drugs* (such as carbamazepine or gabapentin).

Other methods of pain relief include *massage*, *ice-packs*, *poultices*, *TENS*, *acupuncture*, and *hypnosis*. Surgery to destroy pain-transmitting nerves (such as a *sympathectomy*) is occasionally performed in cases where all other appropriate treatments have failed.

palate

The roof of the mouth, which separates the mouth from the nasal cavity. The palate is covered with a *mucous membrane*. At the front is the hard palate, which is a plate of bone forming part of the *maxilla* (upper jaw). At the rear is the soft palate, which is a flap of muscle and fibrous tissue that projects into the *pharynx* (throat). During the process of swallowing, the soft palate presses against the rear wall of the pharynx, thereby preventing food from escaping into the nose. (See also *cleft lip and palate*.)

LOCATION OF THE **PALATE**

The palate forms the floor of the nasal cavity and the roof of the mouth, providing a surface against which the tongue can push during chewing and swallowing.

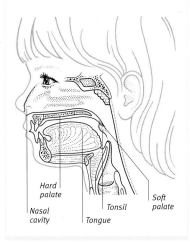

Hard palate

Nasal cavity

Tonsil

Tongue

Soft palate

palliative care

Nursing or medical care that is given to relieve the symptoms of illness rather than to treat the cause. Palliative care is often given to people who are in the last stages of a terminal illness (see *dying, care of the*). In these cases, the aim is to minimize unpleasant symptoms and to provide a comfortable, reassuring environment for the last days or weeks of life. (See also *palliative treatment*.)

palliative treatment

Treatment that relieves the symptoms of a disorder but does not cure it. There is a wide variety of palliative treatments. Examples are *pain relief*; *antiemetic drugs* to relieve nausea and vomiting; *sedative drugs* to relieve insomnia; and other therapies, such as massage and counselling. (See also *dying, care of the*.)

pallor

Abnormal paleness of the *skin* and *mucous membranes*, particularly noticeable in the face. Pallor may have many possible causes and is not always a symptom of disease.

Pallor may be caused by constriction of small blood vessels in the skin, which may occur in response to shock, severe pain, injury, heavy blood loss, or fainting. This restriction of blood flow to the skin ensures that the brain and other vital organs are adequately supplied with blood and that body heat is conserved (at least temporarily).

Less commonly, pallor may be due to a deficiency of the skin pigment *melanin* that may result from spending too little time in daylight. Abnormally pale skin is also a feature of *albinism*.

Disorders that cause pallor include *anaemia*, *kidney failure*, and *hypothyroidism* (underactivity of the thyroid gland). *Lead poisoning* is a rare cause.

palmar erythema

See *liver palms*.

palpation

A technique used in *physical examination* in which parts of the body are felt with the hands to assess the condition of the skin and underlying organs.

palpitation

An awareness or feeling in the chest of the *heartbeat* or a sensation of having a rapid and forceful heartbeat.

CAUSES
Palpitations are usually felt in tense or frightening situations, or following strenuous exercise. When experienced at rest or during a period of calm, they are usually due to *ectopic heartbeats* and are felt as fluttering or thumping in the chest. This condition is usually due to *alcohol* or *caffeine* consumption, or *smoking*, rather than disease. Palpitations may also be due to cardiac arrhythmias (irregularities of the heartbeat; see *arrhythmia, cardiac*); anaemia (a reduced level of the oxygen-carrying pigment haemoglobin in the blood); or *hyperthyroidism* (overactivity of the thyroid gland), which speeds up the heartbeat.

DIAGNOSIS AND TREATMENT
Recurrent palpitations, or those causing chest pain, breathlessness, or dizziness, may indicate an underlying disorder, and need prompt medical attention. They may be investigated by a 24-hour *ECG* and *thyroid function tests*. Treatment depends on the cause.

palsy

A term applied to certain forms of *paralysis*, such as Bell's palsy (the most common form of *facial palsy*).

Paludrine

The brand name for the antimalarial drug *proguanil*.

panacea

A remedy that is claimed to cure all diseases. No such remedy is known.

Panadol

A brand name for the analgesic (pain-killing) drug *paracetamol*.

Pancoast's syndrome

A collection of symptoms that occurs when a growth presses on the *brachial plexus* (the group of major nerves controlling the arm and hand). These symptoms include pain and paralysis in the arm or hand, as well as *Horner's syndrome* if the growth presses on the sympathetic cervical (neck) nerves. Pancoast's syndrome is commonly due to a tumour called Pancoast's tumour, which develops in the upper part of the lung in people with *lung cancer*.

pancreas

A tapered gland that lies across the back of the abdomen, behind the stomach. The broadest part (which is called the head) is on the right-hand side, in the loop of the duodenum (the first part of the small intestine). The main part (which is called the body) tapers from the head and extends horizontally. The narrowest part (the tail) extends leftwards, towards the spleen.

STRUCTURE AND FUNCTION
The major part of the pancreas is made up of exocrine tissue, which release chemicals through ducts. Embedded within these tissues are "nests" of

P

LOCATION OF THE **PANCREAS**

This organ lies behind and under the stomach, except for its head, which lies within the curve of the duodenum.

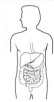

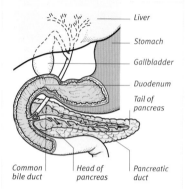

- Liver
- Stomach
- Gallbladder
- Duodenum
- Tail of pancreas
- Common bile duct
- Head of pancreas
- Pancreatic duct

endocrine cells (known as the *islets of Langerhans*), which secrete hormones into the bloodstream.

The exocrine cells secrete digestive enzymes into a network of ducts that meet to form the main pancreatic duct. This duct joins the common bile duct (which carries bile from the *gallbladder*) to form a small chamber, the ampulla of Vater, which opens into the *duodenum*. Also secreted is *sodium bicarbonate*, which neutralizes stomach acid entering the duodenum.

The islets of Langerhans are surrounded by many blood vessels, into which they secrete the hormones *insulin*, *glucagon*, and somatostatin. These hormones regulate the level of *glucose* in the blood. (See also *Disorders of the pancreas* box.)

pancreas, cancer of

A malignant tumour of the *pancreas*. Pancreatic tumours usually arise in the exocrine tissue, which is responsible for producing digestive juices. They may also occasionally arise from parts of the endocrine system or from the ampulla of Vater (the junction of the common bile duct and the pancreatic duct). The cause of cancer of the pancreas is unknown, but smoking, chronic *pancreatitis*, and a high alcohol intake may contribute.

SYMPTOMS

Symptoms and signs of pancreatic cancer include upper abdominal pain that radiates to the back; loss of appetite; weight loss; *jaundice* (yellowing of the skin) if the tumour obstructs the bile ducts; and itching. There may also be indigestion, nausea, vomiting, diarrhoea, and tiredness. In many cases, symptoms do not appear until the cancer has spread (typically to the liver and the lymph nodes in the abdomen).

DIAGNOSIS AND TREATMENT

Diagnosis usually requires ultrasound scanning, *CT scanning* or *MRI* of the upper abdomen, or *ERCP* (endoscopic examination of the pancreatic ducts).

In the early stages, *Whipple's operation* (surgical removal of cancerous tissue), *radiotherapy*, and *anticancer drugs* may provide a cure. In the later stages, little can be done apart from provision of *palliative treatment*, such as pain relief, a *bypass operation* to treat obstruction of the duodenum, or insertion of a *stent* (rigid tube) to relieve jaundice. Most people with advanced pancreatic cancer survive for less than one year.

pancreatectomy

Removal of all or part of the *pancreas*, which may be performed as treatment for *pancreatitis* (inflammation of the pancreas). In rare cases, pancreatectomy is performed as a treatment for *insulinomas* (insulin-producing tumours).

Pancreatectomy may cause a deficiency of pancreatic hormones and digestive enzymes. This situation may lead to *diabetes mellitus*, which needs to receive treatment with insulin therapy, and *malabsorption*, which requires oral supplements of *pancreatin*.

pancreatin

An oral preparation of pancreatic *enzymes* required for digestion. It is used to prevent *malabsorption*, and it may be needed after *pancreatectomy* or by people who have disorders affecting the pancreas, such as chronic *pancreatitis*, cancer (see *pancreas, cancer of*), or *cystic fibrosis*.

pancreatitis

Inflammation of the *pancreas*, a condition that may be acute or chronic. In acute pancreatitis, the pancreas suddenly becomes inflamed, causing severe abdominal pain. This condition can be life-threatening if left untreated. In chronic pancreatitis, the pancreas is persistently inflamed; this condition leads to a progressive loss of function.

CAUSES

The main causes of acute pancreatitis are alcohol abuse, typically a bout of heavy drinking, and *gallstones*. Less common causes are injury (such as a violent blow to the abdomen), viral infections (such as *mumps*), surgery on the *biliary system*, or certain drugs, such as *immunosuppressants* and thiazide *diuretic drugs*.

Chronic pancreatitis is usually due to long-term alcohol abuse. Less common causes include *hyperlipidaemia* (a high level of fat in the blood), *cystic fibrosis*, *haemochromatosis* (a condition in which there is excess iron in the body), and severe acute pancreatitis.

SYMPTOMS

An attack of acute pancreatitis usually lasts about 48 hours. Symptoms are a sudden attack of severe upper abdominal pain, which may spread to the back, often accompanied by vomiting. Movement often makes the pain worse, but sitting may help to relieve it. In severe cases, inflammation may affect the whole abdomen (see *peritonitis*); there is also a risk of *shock* (failure of blood circulation), which may be life-threatening.

Chronic pancreatitis usually develops over several years, and may be symptomless in the early stages. When symptoms do appear they are usually the same as those of acute pancreatitis, although the pain may last from a few hours to several days, and attacks may become more frequent over time. If there is no pain, the principal signs may be of *malabsorption* or *diabetes mellitus* due to reduced levels of pancreatic enzymes and insulin, respectively.

COMPLICATIONS

Acute pancreatitis may recur repeatedly. Severe acute pancreatitis may damage the pancreas and lead to *hypotension* (low blood pressure), *heart failure*, *kidney failure*, *respiratory failure*, pancreatic *cysts*, and *ascites* (accumulation of fluid in the abdomen).

Chronic pancreatitis leads to permanent damage to the gland; the tissue is damaged and gradually replaced by scar tissue, and normal function is progressively impaired. Other possible complications include the development of ascites and cysts, as well as *bile duct obstruction*.

DIAGNOSIS AND TREATMENT

A diagnosis may be made using abdominal *X-rays*, *ultrasound scanning*, or *CT scanning* or *MRI* (techniques that produce cross-sectional or three-dimensional images of body structures). In addition, *blood tests* may be used in cases of suspected acute pancreatitis, to detect pancreatic enzymes that have leaked directly into the blood.

DISORDERS OF THE **PANCREAS**

Serious disruption of pancreatic function occurs only when the secretory tissue of the gland has been damaged or destroyed in advanced disease. The most common pancreatic disorder is *diabetes mellitus*, in which the insulin-producing cells in the gland are destroyed.

Congenital and genetic disorders
About 85 per cent of people with the genetic disorder *cystic fibrosis* produce totally inadequate quantities of pancreatic digestive enzymes, which results in *malabsorption* of fats and proteins. This, in turn, may produce steatorrhoea (excess fat in the faeces) and muscle wasting.

Genetic factors are thought to play some part in diabetes mellitus, although they are not the primary cause of the disease.

Chronic *pancreatitis* (inflammation of the pancreas) may, in rare cases, be hereditary; chronic pancreatitis often causes diabetes.

Infection
Acute pancreatitis may result from certain viral infections, especially with the *mumps* or *hepatitis* viruses. Other viruses, such as coxsackievirus, may also cause pancreatitis. In some cases, coxsackievirus infection may contribute to the development of diabetes.

Tumour
Pancreatic cancer is one of the fairly common cancers (see *pancreas, cancer of*). It is difficult to diagnose and, in most cases, has spread extensively by the time it is detected.

Trauma
Injury to the pancreas – as a result of a blow to the abdomen, for example – may cause acute pancreatitis. The mechanism by which this occurs is not fully established, but it is believed that pancreatic enzymes (most of which are inactive until they reach the intestine) are released within the gland and then activated, with the result that they digest the pancreas.

Poisons and drugs
Excessive alcohol intake is a common cause of pancreatitis. It can also be caused by various drugs, such as sulphonamides, *oestrogen drugs* (including oestrogen-containing contraceptive pills), and thiazide *diuretic drugs*; *corticosteroid drugs* may also cause pancreatitis.

Autoimmune disorders
The cause of the damage to the pancreas in diabetes mellitus remains controversial. However, there is increasing evidence that, possibly in response to a viral infection, the body's immune system produces antibodies (proteins made by the immune system) that inappropriately attack and destroy the pancreatic cells.

Other disorders
The condition most often associated with pancreatitis, other than alcohol overuse, is *gallstones*. these occasionally block the exit of the pancreatic duct into the duodenum, leading to inflammation of the pancreas.

INVESTIGATION

Diagnosis of pancreatic disorders may involve *ultrasound scanning*, *CT scanning*, or *MRI* of the abdomen; tests to measure levels of pancreatic enzymes in the blood or duodenum; and endoscopic examination of the gland (see *ERCP*).

Acute pancreatitis is treated with *intravenous infusion* of fluids and salts and opioid *analgesic drugs* (painkillers). In some cases, the abdominal cavity may be washed out with sterile fluid; *ERCP* (an endoscopic X-ray procedure) may be used to find and remove gallstones; or a *pancreatectomy* (surgical removal of damaged tissue) may be performed.

Treatment for the chronic form is with painkillers, *insulin*, *pancreatin*, and, in some cases, pancreatectomy.

pancreatography

Imaging of the pancreas or its ducts using *CT scanning*, *MRI*, *ultrasound scanning*, *X-ray* (after a radiopaque *contrast medium* is injected into the ducts during exploratory surgery), or with *ERCP* (an endoscopic X-ray procedure).

pancytopenia

A simultaneous and severe reduction in the numbers of red blood cells (causing *anaemia*); white blood cells (a condition called *leucopenia*); and platelets, involved in clotting (*thrombocytopenia*). This condition may be a result of damage to the *bone marrow*, where blood cells are made; such damage may be due to cancer in the marrow, or to destruction of the marrow by *radiotherapy* or *anticancer drugs*. Pancytopenia may also be due to *hypersplenism* (overactivity of the spleen), in which the spleen destroys excessive numbers of blood cells. (See also *aplastic anaemia*; *Fanconi's anaemia*.)

pandemic

A medical term that is applied to a disease that occurs over a large geographical area and that affects a high proportion of the population; a widespread *epidemic*.

panencephalitis

See *subacute sclerosing panencephalitis*.

panic attack

A brief period of acute *anxiety*, often dominated by an intense fear of dying or losing one's reason. Although unpleasant and frightening, panic attacks usually last for only a few minutes, cause no physical harm, and are rarely associated with any serious physical illness.

Panic attacks are generally a feature of an *anxiety disorder*, *agoraphobia*, or other *phobias*. In some cases, however, such attacks are associated with a *somatization disorder* or *schizophrenia*.

Attacks are unpredictable at first, but tend to become associated with specific situations, such as being in a cramped lift. Symptoms begin suddenly. They include a sense of breathing difficulty, chest pains, *palpitations*, feeling light-headed, dizziness, sweating, trembling, and faintness. *Hyperventilation* often also occurs. This condition results in carbon dioxide levels in the blood becoming abnormally low, which leads to a *pins-and-needles* sensation and feelings of *depersonalization* and *derealization*. The attacks end quickly.

The symptoms of hyperventilation may be relieved quickly by covering the mouth and nose with a small paper bag and breathing into the bag for a few minutes; this measure restores carbon

P

dioxide levels to normal. In the longer term, *cognitive–behavioural therapy* and relaxation exercises may be used to help affected people control their anxiety.

panic disorder

A type of *anxiety* disorder characterized by recurrent *panic attacks* that are of intense anxiety and accompanied by distressing physical symptoms.

panniculitis

Inflammation occurring in subcutaneous fat (the layer of fatty tissue just beneath the skin). The inflamed fatty tissue forms multiple tender nodules under the skin. One form of this condition is *erythema nodosum*, in which swellings develop on the legs.

pantothenic acid

A vitamin of the *vitamin B complex*.

papain

A naturally occurring mixture of *enzymes*, including chymopapain, which is found in pawpaws. Papain breaks down proteins and has been used to remove clotted blood and dead tissue from wounds and ulcers.

papilla

Any small, nipple-shaped projection from a tissue's surface, such as the mammary papilla (the breast nipple).

papilloedema

Swelling of the head of the *optic nerve*. This condition is also known as optic disc oedema. The nerve swelling is visible with an *ophthalmoscope*. It usually indicates a dangerous rise in the pressure within the skull, which may sometimes be caused by a *brain tumour*.

papilloma

A noncancerous growth of the *epithelium* (the cell layer that forms the surface of the skin and mucous membranes) that resembles a wart and most commonly affects the skin, tongue, larynx, and urinary and digestive tracts. If it does not disappear spontaneously it can be surgically removed.

Papillon–Lefevre syndrome

A rare *genetic disorder* affecting the skin and gums. Papillon–Lefevre syndrome results in areas of thickened, cracked skin. In addition, it makes the gums prone to infection from very early in life. Severe gum disease (see *periodontal disease*) causes the primary (milk) teeth to be lost prematurely, and may cause all the adult teeth to be lost by age 20.

papovavirus

A family of viruses that includes papillomaviruses (see *human papillomavirus*).

pap smear

See *cervical smear test*.

papule

A small, solid, slightly raised area of skin. Papules are usually less than 5 mm in diameter. They may be raised or flat; rough or smooth; and pigmented or the colour of the surrounding skin.

par-/para-

Prefixes that may mean "beside or beyond", as in the parathyroid glands (which lie behind the thyroid); "closely resembling or related to", as in paratyphoid fever (a disease very similar to typhoid fever); or "faulty or abnormal", as in paraesthesia (abnormal sensation).

para-aminobenzoic acid (PABA)

A biochemical that used to be the active ingredient of many *sunscreen* preparations but is now rarely used because it can cause allergic reactions.

paracentesis

A procedure in which a body cavity is punctured with a needle to remove fluid for analysis, to relieve pressure from excess fluid, or to instil drugs.

paracetamol

An *analgesic drug* that is used to treat mild pain and to reduce fever. Paracetamol may, in rare cases, cause nausea or a rash. An overdose may cause liver damage and can be fatal. An antidote is available, but must be given early.

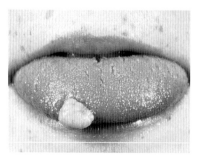

Papilloma on the tongue
This harmless growth, which resembles a wart, may disappear spontaneously but may need to be removed under local anaesthetic.

paraesthesia

Altered sensation in the skin without any stimulus (see *pins-and-needles*).

paraffinoma

A tumourlike swelling under the skin caused by prolonged exposure to paraffin. Paraffinomas may form in the lungs if paraffin is inhaled.

paraffin, white soft

See *petroleum jelly*.

paraldehyde

A *sedative drug* used to stop prolonged epileptic *seizures*. Paraldehyde can be administered as an *enema* or by injection into a muscle.

paralysis

Complete or partial loss of controlled movement caused by the inability to contract one or more *muscles*. Paralysis may be temporary or permanent, and can affect areas of varying sizes, from a small facial muscle to many of the major muscles in the body. There may also be loss of feeling in affected areas. Paralysis is also known as palsy.

TYPES

The types of paralysis are classified by the areas of the body that are affected and by the effect on the muscles. Paralysis of one half of the body is called *hemiplegia*. If corresponding areas on both sides of the body (such as the legs) are affected, it is known as *diplegia*. If all four limbs and the trunk are affected, the paralysis is called *quadriplegia* or tetraplegia. *Paraplegia* is the paralysis of both legs and sometimes part of the trunk. In addition, paralysis may be classified as flaccid, causing floppiness, or spastic, causing rigidity.

CAUSES

The muscles that control body movements are stimulated to contract by impulses originating in the motor cortex of the brain. These impulses travel via the spinal cord and peripheral nerves to reach the muscles. Paralysis may be caused by any form of injury or disorder anywhere along this nerve pathway. Alternatively, it may result from a disorder in the muscle.

Brain disorders A common cause of paralysis is a *stroke*, in which brain tissue is damaged by bleeding from a ruptured blood vessel, or an area of the brain is starved of oxygen due to a clot in the blood vessel supplying that region. The paralysis will occur on the opposite side of the body to the site of the brain damage because the motor nerves cross over in the *brainstem*.

Hemiplegia may be caused by any brain disorder in which the portion of the brain that controls movement is damaged. Examples of such disorders include a *brain tumour*, *brain abscess*, or *brain haemorrhage*.

Some types of paralysis are caused by damage to parts of the nervous system concerned with fine movement control, such as the *cerebellum* and the *basal ganglia*. *Parkinson's disease* is caused by a lack of *dopamine* in the basal ganglia.

Cranial nerve damage may affect a variety of muscles and functions. For example, damage to the *facial nerve* (the seventh cranial nerve) causes weakness of the facial muscles (see *facial palsy*) and loss of taste.

Spinal cord disorders If the spinal cord becomes damaged or diseased, paralysis will develop in muscles that are supplied by nerves below the affected area. Damage to, or pressure on, the spinal cord may result from fracture of one or more *vertebrae* (which may result from severe injury, as in a road traffic accident) or *disc prolapse* (slipped disc). Diseases affecting the spinal cord include *multiple sclerosis* and *poliomyelitis*.

Peripheral nerve disorders Certain nerve disorders, called *neuropathies*, affect the peripheral nerves and may cause varying degrees of paralysis. Neuropathies may be caused by a variety of conditions, such as diabetes mellitus (see *diabetic neuropathy*), vitamin deficiency, liver disease, cancer, and the toxic effects of some drugs or metals (such as lead).

Muscle disorders Certain disorders arising in the muscles, such as *muscular dystrophy*, may cause paralysis. Temporary paralysis sometimes occurs in *myasthenia gravis*.

TREATMENT
The underlying cause is treated, if possible. *Physiotherapy* is given for both temporary and permanent paralysis, to prevent joints from becoming locked in awkward positions. In addition, it retrains and strengthens the muscles and joints in people with temporary paralysis, so that some degree of mobility will be possible after recovery.

For paralysed people who are confined to a bed or a wheelchair, nursing care is essential to avoid the complications that can result from prolonged immobility, such as *bedsores*, *deep vein thrombosis*, *urinary tract infections*, *constipation*, and limb deformities.

paralysis, periodic

A rare, inherited condition that causes intermittent phases of muscle weakness, often associated with raised or lowered blood levels of *potassium*. The disorder shows an autosomal dominant pattern of inheritance (see *genetic disorder*).

Periodic paralysis affects young people, with attacks usually beginning in childhood or adolescence. Episodes of muscle weakness vary in frequency from daily to once every few years and last from a few minutes to a few hours.

Lowered potassium levels may occur after a high-carbohydrate meal or during a period of rest following physical exertion. The diuretic drug *acetazolamide* may be used to prevent attacks; potassium is often given orally to restore muscle strength when an attack occurs.

In other cases, potassium levels are raised; triggers include being cold, having a rest after physical exertion, and pregnancy. *Diuretic drugs* may be given as preventive treatment; a sugary drink may help to relieve an attack.

The condition often clears up without treatment by the age of 40.

paralytic ileus

See *ileus, paralytic*.

paramedic

A term for any healthcare worker who is trained to work in an auxiliary capacity to medical professionals such as doctors and nurses. The term usually refers to ambulance staff who attend accidents or medical emergencies.

paramyxovirus

One of a family of *viruses* that includes the microorganisms which are responsible for *croup*, *mumps*, *measles*, and *parainfluenza* (a mild form of *influenza*).

paranoia

A condition in which the central feature is the *delusion* that people or events are especially connected to oneself. The term "paranoia" may also be used to describe feelings of persecution. A paranoid person builds up an elaborate set of beliefs based on the interpretation of chance remarks or events. Typical themes are persecution, jealousy (see *jealousy, morbid*), love, and grandeur (belief in one's own superior position and powers).

TYPES AND CAUSES
Paranoia may be *chronic* or *acute*. Chronic paranoia may be caused by brain damage, abuse of *alcohol* or *amphetamines*, *bipolar disorder*, or *schizophrenia*. It is also a feature of paranoid *personality disorder*, which is a psychological condition that causes people to be constantly suspicious of the motives of other people.

Acute paranoia, lasting for less than six months, may occur in people who have experienced radical life changes, such as refugees. In shared paranoia (see *folie à deux*), delusion develops because of a close relationship with someone else who has a delusion.

SYMPTOMS
There are usually no other symptoms of mental illness apart from occasional *hallucinations*. In time, however, the anger, suspicion, and social isolation may become severe.

TREATMENT AND OUTLOOK
If acute illness is treated early with *antipsychotic drugs*, the outlook is good. In long-standing cases of paranoia, however, the delusions are usually firmly entrenched, but antipsychotic drugs may make them less debilitating.

paraparesis

Partial *paralysis* or weakness of both legs and sometimes part of the trunk.

paraphimosis

Constriction of the *penis* behind the *glans* (head) by an extremely tight foreskin that has been pulled back, causing swelling and pain. Paraphimosis often occurs as a complication of an abnormally tight foreskin (see *phimosis*).

The problem can often be remedied manually by applying an ice-pack to reduce swelling and then squeezing the glans to return the foreskin to its normal position. Otherwise, an injection or an operation to cut the foreskin may be necessary. *Circumcision* (surgical removal of the foreskin) may be performed to prevent recurrence.

paraplegia

Weakness or *paralysis* of both legs and sometimes of part of the trunk as well, often accompanied by loss of feeling and by loss of urinary control. Paraplegia is a result of nerve damage in the *brain* or *spinal cord*.

parapsychology

The branch of *psychology* dealing with experiences and events that cannot be explained by scientific knowledge. Such phenomena include extrasensory perception (ESP), telepathy (communication

P

PARASITES: ECTOPARASITES (present in skin or on body surface)

Common examples	Activities	How acquired
• Head lice • Ticks • Bedbugs • Cat/Dog fleas • Aquatic leeches	Suck host's blood	Through contact with other people (lice, scabies mites, warts), animals (ringworm fungi, ticks), vegetation (ticks, mites), or water (aquatic leeches). Bedbugs live in bedroom walls or mattresses and visit humans at night. Cat and dog fleas may visit humans when the pet is absent.
• Scabies mites	Burrow in skin	
• Ringworm fungi • Wart viruses	Multiply in skin	

PARASITES: ENDOPARASITES (live within body)

Common examples	Activities	How acquired
• Tapeworms • Flukes • Roundworms • Threadworms • Hookworms	Adults live in human gut, blood vessels, bile ducts, or elsewhere and produce eggs that are passed out of the body.	By eating infected meat, swallowing eggs on food, contaminating fingers with faecal material, or contact with infected water.
• Various disease-causing protozoa, fungi, bacteria, and viruses	Organisms multiply locally or spread throughout the body, causing disease.	By inhalation, water- or food-borne transmission, sexual transmission, or blood-borne infection, among other mechanisms.

of thoughts), telekinesis (movement of objects with the mind), and precognition (being able to see into the future).

Many "paranormal" experiences can probably be explained by mental disturbances; others are probably due to coincidence, self-deception, or fraud.

paraquat

A weedkiller, available in high concentrations for agricultural use, which can be fatal if swallowed, inhaled, or absorbed through the skin. Paraquat poisoning requires urgent medical attention. Symptoms may include breathing difficulty, mouth ulcers, nosebleeds, diarrhoea, and later, respiratory and kidney failure.

Treatments include eating activated charcoal or Fuller's earth, stomach washout (see *lavage, gastric*), and in some cases *haemodialysis* (removal of toxic substances from the blood).

parasite

Any organism living in or on another living creature (the host) and deriving advantage from it, while causing the host disadvantage. In contrast, some organisms live on other creatures but have a symbiotic, or mutually beneficial, rela-

tionship with their host (see *commensal*). Parasites obtain nourishment from the host's blood, tissues, or ingested food. They may spend only part of their lifecycle with the host or remain there permanently. Some cause few symptoms, while others cause disease or even death.

Animal parasites of humans include *protozoa*, *worms*, *flukes*, *leeches*, *lice*, *ticks*, and *mites*. *Viruses* and disease-causing *fungi* and *bacteria* are also parasites.

parasitology

The scientific study of *parasites*. Although viruses and many types of bacteria and fungi are parasites, their study is conducted under the title of *microbiology*.

parasuicide

See *suicide, attempted*.

parasympathetic nervous system

One of the two divisions of the *autonomic nervous system*, which controls the automatic activities of organs, glands, blood vessels, and other tissues throughout the body. In contrast to the function of the sympathetic system, which prepares the body for action, the parasym-

pathetic system controls everyday functions such as breathing, digestion, and excretion of waste products.

parathion

An agricultural *organophosphate* insecticide that is highly poisonous.

parathyroidectomy

Surgical removal of abnormal tissue from the *parathyroid glands*. Parathyroidectomy may be performed to treat *hyperparathyroidism* (excess secretion of parathyroid hormones). Less commonly, it may be used to treat parathyroid cancer.

If hyperparathyroidism is caused by an *adenoma* (a small, benign tumour), usually only one of the parathyroid glands is involved and needs to be removed. If all the glands are enlarged and overactive, more parathyroid tissue may be removed.

parathyroid glands

Two pairs of oval, pea-sized glands that lie behind the *thyroid gland* in the neck. The glands produce parathyroid hormone (PTH), which helps to regulate the level of calcium in the blood.

Blood calcium levels are monitored continuously by the body because even small variations can impair muscle and nerve function. If the calcium levels drop too low, the parathyroid glands

LOCATION OF THE PARATHYROID GLANDS

These glands are embedded in the back of the thyroid gland, in the front of the neck, and are situated on either side of the trachea.

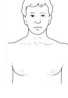

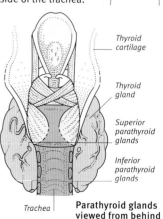

Thyroid cartilage

Thyroid gland

Superior parathyroid glands

Inferior parathyroid glands

Trachea

Parathyroid glands viewed from behind

P

release more PTH (see *feedback*). This response causes the bones to release more calcium into the blood, the intestines to absorb more from food, and the kidneys to conserve calcium; as a result, calcium levels rise rapidly. If the blood level of calcium is too high, the glands reduce their output of PTH.

Some people have only one parathyroid gland or have extra glands in the neck or chest. Rarely, the parathyroid glands may become overactive (a condition called *hyperparathyroidism*), which causes erosion of the bones and stones in the kidneys, ureters, or bladder (see *calculus, urinary tract*). Alternatively, the glands may become underactive (see *hypoparathyroidism*), resulting in *tetany* (painful muscle spasms) or *seizures*.

parathyroid tumour

A growth within a *parathyroid gland*. The tumour may cause excess secretion of parathyroid hormone (PTH), leading to *hyperparathyroidism*. Parathyroid cancers are very rare; most parathyroid tumours are noncancerous *adenomas*. An adenoma that causes hyperparathyroidism will be surgically removed (see *parathyroidectomy*). This usually provides a cure.

paratyphoid fever

An illness identical in most respects to *typhoid fever*, except that it is caused by a different bacterium, SALMONELLA PARA-TYPHI, and is usually less severe.

paraumbilical hernia

A *hernia* occurring near the *navel*. Paraumbilical hernias may occur in obese women who have had several children.

parenchyma

The functional (as opposed to supporting) tissue of an organ.

parenteral

The administration of drugs or other substances by any route other than via the gastrointestinal tract (for example, by injection into a blood vessel).

parenteral nutrition

Intravenous feeding (see *feeding, artificial*).

paresis

Partial *paralysis* or weakness affecting one or more muscles.

parietal

A medical term that is used to refer to the wall of a part of the body.

parity

A term used to indicate the number of pregnancies a woman has undergone that have resulted in the birth of a baby capable of survival.

parkinsonism

Any neurological disorder that is characterized by *tremor* (typically, this is a "pill-rolling" tremor, which occurs when the thumb is rubbed over the index finger); slow movements; and rigidity. The other characteristic features of the disorder of parkinsonism result from the slowness of movement. These features include a masklike face, a *festinating gait* (a shuffling, unbalanced style of walking), a monotonous style of speech, and reduced blinking. The most common type of parkinsonism is known as *Parkinson's disease*.

The known causes of parkinsonism include *cerebrovascular disease* (problems involving the blood vessels in the brain); the use of *antipsychotic drugs*, or the abuse of certain *designer drugs*; *carbon monoxide* poisoning; and, rarely, the infection *encephalitis lethargica*.

CAUSE OF **PARKINSON'S DISEASE**

This disorder results from damage, of unknown origin, to the basal ganglia (nerve cell clusters in the brain). The difference between the healthy state and that of Parkinson's disease is shown in the diagrams below.

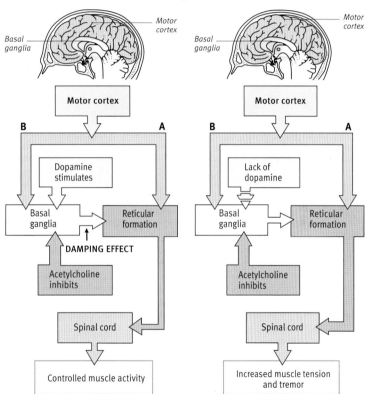

Healthy state
During movement, signals pass from the brain's cortex, via the reticular formation and spinal cord (pathway A), to muscles, which contract. Other signals pass, by pathway B, to the basal ganglia; these damp the signals in pathway A, reducing muscle tone so that movement is not jerky. Dopamine, a nerve transmitter made in the basal ganglia, is needed for this damping effect. Another transmitter, acetylcholine, inhibits the damping effect.

Parkinson's diseaseIn
Parkinson's disease, degeneration of parts of the basal ganglia causes a lack of dopamine within this part of the brain. The basal ganglia are thus prevented from modifying the nerve pathways that control muscle contraction. As a result, the muscles are too tense, causing tremor, joint rigidity, and slow movement. Most drug treatments increase the level of dopamine in the brain or oppose the action of acetylcholine.

P

Parkinson's disease

A neurological disorder that is the most common cause of *parkinsonism*.

CAUSES AND INCIDENCE

Parkinson's disease is caused by degeneration of, or damage to, cells in the *basal ganglia* of the brain. As a result, there is a deficiency of the neurotransmitter *dopamine* (which is needed for the control of movement). The condition occurs mainly in older people and is more common in men.

For further information on the processes leading to Parkinson's disease, see the illustrated box, previous page.

SYMPTOMS AND SIGNS

The main symptoms develop gradually, over several months or even years. The disease usually begins as a slight tremor of one hand, arm, or leg, which is worse when the hand or limb is at rest.

Later, both sides of the body are affected, causing stiffness, weakness, and trembling of the muscles. Symptoms include a stiff, shuffling walk that may break into uncontrolled, tiny running steps; constant hand tremors, sometimes accompanied by shaking of the head; a permanent rigid stoop; and an unblinking, fixed expression. Everyday activities such as eating, washing, and dressing become very difficult.

The intellect is unaffected until late in the disease, although the affected person's speech may become slow and hesitant, and the handwriting usually becomes very small. *Depression* is a common complication.

TREATMENT

There is no cure, but drug treatment, *physiotherapy*, and, rarely, surgery can help to relieve symptoms. In the early stages of Parkinson's disease, exercises, special aids in the home (see *disability*), and support can improve the affected person's morale and mobility. Drug treatment is used to minimize symptoms in later stages. These treatments cannot halt the degeneration of brain cells or progress of the disease, but can minimize symptoms by helping to correct chemical imbalances in the brain.

Levodopa, which the body converts into dopamine, is usually the most effective drug. It may, however, cause side effects such as nausea and vomiting; therefore, the dose is increased gradually, and the drug may be given in combination with benserazide or carbidopa. Levodopa is usually effective for several years, but the effects gradually wear off. Drugs that may be used in conjunction

with levodopa, or as substitutes for it, include *amantadine*, *bromocriptine*, selegiline, and pergolide. In some cases, an *anticholinergic drug* such as trihexyphenidyl (benzhexol) may initially be given to reduce tremor.

Surgical operations on the brain are occasionally performed, if the affected person is young and otherwise in good health. New therapies that are still being assessed include replacement of damaged tissue with transplanted brain cells, and deep brain stimulation with electrical impulses to reduce tremor.

OUTLOOK

If left untreated, the disease progresses over 10 to 15 years, leading to severe weakness and incapacity. Some sufferers eventually develop *dementia*. Modern drug treatments, however, can provide considerable relief from the symptoms and give affected people a much improved quality of life.

paronychia

An infection of the skin fold at the base or side of the *nail*. The affected area becomes swollen and painful, and there may be a buildup of pus.

Paronychia may be acute (caused by bacteria) or chronic (usually caused by CANDIDA ALBICANS). The condition is most common in women, particularly those with poor circulation and whose work involves frequent contact with water. It also affects people with skin disease involving the nail fold.

Treatment is with *antifungal drugs* or *antibiotic drugs*. If pus has collected in the area, it may need to be drained surgically. To prevent the occurrence of paronychia, gloves should be worn for tasks that involve putting the hands in water, and the hands should be dried thoroughly after washing.

parotid glands

The largest of the three pairs of *salivary glands*. The parotid glands are situated on each side of the face, just above the angle of the jaw and in front of the ear. They secrete saliva into the mouth through a duct that opens into the inner cheek, level with the second molar tooth.

The parotid glands may develop various disorders that can affect all of the salivary glands, such as infections, abscesses (collections of pus), or calculi (stones). One disorder that is specific to the parotid glands is *mumps*, which causes inflammation of one or both glands. Another is a form of noncancerous

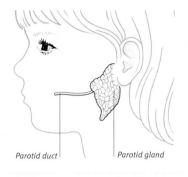

LOCATION OF THE PAROTID GLANDS

The glands are situated deep in the angle of the jaw and secrete saliva into the mouth. Mumps may affect other salivary and exocrine glands.

Parotid duct   Parotid gland

tumour, pleomorphic adenoma, which is slow-growing and painless but may rarely become cancerous.

parotitis

Inflammation of the *parotid glands*, often due to infection with the *mumps* virus.

paroxetine

A *selective serotonin reuptake inhibitor* antidepressant drug. Possible side effects include nausea, indigestion, and appetite loss. It is not usually recommended for those under 18 years old.

paroxysm

A sudden attack, worsening, or recurrence of symptoms or of a disease; a *spasm* or *seizure*.

paroxysmal nocturnal dyspnoea

Acute breathing difficulty that occurs suddenly at night, usually waking the person from sleep. The condition most commonly affects people suffering from congestive *heart failure* with *pulmonary oedema* (a buildup of fluid in the lungs); in these cases, it is caused by fluid leaking out of the blood vessels into the air spaces of the lungs once the person is lying down. It may also occur in people with chronic lung diseases.

paroxysmal tachycardia

A form of tachycardia (abnormally rapid heartbeat) that usually comes on abruptly and stops just as suddenly. It may be due to irregular muscle contractions in one of the chambers of the heart (see *arrhythmia, cardiac*).

parrot fever

The common name for *psittacosis*.

parturition

See *childbirth*.

parvovirus

The virus that causes *fifth disease*.

passive movement

Movement of a person's limbs or body by another person. Passive movement is used in *physiotherapy* to exercise the body if a person has nerve or muscle disorders that prevent voluntary movements.

passive smoking

Also known as secondary *smoking*, the involuntary inhalation of tobacco smoke by people who do not smoke. In adults, passive smoking increases the risk of smoking-related diseases such as *coronary artery disease* and *lung cancer*. In infants and children, it increases the risk of *sudden infant death syndrome (SIDS)* and chest and ear infections; it also makes children more likely to develop *asthma*.

passivity

In *psychology*, a persistent unwillingness or inability to take responsibility for oneself and one's everyday life. Passivity may be a feature of disorders such as *depression* or *dependent personality disorder*. The term has a specific meaning when used in reference to *schizophrenia*: it describes a patient's belief that his or her thoughts, feelings, or actions are controlled by others.

pasteurization

The process of heating foods to destroy disease-causing *microorganisms*, and to reduce numbers of microorganisms that cause fermentation and putrefaction.

Patau's syndrome

A *chromosomal abnormality* in which there are three copies of chromosome 13 rather than the normal two. It is a *congenital* (present from birth) condition and causes low birthweight and a range of deformities including *cleft palate* or *hare lip*; eye deformities; *micrognathia* (undersized jaw); lowset ears; extra digits (see *polydactyly*); and malformation of the genitalia. There may also be serious deformities of the internal organs, such as heart defects, meningomyelocele (see *neural tube defects*), and *exomphalos* (in which part or all of the intestines protrude through the navel).

Most children with Patau's syndrome die before two years of age, and those that survive have *learning difficulties*. Sometimes, affected children may have a mixture of normal and abnormal cells (see *mosaicism*), and they may have milder forms of the condition.

The condition may be diagnosed at an early stage of pregnancy by a test such as *chorionic villus sampling* or *amniocentesis*. In addition, *genetic counselling* may be offered.

patch test

A method that is used to diagnose the substances that are responsible for the skin disorder allergic contact *dermatitis*. A selection of possible *allergens* are put on a patch and taped to the skin. A skin reaction indicates that there is a sensitivity to a particular allergen.

patella

The kneecap (see *knee*).

patent

A term meaning "open" or "unobstructed" (such as in *patent ductus arteriosus*). The term "patent medicine" is sometimes used to refer to proprietary drugs protected by a patent.

patent ductus arteriosus

A defect of the *heart* in which the ductus arteriosus (a channel between the pulmonary artery and the aorta in the fetus) fails to close at birth.

CAUSE

In the fetus, blood that is pumped by the right side of the heart flows through the ductus arteriosus and bypasses the lungs (see *fetal circulation*). Normally, the ductus arteriosus closes at or shortly after birth, and blood passes from the right ventricle (lower chamber) of the heart to the lungs. In some babies this closure may fail to happen, producing a patent ductus arteriosus. In this condition, some of the blood that is pumped by the left side of the heart, and which should go to the rest of the body, is directed via the ductus to the lungs. As a result, the heart has to work harder than normal to pump sufficient blood to the body.

SYMPTOMS

Patent ductus arteriosus usually causes no symptoms, unless a large amount of blood is misdirected, in which case the baby fails to gain weight, becomes short of breath on exertion, and may have frequent chest infections. Eventually, *heart failure* may develop.

DIAGNOSIS AND TREATMENT

Diagnosis is made from hearing a heart *murmur*, from *chest X-rays*, and from an *ECG* and *echocardiography*. The drug indometacin or surgery may be used to close the duct.

paternity testing

The use of tests, including *DNA* tests and blood tests, to help decide whether a particular man is the father of a certain child. This procedure may be requested, or ordered by a court, in legal situations in which the paternity of a child is disputed.

Blood samples or buccal swabs (cell samples taken from rubbing the inside of the cheek) are taken from the child, from the man who is believed to be the father, and from the mother. There are various methods of testing for paternity: blood samples may be tested for *blood groups*, *histocompatibility antigens* (proteins that normally exist within body tissues, and whose form is inherited from the parents), and/or short lengths of DNA (a technique known as *genetic fingerprinting*); buccal swabs may only be used for DNA tests.

Genetic fingerprinting is the most conclusive method of paternity testing. Particular regions of DNA are examined for structures called genetic markers. If certain markers are present in the child's blood but not in the mother's blood, it follows that they must be determined by genes inherited from the child's biological father. If the man being tested has the markers in his blood, there is a high probability that he is the biological father; if he does not, he can be excluded from the paternity of the child. No form of paternity testing is 100 per cent accurate in confirming or excluding someone as the father of a child.

patho-

A prefix denoting a relationship to disease.

pathogen

Any agent, but particularly a *microorganism*, that causes disease.

pathogenesis

The processes by which a disorder originates and develops.

pathognomonic

A medical term applied to a sign or symptom that is characteristic of a disease or disorder and is therefore sufficient by itself to make a diagnosis.

P

PATERNITY TESTING USING DNA ANALYSIS

DNA analysis (commonly referred to as genetic fingerprinting) is replacing older techniques of paternity testing because it gives a decisive result in more cases. Blood samples are taken from the mother, child, and possible father, and some DNA (hereditary material) from each is specially processed.

PATERNITY ESTABLISHED

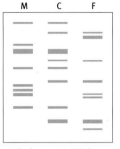

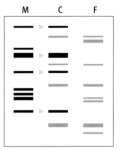

M   C   F   M   C   F   M   C   F

1 Each person's DNA has a unique banding pattern, or "fingerprint", detectable by X-rays after the processing.

2 A child's DNA bands come from the biological parents. First the bands from the mother are identified.

3 The other bands are compared with the suspected father's bands. Here they match, proving paternity.

PATERNITY DISPROVED

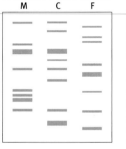

M   C   F   M   C   F   M   C   F

1 The mother's, the child's, and the suspected father's DNA have different banding patterns, shown above.

2 Half the child's DNA bands can be seen to have come from the mother, as in the example above.

3 The other bands are not shared by the suspected father, meaning he is not the biological father.

Key **M** = Mother   **C** = Child   **F** = Father

pathological

Relating to disease or to its study (see *pathology*).

pathological diagnosis

A method of *diagnosis* in which diseases are identified through examination of cells (see *cytopathology*), tissues (see *histopathology*), or body fluids. A clinical diagnosis, based on a patient's symptoms and a physical examination, is also undertaken.

pathological fracture

Fracture of a bone weakened by disease, such as by certain forms of *cancer*, *osteoporosis*, and *Paget's disease*.

pathology

The study of disease, and specifically its causes, mechanisms, and effects on the body. The study of disease-induced changes in cells is called *cytopathology*; the study of such changes in body tissues is called *histopathology*. A doctor who specializes in these subjects is called a pathologist.

Pathologists carry out laboratory studies of cells and tissues that help other doctors to reach accurate diagnoses, and they also supervise other laboratory personnel in the testing and microscopic examination of blood and other body fluids. In addition, pathologists conduct *autopsies* (physical examinations of dead people) to determine causes of death and to determine the effects that a disease or a treatment has had on the body.

pathology, cellular

Also called cytopathology, the branch of *cytology* concerned with the effects of disease on cells.

pathology, chemical

Another name for clinical *biochemistry*, which is the study of abnormalities that occur in the chemistry of diseased body tissues and fluids.

pathophysiology

The study of the effects of disease on body functions.

-pathy

A suffix that is used to denote a disease or disorder.

Paul–Bunnell test

A type of blood test, also called the heterophil agglutination test, that is used to detect infection with the Epstein–Barr virus, which causes glandular fever (see *mononucleosis, infectious*). The Paul–Bunnell test involves detecting particular *antibodies* (proteins produced by the immune system to combat the virus) in a sample of blood.

PCR

The abbreviation for *polymerase chain reaction*.

peak-flow meter

A piece of equipment that measures the maximum speed at which air can flow out of the lungs. A peak-flow meter is useful in assessing the severity of *bronchospasm* (constriction of the airways in the lungs), because narrowed airways slow the rate at which air can be expelled from the lungs. A peak-flow meter is most commonly used to diagnose *asthma*. In people who already have the disorder, it is used to monitor their condition and assess how they respond to treatment.

The peak flow is measured by taking in a deep breath and breathing out with the maximum force possible through the mouthpiece. The meter has a pointer and a scale on the side; the expelled breath moves the pointer to give a reading on the scale – the higher the reading, the greater the speed at which the air is travelling.

P

peau d'orange

A condition in which the skin is a normal colour but looks like orange peel. The skin's dimpled appearance is due to *fluid retention* in the nearby lymph vessels. Peau d'orange is not necessarily a sign of disease, although it is, for example, one of the features of *breast cancer*.

pectin

A form of *polysaccharide* found in apples and in the rinds of citrus fruits. Preparations containing pectins may be used to relieve diarrhoea.

pectoral

A medical term that means "relating to the chest", as in the pectoral muscles on either side of the chest. The pectoralis major is a large muscle covering much of the upper front of the chest. The smaller pectoralis minor lies beneath it.

PECTORAL MUSCLES

The major pectoral draws the arm across the body. The minor, which lies beneath it, moves the shoulder and raises some ribs.

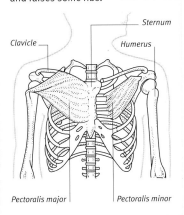

Sternum

Clavicle

Humerus

Pectoralis major

Pectoralis minor

pediculosis

Any type of louse infestation (see *lice*; *pubic lice*).

peer review

Processes by which doctors and scientists review the work of colleagues in the same field, to maintain standards.

pellagra

A potentially fatal disorder due to niacin deficiency (see *vitamin B complex*) resulting in *dermatitis*, diarrhoea, and *dementia*.

CAUSES AND INCIDENCE

Pellagra occurs primarily in poor rural communities in parts of the world, such as areas of India, where people subsist on maize. The body is unable to absorb most of the niacin in maize unless the maize is first treated with an alkali such as limewater. Maize is also low in tryptophan, an amino acid that is converted into niacin in the body.

Disorders such as *carcinoid syndrome* (which increases the breakdown of tryptophan) and *Crohn's disease* (which impairs absorption of tryptophan from the small intestine) may cause pellagra.

SYMPTOMS

The first symptoms are weakness, weight loss, lethargy, depression, irritability, and inflammation and itching of skin that is exposed to sunlight. In acute attacks, weeping blisters may develop on the affected skin, and the tongue becomes bright red, swollen, and painful.

DIAGNOSIS AND TREATMENT

Diagnosis is made from the patient's condition and dietary history. Daily intake of niacin and a varied diet usually bring about a cure.

pelvic abscess

An *abscess* (a collection of pus formed after infection with microorganisms) that develops in one of the structures within the pelvis. Pelvic abscesses may be due to *peritonitis* (inflammation of the membrane lining the abdominal cavity) or to localized inflammation resulting from disorders such as *pelvic inflammatory disease*.

pelvic examination

Examination of a woman's external and internal *genitalia*. After examination of the external genitalia, a *speculum* is inserted into the vagina to allow a clear view of the cervix. A *cervical smear test* may be performed. The doctor also carries out a bimanual examination: he or she inserts two fingers into the vagina, feeling the abdomen with the other hand to evaluate the position and size of the uterus and the ovaries and to detect any tenderness or swelling (see *Procedure for a pelvic examination* box, overleaf).

pelvic floor exercises

A programme of exercises to strengthen the muscles and tighten the ligaments at the base of the abdomen. These tissues make up the pelvic floor, which supports the uterus, vagina, bladder, urethra, and rectum. Slackening of the pelvic floor muscles and ligaments is common following childbirth, and is a part of the aging process.

WHY THEY ARE DONE

Performing pelvic floor exercises, especially during pregnancy and after childbirth, may help to prevent prolapse of the uterus (see *uterus, prolapse of*) and urinary stress incontinence (see *incontinence, urinary*). The exercises may also be of help to women who find achieving *orgasm* difficult.

HOW THEY ARE DONE

The pelvic floor muscles are those that tighten if urine flow is stopped in midstream. The exercises involve contracting (tightening) and relaxing the muscles several times. They can be done anywhere, sitting, standing, or lying down. To perform the exercises, contract the pelvic floor muscles, hold for a few seconds, then relax slowly. Repeat this several times. Gradually build up to ten contractions, taking ten seconds for each and resting for about four or five seconds between contractions. The exercises should be done regularly throughout the day. It may take up to about 12 weeks before any benefit is noticed, and the exercises will need to be continued to prevent symptoms from recurring.

pelvic infection

An infection that affects the female reproductive system. Severe or recurrent pelvic infection is referred to as *pelvic inflammatory disease* (PID).

pelvic inflammatory disease

Inflammation of the internal female reproductive organs. Pelvic inflammatory disease (PID) is usually due to an infection. It is most common in young, sexually active women. PID is a common cause of lower abdominal pain in women. In some cases, however, there are no obvious symptoms, and affected women may be unaware that they have had the condition until they undergo an examination to assess their fertility.

CAUSES

Pelvic inflammatory disease may not have any obvious cause, but it usually occurs as a result of a sexually transmitted infection such as *chlamydial infection* or *gonorrhoea*. It may also occur after a *miscarriage*, abortion (see *abortion, induced*), or *childbirth*. Use of an *IUD* increases the risk of developing pelvic inflammatory disease, particularly soon after the device has been inserted.

P

PROCEDURE FOR **PELVIC EXAMINATION**

The examination is usually performed with the woman lying on her back with her knees bent. If the examination is carried out because of uterine prolapse or incontinence, the woman may be asked to lie on her side. The doctor usually begins by inspecting the external genitals for ulceration or swelling and then does an internal examination.

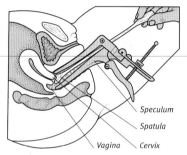

Use of speculum
A speculum is inserted into the vagina to hold the vaginal walls apart; this gives the doctor a clear view of both the vagina and cervix. A *cervical smear test*, in which cells are removed with a spatula, may also be performed.

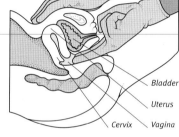

Manual examination
The doctor inserts two fingers into the vagina and palpates (feels) the abdomen with the other hand to evaluate the size and position of the uterus and ovaries, and to detect any abnormal pelvic swelling or tenderness.

SYMPTOMS AND COMPLICATIONS
Common symptoms of PID include pain and tenderness in the lower abdomen, fever, and irregular menstrual periods. There may also be a profuse vaginal discharge consisting of blood and/or pus. Pain often occurs after *menstruation* and may be worse during sexual intercourse (see *intercourse, painful*). There may also be malaise, vomiting, or backache. PID may be acute or chronic.

DIAGNOSIS AND TREATMENT
Diagnosis of pelvic inflammatory disease is usually made by an internal *pelvic examination* and examination of swabs from the vagina or cervix to look for infectious organisms. *Laparoscopy* (examination of the abdominal cavity using a viewing instrument) can confirm the diagnosis.

Antibiotic drugs are prescribed to clear the infection, and sometimes *analgesic drugs* (painkillers) may be given. If an IUD is the suspected cause of PID, the device may need to be removed.

OUTLOOK
If PID is detected and treated early, the patient should recover fully. Some affected women, however, have repeated attacks with or without reinfection. A *pelvic abscess* may develop as a complication of the condition. PID may cause *infertility* or increase the risk of *ectopic pregnancy*; this is primarily due to scarring of the fallopian tubes, which prevents eggs from travelling down the tubes to the uterus.

pelvic pain

See *abdominal pain*.

pelvimetry

Assessment of the shape and dimensions of a woman's pelvis. Pelvimetry may be carried out a couple of weeks before *childbirth*, to determine whether a woman is likely to have difficulty in delivering a baby vaginally. The procedure may also be performed after a vaginal delivery has been unsuccessful and a *caesarean section* has been carried out, to assist in planning a future pregnancy and delivery.

Medical staff can obtain a rough indication of the size of the pelvic outlet by manually checking the distance between the ischial tuberosities (the prominent bones in the lower pelvis) during a pelvic examination. More precise information may be obtained by taking an *X-ray* of the pelvis and then making measurements from the resulting image. However, excessive exposure to X-rays in pregnancy may increase the risk of subsequent *leukaemia* or other cancers in the unborn child, and therefore this procedure is carried out only in rare circumstances.

pelvis

The ring of bones in the lower trunk that supports the trunk, protects the lower abdominal organs, and forms part of the hip joints. Attached to the pelvis are the muscles of the abdominal wall, the buttocks, the lower back, and the insides and backs of the thighs.

STRUCTURE
The pelvis consists of two innominate bones (hip-bones). At the back, the hip-bones are joined by rigid joints (the *sacroiliac joints*) to the *sacrum* (the triangular spinal bone below the lumbar vertebrae). At the front, they curve forwards to join at a central point known as the pubic symphysis.

Each innominate bone consists of three fused bones: the ilium, ischium, and pubis. The ilium, the largest and uppermost of these bones, consists of a wide, flattened plate with a long, curved ridge (the iliac crest) along its upper border. The ischium is the bone that bears much of the body weight when sitting. The pubis is the smallest of the pelvic bones; from the ischium it extends forwards and round to the pubic symphysis, where it is joined to the other pubis bone by tough fibrous tissue. All three bones meet in the acetabulum, the cup-shaped cavity that forms the socket of the hip joint.

In women, the pelvis is generally shallow and broad, and the pubic symphysis joint is less rigid than a

P

STRUCTURE OF THE **PELVIS**

A basin-shaped bony structure at the base of the trunk, the pelvis consists of the sacrum and coccyx at the back and, on either side, the hips (each comprising three fused bones: the ilium, ischium, and pubis), which curve round to meet at the front. The pelvis supports the upper half of the body and protects the lower abdominal organs. The female pelvis is shallower and wider.

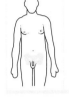

Male pelvis

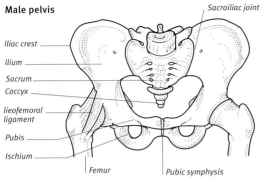

Sacroiliac joint
Iliac crest
Ilium
Sacrum
Coccyx
lieofemoral ligament
Pubis
Ischium
Femur
Pubic symphysis

Female pelvis

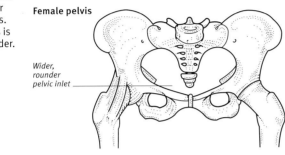

Wider, rounder pelvic inlet

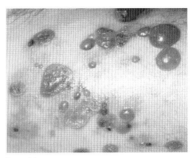

Pemphigus
The fragile blisters, as seen in this photograph, break down, leaving numerous large, raw areas of skin that are typical of this condition.

man's. These differences facilitate childbirth. In men, the greater body weight needs a larger and more heavily built pelvis for support.

DISORDERS
Fractures of the pelvis may be caused by a direct blow, or by a force transmitted through the femur (thigh-bone). Considerable force is required to cause such a fracture, and it is usually the result of a road traffic accident; motorcycle riders are particularly at risk. The fracture itself often heals without any problems, but it is frequently accompanied by damage to internal organs within the pelvis, and especially to the bladder; such damage may require immediate surgical treatment.

Osteitis pubis (inflammation of the pubic symphysis) is usually caused by repeated stress on the pelvis. It occurs in soccer players due to continually kicking a ball. The symptoms include pain in the groin and tenderness over the front of the pelvis. In most cases, the condition clears up with rest.

pelviureteric junction

The point at which the renal pelvis (the main collecting duct of the *kidney*) narrows to become the *ureter* (the tube that carries urine from the kidney to the bladder). Obstruction to the flow of urine may occur at the pelviureteric junction, and this can result in damage to the kidneys.

pemphigoid

An uncommon, chronic skin disease, mainly affecting elderly people, in which large, sometimes itchy, blisters form on the skin. Pemphigoid is thought to be an *autoimmune disorder* (one in which the body reacts against its own tissues).

Diagnosis is made with a skin *biopsy*. Treatment of the disease is usually with a long-term course of *corticosteroid* or *immunosuppressant drugs*.

pemphigus

A rare, serious skin disease in which numerous *blisters* develop on the skin and in the mouth. Pemphigus primarily affects people aged between 40 and 60. The blisters usually develop in the mouth, then appear on the skin. They rupture to form raw areas that may become infected and later crust over. Skin that appears unaffected may also blister after gentle pressure is applied. If a large area of the body is affected by the disease, there may be severe skin loss, which can lead to bacterial infection and, sometimes, death.

The diagnosis is confirmed by a skin *biopsy*. Treatment of pemphigus is with a long-term course of *corticosteroid drugs* and, in some cases, with *immunosuppressants*. *Antibiotics* may also be prescribed.

penciclovir

An *antiviral* drug. Penciclovir is commonly used in the form of a cream to treat cold sores (see *herpes simplex*).

penicillamine

A *disease-modifying antirheumatic drug* sometimes used to treat acute, progressive *rheumatoid arthritis*. Penicillamine is also used to treat copper, mercury, lead, or arsenic poisoning; *Wilson's disease* (a rare brain and liver disorder caused by a buildup of copper); and primary *biliary cirrhosis* (a liver disorder).

The possible adverse effects of penicillamine can include allergic rashes, itching, nausea, vomiting, abdominal pain, loss of taste, blood disorders, and impaired kidney function.

penicillin drugs

COMMON DRUGS
- Amoxicillin • Ampicillin • Benzylpenicillin
- Co-amoxiclav • Co-fluampicil • Flucloxacillin
- Phenoxymethylpenicillin

A group of *antibiotic drugs*. Natural penicillins are derived from the mould PENICILLIUM; others are synthetic preparations. Penicillins are used to treat many infective conditions, including *tonsillitis*, *bronchitis*, bacterial *endocarditis*, *gonorrhoea*, *osteomyelitis*, and *pneumonia*. They are also given to prevent *rheumatic fever* from recurring.

POSSIBLE ADVERSE EFFECTS
Diarrhoea is a common adverse effect of penicillin drugs. Penicillins may also provoke an allergic reaction (see *allergy*) in susceptible individuals. Allergic symp-

P

toms appear immediately after the drug is taken and include *urticaria* (nettle rash), wheezing, and *angioedema* (swelling of body tissues, occurring especially around the mouth and eyes). In rare cases, penicillins may cause the life-threatening allergic reaction *anaphylactic shock*. Reaction to a penicillin drug requires immediate discontinuation of the drug; urgent medical advice should be sought.

penile implant

A *prosthesis* inserted into the *penis* to help a man suffering with permanent *erectile dysfunction* to achieve sexual intercourse. The various types include a silicone splint inserted in the tissues of the upper surface of the penis, and an inflatable prosthesis that is inflated by squeezing a small bulb in the scrotum.

penile warts

See *warts, genital*.

penis

The male sex organ, through which *urine* and *semen* pass.

STRUCTURE AND FUNCTION

The penis consists of three cylindrical bodies of erectile tissue (spongy tissue full of blood vessels) that run along its length. Two of these bodies, the corpora cavernosa, lie side by side along the upper part of the penis. The third body,

ANATOMY OF THE PENIS

The corpora cavernosa and the spongiosum are the erectile tissues of the penis. A network of nerves controls the blood flow into them.

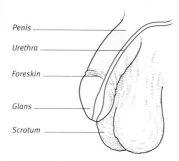

Penis
Urethra
Foreskin
Glans
Scrotum

Cross-section of penis

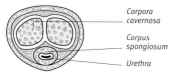

Corpora cavernosa
Corpus spongiosum
Urethra

the corpus spongiosum, lies centrally beneath them and expands at the end to form the *glans*. Around the erectile tissue is a sheath consisting of fibrous connective tissue that is enclosed by skin. Over the glans, the skin forms a fold called the *foreskin*.

Through the centre of the corpus spongiosum runs the *urethra*, which is a narrow tube that carries urine and semen out of the body through an opening at the tip of the glans.

The principal functions of the penis are the excretion of urine and the discharge of semen during sexual intercourse (see *erection*; *ejaculation*).

DISORDERS

One common problem is *erectile dysfunction* (failure to attain or maintain an erection). This condition affects most men at some point in their lives, and is usually psychological in origin. However, persistent erectile dysfunction may be caused by nerve damage associated with *diabetes mellitus*, *alcohol* dependence, *atherosclerosis*, or spinal cord injury.

Balanitis (inflammation of the glans and foreskin) is usually caused by *candidiasis*, although other organisms, including those that cause *gonorrhoea* and *syphilis*, may cause inflammation. Balanitis may lead to *phimosis*, in which the foreskin is abnormally tight, or *paraphimosis*, in which the foreskin retracts at erection but is too tight to move back over the glans.

Penile warts (see *warts, genital*) are caused by a sexually transmitted virus. Cancer of the penis (see *penis, cancer of*) is a rare disorder; the incidence is higher in men who have not been circumcised than in those who have.

The most common congenital abnormality of the penis is *hypospadias*, a condition in which the opening to the urethra is located on the underside of the penis. In male *pseudohermaphroditism*, which is also congenital, the penis is very small and there is usually also hypospadias.

Other disorders of the penis include *priapism*, in which an erection is painful and abnormally prolonged, and a condition called *Peyronie's disease*, in which the erect penis bends.

penis, cancer of

A rare type of cancerous tumour that is more common in uncircumcised men with poor personal hygiene. Viral infection and smoking have both been shown to be additional risk factors. The tumour usually starts on the *glans* or on

the foreskin as a painless, wartlike lump or a painful ulcer, and develops into a cauliflowerlike mass. The growth usually spreads slowly, but in some cases it can spread to the *lymph nodes* in the groin within a few months.

Diagnosis is made by a *biopsy* (tissue sample). If the tumour is detected early, surgical removal is usually successful. Otherwise, removal of part or all of the penis may be necessary. *Radiotherapy* and *chemotherapy* may also be used.

pentamidine

An antiprotozoal drug (see *protozoa*) administered by intravenous infusion or nebulizer to prevent and treat *pneumocystis pneumonia* in immunosuppressed people. Pentamidine is also used to treat the tropical diseases *leishmaniasis* and *trypanosomiasis*. Side effects may include nausea and vomiting, dizziness, flushing, rash, and taste disturbances.

pentazocine

An opioid *analgesic drug* used to relieve moderate or severe pain caused by injury, surgery, cancer, or childbirth. It is rarely used because of its adverse affects, which include dizziness, drowsiness, nausea, vomiting, and, rarely, hallucinations. *Drug dependence* may develop if high doses are taken for prolonged periods.

peppermint oil

An oil obtained from the peppermint plant MENTHA PIPERITA. It is prescribed to relieve abdominal colic but may cause heartburn. Peppermint oil is also used as a flavouring in some drug preparations.

peptic ulcer

A raw area that develops in the gastrointestinal tract due to erosion by acidic gastric juice. A peptic ulcer most commonly occurs in the stomach, where it is called a gastric ulcer, or the *duodenum* (the first part of the small intestine), where it is known as a duodenal ulcer.

CAUSES

The lining of the stomach and duodenum is usually protected from the acid gastric juice by a layer of mucus. If this layer is damaged, the acid can come into contact with the tissues, causing inflammation and erosion. Ulcers can also form in the *oesophagus*, when acidic juice from the stomach enters it (see *gastro-oesophageal reflux disease*).

The major cause of peptic ulcers is infection with HELICOBACTER PYLORI bacteria, which can damage the lining of the stomach and duodenum, allowing the acid stomach contents to attack it. The long-term use of *nonsteroidal anti-inflammatory drugs* (NSAIDs), smoking, alcohol consumption, and excess acid production can also damage the stomach lining. In some cases, there is a family history of peptic ulcers, indicating that a genetic factor may be involved. A *stress ulcer* is a peptic ulcer caused by severe physiological stress, such as that due to neurosurgery or to burns (for example, a *Curling's ulcer*). Psychological stress is thought to aggravate an existing ulcer. For further information on ulcer formation and sites, see the illustrated box (below).

SYMPTOMS

There may be no symptoms, or there may be burning or gnawing pain in the upper abdomen when the stomach is empty. The pain of a duodenal ulcer is often relieved by eating, but usually recurs a few hours later. The pain of a gastric ulcer may be worsened by food.

Other possible symptoms of a peptic ulcer include a loss of appetite, a bloated or full feeling in the abdomen, nausea, and, sometimes, vomiting.

COMPLICATIONS

The most common complication of a peptic ulcer is bleeding as the ulcer penetrates deeper and damages blood vessels. If severe, bleeding may result in haematemesis (vomiting of blood) and *melaena* (black faeces) and is a medical emergency. Chronic bleeding may cause

SITES AND CAUSES OF **PEPTIC ULCER**

A peptic ulcer develops in about one in eight people in the UK at some time in their lives. Some of the mechanisms that are involved in causing ulcers are shown below. A peptic ulcer is investigated using endoscopy, which involves passing a gastroscope (a type of endoscope) through the mouth to view the stomach and duodenum. A sample of the stomach lining may be taken at the same time to look for evidence of HELICOBACTER PYLORI infection, the major cause of peptic ulcers; blood tests (to check for antibodies against HELICOBACTER PYLORI) and *breath tests* are also used to confirm its presence.

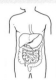

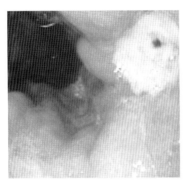

Gastric ulcer
This photograph of an ulcer in the wall of the stomach was taken using a gastroscope passed through the mouth into the stomach.

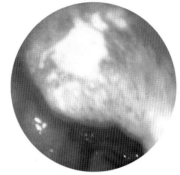

Duodenal ulcer
In this gastroscopic view of the top of the duodenum, an ulcer is clearly visible as a smooth white area.

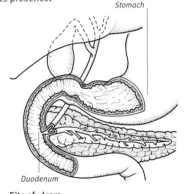

Stomach

Duodenum

Site of ulcers
Peptic ulcers are most common in the first part of the duodenum or lower half of the stomach; oesophageal ulcers also occur.

HOW AN ULCER FORMS

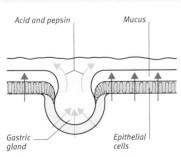

Acid and pepsin   Mucus

Gastric gland   Epithelial cells

1 Gastric glands in the lining of the stomach secrete acid and the enzyme pepsin, which help to break down food. The acid and pepsin would quickly eat away the stomach and duodenum if other cells in the lining did not secrete a protective mucus.

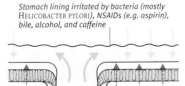

Stomach lining irritated by bacteria (mostly HELICOBACTER PYLORI), NSAIDs (e.g. aspirin), bile, alcohol, and caffeine

Increased acid secretion

Reduced mucus production

2 Most peptic ulcers are due to bacterial infection of the stomach lining, which damages its mucous layer (making it vulnerable to acid) and the cells that control excess acid production. Ulcers can also be caused by NSAIDs or excess alcohol combined with excess production of acid. Smoking is another important irritant factor.

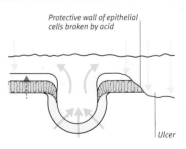

Protective wall of epithelial cells broken by acid

Ulcer

3 If damaging influences overcome the protective factors in the stomach or duodenal lining, the mucous layer and mucus-secreting cells are eroded and an ulcer forms. Stress is probably not a prime cause of ulcers but it is possible it may aggravate an existing ulcer.

P

iron-deficiency *anaemia*. Rarely, an ulcer may perforate the wall of the digestive tract and lead to *peritonitis* (inflammation of the abdominal cavity's lining).

Another rare complication is scarring of the tissues that occurs as a result of chronic ulcers. Scar tissue around the pyloric sphincter (the outlet where the stomach opens into the duodenum) may cause narrowing of the outlet. This condition, which is called *pyloric stenosis*, may obstruct the passage of food from the stomach to the duodenum, resulting in vomiting and weight loss.

DIAGNOSIS AND TREATMENT

An ulcer is usually diagnosed by *endoscopy* of the stomach and duodenum, or, less commonly, a barium meal (see *barium X-ray examination*). Blood and breath tests are carried out to see whether the person is infected with the HELICOBACTER bacterium. If so, a combination of *antibiotics* and an *ulcer-healing drug* will be given as treatment. A further test may be carried out to check that the treatment has been successful.

If HELICOBACTER is not detected, however, (for example, in cases where the ulcer was the result of the use of NSAIDs), the NSAIDs will be stopped and treatment with *proton pump inhibitors* or H_2-blockers will be given.

Surgery is now rarely needed for peptic ulcers, except to treat complications such as bleeding or perforation.

Stopping smoking and reducing alcohol consumption reduce the likelihood of an ulcer recurring.

peptide

A protein fragment consisting of two or more *amino acids*. Peptides that consist of very many linked amino acids are called polypeptides; chains of polypeptides are called *proteins*. In the body, peptides occur in forms such as *hormones* and *endorphins*.

perception

The interpretation of a *sensation*. Information is received through the five senses (taste, smell, hearing, vision, and touch), then identified and organized into a pattern by the brain. Factors such as attitude, mood, and expectations affect the final interpretation; for example, a person who is hungry is more likely to notice the sight and smell of food than someone who has just eaten.

Hallucinations are false perceptions that occur in the absence of any type of sensory stimuli.

percussion

A diagnostic technique that involves tapping the chest or abdomen with the fingers and listening to the sound that is produced. From this sound, the doctor can deduce the condition of the internal organs. (See also *examination, physical*.)

percutaneous

A term meaning "through the skin".

perforation

A hole made in an organ or tissue by disease or injury.

pergolide

A drug used to treat *Parkinson's disease*, a neurological disorder resulting from a lack of the neurotransmitter *dopamine*. The drug works by stimulating the *receptors* for dopamine in the brain.

peri-

A prefix meaning "around", as in pericardium, the membranous sac that surrounds the heart.

perianal haematoma

A *haematoma* (collection of blood) under the skin around the anus. A perianal haematoma is painful and of sudden onset. It usually disappears with no treatment, but minor surgery may be required to drain the blood.

periapical abscess

See *abscess, dental*.

pericarditis

Inflammation of the *pericardium* (the double-layered membrane surrounding the heart). This disorder often leads to chest pain and fever. There may also be an increased amount of fluid (see *effusion*) in the pericardial space, which separates the two smooth layers of the pericardium. The excess fluid may compress the heart and restrict its action.

Long-term inflammation of the pericardium can cause a condition called constrictive pericarditis, in which the pericardium becomes scarred, thickens, and contracts, and as a result impedes the heart's action.

CAUSES

Causes of pericarditis include infection; *myocardial infarction* (heart attack); cancer spreading from another site; and injury to the pericardium. The disorder may accompany the autoimmune conditions *rheumatoid arthritis* and systemic *lupus erythematosus*, or *kidney failure*.

SYMPTOMS

The main symptom is sharp pain behind the sternum (breastbone) and sometimes in the neck and shoulders, which may be more severe if the person takes a deep breath, changes position, or swallows. The pain may be relieved by sitting up and leaning forward. There may also be fever. Constrictive pericarditis causes *oedema* (swelling due to accumulation of fluid) of the legs and abdomen.

DIAGNOSIS AND TREATMENT

Diagnosis is made from a *physical examination*, from an *ECG* (which records the electrical activity in the heart) and *chest X-rays* or *echocardiography*, which will show any excess fluid around the heart.

If possible, treatment is aimed at the cause. *Analgesic drugs* or *anti-inflammatory drugs* may be given. If there is an effusion, the excess fluid may be drawn off through a needle. In severe constrictive pericarditis, the thickened part of the pericardium may be surgically removed so that the heart can pump freely.

pericardium

The membranous bag that surrounds the *heart* and the roots of the major blood vessels that emerge from it.

The pericardium is made up of two layers. The outer layer is tough, inelastic, and fibrous. It is attached to the diaphragm below and to the sternum (breastbone) in front. The inner layer is separated into two sheets; the innermost one is firmly attached to the heart, and the outer one is attached to the fibrous layer. The smooth inner surfaces of these sheets are separated by a space called the pericardial space, which contains a small amount of fluid that lubricates the heart.

perimenopause

The period immediately preceding the *menopause* (when the ovaries stop producing eggs and *menstruation* ceases). During the perimenopause, levels of *oestrogen* begin to fall. Fluctuations in hormone levels cause menstrual periods to become irregular and results in symptoms such as hot flushes.

perimetry

A visual field test to determine the extent of peripheral vision. (See *eye, examination of*).

perinatal

A term used to describe the period that extends from just before the birth of a baby to just after. The perinatal period

P

is often defined as the period lasting from the 24th week of pregnancy to the end of the first week after birth.

perinatology

A branch of *obstetrics* and *paediatrics* concerned with the study and care of the mother and baby during pregnancy and just after birth.

Perinatologists are specialists in the management of high-risk pregnancies and births, and in the investigation and treatment of prenatal conditions that might endanger the life or health of the fetus, such as *rhesus incompatibility*, *spina bifida*, or biochemical disorders. These doctors are also skilled in assessing the function of the placenta and maintaining the health of an expectant mother who may herself be at risk of health problems.

perindopril

One of a class of drugs called *ACE inhibitors*, which act by widening the blood vessels and thereby ease the workload on the heart. Perindopril may be used to relieve *hypertension* (high blood pressure) or congestive heart failure.

The drug may have side effects related to widening of the blood vessels, such as *hypotension* (low blood pressure), which may lead to dizziness or fainting; flushed skin; and headaches.

perineum

The area that is bounded internally by the bony structures that surround the pelvic floor (the muscles that support the pelvis). Internally, the perineum extends from the coccyx (the "tailbone" of the spine) at the back to the pubic symphysis, where the pelvic bones meet at the front of the body, and incorporates the lower parts of the genitourinary and gastrointestinal tracts. Outside the body, the perineum is the area that extends from the genitals to the anus.

periodic fever

An inherited condition that causes recurrent bouts of fever (see *familial Mediterranean fever*).

periodic paralysis

See *paralysis, periodic*.

period, menstrual

See *menstruation*.

periodontal abscess

See *abscess, dental*.

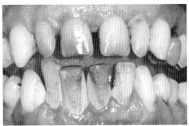

Periodontal disease
The gums are inflamed and have receded. Many of the teeth are eroded at the base; and the tooth sockets may also be decayed.

periodontal disease

Any disorder of the periodontium (the tissues that surround and support the *teeth*). The most common type of periodontal disease is *gingivitis* (inflammation of the gums). Gingivitis can lead to marginal *periodontitis*, which often causes the development of a periodontal abscess (see *abscess, dental*).

periodontics

The branch of dentistry concerned with the structures that surround and support the teeth, particularly the gums.

periodontitis

Inflammation of the periodontium (the tissues surrounding the *teeth*). There are two types: periapical and marginal.

CAUSES

Periapical periodontitis results from neglected tooth decay (see *caries, dental*). If dental caries is left untreated, areas of enamel and the dentine (softer tissue) beneath are eventually destroyed, allowing bacteria to enter the tooth pulp and then spread to the root tip and into the surrounding tissues, sometimes causing an abscess (see *abscess, dental*), *granuloma*, or *cyst*.

Marginal periodontitis is the major cause of tooth loss in adults. It is a result of untreated *gingivitis* (gum disease), which in turn is usually due to poor *oral hygiene*. In gingivitis, neglected, inflamed gum tissue at the base of the teeth becomes damaged, and pockets form between the gums and the teeth. Plaque (see *plaque, dental*) and a hard, mineralized coating (see *calculus, dental*) then collect in these pockets. The bacteria in the plaque and calculus attack the periodontal tissues, causing them to become inflamed and then detached from the teeth. The bacteria also eventually erode the bones around the teeth. As a result, the teeth become loose in their sockets and fall out.

SYMPTOMS

Periapical periodontitis may cause localized toothache, especially on biting. An abscess may damage bone and periodontal ligaments, causing the tooth to become loose; a large dental cyst may cause swelling of the jaw.

In marginal periodontitis there are signs of gingivitis, such as red, soft, shiny, tender gums that bleed easily. There is also an unpleasant taste in the mouth and bad breath. The deepening pockets in the gums gradually expose the sensitive dentine in the roots of the teeth, causing the teeth to ache when hot, cold, or sweet foods or liquids are consumed. Occasionally, there is a discharge of pus from the gums, or a periodontal abscess develops.

DIAGNOSIS AND TREATMENT

The diagnosis of periodontitis is by a dental examination to find any pockets and assess their size and depth, and dental *X-rays* to check for bone loss.

Periapical periodontitis is treated by draining the pus and filling the tooth or alternatively by *root-canal treatment*, in which decayed pulp is removed from a tooth and its root and the cavity is then filled. If the tooth cannot be saved, however, *extraction* is performed.

In the early stages of marginal periodontal disease, regular, scrupulous teeth cleaning can prevent further plaque and calculus formation and thus halt destruction of the tissues surrounding the teeth. For more severe periodontitis, the dentist will remove existing plaque and calculus by *scaling* and root planing (smoothing the surface of an exposed root). In some cases, *gingivectomy* (surgical trimming of the gums) may be performed to reduce the size of gum pockets. Surgery may also be carried out in order to remove the diseased lining from the pocket (see *curettage, dental*), so that healthy underlying tissue will reattach itself to the tooth; and the damaged, irregular bone is smoothed. Loose teeth can sometimes be anchored to firmer ones by a method called splinting (see *splinting, dental*).

period pain

See *dysmenorrhoea*.

periosteum

The layer of connective tissue that coats all of the *bones* in the body except the joint surfaces. The periosteum contains small blood vessels and nerves. It produces new bone in the initial stages of healing following a *fracture*.

P

periostitis

Inflammation of the *periosteum* (connective tissue covering bone). The usual cause is a blow that presses directly on to bone. Symptoms include pain, tenderness, and swelling over the affected area.

peripheral nerves

Nerves that run between the *central nervous system* (brain and spinal cord) and body tissues. Of these, 12 pairs are *cranial nerves* and 31 pairs are *spinal nerves*. Some peripheral nerves are sensory, carrying messages from sensory organs and nerve endings (see *receptor*) towards the brain and spinal cord; others are motor nerves, carrying signals away from the CNS to stimulate responses in the tissues.

peripheral nervous system

The system of *peripheral nerves*, which fan out from the *central nervous system* (the brain and spinal cord) to the muscles, skin, internal organs, and glands.

peripheral vascular disease

Narrowing of arteries in the legs, and sometimes in the arms, which restricts blood flow and causes pain. In severe cases, *gangrene* may develop.

CAUSES

In most affected people, peripheral vascular disease is caused by *atherosclerosis*, in which fatty deposits form on the inner walls of arteries. The principal risk factors for atherosclerosis (and therefore peripheral vascular disease) are *smoking*, *hyperlipidaemia* (high blood lipid levels), *hypertension* (high blood pressure), poorly controlled *diabetes mellitus*, a high-fat diet, and lack of exercise. Diseases of the peripheral arteries that are not caused by atherosclerosis include *Buerger's disease* and *Raynaud's disease*.

SYMPTOMS AND COMPLICATIONS

The first symptom is usually aching in the leg muscles (usually in the calf) when walking. The pain may be relieved by resting for a few minutes, but recurs after the same amount of walking as before. Prolonged use of the arms may also cause pain. Symptoms then become worse until eventually pain is present even at rest. The pain may be severe and continuous, even disrupting sleep. By this stage, the blood supply to the affected leg is dangerously low. The affected limb is cold and numb, with dry, scaly skin, and *leg ulcers* may develop after even minor injuries. In the final stage, *gangrene* (tissue death) develops, initially appearing in the toes and then spreading up the leg.

Sudden arterial blockage sometimes occurs, causing acute *ischaemia* (insufficient blood supply to an organ or tissue). This arterial blockage may be due to the rapid development of a clot on top of a plaque of atherosclerosis, by a dissecting aneurysm (splitting of an arterial wall), or by an embolism arising from a clot formed in the heart and carried to a peripheral artery. It causes sudden, severe pain. The affected limb becomes cold and pale or blue, with no pulse. Movement and feeling in the limb are lost.

DIAGNOSIS AND TREATMENT

A diagnosis is often based on the results of *Doppler ultrasonography*, which shows blood flow through the affected vessels, or *angiography*, which will reveal narrowing or other structural abnormalities.

Exercise and giving up smoking are important aspects of treatment. *Antiplatelet drugs*, *lipid-lowering drugs*, and peripheral vasodilator drugs (which widen peripheral blood vessels) such as naftidrofuryl may be prescribed. For peripheral vascular disease of the legs, the affected person needs to take scrupulous care of the feet to prevent infection and minimize the risk of gangrene. *Arterial reconstructive surgery*, *bypass surgery*, or balloon *angioplasty* may be needed to widen or bypass the affected blood vessels. Amputation is necessary if gangrene has developed.

peristalsis

Wavelike movement caused by the rhythmic contraction and relaxation of the smooth muscles in the walls of the

---

PERIPHERAL VASCULAR DISEASE

The disease usually starts with the formation of atheroma (fatty plaques) in the lining of artery walls. Smokers are among those at highest risk.

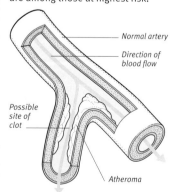

Normal artery
Direction of blood flow
Possible site of clot
Atheroma

Clot formation
Clots may form on top of the atheroma (plaques), restricting blood flow to tissues, which may lead to pain and tissue death.

PERISTALSIS

The walls of many body passages contain a special type of muscle called smooth muscle. The muscle fibres contract in sequence, sending waves of contraction along the walls of the passage.

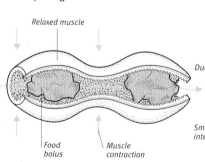

Relaxed muscle
Food bolus
Muscle contraction

Effect of peristalsis
As each group of muscle fibres in the wall of the intestinel contracts, it narrows that part of the passage, squeezing the food bolus into an adjoining section where the muscle fibres are relaxed.

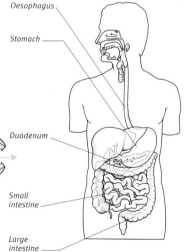

Oesophagus
Stomach
Duodenum
Small intestine
Large intestine

Sites of peristaltic action
Peristalsis occurs most obviously in the digestive tract, shown above, but it also moves urine through the ureters.

P

digestive tract and the ureters. Peristalsis is responsible for the movement of food and waste products through the digestive system and for transporting urine from the kidneys to the bladder.

In the digestive system, peristalsis in the oesophagus (gullet) moves food towards the stomach, even if the body is turned upside down. In the stomach, similar muscle movements help to mix food with gastric juices and move the partly digested food into the duodenum (the first part of the small intestine). The muscles of the small intestine move in a slow, back-and-forth churning motion that allows more time for the intestine to absorb nutrients. In the large intestine, peristaltic contractions occur only about once every 30 minutes. Two or three times a day, however, usually following a meal, a strong, sustained wave of peristalsis in the colon forces the contents into the rectum, and may prompt the urge to defaecate. (See also the illustrated box.)

peritoneal dialysis

See *dialysis*.

peritoneum

The two-layered membrane that forms a lining in the abdominal cavity and covers and supports the abdominal organs. The peritoneum contains blood vessels, lymph vessels, and nerves. The surface area of the peritoneum is equal to that of the entire skin.

The peritoneum produces a lubricating fluid that allows the abdominal organs to glide smoothly over each other. It also protects the organs against infection. In addition, the membrane absorbs fluid and acts as a natural filtering system; this function is utilized in one form of *dialysis*. The peritoneum may become inflamed as a complication of an abdominal disorder (see *peritonitis*).

peritonitis

Inflammation of the *peritoneum* (the membrane lining the abdominal wall and covering the abdominal organs). Peritonitis is a serious condition.

CAUSES

The inflammation is almost always due to irritation and bacterial infection caused by another abdominal disorder. The most common cause is *perforation* of the stomach or intestine wall, which allows bacteria and digestive juices to move into the abdominal cavity. Perforation is usually the result of a *peptic ulcer*, *appendicitis*

(acute inflammation of the appendix), or *diverticulitis* (inflammation of abnormal pouches in the wall of the intestine).

Peritonitis may also be associated with acute *salpingitis* (inflammation of a fallopian tube), *cholecystitis* (inflammation of the gallbladder), or *septicaemia*.

SYMPTOMS

There is usually severe abdominal pain over part or all of the abdomen. After a few hours, the abdomen feels hard, and *peristalsis* (wavelike contractions of the intestinal muscles) stops (see *ileus, paralytic*). Other symptoms include fever, bloating, nausea, and vomiting. *Dehydration* and *shock* may occur.

DIAGNOSIS AND TREATMENT

Diagnosis is made from a *physical examination*. The affected person will need to be admitted to hospital without delay. Surgery may be necessary to deal with the cause. If the cause is unknown, a *laparoscopy* or an exploratory *laparotomy* may be performed. *Antibiotic drugs* are often given to destroy bacteria, and *intravenous infusions* of fluid may be given to treat dehydration.

OUTLOOK

In most cases, a full recovery is made. Rarely, however, intestinal obstruction, caused by *adhesions* (bands of scar tissue between loops of intestine), may occur at a later stage.

peritonsillar abscess

An abscess (collection of pus) in the soft tissue around the tonsils that occurs as a complication of *tonsillitis*. A peritonsillar abscess, also known as quinsy, causes pain, swallowing difficulties, and jaw stiffness. The tonsils appear asymmetrical. *Antibiotic drugs* and *analgesic drugs* (painkillers) are usually given to help relieve the symptoms, and in some cases a small surgical incision may be made to drain the abscess.

permanent teeth

The second set of *teeth*, which usually start to replace the primary teeth at about the age of six. There are 32 permanent teeth: 16 in each jaw. Each set of 16 consists of four incisors, two canines, four premolars and six molars. (See also *eruption of teeth*.)

permethrin

A substance included in preparations used to treat *pubic lice* and *scabies*. Permethrin can also be used as an insecticide: sprayed on to mosquito nets and clothing, it repels mosquitoes and ticks.

pernicious anaemia

A type of *anaemia* (reduced blood levels of the oxygen-carrying pigment *haemoglobin*) caused by the stomach lining failing to produce intrinsic factor – which is necessary for absorption of vitamin B_{12}. The resulting deficiency of vitamin B_{12} prevents bone marrow from producing normal red blood cells (see *anaemia, megaloblastic*).

pernio

An alternative term for *chilblain*.

peroneal muscular atrophy

A rare, inherited disorder characterized by muscle wasting in the feet and calves and then in the hands and forearms. The condition, which is also known as Charcot–Marie–Tooth disease, is caused by degeneration of some peripheral nerves. It usually appears in late childhood or adolescence.

Muscle wasting stops halfway up the arms and legs, making them look like inverted bottles; sensation may be lost. There is no treatment for the disorder, but it is rare for the sufferer to become totally incapacitated because the disease usually progresses at a very slow rate. Life expectancy is normal.

perphenazine

A *phenothiazine*-type *antipsychotic drug* that is used to relieve symptoms in psychiatric disorders, such as *schizophrenia*; to sedate agitated or anxious patients; and sometimes for the relief of severe nausea and vomiting.

Possible adverse effects include abnormal movements of the face and limbs, drowsiness, blurred vision, stuffy nose, and headache. Long-term use of the drug may cause the movement disorder *parkinsonism*.

persistent vegetative state

A term used to describe a type of indefinite, deep *coma* (unconsciousness and unresponsiveness to stimuli). The condition is caused by damage to areas of the brain that control higher mental functions. Although the eyes may open and close and there may be random movements of the head and limbs, there is no response to stimuli such as pain. Only basic functions, such as breathing and heartbeat, are maintained due to functioning of the *brainstem*. There is no treatment to reverse the situation; with good nursing care, survival for several years is possible.

P

personality

A term that is used to describe the sum of a person's traits, habits, and experiences. Temperament, intelligence, emotion, and motivation are important aspects. The development of personality seems to depend on the interaction of heredity and environment.

personality disorders

A group of conditions characterized by a failure to learn from experience or to adapt appropriately to changes, resulting in distress, impaired social functioning, and, in some cases, occupational problems. Personality disorders are patterns of abnormal behaviour that may become especially obvious during periods of stress. They are usually first recognizable in adolescence and may continue throughout life, often leading to *depression* or *anxiety*. Personality disorders are not the result of another psychiatric disorder or a result of substance abuse.

TYPES

Specific types of personality disorders are divided into three groups, but there is often overlap between them.

The first group is characterized by eccentric behaviour. Paranoid people show suspicion and mistrust of others; schizoid people are cold emotionally; and schizotypal personalities have behavioural oddities similar to, but less severe than, those of *schizophrenia*.

In the second group, behaviour tends to be dramatic. Histrionic people are excitable and constantly crave stimulation. Narcissists have an exaggerated sense of self-importance (see *narcissism*). People with antisocial personality disorder (formerly called psychopaths) disregard accepted standards of behaviour and show no concern for other people's feelings and rights. People with borderline personality disorder behave very impulsively; their self-image, relationships, and emotions are unstable.

People in the third group show anxiety and fear. Dependent personalities lack the self-confidence to function in an independent way (see *dependence*). People who have avoidant personalities are hypersensitive to criticism and rejection and cautious about new experiences. Those with obsessive–compulsive personalities are very rigid in their habits (see *obsessive–compulsive disorder*).

TREATMENT

Personality disorders are generally difficult to treat. Treatment options include *counselling*, *psychotherapy*, and *behaviour therapy*. The treatment may need to be prolonged, however, and affected people may not always comply with guidance from doctors or therapists.

personality tests

Questionnaires designed to define various personality traits or types. Tests may be used to detect psychiatric symptoms, various underlying traits, how outgoing or reserved a person is, and predisposition to developing neurotic illness.

perspiration

The production and excretion of sweat from the *sweat glands*. Perspiration is another name for sweat.

Perthes' disease

Inflammation of an *epiphysis* (growing area) of the head of the *femur* (thigh bone). The disease is a type of *osteochondritis juvenilis*, thought to be due to disrupted blood supply to the bone.

The condition is most common in boys aged between five and ten years, and usually affects one hip. Symptoms include pain in the thigh and groin, and a limp on the affected side. Movement of the hip is restricted and painful.

Diagnosis is made with *X-rays*, which may show flattening, fragmentation, and (in later stages) shrinking of the head of the femur. Treatment of the disease may be rest for a few weeks, followed by splinting of the hip, or surgery to fit the head of the femur more securely into the pelvis. The disease usually clears up by itself within three years, but the hip may be permanently deformed.

pertussis

A highly contagious infectious disease, also called whooping cough. It mainly affects infants and young children and is most dangerous in newborn babies. The main features are bouts of coughing, often followed by a "whoop" as air is drawn back into the lungs.

CAUSE

The main cause is infection with BORDETELLA PERTUSSIS bacteria, which are spread in airborne droplets. In affluent countries such as the UK, however, the incidence of pertussis has been greatly reduced by *immunization*.

SYMPTOMS

After an *incubation period* of seven to ten days, the illness starts with a mild cough, sneezing, nasal discharge, fever, and sore eyes. After a few days, the cough becomes worse. Whooping occurs in most cases. Sometimes the cough can cause vomiting. In infants, there is a risk of temporary *apnoea* (cessation of breathing) following a coughing spasm. The illness may last anything from a few weeks up to three months, although the child is usually only infectious for about three weeks.

COMPLICATIONS

Coughing may cause nosebleeds and bleeding from ruptured blood vessels on the surface of the eyes or *petechiae* (red, flat, pinhead spots) on the face. Other possible complications include *dehydration* from repeated vomiting; *pneumonia*; *pneumothorax* (a form of collapsed lung); *bronchiectasis* (permanent widening of the airways); and *seizures*. Untreated, pertussis may prove fatal.

DIAGNOSIS AND TREATMENT

Pertussis is usually diagnosed from the symptoms. In the early stages of the illness, the antibiotic *erythromycin* is often given to reduce the child's infectivity. Treatment consists of keeping the child warm, giving small, frequent meals and plenty to drink, and protecting him or her from stimuli, such as smoke, that can provoke coughing. If the child becomes blue or persistently vomits after coughing, he or she must be admitted to hospital.

PREVENTION

In the UK, vaccination against pertussis is usually given at two, three, and four months of age, with a booster dose at between three years four months and five years of age.

Possible complications of vaccination include mild fever and fretfulness. Very rarely, an infant may react severely, with high-pitched screaming or seizures.

Communities need to maintain a high level of immunity, through immunization, to protect infants. It should be remembered that the risks from the disease itself are far greater than any risk from the pertussis vaccine.

perversion

See *deviation, sexual*.

pes cavus

See *claw-foot*.

pessary

Any of a variety of devices placed in the vagina. Some types are used to correct the position of the uterus (see *uterus, prolapse of*); others are used as contraceptive devices. The term "pessary" is also used to refer to a dose of medication, in solid form, that is inserted into the vagina, where it dissolves to release the drug.

pesticides

Poisonous chemicals used to eradicate pests. Different types of pesticide include herbicides, insecticides, and fungicides. Pesticide poisoning, particularly in children, may result from swallowing an insecticide or a garden herbicide (see *chlorate poisoning*). Poisoning may also occur in agricultural workers, often due to inhalation or absorption through the skin. Exposure to pesticides can also occur indirectly, through eating food in which chemicals have accumulated as a result of crop spraying. (See also *DDT*; *defoliant poisoning*; *organophosphates*; *paraquat*; *parathion*.)

petechiae

Red or purple, flat, pinhead-sized spots that occur in the skin or mucous membranes. They do not blanch (go pale) when pressure is applied to them. Petechiae are caused by a localized *haemorrhage* (leakage of blood) from small blood vessels. They occur in *purpura* (a group of bleeding disorders) and, sometimes, in bacterial *endocarditis* (infection of the inner lining of the heart). Petechiae may also arise after periods of excessive straining; in conditions such as *pertussis* (whooping cough), for example.

pethidine

A synthetic opioid *analgesic drug* similar to, but less powerful than, *morphine*. Pethidine is used as a *premedication* and to relieve severe pain after operations or during childbirth. The drug may cause nausea and vomiting, so it is usually given with an *antiemetic drug*. Pethidine can be addictive, making it unsuitable for treating continuing pain.

petit mal

A type of generalized seizure that occurs in *epilepsy*. Petit mal attacks affect children and adolescents but rarely persist into adulthood. Attacks may take place many times a day, and they may sometimes last as long as 30 seconds each. The signs include a momentary loss of awareness, occasionally with drooping eyelids. Treatment for petit mal attacks is with an *anticonvulsant drug*.

petroleum jelly

A greasy substance, also known as petrolatum or soft paraffin, that is obtained from petroleum. The jelly is commonly used as an *ointment* base, a protective dressing, and an *emollient*.

PET scanning

The abbreviation for positron emission tomography. This imaging procedure is a diagnostic technique that is based on the detection of positrons (a type of subatomic particle) emitted by radioactively labelled substances introduced into the body. PET scanning produces images of the metabolic and chemical activity of tissues.

HOW IT WORKS

Certain substances used in biochemical processes in the body, such as glucose or oxygen, are labelled with radioisotopes and then injected into the bloodstream. They are taken up in greater concentrations by tissues that are more active or overactive metabolically. The substances emit positrons, which release photons that are detected by the scanner. A computer then converts this information into images, which are colour-coded to show different levels of tissue activity.

WHY IT IS DONE

PET scans are used to detect brain tumours, locate epileptic activity within the brain, and examine brain function in *Alzheimer's disease* and in mental illnesses such as *depression*.

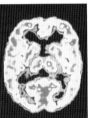

Normal brain   Alzheimer"s disease

PET scans of the brain
A scan of a normal brain (left) can be compared to that of a patient with Alzheimer"s disease, in which the dark areas on both sides of the brain indicate reduced function and blood flow.

Peutz–Jeghers syndrome

A rare, inherited condition in which *polyps* occur in the gastrointestinal tract and small, flat, brown spots appear on the lips and in the mouth. Occasionally, the polyps bleed or cause abdominal pain or *intussusception* (the intestine telescopes in on itself, causing obstruction).

Tests for the condition include *barium X-ray examination* and *endoscopy*. Bleeding polyps may be removed.

Peyer's patches

Areas of mucosa-associated lymphoid tissue (MALT) situated in the mucous membrane lining the ileum (the last portion of the small intestine). Peyer's patches form part of the *lymphatic system*, which helps to fight infection.

peyote

A cactus plant found in northern Mexico and the southwest of the United States. Dried blossoms are used to prepare the hallucinogenic drug *mescaline*.

Peyronie's disease

A disorder of the *penis* in which part of the sheath of fibrous connective tissue thickens, causing the penis to bend during erection. The problem commonly makes intercourse difficult and painful. The thickened area can be felt as a firm nodule when the penis is flaccid. Eventually, some of the erectile tissue may also thicken. Men over 40 are most often affected. The cause is unknown.

The disease may improve without treatment. Otherwise, surgical removal of the thickened area and replacement with normal tissue may be carried out.

pH

A measure of the acidity or alkalinity of a solution. The pH scale ranges from 0–14, 7 being neutral; values smaller than this are acid, and values that are larger are alkaline.

The pH of body fluids must be close to 7.4 for metabolic reactions to proceed normally (see *acid–base balance*). If it falls lower than 7.35, the resulting acidity is called *acidosis*; if it rises above 7.45, the result is *alkalosis*.

phacoemulsification

A surgical procedure used to treat *cataract* (an opacity in the lens of the eye). In this procedure, *ultrasound* waves are used in order to break down the lens tissue, and then the broken-down material is removed through a tiny incision in the eye. An artificial lens implant may then be inserted to improve vision. (See also *cataract surgery*.)

phaeochromocytoma

A rare, usually noncancerous, tumour arising in cells in the *medulla* (core) of the *adrenal glands*. These cells secrete the hormones *adrenaline* (epinephrine) and *noradrenaline* (norepinephrine). The tumour causes increased production of the two hormones, which leads to *hypertension* (high blood pressure) and signs of stress, such as anxiety. The disorder is most common in young to middle-aged adults.

P

SYMPTOMS AND SIGNS

Hypertension is usually the only sign. However, certain conditions or situations (such as pressure on the tumour, emotional upset, change in posture, or taking *beta-blocker drugs*) can cause a surge of hormones. This surge brings on a sudden rise in blood pressure, *palpitations*, headache, nausea, vomiting, facial flushing, sweating, and, sometimes, a feeling of impending death.

DIAGNOSIS AND TREATMENT

Blood tests and *urinalysis* are used to detect excessive levels of adrenaline and noradrenaline and thus make a diagnosis. *CT scanning*, *MRI*, and *radioisotope scanning* may be used to locate the tumours, and they are then usually removed surgically. Follow-up medical checks are required because the condition occasionally recurs.

phagocyte

A type of cell in the *immune system* that can surround, engulf, and digest *microorganisms*, foreign particles, and cellular debris. Phagocytes are found in the blood, *spleen*, *lymph nodes*, and alveoli (small air sacs) within the lungs. Some types of white *blood cell*, especially granulocytes and some monocytes, are "free" phagocytes, which are able to migrate through the tissues and engulf harmful organisms and debris.

phalanges

The small bones that make up the fingers, thumb, and toes. The thumb and big toe have two phalanges; all the other fingers and toes have three.

phalanx

A term for any of the bones in the fingers or the toes.

phallus

Any object that may symbolize the *penis*.

phantom limb pain

The *perception* that a limb is still present after it has been amputated. The sensation occurs because impulses from the nerves in the stump are interpreted by the brain as coming from the limb.

phantom pregnancy

See *pregnancy, false*.

pharmaceutical

Any medicinal drug. The term is also used with reference to the manufacture and sale of drugs.

pharmacognosy

The study or knowledge of the pharmacologically active ingredients of plants.

pharmacokinetics

The term that is used to describe how the body deals with a *drug*. It covers the way in which the drug is absorbed into the bloodstream, how the drug is distributed to different body tissues, and how the drug is broken down for excretion from the body.

pharmacology

The branch of science that is concerned with the discovery and development of *drugs*; their chemical composition; their actions; their uses; and their toxicity. Pharmacodynamics involves the study of the drugs' interactions with, and effects on, living organisms.

pharmacopoeia

Any book that lists and describes most medicinal drugs, especially an official publication. One such example is the British Pharmacopoeia (BP).

A pharmacopoeia provides a description of the sources, preparations, and doses of drugs. There may also be information on how drugs work and on possible adverse effects.

pharmacy

The practice of preparing drugs, and making up and dispensing prescriptions. The term is also used to describe the place, in a hospital for example, where these activities are carried out.

pharyngeal diverticulum

An alternative term for a pharyngeal pouch (see *oesophageal diverticulum*).

pharyngeal pouch

See *oesophageal diverticulum*.

pharyngitis

Acute or chronic inflammation of the *pharynx* (the part of the throat that is situated between the tonsils and the voicebox), causing a sore throat.

CAUSES

The most common cause is a viral infection. Pharyngitis often occurs as part of a cold (see *cold, common*) or *influenza*. It may also be an early feature of glandular fever (see *mononucleosis, infectious*) or *scarlet fever*. Sometimes, the condition is due to a bacterial infection, such as a *streptococcal infection*; a rare but serious bacterial cause is *diphtheria*.

Swallowing substances that can scald, corrode, or scratch the lining of the throat, smoking, and excessive consumption of alcohol may also be the causes of pharyngitis.

SYMPTOMS

As well as a sore throat, there may be discomfort when swallowing, slight fever, earache, and swollen *lymph nodes* in the neck. In severe cases of pharyngitis, there may be a high fever, and the soft palate and throat may swell so much that breathing and swallowing can become difficult.

TREATMENT

Gargling with warm salt water and taking *analgesic drugs (painkillers)* is usually the only treatment needed. If the sore throat is severe or prolonged, a doctor may take a throat *swab* and prescribe *antibiotic drugs*.

pharynx

The passage that connects the back of the mouth and nose to the *oesophagus*. The upper part of the passage, or *nasopharynx*, connects the nasal cavity to the area situated behind the soft *palate*. The middle part, the oropharynx, runs from the nasopharynx to below the tongue. The lower part, called the laryngopharynx, lies behind and to each side of the *larynx* (voicebox).

LOCATION OF THE **PHARYNX**

The pharynx, or throat, plays an essential part in breathing and eating and can change shape to help form vowel sounds in speech. It has a mucous membrane lining.

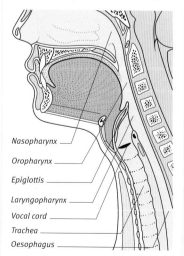

Nasopharynx

Oropharynx

Epiglottis

Laryngopharynx

Vocal cord

Trachea

Oesophagus

P

PHENYLKETONURIA

DISORDERS

The most common disorder affecting the pharynx is acute *pharyngitis* (inflammation of the pharynx), which causes a sore throat. Another common problem is choking due to the presence of a foreign body, such as a fish-bone, that has become lodged in the pharynx.

A rare disorder is *oesophageal diverticulum*. In this condition, a small sac (a pharyngeal pouch) develops in the rear wall of the laryngopharynx.

Cancerous tumours (see *nasopharynx, cancer of*; *pharynx, cancer of*) are relatively rare in Western countries, but more common in the Far East. Some forms of cancer have been linked with smoking and excessive drinking.

pharynx, cancer of

A cancerous tumour of the *pharynx* (the part of the throat between the tonsils and the voicebox). Pharyngeal cancer usually develops in the *mucous membrane* lining the throat.

CAUSES AND INCIDENCE

In the West, almost all cases of pharyngeal cancer are related to smoking and alcohol. The disorder is more common in men, and incidence rises with age.

Tumours of the nasopharynx (see *nasopharynx, cancer of*) have different causes and symptoms from those that arise lower in the pharynx.

SYMPTOMS

Cancerous tumours of the oropharynx (the middle section of the pharynx) usually cause difficulty in swallowing, often accompanied by a sore throat and earache. Bloodstained sputum may be coughed up. Sometimes, there is only the feeling of a lump in the throat or a visibly enlarged *lymph node* in the neck.

Cancer of the laryngopharynx (the lowermost part of the pharynx) initially produces a sensation of incomplete swallowing; symptoms that develop in the later stages include a muffled voice, hoarseness, and also an increased difficulty in swallowing.

DIAGNOSIS AND TREATMENT

Diagnosis is made by *biopsy*, which is often performed in conjunction with *laryngoscopy*, *bronchoscopy*, or *oesophagoscopy*. The growth may be removed surgically or treated with *radiotherapy*. *Anticancer drugs* may also be given.

phencyclidine

A drug of abuse, commonly known as angel dust or PCP. It produces euphoria, which sometimes leads to anxiety or depression. Coordination, speech, and thinking are impaired; the user may have *hallucinations*, and may become violent. Other possible effects include increases in blood pressure and heart rate, dilated pupils, tremor, and reduced sensitivity to pain. High doses of phencyclidine may cause *coma*.

Long-term effects include violent behaviour, anxiety, and mental disorders such as severe *depression*, *paranoia*, and *schizophrenia* (see *drug-induced psychosis*). There is also a risk of brain damage, and of death due to *seizures* or cardiac or respiratory arrest.

phenelzine

A monoamine oxidase inhibitor *antidepressant drug* usually used only when other antidepressant drugs have been ineffective. Possible side effects include dizziness, drowsiness, and rash. When taken with some other drugs or certain foods, such as mature cheese, broad beans, and yeast extract, phenelzine can cause a dangerous rise in blood pressure.

Phenergan

A brand name for the antihistamine drug *promethazine*.

phenobarbital

A *barbiturate drug* that is used mainly as an *anticonvulsant*. Phenobarbital may be used with *phenytoin* in the treatment of *epilepsy*. Possible side effects of the drug include drowsiness, clumsiness, dizziness, excitement, and confusion.

phenol

A strong *antiseptic*, also called carbolic acid. Liquids or ointments that contain phenolic compounds are used to cleanse wounds and inflamed skin, while phenol in an oil base can be injected into haemorrhoids in order to shrink them. Phenol is also found in chemical substances such as *disinfectants*; in this form, it is highly toxic.

phenothiazine drugs

COMMON DRUGS

- Chlorpromazine • Fluphenazine
- Methotrimeprazine • Perphenazine
- Pipotiazine • Trifluoperazine

A group of drugs that are used in the treatment of psychotic illnesses (see *antipsychotic drugs*) and severe agitation, Some phenothiazine drugs are also used to relieve severe nausea and vomiting (see *antiemetic drugs*).

phenotype

The physical appearance, form, and biochemical make-up of an individual. (In contrast, the *genotype* is an individual's genetic make-up.) The phenotype is influenced by the *genes* that a person possesses and by environmental factors (such as diet).

phenoxymethylpenicillin

Also known as penicillin V, a synthetic *penicillin drug* that is used to treat a wide range of bacterial infections. Various respiratory tract infections, including tonsillitis, pharyngitis, dental abscesses, and *otitis media* (middle-ear infection), often respond well to treatment with the drug.

Phenoxymethylpenicillin is also used to treat *Vincent's disease* (a severe form of the gum disease, *gingivitis*) and less common infections caused by the STREPTOCOCCUS bacterium.

Possible common adverse effects of phenoxymethylpenicillin include nausea and vomiting. As with other penicillin antibiotics, a rare but serious allergic reaction may occur that may cause a rash, itching, and breathing difficulties in susceptible people.

phenylephrine

A constituent of eye-drops used to dilate the pupils for eye examinations. Side effects include eye pain, blurred vision, and photophobia (oversensitivity of the eyes to light). Rarely, phenylephrine may be given by injection to treat severe *hypotension* (low blood pressure) when other measures have failed.

phenylketonuria

An inherited metabolic disorder (see *metabolism, inborn error of*) in which the *enzyme* that converts the *amino acid* phenylalanine into tyrosine (another amino acid) is defective. As a result, unless phenylalanine is excluded from the diet it builds up in the body and causes severe *learning difficulties*. All newborn babies are given a *blood spot screening test* to check for phenylketonuria.

SYMPTOMS

Affected babies show few signs of abnormality, but, if phenylalanine is not excluded from the diet, they develop neurological disturbances including *epilepsy*. The babies tend to have blonde hair and blue eyes, and their urine may have a musty odour. Many have the skin condition *eczema*.

P

P

TREATMENT AND PREVENTION

Phenylalanine is found in most foods that contain protein, and also in artificial sweeteners. A specially modified diet is generally recommended throughout life, and sticking to this diet is especially important during pregnancy, because high levels of phenylalanine in the mother can damage the fetus.

phenytoin

An *anticonvulsant drug* used in the treatment of *epilepsy*. Side effects may include nausea, dizziness, tremor, and overgrown and tender gums.

pheromone

A substance with a particular odour that, when released in minute quantities by an animal, affects the behaviour or development of other individuals of the same species.

Philadelphia chromosome

A *chromosomal abnormality* that is associated with one form of leukaemia (see *leukaemia, chronic myeloid*). In this abnormality, one copy of *chromosome* 22 has a missing section, which has become detached and then reattached to a copy of chromosome 9. (See also *karyotype*.)

phimosis

Tightness of the foreskin, preventing it from being drawn back over the *glans* (head) of the penis. In uncircumcised babies, some degree of phimosis is normal, but it usually improves by the age of three or four. In some boys, the condition persists and may cause the foreskin to balloon out on urination. Attempts to retract a tight foreskin may make the condition worse.

Phimosis may also develop in adult men, causing painful erection and it may lead to *paraphimosis* (constriction of the penis behind the glans). Proper cleaning of the glans may not be possible, as a result of which *balanitis* (infection of the glans) may develop.

The treatment for both adults and children is *circumcision*.

phlebitis

Inflammation of a vein. A clot often develops, in which case the condition is termed *thrombophlebitis*.

phlebography

The obtaining of *X-ray* images of veins that have been injected with a *radiopaque* substance. An alternative name is *venography*.

phlebotomy

Puncture of a vein to remove blood (see *venepuncture*; *venesection*).

phlegm

See *sputum*.

phobia

A persistent, irrational fear of a certain object or situation. Many people have minor phobias, which may cause distress but do not affect everyday life. A phobia is considered a psychiatric disorder when it interferes with normal social functioning.

TYPES

Simple phobias (specific phobias) are the most common. These problems may involve fear of particular animals or situations, such as enclosed spaces (*claustrophobia*). Animal phobias usually start in childhood, but other types of phobia can develop at any time.

More severe, pervasive fears are called complex phobias. One form is *agoraphobia*, which often causes severe impairment. The disorder usually starts in the late teens or early 20s. Another complex phobia is social phobia – fear of being exposed to scrutiny, such as a fear of eating or speaking in public. The onset of this disorder usually occurs in late childhood or early adolescence.

CAUSES

The causes of phobias are unknown. Simple phobias are thought by some to be a form of *conditioning*. For example, a person with a fear of dogs may have been frightened by a dog in childhood.

SYMPTOMS AND COMPLICATIONS

Exposure to the feared object or situation causes intense *anxiety* and, in some cases, may lead to a *panic attack*. The person may start to avoid any situation that might involve contact with the trigger for the fear, and this may adversely affect his or her lifestyle. Phobias may also be associated with *depression* or with *obsessive–compulsive behaviour*. In addition, the person may attempt to relieve the fear by using drugs or drinking alcohol to excess.

TREATMENT

Treatment depends on the severity of the condition and the wishes of the individual. For simple phobias, no treatment may be necessary unless the feared object is so common that it cannot easily be avoided (for example, if a person lives in the city but has a fear of lifts). Treatment is more commonly sought for complex phobias. It may involve *cognitive–behavioural therapy* and sometimes *antidepressant drugs*.

phocomelia

A limb defect in which the feet and/or the hands are joined to the trunk by short stumps. The condition is extremely rare, but used to occur as a side effect of women taking the drug *thalidomide* in early pregnancy.

pholcodine

A *cough* suppressant.

phosphates

Salts containing *phosphorus* and *oxygen*. Phosphates are an essential part of the diet and are present in many foods, including cereals, dairy products, eggs, and meat.

FUNCTION

Most of the phosphorus in the body is combined with *calcium* to form the structure of bones and teeth. The remainder is present in small amounts in most of the body's tissues, and plays a part in maintaining the *acid–base balance* of the blood, urine, saliva, and other body fluids. *ATP* (adenosine triphosphate) is a phosphate compound that stores the energy for chemical reactions in cells.

DISORDERS

In most people, the kidneys maintain a constant level of phosphates in the body by regulating the amount that is excreted in the urine. They can compensate for a slight deficiency of phosphates in the diet by reducing the amount that is lost in the urine.

Hypophosphataemia (an abnormally low level of phosphates in the blood) may occur in some forms of kidney disease, *hyperparathyroidism*, long-term treatment with *diuretic drugs*, *malabsorption*, or prolonged starvation. It causes bone pain, weakness, *seizures*, and, in severe cases, *coma* and death.

DRUG THERAPY

Phosphates may be taken by mouth in the form of drug preparations or milk to treat hypophosphataemia. They are also used to treat *hypercalcaemia* (abnormally high levels of calcium in the blood). Diarrhoea is a possible side effect of phosphate drugs.

phospholipid

A compound formed from one or more lipids (fats), phosphate, and, usually, glycerol. They are manufactured in the liver and small intestine. Examples of phospholipids include *lecithins*.

Phospholipids are important constituents of cell membranes and nerve tissues, particularly in the brain. In addition, those existing on the surfaces of blood platelets play a part in *blood clotting*. In an *autoimmune disorder* called *Hughes' syndrome*, the immune system may form antibodies to phospholipids and thus disrupt the clotting process, causing abnormal clot formation.

phosphorus

An essential *mineral* present in many foods, including cereals, dairy products, and meat. In the body, phosphorus is combined with *calcium* to form the bones and teeth. (See also *phosphates*.)

photocoagulation

The destructive heating of tissue by intense light focused to a fine point, as in *laser treatment*.

photophobia

An uncomfortable sensitivity or intolerance to light. It occurs with certain eye disorders, such as *corneal abrasion*, and is a feature of *meningitis* (inflammation of the membranes that surround the brain and spinal cord).

photorefractive keratectomy

A surgical treatment for *astigmatism* (a vision disorder resulting from uneven curvature of the front of the eye), *myopia* (shortsightedness), and *hypermetropia* (longsightedness) in which areas of the *cornea* are shaved away by *laser*.

photosensitivity

An abnormal reaction to light. Photosensitivity usually causes a rash on skin exposed to sunlight or artificial *ultraviolet light*. It often occurs because a photosensitizer (a substance such as a particular dye, chemical in perfume or soap, a plant such as mustard, or some drugs such as *tetracyclines* and *phenothiazines*) has been ingested or applied to the skin. Photosensitivity is also a feature of disorders such as systemic *lupus erythematosus*.

People who are susceptible to photosensitivity reactions should avoid being exposed to sunlight and known photosensitizers and should use *sunscreens*.

phototherapy

Treatment that uses light, including sunlight, *ultraviolet light*, and blue light. Moderate exposure to sunlight is the most basic form and is often helpful in treating the skin disorder *psoriasis*. PUVA is another form of phototherapy. Phototherapy may also be used to treat *seasonal affective disorder*.

PUVA

This therapy combines the use of long-wave ultraviolet light (UVA) with a *psoralen drug*, which sensitizes the skin to light. The procedure is used to treat psoriasis and certain other skin diseases, such as *vitiligo*. Psoriasis may also be treated using medium-wave ultraviolet light (UVB), sometimes combined with the application of coal tar.

BLUE LIGHT

Visible blue light is used to treat neonatal jaundice (see *jaundice, neonatal*), which is due to high levels of the pigment *bilirubin* in the blood. The light is thought to cause the conversion of bilirubin into a harmless substance that can be excreted. To maximize exposure, the baby is undressed and placed under the lights in an incubator (with his or her eyes shielded).

phrenic nerve

One of the pair of main nerves that supply the *diaphragm*. The phrenic nerves branch from the third, fourth, and fifth cervical nerves in the neck (see *spinal nerves*) and then pass down through the chest to each side of the diaphragm. Each of the phrenic nerves carries motor impulses to one half of the diaphragm and plays a part in the control of breathing. Damage to either of the nerves, including invasion by a tumour (as may occur in *lung cancer*), results in *paralysis* of that half of the diaphragm.

LOCATION OF **PHRENIC NERVES**

There are two phrenic nerves, one on each side of the body. Each follows a tortuous course from its origin in the neck, through the chest, to the diaphragm.

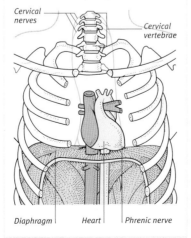

Cervical nerves
Cervical vertebrae
Diaphragm | Heart | Phrenic nerve

physical examination

See *examination, physical*.

physiological saline

An *isotonic* solution of 0.9% sodium chloride in water, also called normal saline, used to replace body fluids and rehydrate tissues. Physiological saline is given by intravenous infusion.

physiology

The study of body functions, including physical and chemical processes of cells, tissues, organs, and systems, and their various interactions.

physiotherapy

Treatment with physical methods, such as exercise or physical agents. It can prevent or reduce joint stiffness and restore muscle. It is also used to reduce pain, inflammation, and muscle spasm, and to retrain joints and muscles, after *stroke* or nerve injury, for example. Methods include active exercises and passive movement, *heat treatment*, *massage*, *ice-packs*, *hydrotherapy*, and *TENS* (therapeutic use of electrical currents).

Physiotherapy is also used to maintain breathing in people with impaired lung function, and to prevent and treat pulmonary complications after surgery. Techniques for doing this include *postural drainage*, *breathing exercises*, and administration of oxygen, drugs, or moisture through a *nebulizer*.

phyto-

A prefix meaning of plant origin.

phytomenadione

A form of *vitamin K*.

phyto-oestrogens

Oestrogens that occur naturally in plants.

pia mater

The innermost of the three membranes of the *meninges*, lying next to the brain.

pica

A craving to eat non-food substances such as earth or coal. Pica is common in early childhood and may occur during pregnancy. It may also occur in nutritional or iron-deficiency disorders, and in severe psychiatric disorders.

Pickwickian syndrome

An uncommon disorder characterized by extreme *obesity*, shallow breathing, excessive sleepiness, and *obstructive sleep*

P

apnoea. Pickwickian syndrome is of unknown cause. The symptoms usually improve with weight loss; specific treatment for sleep apnoea may be required.

PID

The abbreviation for *pelvic inflammatory disease*.

piebaldism

A rare *genetic disorder* in which a patchy absence of the dark pigment *melanin* results in areas of skin and sometimes hair that lack pigmentation. In many cases, there is a white panel in the centre of the face, which may include the hair and eyebrows as well as the skin. Piebaldism shows an autosomal dominant pattern of inheritance.

piercing

See *ear piercing*.

Pierre Robin's syndrome

A disorder causing abnormalities of the lower jaw and throat. The condition may occur by itself, or may be associated with other problems. It is *congenital* (present at birth).

The main structural malformations are micrognathia (an abnormally small lower jaw) and cleft palate (or an unusually arched palate). Functional defects include a tendency for the tongue to fall backwards into the throat, causing breathing difficulty and a tendency to choke.

Affected babies may have difficulty in feeding. Micrognathia may disappear as the child grows, but cleft palate and airway obstruction may require surgery.

pigeon toes

A minor abnormality in which the leg or foot is rotated, forcing the foot and toes to point inwards. Although the condition occurs commonly in toddlers, it has usually corrected itself by the time the child is seven years old.

pigmentation

Coloration of the skin, hair, and *iris* of the eyes by *melanin*, a brown or black pigment produced by cells called melanocytes. The more melanin, the darker the coloration (the amount produced is determined by heredity and exposure to sunlight). Blood pigments can also colour skin (as in a bruise).

There are many defects of pigmentation, which may cause abnormally pale or dark skin, or may produce areas of discoloured skin.

REDUCED PIGMENTATION

Patches of pale skin occur in the skin disorders *psoriasis*, *pityriasis alba*, and *pityriasis versicolor*; these disorders cause skin scales to flake off, resulting in a loss of melanin. In *vitiligo*, areas of skin stop producing melanin.

In the genetic disorder *albinism* there is a generalized deficiency of melanin, resulting in very pale skin and white hair. Another genetic condition, *phenylketonuria*, results in a reduced level of melanin, making people with the condition more pale-skinned and fair-haired than other members of their family.

INCREASED PIGMENTATION

Areas of dark skin may appear temporarily following disorders such as *eczema* or psoriasis, pityriasis versicolor, or *chloasma* (development of dark patches on the face due to hormonal changes). Such areas of dark pigmentation may also appear after the use of perfumes and cosmetics containing chemicals that cause *photosensitivity*.

Permanent areas of deep pigmentation, such as freckles, moles, or some types of naevi (see *naevus*), are usually due to an abnormality in some of the melanocytes. *Acanthosis nigricans*, a condition that may be either inherited or acquired, is characterized by dark patches of velvetlike, thickened skin. Darkening of the skin that is unrelated to sun exposure may occur in certain hormonal disorders, such as *Addison's disease* and *Cushing's syndrome*.

ABNORMAL COLORATION

Some forms of abnormal colouring result from excessive levels of certain pigments or other substances in the blood. An excess of the bile pigment bilirubin in *jaundice* turns the skin yellow, and an excessive blood level of iron in *haemochromatosis* turns the skin bronze. Discoloration may also be caused by an abnormal collection of blood vessels, as in a *haemangioma*, or may occur temporarily in a bruise, when blood collects under the skin.

piles

A common name for *haemorrhoids*.

pill, contraceptive

See *oral contraceptives*.

pilocarpine

A drug used in the form of eye-drops to treat *glaucoma* (raised pressure in the eyeball). Pilocarpine may initially cause blurred vision, headache, and eye irrita-

tion. In tablet form, the drug is used to treat *dry mouth* due to *Sjogren's syndrome* or *radiotherapy* to the head and neck.

pilonidal sinus

A pit in the skin, often containing hairs, in the upper part of the buttock cleft. The cause is probably hair fragments growing inwards. Although the condition is usually harmless, infection may occur, causing recurrent, painful abscesses.

If a pilonidal sinus is infected, the sinus and a wide area around it will be surgically removed. The resulting wound will usually be left open to allow slow healing from the skin layers below. Recurrence of infection is common, and plastic surgery is sometimes required.

pimozide

An *antipsychotic drug* used to treat *schizophrenia* and other psychoses, and also sometimes *Gilles de la Tourette's syndrome*. It may cause sedation, dry mouth, constipation, and blurred vision. An *ECG* (electrocardiogram) is recommended before and during treatment because the drug has been associated with abnormalities of the heart's electrical activity.

pimple

A small *pustule* or *papule*.

pindolol

A *beta-blocker drug* used to treat *angina pectoris* (chest pain due to inadequate blood supply to the heart) and *hypertension* (high blood pressure). Possible side effects are typical of other beta-blocker drugs, except that pindolol is less likely than some others to cause *bradycardia* (abnormally slow heartbeat).

pineal gland

A tiny, cone-shaped structure deep within the *brain*. The pineal gland is situated just below the back of the corpus callosum, the band of nerve fibres that connects the two halves of the cerebrum (the topmost, and largest, area of the brain).

The sole function of the gland appears to be secretion of the hormone *melatonin* in response to changes in light. The amount of melatonin secreted varies over a 24-hour cycle, being greatest at night. Hormone secretion is thought to be controlled through nerve pathways from the retina in the eye; a high light level seems to inhibit secretion. The exact function of melatonin is not understood, but it may help to synchronize circadian (24-hour) and other *biorhythms*.

LOCATION OF **PINEAL GLAND**

The pineal gland is situated in the brain, below the rear part of the corpus callosum.

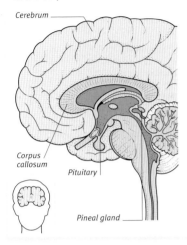

Cerebrum

Corpus callosum

Pituitary

Pineal gland

pinguecula

A small, noncancerous, yellowish spot that occurs on the *conjunctiva* over the white of the eye. These spots are common in elderly people and may be removed purely for cosmetic reasons. If a pinguecula encroaches on the cornea, it may lead to *pterygium*.

pink-eye

A common name for *conjunctivitis*.

pinna

The fleshy part of the outer ear, consisting of a flap of cartilage and skin. It is also called the auricle.

pins-and-needles

A tingling or prickly feeling in an area of skin that is usually associated with *numbness* and, sometimes, a burning feeling. The medical term for this phenomenon is paraesthesia. Transient pins-and-needles is due to a temporary disturbance in the conduction of nerve signals from the skin to the brain. Persistent pins-and-needles may be caused by a nerve disorder, or *neuropathy*.

pinta

A bacterial skin infection, caused by TREPONEMA CARATEUM, occurring in remote areas of tropical America. A large spot surrounded by smaller ones appears on the face, neck, buttocks, hands, or feet. After one to twelve months, it is followed by red skin patches that turn blue, then brown, and finally white. A *penicillin drug* usually clears up the infection, but the skin may be permanently disfigured.

pinworm infestation

An alternative name for *threadworm infestation*.

pioglitazone

An oral hypoglycaemic drug (see *hypoglycaemics, oral*) that is used in combination with other oral hypoglycaemics (either *metformin* or a sulphonylurea) in the treatment of type 2 *diabetes mellitus*. Pioglitazone acts by reducing resistance to insulin in the body tissues. Side effects may include gastrointestinal disturbances, weight gain, and anaemia. Rarely, pioglitazone may cause liver problems, and blood tests may therefore be done before and during treatment,

piperazine

An *anthelmintic drug* used to treat *infestation* by *roundworms* and *threadworms*. Possible side effects include abdominal pain, nausea, vomiting, and diarrhoea.

piroxicam

A type of *nonsteroidal anti-inflammatory drug* (NSAID) used to relieve the symptoms of types of *arthritis*, and to relieve pain in *bursitis*, *tendinitis*, acute *gout*, and after minor surgery. Possible adverse effects of the drug include nausea, indigestion, abdominal pain, swollen ankles, *peptic ulcer*, and liver problems.

pituitary gland

Sometimes referred to as the master gland, the pituitary is the most important of the *endocrine glands* (glands that release hormones directly into the bloodstream).

LOCATION OF **PITUITARY GLAND**

This master gland is itself controlled by the hypothalamus, located immediately above it.

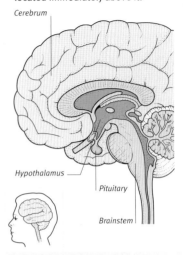

Cerebrum

Hypothalamus

Pituitary

Brainstem

P

HORMONES SECRETED BY THE **PITUITARY GLAND**

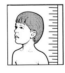

Growth hormone stimulates cell division and protein synthesis in tissues such as bone and cartilage, leading to growth.

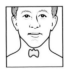

Thyroid-stimulating hormone (TSH) stimulates the thyroid gland to secrete various hormones vital to body metabolism.

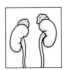

Adrenocorticotrophic hormone (ACTH) stimulates the adrenal glands to secrete hormones, with multiple effects on metabolism.

Prolactin stimulates milk production, particularly in response to the infants' sucking.

Luteinizing and follicle-stimulating hormones (LH and FSH) help control the function of male and female sex organs.

Melanocyte-stimulating hormone (MSH) controls skin darkening by stimulating pigment cells (melanocytes).

Antidiuretic hormone (ADH) acts on the kidneys to decrease water loss in the urine and thus reduces urine volume.

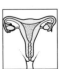

Oxytocin stimulates contraction of the uterus during childbirth and milk release from the breasts.

DISORDERS OF THE **PITUITARY GLAND**

Any abnormality of the pituitary gland usually means that it produces either too much or too little of one or more hormones, causing changes elsewhere in the body. Locally, serious effects may be caused by enlargement of the gland; for example, it may press on the nearby optic nerves and cause visual defects.

Congenital and genetic disorders

Deficiency of *growth hormone* may be a genetic disorder, or it may be due to congenital absence or undergrowth of the pituitary or to damage to the gland sustained during birth. Whatever the cause, deficiency of growth hormone leads to *short stature*.

Congenital growth hormone deficiency may also be associated with deficiency of other pituitary hormones, notably *ACTH* (adrenocorticotrophic hormone), *gonadotrophin hormones*, and thyroid-stimulating hormone (TSH).

Tumours

Pituitary tumours are usually noncancerous but may cause either overproduction of pituitary hormones (hyperpituitarism) or underproduction (hypopituitarism), as well as headaches and loss of the visual field.

Injury

Birth injury may cause loss of pituitary function, as may head injuries at any age.

Impaired blood supply

Rarely, the pituitary may suffer deprivation of its blood supply as a result of pressure exerted on its blood vessels from a growing tumour. This may cause a sudden loss of pituitary function, which may be fatal, or a more gradual loss, which produces signs of general underactivity of the gland.

A similar deprivation of blood supply may occur as a complication of massive blood loss associated with childbirth (Sheehan's syndrome). This may lead to failure of milk production, and a wide range of secondary effects due to the resultant underactivity of other endocrine glands. Impaired blood supply may also occur due to *vasculitis* or pressure on the gland from an *aneurysm* of a nearby artery.

Radiation

Radiotherapy for a pituitary tumour may cause general underactivity of the gland.

INVESTIGATION

Techniques include analysis of pituitary hormones in the blood or urine, and of hormones from other endocrine glands under pituitary control; pituitary *X-rays*, *CT scanning*, or *MRI*; *angiography*, to show blood-vessel displacement by a pituitary tumour; and, possibly, a visual field test (see *vision tests*).

It regulates the activities of other endocrine glands and many body processes (see *endocrine system*).

For information on disorders that can affect the pituitary gland, see the pituitary gland disorders box, above.

STRUCTURE
The pituitary gland is a pea-sized structure attached by a stalk of nerve fibres to the *hypothalamus*, a region of the brain just above the gland. The hypothalamus controls pituitary function by nervous stimulation and by secreting substances called hormone-releasing factors.

The pituitary gland consists of three lobes: the anterior, the intermediate, and the posterior.

FUNCTIONS
The three lobes of the pituitary produce a range of hormones. For further information on the individual pituitary hormones and their effects, see the illustrated box, previous page.

The anterior lobe produces most of the pituitary hormones, including *growth hormone*, *prolactin*, *ACTH* (adrenocorticotrophic hormone), the *gonadotrophins* FSH (follicle-stimulating hormone) and LH (luteinizing hormone), and TSH (thyroid-stimulating hormone). The intermediate lobe secretes MSH (melanocyte-stimulating hormon). The secretion of hormones is triggered by hormone-releasing factors from the hypothalamus.

The posterior pituitary lobe secretes *ADH* and *oxytocin*. These hormones are actually produced in the hypothalamus, and pass down nerve fibres to be stored in the posterior lobe until they are needed.

pituitary tumours

Growths in the *pituitary gland*. Pituitary tumours are rare, and usually noncancerous, but they can put pressure on the *optic nerves*, causing visual defects.

CAUSES AND SYMPTOMS
The causes of pituitary tumours are unknown. One type, called an endocrine inactive tumour, causes the destruction of some of the hormone-secreting cells in the pituitary gland. This leads to inadequate hormone production, causing problems such as tiredness, loss of appetite, symptoms of *hypothyroidism* (underactivity of the thyroid gland), and cessation of menstrual periods or reduced sperm production.

Tumours may also cause the gland to produce excessive amounts of certain hormones. Tumours of the anterior lobe can cause various disorders. Overproduction of growth hormone causes *gigantism* or *acromegaly*. Excess thyroid-stimulating hormone (TSH) can lead to *hyperthyroidism*. Excess adrenocorticotrophic hormone (ACTH) can cause Cushing's disease (see *Cushing's syndrome*). An increase in prolactin can cause *galactorrhoea* (abnormal milk production), *amenorrhoea* (absence of menstrual periods), and *infertility* in women. In men, it can cause *erectile dysfunction*, infertility, *feminization*, and galactorrhoea. Tumours that affect the posterior pituitary may disrupt the production of antidiuretic hormone (ADH) and lead to *diabetes insipidus*.

Pressure from tumour enlargement may cause headaches, cranial nerve *paralysis*, and defects of vision.

DIAGNOSIS AND TREATMENT
Diagnosis is made using *blood tests* to measure hormone levels; X-rays; *MRI* or *CT scanning* of the pituitary; and, often, *vision tests*. Treatment may consist of surgical removal of the tumour, *radiotherapy*, hormone replacement, or a combination of these techniques. The drug *bromocriptine* may be used; it can reduce production of certain hormones and shrink some tumours.

pityriasis alba

A common skin condition occurring in childhood and adolescence, particularly in dark-skinned children, that is caused by mild *eczema*. Irregular, fine, scaly, pale patches appear on the face; the patches may be more noticeable after exposure to the sun, because they tan poorly. The condition can usually be cleared up with *emollients*.

P

pityriasis rosea

A common, mild skin disorder in which a rash of flat, scaly-edged, pink spots or patches appears on the trunk and upper arms. It is not contagious and mainly affects children and young adults. Its cause is unknown, but may be associated with a viral infection.

The first sign is a large, round spot, called a herald patch, on the trunk. The rash appears about a week later. It lasts for four to eight weeks, may cause itching, and usually clears up without treatment. Calamine lotion or *antihistamine drugs* may relieve any itching.

pityriasis versicolor

A common skin condition, also known as tinea versicolor, in which patches of white, brown, or salmon-coloured flaking skin appear on the trunk and neck. The patches are more noticeable on suntanned skin; they may be either paler or darker than the surrounding skin. Pityriasis versicolor mainly affects young and middle-aged adults. It is caused by an overgrowth of PITYROSPORUM, a fungus that exists on most people's skin and normally produces no symptoms. The condition is not contagious.

Treatment is with *selenium* sulphate shampoo, used as a lotion, or with *antifungal drugs* in the form of a cream or lotion. The whole of the affected area must be treated thoroughly, to prevent the infection from recurring. With careful treatment, the infection will clear up in two to three weeks, but the spots may take months to disappear. Antifungal tablets may be needed if the rash does not improve or is very widespread.

Pityrosporum

A group of fungi that normally live on the skin or the scalp, but which may sometimes cause *pityriasis versicolor* or may multiply excessively resulting in a condition called *folliculitis* (inflammation of the hair follicles). This overgrowth of fungi may occur in people with lowered resistance to infection; people taking *antibiotic drugs*, *corticosteroids*, or *oral contraceptives*; those with *diabetes mellitus*; and those under emotional stress. It may also be associated with a predisposition to severe dandruff or *seborrhoeic dermatitis*.

Treatment includes addressing any underlying cause and using solutions or creams containing *antifungal drugs*.

pivmecillinam

A type of *penicillin drug*.

pivot joint

A form of *joint* that allows only rotation, such as the joint between the top of the spine and the skull.

pizotifen

A drug used to prevent migraine in people who have frequent, disabling attacks. Possible adverse effects of pizotifen may include nausea, dizziness, drowsiness, dry mouth, and muscle pains. Prolonged use of the drug may cause weight gain in some cases.

PKU

The abbreviation for *phenylketonuria*.

placebo

A chemically inert substance given instead of a drug. Benefit may be gained from a placebo because the person taking it believes it will have a positive effect. As the effectiveness of any drug may be partly due to this "placebo effect", many new drugs are tested against a placebo preparation.

placenta

The organ that develops inside the uterus during pregnancy and that is the link between the blood supplies of the mother and the baby.

STRUCTURE

The placenta develops from the *chorion* (the outermost layer of cells that develops from the fertilized egg). It is attached to the uterus lining and connected to the baby by the *umbilical cord*. The placenta, and the other uterine tissues, which are all expelled at birth, are collectively known as the afterbirth.

FUNCTION

The placenta transfers oxygen, nutrients, and protective *antibodies* from the mother's circulation to the fetus's circulation and removes waste products from the fetal blood into the mother's blood for excretion by her lungs and kidneys.

The organ also produces hormones such as *oestrogen*, *progesterone*, and *human chorionic gonadotrophin* (HCG). These hormones enter the mother's blood to help her body adapt to the conditions of pregnancy; they also prepare the breasts for *breast-feeding*. High levels of HCG appear in the woman's urine during early pregnancy, and detection of them in the urine forms the basis of *pregnancy tests*.

placental abruption

Separation of all or part of the placenta from the wall of the uterus before the baby is delivered.

FUNCTION OF THE **PLACENTA**

The mother's and baby's blood do not mix in the placenta, but are separated from each other by such a thin layer of cells that exchange of nutrients and oxygen (from mother to baby) and waste products (from baby to mother) can occur between the two blood circulations.

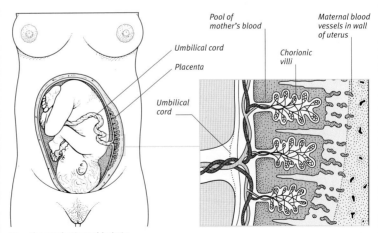

Umbilical cord
Placenta
Umbilical cord
Pool of mother's blood
Maternal blood vessels in wall of uterus
Chorionic villi

How the mother's and baby's blood are brought together
The baby's blood flows via the umbilical cord to the placenta, where it enters numerous tiny blood vessels arranged in "fingers" (chorionic villi). These are surrounded by a pool of maternal blood brought to the placenta by a major artery.

P

CAUSES
The exact cause of placental abruption is not known, but it is more common in women who have long-term *hypertension* (high blood pressure) and in those who have previously had the condition or who have had several pregnancies. Smoking and high alcohol intake may also contribute to the risk of placental abruption.

SYMPTOMS
Symptoms usually occur suddenly and depend on how much of the placenta has separated from the wall of the uterus. They include vaginal bleeding, which can be severe haemorrhaging in complete separation; abdominal cramps or backache; severe, constant abdominal pain; and reduced fetal movements.

TREATMENT
If the bleeding does not stop, or if it starts again, it may be necessary to induce labour (see *induction of labour*). A small placental abruption is usually treated with bed-rest in hospital. In more severe cases of placental abruption, an emergency *caesarean section* is often necessary to save the the the life of the fetus. A *blood transfusion* is also sometimes required.

placenta praevia
Implantation of the *placenta* in the lower part of the uterus, near or over the cervix. The condition varies in severity from marginal placenta praevia, when the placenta reaches the edge of the cervical opening, to complete placental praevia, when the entire opening of the cervix is covered.

SYMPTOMS
Marginal placenta praevia may have no adverse effect. More severe cases often cause painless vaginal bleeding in late pregnancy, as placental tissue separates from the wall of the uterus.

TREATMENT
If the bleeding is slight and the pregnancy still has several weeks to run, bed rest in hospital may be all that is necessary. The baby will probably be delivered by *caesarean section* at the 38th week. If the bleeding is heavy or if the pregnancy is near term, an immediate delivery is carried out.

placenta, tumours of
See *choriocarcinoma*; *hydatidiform mole*.

plagiocephaly
Any asymmetry or distortion in the shape of the head. Plagiocephaly is usually due to irregularity in the closure of the *sutures* (fixed joints) between the skull bones.

SPREAD OF **PLAGUE**

Stage 1
The bacterium that causes plague (Yersinia pestis) circulates mainly among wild rodents; the bacterium is spread from one rodent to another by rodent fleas.

Stage 2
Sometimes so many wild rodents die that the fleas transfer to and infest new wild hosts, such as rats, or even humans who enter plague-affected areas.

Stage 3
The real danger is of plague spreading to, and killing, large numbers of urban rats; rat fleas might then transfer from dead rats to humans en masse, causing an epidemic.

plague
A serious infectious disease caused by the bacterium YERSINIA PESTIS. It mainly affects rodents but can be transmitted to humans by flea bites. Plague caused one of the largest pandemics (worldwide epidemics) in history: the "Black Death" of the 14th century, which killed 25 million people in Europe alone. Today, human plague occurs sporadically in parts of the world, but not in Europe.

CAUSES, TYPES, AND SYMPTOMS
There are two main types: bubonic and pneumonic. Bubonic plague is caused by a bite from an infected flea. Pneumonic plague can be a complication of bubonic plague or can be transmitted in infected droplets expelled in coughing.

Bubonic plague is characterized by swollen *lymph nodes* (which are called "buboes"). Symptoms usually start two to five days after infection, with fever, shivering, and severe headache. Soon, the smooth, red, painful buboes appear, usually in the groin. There may be bleeding into the skin around the buboes, causing dark patches. The victim may have *seizures*. Without prompt treatment, the person may die. Occasionally, *septicaemia* (blood poisoning) may cause death before buboes appear.

Pneumonic plague affects the lungs. The symptoms are severe coughing that produces a bloody, frothy *sputum* and laboured breathing. Without early treatment, death is almost inevitable.

DIAGNOSIS AND TREATMENT
A sample of fluid from a bubo, or a sputum sample, is taken to establish the presence of plague bacteria and confirm the diagnosis. Treatment is with *antibiotic drugs*, which should be started as soon as possible.

plantar fasciitis
Fasciitis (inflammation of a layer of connective tissue) affecting the sole of the foot, especially the heel.

plantar wart
See *wart, plantar*.

plants, poisonous
Several species of plant, including foxglove, holly, deadly nightshade, and laburnum, are poisonous or can cause severe allergic reactions.

Paradoxically, many poisonous plants are also sources of useful drugs. Examples include deadly nightshade, from which *atropine* is made, and foxglove, from which *digitalis drugs* are created.

CAUSES AND SYMPTOMS OF POISONING
Toxins from plants can cause poisoning either through skin contact, if a person touches the plants, or internally, if a person (usually a child) ingests them.

Skin contact Nettles, hogweed, poison ivy, and primula cause skin reactions, including rash, itching, and blistering, on contact. In some people, these reactions can be extremely severe.

Internal poisoning Plants that are poisonous to eat include foxglove, aconite, hemlock, laburnum seeds, and holly and deadly nightshade berries. Internal poisoning most commonly affects young children who have consumed colourful berries. Symptoms of poisoning vary according to the plant but may include abdominal pain, vomiting, flushing, breathing difficulty, *delirium*, and *coma*. Urgent medical attention is required.

TREATMENT
Skin reactions can be treated by washing the area affected (and any clothes that have come into contact with the plant), and applying *calamine* lotion. *Corticosteroid drugs* may be prescribed for severe reactions. Internal poisoning usually requires gastric *lavage* (stomach washout). Fatal poisoning is rare. (See also *mushroom poisoning*.)

plaque
The term given to an area of *atherosclerosis* (fatty deposits within arteries). The plaques are symptomless until they

DEVELOPMENT OF **PLAQUE**

Plaque starts with a deposit of salivary mucus on the teeth. The mucus is colonized by various types of bacteria. Initially, the predominant bacteria are spherical cocci. After a day or two, long filamentous colonies of bacteria spread over the surface of the teeth.

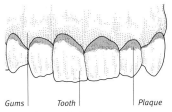

Gums | Tooth | Plaque

Areas of plaque buildup
Plaque develops predominantly at the margin of teeth and gums. If the gums are inflamed or otherwise unhealthy, the plaque tends to develop more rapidly.

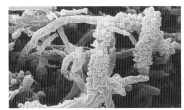

Mature plaque
This picture, taken with a scanning electron microscope (SEM), shows a mass of filamentous bacterial colonies in plaque, magnified about 3,000 times.

are large enough to reduce blood flow or until the surface of a plaque is disturbed, causing *thrombosis* (clotting of blood). Plaques in coronary arteries, which supply blood to the heart, cause *coronary artery disease*.

plaque, dental

A rough, sticky coating on the teeth consisting of saliva by-products, food deposits, bacteria, and dead cells from the lining of the mouth. It is the chief cause of tooth decay (see *caries, dental*) and *gingivitis* (gum disease), and forms the basis of a hard deposit (see *calculus, dental*) that forms on teeth.

Some of the *microorganisms* found in plaque, particularly the bacterium STREPTOCOCCUS MUTANS, break down sugar in the remains of *carbohydrate* food that sticks to the mucus, creating an acid that can erode tooth enamel.

plasma

The fluid part of *blood* that remains if the blood cells are removed. Plasma is a solution that contains many nutrients, salts, and proteins.

plasma D-dimers

Substances formed in the body by the breakdown of blood clots (see *blood clotting*); for example, when the body clears blocked blood vessels. Tests that can detect plasma D-dimers can be helpful in monitoring conditions such as *disseminated intravascular coagulation* or in deciding whether someone may have had a pulmonary embolism or deep vein thrombosis (see *thrombosis,*

deep vein). These tests are not used to make or confirm a diagnosis, but the possibility of pulmonary embolism or deep vein thrombosis may be ruled out if plasma D-dimers are not present.

plasmapheresis

A procedure for removing, or reducing the concentration of, unwanted substances in the blood; it is also known as plasma exchange.

Blood is withdrawn from the body in the same way as for a *blood donation* and the plasma portion of the blood is removed by machines known as cell separators. The blood cells are mixed with a plasma substitute and returned to the circulation in the same way as for a *blood transfusion*.

Plasmapheresis is used to remove damaging *antibodies* or *immune complexes* (antibody–antigen particles) from the circulation in various *autoimmune disorders* such as *myasthenia gravis* and *Goodpasture's syndrome*.

plasma proteins

Proteins that are present in blood *plasma*. These proteins include *albumin*, *blood clotting* proteins, and *immunoglobulins* (which are active in the immune system). In addition to their specific roles, the plasma proteins help to maintain blood volume by preventing loss of water from the blood into the tissues. The proteins keep the water in the blood by osmotic pressure (see *osmosis*). If proteins are lost from the plasma, excessive amounts of fluid may build up in the tissues (a condition called *oedema*).

plasminogen activator

See *tissue plasminogen activator*.

Plasmodium

A group of protozoa (single-celled organisms) including the microorganisms that are responsible for *malaria*. Once they are introduced into the body, usually via a mosquito bite, plasmodia live in liver cells, *red blood cells*, and in the bloodstream.

plaster cast

See *cast*.

plaster of Paris

A white powder that is made of a calcium compound that, when mixed with water, produces a paste that can be shaped before it sets. Plaster of Paris is used for constructing *casts* and making dental models (see *impression, dental*).

plastic surgery

Any operation carried out to repair or reconstruct skin and tissue that has been damaged or lost, is malformed, or has changed with aging. (Any procedures that are performed mainly to improve the appearance of a healthy person are described as *cosmetic surgery*.)

Plastic surgery is often performed to repair damage caused by severe burns or injuries, cancer, or some operations, such as *mastectomy* (removal of breast tissue). Some congenital conditions may also require plastic surgery; these include *cleft lip and palate*, *hypospadias* (a defect in the penis), and imperforate anus (see *anus, imperforate*).

Techniques that are used in plastic surgery include *skin grafts*, *skin flaps*, and *Z-plasty*; these may be combined with *implants* or a *bone graft*.

-plasty

A suffix meaning "shaping by surgery". The term is usually used to describe various procedures in *plastic surgery*, such as *rhinoplasty* (surgery on the nose) and *mammoplasty* (reshaping or reconstruction of the breast).

platelet

The smallest type of *blood cell*; also called a thrombocyte. Platelets play a major role in *blood clotting*. When they are activated, for example by contact with damaged blood-vessel walls, they clump together at injury sites, releasing chemicals that constrict the damaged blood vessels and trigger the process of

P

Scanning electron micrograph of platelets
This SEM shows activated platelets (also called thrombocytes) magnified 13,000 times. Platelets play an important role in blood clotting.

clot formation. A deficiency of platelets (a condition called *thrombocytopenia*) can cause certain *bleeding disorders*.

platyhelminth

A flat or ribbon-shaped parasitic worm (see *liver fluke*; *schistosomiasis*; *tapeworm*).

play therapy

A method used in the *psychoanalysis* of young children, based on the idea that play has symbolic significance. Watching a child at play helps a therapist diagnose the source of the child's problems; the child is then helped to act out thoughts and feelings that are causing anxiety.

plethora

A florid, bright-red, flushed complexion. It may be caused by dilation of blood vessels, or, less commonly, by *polycythaemia* (excessive numbers of red blood cells).

pleura

A thin, two-layered membrane, one layer covering the outside of the lungs, the other lining the inside of the chest cavity. Fluid in the pleural cavity between the two layers provides lubrication, allowing smooth expansion and contraction of the lungs during breathing.

DISORDERS
Pleurisy (inflammation of the pleura) is usually due to a lung infection, such as *pneumonia* or *tuberculosis*, and may lead to *pleural effusion* (excess fluid between the layers of the pleura). *Pneumothorax* (air in the pleural cavity) may result in collapse of a lung; this may occur spontaneously or result from a penetrating injury. Cancerous tumours (see *mesothelioma*) may also develop in the pleura.

pleural effusion

An accumulation of fluid between the layers of the *pleura* (the membrane lining the lungs and chest cavity). Pleural effusion may be caused by lung infections such as *pneumonia* or *tuberculosis*, or other lung disorders such as *pulmonary embolism* or *mesothelioma* (a tumour of the pleura). It may also result from *heart failure* or *cancer*. Pleural effusion may affect one or both sides of the chest. The excess fluid compresses the lung beneath, making breathing difficult.

Diagnosis is confirmed by *chest X-ray*. Some fluid may be removed with a needle and syringe and examined to find the cause of the condition. A *biopsy* (tissue sample) of the pleura may also be needed. The underlying cause is treated; fluid may also be drained off to relieve breathing problems.

pleurisy

Inflammation of the *pleura* (the membrane lining the lungs and chest cavity). Causes include lung infections, such as *pneumonia*, or, more rarely, *pulmonary embolism*, *lung cancer*, or *rheumatoid arthritis*. Pleurisy causes a sharp chest pain, which is worse when breathing in; this pain is due to the inflamed layers of the membrane rubbing together. Treatment is aimed at the underlying cause, and *analgesic drugs* are also given.

pleurodynia

Pain in the chest, also known as Bornholm disease. Pleurodynia is caused by *coxsackievirus* B infection. It often occurs in epidemics and usually affects children.

There is sudden severe pain in the lower chest or upper abdomen, with fever, sore throat, headache, and malaise. The disease usually settles in three to four days without treatment.

plexus

A network of interwoven nerves or blood vessels. Examples include the *solar plexus* (the large network of nerves just behind the stomach) and the *brachial plexus* (a network of nerves in the neck and upper arm).

plication

A surgical procedure in which tucks are made in the walls of a hollow organ and then stitched in order to decrease the size of the organ.

Plummer–Vinson syndrome

Difficulty in swallowing due to webs of tissue forming across the upper *oesophagus*. The syndrome often occurs along with severe iron-deficiency *anaemia* and affects middle-aged women.

plutonium

A radioactive metallic element which occurs naturally only in *uranium* ores; it is produced artificially in breeder reactors. It is used as a fuel in nuclear reactors and nuclear weapons. The element is highly toxic if it enters the body, because it emits high levels of radiation and is absorbed into the bone marrow, where it may remain for many years.

PMS

The abbreviation often used for *premenstrual syndrome*.

PMT

The abbreviation for premenstrual tension, an alternative name for *premenstrual syndrome*.

pneumaturia

The presence of gas, including air, in the *urine*. Pneumaturia usually indicates that a *fistula* (abnormal channel) has developed between the bladder and the intestine.

pneumo-

A prefix meaning related to the lungs, to air, or to the breath.

pneumococcus

A common name for STREPTOCOCCUS PNEUMONIAE, a bacterium that can cause various diseases, including *meningitis*, *pneumonia*, and *sinusitis*. Vaccination against pneumococcal infection is given at 2, 4, and 13 months as part of the childhood immunization schedule Vaccination is also recommended for those over 65 and various groups at special risk, including those with chronic respiratory disease, chronic heart disease, chronic kidney disease, chronic liver disease, diabetes mellitus, a suppressed immune system, coeliac disease, and people who have had their spleen removed or have a disorder of the spleen.

pneumoconiosis

Any of a group of lung diseases that are caused by the inhalation of certain mineral dusts. Dust particles of less than 0.005 mm across can reach the air sacs in the lungs (see *alveolus, pulmonary*); they may accumulate and cause thickening and scarring. As a result, the lungs may become less efficient at supplying oxygen to the blood.

TYPES AND CAUSES
The main types of pneumoconiosis are asbestosis (see *asbestos-related diseases*), coal workers' pneumoconiosis, and

P

silicosis, caused by silica dust. These primarily affect workers over 50 years of age. However, the incidence is falling due to better preventive measures.

SYMPTOMS AND COMPLICATIONS

The main symptom of pneumoconiosis is shortness of breath. In severe cases, *cor pulmonale* (right-sided heart failure due to lung damage) or *emphysema* (destruction of the air sacs in the lungs) may develop. The risk of *tuberculosis* is increased in coal workers' pneumoconiosis and silicosis; the risk of *lung cancer* is increased in asbestosis. Smoking further increases the risk.

DIAGNOSIS AND TREATMENT

Pneumoconiosis is often detected by a *chest X-ray* before symptoms develop. Diagnosis is also based on a history of exposure to dusts, medical examination, a *CT scan*, and *pulmonary function tests*.

There is no treatment for the condition apart from treating any complications. Further exposure to any dust must be avoided.

pneumocystis pneumonia

A lung infection caused by the *protozoa* PNEUMOCYSTIS JIROVECI (formerly known as PNEUMOCYSTIS CARINII). Pneumocystis pneumonia is an *opportunistic infection*, which is dangerous only to people with impaired resistance to infection. It is particularly common in those with *AIDS*. Symptoms include fever, dry cough, and shortness of breath, and may last for several weeks or months.

Diagnosis is made by *chest X-ray*, examination of sputum, or a lung *biopsy* (tissue sample). High doses of *antibiotic drugs* (commonly co-trimoxazole) may

eradicate the infection; lower doses are used in the long term to prevent infection in people at increased risk.

pneumonectomy

Surgery carried out to remove a *lung*.

pneumonia

Inflammation of the lungs usually due to infection. There are two main types: lobar pneumonia and bronchopneumonia. Lobar pneumonia first affects one lobe of a lung. In the condition bronchopneumonia, inflammation initially starts in the bronchi and bronchioles (airways), then spreads to affect patches of tissue in one or both lungs.

CAUSES

Pneumonia is usually caused by various types of infection. Most cases are due either to viruses, such as adenovirus or respiratory syncytial virus, or to bacteria, such as STREPTOCOCCUS PNEUMONIAE, HAEMOPHILUS INFLUENZAE, STAPHYLOCOCCUS AUREUS, and MYCOPLASMA PNEUMONIAE.

Another form is aspiration pneumonia, due to accidental inhalation of vomit. Aspiration pneumonia usually occurs in people whose cough reflex is not functioning, such as those who have drunk excessive amounts of alcohol or taken certain illegal drugs, or people who have suffered a head injury.

SYMPTOMS AND COMPLICATIONS

Symptoms usually include fever, chills, shortness of breath, a sharp chest pain, and a cough that produces yellow-green *sputum* and occasionally blood.

Potential complications include *pleural effusion* (fluid around the lung), *pleurisy* (inflammation of the membrane lining

the lungs and chest cavity), a lung *abscess* (collection of pus), and *septicaemia* (blood poisoning).

DIAGNOSIS AND TREATMENT

Diagnosis is made by physical examination, *chest X-ray*, and examining sputum and blood for microorganisms. Treatment depends on the cause, and usually includes *antibiotic drugs*. *Paracetamol* or *ibuprofen* may be given to reduce fever, and, in severe cases, *oxygen therapy* and artificial *ventilation* may be needed. In most cases, recovery usually occurs within about two weeks.

Vaccination against *influenza* and *pneumococcus* can help to prevent pneumonia, as can stopping smoking.

pneumonitis

Inflammation of the lungs that may cause coughing, breathing difficulty, and wheezing. Causes include an allergic reaction to dust containing animal or plant material (see *alveolitis*) and exposure to radiation (see *radiation hazards*). Pneuomonitis may also occur as a side effect of drugs, such as *amiodarone* and *azathioprine*.

pneumothorax

A condition in which air enters the pleural cavity (the space between the layers of membrane lining the lung), causing partial or total collapse of the lung. The air may enter the lungs from the airways or from outside the body.

CAUSES

The most common cause is the spontaneous rupture of an enlarged alveolus (air sac). This occurrence is much more common in men than in women; it

P

PNEUMONIA

Pneumonia is not a single disease, but the name for several types of lung inflammation usually caused by infectious organisms. In some cases, accidental inhalation of vomit or a liquid may start an infection. The symptoms, treatment, and outcome vary greatly, depending on the cause and on the general health of the patient.

Lobar pneumonia
In this type of pneumonia, the inflammation is usually confined to just one lobe of one lung, often a lower lobe.

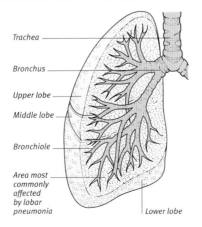

Trachea
Bronchus
Upper lobe
Middle lobe
Bronchiole
Area most commonly affected by lobar pneumonia
Lower lobe

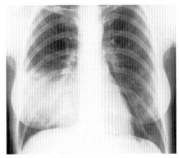

Chest X-ray in lobar pneumonia
The X-ray clearly shows lobar pneumonia in the patient's right lung (on the left in the image). The blotchy white areas within the darker areas correspond to patches of inflamed lung.

usually affects tall, thin young men who have no underlying lung disease. Other possible causes include a penetrating chest wound that allows air into the pleural cavity, or a fractured rib that tears the lung beneath it.

SYMPTOMS

The main symptoms of pneumothorax are chest pain or shortness of breath, which varies depending on the size of the pneumothorax. If air continues to leak, the pneumothorax may grow to produce a tension pneumothorax. This condition may be life-threatening. It causes an area of high pressure that compresses the lung and heart tissues, preventing the passage of oxygen-rich blood from the lungs to the heart.

DIAGNOSIS AND TREATMENT

Diagnosis is confirmed by *chest X-ray*. A small pneumothorax may disappear in a few days without treatment. A larger one, or one associated with underlying lung disease, may need hospital treatment. This involves removing the air through a tube with a one-way valve, known as a chest drain, to allow the lung to reinflate fully.

pocket, gingival

A feature of marginal *periodontitis*.

podiatry

Another name for *chiropody*, a paramedical speciality concerned with the feet.

podophyllin

A drug used to treat genital warts (see *warts, genital*). Podophyllin may cause irritation of the treated area and severe toxicity on excessive application.

poison

A substance that, in small amounts, disrupts the structure and/or function of cells. (See also *drug poisoning*; *poisoning*.)

poisoning

Poisons may be swallowed, inhaled, absorbed through the skin, or injected under the skin (as with an insect sting). They may also originate within the body, for example when bacteria produce *endotoxins*, or when *metabolic disorders* produce poisonous substances or allow them to accumulate. Poisoning may be acute, if a large amount of poison enters the body in a short time, or chronic, resulting from a gradual accumulation of poison that is not quickly eliminated from the body.

Unintentional poisoning occurs most commonly in young children. Adults may be poisoned by mistaking the dosage of a prescribed drug (see *drug poisoning*), by taking very high doses of vitamin or mineral supplements, by exposure to poisonous substances in industry, or by *drug abuse*. Poisoning may also be a deliberate attempt to commit *suicide*.

Antidotes may be available to counteract the effects of the poison.

polio

An abbreviation for *poliomyelitis*.

poliomyelitis

Also called polio, a highly infectious disease caused by the polio virus. It is usually mild, but in serious cases, it attacks the brain and spinal cord, sometimes causing paralysis or death.

CAUSE AND INCIDENCE

The virus is spread from the faeces of infected people to food. Airborne transmission also occurs. In countries with poor hygiene and sanitation, most children develop immunity through being infected early in life, when the infection rarely causes serious illness. In countries with better sanitation, this does not occur and, if children are not vaccinated, epidemics can occur.

SYMPTOMS

Most infected children have no symptoms at all. In others, however, there is usually an *incubation period* of seven to 14 days, after which a slight fever, sore throat, headache, and vomiting occur.

Most children recover completely after a few days. In some, however, inflammation of the *meninges* (membranes surrounding the brain and spinal cord) may develop. This condition causes fever, severe headache, stiff neck and back, and aching muscles, sometimes with widespread twitching. In a few cases, extensive paralysis, usually of the legs and lower trunk, then develops within a few days. If the infection spreads to the *brainstem*, the affected person may find it difficult or impossible to breathe and swallow.

DIAGNOSIS

Diagnosis is made from a sample of cerebrospinal fluid (see *lumbar puncture*), a throat *swab*, a faeces sample, or *blood tests* for antibodies to the virus. Paralysis occurring with an acute feverish illness is characteristic of severe polio, and an immediate diagnosis can often be made.

TREATMENT

There is no effective drug treatment for polio. Nonparalytic patients usually need bed rest and *analgesic drugs* (painkillers). If the person is paralysed, *physiotherapy* and, in some cases, *catheterization*, *tracheostomy* (surgical creation of an opening in the windpipe for a breathing tube), and artificial *ventilation* are needed.

OUTLOOK

Recovery from nonparalytic polio is complete. More than half of those with paralysis make a full recovery, fewer than a quarter are left with severe disability, and fewer than 1 in 10 dies.

PREVENTION

In the UK, vaccination against polio is given at ages two, three, and four months, with booster doses given between the ages of three years four months and five years, and again at 13 to 18 years. The polio vaccine is combined with other vaccines and given as part of the routine childhood immunization programme. Since 2004 inactivated polio vaccine (which is given by injection) has been used; this is safer than the previously used oral vaccine.

pollen

Dustlike grains produced by the male sexual organs of plants for fertilizing the female organs. Pollen may produce allergic reactions (see *allergy*) and cause hay fever (see *rhinitis, allergic*).

poly-

A prefix meaning "many" or "much".

polyarteritis nodosa

Also called periarteritis nodosa, an uncommon form of *vasculitis* (inflammation of blood vessels), affecting medium-sized arteries. Areas of arterial wall become inflamed, weakened, and liable to *aneurysms* (ballooned-out segments). The severity of the condition depends on the arteries that are affected and how much they are weakened.

CAUSE AND INCIDENCE

The cause seems to be an *immune system* disturbance, sometimes triggered by exposure to the *hepatitis B* virus. It is most common in adults and affects men more than women.

SYMPTOMS

Early symptoms of polyarteritis nodosa include fever, aching muscles and joints, general malaise, loss of appetite and weight, and, sometimes, nerve pain. There may also be *hypertension* (high blood pressure), skin ulceration, and *gangrene* (localized tissue death). If the coronary arteries are affected, *myocardial infarction* (heart attack) may occur. Many people with polyarteritis nodosa also suffer abdominal pain, nausea, vomiting, diarrhoea, and blood in the faeces. The condition may occasionally lead to *kidney failure*.

DIAGNOSIS, TREATMENT, AND OUTLOOK

Diagnosis is made by *biopsy* (tissue sampling) and *angiography*. Large doses of *corticosteroids*, and in some cases *immunosuppressants*, may allow survival for at least five years. Without treatment, few patients survive for this length of time.

polyarthritis

Any form of *arthritis* (joint inflammation) that affects several joints at once. It may be a complication of infections such as *rubella*, *gastroenteritis*, or sexually transmitted infections (see *reactive arthritis*). Other arthritic conditions that can cause polyarthritis include *rheumatoid arthritis*, *osteoarthritis*, and *juvenile chronic arthritis*.

polycystic kidney

See *kidney, polycystic*.

polycystic ovary syndrome

A condition, previously known as Stein–Leventhal syndrome, that is characterized by multiple *ovarian cysts* together with various other symptoms. Most women with the syndrome begin menstruation at a normal age, but between the ages of about 15 and 30 periods become irregular or light and sometimes cease altogether (*amenorrhoea*). In addition, affected women may become infertile, gain weight, and develop acne and *hirsutism* (excessive hairiness).

CAUSES

The condition is thought to result from *insulin* resistance, which leads to overproduction of insulin. This situation is associated with increased levels of *androgen hormones*, giving rise to symptoms. Polycystic ovary syndrome may also have a genetic element.

DIAGNOSIS AND TREATMENT

A diagnosis of polycystic ovary syndrome is based on the patient's history, measurement of hormone levels, and *ultrasound scanning* of the ovaries. Treatment depends on which aspect of the condition most concerns the patient. Weight reduction often brings about an improvement in all other symptoms and the return of regular periods. *Metformin*, an *oral hypoglycaemic* drug, may be used to reduce insulin resistance and as an aid to weight loss; hirsutism may respond to treatment with an anti-androgen drug, such as cyproterone; fertility treatment with the anti-oestrogen drug *clomifene* is often successful.

OUTLOOK

In the long term, women with polycystic ovary syndrome are at an increased risk of developing *diabetes mellitus* during pregnancy and in later life. Obesity leads to a greater risk of *atherosclerosis* and *hypertension* (high blood pressure). High levels of oestrogen may also increase the risk of developing endometrial cancer (see *uterus, cancer of*).

polycythaemia

A condition in which an increased production of red *blood cells* leads to an unusually large number of them in the blood. This disorder is usually caused by another disorder or by *hypoxia* (reduced oxygen in the blood and body tissues), in which cases it is called secondary polycythaemia. If the increase in red blood cells occurs for no apparent reason, it is called polycythaemia vera or primary polycythaemia.

SECONDARY POLYCYTHAEMIA

Secondary polycythaemia occurs naturally at high altitudes due to the reduced oxygen level. It can also result from a disorder that impairs the oxygen supply to the blood, such as chronic bronchitis (see *pulmonary disease, chronic obstructive*). In these cases, the low level of oxygen in the blood stimulates the kidneys to produce a hormone called erythropoietin, which in turn stimulates the bone marrow to produce more red cells and thus compensate for the lack of oxygen. Secondary polycythaemia may also be secondary to *liver cancer*, some kidney disorders, or heavy smoking.

Descending to sea level, or effective treatment of an underlying disorder, returns the blood to normal.

POLYCYTHAEMIA VERA

Polycythaemia vera is a rare disorder that mainly affects people over the age of 40. The large number of red blood cells causes increased volume and thickening of the blood, which may lead to headaches, blurred vision, and *hypertension* (high blood pressure). There may also be flushed skin, dizziness, night sweats, and widespread itching. The *spleen* is often enlarged.

Possible complications include a tendency to bleed easily or for the blood to clot; *stroke*; and disorders affecting the bone marrow, such as *myelofibrosis* or acute leukaemia (see *leukaemia, acute*).

Diagnosis is made from a physical examination and *blood tests* and by ruling out other possible causes of poly-

cythaemia. Treatment is by *venesection* (bloodletting) sometimes in combination with *anticancer drugs* or with radioactive phosphorus. This enables most patients to survive for 10 to 15 years.

polydactyly

A birth defect in which there is an excessive number of fingers or toes. The extra digits may be fully formed or they may be fleshy stumps. Polydactyly often runs in otherwise normal families; however, it may also occur as part of *Laurence–Biedl–Moon syndrome* or some other congenital syndromes.

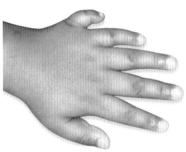

Polydactyly
Polydactylic digits are sometimes fully formed but are most often rudimentary (undersized). They are usually removed surgically during childhood.

polydipsia

Persistent excessive thirst (see *thirst, excessive*). Examples of conditions that can cause polydipsia include *diabetes mellitus* and *diabetes insipidus*.

polyhydramnios

Excess *amniotic fluid* surrounding the fetus during pregnancy. The condition often has no known cause. It sometimes occurs if the fetus has a malformation that makes normal swallowing impossible, in multiple pregnancy, or if the pregnant woman has *diabetes mellitus*.

SYMPTOMS

The excess amniotic fluid usually accumulates during the second half of pregnancy, producing symptoms from about week 32. The main symptom is abdominal discomfort. Other possible symptoms are breathlessness and swelling of the legs (see *oedema*). The uterus is larger than expected. Polyhydramnios may also be associated with an increased risk of abnormal fetal presentation (see *malpresentation)*, *placental abruption*, and haemorrhage after delivery.

Occasionally, acute polyhydramnios occurs. Fluid collects rapidly, causing abdominal pain, breathlessness, nausea,

P

vomiting, and leg swelling. The abdomen becomes tense, and the skin is shiny. Premature labour may occur.

DIAGNOSIS AND TREATMENT
The condition is usually evident from a physical examination, but *ultrasound scanning* may be needed. In mild cases, only rest is needed. In more severe cases, amniotic fluid may be withdrawn using a needle. In late pregnancy, *induction of labour* may be performed.

polymerase chain reaction (PCR)

A method of rapidly copying *DNA* sequences so that they can be analysed.

polymorphic light eruption (PLE)

A common skin condition that occurs in people who are sensitive to light (see *photosensitivity*) and results from exposure to *ultraviolet light* rays in sunlight. PLE is thought to be a form of delayed *allergy*, but the cause is unknown.

Light causes an itchy rash of papules (raised bumps) to develop on exposed areas of skin. The rash may last for several days. Sunblock should be used as a preventive measure. A mild case of PLE may be treated by applying a topical *steroid*. In severe cases, a short course of oral steroids can be used to prevent or treat an attack. Controlled exposure to ultraviolet light (see *phototherapy*) may reduce the symptoms in resistant cases.

polymyalgia rheumatica

An uncommon disease that occurs in older people, which is marked by pain and stiffness in the muscles of the hips, thighs, shoulders, and neck. Symptoms are worse in the mornings. The cause is unknown, but the condition may be associated with *temporal arteritis*. It is unusual before the age of 50 and is more common in women.

The diagnosis is often difficult to confirm; it is based on the patient's history, a physical examination, and *blood tests* (notably an *ESR*). If temporal arteritis is suspected, a *biopsy* (removal of a tissue sample for analysis) may be performed on an artery at the side of the scalp.

Treatment is with *corticosteroid drugs*, which usually improve the condition within a few days. Drug treatment usually needs to be continued for about two years to prevent symptoms from recurring, although some people need to continue treatment for longer, sometimes for life.

polymyositis

A rare disease in which the muscles are inflamed and weak.

polymyxins

A group of *antibiotic drugs* derived from the bacterium BACILLUS POLYMYXA. Polymyxins, which include the drug *colistin*, are given to treat eye and skin infections.

polyp

A growth that projects, usually at the end of a stalk, from the lining of the nose, cervix, intestine, larynx, or from any other *mucous membrane*. Some types of polyp are liable to develop into cancer; these types are surgically removed.

polypeptide

A compound made up of many *peptides*.

polypharmacy

The practice of prescribing several drugs to one person at the same time. Combinations of drugs may be more effective than single drugs and may reduce the risk of drug resistance. However, polypharmacy increases the risk of drug interactions and, as a result, the risk of adverse effects.

polyposis, familial adenomatous

A rare, inherited disorder, also known as polyposis coli, in which many *polyps* are present throughout the large intestine, but mainly in the colon. If familial adenomatous polyposis (FAP) is not treated, cancer of the colon (see *colon, cancer of*) is almost certain to develop.

The polyps may appear from the age of ten. They may cause bleeding and diarrhoea; however, there are often no symptoms until cancer has developed. The polyps are detected by *colonoscopy* (examining the interior of the colon with a viewing instrument).

There is a 50 per cent chance that a child of an affected person will inherit the disease, so medical surveillance with colonoscopy is necessary from about the age of 12. Individual polyps may be heat-treated (see *cauterization*). Since there is a high risk of developing cancer; a *colectomy* and *ileostomy* are often performed.

polysaccharide

A *carbohydrate* that is formed from many *monosaccharides* (simple sugar molecules) joined together. Examples of polysaccharides include *glycogen* (the main form in which carbohydrates are stored in the body); *starch*, a form of carbohydrate obtained from fruits, vegetables, and cereals; and *cellulose*, an indigestible material found in plant-based foods (see *fibre, dietary*).

polyunsaturated fats

Fats (see *fats and oils*) with relatively few hydrogen atoms in their chemical structure. Polyunsaturated fats tend to protect against cardiovascular disease.

polyuria

See *urination, excessive*.

PoM

The abbreviation for *prescription-only medicine*.

pompholyx

An acute form of *eczema* in which itchy blisters form on the palms and/or soles. The condition, also called dyshydrotic eczema, is sometimes due to an allergic response. Rarely, pompholyx is associated with *fungal infections* of the skin. Treatment includes an *astringent* and topical application of a *corticosteroid drug*. Antibiotics may be prescribed if secondary infection develops.

pons

The middle part of the *brainstem*.

POP

An abbreviation for "progestogen-only pill" (see *minipill*; *oral contraceptives*) and for "plaster of Paris" *cast*.

popliteal cyst

A fluid-filled sac that develops at the back of the knee. The cysts may occur in both adults and children, but for different reasons.

In children, the condition may be due to a swollen *bursa* (fluid-filled pad) behind the knee; the cause is unknown, but not related to any knee problem. These cysts usually cause no symptoms and disappear spontaneously.

In adults, the cysts usually result from conditions that cause chronic swelling or an accumulation of fluid in the knee joint. One possible cause is *osteoarthritis*; others include injuries to the *meniscus* (cartilage inside the knee) or to the ligaments, which allow *synovial fluid* (which lubricates joints) to escape from the joint capsule.

Most popliteal cysts disappear without treatment, although some may rupture, resembling a *deep vein thrombosis* (DVT). A diagnosis of DVT must be excluded before treatment with rest and *analgesic drugs*. In some cases, the cyst may need to be removed surgically.

pore

A tiny opening, usually in the skin.

porphyria

Any of a group of rare, often inherited disorders caused by the accumulation of substances called porphyrins.

CAUSES

Porphyrins are chemicals formed in the body during the manufacture of haem (a component of *haemoglobin*, the oxygen-carrying pigment in red blood cells). A block in this process causes a buildup of porphyrins, which can act as a poison. Such blocks may result from various genetic *enzyme* deficiencies. Porphyria may also be due to poisoning.

TYPES AND SYMPTOMS

There are six types of porphyria, each of which has different symptoms. Sufferers often have a rash or blistering brought on by sunlight, and may have abdominal pain and nervous system disturbances due to the effects of certain drugs or alcohol.

Acute intermittent porphyria This form usually appears in early adulthood, causing abdominal pain, and often limb cramps, muscle weakness, and psychiatric disturbances. The patient's urine turns red when left to stand. *Barbiturate drugs*, *phenytoin*, *oral contraceptives*, and certain other drugs precipitate attacks.

Variegate porphyria This condition has similar effects to acute intermittent porphyria, and may be caused by the same drugs. An additional symptom is blistering on skin that is exposed to sunlight.

Hereditary coproporphyria This form also has similar effects to acute intermittent porphyria, and may cause additional skin symptoms.

Protoporphyria In this form of porphyria, mild skin symptoms appear after exposure to sunlight.

Porphyria cutanea tarda This condition causes blistering of skin that is exposed to the sun, but with no disturbances of the digestive or nervous systems. Wounds are slow to heal, and urine is sometimes pink or brown. Many cases are precipitated by liver disease.

Congenital erythropoietic porphyria This is the rarest and most serious form of porphyria. It causes red discoloration of urine and teeth, excessive hair growth, severe skin blistering and ulceration, and haemolytic *anaemia*. Death may occur in childhood.

DIAGNOSIS AND TREATMENT

Diagnosis is made from abnormal levels of porphyrins in the urine and faeces. Treatment of porphyria is difficult. Avoiding sunlight and/or precipitating drugs is the most important measure. Acute intermittent porphyria, hereditary coproporphyria and variegate porphyria may be helped by the administration of *glucose* or hemin (a substance that is chemically related to haem). Cases of porphyria cutanea tarda may sometimes be helped by *venesection* (withdrawing blood from a vein).

portal hypertension

Increased blood pressure in the portal vein, which carries blood from the stomach, intestines, and spleen to the liver. The pressure causes *oesophageal varices* (widened veins in the oesophagus), which may rupture and cause internal bleeding. In addition, fluid is forced out of the overloaded portal vein, resulting in *ascites* (accumulation of fluid in the abdomen).

CAUSES

The most common cause is *cirrhosis* of the liver, in which areas of scar tissue in the liver obstruct the portal vein. Another possible cause is *thrombosis* (abnormal blood clotting) due to narrowing of the portal vein. The narrowing may be present from birth, appear shortly after birth, or develop later in life (due to compression of the vein by enlarged *lymph nodes*, or to inflammation resulting from an infection). In tropical areas, a common cause is disease that causes the spleen to enlarge and results in an increased blood flow from the spleen through the portal vein.

A rare cause of portal hypertension is an abnormal connection that occurs between the portal vein and an artery (see *arteriovenous fistula*); this is usually the result of injury.

SYMPTOMS

Symptoms may only appear once complications have developed. Ruptured oesophageal varices lead to massive, recurrent vomiting of blood and produce black faeces (*melaena*). Ascites results in abdominal swelling and discomfort, and sometimes difficulty breathing. The veins just under the skin of the abdomen may also be visibly swollen.

DIAGNOSIS

Diagnosis is usually made from the symptoms and signs. *Doppler ultrasound scanning* may be used to assess the pressure in the portal vein.

TREATMENT

Various treatments may be used to reduce blood pressure and to stop bleeding or prevent further bleeding. For example,

P

PORTAL HYPERTENSION

The most common cause of portal hypertension is cirrhosis of the liver or some other obstruction to the blood flow through the liver. The portal vein becomes congested with blood, with the result that back pressure develops through the system of veins that join the portal vein.

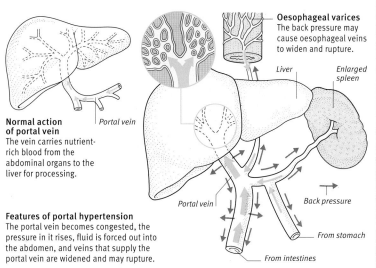

Normal action of portal vein
The vein carries nutrient-rich blood from the abdominal organs to the liver for processing.

Portal vein

Oesophageal varices
The back pressure may cause oesophageal veins to widen and rupture.

Liver

Enlarged spleen

Portal vein

Back pressure

From stomach

Features of portal hypertension
The portal vein becomes congested, the pressure in it rises, fluid is forced out into the abdomen, and veins that supply the portal vein are widened and may rupture.

From intestines

ruptured blood vessels may be treated by sclerotherapy, in which a chemical is injected into the veins to block them. A *shunt* is sometimes carried out to prevent further bleeding. Ascites is controlled by restriction of salt and with *diuretic drugs*.

port-wine stain

A purple-red birthmark that is a permanent, non-raised type of *haemangioma*. Port-wine stains are one of the features of *Sturge–Weber syndrome*.

positron emission tomography

See *PET scanning*.

posseting

The regurgitation of small quantities of milk by infants after they have been fed. Posseting is common and harmless.

postcoital contraception

See *contraception, emergency*.

posterior

Relating to the back of the body, or referring to the rear part.

postherpetic neuralgia

Burning pain due to nerve irritation (see *neuralgia*) occurring at the site of a previous attack of *herpes zoster* (shingles).

postmaturity

A condition in which a pregnancy persists for longer than 42 weeks; the average length of a normal pregnancy is 40 weeks (see *gestation*). Postmaturity may be associated with a family tendency to prolonged pregnancy.

Postmaturity is associated with a prolonged labour and an increased risk of a difficult delivery; this is because a postmature fetus is larger than average, and the skull bones are harder and mould less readily to fit through the birth canal. The risk of fetal death increases after 42 weeks because the *placenta* becomes less efficient, causing the fetus to be starved of oxygen and nutrients. Postmature infants tend to have dry skin and may be more susceptible to infection.

Many obstetricians attempt to prevent postmaturity by *induction of labour* as the pregnancy nears 42 weeks.

postmenopausal bleeding

Any vaginal bleeding in women who have already gone through the *menopause* (the period during which *ovulation* and *menstruation* cease). The bleeding may be a result of taking *hormone* *replacement therapy (HRT)*. It may also be a symptom of various disorders of the reproductive organs. The most common, and least serious, is irritation of the genital tissues (see *vulvovaginitis*). Other causes include atrophic *vaginitis*; cervical cancer (see *cervix, cancer of*); growths in the uterus (see *uterus, cancer of*; *polyp*); or, rarely, cancer of the vulva or the vagina. All postmenopausal bleeding must be investigated in order to exclude the possibility of cancer.

postmenopausal osteoporosis

Osteoporosis (loss of bone density) in women who have gone through the *menopause* (the time when *ovulation* and *menstruation* cease). In postmenopausal women, thinning of the bones is due to the sharp decrease in levels of *oestrogen hormones*, which normally help to maintain bone mass.

postmenopause

The period of a woman's life following the *menopause* (the time when *ovulation* and *menstruation* cease).

postmortem examination

An alternative term for an *autopsy*.

postmyocardial infarction syndrome

Another name for *Dressler's syndrome*.

postnasal drip

A watery or sticky discharge from the back of the nose into the *nasopharynx* (the uppermost part of the throat, behind the nose), particularly at night when a person is lying down. The fluid may cause a cough, hoarseness, or the feeling of a foreign body. The usual causes are allergic *rhinitis* (inflammation of the mucous membrane in the nose) and the common cold. Another cause, in young children, is enlarged *adenoids*.

postnatal care

Care of the mother after *childbirth* until about six weeks later.

After delivery, the mother's temperature, pulse, and blood pressure are monitored, especially after a *caesarean section* or if there have been complications, such as *pre-eclampsia* or bleeding.

The length of stay in hospital depends on whether or not there have been any complications. Women used to remain in hospital for up to a week after delivery, but now the length of stay after a straightforward delivery may be only 48 hours or even less. During the hospital stay, a daily check is made for any signs of *puerperal sepsis* (infection of the genital tract after childbirth), including inspection of the *lochia* (vaginal discharge after childbirth). If the woman has had an *episiotomy* or if she has torn tissue around the vagina, the wounds are checked daily.

The woman is encouraged to walk as soon as possible after the delivery to reduce the risk of *thrombosis* (abnormal blood clotting). If necessary, help is given with feeding techniques (see *bottle-feeding*; *breast-feeding*). There may also be instruction on various abdominal exercises and *pelvic floor exercises*, which can help to restore muscle tone.

A final postnatal check-up usually takes place about six weeks after delivery. The obstetrician or GP may check the woman's blood pressure, weight, breasts, haemoglobin levels, and emotional state; may examine the uterus and bladder to make sure they are in the correct positions; may check for urinary incontinence (see *incontinence, urinary*); may take a smear; and ensures that any wounds are healing properly. Advice on *contraception* may also be given.

postnatal depression

Depression in a woman after *childbirth*. The cause is probably a combination of sudden hormonal changes and psychological and environmental factors. The depression ranges from an extremely common and mild, shortlived episode ("baby blues") to a rare, severe depressive illness: *puerperal psychosis*.

MILD DEPRESSION

Most mothers first get the "blues" four to five days after childbirth and may feel miserable, irritable, and tearful. The feeling is caused by hormonal changes, perhaps coupled with a sense of anticlimax after the birth or an overwhelming sense of responsibility for the baby. With reassurance and support, the depression usually passes in two to three days.

MORE SEVERE DEPRESSION

In some women, postnatal depression lasts for several weeks and causes a constant feeling of tiredness, difficulty in sleeping, loss of appetite, and restlessness. The condition usually clears up of its own accord or is treated with *antidepressant drugs* and emotional support.

PUERPERAL PSYCHOSIS

This condition causes severe mental confusion, feelings of worthlessness, threats of suicide or harm to the baby,

P

and sometimes *delusions*. Admission to hospital, ideally with the baby, and anti-depressant drugs are often needed.

postpartum depression

See *postnatal depression*.

postpartum haemorrhage

Excessive blood loss after *childbirth*. It is more common after a long labour or after a multiple birth.

CAUSES AND SYMPTOMS
Most cases occur immediately after delivery (primary postpartum haemorrhage) and are due to excessive bleeding from the site where the *placenta* was attached to the uterus. Normally, once the placenta is delivered, contractions of the uterus constrict the blood vessels at the site, and stop the bleeding. Excessive bleeding may be caused by failure of the uterus to contract efficiently after delivery. It may also be due to the retention of placental tissue within the uterus.

Haemorrhaging immediately after delivery may also be caused by tears anywhere along the birth canal. Tearing is more likely to occur during a *forceps delivery* or a *breech delivery*. In some cases, however, postpartum haemorrhage occurs because the mother has a bleeding disorder.

Occasionally, haemorrhage occurs with pain and fever between five and 10 days after delivery (secondary postpartum haemorrhage). In these cases of haemorrhage, the cause is usually infection of a retained fragment of placenta.

TREATMENT
A blood transfusion may be given to replace lost blood, and emergency treatment may be needed for *shock* (a severe drop in blood pressure, which may be due to heavy blood loss). Other treatment depends on the cause of the haemorrhage. Any retained placental tissue may need to be removed; an injection of a drug such as *ergometrine* may be given to stimulate uterine contractions; and any lacerations that have been made in the vagina or on the cervix are sutured (stitched). *Antibiotic drugs* are used to treat infection and iron supplements may be needed to counteract iron deficiency due to blood loss.

post-traumatic stress disorder

A form of *anxiety* that develops after a stressful or traumatic event. Common causes include natural disasters, violence, *rape*, torture, serious physical injury, and military combat.

Symptoms, which may develop many months after the event, include recurring memories or dreams of the event, a sense of personal isolation, and disturbed sleep and concentration. There may be a deadening of feelings, or irritability and feelings of guilt, sometimes building up to depression. The symptoms may be worsened by any reminder of the trauma.

Most people recover, in time, with emotional support from family and friends. However, some people may require specialized trauma *counselling* or *cognitive-behavioural therapy*.

postural drainage

A technique that enables sputum (phlegm) or other secretions to drain from a person's lungs in order to clear the lungs and so ease breathing.

Postural drainage is used in the treatment of *cystic fibrosis* and *bronchiectasis*, a lung disorder. The person lies on his or her front or side, with the head lower than the chest. This position allows the secretions to drain by gravity, into the *trachea* (windpipe), from where they can be coughed up. Tapping the person's chest with cupped hands can help to loosen sticky secretions.

postural hypotension

See *hypotension*.

posture

The relative positions of different parts of the body when a person is at rest or during movement. Good posture consists of balancing the body weight around the body's centre of gravity, which is in the lower spine and pelvis. Maintaining good posture helps prevent neck pain and back pain.

post-viral fatigue syndrome

See *chronic fatigue syndrome*.

potassium

A metallic *mineral* needed to help maintain normal heart rhythm, regulate the body's water balance, conduct nerve impulses, and contract muscles.

Many foods contain potassium; particularly rich dietary sources include lean meat, whole grains, green leafy vegetables, beans, and various fruits, such as apricots, dates, and peaches.

POTASSIUM DEFICIENCY
When there is a low level of potassium in the blood, the condition is known as hypokalaemia. This condition usually results from loss of fluids through diarrhoea and/or vomiting, and causes fatigue, drowsiness, dizziness, and muscle weakness. Children are particularly susceptible to this form of potassium loss. In more severe cases of hypokalaemia, there may be abnormal heart rhythms and muscle paralysis.

Other potential causes of hypokalaemia include any prolonged treatment that involves taking *diuretic drugs* or *corticosteroid drugs*; the overuse of *laxative drugs*; *diabetes mellitus*; *aldosteronism* (overproduction of the hormone aldosterone by the adrenal glands); *Cushing's syndrome* (overproduction of corticosteroid hormones by the adrenal glands); certain kidney diseases; excessively high intake of coffee or alcohol; and extremely profuse sweating.

POTASSIUM EXCESS
Excess potassium in the blood is known as hyperkalaemia and is much less common than hypokalaemia. It may be due to excessive intake of potassium supplements, severe *kidney failure*, *Addison's disease*, or prolonged treatment with potassium-sparing *diuretics*. The effects of high potassium levels in the blood can include numbness and tingling, disturbances of the heart rhythm, and muscle paralysis. In severe cases, there may be *heart failure*.

potassium channel activators

A class of drugs that are used in the prevention and long-term treatment of *angina* (chest pain due to inadequate blood supply to the heart). Nicorandil is a potassium channel activator that acts in a similar way to *nitrates*, and widens both arteries and veins. Possible side effects of taking potassium channel activators include flushing, headaches, nausea, vomiting, and dizziness.

potassium citrate

A substance used to relieve discomfort in mild *urinary tract infections* by making the urine less acid.

potassium permanganate

A drug that has an *antiseptic* and *astringent* effect and is used to treat *dermatitis*. Potassium permanganate can occasionally cause irritation and can also stain skin and clothing.

potency

The ability of a man to perform *sexual intercourse*; or the ability of a drug to cause desired effects.

P

P

Pott's fracture

A combined fracture and dislocation of the ankle caused by excessive or violent twisting. The *fibula* (the outer of the two bones of the lower leg) breaks just above the ankle; in addition, the *tibia* (shin) breaks or the *ligaments* tear, resulting in dislocation.

poultice

A warm pack consisting of a soft, moist substance (such as *kaolin*) that is spread between layers of soft fabric. Poultices are applied to the skin. They were once widely used for the reduction of localized pain or inflammation, bringing *boils* to a head, and improving circulation in a specific area.

pox

Any of various infectious diseases characterized by blistery skin eruptions (for example *chickenpox*). Pox is sometimes used as a slang word for *syphilis*.

Prader–Willi syndrome

A rare *genetic disorder* that is believed to result from a *chromosomal abnormality* affecting chromosome 15. The condition is congenital (present at birth).

The physical features of this condition include *short stature*; *hypogonadism* (underdeveloped testes or ovaries); a small penis, in males; very small hands and feet; almond-shaped eyes; and a *squint*. Mental characteristics include specific *learning difficulties*.

Affected babies have *hypotonia* (floppy muscles), feeding difficulties, and are abnormally sleepy; these problems lessen after about six months. Young children may be slow learning to walk and talk (see *developmental delay*).

Affected children develop an uncontrollable hunger and an obsession with eating. If their food intake is not controlled, they will eat continually. This can lead to *obesity*, which may in turn cause other disorders, such as *diabetes mellitus* and *heart failure*. The desire for food may cause behavioural problems if a child is prevented from eating; in addition, he or she may suffer from *anxiety* and show harmful behaviour, such as picking at the skin. In most other aspects, affected children are generally good-natured, although their problems may cause them to be socially isolated.

Treatment is for the symptoms. Parents, teachers, and carers must ensure that the child does not eat too much. Underdevelopment of sexual organs, especially in boys, may be corrected by treatment with *sex hormones*. *Growth hormone* may be given for short stature. Learning difficulties are treated with appropriate education or therapy.

pravastatin

A *lipid-lowering drug*.

praziquantel

An *anthelmintic drug* used to treat *tapeworm infestation* and *schistosomiasis*. Side effects may include dizziness, drowsiness, and abdominal pain.

prazosin

A *vasodilator drug* used to treat *hypertension* (high blood pressure), *heart failure*, *Raynaud's disease*, and urinary symptoms resulting from an enlarged prostate gland (see *prostate, enlarged*). Side effects include dizziness and fainting, nausea, headache, and dry mouth.

precancerous

A term applied to any condition in which there is a tendency for *cancer* to develop. Such conditions are characterized by abnormal changes in cells; the affected areas may need to be removed in order to prevent cancer.

Examples of precancerous conditions are *cervical intraepithelial neoplasia*, the pre-invasive stage of cervical cancer (see *cervix, cancer of*); *leukoplakia* of the mouth, vulva, or penis, which can develop into *squamous cell carcinoma*; and familial adenomatous polyposis (growth of multiple polyps in the intestine; see *polyposis, familial adenomatous*), which may also become cancerous.

Certain other disorders carry a risk of cancerous changes, but such changes are less inevitable than with precancerous conditions. These disorders may require monitoring but do not always need treatment. Examples include *ulcerative colitis*, carrying an increased risk of tumours in the colon and rectum, and atrophic *gastritis*, with an increased risk of stomach cancer.

precocious puberty

The development of *secondary sexual characteristics* that occurs before age eight in girls and nine in boys.

CAUSES

Precocious puberty is uncommon. It may be due to various disorders that can cause the production of *sex hormones* at an abnormally early age. Some possible underlying causes include a *brain tumour* or other brain abnormalities; abnormality of the adrenal glands (for example, *congenital adrenal hyperplasia*); *ovarian cysts*, and *tumours*, or a tumour in the testes. In some cases, no underlying cause can be identified.

SYMPTOMS

The hormones may cause a premature growth spurt followed by early fusion of the bones. As a result, affected children may initially be tall but, if untreated, final height is often greatly reduced.

INVESTIGATION AND TREATMENT

The child's pattern of pubertal development is assessed by a doctor. *Blood tests* are performed to measure hormone levels. *Ultrasound scanning* of the ovaries and testes, and *CT scanning* of the adrenal glands or brain, may also be carried out, depending on the suspected cause.

Treatment is of the underlying cause, and hormone drugs may be given to delay puberty and increase final height.

predisposing factors

Factors that lead to increased susceptibility to a disease.

prednisolone

A *corticosteroid drug* used in the treatment of a wide variety of disorders.

pre-eclampsia

A serious condition that can arise from 20 weeks of pregnancy. Features of pre-eclampsia include *hypertension* (high blood pressure), *oedema* (accumulation of fluid in tissues), and *proteinuria* (protein in the urine). If severe, symptoms may include headache, nausea and vomiting, abdominal pain, and visual disturbances. The cause is not fully understood.

The condition, which is sometimes called pre-eclamptic toxaemia or PET, is more common in first pregnancies and if the mother suffers from *diabetes mellitus*, hypertension, or kidney disease. Pre-eclampsia may cause liver, kidney, or *blood clotting* problems. Untreated pre-eclampsia may lead to *eclampsia*, which can cause *seizures* in the mother and even death of the mother and/or fetus.

For some cases, treatment is with bed rest and *antihypertensive drugs*, and hospital admission is usually advised so that health of the fetus and functioning of the placenta can be monitored carefully. However, the only complete cure is delivery of the baby, therefore *induction of labour* or a *caesarean section* may be performed in late pregnancy or if pre-eclampsia is severe. An *anticonvulsant drug* may be given to the mother around the time of delivery to help prevent eclampsia from developing.

Regular blood pressure checks and *urinalysis* (to look for protein in the urine) during *antenatal care* can help identify women who are at risk of developing pre-eclampsia.

pregnancy

The period from *conception* to birth. Pregnancy begins with *fertilization* of an ovum (egg) and its implantation. The egg develops into the *embryo*, which becomes the *fetus*, and the *placenta*, the organ that nourishes the embryo and then the fetus.

Most eggs implant into the uterus. Very occasionally, an egg implants into an abnormal site, such as a fallopian tube, resulting in an *ectopic pregnancy*.

STAGES AND FEATURES OF PREGNANCY

Pregnancy is traditionally dated from the first day of a woman's last menstrual period (LMP), although conception would not have taken place until two weeks after this. A normal pregnancy is considered to last between 37 and 42 weeks; it is divided into three stages (trimesters) of three months each. For the first eight weeks of pregnancy, the developing baby is called an embryo; thereafter it is called a fetus.

In the first trimester the breasts start to swell and may become tender. Morning sickness (see *vomiting in pregnancy*) is common. The baby's major organs have developed by the end of this stage. During the second trimester, the mother's nipples enlarge and darken and weight rises rapidly. The baby is usually felt moving by 16–22 weeks. During the third trimester, stretch marks and *colostrum* (nipple secretions) may appear, and *Braxton Hicks' contractions* may be felt. The baby's head engages at about 36 weeks. (See also box, below, and, for information on the hormones involved in pregnancy, see the box overleaf.)

STAGES AND FEATURES OF **PREGNANCY**

Pregnancy typically lasts 40 weeks, counted from the first day of the pregnant woman's last menstrual period, and is conventionally divided into three trimesters, each lasting three months. For the first eight weeks following conception, the developing baby is referred to as an embryo; thereafter, it is known as a fetus. It is during the early part of pregnancy (first trimester), while the growing baby is still an embryo, that it is at its most vulnerable to damage.

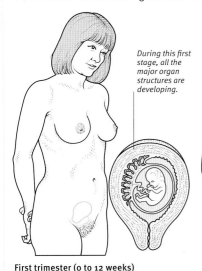

During this first stage, all the major organ structures are developing.

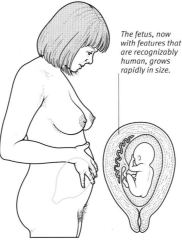

The fetus, now with features that are recognizably human, grows rapidly in size.

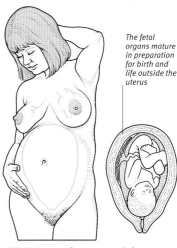

The fetal organs mature in preparation for birth and life outside the uterus

First trimester (0 to 12 weeks)

The first sign of pregnancy is usually the absence of a menstrual period, although some women have breakthrough bleeding. The breasts start to swell and may become tender as the mammary glands develop to prepare for breast-feeding. The nipples start to enlarge and the veins over the surface of the breasts become more prominent. A supportive bra should be worn.

Nausea and vomiting are common, and are often worse in the morning; these problems usually persist for six to eight weeks (see *vomiting in pregnancy*). There is a need to pass urine more frequently and there is often a creamy white discharge from the vagina. Many women feel unusually tired during the early weeks of pregnancy. Some notice a metallic taste in the mouth or a craving for certain foods or non-edible products. Weight begins to increase towards the end of this stage.

Second trimester (13 to 28 weeks)

From 16 weeks, the enlarging uterus is easily felt from the outside and the woman begins to look noticeably pregnant. The nipples enlarge and darken, and skin pigmentation may deepen. Some women may feel warm and flushed. Appetite tends to increase and weight rises rapidly. The woman's facial features tend to become heavier. By 22 weeks (and usually between the 16th and 20th weeks), most pregnant women have felt the baby moving around (a sensation that is sometimes known as "quickening").

During the second trimester, nausea, vomiting, and frequency of urination diminish, and the woman may feel generally better and more energetic than she did during the early weeks. The heart-rate increases, as does the volume of blood pumped by the heart; these changes allow the fetus to develop properly. However, they put an extra strain on the heart of women who have pre-existing heart disease.

Third trimester (29 to 40 weeks)

In some women, stretch marks develop on the abdomen, breasts, and thighs. Also, a dark line may appear that runs from the umbilicus to the pubic hair. Colostrum (secretions from the nipples) can be expressed from the nipples.

Minor problems are common. Many women become hot and sweat easily because body temperature rises slightly. More rest may be needed at this stage, although for many women it is difficult to find a comfortable position. Braxton Hicks' contractions may start to get stronger.

The baby's head engages (drops down low into the pelvis) around the 36th week in a first pregnancy, but not until a few weeks later in subsequent pregnancies. This so-called "lightening" may relieve pressure on the upper abdomen and on breathing, but it increases pressure on the bladder and may result in a more copious vaginal discharge.

P

PROBLEMS IN PREGNANCY

In addition to the expected features of pregnancy, such as experiencing nausea and tiredness, some women experience certain common, minor health problems. Although these conditions may be uncomfortable or troublesome, they usually disappear after delivery.

During pregnancy, food passes through the intestine more slowly than normal. This enables more nutrients to be absorbed for the baby, but also tends to cause constipation. *Pica* (craving to eat substances other than foods) is another common condition. In late pregnancy, the growing fetus puts pressure on the internal organs; this pressure may result in *haemorrhoids*, *heartburn* (due to acid reflux), swollen ankles, and *varicose veins*. Other common disorders during pregnancy include *urinary tract infections*, stress incontinence (see *incontinence, urinary*), and vaginal *candidiasis*.

EFFECTS OF **HORMONES DURING PREGNANCY**

A pregnant woman undergoes many changes that enable her to maintain the pregnancy, nourish the baby, and prepare for breast-feeding. These adaptations are brought about by increased levels of the female sex hormones oestrogen and progesterone, and by the action of two other hormones, human chorionic gonadotrophin (HCG) and human placental lactogen (HPL), produced only by the placenta.

Hormone	Effect
Progesterone	Decreases the excitability of smooth muscle, thereby helping to prevent uterine contractions and premature labour.
	Causes constipation and oesophageal acid reflux as a result of its effects on smooth muscle.
	Increases body temperature.
	Affects mood.
	Increases breathing rate.
Human placental lactogen (HPL)	Increases energy production necessary for fetal development.
	Causes enlargement of breasts and development of milk glands.
	Induces temporary diabetes mellitus (gestational diabetes) in susceptible women as a result of its effects on metabolism.
Human chorionic gonadotrophin (HCG)	Increases energy production necessary for fetal development.
	Induces gestational diabetes in susceptible women.
Oestrogens	Are important for the development of the reproductive system and breasts.
	Stimulate growth of the uterine muscle to enable the powerful contractions of labour.
	Increase vaginal secretions.
	Increase the size of the nipples and help the development of milk glands in the breasts.
	Increase the production of protein, which is essential for healthy growth of the woman and fetus.
	Alter collagen and other substances to allow body tissues to soften and stretch in preparation for labour.
	Relax ligaments and joints.
	May cause sciatica and backache, and may also contribute to the formation of varicose veins as a result of their effects on body tissue.
Melanocyte-stimulating hormone	Stimulates pigmentation (in combination with oestrogens), particularly of the nipples. May also produce chloasma (darkening of the facial skin).

Complications of pregnancy and disorders that affect it include *antepartum haemorrhage*; *diabetic pregnancy*; *miscarriage*; *polyhydramnios*; *pre-eclampsia*; *prematurity*; and *rhesus incompatibility*. (See also *childbirth*; *fetal heart monitoring*; *pregnancy, multiple*.)

pregnancy, drugs in

If certain drugs, such as *isotretinoin*, are taken during *pregnancy*, they may pass from the mother to the fetus through the *placenta*. They may interfere with fetal development, leading to *birth defects*. Relatively few drugs have been proved to cause harm to a developing baby but no drug should be considered completely safe, especially in early pregnancy. Pregnant women should seek medical advice before taking any drug, including over-the-counter preparations. However, if the benefits of a drug to the mother outweigh the risks to the fetus, the drug may be recommended.

Problems may also be caused in a developing baby if a pregnant woman drinks *alcohol*, smokes tobacco (see *smoking*), or takes drugs of abuse. The babies of women who use *heroin* during pregnancy tend to have a low birthweight and a higher death rate than normally expected during the first few weeks of life. Babies of women who abuse drugs intravenously are at high risk of *HIV* infection.

pregnancy, false

An uncommon psychological disorder, which is also known as pseudocyesis. In false pregnancy, a woman has many of the physical signs of pregnancy, including morning sickness (see *vomiting in pregnancy*), *amenorrhoea* (absence of periods), enlarged breasts, and abdominal swelling, but is not pregnant. The woman is convinced that she is pregnant. Treatment for false pregnancy may involve *counselling* or *psychotherapy*. (See also *conversion disorder*.)

pregnancy, multiple

More than one *fetus* in the uterus. Multiple *pregnancy* can occur if two or more ova (eggs; see *ovum*) are fertilized at the same time or if a single egg divides early in development.

CAUSES AND INCIDENCE

Twins are the most common type of multiple pregnancy and occur in about 1 in 80 pregnancies; triplets occur in about 1 in 8,000, and quadruplets in about 1 in 500,000. Multiple pregnancies are

P

more common in women who are treated with *fertility drugs*, or if a number of fertilized ova are implanted in the uterus during *in vitro fertilization*.

SYMPTOMS AND COMPLICATIONS

The common problems that are associated with normal pregnancy may be more severe in a multiple pregnancy. There is also an increased risk of severe morning sickness, *anaemia*, and *antepartum haemorrhage*. *Hypertension* (high blood pressure), *polyhydramnios* (an excess of amniotic fluid), *postpartum haemorrhage*, and *malpresentation* (abnormal positioning of a fetus just before birth) all occur more frequently in a multiple pregnancy. *Prematurity* is a common complication, and the weight of each baby is usually less than the weight of a single baby. *Caesarean section* is required more frequently than for single pregnancies.

DIAGNOSIS AND TREATMENT

During the woman's antenatal examination, the doctor or midwife may be able to feel more than one fetus, and may find that the abdomen is larger than expected for the stage of gestation. The doctor or midwife may also be able to hear more than one fetal heartbeat. Ultrasound scanning is used to confirm the diagnosis.

The woman is advised to take more rest during pregnancy and to increase her intake of protein. Supplements of *iron* and *folic acid* are also recommended in order to prevent iron-deficiency anaemia in the mother and *neural tube defects* in the fetuses, respectively.

pregnancy tests

Tests on urine or blood performed to determine whether a woman is pregnant. Pregnancy testing kits are available over the counter from pharmacies.

All pregnancy testing kits are designed to test for the presence of *human chorionic gonadotrophin* (HCG) in a sample of urine. This hormone is normally produced only by a developing placenta. The tests are extremely accurate (about 97 per cent accurate for a positive result, and about 80 per cent accurate for a negative result) and can be reliably used from the first day of a missed period. The tests can, however, misdiagnose pregnancy in cases of *hydatidiform mole* due to the very high levels of HCG that occur in this disorder.

Different brands of test vary, but all involve introducing a sample of urine to a test stick that has been treated with a chemical that reacts with HCG. *Blood tests* for detecting pregnancy can be used from 9 to 12 days after conception (even before a period is missed).

premature aging syndrome

See *progeria*.

premature ejaculation

See *ejaculation, disorders of*.

premature menopause

Menopause (cessation of ovulation and menstruation) that occurs before the age of 40. Premature menopause can be caused by any disorder or treatment in which the ovaries are destroyed or removed or ovarian functions are permanently disrupted (*radiotherapy* of the pelvic region, for example). *Hormone*

PREGNANCY TEST KIT

The pregnancy test shown here is one of a variety that are available over the counter at chemists' shops, allowing pregnancy testing to be carried out at home. All of the kits test for the presence of the hormone human chorionic gonadotropin (HCG) in a sample of urine. HCG is normally produced only by a developing placenta, which makes the tests very accurate, even if they are carried out early in a pregnancy.

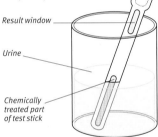

Result window

Urine

Chemically treated part of test stick

1 The indicator stick is dipped into a container of urine (as shown here). Alternatively, the user can place it directly into the urine flow while passing urine normally.

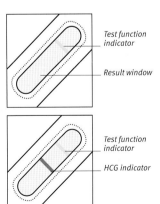

Test function indicator

Result window

Test function indicator

HCG indicator

2 The first line that becomes visible in the result window shows that the test is working. If HCG is present, this line is quickly followed by a second, different coloured line, which signifies pregnancy. A result can be obtained within a few minutes.

MULTIPLE PREGNANCY

About one pregnancy in 80 is multiple (e.g. twins or triplets). The rate is highest among women in their 30s. Problems arise more often in multiple pregnancies than in single pregnancies. For example, twins are much more likely than single babies to be born prematurely.

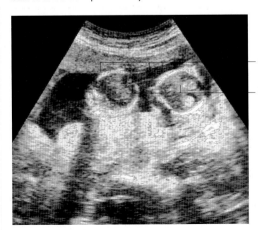

Amniotic sacs

Fetal heads

Ultrasound scan revealing twins
Ultrasound scanning of the woman's uterus can reveal the presence of twins within the first several weeks of pregnancy. Here, two fetal heads and a limb that belongs to the fetus on the right can be seen.

P

replacement therapy can relieve symptoms and reduce the risk of *osteoporosis* (loss of bone tissue). For women who want to conceive, *in vitro fertilization* (IVF) is possible, using donor eggs.

premature sexual maturation

See *precocious puberty*.

prematurity

The birth of a baby before 37 weeks' *gestation*. The premature infant may not be sufficiently developed to cope with independent life and needs special care.

CAUSES

Nearly 50 per cent of premature deliveries occur for no known reason. The remainder are due to conditions such as *pre-eclampsia*, *hypertension*, *diabetes mellitus*, long-standing kidney disease, and heart disease. Other causes include *antepartum haemorrhage*, intrauterine infection, premature rupture of the membranes, and multiple pregnancy (see *pregnancy, multiple*).

FEATURES AND COMPLICATIONS

A premature infant is smaller than a full-term baby. He or she lacks subcutaneous fat, is covered with downy hair (*lanugo*), and has very thin skin.

The baby's internal organs are also immature. The major complication is *respiratory distress syndrome*, which may occur because the lungs are insufficiently developed. There are also increased risks of brain haemorrhage, *jaundice*, and *hypoglycaemia* (low blood sugar). The baby has a limited ability to suck and to maintain a normal body temperature, and he or she is also prone to infection due to a poorly developed immune system. The earlier a baby is born, the more likely it is that he or she will have such problems.

TREATMENT AND OUTLOOK

Premature infants are usually nursed in a special baby unit that provides intensive care. The baby is placed in an *incubator*. He or she may have artificial *ventilation* to assist breathing, artificial feeding through a stomach tube or into a vein, and treatment with *antibiotic drugs* and *iron* and *vitamin supplements*. The baby is usually kept in hospital until he or she has reached a weight of at least 2.25 kg, is growing sufficiently, and is feeding well.

With the modern techniques that are now generally available, some infants survive even if they are born as early as 24 weeks' gestation. Most babies that are born after 28 weeks, and given specialist

PREMATURITY

A premature baby may need to be nursed in an incubator where the temperature and humidity are carefully controlled and the baby can be closely observed. If breathing difficulties develop, they may be treated by artificial ventilation. Very small babies cannot suck so they must be fed intravenously or via a tube passed into the stomach. If jaundice develops, they may be treated by phototherapy (light therapy), which breaks up the bilirubin that causes the yellow discoloration of the skin.

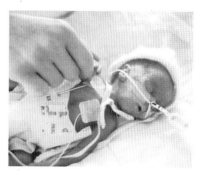

Premature infant
This baby was born several weeks prematurely and is being fed via a flexible tube that passes through the nose and oesophagus into the stomach.

FEATURES AND COMPLICATIONS OF PREMATURITY

Physical features

- Low birthweight (often less than 2.5kg)
- Small size
- Relatively large head and hands
- Thin, smooth, shiny skin
- Veins visible under the skin
- Little fat under the skin
- Wizened, wrinkled features
- Soft, flexible ear cartilage
- Short toenails (but normal length fingernails)
- Downy (lanugo) hair
- Reduced vernix (greasy substance that covers the newborn)
- Protuberant abdomen
- Enlarged clitoris (girls)
- Small scrotum (boys)
- Feeble, whining cry
- Irregular breathing
- Poor sucking and swallowing ability
- Tendency to regurgitate

Complications

- Increased risk of birth injury
- Respiratory distress syndrome
- Recurrent episodes of breathing stoppage
- Jaundice
- Infection
- Poor temperature control
- Anaemia
- Hypoglycaemia (low blood sugar level) and other disturbances of body chemicals
- Rickets
- Increased bleeding tendency
- Brain haemorrhage
- Necrotizing enterocolitis (severe intestinal inflammation that may lead to death of intestinal tissue)

care, survive. The majority of premature babies catch up with full-term babies, in terms of their development, before the end of their first year.

premedication

The term applied to drugs that are given, usually by injection, one to two hours before an operation in order to prepare a person for surgery. The pre-

medication injection usually contains an opioid *analgesic drug* (painkiller), and often an *anticholinergic drug* (which reduces the secretions in the airways and protects the heart).

premenstrual syndrome

The combination of physical and emotional symptoms that occurs in many women in the week or so running up to

P

menstruation. Premenstrual syndrome (commonly known as PMS) begins at or after *ovulation* (the mid-point of the menstrual cycle, when an egg is released from an ovary) and continues up until the onset of menstruation. In some women, the condition may be so severe that work and social relationships are seriously disrupted.

CAUSES
Theories for the cause of PMS include hormonal changes and vitamin or mineral deficiencies, but none of these has been confirmed.

SYMPTOMS
The most common emotional symptoms are fatigue, irritability, tension, aggression, tearfulness, and depression. Physical symptoms include breast tenderness, fluid retention, headache, backache, and lower abdominal pain.

TREATMENT
No single treatment has proved completely successful. Remedies for specific symptoms include dietary changes, relaxation techniques, and regular physical exercise. Pyridoxine (vitamin B_6) may help to relieve some symptoms in some women. *Oral contraceptives* can relieve symptoms by suppressing the normal menstrual cycle. Progesterone supplements may sometimes be used but are not always effective.

premenstrual tension
See *premenstrual syndrome*.

premolar
One of eight permanent grinding teeth. On each side of the mouth, there are two premolars in the upper jaw, and two in the lower. The premolars are located between the canine and the molar teeth. (See also *permanent teeth*; *eruption of teeth*.)

Prempak-C
A brand-name drug that is used in *hormone replacement therapy (HRT)* to relieve symptoms of the *menopause* and, in some cases, to prevent *osteoporosis* (thinning of the bones). Prempak-C contains conjugated oestrogens (see *oestrogen drugs*) and the *progestogen drug* norgestrel.

prenatal
A term referring to the period of pregnancy; a synonym for antenatal.

prepuce
See *foreskin*.

presbyacusis
The progressive loss of hearing that occurs with age. Presbyacusis is a form of sensorineural *deafness* (degeneration of the hair cells and nerve fibres in the inner ear), which makes sounds less clear and tones less audible.

SYMPTOMS AND CAUSES
Symptoms develop gradually. People with presbyacusis often find it difficult to understand speech and cannot hear well when there is background noise. The severity and progression of the disorder vary considerably from person to person.

Presbyacusis may be exacerbated by exposure to high *noise* levels, diminished blood supply to the inner ear due to *atherosclerosis* (the buildup of fatty deposits on artery walls), and damage to the inner ear from drugs such as *aminoglycoside drugs*.

DIAGNOSIS AND TREATMENT
Diagnosis is by physical examination using an otoscope, and by various *hearing tests* to determine the type and degree of hearing loss. *Hearing-aids* help most affected people.

presbyopia
The progressive loss of the power of adjusting the eye (see *accommodation*) for near vision. The focusing power of the eyes weakens with age. Presbyopia is usually noticed around the age of 45 when the eyes cannot accommodate to read small print at a normal distance. Reading *glasses* with convex lenses are used to correct presbyopia.

prescribed diseases
A group of industrial diseases that give sufferers legal entitlement to financial benefit. To be eligible, a claimant has to have worked in an occupation that is recognized to increase the risk of developing a particular disease. Examples include asbestosis (see *asbestos-related diseases*), work-related chronic bronchitis (see *bronchitis, chronic*), work-related *asthma*, work-related *deafness*, and vibration white finger (see *Raynaud's phenomenon*). (See also occu*pational disease and injury*.)

prescription
An instruction written by a doctor, dentist, or specially trained nurse that directs a pharmacist to dispense a particular drug in a specific dose. A prescription details how often the drug must be taken, how much is to be dispensed, and other relevant facts.

prescription-only medicine (PoM)
Drugs and medicines that are not available over the counter and can only be obtained by *prescription*. PoMs are those whose safe use is hard to ensure without medical supervision. Some drugs are available over the counter in low-dose preparations but require a prescription for high-dose preparations.

presenile dementia
A general term for *dementia* (a deterioration in brain function) that occurs in a person under the age of 65.

presentation
A term describing the position of the fetus before *childbirth*. The presentation is classified by the part of the fetus that is closest to the cervix and will emerge first. The cephalic (head) presentation is normal. Forms such as the breech presentation (in which the buttocks lie over the cervix) and the shoulder presentation may cause problems during delivery (see also *breech delivery*). The term presentation is also used to describe how an illness or condition manifests itself.

preservative
A substance that inhibits the growth of bacteria, yeasts, and moulds and therefore protects foods from putrefying and fermenting. Examples include sulphur dioxide, benzoic acid, salt, sugar, and nitrites. (See also *food additives*.)

pressure points
Places on the body where pressure can be applied by hand to limit severe arterial bleeding (in which bright red blood is pumped out in regular spurts with the heartbeat). At these points, arteries lie near the surface of the body and can easily be compressed against a bone to stop the blood flow.

Major pressure points of the body include the brachial pressure point in the middle part of the upper arm and the carotid pressure point at the side of the neck, below the jaw.

pressure sore
See *bedsore*.

prevalence
The total number of cases of a disease in existence at any one time in a defined population. Prevalence is often expressed as the number of cases per 100,000 people. (See also *incidence*.)

P

preventive dentistry

An aspect of dentistry concerned with the prevention of tooth decay and gum disease. It consists of the encouragement of good *oral hygiene*, *fluoride* treatment, and *scaling*.

preventive medicine

The branch of medicine that deals with disease prevention. It involves public health measures, such as the provision of pure water supplies and sanitation; health education and promotion; specific preventive measures, such as *immunization* against infectious diseases; and *screening* programmes to detect diseases before they cause symptoms.

In affluent countries, the main objective of preventive medicine is to educate the adult population to adopt a healthier lifestyle. In the UK, many of the deaths that occur in adults before the age of 65 are preventable, being due to accidents and/or linked to such factors as *smoking*, an unhealthy diet, excessive *alcohol* consumption, and insufficient exercise. Adoption of a healthier lifestyle, the wider use of screening for various cancers, and measures to reduce accidents could all lead to substantial improvements in health.

priapism

Persistent, painful *erection* of the *penis* that occurs without sexual arousal. This is a dangerous condition that requires emergency treatment.

Priapism occurs when the penis has become erect but blood cannot drain from the spongy tissue, and as a result the erection cannot subside. Possible causes of the condition include a blockage in the penile blood vessels due to a blood disorder such as *sickle cell anaemia*; damage to nerves supplying the penis; or, rarely, the effects of treatment for *erectile dysfunction*.

Urgent treatment is needed to avoid permanent damage to the tissues of the penis. Blood may be withdrawn from the penis with a needle.

prickly heat

An irritating skin rash that is associated with profuse sweating. The medical name is miliaria rubra. Multiple tiny, red, itchy spots cover the affected areas of skin and are accompanied by prickling sensations. The irritation tends to affect areas where sweat collects, such as the armpits. The cause is not fully known, but unevaporated sweat is an important contributory factor; the ducts from sweat glands become blocked with debris and leak sweat into the skin. Frequent cool showers and sponging of the affected areas relieve the itching.

primaquine

A drug used to treat vivax and ovale *malaria*. It is given after treatment with *chloroquine*. Side effects include nausea, vomiting, and abdominal pain. In people with *G6PD deficiency*, primaquine may cause haemolytic anaemia (see *anaemia, haemolytic*).

primary

A term used to describe a disease that has originated within the affected organ or tissue and is not derived from any other cause or source; an example is primary *cancer*. The term "primary" is also applied to the first of several diseases that may affect a tissue or organ. The preventive measures taken before an illness has manifested itself are known as primary prevention; secondary prevention is used to prevent recurrence.

primary biliary cirrhosis

See *biliary cirrhosis*.

primary care

Health care that is provided by a general practitioner (GP) or other healthcare professional who is the first point of contact for a patient.

primary central nervous system lymphoma (PCNSL)

A form of non-Hodgkin's lymphoma (see *lymphoma, non-Hodgkin's*) affecting the brain or spinal cord. The cancer occurs most commonly in *immunocompromised* people, such as people with *AIDS* and those who are taking *immunosuppressant drugs*.

primary teeth

The first teeth to erupt (also known as milk teeth), which usually start to appear around the age of six months. The primary teeth are replaced by the *permanent teeth* from about the age of six years. There are 20 primary teeth in total, ten of which are in the upper jaw and ten in the lower jaw. (See also *teeth*; *eruption of teeth*; *teething*.)

primidone

An *anticonvulsant drug* that is used to treat *epilepsy* and, occasionally, *tremor*. It is usually prescribed together with another anticonvulsant. Possible adverse effects of primidone may include drowsiness, clumsiness, and dizziness.

primitive reflex

See *reflex, primitive*.

Prinzmetal's angina

See *variant angina*.

prion

A tiny, protein-based infectious particle. Prions transmit diseases that cause degeneration of the central nervous system, including *Creutzfeldt–Jakob disease* in humans and *bovine spongiform encephalopathy (BSE)* in cattle. Prions do not contain *nucleic acids* (unlike viruses) and are difficult to destroy because they are highly resistant to heat and disinfectants. There is currently no effective treatment for prion diseases. (See also *spongiform encephalopathy*.)

PRK

The abbreviation for *photorefractive keratectomy* (laser reshaping of the cornea).

probenecid

A drug used to prevent kidney damage in AIDS patients who are taking the drug cidofovir for the treatment of cytomegalovirus retinitis. Probenecid may cause nausea and vomiting. Other possible side effects of probenecid include flushing and dizziness.

probiotic bacteria

Species of microorganisms that inhabit the digestive tract, guarding it against harmful microorganisms such as *bacteria*, *yeasts*, and *viruses*. Some drinks are manufactured using probiotic bacteria; they are thought to protect the health of the *digestive system*.

procainamide

An *antiarrhythmic drug* that is used to treat certain types of *tachycardia* (abnormally rapid heartbeat). Procainamide include nausea, vomiting, loss of appetite, and, rarely, confusion. Prolonged treatment with this drug may induce *lupus erythematosus*.

procaine

A local anaesthetic (see *anaesthesia, local*).

procarbazine

An *anticancer drug* used most often in *Hodgkin's disease*. Side effects are typical of anticancer drugs.

prochlorperazine

A *phenothiazine*-type *antipsychotic drug* used to relieve symptoms of certain psychiatric disorders, such as *schizophrenia* and *mania*. Prochlorperazine is also used in small doses as an *antiemetic drug*. It may in some cases cause involuntary movements of the face and limbs, lethargy, dry mouth, blurred vision, and dizziness.

procidentia

Severe *prolapse*, usually of the uterus.

proctalgia fugax

A severe cramping pain in the *rectum* unconnected with any disease. It may be due to muscle spasm. The pain is usually of short duration and subsides without any treatment.

proctitis

Inflammation of the *rectum*, causing soreness and bleeding, sometimes with a mucus and pus discharge. Proctitis commonly occurs as a feature of certain diseases including *ulcerative colitis*, *Crohn's disease*, or *dysentery*. In cases where inflammation is confined to the rectum, the cause is often unknown. Proctitis is sometimes due to *gonorrhoea* or another sexually transmitted infection, especially in male homosexuals. Rare causes of proctitis include *tuberculosis*, *amoebiasis*, and *schistosomiasis*.

Diagnosis is made by *proctoscopy*. A *biopsy* (collection of a tissue sample) is sometimes done at the same time. Treatment depends on the underlying cause. When the cause is unknown, treatment is directed towards relieving symptoms.

proctoscopy

Examination of the *anus* and *rectum* using a proctoscope (a rigid viewing instrument).

procyclidine

An *anticholinergic drug* that is used to treat *Parkinson's disease*. It is also used to minimize the side effects of some *antipsychotic drugs*. The possible adverse effects of procyclidine include a dry mouth and blurred vision.

prodrome

An early warning symptom of illness. One example of a prodrome is an aura, which is a particular set of physical and mental symptoms that may occur immediately before an attack of *migraine* or *epilepsy*.

progeria

Premature aging. There are two forms of progeria, and both are very rare.

In Hutchinson-Gilford syndrome, premature aging starts at about four years old, and many features of old age, including grey hair, balding, sagging skin, and *atherosclerosis* (buildup of fatty deposits on artery walls), have developed by the age of ten to twelve. Death usually occurs at puberty. Werner's syndrome (adult progeria) starts in adolescence or early adulthood and follows the same course.

The cause of Hutchinson-Gilford syndrome is a gene mutation. The cause of Werner's syndrome is unknown.

progesterone hormone

A female sex hormone essential for the functioning of the female reproductive system. Progesterone is made in the *ovaries* during the second half of the menstrual cycle (see *menstruation*), and by the *placenta* during *pregnancy*. Small amounts are also produced by the *adrenal glands* and, in men, by the *testes*.

During the menstrual cycle, increasing progesterone levels after *ovulation* (the release of an egg from an ovary) cause the endometrium (uterine lining) to thicken in preparation for receiving a fertilized egg. If fertilization does not occur, the production of progesterone and *oestrogen hormones* falls to a level that results in a *menstrual period*, during which the uterine lining is expelled from the body.

If pregnancy occurs, progesterone is produced by the *placenta*. The progesterone causes a number of changes in the mother's body, one of which is enlargement of the breasts. In late pregnancy, the mother's progesterone level fall, and this fall helps to initiate labour (see *childbirth*).

Other effects of progesterone in women include increased fat deposition and increased *sebum* production by glands in the skin.

progestogen drugs

COMMON DRUGS

- Desogestrel • Dydrogesterone
- Levonorgestrel • Medroxyprogesterone
- Norethisterone • Norgestimate • Norgestrel
- Progesterone

A group of drugs that are similar to *progesterone hormone*. They include both natural progesterone and synthetic progesterone derivatives.

Progestogen drugs are used in *oral contraceptives*. They may be used on their own in, for example, the progestogen-only pill (POP), as *contraceptive implants*, or as contraceptive injections (see *contraceptives, injectable*); progestogen drugs may also be used in combination with *oestrogen drugs* in the combined pill (COC). Progestogens work by making the cervical mucus too thick for sperm to penetrate and the lining of the uterus thinner so that implantation of a fertilized ovum is less likely. They also reduce the movement of an egg along the fallopian tube, which may lead to an increased risk of an *ectopic pregnancy*. One progestogen preparation of *desorgstrel* (Cerazette) also inhibits ovulation.

Another use for progestogens is in *hormone replacement therapy (HRT)*. A progestogen drug is used in combination with an oestrogen drug to reduce the risk of uterine cancer (see *uterus, cancer of*), which may occur if oestrogens alone are taken over a long period of time. The progestogens induce a monthly shedding of the uterine lining, if taken cyclically (for the last 10–13 days of the cycle).

Progestogen drugs are also prescribed as a treatment for various menstrual problems (see *menstruation, disorders of*). In addition, they are used to treat *endometriosis* (in which fragments of uterine lining are found elsewhere in the pelvic cavity), and are sometimes used as *anticancer drugs*.

Adverse effects of taking progestogen drugs are weight gain, *oedema* (accumulation of fluid in body tissues), headache, dizziness, rash, irregular periods, breast tenderness, and *hirsutism*. (See also *contraception, hormonal methods of*.)

progestogen-only pill (POP)

Also known as the *minipill*, the POP is an *oral contraceptive* that contains only a *progestogen drug*.

prognathism

Abnormal protrusion of the lower jaw or both jaws.

prognosis

An assessment of the probable course and outcome of a disease.

progressive

A term that is used to describe a condition that becomes more severe and/or extensive over time.

P

progressive muscular atrophy

A type of *motor neuron disease* in which the muscles of the hands, arms, and legs become weak and wasted and twitch involuntarily. As the muscular atrophy advances, it eventually spreads to other muscles.

proguanil

An antimalarial drug that is used in the prevention of *malaria*. Side effects of the drug are rare. Indigestion, nausea, or vomiting may occur but usually disappear as treatment continues.

prolactin

A *hormone* produced by the *pituitary gland*. Prolactin helps to stimulate the development of the mammary glands (see *breast*), and to initiate and maintain milk production for *breast-feeding*. (See also *prolactinoma*.)

prolactinoma

A noncancerous tumour of the *pituitary gland* that causes overproduction of the hormone *prolactin*. In women, this may result in *galactorrhoea* (breast secretion at any time other than during breast-feeding), *amenorrhoea* (absence of menstrual periods), or *infertility*. In men, it may lead to *erectile dysfunction* and *gynaecomastia* (development of breasts). In either sex, it may cause headaches, *diabetes insipidus*, and, if the tumour presses on the optic nerves, loss of the outer *visual field*.

Diagnosis of the condition is made from *blood tests* and *CT scanning* or *MRI* of the brain. Treatment of prolactinoma may involve removal of the tumour, *radiotherapy*, or the drug *bromocriptine*.

prolapse

The displacement of part or all of an organ or tissue from its normal position in the body (see *disc prolapse*; *mitral valve prolapse*; *rectal prolapse*; *uterovaginal prolapse*; *uterus, prolapse of*).

promazine

A *phenothiazine*-type drug that is used to treat agitation and restlessness. Possible adverse effects include abnormal movements of the face and limbs, drowsiness, lethargy, constipation, dry mouth, and blurred vision. Long-term treatment may cause *parkinsonism*.

promethazine

An *antihistamine drug* used to relieve itching in a variety of skin conditions, such as *eczema*. It is also used as an *antiemetic drug*, and sometimes as a *premedication*. Possible adverse effects of promethazine include a dry mouth, blurred vision, and drowsiness.

pronation

The act of turning the body to a prone (face-down) position, or the hand to a palm-backwards position.

propantheline

An *antispasmodic drug* used to treat *irritable bowel syndrome* and forms of *urinary incontinence*. Possible adverse effects of propantheline include a dry mouth, blurred vision, and retention of urine.

Propecia

A brand name for *finasteride*, an anti-androgen drug (one that blocks the effects of male sex hormones). This preparation is used to treat male-pattern baldness (see *alopecia*).

prophylactic

A drug, procedure, or piece of equipment that is used to prevent disease. The term is also used to describe a *condom*.

prophylactic antibiotics

Antibiotic drugs that are used to prevent the development of bacterial infections. They are used, for example, in people who are undergoing surgery or in those with recent, serious injuries. They are given, for example, to prevent *endocarditis* in patients who have replacement *heart valves* or heart-valve lesions who are undergoing dental procedures. They may also be given to people who are in close contact with a source of meningococcal *meningitis* to prevent contraction of the disease, as well as to prevent infection following a bite (see *bites, animal*; *bites, human*).

propranolol

A *beta-blocker drug* used to treat *hypertension* (high blood pressure), *angina pectoris* (chest pain due to inadequate blood supply to the heart), and cardiac *arrhythmias* (irregular heartbeats). It may also be used to reduce the risk of further heart damage after *myocardial infarction* (heart attack). In addition, it relieves symptoms of *hyperthyroidism* (overactivity of the thyroid gland) and *anxiety*, and can prevent *migraine* attacks.

Possible adverse effects of propranolol are typical of most beta-blocker drugs; they include fatigue, nausea, and cold hands and feet. As with other beta-blockers, propranolol is not usually prescribed for people with a history of *asthma* or *bronchospasm*.

proprietary

A term for a drug patented for production by one company.

proprioception

The body's internal system for collecting information about its position and the state of contraction of its muscles.

Information originating from proprioceptors (sensory nerve endings in the muscles, tendons, joints, and inner ear) passes to the brain and spinal cord. The information is used to make adjustments to maintain posture and balance. During movement, there is a constant feedback of information from the proprioceptors and the eyes to the brain. This helps the brain to ensure that actions are smooth and coordinated.

proptosis

A term meaning protrusion, especially of the eyeballs (see *exophthalmus*).

propylthiouracil

A drug used to treat *hyperthyroidism* (overactivity of the thyroid gland) or to control its symptoms before a *thyroidectomy* (surgical removal of thyroid tissue). Possible side effects are itching, headache, rash, joint pain, and decreased production of *white blood cells*.

prostaglandin

One of a group of *fatty acids* that is made naturally in the body and acts in a similar way to *hormones*. Prostaglandins were first discovered in semen but are now known to occur in many different body tissues, including the uterus, brain, and kidneys. Prostaglandins are divided into broad groups according to their chemical structure.

Prostaglandins produce a wide range of effects on the body. These actions include causing pain and inflammation in damaged tissue; protecting the lining of the stomach and duodenum against ulceration; lowering blood pressure; and stimulating contractions in labour. (These effects may also be achieved by the use of *prostaglandin drugs*.) For further information describing the effects of various prostaglandins, see the box opposite.

Certain drugs counteract the effects of prostaglandin in the body. Examples of these drugs are *aspirin*, *nonsteroidal*

P

anti-inflammatory drugs (NSAIDs), and *corticosteroids*, which relieve pain and inflammation by reducing prostaglandin production in the tissues. If taken for a long period, however, NSAIDs and aspirin may increase the risk of a peptic ulcer, in part by reducing the production of the prostaglandins that protect the stomach lining.

prostaglandin drugs

Synthetically produced *prostaglandins*. Dinoprostone is used with synthetic *oxytocin* for *induction of labour*. *Mifepristone* may be taken orally to induce an *abortion*; this is followed by insertion of a gemeprost suppository, which softens and helps to dilate the cervix. Alprostadil is used to treat newborn infants who are awaiting surgery for certain congenital heart diseases. It is also used in the treatment of some cases of *erectile dysfunction*.

EFFECTS OF SOME PROSTAGLANDINS

Type	Effect
PGA1	• Lowers blood pressure.
	• May protect against peptic ulcer.
PGD2	• Causes inflammation.
	• Involved in asthma.
PGE1	• Stimulates contractions of the uterus.
	• Lowers blood pressure.
	• Reduces stickiness of platelets in blood.
PGE2	• Causes inflammation.
	• Widens airways.
	• Increases stickiness of platelets in blood.
	• Stimulates contractions of the uterus.
	• Protects against peptic ulcer.
PGF2 alpha	• Stimulates contractions of the uterus.
	• Narrows airways.
PGG2	• Causes inflammation.
PGI2	• Reduces stickiness of platelets in blood.

prostate, cancer of

A cancerous growth in the *prostate gland*. It is one of the most common types of cancer in men and most frequently affects elderly men. The cause of the cancer is unknown, but the male sex hormone *testosterone* has been found to influence the growth rate and spread of the tumour. Men with a family history of prostate cancer are at increased risk of developing the disease.

SYMPTOMS

An enlarged prostate (see *prostate, enlarged*) may cause symptoms that include difficulty in starting to pass urine, poor urine flow, blood in the urine, and increased frequency of urination. If a tumour blocks the *urethra* (the passage from the bladder to outside the body) or the cancer spreads to the *ureters* (the tubes linking each kidney to the bladder), urine flow may eventually cease altogether (see *urinary retention*).

In some cases, there are no urinary symptoms and the first signs may only appear once secondary cancers have arisen. Such signs may include pain in the bones, enlarged *lymph nodes*, shortness of breath (due to spread of the cancer to the lungs), and weight loss.

SCREENING AND DIAGNOSIS

Men with symptoms of an enlarged prostate and those at risk of prostate cancer are screened for the disorder. This procedure involves tests to detect blood levels of a protein called *prostate-specific antigen (PSA)*, as well as a *rectal examination*. Raised blood levels of PSA may be an early sign of prostate cancer (although a raised PSA level is not a definitive sign of cancer); a rectal examination allows a doctor to assess the size and hardness of the gland.

Transrectal *ultrasound* (a procedure in which an ultrasound probe is inserted into the rectum) and a *biopsy* (removal of a tissue sample for analysis) are used to confirm a diagnosis. *Blood tests*, *CT scanning*, *MRI* scanning, and *bone imaging* may also be carried out.

TREATMENT

Medical opinions vary regarding the appropriate treatment for localized prostate cancer. If the man is elderly and has a small prostate cancer that has not spread, no treatment may be recommended although the man's condition will be monitored. For younger men, *prostatectomy* (removal of the prostate gland), *brachytherapy* (internal radiotherapy), or external *radiotherapy* may be performed.

In many cases, widespread disease is controllable for some years with the use of *anticancer drugs* or with *orchidectomy* (removal of part or all of the testes).

prostatectomy

The surgical removal of part or all of the *prostate gland*. Prostatectomy is performed to treat enlargement of the prostate (see *prostate, enlarged*), in cases where the enlarged prostate is obstructing the flow of urine, and cancer (see *prostate, cancer of*).

The most common method is transurethral prostatectomy (TURP), in which the prostate is accessed via the urethra (the channel in the penis through which urine is excreted), thereby avoiding open surgery. If the prostate gland is very enlarged, retropubic prostatectomy may be performed: an incision is made to expose the prostate and the tissue is removed. These techniques are shown in the illustrated box overleaf.

In some cases, a newer method called laser prostatectomy may be used. In this procedure, a *cystoscope* (a type of endoscope) is inserted into the urethra. A laser is passed along the cystoscope to the prostate and used to destroy prostate tissue. Because laser prostatectomy destroys prostate tissue, a sample cannot be taken to check for cancer, therefore this method is only suitable when prostate cancer has been ruled out.

Prostatectomy may result in sexual or urinary complications. Prostate surgery often causes retrograde *ejaculation*, in which semen is expelled backwards into the bladder rather than out of the penis; this condition is harmless but reduces fertility. Surgery may also cause *erectile dysfunction* and urinary incontinence. In addition, a small proportion of men require a repeat prostatectomy in the future.

prostate, enlarged

Increased size of the inner zone of the *prostate gland*, caused by benign prostatic hypertrophy (see *prostatic hypertrophy, benign*), *prostate cancer*, or *prostatitis* (inflammation of the prostate gland). Enlargement of the prostate can cause obstruction to the flow of urine from the bladder to the urethra, leading to *prostatism* and *urinary retention* (the inability to pass urine). The size of the gland can be assessed by a *rectal examination* and transrectal *ultrasound* (in which an ultrasound probe is inserted into the rectum).

P

PROSTATECTOMY: REMOVAL OF THE PROSTATE GLAND

Two of the possible methods of removal are shown. The transurethral method (TURP) is the most commonly used. It avoids the disadvantages of an abdominal incision and usually permits a shorter stay in hospital. The retropubic method may be necessary if the prostate is very enlarged or if surgery is a treatment for prostate cancer.

TRANSURETHRAL PROSTATECTOMY

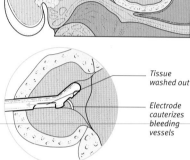

1 Under general or spinal anaesthesia, a special type of cystoscope (bladder viewing tube) called a resectoscope is passed up the urethra so that the prostate can be seen.

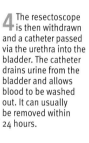

2 A heated wire loop, or sometimes a cutting edge, is inserted through the resectoscope and used to cut away as much of the prostatic tissue as possible.

3 The pieces of tissue are washed out through the resectoscope and any bleeding vessels are cauterized by means of an electrode passed up the tube.

4 The resectoscope is then withdrawn and a catheter passed via the urethra into the bladder. The catheter drains urine from the bladder and allows blood to be washed out. It can usually be removed within 24 hours.

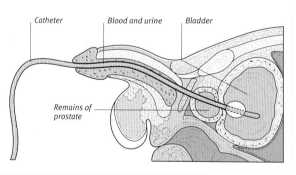

RETROPUBIC PROSTATECTOMY

Site of incision

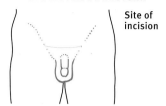

1 Under general anaesthesia, an incision is made in the abdomen to expose the bladder and prostate. The surgeon cuts open the capsule containing the gland.

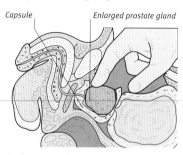

2 The surgeon then removes the prostatic tissue. Once it is removed, bleeding vessels are cauterized and a catheter is then passed up the urethra in order to drain urine from the bladder.

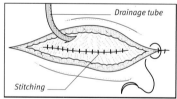

3 A tube is inserted beside the empty capsule to drain any fluid and blood that may collect; the abdomen is sewn up. The tube and catheter are left in for a few days.

prostate gland

A solid, chestnut-shaped organ that surrounds the first part of the male *urethra*. The prostate gland is situated just underneath the *bladder*. It produces secretions that form part of the seminal fluid during *ejaculation*.

The prostate gland consists of two distinct zones: an inner zone, which produces secretions that keep the lining of the urethra moist, and an outer zone, which produces seminal secretions. Two ejaculatory ducts pass from the seminal vesicles through the prostate gland to enter the urethra; the ducts carry fluid and nutrients from the vesicles to be added to the semen. The prostate gland weighs only a few grams at birth. At puberty, *androgen hormones* cause the gland to enlarge, and it reaches adult size at around age 20. In most men, the prostate begins to enlarge further after the age of 50.

There are a number of disorders that affect the prostate gland. These include benign prostatic hypertrophy (see *prostatic hypertrophy, benign*), cancer (see *prostate, cancer of*), and *prostatitis* (inflammation of the prostate gland).

prostate-specific antigen (PSA)

An *enzyme* that is normally produced by the prostate gland. If the enzyme is produced in excess, it may indicate the presence of *prostate cancer*. Tests to measure blood levels of PSA therefore help detect early prostate cancer and may be used to monitor cancer treatment. However, the PSA blood test is

LOCATION OF PROSTATE GLAND

Located under the bladder and in front of the rectum, the prostate gland secretes substances into the semen as the fluid passes through ducts leading from the seminal vesicles into the urethra.

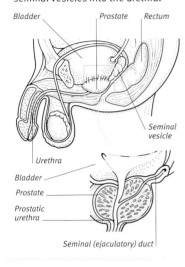

not a definitive test for prostate cancer because, in a few cases, PSA levels may be normal even when prostate cancer is present and, conversely, PSA levels may be raised in other, noncancerous prostate conditions, such as benign prostatic hypertrophy (see *prostatic hypertrophy, benign*) and *prostatitis* (inflammation of the prostate gland).

prostatic hypertrophy, benign

An increase in size of the *prostate gland*, which is most common in men over the age of 50. The cause is unknown.

SYMPTOMS

The enlarging prostate compresses and distorts the *urethra* (the passage from the bladder to outside the body), impeding the flow of urine from the bladder (known as outflow obstruction). This causes symptoms of *prostatism*, such as frequent urination and dribbling at the end of the urine stream. There may also be incontinence (see *incontinence, urinary*). Eventually the bladder is unable to expel all the urine (see *urinary retention*) and becomes distended, causing swelling, which may be painful. The bladder's inability to empty completely each time urine is passed may lead to *urinary tract infections*. *Kidney failure* may occur as a complication of outflow obstruction.

DIAGNOSIS AND TREATMENT

Prostate enlargement is detected by a *rectal examination*. Tests may include *blood tests*, *ultrasound scanning*, and recording the strength of urine flow. Tests to exclude *prostate cancer* as a cause of enlargement may be needed.

Mild cases do not require treatment, but severe abdominal pain due to blockage of the urine flow needs immediate treatment. Men with a severely enlarged prostate usually require *prostatectomy* (surgical removal of part or all of the prostate gland). Alternatively, *alpha-blocker drugs* may be given to improve the flow of urine or antiandrogen drugs, such as *finasteride*, may be used to counteract the effects of testosterone.

prostatism

Symptoms that arise from the enlargement of the prostate gland (see *prostate, enlarged*) due to its compression and distortion of the *urethra*, which impedes the flow of urine from the bladder (outflow obstruction). Symptoms of prostatism often include frequent urination (see *urination, frequent*), getting up at night to urinate, delay before the urine stream starts, dribbling at the end of the stream, and incontinence (see *incontinence, urinary*).

prostatitis

Inflammation of the *prostate gland*, usually affecting men aged between 30 and 50. It is often caused by a bacterial infection that has spread from the *urethra*. The presence of a urinary *catheter* increases the risk of prostatitis.

The main symptoms of prostatitis are fever, flulike symptoms, and pain in the lower back. There may also be pain around the rectum, which is particularly troublesome on passing faeces. Diagnosis is made by *rectal examination* and tests on urine samples. Treatment is with *antibiotic drugs*. The condition may be slow to clear up and tends to recur.

prosthesis

An artificial replacement for a missing or diseased part of the body; for example, artificial limbs (see *limb, artificial*), heart valves (see *heart-valve surgery*), or glass eyes (see *eye, artificial*).

prosthetics, dental

The branch of *dentistry* that is concerned with the replacement of missing teeth and their supporting structures. dental prosthetics includes *dentures*, overdentures (semipermanent fittings over existing teeth), crowns (see *crown, dental*), and bridges (see *bridge, dental*).

protease inhibitors

A type of *antiretroviral drug* that is used to delay the progression of *HIV* infection. (See also *AIDS*.)

proteins

Large molecules consisting of hundreds or thousands of *amino acids* linked into long chains. Proteins may be combined with sugars (glycoproteins) and *lipids* (lipoproteins).

There are two main types of proteins. The first type, fibrous proteins, are insoluble and form the structural basis of many body tissues. The second type, lobular proteins, are soluble and include all *enzymes*, many *hormones*, and some blood proteins, such as *haemoglobin*. In addition, the *chromosomes* in cell nuclei are formed from proteins linked with *nucleic acids*, and cell walls are formed in part from proteins linked with lipids (see *cell*).

Dietary proteins are needed mainly to supply the body with amino acids. Ingested proteins are broken down in the digestive system into amino acids, which are absorbed and rebuilt into new body proteins (see *protein synthesis*).

protein synthesis

The formation of protein molecules through the joining of *amino acids*. Proteins provide many of the structural components and the enzymes that promote biochemical reactions in the body, so their manufacture is essential for development and growth.

Different cells manufacture various ranges of proteins. The instructions for these processes are held by the *DNA* (deoxyribonucleic acid) in the nucleus of the cell. Protein synthesis starts when a *gene* (a particular length of DNA) acts as a template to form a strand of a substance called messenger *RNA*. Like DNA, RNA consists of a string of building blocks, which are called nucleotide bases; the sequence of bases provides the genetic code for making whichever protein is required.

The strand of messenger RNA passes out of the cell nucleus, where it is then decoded (see the illustrated box overleaf) to form a polypeptide chain (a string of amino acids). Several polypeptide chains may be combined to form one protein molecule.

P

STEPS IN **PROTEIN SYNTHESIS**

Proteins consist of one or more subunits, which are called polypeptides. These are formed, within cells, from building blocks called amino acids, which are provided to each cell as raw materials. The instructions for making polypeptides are encoded in the DNA that is present within the cell nucleus.

1 To make a specific protein or polypeptide, DNA separates into two strands and acts as a template to make a strand of a substance called messenger RNA. Like DNA, this consists of a string of substances called nucleotide bases.

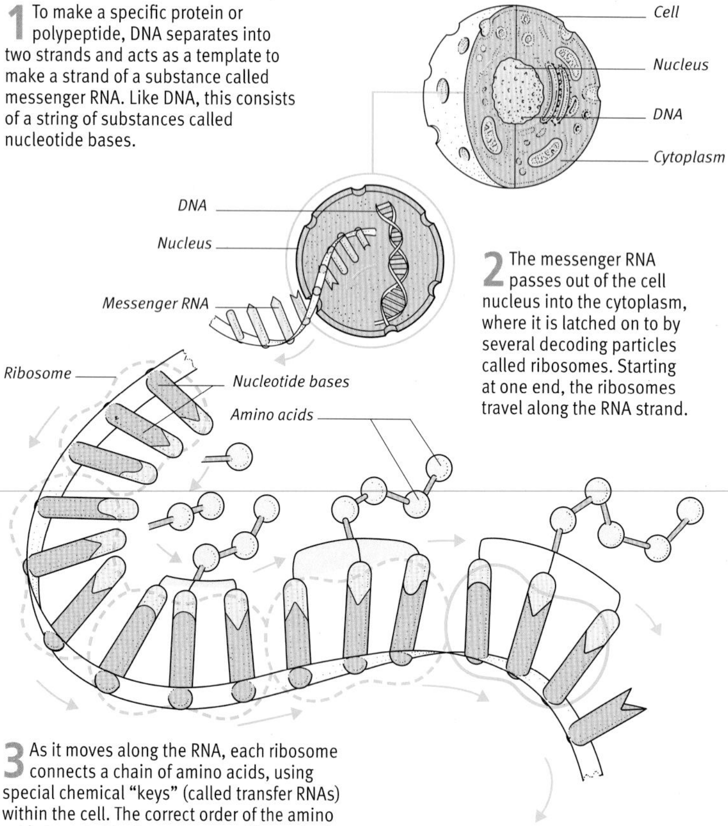

Cell

Nucleus

DNA

Cytoplasm

DNA

Nucleus

Messenger RNA

2 The messenger RNA passes out of the cell nucleus into the cytoplasm, where it is latched on to by several decoding particles called ribosomes. Starting at one end, the ribosomes travel along the RNA strand.

Ribosome

Nucleotide bases

Amino acids

3 As it moves along the RNA, each ribosome connects a chain of amino acids, using special chemical "keys" (called transfer RNAs) within the cell. The correct order of the amino acids is coded by the sequence of bases in the messenger RNA.

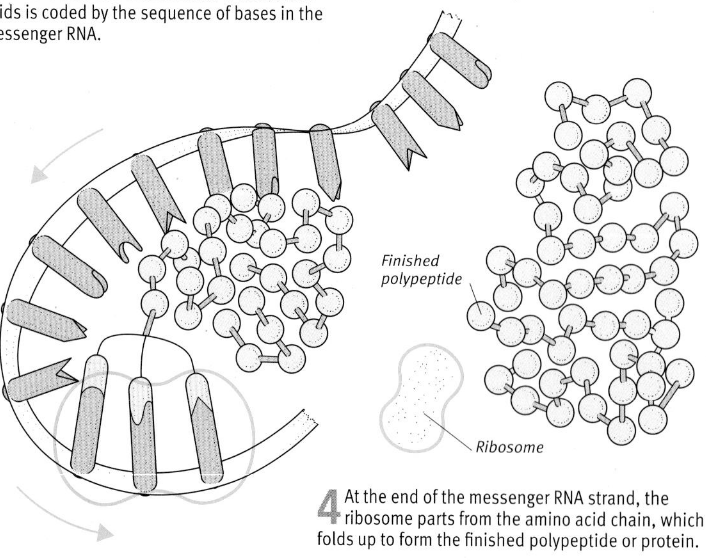

Finished polypeptide

Ribosome

4 At the end of the messenger RNA strand, the ribosome parts from the amino acid chain, which folds up to form the finished polypeptide or protein.

P

The rate of protein synthesis is regulated by adjustments in the amount of messenger RNA formed in the nucleus of the cell. Highly complex mechanisms operate in order to ensure that the cell manufactures the correct type of proteins, in the required quantities, and at exactly the right time.

proteinuria

The presence of *protein* in the *urine*. It may result from kidney disorders, such as *glomerulonephritis* and *urinary tract infection*. Proteinuria may also occur because of a generalized disorder that causes increased protein in the blood. It is diagnosed by *urinalysis*.

prothrombin time

A form of *blood-clotting test*. The conversion of prothrombin to thrombin is one of the chemical reactions that takes place during the process of *blood clotting*. This reaction depends on the presence of clotting factors together with calcium and a substance called thromboplastin. If calcium and thromboplastin are added to a sample of blood, it should clot within a certain time. A clotting time that is abnormally slow indicates a deficiency of clotting factors, as occurs in some liver diseases and in vitamin K deficiency. Tests to measure prothrombin time are used to monitor people undergoing treatment with *warfarin* (an *anticoagulant drug*). (See also *International Normalized Ratio*.)

proton pump inhibitors

A type of *ulcer-healing drug* used in the treatment of *peptic ulcers*.

protoplasm

A term for the entire contents of a *cell*.

protozoa

The simplest, most primitive type of animal, consisting of a single cell. Protozoa are bigger than *bacteria* but still microscopic. About 30 types are human parasites, including those responsible for *malaria*, *amoebiasis*, *giardiasis*, *sleeping sickness*, *trichomoniasis*, *toxoplasmosis*, and *leishmaniasis*.

proximal

A term describing a part of the body nearer to a central point of reference, such as the trunk. (See also *distal*.)

Prozac

A brand name for the antidepressant drug *fluoxetine*.

PSORIASIS

prurigo

Thickening and *itching* of the skin due to repeated scratching.

pruritus

The medical term for *itching*.

pruritus ani

Itching of the *anus*. Causes of pruritus ani may include an *anal fissure*, *haemorrhoids*, or *threadworm infestation*.

PSA

The abbreviation for *prostate specific antigen*.

pseud-/pseudo-

Prefixes meaning false.

pseudarthrosis

A term meaning "false joint", which is used to describe an operation in which the ends of the two opposing bones in a joint are removed and a piece of tissue is fixed in the gap as a cushion. The term also describes a rare childhood condition in which congenital abnormality of the lower half of the *tibia* leads to spontaneous *fracture*.

pseudoacanthosis nigricans

The most common form of *acanthosis nigricans*, a condition in which dark patches of thickened skin appear in the body's various skin folds.

pseudocyesis

See *pregnancy, false*.

pseudodementia

Severe *depression* in elderly people that mimics *dementia*. Symptoms of pseudodementia include impairment of the intellect and loss of memory.

pseudoephedrine

A *decongestant drug* used to relieve *nasal congestion*. High doses may cause anxiety, nausea, and dizziness. Occasionally, *hypertension* (high blood pressure), headache, and *palpitations* occur. Pseudoephedrine should not be used by people who are taking *monoamine oxidase inhibitors* (MAOIs) because the interaction may cause a dangerous rise in blood pressure.

pseudoepidemic

An outbreak of an illness in a community or in an institution that is thought to be due to a form of *hysteria*. The typical symptoms are a headache and a general feeling of sickness.

pseudogout

A form of *arthritis* that results from deposition of calcium crystals in a joint. The underlying cause is unknown; in rare cases, it is a complication of *diabetes mellitus*, *hyperparathyroidism*, and *haemochromatosis*. Symptoms are similar to *gout*. Diagnosis is from a sample of joint fluid. Treatment is with *nonsteroidal anti-inflammatory drugs*.

pseudohermaphroditism

A *congenital* abnormality in which the external genitalia resemble those of the opposite sex, but ovarian or testicular tissue is present as normal. A female with pseudohermaphroditism may have an enlarged *clitoris* that resembles a *penis* and enlarged *labia* resembling a *scrotum*. A male may have a very small penis that may resemble a clitoris and a divided scrotum resembling labia. (See also *hermaphroditism*; *sex determination*.)

Pseudomonas

Rodlike *bacteria* that are inhabit soil and decomposing matter. PSEUDOMONAS AERUGINOSA can cause disease in humans and is present in pus from wounds.

psilocybin

An *alkaloid* present in certain types of mushrooms. It is a *hallucinogenic drug* with properties similar to those of *LSD*.

psittacosis

A rare illness resembling *influenza* that is caused by the microorganism CHLAMYDIA PSITTACI. The disease is contracted by inhaling dust containing the droppings of infected birds. Most cases occur among poultry farmers, pigeon owners, and people working in pet shops. Common symptoms are severe headache, fever, and cough, developing a week or more after infection. Other symptoms may include muscle pains, sore throat, nosebleed, lethargy, and depression. In some cases, breathing difficulty may also occur.

Diagnosis is made by confirming the presence of *antibodies* against CHLAMYDIA PSITTACI in the blood. Treatment is with *tetracycline* antibiotic drugs. If no treatment is given, death may result.

psoas muscle

A muscle that bends the hip upwards towards the chest. There are two parts: psoas major and psoas minor. The psoas major acts to flex the hip. The psoas minor bends the spine down to the pelvis.

psoralen drugs

Drugs containing chemicals called psoralens, which occur in some plants and are present in some perfumes. When absorbed into the skin, psoralens react with *ultraviolet light* to cause skin darkening or inflammation. Psoralen drugs may be used in conjunction with ultraviolet light (a combination called *PUVA*) to treat *psoriasis* and *vitiligo*.

Overexposure to ultraviolet light during treatment, or to too high a dose of a psoralen drug, may cause redness and blistering of the skin. Psoralens in perfumes may cause *photosensitivity*.

psoriasis

A common skin disease characterized by thickened patches of red, inflamed skin, often covered by silvery scales. The disease usually appears between the ages of 10 and 30, tends to run in families, and affects both men and women. The exact cause of the disease is unknown, although one form (guttate psoriasis) may be caused by a *streptococcal infection*, such as *tonsillitis*.

SYMPTOMS AND TYPES
In psoriasis, new skin cells are made about ten times faster than normal. The excess cells accumulate, forming thickened patches covered with dead, flaking skin. Some people also develop painful inflammation and stiffness in the joints (commonly finger and toe joints), a

LOCATION OF **PSOAS MUSCLE**

The muscle has two parts – major and minor. The psoas major acts to flex the hip (bend it up towards the trunk) and rotates the thigh inwards. The psoas minor acts to bend the spine down towards the pelvis.

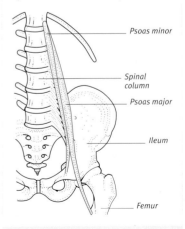

P

635

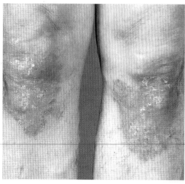

Front view   **Rear view**

Psoriasis on the knees

Distribution and appearance of psoriasis
The knees, elbows, scalp, trunk, and back are common sites for psoriasis. The usual appearance is of patches of thickened skin covered by dry, silvery, adherent scales.

P

condition known as psoriatic arthritis. Psoriasis tends to recur in attacks, which may be triggered by factors such as emotional stress, skin damage, and physical illness.

There are different forms of the disease, and the most common of which is discoid, or plaque, psoriasis, in which patches appear on the trunk, limbs, and scalp. Another type, guttate psoriasis, occurs most often in children, and consists of many small patches that develop over a wide area of skin. Pustular psoriasis is characterized by small *pustules* over part or all of the body.

TREATMENT
In most cases, psoriasis can be improved with topical treatments, such as those containing *corticosteroid drugs*, coal tar, *calcipotriol* and other *vitamin D* analogues, or dithranol. In some cases, *PUVA* (ultraviolet light plus a psoralen drug) may be used. For severe psoriasis, treatment may include *immunosuppressant drugs* such as *methotrexate* and *ciclosprin*. Psoriasis is usually a long-term condition.

psych-

A prefix meaning mental processes or activities, as in psychology.

psyche

A term meaning mind. (See also *psychoanalytic theory*.)

psychiatry

The branch of medicine concerned with the study, prevention, and treatment of mental illness and emotional and behavioural problems. Psychiatrists conduct examinations of physical and mental state and trace the patient's personal and family history. Treatment may include medication, *counselling*, *psychotherapy*, *cognitive–behavioural therapy*, *psychoanalysis*, or, rarely, *ECT*.

psychoanalysis

A treatment that is based on *psychoanalytic theory* that is used to help people who have *neuroses* and *personality disorders*. A modified approach may also be used in the treatment of *psychosis*. Psychoanalysis aims to help the patient to understand his or her emotional development and to make adjustments in particular situations. Interpretation of the patient's dreams is another aspect of the treatment (see *dream analysis*).

psychoanalytic theory

A system of ideas developed by Sigmund Freud that explains personality and behaviour in terms of unconscious wishes and conflicts. The main emphasis was on sexuality. Freud believed that a child passes through three stages in the first few years of life: oral, anal, and genital. After this, the child develops a sexual attraction to the parent of the opposite sex and wants to eliminate the other parent (*Oedipus complex*). Sexual feelings become latent around the age of five but re-emerge at puberty. Psychological problems may develop if *fixation* occurs at a primitive stage.

Modern psychoanalysis is generally based on the idea that most emotional problems are caused by childhood experiences. The aim of psychoanalysis is to free the person from the past, thereby helping him or her adjust to the present.

psychodrama

An aid to treatment with *psychotherapy* in which the patient acts out certain roles or incidents. Psychodrama is often carried out with a partner or in a group, and often uses music, dance, and mime.

psychogenic

A term used to describe a symptom or disorder that is caused by psychological or emotional problems.

psychology

The scientific study of mental processes. Psychology deals with all internal aspects of the mind, such as *memory*, feelings, *thought*, and *perception*, as well as external manifestations, such as *speech* and behaviour. In addition, psychology is concerned with *intelligence*, *learning*, and *personality* development.

psychometry

The measurement of psychological functions with the use of *intelligence tests*, *personality tests*, and tests for specific aptitudes, such as *memory*, logic, concentration, and speed of response.

psychoneurosis

A term that can be used interchangeably with *neurosis*.

psychopathology

The study of abnormal mental processes. There are two main approaches: the descriptive, which aims to record symptoms that make up a diagnosis of mental illness; and the psychoanalytic, which is concerned with a person's unconscious feelings and motives.

psychopathy

An outdated term for an *antisocial personality disorder*.

psychopharmacology

The study of drugs that affect mental states, such as *antipsychotic drugs*, *antidepressant drugs*, and *anti-anxiety drugs*.

psychosexual disorders

A range of disorders related to sexual function. Psychosexual disorders include *transsexualism*, *psychosexual dysfunction*, and sexual *deviation*.

psychosexual dysfunction

A disorder in which there is interference with the sexual response for no physical cause. (See also *sex therapy*.)

psychosis

A severe mental disorder in which the individual loses contact with reality and develops a distorted view of life. Unlike *neurotic* people, who know they have a problem, those with psychoses may be unaware they are ill. The cause is most likely to be a disorder of brain function. *Drug abuse* may also precipitate psychosis, which can be acute or chronic.

Psychosis is divided into three main categories, namely *schizophrenia*, *bipolar disorder*, and organic brain syndrome (see *brain syndrome, organic*). *Paranoia* may be considered to constitute a fourth category. Symptoms of psychosis include *delusions*, *hallucinations*, and alterations in affect (mood), including *mania* and *depression*.

Episodes of acute psychosis may improve with or without drug treatment. *Antipsychotic drugs* are usually effective in controlling the symptoms. Long-term treatment, *rehabilitation*, and support are often needed. (See also *puerperal psychosis*.)

psychosomatic

A term that describes physical disorders that seem to be caused, or made worse, by psychological factors. Common examples of conditions that may be psychosomatic are headache, breathlessness, nausea, *asthma*, *irritable bowel syndrome*, *dyspepsia*, and some types of *eczema*. (See also *somatization disorder*.)

psychosurgery

Any operation on the brain carried out as a treatment for serious mental illness. It is performed only as a last resort when other treatments have failed.

psychotherapy

Treatment of mental and emotional problems by the use of psychological methods. Patients talk to a therapist about their symptoms and problems, with the aim of learning about themselves, developing insights into their relationships, and, ultimately, changing their behaviour patterns. Examples of psychotherapy include *psychoanalysis* and *cognitive-behavioural therapy*.

psychotropic drugs

Drugs that have an effect on the mind, including *hallucinogenic drugs*, *sedative drugs*, *sleeping drugs*, *tranquillizer drugs*, and *antipsychotic drugs*.

pterygium

A wing-shaped thickening of the *conjunctiva* that extends from either side of the eye towards the centre. Pterygium is attributed to prolonged exposure to bright sunlight and is common in tropical areas. It is surgically removed if it threatens vision or causes discomfort.

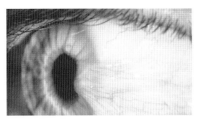

Appearance of pterygium
The conjunctiva has extended beyond the white of the eye to encroach on the cornea (the transparent front part of the eye).

ptosis

Drooping of the upper eyelid. It may be *congenital*, occur spontaneously, or be due to injury or disease, such as *myasthenia gravis*. It may be due to weakness of the levator muscle of the eyelid or interference with nerve supply. Severe congenital ptosis is corrected surgically.

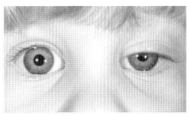

Congenital ptosis in a child
This condition, which is present from birth, should be corrected surgically in order to prevent any disturbance of visual development.

ptyalism

See *salivation, excessive*.

puberty

The period during which adult body features (see *sexual characteristics, secondary*) develop and the sexual organs mature, making reproduction possible.

CHANGES OF **PUBERTY**

There is considerable variation in the age of onset of puberty, but girls, on average, undergo puberty at an earlier age than boys. The entire process takes about three to four years to reach completion. In addition to the changes specific to each sex, height and weight of both girls and boys increase rapidly.

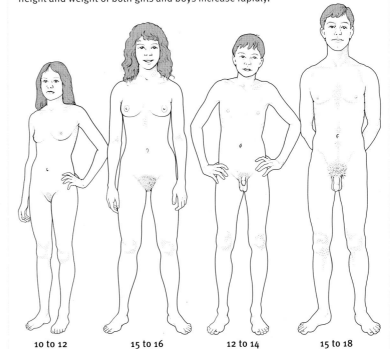

10 to 12   15 to 16   12 to 14   15 to 18

Girls
Puberty most often starts between the ages of 10 and 12 in girls. Major changes include growth of breasts and pubic hair, widening of the hips, enlargement of the uterus, and the onset of menstruation.

Boys
The main changes are enlargement of the sex organs, widening of the shoulders, deepening of the voice, and the growth of facial and pubic hair. The onset is usually between the ages of 12 and 14.

P

Puberty usually occurs between the ages of 10 and 15. It is initiated by the pituitary gland producing *gonadotrophin hormones*, which in girls stimulate the ovaries to increase secretion of oestrogen hormones and in boys the testes to increase secretion of testosterone.

Puberty is accompanied by a significant growth spurt. Body weight may double during this period, primarily due to muscle growth in boys and increased fat in girls. The growth spurt occurs later in boys.

PUBERTY IN GIRLS

The first sign of puberty in girls is usually breast budding, which occurs around the age of 11; in about one third of girls, pubic hair appears first. The breasts may grow at unequal rates, but any difference usually disappears by the time full maturity is reached. Other secondary sexual characteristics, such as the wider pelvis, the female distribution of fat, and the growth of pubic and underarm hair, develop progressively during this period.

The first menstrual period (see *menstruation*) usually occurs a year or more after the start of puberty. The process of puberty is considered complete when periods occur at regular, predictable intervals. The age at which menstruation starts has decreased during the past century, probably because of an improvement generally in nutrition and living standards, but is now stable. Strenuous sports or other hard physical activity (such as ballet), and debilitating disease, can also delay the onset of menstrual periods.

PUBERTY IN BOYS

In boys, puberty is heralded by a sudden increase in the growth of the testes and scrotum, followed by the appearance of pubic and facial hair. The penis begins to grow around the age of 13 and reaches its adult size about two years later; however, there is a wide variation, so that, at the age of 14, some boys may be fully grown while others still have immature genitals.

Secretion of the male sex hormone *testosterone* increases; this stimulates sperm production and causes the *prostate gland* and *seminal vesicles* to mature. It leads to the development of the typical male distribution of hair on the face, chest, and abdomen. The larynx enlarges and the vocal cords become longer and thicker, causing the pitch of the voice to drop. (See also *delayed puberty*; *precocious puberty*.)

pubic bone

The front part of each of the two hip bones (see *pelvis*). The two pubic bones meet at the pubic *symphysis*, which is situated at the front of the pelvis.

pubic lice

Small, wingless insects (PHTHIRUS PUBIS), also called crab lice or crabs, that live in the pubic hair and feed on blood. A louse has a flattened body, up to 2 mm across. Female lice lay eggs (nits) on the hair, where they hatch about eight days later. On men, the lice may also be found in hair around the anus, on the legs, on the trunk, and on the face. The bites sometimes cause itching.

The lice are usually spread from person to person by sexual contact. Children can become infested by transmission from parents, and the lice may live on the eyelids.

Treatment is by applying a topical insecticide medication (containing permethrin, phenothrin, or malathion) to the entire body, including all parts of the head, face and neck; a repeat treatment is necessary seven days later to eradicate any lice newly hatched from nits. In addition, anyone in close personal contact with the infested person should be treated, and clothes, bedding, and bath linen should be washed in very hot water (60°C or above) then put in the hot cycle of a dryer for at least 20 minutes. Items that cannot be washed should be dry-cleaned or, if that is not possible, put in an airtight bag for two weeks.

public health

The branch of medicine concerned with prevention of disease through measures such as health education, provision of clean water supplies, sewage disposal, safer working conditions, infection control, immunizations, and care of pregnant women and young children.

pudenda

The external *genitalia*.

pudendal block

A type of *nerve block* used to provide pain relief for a *forceps delivery*. A local anaesthetic (see *anaesthesia, local*) is injected into either side of the *vagina* near the pudendal nerve.

puerperal psychosis

A severe mental illness that follows *childbirth*. Symptoms of *psychosis* usually develop within two weeks of delivery of the baby and include confusion and mood swings, together with disordered thinking and behaviour, for example believing that the baby is abnormal. *Hallucinations* and *delusions* also occur. There may be very severe *depression*, including thoughts of suicide and/or of harming the baby. Many women who suffer from puerperal psychosis have a family history of psychotic illness or have had such an illness themselves.

Puerperal psychosis requires urgent psychiatric assessment and hospitalization, ideally in a mother and baby psychiatric unit. Treatment of the condition is with *antipsychotic drugs* and *antidepressant drugs*.

puerperal sepsis

An infection that originates in the genital tract within the first ten days after *childbirth*, *miscarriage*, or *abortion*. Formerly a common cause of death, puerperal sepsis is now easily treated with *antibiotic drugs*.

puerperium

The period of time after *childbirth* during which the *uterus* and genitals return to their pre-pregnancy state.

pulmonary

Relating to the *lungs*.

pulmonary disease, chronic obstructive

A combination of the two lung conditions chronic *bronchitis* and *emphysema*. Chronic obstructive pulmonary disease (COPD) severely restricts air flow in or out of the lungs. Bronchitis causes inflammation and narrowing of the airways, while emphysema results in damage to the alveoli (tiny air sacs) in the lungs, making them much less effective at transferring oxygen from the lungs to the bloodstream.

The major cause of COPD is *smoking*. Atmospheric pollution is a contributory factor, and occupational exposure to dusts and certain other irritants can worsen pre-existing COPD.

SYMPTOMS

Some affected people (so-called "pink puffers") maintain adequate oxygen in their bloodstream through an increase in their breathing rate; however, they suffer from almost constant shortness of breath. Others ("blue bloaters") have cyanosis (a bluish discoloration of the skin and mucous membranes), and sometimes *oedema* (an accumulation of

P

fluid in tissues), mainly due to *heart failure* resulting from the lung damage. Other symptoms include wheezing and weight loss. The symptoms tend to be worse in winter.

DIAGNOSIS AND TREATMENT

COPD may be diagnosed from the symptoms and a physical examination. The diagnosis of COPD is confirmed by procedures such as *pulmonary function tests*, *chest X-rays*, *blood gases*, *CT scans*, and *echocardiography*.

Lung damage that is pre-existing is irreversible, but the affected person must stop smoking immediately in order to prevent further damage. Also, exposure to smoke, pollution, dust, damp, and cold should be minimized.

Drug treatment for COPD may include *bronchodilator drugs* to widen the airways, *diuretic drugs* to remove excess fluid, and *antibiotic drugs* for chest infections. Some people may need *oxygen therapy* for the relief of severe shortness of breath.

pulmonary embolism

Obstruction that affects the pulmonary artery or one of its branches in the lung by an *embolus*, usually a blood clot that has formed as a result of deep vein thrombosis (see *thrombosis, deep vein*). In cases in which the embolus is large enough to block the main pulmonary artery or if there are many clots, it may lead to *cardiac arrest* and require emergency resuscitation (see *cardiopulmonary resuscitation*).

CAUSES AND SYMPTOMS

Pulmonary embolism is more likely to occur in the elderly; people who are obese; and after recent surgery, pregnancy, oestrogen treatment – for example, with the combined pill (see *contraceptives, oral*) or *hormone replacement therapy (HRT)* – and immobility, including long-haul flights. Pulmonary embolism may also be linked to *thrombophilia* (a genetic tendency for blood to clot too readily).

A massive pulmonary embolus can cause sudden death. Smaller emboli may cause severe shortness of breath, rapid pulse, dizziness, chest pain that is made worse by breathing, and coughing up of blood. Tiny emboli may not produce any symptoms, but, if recurrent, they may eventually lead to *pulmonary hypertension* (high blood pressure in the arteries that supply the lungs). After having a first embolism, the risk of developing further emboli is significantly increased.

DIAGNOSIS

A diagnosis may be made using procedures including *chest X-rays*, *radionuclide scanning*, pulmonary *angiography*, and *ECG* (electrocardiography). Analysis of arterial *blood gases* and *pulmonary function tests* may also be performed.

TREATMENT

Normally, treatment is with *anticoagulant drugs*. In cases where there is a large embolism, *thrombolytic drugs* may be given. If the condition recurs, tests are needed to investigate the possibility of *blood clotting* disorders. Affected females should stop using combined oral contraceptives and HRT.

pulmonary fibrosis

Scarring and thickening of lung tissue, usually as a result of previous lung inflammation. It may be confined to an area of the lung affected by a condition such as *pneumonia* or *tuberculosis*, or it may be widespread through the lungs (see *fibrosing alveolitis*). Shortness of breath is a common symptom.

Diagnosis is confirmed by *chest X-ray*. Treatment depends on the cause, but in most cases the fibrosis is irreversible and treatment aims to prevent the condition from progressing.

pulmonary function tests

A group of procedures that are used to evaluate lung function, to confirm the presence of lung disorders, or to ensure that surgery on the lungs will not disable the patient. Pulmonary function tests include an assessment of the degree of *bronchospasm* (narrowing of the airways due to muscle contraction) with a *peak-flow meter*, *spirometry*, measurement of lung volume, a test of *blood gases*, and measurement of the exchange of gases across the alveoli (the tiny air sacs in the lungs).

pulmonary hypertension

A disorder in which the blood pressure in the arteries supplying the lungs is abnormally high, which develops in response to increased resistance to blood flow through the lungs. In order to maintain an adequate blood flow, the right-hand side of the heart needs to contract more vigorously than previously. As a consequence of this extra work for the heart, right-sided *heart failure* may later develop. (See also the illustrated box, overleaf.)

CAUSES

Causes of pulmonary hypertension may include chronic obstructive pulmonary disease (COPD) (see *pulmonary disease, chronic obstructive*), a *pulmonary embolism*, *pulmonary fibrosis*, and some congenital heart diseases (see *heart disease, congenital*), but it can also develop without there being an obvious cause.

P

PULMONARY EMBOLISM

This condition results when one or more emboli (fragments of material) break off from a blood clot, usually in a vein, and are carried, via the heart, to the lungs. The effects mainly depend on the size and numbers of emboli but also on the general health of the person's lungs and heart.

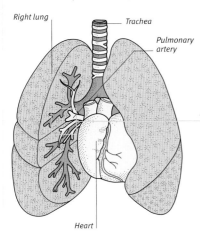

Right lung
Trachea
Pulmonary artery
Heart

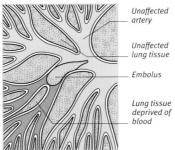

Unaffected artery
Unaffected lung tissue
Embolus
Lung tissue deprived of blood

Site of obstruction
Emboli are carried into the lungs by the pulmonary artery. They may lodge within one of the larger or medium-sized arteries and partially deprive a section of lung tissue of a blood supply.

PULMONARY HYPERTENSION

In this condition, there is increased resistance to blood flow through the lungs (coloured arrows), usually due to lung disease. The result is a rise in pressure in the pulmonary artery, the right side of the heart (black lines and arrows), and in the veins that bring blood to the heart.

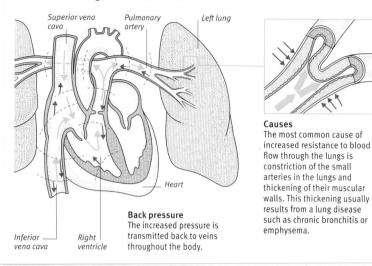

Superior vena cava · Pulmonary artery · Left lung · Inferior vena cava · Right ventricle · Heart

Back pressure
The increased pressure is transmitted back to veins throughout the body.

Causes
The most common cause of increased resistance to blood flow through the lungs is constriction of the small arteries in the lungs and thickening of their muscular walls. This thickening usually results from a lung disease such as chronic bronchitis or emphysema.

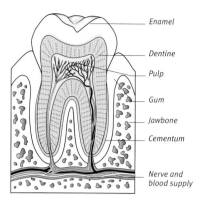

Enamel · Dentine · Pulp · Gum · Jawbone · Cementum · Nerve and blood supply

Location of the dental pulp
The pulp is the soft core at the centre of a tooth. If tooth decay reaches as far as the pulp, the latter degenerates rapidly and must be removed in order to save the tooth.

DIAGNOSIS AND TREATMENT
Diagnosis of pulmonary stenosis is made by a *chest X-ray*, *ECG*, *echocardiography*, and Doppler *ultrasound* scanning. A *balloon catheter* may relieve the narrowing. In more serious cases, *heart valve surgery* or other types of *open heart surgery* are often very successful.

pulp, dental
The soft tissue containing blood vessels and nerves that is situated in the middle of each tooth (see *teeth*).

pulpectomy
The removal of the tooth *pulp*. Pulpectomy is part of *root-canal treatment*.

pulpitis
Inflammation of the dental *pulp*, which most commonly occurs as a result of dental *caries*. Pulpitis can lead to periapical *periodontitis* and a periapical abscess (see *abscess, dental*).

pulpotomy
Removal of the coronal part of the *pulp* of a tooth (the part of the pulp under the crown of a tooth) after it has become inflamed, usually by infection. Infection of the pulp is most often caused by extensive tooth decay (see *caries, dental*) or to dental fractures (see *fracture, dental*). Pulpotomy prevents further degeneration of the tooth's pulp. If pulpotomy is unsuccessful, *root-canal treatment* may be required.

pulse
The rhythmic expansion and contraction of an artery as blood is pumped through it by the heart. The pulse can be felt at

SYMPTOMS
Symptoms, which include enlarged veins in the neck, enlargement of the liver, and generalized *oedema*, only develop when heart failure occurs.

TREATMENT
Treatment is aimed at the underlying disorder (if this is known) and the relief of the heart failure. *Diuretic drugs* or other drugs may be given, and *oxygen therapy* may also be necessary.

pulmonary incompetence
A rare defect of the pulmonary *valve* at the exit of the heart's right *ventricle* (lower chamber). The valve fails to close properly, allowing blood to leak back into the heart. The usual causes are *rheumatic fever*, *endocarditis* (inflammation of the inner lining of the heart), or severe *pulmonary hypertension*.

pulmonary oedema
Accumulation of fluid in the lungs, which is usually due to left-sided *heart failure*. The buildup of fluid may also be due to a chest infection, to inhalation of irritant gases, or to any of the problems that cause generalized *oedema* (fluid accumulation in tissues).

The main symptom of pulmonary oedema is breathlessness, which is usually worse when the person is lying flat and may disturb sleep (see *paroxysmal*

nocturnal dyspnoea). There may also be a cough that produces frothy sputum, which is sometimes pink coloured. In some cases breathing may sound bubbly or possibly wheezy.

A diagnosis of pulmonary oedema is made by a *physical examination* and by a *chest X-ray*. Treatment of the condition may include *morphine*, *diuretic drugs*, *ACE inhibitor drugs*, and *oxygen therapy*; artificial *ventilation* may also be given.

pulmonary stenosis
A *heart* condition in which the outflow of blood from the right *ventricle* (lower heart chamber) is obstructed, causing the heart to work harder in order to pump blood to the lungs.

CAUSES
The obstruction may be caused by narrowing of the pulmonary *valve* at the exit of the ventricle; by narrowing of the pulmonary artery, which carries blood to the lungs; or by narrowing of the upper part of the ventricle.

SYMPTOMS
Pulmonary stenosis is usually *congenital* (present from birth), and it may occur on its own or with a set of heart defects that collectively are called the *tetralogy of Fallot*. In rare cases, pulmonary stenosis develops later in life, after *rheumatic fever*, and in such cases it may cause symptoms of heart failure.

various points on the body where arteries lie just below the skin's surface, such as the inside of the wrist, the side of the neck, and the top of the thigh.

pump, infusion

A machine that is used to administer a continuous and controlled amount of a drug (in liquid form) or sometimes of another fluid. The drug or fluid is delivered through a needle inserted into a vein or under the skin.

pump, insulin

A type of infusion pump (see *pump, infusion*) that is used to administer insulin to some patients who have *diabetes mellitus*. The rate of flow of insulin is adjusted so that the level of blood glucose (sugar) remains constant.

PUO

See *pyrexia of unknown origin*.

LOCATION OF THE **PUPIL**

The pupil is the circular opening in the centre of the iris. It can be widened or narrowed by muscles in the iris to adjust the amount of light entering the eye.

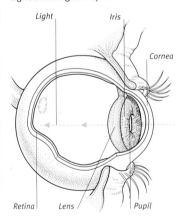

pupil

The circular opening in the centre of the *iris*. In bright conditions, the pupil constricts; in dim light, it dilates.

purine

Any of a group of nitrogen-containing compounds synthesized in the body or produced by the digestion of certain proteins. Increased levels of purine can cause *hyperuricaemia*, which may lead to *gout*. Foods that have a high purine con-tent include sardines, liver, kidneys, pulses, and poultry. Purine is also a component of adenine and guanine, two *nucleotide* bases found in the *nucleic acids* DNA and RNA.

purpura

Any of a group of disorders that are characterized by purple to red-brown areas (or spots) on the skin, caused by bleeding within the skin or mucous membranes. The term purpura also refers to the discoloured areas themselves, which do not blanch (go pale) when pressure is applied to the skin (see *glass test*).

There are many different types and causes of purpura. Common purpura, also known as senile purpura, mostly affects middle-aged or elderly women. Large discoloured areas, caused by thinning of the tissues supporting blood vessels under the skin, appear on the thighs or back of the hands and forearms. *Henoch–Schönlein purpura* is caused by inflammation of the blood vessels that lie just beneath the skin. Purpura can also occur as a result of *thrombocytopenia* (a bleeding disorder), and can be associated with *septicaemia* (blood poisoning) and with *meningitis* (inflammation of the membranes that cover the brain and the spinal cord).

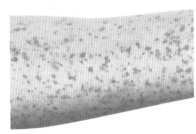

Appearance of Henoch–Schönlein purpura
This condition can occur following an infection, or it may be caused by an allergic reaction. Here, a raised rash has appeared on the arm.

purulent

A term that means containing, producing, or consisting of *pus*.

pus

A pale yellow or green, creamy fluid that is found at the site of a bacterial infection. The creamy fluid is composed of many millions of dead white *blood cells*, as well as partly digested tissue, dead and living bacteria, and some other substances. When a collection of pus occurs within a solid area of tissue, this is called an *abscess*.

pustule

A small skin *blister* that contains *pus*.

PUVA

A type of *phototherapy* that is used to treat a variety of skin conditions, in particular *psoriasis*. PUVA is a combination of a *psoralen drug* and a controlled dose of long-wavelength *ultraviolet light*.

pyelitis

See *pyelonephritis*.

pyelography

Another term for urography (see *intravenous urography*).

pyelolithotomy

An operation that is performed in order to remove a kidney stone (see *calculus, urinary tract*). Pyelolithotomy has been largely replaced by other procedures that are less invasive. One example is *lithotripsy*, which uses ultrasonic waves to break up the stones.

pyelonephritis

Inflammation of the *kidney*, which is usually the result of a bacterial infection. Pyelonephritis is more common in women and is most likely to occur during pregnancy. Symptoms include high fever, chills, and back pain. *Septicaemia* (blood poisoning) may be a complication. Treatment of pyelonephritis is with *antibiotic drugs*. Recurrent pyelonephritis can lead to *kidney failure*. (See also *vesicoureteric reflux*.)

pyeloplasty

A surgical procedure that is used to relieve hydronephrosis (a buildup of fluid in the *kidney*) that results from structural defects in the renal pelvis (the part of the kidney involved in collecting urine) or in the *ureter* (the tube carrying urine from the kidney to the bladder). The operation involves reshaping the affected areas.

pyloric sphincter

The valve situated at the base of the *stomach*; its function is to control movement of food into the *duodenum*.

pyloric stenosis

A condition that is characterized by narrowing of the pylorus (the lower outlet from the stomach). Pyloric stenosis causes an obstruction to the passage of food into the *duodenum* (the first part of the small intestine).

P

CAUSES

Pyloric stenosis occurs in babies as a result of thickening of the pyloric muscle. When it occurs in adults, however, the condition is due to scarring from a *peptic ulcer* or *stomach cancer*.

SYMPTOMS

Babies start projectile vomiting (profuse vomiting in which the stomach contents may be ejected several feet) two to five weeks after birth. Adults with the disorder vomit undigested food several hours after a meal.

DIAGNOSIS

In infants, *ultrasound scanning* is the procedure used for confirmation of the diagnosis. In adults, however, diagnosis is likely to be made by means of a *barium X-ray examination* and a *gastroscopy* (examination of the stomach using a viewing instrument).

TREATMENT

In infants, surgical treatment involves making an incision along the thickened muscle. In adults, surgery is carried out to correct the underlying cause.

PYLORIC STENOSIS IN INFANTS

In infantile pyloric stenosis, the muscle surrounding the outlet from the stomach is abnormally thickened, as shown in the enlarged drawing (below). The condition occurs more often in male than female babies and tends to run in families – infants of a woman who was affected with pyloric stenosis as a baby may develop it.

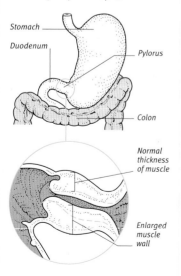

Stomach

Duodenum

Pylorus

Colon

Normal thickness of muscle

Enlarged muscle wall

pyloroplasty

An operation in which the pylorus (the outlet leading from the stomach) is widened to allow free passage of food into the intestine. Pyloroplasty may be performed as part of the surgery for a *peptic ulcer*, or in order to prevent tightening of the pyloric muscles after *vagotomy* (cutting of the vagus nerve to reduce stomach acid production).

pyo-

A prefix that is used to denote a relationship to *pus*. The prefix "py" is also used in the same way.

pyoderma gangrenosum

A rare condition that is characterized by ulcers, usually on the legs, that turn into hard, painful areas surrounded by discoloured skin. Pyoderma gangrenosum occurs as a rare complication in *ulcerative colitis*.

pyogenic granuloma

A common, noncancerous skin tumour that develops on exposed areas after minor injury. The tumour can be removed surgically, by *electrocautery*, or by *cryosurgery*.

pyrazinamide

A drug sometimes used in combination with other drugs to treat *tuberculosis*. Possible adverse effects are nausea, joint pains, *gout*, and liver damage.

pyrexia

A medical term for *fever*.

pyrexia of unknown origin

Persistent fever that has no apparent cause. It is usually due to an illness that is difficult to diagnose or a common disease that appears in an unusual way. Such illnesses include viral infections; *tuberculosis*; cancer, particularly *lymphoma*; and *connective tissue diseases*, such as systemic *lupus erythematosus* and *temporal arteritis*. Another possible cause of pyrexia of unknown origin is a reaction to a *drug*.

pyridoxine

Vitamin B_6 (see *vitamin B complex*). Dietary deficiency of this vitamin is very rare but can be induced by some drugs. Pyridoxine is sometimes used to treat *premenstrual syndrome*. The long-term use of high-dose pyridoxine has been associated with disorders of the peripheral nerves.

pyrimethamine

A drug that is used in combination with other drugs to treat resistant *malaria*.

pyrogen

A substance that produces *fever*. The term is usually applied to proteins released by white *blood cells* in response to infections. The word is also sometimes used to refer to chemicals released by microorganisms.

pyromania

A persistent impulse to start fires. It is more often seen in males, and may be associated with a low IQ, alcohol abuse, and a *psychosexual disorder*.

pyruvate kinase deficiency

A disorder in which there are abnormally low levels of an *enzyme* called pyruvate kinase, which is carried in *red blood cells*. Normally, pyruvate kinase aids the breakdown of glucose to create energy in *anaerobic* (low-oxygen) conditions. If there is a deficiency of the enzyme, the red cells cannot generate enough energy for themselves; they also develop chemical imbalances that cause them to be destroyed prematurely by the spleen, thereby causing anaemia (see *anaemia, haemolytic*) and enlargement of the spleen. The disorder is usually the result of an autosomal recessive gene defect (see *genetic disorders*).

The severity of the disease varies. Most people require no treatment. *Blood transfusions* may be needed in some cases, particularly when the person is under physiological stress (such as acute illness or pregnancy), at which times the disease tends to be worse. *Splenectomy* (removal of the spleen) may be recommended in severe cases.

pyuria

The presence of *white blood cells* in the *urine*, which is often an indication of an infection of a *kidney* or *urinary tract infection* and inflammation.

P

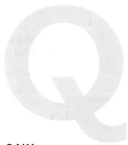

QALY

A quality-adjusted life year. QALY is used by health economists to compare the relative costs and outcomes of treatment for various diseases. Each year of life saved or prolonged is adjusted by a factor, Q, which takes account of how close to normal the individual's lifestyle is before and after treatment.

Q fever

An uncommon illness causing symptoms that are similar to those of *influenza*. Q fever occurs throughout the world.

CAUSES

Q fever is caused by the *rickettsia* (a type of small bacterium) COXIELLA BURNETII and may be contracted by inhaling dust contaminated with faeces, urine, or birth products from infected farm animals. Rarely, it is spread by tick bites.

SYMPTOMS

Symptoms develop suddenly about 20 days after infection. They include high fever (lasting up to two weeks), severe headache, muscle and chest pains, and a cough. A form of *pneumonia* subsequently occurs. Most people recover, but the disease is sometimes prolonged: occasionally, *hepatitis* (liver inflammation) or *endocarditis* (inflammation of the inner lining of the heart) may develop.

DIAGNOSIS AND TREATMENT

After diagnosis is confirmed by a *blood test*, treatment is with *antibiotic drugs*. A vaccine is available for people at risk.

quackery

A false claim by someone to have the ability to diagnose and treat disease.

quadrantectomy

A surgical procedure that involves the removal of tissue in one quadrant of a breast in order to treat *breast cancer*. (See also *lumpectomy*; *mastectomy*.)

quadriceps muscle

A large muscle with four distinct parts, located at the front of the thigh. The quadriceps muscle straightens the knee.

LOCATION OF THE QUADRICEPS MUSCLE

One upper end attaches to the pelvis; the other two ends attach to the femur. The lower ends merge into a tendon that surrounds the patella and attaches to the tibia.

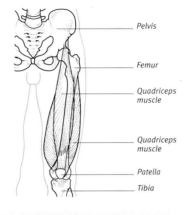

Pelvis
Femur
Quadriceps muscle
Quadriceps muscle
Patella
Tibia

DISORDERS

The most common quadriceps disorder is a *haematoma* (collection of blood), due to a direct blow. Bruising may follow after a few days. Rarely, bone forms in the haematoma, restricting movement.

Sudden stretching of the leg may tear the muscle, especially in middle-aged or elderly people. Rupture of the quadriceps tendon can be caused by a direct blow to the leg or stumbling. Knee disorders that cause pain or swelling, limiting full extension of the leg, cause the muscle to begin to waste away within 48 hours, making the knee feel as if it is giving way when weight is placed on the affected leg. Exercises to strengthen the quadriceps are used to treat certain knee disorders.

quadriparesis

Muscle weakness in all four limbs and the trunk. (See also *quadriplegia*.)

quadriplegia

Paralysis of all four limbs and the trunk, also known as tetraplegia. Quadriplegia may be caused by damage to the *spinal cord* in the neck region. The condition results in loss of feeling and power in the affected parts. (See also *paraplegia*.)

quarantine

The isolation of a person or animal recently exposed to a serious infectious disease in order to prevent the spread of the disease by symptomless individuals.

Quarantine procedures are now rarely used due to the reduced incidence of serious infectious diseases and the availability of *vaccinations* for many of them. The principal remaining quarantine regulations apply to animals imported into countries that are free from *rabies*.

quickening

The first fetal movements felt by a pregnant woman, which usually occur after about 18 weeks' gestation.

quinapril

An *ACE-inhibitor drug* used in the treatment of *hypertension* and *heart failure*.

quinine

The oldest drug treatment for *malaria*. Quinine is mainly used in large doses to treat strains that are resistant to other antimalarials. There is a high risk of side effects such as headache, nausea, ringing in the ears, hearing loss, and visual disturbance. It is also prescribed in low doses to help prevent leg cramps at night; side effects in this case are rare.

quinolone drugs

COMMON DRUGS

• Ciprofloxacin • Levofloxacin • Nalidixic acid • Norfloxacin • Ofloxacin

A group of *antibiotic drugs* used to treat bacterial infections. Quinolones are derived from chemicals, rather than living organisms. They are used to treat a range of conditions, including *prostatitis* (inflammation of the prostate), *urinary tract infections*, *gonorrhoea*, acute diarrhoeal diseases (such as those caused by *salmonella infections*), and *enteric fever*. Ciprofloxacin may also be used as an initial treatment for *anthrax*. Absorption of quinolones is reduced by *antacid drugs*.

POSSIBLE ADVERSE EFFECTS

Side effects include nausea, diarrhoea, headache, sleep disorders, rash, and blood disorders. Rarely, there is tendon damage (especially in the elderly and those taking corticosteroid drugs).

WARNING

Quinolones should be used with caution by people with *epilepsy*, during pregnancy and breast-feeding, and by children and adolescents. Swelling and pain in the tendons should be reported.

quinsy

Another name for a *peritonsillar abscess* (an abscess in the soft tissue around the tonsils), a complication of *tonsillitis*.

Q

R

rabies

An acute viral infection of the nervous system, once known as hydrophobia, that affects mammals, including bats. The virus travels along nerve pathways to the brain; once symptoms develop, rabies is usually fatal.

CAUSES AND INCIDENCE

Rabies can be transmitted from a rabid animal to a human by a bite or a lick over broken skin; most human cases result from being bitten by a rabid dog. Rabies is an extremely rare disease in the UK.

SYMPTOMS

The average *incubation period* is three to twelve weeks, depending on the site of the bite. The first symptoms of rabies are slight fever and headache. These are followed by restlessness, hyperactivity, and, in some cases, strange behaviour, hallucinations, and paralysis. The victim develops *seizures*, arrhythmias (see *arrhythmia, cardiac*), and paralysis of the respiratory muscles. There is often intense thirst but drinking induces painful spasms of the throat. Death usually occurs 10 to 14 days after the onset of symptoms.

TREATMENT AND PREVENTION

Following an animal bite, the wound should be cleaned thoroughly and immediate medical advice should be sought. *Immunization* with human rabies immunoglobulin and a course of rabies vaccine is necessary; this may prevent the onset of rabies. If symptoms appear, they are treated with sedative drugs and *analgesics* (painkillers).

Emphasis is placed on preventing rabies through *quarantine* and human and animal immunization. Prophylactic immunization is recommended for certain people, for example wild animal handlers and travellers to areas where rabies is endemic. (See also *bites, animal.*)

rachitic

A term that is used to describe abnormalities associated with *rickets* (a bone disease caused by a deficiency of vitamin D) or to refer to people or populations particularly afflicted by rickets.

rad

A unit of absorbed dose of ionizing radiation (see *radiation unit*), which has been superseded by the gray (Gy). "Rad" stands for radiation absorbed dose.

radial keratotomy

See *keratotomy, radial.*

radial nerve

A branch of the *brachial plexus*. The radial nerve, one of the main nerves of the arm, runs from the shoulder to the hand. The radial nerve controls the muscles that straighten the wrist. It conveys sensation from the back of the forearm; the thumb, second, and third fingers; and the base of the thumb.

The radial nerve may be damaged by a fracture of the *humerus* (upper-arm bone) or by persistent pressure on the armpit, such as from the use of a crutch. Such damage may result in *wrist-drop* (an inability to straighten the wrist) and numbness in the areas of skin supplied by the radial nerve.

radiation

The emission of energy (as electromagnetic waves) or matter (as particles) from unstable atoms, which turns them into a more stable form. Some types of radiation are harmful to life; other types are essential, such as light and heat energy radiated from the sun. Even harmful radiation may be used for beneficial purposes. In treatment by *radiotherapy*, for example, the biologically damaging effects of radiation are used to destroy cancerous cells.

IONIZING RADIATION

Four significant types of harmful radiation are gamma radiation, *X-rays*, alpha particles, and beta particles. Gamma radiation and X-rays are types of electromagnetic waves and are similar to more energetic forms of light. The principal difference between the two is that gamma rays are produced by the spontaneous decay of radioactive materials whereas X-rays are produced by a machine. Particle radiation may be produced either during the decay of radioactive atoms or by machine.

All four types of harmful radiation cause damage by ionization: the waves or particles knock out electrons from atoms in the matter that they pass through, turning them into highly reactive *ions*. In the case of living tissue, the ions formed can cause biological damage. Radioactive substances that emit any of these types of radiation constitute a health hazard. However, alpha particles cannot penetrate the skin, and therefore sources of alpha radiation are only dangerous if they are ingested or inhaled. Gamma radiation can travel large distances through many substances; even distant gamma sources can pose a risk to humans.

Most sources of radiation are natural. Natural sources of ionizing radiation include cosmic rays from space and radioactive minerals. In some areas, the gas *radon*, which is found in soil, rocks, or building materials, is a major source of ionizing radiation. Sources of ionizing radiation that are artificial include X-ray machines, radioactive isotopes used in diagnosis and treatment (see *radionuclide scanning*), and nuclear reactors.

NONIONIZING RADIATION

Less energetic types of radiation, such as *ultraviolet light*, infra-red radiation (radiant heat), and microwaves, may cause biological damage by mechanisms other than ionization. Ultraviolet radiation from the sun does not penetrate the body deeply but can damage genetic material in cells and may lead to *skin cancer*. Certain wavelengths of microwaves and infra-red radiation can cause burns.

The other type of nonionizing radiation to which people are subjected are radio waves, which are generated during *MRI* (magnetic resonance imaging). MRI is not thought to have any adverse side effects. *Ultrasound* uses sound waves, not electromagnetic waves or particles, and is therefore not usually classed as a source of radiation; ultrasound is also thought to have no adverse effects. (See also *radiation hazards; radiation sickness; radiation unit*).

radiation dermatitis

A type of *dermatitis* (inflammation of the skin) that may be caused by single exposure to a high dose of *radiation*.

radiation enteritis

A potentially long-standing form of *enteritis* (inflammation of the small intestine) that is caused by exposure of the intestine to *radiation*, including the use of *radiotherapy*. The symptoms of radiation enteritis include nausea, vomiting, and diarrhoea.

radiation fibrosis

Scarring and thickening of the tissues around an area of the body that has been treated with *radiotherapy*.

radiation hazards

Hazards brought about by *radiation* (the emission of energy in the form of waves or particles) that may arise either from external sources of radiation, such as *X-rays* or gamma rays, or from radioactive materials taken into the body. The effects of radiation depend on the dose, the duration of exposure, and the organs exposed.

With some forms of radiation, damage occurs only when the radiation dose exceeds a certain limit – this is usually 1 sievert (Sv) (see *radiation unit*). Examples of such damage are *radiation dermatitis*, *cataract*, organ failure (which may occur many years later), or *radiation sickness* (an early reaction to massive irradiation).

For other types of radiation damage, the risk that damage will occur increases with repeated doses of radiation. *Cancer* that is caused by radiation-induced *mutation* (a change in the genetic material of cells) is an example of this type of damage. Radioactive leaks from nuclear reactors can cause a rise in mutation rates, which may lead to an increased incidence of cancers such as *leukaemias*; *birth defects* in succeeding generations; and hereditary diseases. Cancer usually develops years after exposure.

Damage can be controlled by limiting exposure to radiation. People exposed to radiation at work should have their exposure monitored to ensure it does not exceed safe limits. People of reproductive age or younger should have their reproductive organs shielded when having X-rays or undergoing *radiotherapy*.

There is no evidence of radiation hazards arising from visual display units (VDUs) or the *irradiation of food*.

radiation sickness

The term applied to the acute effects of ionizing *radiation* on the whole, or a major part, of the body when the dose exceeds 1 gray (Gy) of *X-rays* or gamma rays or 1 sievert (Sv) of other types of radiation (see *radiation unit*).

The effects of radiation depend on the dose and the duration of exposure. Total-body doses of less than 2 Gy are unlikely to be fatal to a healthy adult. At doses of 1 to 10 Gy, transient nausea and occasional vomiting may occur, but these usually disappear rapidly and are often followed by a two- to three-week period of relative wellbeing. By the end of this period, the effects of radiation damage to the bone marrow and *immune system*

begin to appear, with repeated infections (which may be fatal unless treated with *antibiotic drugs*) and petechiae (pinpoint spots of bleeding under the skin). Some people are successfully treated with a *stem cell* or *bone marrow transplant* or by isolation in a sterile environment until the bone marrow recovers.

With a dose of 10 to 30 Gy there is also an early onset of nausea and vomiting, but these symptoms tend to disappear a few hours later. However, damage to the gastrointestinal tract, which causes severe and frequently bloody *diarrhoea* (known as the gastrointestinal syndrome), and overwhelming infection due to damage to the immune system are likely to result in death between four and 14 days after exposure.

Acute exposures of 30 to 100 Gy cause the rapid onset of nausea, vomiting, anxiety, and disorientation. Within hours, the victim usually loses consciousness and dies due to damage to the *nervous system* and *oedema* (accumulation of fluid) of the brain; these combined effects are known as the central nervous system syndrome.

radiation unit

Several different internationally agreed units (called SI units) are used to measure ionizing *radiation*. For example, the becquerel (symbol Bq) is the SI unit of spontaneous activity of a radioactive source such as uranium. In medicine, the most commonly used units are the gray (symbol Gy) and sievert (symbol Sv).

The gray is the SI unit of radiation that is actually absorbed by any tissue or substance as a result of exposure to radiation. One Gy is the absorption of one joule of energy (from gamma radiation or X-rays) per kilogram of irradiated matter. The gray supersedes an older unit called the rad (1 Gy = 100 rads).

Because some types of radiation affect biological organisms more than others, the sievert is used as a measure of the impact of an absorbed dose. It uses additional factors, such as the kind of radiation and its energy, to quantify the effects on the body of equivalent amounts of different types of absorbed energy. (See also *Radiation units* box, overleaf.)

radical surgery

Extensive surgery that is aimed at eliminating a major disease, usually *cancer*, by removing all the affected tissue and any surrounding tissue that might also be diseased.

Some examples of radical surgery are radical *mastectomy* performed to treat *breast cancer*, which involves removing the entire affected breast along with chest muscles, underarm *lymph nodes*, and other tissue; radical neck dissection (see *neck dissection, radical*), in which the lymph nodes in the neck are removed; and *amputation*, which is usually performed to prevent the spread of *gangrene* (tissue death).

radiculopathy

Damage to the *nerve* roots that enter or leave the *spinal cord*. Radiculopathy may be caused by *disc prolapse*, spinal *arthritis*, *diabetes mellitus*, or ingestion of heavy metals, such as lead. Symptoms of radiculopathy are severe pain and, occasionally, loss of feeling in the area supplied by the affected nerves. There may also be weakness, *paralysis*, and wasting of the muscles that are supplied by the nerves.

Where possible, the underlying cause is treated; otherwise, symptoms may be relieved by *analgesic drugs* (painkillers), *physiotherapy*, or, in some cases, surgery.

radioactivity

The emission of alpha particles, beta particles, and/or gamma *radiation* that occurs during the spontaneous disintegration of the nuclei (see *nucleus*) of unstable atoms.

Many radioactive substances, such as uranium ores, are naturally occurring. However, the majority of elements can be made radioactive by bombarding them with high-energy particles, such as neutrons.

radioallergosorbent test

See *RAST*.

radiofrequency ablation

A minimally invasive procedure in which radiofrequency alternating electric current is used to destroy diseased or abnormal tissue. The procedure, which may be carried out under local or general anaesthesia, involves applying the electric current using electrodes inserted into the affected tissue. Radiofrequency ablation may be used to treat some tumours and certain abnormal heart rhythms

radiography

The use of *radiation* to obtain images of parts of the body. Radiographers prepare patients for *X-ray* examinations,

R

RADIATION UNITS

In the SI system (the internationally agreed system of units), three main units are used to measure radiation levels – the becquerel, the gray, and the sievert. These three units are defined below, along with two other radiation units (the rad and rem) that have now been largely superseded but are still occasionally used for some purposes.

Becquerel
The SI unit of radioactivity. One becquerel (symbol Bq) is defined as one disintegration (or other nuclear transformation) per second. Although the number of becquerels is a measure of how strongly radioactive a particular source is, it takes no account of the different effects of different types of radiation on tissue; for medical purposes, the sievert is generally more useful.

Gray
The SI unit of absorbed dose of ionizing radiation, the gray (symbol Gy) has superseded the rad. One gray is defined as an energy absorption of 1 joule per kilogram of irradiated material. One gray is equivalent to 100 rads.

Rad
An acronym for radiation absorbed dose, the rad is a unit of absorbed dose of ionizing radiation. One rad is equal to an energy absorption of 100 ergs (an erg is a unit of work or energy) per gram of irradiated material. The rad has been superseded by the gray (the corresponding SI unit); 1 rad is equivalent to 0.01 grays.

Rem
An acronym for roentgen equivalent man, the rem is the absorbed dose of ionizing radiation that produces the same biological effect as 1 rad of X-rays or gamma rays. The rem was introduced as a result of the observation that some types of ionizing radiation, such as neutrons, produce a greater biological effect for an equivalent amount of absorbed energy than X-rays or gamma rays. In short, the rem is a measure of the biological effectiveness of irradiation. For X-rays and gamma rays, the rem is equal to the rad. For other types of radiation, the number or rems equals the number of rads multiplied by a special factor (called the quality factor or relative biological effectiveness) that depends on the type of radiation involved. The rem has been superseded by the sievert in the SI system of units; 1 rem is equivalent to 0.01 sieverts.

Sievert
The SI unit of equivalent absorbed dose of ionizing radiation, the sievert (symbol Sv) has superseded the rem. One sievert is the absorbed dose of radiation that produces the same biological effect as 1 gray of X-rays or gamma rays. One sievert is equivalent to 100 rems.

take and develop X-ray pictures, and assist with other *imaging techniques*, such as *radionuclide scanning*, *ultrasound scanning*, and *MRI* (magnetic resonance imaging). (See also *radiology*).

radioimmunoassay

A sensitive laboratory technique that uses radioactive isotopes to measure the concentration of specific proteins, such as hormones or antibodies, in a person's blood. (See also *immunoassay*).

radioisotope scanning

See *radionuclide scanning*.

radiology

The medical speciality that uses *X-rays*, *ultrasound scanning*, *MRI* (magnetic resonance imaging), and *radionuclide scanning* to investigate, diagnose, and treat disease.

Radiological methods provide images of the body in a *noninvasive* way so that exploratory surgery is not required. The techniques also enable instruments (such as needles and *catheters*) to be accurately guided into different parts of the body both for diagnosis and for treatment, a subspecialty known as interventional radiology.

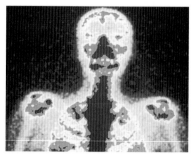

Radionuclide bone scan
Here, the radionuclide has been absorbed by bone. Abnormalities (such as metastases) absorb it in greater amounts and appear as 'hot spots'.

radiolucent

A term referring to anything that is almost transparent to *radiation*, especially to *X-rays* and gamma rays. Some X-ray imaging procedures require the introduction of *radiopaque* substances into the body to make *radiotransparent* and radiolucent organs and/or body tissues stand out more clearly.

radionuclide scanning

A diagnostic technique that is based on the detection of *radiation* emitted by radioactive substances introduced into the body. Different substances are taken up in different concentrations by different tissues, allowing specific organs to be studied. For example, iodine is taken up mainly by the thyroid gland, so by "tagging" a sample of iodine with a radioactive marker (radionuclide), the thyroid gland's uptake of iodine can be monitored to investigate the functioning of the gland.

HOW IT WORKS
The radionuclide is swallowed or alternatively injected into the bloodstream and then accumulates in the target organ. The organ emits radiation in the form of gamma radiation, which is detected by a gamma camera and then an image is produced.

Cross-sectional images ("slices") can be obtained by using a computer-controlled gamma camera that rotates around the patient. This specialized form of radionuclide scanning is known as SPECT (single photon emission computed tomography). Moving images can also be taken with the use of a computer; a series of images is recorded immediately following the administration of the radionuclide.

WHY IT IS DONE
Radionuclide scanning is capable of detecting some disorders at an earlier stage than other *imaging techniques* because changes in the functioning of an organ often occur before the structure of the organ is affected. The technique is also used to detect disorders that affect only the function of an organ. Moving images can provide information about blood flow, the movement of the heart walls, the flow of urine through the kidneys, and bile flow through the liver.

RISKS
Radionuclide scanning is a safe procedure, requiring only minute doses of radiation that are excreted within hours. The radionuclides carry virtually no risk of toxicity or *hypersensitivity*.

radiopaque

A term describing anything that can block *radiation*, especially *X-rays* and gamma rays. As many body tissues are *radiolucent* (almost transparent to X-rays), some X-ray imaging procedures require the introduction of radiopaque substances into the body to make organs clearly visible. (See also *radiotransparent*.)

radiotherapy

Treatment of *cancer* and, occasionally, some noncancerous tumours, by the use of *X-rays* or other *radiation*. Radioactive sources produce ionizing radiation, which destroys or slows down the development of abnormal cells. Normal cells should suffer little or no damage in the long term, but short-term damage is a side effect of radiotherapy.

WHY IS IT DONE

Radiotherapy may be used on its own in an attempt to destroy all the abnormal cells in various types of cancer, such as *squamous cell carcinoma* (a type of skin cancer), *Hodgkin's disease* (a cancer of lymphoid tissue), *prostate cancer*, and cervical cancer (see *cervix, cancer of*). It may also be used in conjunction with other cancer treatments. For example, surgical excision of a cancerous tumour is often followed by radiotherapy to destroy any remaining tumour cells, as in the treatment of *breast cancer*.

Radiotherapy may also be used to relieve symptoms of a cancer that is too advanced to be cured. An example of such *palliative* treatment is radiotherapy to shrink a *brain tumour* to relieve headaches and paralysis.

Total body irradiation is often carried out before a *stem cell* or *bone marrow transplant* in order to destroy all abnormal cells before they are replaced with healthy transplanted ones.

USE OF **RADIOTHERAPY**

Radiotherapy destroys cancer cells using radiation. A linear accelerator is used for external radiation (right). The position and dose of radiation are carefully calculated to minimize exposure of normal cells to the radiation, allowing them to recover with little or no long-term damage.

Internal radiation (below) involves placing radioactive materials in the body, directly into or around a cancer.

External radiation

The patient lies still on a table under the machine. A radiographer operates the machine, which sends X-rays, in the predetermined directions and amounts, through the diseased areas of the patient's body. The machine can be tilted to irradiate the cancer from different angles (see below, centre). The procedure causes no discomfort, and usually lasts a few minutes, but setting up the equipment may take 30 minutes.

Radiation source

Beam of radiation

Adjustable table

INTERNAL RADIATION

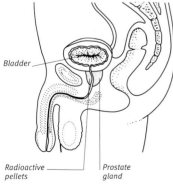

Bladder

Radioactive pellets

Prostate gland

Use of radioactive pellets

Tiny radioactive pellets are inserted, via a hollow needle, directly into the organ or tissue to be treated (here, the prostate gland).

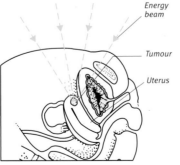

Energy beam

Tumour

Uterus

Rays from different directions

By aiming relatively low-energy rays coming from many directions at a tumour, a large enough dose of radiation is achieved in the locality of the tumour to destroy it completely (see above).

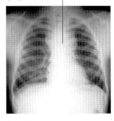

Lymphoid tissue

Before treatment
There is a proliferation of lymphoid tissue in this lung X-ray of a patient with Hodgkin's disease.

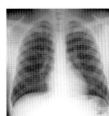

After treatment
The invading lymphoid tissue has diminished following radiotherapy.

R

If the benefits of destroying diseased tissue outweigh the risks of damage to healthy tissue, radiotherapy may be used to treat noncancerous diseases; for example, part of an overactive thyroid gland (see *thyrotoxicosis*) may be destroyed using radioactive iodine.

HOW IT IS DONE

Radiotherapy is usually performed on an outpatient basis. *X-rays* (or sometimes electrons), which are produced by a machine called a linear accelerator, are aimed at the tumour from many directions. Alternatively, a source of radiation, in the form of tiny pellets, is inserted into the tumour through a hollow needle (see *interstitial radiotherapy*) or into a body cavity (see *intracavitary therapy*). These techniques are both types of brachytherapy. Radioactive iodine used to treat thyrotoxicosis is given by mouth.

COMPLICATIONS AND RESULTS

There may be some unpleasant side effects of radiotherapy, such as fatigue, nausea and vomiting (for which *antiemetic drugs* may be prescribed), and loss of hair from irradiated areas. Rarely, there may be reddening and blistering of the skin.

Radiotherapy can be used successfully to treat many types of cancer; the likelihood of success increases the earlier the treatment is started.

radiotransparent

A term referring to anything that is entirely transparent to *radiation*, especially to *X-rays* and gamma rays. Some X-ray imaging procedures require the introduction of *radiopaque* substances into the body to make radiotransparent and *radiolucent* organs and/or body tissues stand out more clearly.

radium

A rare, radioactive, metallic element that occurs naturally only as compounds in *uranium* ores. Radium has four naturally occurring isotopes (varieties of the element that are chemically identical but differ in some physical properties): radium 226, radium 228, radium 224, and radium 223. Radium 226 was used to treat tumours but it has been superseded by other radioisotopes, such as cobalt 60.

radius

The shorter of the two long bones of the forearm; the other is the *ulna*. The radius is the bone on the thumb side of the arm, which articulates with the humerus (the upper-arm bone) at the elbow and the upper carpal bones (upper wrist bones) at the wrist.

The radius takes most of the strain when weight is placed on the wrist, and it is a common site of fractures (see *Colles' fracture*; *radius, fracture of*). A fall or a blow may sometimes cause dislocation of the radius from the elbow joint, along with fracture of the ulna, a condition that is known as Monteggia's fracture.

radius, fracture of

A common type of fracture that may affect the lower end, upper end, or shaft of the *radius* (the shorter of the two long bones in the forearm).

Fracture of the radius just above the wrist (see *Colles' fracture*) is the most common of all fractures in people over 40. It is usually caused by falling on the palm of a hand, resulting in backward displacement of the wrist and hand.

Fracture of the disc-shaped head of the radius, just below the elbow, is one of the most common fractures in young adults. Treatment depends on the type and severity of the fracture. A minor fracture may heal if placed in a soft, supportive bandage; others may require surgical correction. If the head of the bone is crushed or splintered, it may need to be removed.

Fracture of the shaft of the radius may result in displacement of the broken ends of the bone. An operation may be required in order to reposition the

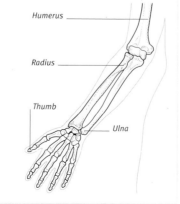

LOCATION OF THE RADIUS

The radius bone is on the outside of the forearm (here, the right), with the palm facing forwards, or on the inside with the palm facing backwards.

Humerus

Radius

Thumb

Ulna

bone ends and fix them together before the limb is immobilized. Fractures of the radius usually take approximately six weeks to heal.

radon

A colourless, odourless, tasteless, radioactive gaseous element produced by the radioactive decay of *radium*.

raloxifene

A drug that is prescribed to prevent and treat postmenopausal *osteoporosis*. Raloxifene has no beneficial effect on other menopausal problems, such as hot flushes. The drug may carry an increased risk of developing a deep vein thrombosis (see *thrombosis, deep vein*).

ramipril

An *ACE inhibitor drug* used in the treatment of *hypertension* (high blood pressure) and *heart failure* (reduced pumping efficiency). Ramipril is also used to prevent or delay kidney damage in patients with *diabetes mellitus*. Side effects may include a persistent dry cough, a disturbance in taste, *hypotension* (low blood pressure), and other effects common to all ACE inhibitors.

Ramsay–Hunt syndrome

A type of *herpes zoster* (shingles) that affects the *facial nerve*. Symptoms of Ramsay–Hunt syndrome include facial paralysis, intense ear pain, hearing loss, loss of taste, a painful rash on the affected part of the face, and pain in other parts of the body supplied by the facial nerve. Treatment of the condition is with *antiviral drugs* and, sometimes, *anti-inflammatory drugs*.

randomized controlled trial

A type of *controlled trial* used to evaluate the effectiveness of a drug or treatment in which subjects are randomly allocated to one of the study groups. This random allocation means an individual is equally likely to be selected to receive the treatment being investigated as to be part of the control group of the trial, which may be given a placebo (a chemically inert substance). A comparison is made between various results of the two groups to assess the benefit of the treatment in question.

ranitidine

An *ulcer-healing drug* belonging to the H_2-receptor antagonist group. Ranitidine is used to prevent and treat *peptic ulcers* and to treat *gastro-oesophageal reflux disease*. Side effects may include headache, rash, nausea, constipation, and lethargy.

ranula

A *cyst* in the floor of the mouth, which produces a translucent bluish swelling. Ranulas probably arise from damage to a *salivary gland*. Treatment of the ranula is by surgical removal.

rape

Sexual intercourse with an unwilling partner, achieved by the use or the threat of force or violence. Rape is rarely sexually motivated; it is a crime of dominance, anger, and hostility, not a crime of passion. Rape is a criminal offence.

EFFECTS
The rape victim may suffer a variety of physical injuries. Severe injury to the genitals is rare, but there may be swelling of the labia (folds of skin), bruising of the vaginal walls or cervix, and possibly tearing of the anus or the perineum (the area between the genitals and the anus).

The psychological effects of rape are often severe and may include significant *anxiety*, *depression*, or *post-traumatic stress disorder*. Nightmares or flashbacks of the event may also occur.

FORENSIC TESTS
Physical examination of a rape victim involves noting signs of bruising or injury, particularly to the genital area, and visual inspection of the vaginal canal. The doctor collects *swabs* from suspected bite marks, soiled areas of the body, and the vagina, anus, or throat, as well as fingernail scrapings or clippings and any loose strands of hair. Such specimens are analysed in a laboratory and *DNA* tests are performed on them. The results of these tests may be compared with test results on samples that are taken from a suspect.

TREATMENT
Physical injuries are treated as required. Emergency contraception (see *contraception, emergency*), *hepatitis B* vaccination, and screening for *sexually transmitted infections*, including *HIV*, are offered, and the appropriate treatment given if the tests prove positive. The victim may also be offered prophylactic antibiotics and prophylactic HIV medication.

In the treatment of psychological trauma, *counselling* may be beneficial. In some cases, psychiatric help may also be required. Many victims also find rape support groups helpful.

rash

A group of spots or an area of red, inflamed skin. A rash is usually temporary and is only rarely a sign of a serious underlying problem. A rash may be accompanied by itching or fever.

TYPES
Rashes are classified according to whether they are localized (affecting a small area of skin) or generalized (covering the entire body) and also by the type of spots present.

A macular rash consists of spots that are level with the surrounding skin and discernible from it only by a difference in colour or texture. Nodular and papular rashes are composed of small, raised bumps, which may or may not be the same colour as the surrounding skin. A bullous rash has large blisters, a vesicular rash has small blisters, and a pustular rash has blisters filled with pus. A butterfly rash is a skin eruption across the cheeks with a narrow connecting band across the nose; it is characteristic of systemic *lupus erythematosus*.

CAUSES
Rashes are the main sign of many infectious diseases, such as *chickenpox*, and are a feature of many *skin disorders*, such as *eczema* and *psoriasis*. A rash may also indicate an underlying medical problem, such as the rashes of *scurvy* or *pellagra*, which are caused by vitamin deficiency. The rashes that are characteristic of *urticaria* (nettle rash) or contact *dermatitis* may be caused by an allergic reaction (see *allergy*). Drug reactions, particularly those to *antibiotic drugs*, are another common cause.

DIAGNOSIS AND TREATMENT
Diagnosis is based on the appearance and distribution of the rash, the presence of any accompanying symptoms, and the possibility of allergy.

Any underlying cause of the rash is treated where possible. An itching rash may be relieved by a soothing lotion, such as *calamine*, or an *antihistamine drug*. (See also *meningococcal rash*.)

RAST

An abbreviation for radioallergosorbent test. RAST is a type of *radioimmunoassay* used to detect antibodies to specific *antigens* (substances that can trigger an *immune response*).

rats, diseases from

Rats live close to human habitation and can damage and contaminate crops and food stores, and can also spread disease.

The organisms responsible for *plague* and one type of *typhus* are transmitted to humans by the bites of rat fleas. *Leptospirosis* (Weil's disease) is caused by contact with anything contaminated with rat's urine.

Rat-bite fever is a rare infection transmitted directly by a rat bite. There are two types of rat-bite fever, each caused by different bacteria. Symptoms include inflammation at the site of the bite and in nearby *lymph nodes* and vessels; bouts of fever; a rash; and, in one type, painful joint inflammation. Treatment for both types is with *antibiotic drugs*.

The *rabies* virus can be transmitted by the bites of infected rats. *Lassa fever*, another viral disease, may be contracted from the urine of infected rats in West Africa. Rats also carry the viral infection lymphocytic choriomeningitis, as well as the bacterial infection *tularaemia*.

Raynaud's disease

A disorder of the blood vessels in which exposure to cold causes the small arteries supplying the fingers and toes to contract suddenly. This action cuts off blood flow to the digits, which become pale. The fingers are more frequently affected than the toes. The cause of Raynaud's disease is unknown, but young women are most commonly affected.

Symptoms develop with no known cause. On exposure to cold, the digits turn white due to lack of blood. As sluggish blood flow returns, the digits become blue; when they are warmed and normal blood flow returns, they turn red. During an attack, there is often tingling, numbness, or a burning feeling in the affected fingers or toes. In rare cases, the artery walls gradually thicken, permanently reducing blood flow, leading to painful ulceration or even *gangrene* (tissue death) at the tips of the affected digits.

Treatment involves keeping the hands and feet as warm as possible; it is also important to stop smoking. *Vasodilator drugs* or *calcium channel blockers* may be prescribed in severe cases. (See also *Raynaud's phenomenon*).

Raynaud's phenomenon

A circulatory disorder affecting the fingers and toes that shares the mechanism, symptoms, and signs of *Raynaud's disease* but which results from a known underlying disorder. Possible causes of Raynaud's phenomenon include arterial diseases, such as *atherosclerosis* (fat

R

deposits on the artery walls); connective tissue diseases, such as *rheumatoid arthritis*; and various drugs, such as *beta-blocker drugs*. Raynaud's phenomenon is a recognized occupational disorder (commonly known as vibration white finger) of people who use pneumatic drills, chain saws, or other vibrating machinery, and other people whose fingers suffer repeated trauma.

Treatment is the same as for Raynaud's disease, along with treatment of the underlying disorder.

reactive arthritis

Inflammation of the joints due to an abnormal *immune response* (the body's defensive response to foreign substances) that occurs after an infection of the genital tract, such as *chlamydial infection*, or of the intestinal tract, such as *gastroenteritis*. If there is additional inflammation elsewhere in the body, such as in the eyes, the condition is known as *Reiter's syndrome*.

reactive depression

A term that was formerly used to describe a type of *depression* (feelings of sadness, hopelessness, and a lack of interest in life) resulting from a stressful or emotional event or period of life. In contrast, another type of depression known as "endogenous depression" was seen to originate from biological factors within an individual. In the majority of cases, however, depression is a combination of these two types.

reactive hypoglycaemia

A form of *hypoglycaemia* (low blood glucose levels) that occurs within a few hours of eating foods that are rich in glucose. In reactive hypoglycaemia, the body overreacts to the sudden rise in blood sugar by releasing large amounts of *insulin*. This results in a rapid and excessive drop in the blood sugar level causing hypoglycaemic symptoms.

reagent

A term that is used for any chemical substance that takes part in a chemical reaction. The term usually refers to a chemical or a mixture of chemicals that are used in chemical analysis (see *analysis, chemical*) or used to detect a biological substance.

TYPES OF **RECEPTOR**

Stimuli are detected by the free endings of sensory nerve cells or by special structures forming the endings of these cells. These respond to specific stimuli (such as light of a certain wavelength) and send a signal indicating the presence of the stimulus to the spinal cord and/or the brain. Cell surface or chemical receptors (right) are tiny structures on the outer surface of a cell. They allow certain chemicals to bind to the cell and trigger some change within it.

Skin receptors
The skin contains many types of receptor that respond to stimuli such as pressure, cold, heat, and hair movement, allowing the sensations of touch, temperature, and pain. They include such structures as pacinian corpuscles and Merkel's discs and are all special types of nerve cell ending.

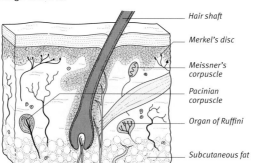

Hair shaft
Merkel's disc
Meissner's corpuscle
Pacinian corpuscle
Organ of Ruffini
Subcutaneous fat

Receptors in tongue
Each taste-bud (below) consists of many receptor cells. Each has surface receptors that respond to chemicals in food.

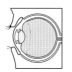

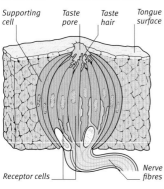

Supporting cell
Taste pore
Taste hair
Tongue surface
Receptor cells
Nerve fibres

Receptors in eye
The retina, located at the back of the eye, contains receptor cells, called rods and cones, which are responsive to light.

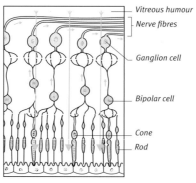

Vitreous humour
Nerve fibres
Ganglion cell
Bipolar cell
Cone
Rod

HOW CELL SURFACE OR CHEMICAL RECEPTORS WORK

Most cells have many surface receptors (only one is shown below). Their existence allows the activity of the cell to be influenced from outside.

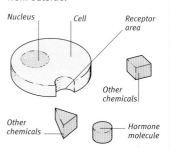

Nucleus
Cell
Receptor area
Other chemicals
Other chemicals
Hormone molecule

1 A receptor allows only one specific chemical (which may be a hormone or a neurotransmitter substance) to bind to it. The chemical must have a configuration that "fits" the receptor.

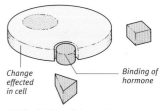

Change effected in cell
Binding of hormone

2 The binding of chemical to receptor alters the outer cell membrane and triggers a change, such as contraction by a muscle cell or increased activity in an enzyme-producing cell.

R

reboxetine

An *antidepressant drug* that blocks the reuptake of *noradrenaline* (norepinephrine) within the nervous system. Side effects of reboxetine include insomnia, sweating, and dizziness on standing.

receding chin

Underdevelopment of the lower jaw. The condition can be corrected by the use of *orthodontic appliances* if used in the growth spurt at adolescence or by *cosmetic surgery*.

receding gums

Withdrawal of the gums from around the teeth, resulting in the exposure of part of the roots. The teeth may become sensitive to hot and cold substances and the attachment of the tooth in the socket may weaken, causing the tooth to become loose. Severe cases of receding gums are usually a sign of gum disease (see *gingivitis*; *periodontitis*).

receding hairline

A feature that is characteristic of male-pattern baldness (see *alopecia*).

receptor

A general term for any sensory nerve cell (one that converts stimuli into nerve impulses). The term receptor is also used to refer to specific structures that occur on the surface of a cell (see *Types of receptor* box, left) that allow chemicals to bind with the cell in order to exert their effects.

recessive

A term used in *genetics* to describe a gene that shows its effects only when it is present in a double dose in the genotype: that is, when there is a pair of the recessive gene. If a recessive gene is not paired, its effects are overridden by the corresponding *dominant* gene. For example, the gene for blue eye colour is recessive and the gene for brown eyes is dominant; therefore if a child inherits the gene for brown eyes from one parent and the gene for blue eyes from the other, the "blue eye" gene is overridden by the "brown eye" gene and the child has brown eyes. The child must inherit two of the recessive blue eye genes, one from each parent, to have blue eyes. Many genetic disorders, such as *cystic fibrosis* and *sickle cell anaemia*, are determined by recessive genes. A child will only have the disease if he or she inherits the gene from both parents.

recombinant DNA

A section of *DNA* (genetic material) from one organism that has been artificially spliced into the DNA of another organism, often that of a viral or bacterial cell. This procedure may be carried out in order to make the recipient cell produce a substance that it would not normally be able to produce. An example of this technique is the addition of a DNA section containing the genetic code for the hormone *insulin* into a recipient cell. If this cell can be encouraged to replicate, it is possible for large amounts of the hormone to be obtained. (See also *genetic engineering*.)

reconstructive surgery

See *arterial reconstructive surgery*; *plastic surgery*.

recovery position

The position in which to place an unconscious, breathing casualty, while waiting for medical help to arrive.

The body is placed on its side with the upper leg bent at a right angle; the lower leg is kept straight. The lower arm is bent at a right angle; the upper arm is bent with the back of the hand placed against the lower cheek to support the head, which is tilted back to keep the airway open. Casualties with suspected spinal injuries should not be placed in the recovery position.

recovery room

A hospital unit situated near operating theatres and delivery rooms that contains specialized equipment and staff who have been trained in the monitoring and care of postoperative patients and women who have recently given birth. Patients leave the recovery room to return to general nursing care as soon as they are considered to be in a sufficiently safe and stable condition. (See also *intensive care unit*.)

rectal bleeding

The passage of blood from the *rectum* or *anus*. The blood may range in colour from bright red to dark brown or black. It may be mixed with, or on the surface of, *faeces* or passed separately. Rectal bleeding may or may not be accompanied by pain.

Haemorrhoids (swollen veins in the lining of the anus) are the most common cause of rectal bleeding. Small amounts of bright red blood appear on the surface of faeces or on toilet paper. *Anal fissure* (a tear at the margin of the

RECOMBINANT DNA AND GENETICALLY ENGINEERED INSULIN

Genetic engineering can force bacteria to produce human insulin. The insulin gene is obtained (by removing it from human DNA, then purifying it) and spliced into the DNA of a bacterium, causing it to produce human insulin. The bacterium is then cultured for large-scale insulin extraction.

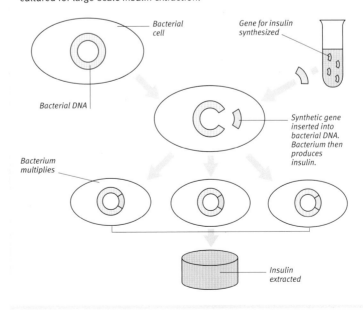

Bacterial cell

Gene for insulin synthesized

Bacterial DNA

Synthetic gene inserted into bacterial DNA. Bacterium then produces insulin.

Bacterium multiplies

Insulin extracted

R

anus), *anal fistula* (an abnormal anal channel), *proctitis* (inflammation of the rectum), or *rectal prolapse* (protrusion of the rectal lining) may also cause bleeding from the rectum.

Cancer of the colon (see *colon, cancer of*) or the rectum (see *rectum, cancer of*) or *polyps* (grape-like growths) can also cause bleeding. Disorders of the colon, such as *diverticular disease*, may cause dark red faeces. Black faeces (see *melaena*) may be due to bleeding from high in the digestive tract. Bloody diarrhoea may be caused by *ulcerative colitis, amoebiasis,* or *shigellosis.*

Diagnosis may be made from a *rectal examination, proctoscopy, sigmoidoscopy,* or *colonoscopy* (internal examination using a rigid or flexible viewing instrument), or a double-contrast *barium X-ray examination.* Rectal bleeding in anyone over the age of 40 should be carefully investigated to rule out the possibility of colorectal cancer.

rectal examination

Examination of the *anus* and *rectum,* which may be performed as part of a general *physical examination.* A rectal examination is usually used to assess symptoms of pain, changes in bowel habits, the size of the prostate gland, or to check for the presence of *tumours* of the rectum or *prostate gland.*

rectal prolapse

Protrusion outside the *anus* of the lining of the *rectum,* usually brought on by straining to defaecate. The condition commonly causes discomfort, a mucus discharge, and *rectal bleeding.*

Rectal prolapse is usually temporary in young children, but it is often permanent in elderly people due to a weakening of the tissues that support the perineum (the area between the anus and the external genitals). In cases in which the prolapse is large, leakage of *faeces* may occur.

Treatment is with a fibre-rich diet. Surgery may also be performed, especially on older people.

rectocele

A bulging inwards and downwards of the back wall of the *vagina,* which occurs as a result of the *rectum* pushing against weakened tissues in the vaginal wall. A rectocele is usually associated with a *cystocele* (protrusion of the bladder into the front wall of the vagina) or a prolapsed uterus (see *uterus, prolapse of*).

STRUCTURE OF THE **RECTUM**

The rectum is about 12 cm long; its wall consists mainly of longitudinal and circular muscle. An inner, mucous layer provides lubrication.

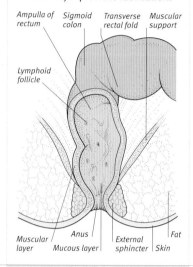

There may be no symptoms or the rectocele may cause *constipation. Pelvic floor exercises* may help to relieve symptoms. If the exercises do not help, an operation to tighten the tissues at the back of the vagina may be recommended.

rectum

A short, muscular tube that forms the lowest part of the large intestine and connects it to the *anus.*

STRUCTURE

The first part of the rectum consists of four layers: an outermost serous layer; a muscular layer; a submucous layer; and an innermost mucous layer that lubricates the rectum. There is no serous layer in the last third of the rectum.

FUNCTION

The rectum collects *faeces* that have formed in the alimentary tract (the tubelike structure that extends from the mouth to the anus). Pressure on the rectal wall causes nerve impulses to pass to the brain; the urge to defaecate occurs when the collected faeces distend (stretch) the rectum.

DISORDERS

Rarely, a baby is born with no rectum or anus (see *anus, imperforate*). There are various diseases and disorders that affect the rectum, including *proctitis* (inflammation), *polyps* (grapelike growths), and cancer (see *rectum, cancer of*).

The rectum can become obstructed as a result of narrowing, which may be caused by *radiotherapy, granuloma inguinale* (a sexually transmitted infection), or a pelvic infection. In rare cases, an *ulcer* develops in the rectum, causing bleeding and a discharge.

Rectal prolapse occurs when the lining of the rectum protrudes outside the anus. In a *rectocele,* the rectum and rear wall of the vagina bulge downwards into the vagina.

Rectal disorders are usually diagnosed by means of *rectal examination* and *proctoscopy* or *sigmoidoscopy* (internal examination using a rigid or flexible viewing instrument).

rectum, cancer of

A malignant *tumour* in the *rectum* (the muscular tube that forms the last part of the large intestine). There may be a genetic basis for some types of rectal cancer. In particular, an inherited disorder called familial adenomatous *polyposis* (in which large numbers of polyps develop in the large intestine) increases the risk. In most cases, however, the precise cause is unknown. Dietary factors, such as eating a lot of meat and fatty foods and not enough fibre, may also increase the risk. Cancer of the rectum is most common between the ages of 50 and 70.

SYMPTOMS

Early symptoms of cancer of the rectum are *rectal bleeding* during defaecation and diarrhoea or constipation. Later, pain may occur. Left untreated, the cancer may eventually cause severe bleeding and pain and block the intestine, preventing the passage of faeces. The cancer may also spread to other organs.

DIAGNOSIS AND TREATMENT

Most cases can be diagnosed by a *rectal examination* and confirmed by means of *proctoscopy* or *sigmoidoscopy* (internal examination using a rigid or flexible viewing instrument) and a *biopsy* (removal of a sample of tissue for microscopic analysis). A barium enema (see *barium X-ray examinations*) may also be done in some cases.

Treatment is usually with surgery. For a tumour in the upper rectum, the affected area and the last part of the colon are removed and the two free ends of the intestine are sewn together. To promote healing, a temporary *colostomy* (which diverts faeces through a surgical opening in the abdomen) may be made. For a growth in the lower rectum, the entire

R

rectum and anus are removed. Because there is no outlet for faeces, a permanent colostomy is created. *Radiotherapy* and *anticancer drugs* may be used in addition to, or instead of, surgery. The outlook depends on how widespread the cancer is at the time treatment is started.

recurrent pregnancy loss

Another term for *habitual miscarriage*.

red blood cell

Also known as an erythrocyte, a *blood cell* containing the red, oxygen-carrying pigment *haemoglobin*. The main function of red blood cells is to transport oxygen around the body. A mature red blood cell is a biconcave disc shape and does not have a nucleus. (See also *white blood cell*.)

red-eye

Another name for *conjunctivitis*.

reduction

The process of manipulating a displaced part of the body back into its original position. Reduction may be carried out to realign fractured bone ends (see *fracture*), to replace a dislocated joint in its socket (see *dislocation, joint*), or to treat an abdominal *hernia* by pushing the protruding intestine back through the abdominal wall.

Reference Nutrient Intake (RNI)

Figures, based on the needs of a healthy individual, that establish the minimum daily requirements of vitamins and minerals. Requirements of certain vitamins and minerals may differ according to factors such as age, gender, and stage of life.

referred pain

Pain felt in a part of the body at some distance from its cause. Referred pain occurs because some remote parts of the body are served by the same *nerve* or group of nerves. Occasionally, nerve impulses that reach the brain from one of these areas may be misinterpreted as coming from another.

Examples of referred pain are *sciatica* and the pain down the inside of the left arm caused by *angina pectoris* (pain due to impaired blood supply to the heart) or a *myocardial infarction* (heart attack).

reflex

An action that occurs automatically and predictably in response to a particular stimulus; a reflex is independent of the will of the individual.

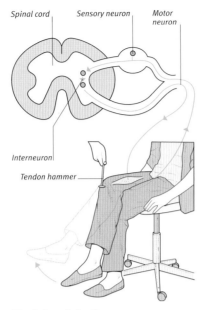

Simple knee-jerk reflex
A tap with a rubber hammer just below the kneecap stretches a tendon of one of the thigh muscles. A signal passes via a sensory neuron (nerve cell) to the spinal cord, activating a motor neuron, which contracts the muscle, jerking the lower leg upwards.

In the simplest reflex, a sensory nerve cell reacts to a stimulus, such as heat or pressure, and sends a signal along its nerve fibre to the *central nervous system* (the brain and spinal cord). There, another nerve cell becomes stimulated and causes a muscle to contract or a gland to increase its secretory activity. The passage of the nerve signal from original sensation to final action is known as a reflex arc.

Reflexes may be inborn or conditioned. Some inborn reflexes occur only in babies (see *reflex, primitive*), such as the grasp reflex that occurs when an adult's finger is placed in the baby's palm. Inborn reflexes include those that control basic body functions, such as contraction of the bladder after it has filled beyond a certain point. Such inborn reflexes are managed by the *autonomic nervous system*.

Conditioned reflexes are acquired through experience in a process called *conditioning*. For example, a person may follow a familiar route home from work without making a conscious effort.

Several simple reflexes, such as the knee-jerk reflex and constriction of the pupil in response to light, are tested in a *physical examination*. Changes in reflexes may indicate damage to the nervous

system. The examination of vital reflexes that are controlled by the brainstem is the basis for diagnosing *brain death*.

reflexology

A form of *complementary medicine* in which the practitioner massages parts of the patient's feet in an attempt to treat disorders affecting other areas of the body.

reflex, primitive

An automatic movement in response to a stimulus that is present in newborn infants but disappears during the first few months after birth. Primitive reflexes are believed to represent actions that may have been important for survival in earlier stages of human evolution.

Primitive reflexes include the grasp reflex, which occurs when something is placed in the baby's hand, and the rooting reflex, which enables a baby to find the nipple (see *Types of primitive reflex* box, overleaf).

Primitive reflexes are tested after birth to give an indication of the condition of an infant's nervous system. Their persistence beyond the expected stage of development may point to a disorder of the developing brain.

reflux

Abnormal backflow of fluid in a body passage, which may result from failure of the passage's exit to close properly. A common type is the *regurgitation* of acidic fluid from the stomach into the oesophagus (see *gastro-oesophageal reflux disease*). (See also *vesicoureteric reflux*.)

reflux oesophagitis

A type of *oesophagitis* (inflammation of the oesophagus) that is caused by poor functioning of the muscles in the lower oesophagus, leading to *gastro-oesophageal reflux disease*.

reflux, vesicoureteric

See *vesicoureteric reflux*.

refraction

The bending of light rays as they pass from one substance to another. Refraction is the mechanism by which images are focused on the *retina* in the eye.

Refsum's disease

A rare *genetic disorder* that affects lipid metabolism (the processing of fats by the body). Refsum's disease causes excessively high levels of phytanic acid, a fatty acid, in the body.

R

TYPES OF PRIMITIVE **REFLEX**

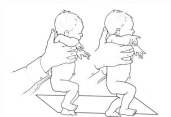

Grasping reflex
Certain automatic reflexes are present early in life before the baby becomes capable of voluntary movement. These reflexes disappear as the nervous system matures. For about the first four months, any object placed in the infant's palm will be firmly grasped.

Tonic neck reflex
When the young baby turns the head, the arm, and leg of that side are stretched out while on the other side the arm and leg bend. This reflex normally disappears after the first few months except in premature babies. A strong reflex, persisting for longer than three months, suggests brain damage.

Walking reflex
When the baby is held upright with a foot touching the ground, a forward stepping movement is made by each leg as the weight is placed on the other foot. This occurs during the first two months of life and is then lost.

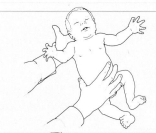

Moro reflex
If the baby's head is momentarily left unsupported, the arms will be swung outwards and then brought together in an embracing movement. At the same time the legs are extended and the baby cries. This symmetrical reflex disappears two or three months after birth.

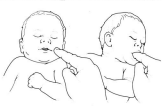

Rooting reflex
This reflex enables the baby to find the nipple. It is evoked by touching the baby's cheek near the corner of the mouth. The baby's head turns and the mouth opens. The reflex is best shown if tried when the baby is hungry.

One major symptom is *polyneuritis* (inflammation of nerves). This may result in weakness and numbness, often affecting the limbs. Other common features are a visual defect called *retinitis pigmentosa* and *ataxia* (unsteady gait caused by damage to the brain's *cerebellum*). Symptoms usually appear before the age of 20. The disease is progressive, although there are periods of remission.

People with Refsum's disease are advised to avoid all foods containing phytanic acid. The main dietary sources of this substance are meat from animals that feed on grass (cows, sheep, and goats) and dairy products.

Regaine

A brand name for *minoxidil*. Regaine is used as a topical lotion in the treatment of male-pattern baldness (see *alopecia*).

regression

A term used in *psychoanalytic theory* to describe the process of returning to a childhood level of behaviour, such as thumb-sucking. (See also *fixation*.)

regurgitation

A backflow of fluid. In medicine, the term is commonly used to describe the return of swallowed food or drink from the stomach into the *oesophagus* and

mouth. The term is also used to describe the backflow of blood through a *heart valve* that does not close fully because of a disorder such as *mitral incompetence*. (See also *reflux*.)

rehabilitation

Treatment aimed at enabling a person to live an independent life following injury (such as *spinal injury*), illness (such as a *stroke*), *alcohol dependence*, or *drug dependence*. Treatment may include *physiotherapy*, *occupational therapy*, *psychotherapy*, or *speech therapy*.

In a rehabilitation centre, a person's *disability* or dependence is assessed by a doctor who specializes in rehabilitation medicine, and a treatment programme is developed. Industrial rehabilitation centres provide retraining for those who cannot return to their previous job. Drug and alcohol rehabilitation centres help people through *withdrawal* and provide psychological support to reduce the risk of a relapse (the recurrence of a condition after apparent recovery).

rehydration, oral

See *rehydration therapy*.

rehydration therapy

The treatment of *dehydration* by administering fluids, salts, and sugars usually by mouth (oral rehydration) or by *intravenous infusion*. The amount of fluid needed depends on the patient's age and weight and the degree of dehydration.

Mild dehydration, which occurs in many young children with diarrhoea, can usually be treated with oral solutions, which are available as an effervescent tablet or powder to be made up at home. In severe dehydration, or if the patient cannot take fluids by mouth because of nausea or vomiting, an *intravenous infusion* of *saline* and/or *glucose* solution may be given in hospital.

reimplantation, dental

The replacement of a *tooth* in its socket after an accident so that it can become reattached to supporting tissues. The front teeth are those that are most commonly reimplanted. Primary teeth should not be reimplanted, only secondary (adult) teeth.

The tooth needs to be reimplanted soon after the accident; it is then maintained with the help of a splint (see *splinting, dental*) while healing takes place. If the tooth cannot be replaced in its socket immediately, it should be put

R

in milk or in the injured person's mouth between the cheek and gum, and a dentist should be seen as soon as possible.

Reiter's syndrome

A condition in which there is a combination of *urethritis*, *reactive arthritis*, and *conjunctivitis*. There may also be *uveitis*. Reiter's syndrome is more common in men than in women.

It is caused by an *immune response* and usually develops only in people with a genetic predisposition. Most patients have the HLA-B27 tissue type (see *histocompatability antigens*). The syndrome's development is induced by infection: usually by *nongonococcal urethritis*, but sometimes by bacillary *dysentery*.

Reiter's syndrome usually starts with a urethral discharge, followed by conjunctivitis, and then arthritis. The arthritis usually affects one or two joints (generally the knee and/or ankle) and is often associated with *fever* and malaise. Attacks can last for several months. Tendons, ligaments, and tissue in the soles of the feet may also become inflamed. Skin rashes are common.

Diagnosis is from the symptoms. *Analgesic drugs* (painkillers) and *nonsteroidal anti-inflammatory drugs* (NSAIDs) relieve pain and inflammation but may have to be taken long term. The urethritis is treated with antibiotics. Relapses occur in about one third of cases.

rejection

An *immune response* that is aimed at destroying organisms or substances recognized as foreign by the body's *immune system*. Rejection also refers to nonacceptance of tissue grafts (see *grafting*) or organ transplants (see *transplant surgery*).

To avoid rejection, donor tissues are closely matched to recipient ones (see *tissue-typing*). *Immunosuppressant drugs*, such as *corticosteroid drugs* and *ciclosporin*, are given to organ transplant recipients to suppress rejection.

relapse

The recurrence of a disease after an apparent recovery, or the return of symptoms after a period of *remission*.

relapsing fever

An illness that is caused by infection with *spirochaetes* (spiral-shaped bacteria). Relapsing fever is transmitted to humans by *ticks* or *lice* and is characterized by high fever. The condition does not occur in the UK.

A high fever of up to 40°C suddenly develops, with shivering, headache, muscle pains, nausea, and vomiting. The symptoms persist for three to six days, culminating in a *crisis* with a risk of collapse and death. The affected person then seems to recover but suffers another attack seven to ten days later. If the fever is tick-borne, there may be several such relapses, each progressively milder.

The spirochaetes can be seen in a blood film and they can be eliminated with antibiotic drugs.

relationship counselling

Formerly known as marriage guidance, a type of professional therapy for established partners aimed at resolving the problems within their relationship. The couple attends regular sessions together in which the counsellor promotes communication and attempts to help resolve differences. Relationship counselling is largely based on the ideas and methods of *behaviour therapy*. If some of the couple's problems are sexual, the counsellor may also refer them for *sex therapy*.

relaxation techniques

Methods of consciously releasing muscular tension to achieve a state of mental calm. Relaxation techniques can assist people with symptoms of *anxiety*, help to reduce *hypertension* (high blood pressure), and relieve stress. They may also be used to help pregnant women to cope with labour pains (see *childbirth, natural*).

Active relaxation consists of tensing and relaxing each of the body's muscles in turn. Passive relaxation involves clearing the mind and concentrating on a single phrase or sound. *Breathing exercises* help to prevent *hyperventilation*, which often brings on or worsens anxiety. Traditional methods, such as *yoga* and *meditation*, employ similar techniques.

releasing factors

A group of *hormones* produced by the *hypothalamus* in the brain that stimulate the release of other hormones. *Luteinizing hormone-releasing hormone* is an example.

Relenza

The brand name for *zanamivir*, an *antiviral drug* used to treat at-risk people who develop influenza.

rem

An outdated unit of absorbed *radiation* dose, now superseded by the *sievert*. (See also *radiation unit*.)

remission

A temporary disappearance of the symptoms of a disease, or a reduction in their severity. The term may also refer or the period during which this occurs.

REM sleep

The abbreviation for rapid eye movement *sleep*, the period of sleep during which the brain is more active and *dreaming* takes place. REM sleep alternates with non-REM (NREM) sleep during the course of the night.

renal

Related to the *kidney*.

renal biopsy

See *kidney biopsy*.

renal calculus

A kidney stone (see *calculus, urinary tract*).

renal cell carcinoma

The most common type of *kidney cancer*.

renal colic

Spasms of severe pain on one side of the back, extending down to the groin, that are usually caused by a kidney stone (see *calculus, urinary tract*) passing down the *ureter* (a tube that carries urine from the kidney to the bladder). There may also be nausea, vomiting, sweating, and blood in the urine.

The treatment of renal colic usually consists of bed rest and plenty of fluids. Injections of a strong *analgesic drug* (painkiller), such as *diclofenac* or *pethidine*, help to ease the pain.

renal failure

See *kidney failure*.

renal tubular acidosis

A condition in which the *kidneys* are unable to excrete normal amounts of acid made by the body. In renal tubular acidosis, the blood is more acidic than normal, and the urine less acidic.

Possible causes of renal tubular acidosis include kidney damage that may be due to disease, drugs, or a *genetic disorder*. However, in many cases the cause of the condition is unknown.

The acidosis may result in *osteomalacia* (softening of the bones), kidney stones (see *calculus, urinary tract*), *nephrocalcinosis* (calcification of the kidney), and *hypokalaemia* (an abnormally low level of potassium in the blood).

renin

An *enzyme* that is involved in the regulation of *blood pressure*. When the blood pressure falls, the *kidneys* release renin, which changes a substance called angiotensinogen into angiotensin I. This is rapidly converted into angiotensin II, which acts to increase blood pressure by constricting (narrowing) blood vessels and stimulating the release of *aldosterone*, a hormone that causes the kidneys to retain *sodium* in the body.

Blood pressure can be lowered by drugs that affect the renin–angiotensin system, such as *beta-blocker drugs*, which inhibit the production of renin, and *ACE inhibitor drugs*, which interfere with the conversion of angiotensin I to angiotensin II.

renography

A technique, also known as renal scintigraphy, that uses a radioactive substance to measure *kidney* function. Renography is quick and painless and is used, for example, when obstruction of the passage of *urine* is suspected.

The radioactive substance is injected into the blood and passes via the kidneys into the urine. Radiation counts are taken throughout the procedure and both kidneys are examined to compare their function. Normally, the radiation count rises and then falls as the substance passes into the bladder. If an obstruction is present, the substance accumulates in the kidneys and the count continues to rise. (See also *kidney imaging*.)

repaglinide

An oral hypoglycaemic drug (see *hypoglycaemics, oral*) that is used either alone or in combination with *metformin* in the treatment of type 2 *diabetes mellitus*. Repaglinide stimulates the release of *insulin* (a hormone that regulates the blood level of glucose). Side effects may include abdominal pain, diarrhoea or constipation, nausea, and vomiting.

repetitive strain injury (RSI)

An *overuse injury* that affects people who do repetitive movements for long periods, such as keyboard workers and musicians, causing pain and weakness in the wrists, fingers, or arms. RSI can become chronic, with continuous pain that does not cease when the causative activity is stopped.

repression

A term used in *psychoanalysis* to refer to the burial of an unacceptable idea or memory deep from an individual's consciousness. The data that has been repressed is generally out of the reach of voluntary recall. One of the aims of psychoanalysis is to return repressed material to conscious awareness in order that it can be accepted and therefore dealt with in a rational manner.

reproduction, sexual

The process of producing offspring by the fusion of two cells from different individuals; this is achieved in humans by the fusion of one *sperm* and one *ovum*. This fusion (which is known as *fertilization*) may be achieved by *sexual intercourse* or *artificial insemination*.

reproductive system, female

The female organs involved in *ovulation*, *sexual intercourse*, nourishing a fertilized *ovum* (egg) until it has developed into a full-grown *fetus*, and *childbirth*. Apart from the *vulva* (the external genitalia that protect the opening of the *vagina*), these organs lie within the pelvic cavity.

An ovum is released each month from one of the two *ovaries*, which also secrete *oestrogen hormones* and *progesterone hormones* – hormones involved in the control of the reproductive cycle, together with *follicle-stimulating* hormone and *luteinizing* hormone. The ovum travels through the *fallopian tubes* to the *uterus*. *Fertilization* takes place if a *sperm* released into the vagina during *sexual intercourse* or *artificial insemination* travels through the *cervix* and uterus to penetrate the ovum while it is in the fallopian tube.

The normal functioning of the female reproductive system begins at *puberty* with the onset of *menstruation*; the potential for reproduction ends at the time of the *menopause*.

reproductive system, male

The male organs involved in the production of *sperm* and in *sexual intercourse*. Sperm and male sex hormones (see *androgen hormones*) are produced in the testes (see *testis*), which are suspended in the *scrotum*. From each testis, sperm pass into an *epididymis* (a long coiled tube behind the testis), where they mature and are stored. Shortly before *ejaculation*, sperm are propelled into a duct (called the *vas deferens*), which carries them to the *seminal vesicles* behind the *bladder*. These two sacs produce *seminal fluid*, which is added to the sperm to produce *semen*.

Semen travels along two ducts to the *urethra* (a tube that is a passage for urine and semen). The two ducts pass through the *prostate gland*, which produces secretions that are added to the semen. At *orgasm*, semen is ejaculated from the urethra through the erect *penis*, which is placed in the woman's *vagina* during sexual intercourse. (See also *fertilization*.)

rescue breathing

The forced introduction of air into the lungs of someone who has stopped breathing (see *respiratory arrest*) or who

FEMALE REPRODUCTIVE SYSTEM

Each month an ovum from one ovary is carried along the fallopian tube. If fertilized, it begins to divide and implants into the endometrium (lining of the uterus) to develop into an embryo. If the ovum is not fertilized, the endometrium is shed in the form of menstrual bleeding.

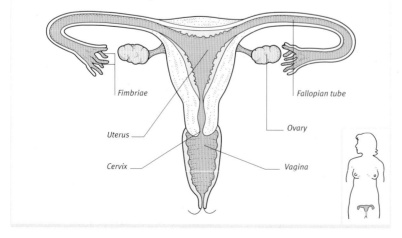

Fimbriae

Fallopian tube

Uterus

Ovary

Cervix

Vagina

MALE REPRODUCTIVE SYSTEM

Sperm made in the testes pass via the vas deferens to the seminal vesicle. Secretions from the prostate increase the volume of the semen, which is ejaculated from the penis via the urethra during orgasm.

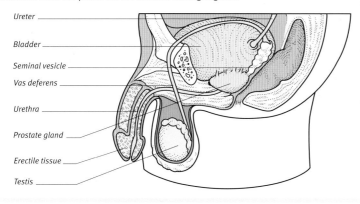

Ureter
Bladder
Seminal vesicle
Vas deferens
Urethra
Prostate gland
Erectile tissue
Testis

has inadequate breathing. Rescue breathing was known as artificial respiration. As an emergency first-aid measure, rescue breathing can be given mouth-to-mouth or mouth-to-nose in order to prevent brain damage due to oxygen deprivation; a delay in breathing for more than three minutes can cause death. Cardiac compressions may also be necessary if the heartbeat stops (see *cardiopulmonary resuscitation*).

Mouth-to-mouth resuscitation involves opening the victim's airway, pinching the nose shut, and blowing air into his or her mouth until help arrives or the victim begins breathing unaided. Mouth-to-nose resuscitation is an alternative if the victim has a facial injury. If there are no signs of circulation after rescue breathing has been given, cardiopulmonary resuscitation may also be required.

An alternative to rescue breathing that is commonly used by healthcare professionals is the "bag and mask" system. A mask is placed over the patient's face and the attached bag (which may be linked to a supply of oxygen) is squeezed hard to inflate the lungs.

resection

Surgical removal of all or part of a diseased or injured organ. An anterior resection is an operation that removes part of the large intestine as a treatment for colorectal cancer (see *colon, cancer of*; *rectum, cancer of*).

resistance

The ability to oppose. In medicine, the term resistance has several different meanings. For example, a resistance to

the flow of blood is exerted by the blood vessel walls. This resistance increases as the diameter of the blood vessels decreases, whether due to normal physiological processes or to narrowing as a result of disease. An increased resistance leads to raised blood pressure.

In *psychoanalysis*, resistance refers to the blocking off from consciousness of repressed memories or emotions (see *repression*). The psychoanalyst helps the patient to break down this resistance.

Resistance may also refer to an ability to withstand attack from poisons, irritants, or *microorganisms*. An individual's resistance to infection is called *immunity*.

Drug resistance is the ability of some microorganisms to resist attack from previously effective drug treatments. Certain bacteria have acquired *genes* (units of hereditary material) that confer protection against certain *antibiotic drugs*. Overuse of these antibiotics encourages the spread of resistant strains, so doctors now try to avoid the indiscriminate prescription of these drugs.

resorption, bone

Loss of substance from *bone*. Bone resorption and new bone formation are a normal part of bone physiology. In conditions such as *osteoporosis* (loss of bone tissue), however, the rate of bone resorption exceeds that of bone formation.

resorption, dental

The loss of substance from *teeth*. The loss may be external (affecting the surface of the root) or internal (affecting the wall of the pulp cavity).

External resorption is part of the process by which *primary teeth* are lost and is thought to be activated by pressure from the underlying *permanent teeth* as they erupt (see *eruption of teeth*). Some degree of external resorption also occurs as part of the aging process and may also be due to injury, inflammation of surrounding tissues (see *periodontitis*), or pressure, for example from an impacted tooth (see *impaction, dental*). Internal resorption is rare, occurring in only about one per cent of adults, and is of unknown cause.

Resorption is usually detected from a *dental X-ray*. Treatment of external resorption depends on the underlying cause. Internal resorption can usually be halted by *root-canal treatment*.

respiration

A term for the processes by which *oxygen* reaches body cells and is utilized by them (see *metabolism*) and by which *carbon dioxide* is eliminated.

Air, containing oxygen, is breathed into the *lungs* and enters the alveoli (tiny, balloonlike sacs; see *alveolus, pulmonary*). Oxygen diffuses into the blood, which then carries it to cells in the body, where it is used to metabolize *glucose* to provide energy. Carbon dioxide is produced as a waste product and passes into the blood from the body cells. It is transported via the blood to the lungs to be breathed out.

Respiration is controlled automatically by the respiratory centre in the *brainstem* (see *Respiration* box, overleaf). (See also *respiratory system*.)

respirator

See *ventilator*.

respiratory arrest

Sudden cessation of *breathing* that may be due to problems affecting the respiratory apparatus, such as severe *asthma*, sudden exacerbation of chronic obstructive pulmonary disease (see *pulmonary disease, chronic obstructive*), or obstruction of the airways; to any process that depresses the function of the respiratory centre in the *brainstem*, including prolonged *seizures*, an overdose of opioid *analgesic drugs*, *electrical injury*, serious *head injury*, or *stroke*; or to *cardiac arrest*.

Respiratory arrest leads rapidly to *anoxia* (lack of oxygen to tissues) and, if the condition is left untreated, it will progress to cardiac arrest (due to a reduced oxygen supply to the coronary

R

RESPIRATION

The function of respiration is to provide the energy needed by body cells. Cells obtain this energy mainly by metabolizing glucose with oxygen, and so they require a constant supply of oxygen. In addition, the waste products of the metabolic process (mainly carbon dioxide) must be carried away from the cells.

Respiration includes the breathing of air into the lungs, the transfer of oxygen from the air to the blood, the transport of oxygen in the blood to the body cells, the metabolism of glucose with oxygen in the cells, and the transport of carbon dioxide to the lungs to be breathed out.

During exercise, respiration increases to compensate for higher energy demands by muscle cells.

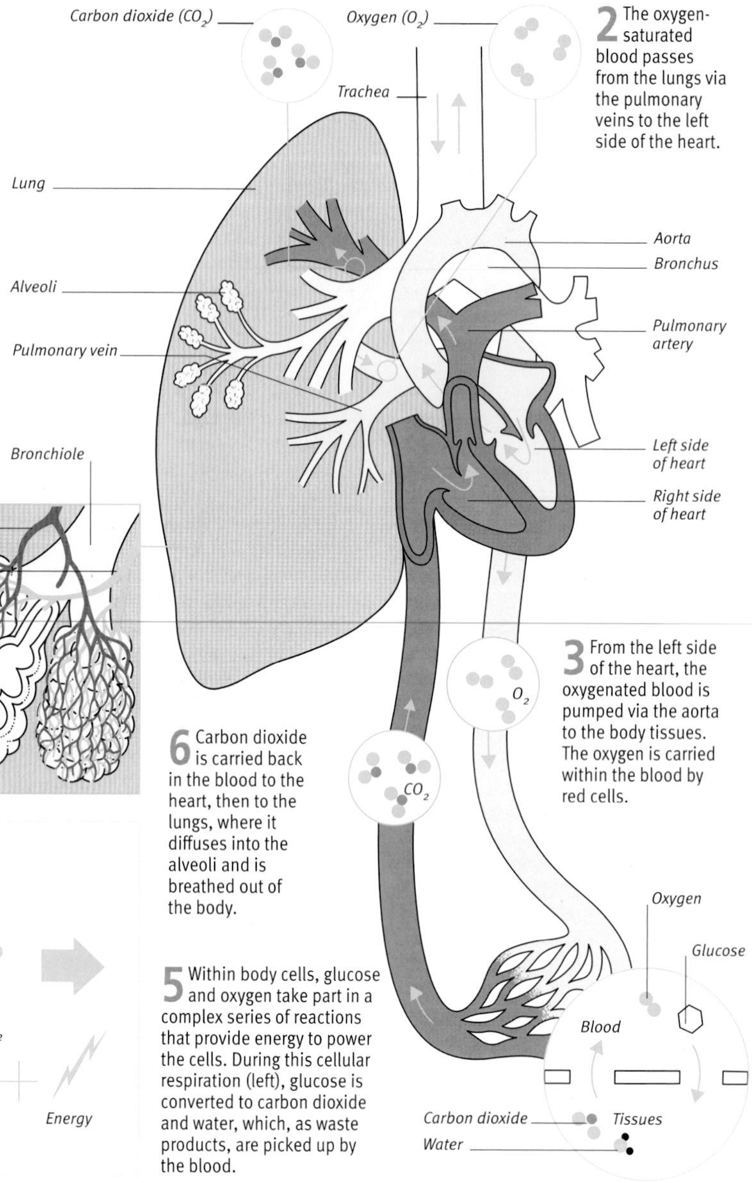

Carbon dioxide (CO₂) — $Carbon\ dioxide\ (CO_2)$

Oxygen (O₂) — $Oxygen\ (O_2)$

Trachea

Lung

Alveoli

Pulmonary vein

Bronchiole

Artery

Vein

Alveolus

Network of capillaries

Aorta

Bronchus

Pulmonary artery

Left side of heart

Right side of heart

2 The oxygen-saturated blood passes from the lungs via the pulmonary veins to the left side of the heart.

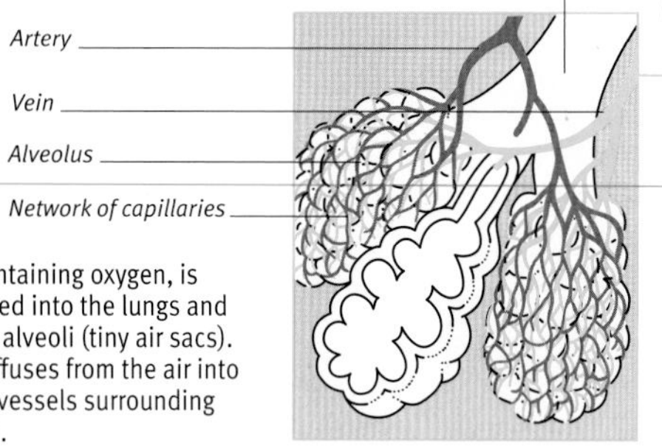

1 Air, containing oxygen, is breathed into the lungs and enters the alveoli (tiny air sacs). Oxygen diffuses from the air into the blood vessels surrounding the alveoli.

CELLULAR RESPIRATION

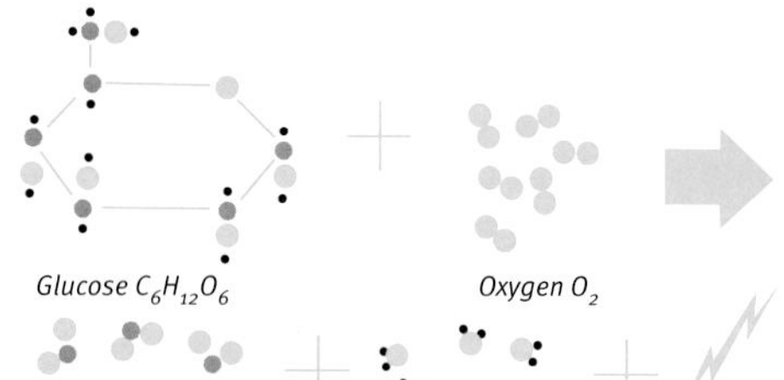

Glucose $C_6H_{12}O_6$

Oxygen O_2

Carbon dioxide CO_2

Water H_2O

Energy

6 Carbon dioxide is carried back in the blood to the heart, then to the lungs, where it diffuses into the alveoli and is breathed out of the body.

5 Within body cells, glucose and oxygen take part in a complex series of reactions that provide energy to power the cells. During this cellular respiration (left), glucose is converted to carbon dioxide and water, which, as waste products, are picked up by the blood.

3 From the left side of the heart, the oxygenated blood is pumped via the aorta to the body tissues. The oxygen is carried within the blood by red cells.

O_2

CO_2

Oxygen

Glucose

Blood

Carbon dioxide

Water

Tissues

4 As the blood passes through tissue capillaries, it gives up oxygen (and nutrients such as glucose) to the body tissues and cells.

BREATHING VOLUMES

One way the body copes with varied demands for oxygen is through changes in breathing volume. The tidal volume – the amount breathed into and out of the lungs at each breath – may vary from 0.5 litre at rest, up to 4.5 litres (near the maximum or vital capacity) during heavy exercise.

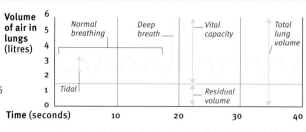

Volume of air in lungs (litres)

Normal breathing

Deep breath

Vital capacity

Total lung volume

Tidal

Residual volume

Time (seconds)   10   20   30   40

R

arteries), brain damage, *coma*, and death. The patient should be given *rescue breathing* and, if necessary, placed on a *ventilator* without delay. The cause of the respiratory arrest will be treated.

respiratory distress syndrome

An acute lung disorder that makes breathing difficult and leads to *respiratory failure*, resulting in life-threatening *hypoxia* (an inadequate supply of oxygen to the tissues). The condition may also cause failure of other systems; for example, *heart failure* or *kidney failure*.

There are two types of respiratory distress syndrome. The first is seen in premature babies (see *prematurity*): the lungs are stiff and do not inflate easily due to a lack of *surfactant*, a group of chemicals that keep the alveoli (tiny air sacs in the lungs; see *alveolus, pulmonary*) open. In adults, the condition is known as acute respiratory distress syndrome (ARDS) and may develop as a result of a severe injury or overwhelming infection (particularly *septicaemia*).

Breathing becomes laboured and more rapid as the condition develops. Affected babies make grunting noises and the chest wall is drawn in when they breathe. If the condition worsens, progressive deoxygenation of the blood makes the sufferer turn blue (see *cyanosis*). Without any treatment, death may eventually occur.

Treatment is for the underlying cause, as well as with artificial *ventilation* and oxygen; inhaled surfactant is given to babies thought to be at risk of respiratory distress syndrome. In cases in which premature delivery is seen to be inevitable, the mother is given corticosteroid injections in order to promote the production of fetal lung surfactant.

respiratory failure

A condition in which there is a fall in the blood oxygen level (see *hypoxia*) caused by the inadequate exchange of gases in the lungs. Respiratory failure may have a number of causes: lung disorders, such as severe *asthma* or *pneumonia*; depression of the respiratory centre in the brainstem due, for example, to an overdose of opioid *analgesic drugs*, a *stroke*, or a *head injury*; damage to the chest wall, such as *flail chest*; and nerve and muscle diseases that affect breathing, including *poliomyelitis*.

The symptoms of respiratory failure include breathlessness, *cyanosis* (bluish coloration of the skin), confusion, and agitation. Treatment is for the underlying cause, and oxygen and/or assisted *ventilation* may also be given if required. In some cases, a respiratory stimulant drug may be prescribed.

respiratory function tests

See *pulmonary function tests*.

respiratory syncytial virus (RSV)

A *paramyxovirus* that is responsible for some nose and throat infections. The RSV is one of the principal causes of *bronchiolitis* (inflammation of the bronchioles in the lungs) and *pneumonia* (inflammation of the lungs) in babies and young children.

respiratory system

The organs responsible for carrying *oxygen* from the air to the blood and expelling *carbon dioxide*.

The upper part of the respiratory system consists of two nasal passages, the *pharynx* (throat), the larynx (voicebox), and the *trachea* (windpipe). The lower part of the respiratory system consists of two *lungs*, which are enclosed in a double membrane called the *pleura*, and the lower airways (the *bronchi* and smaller bronchioles). These structures are encased in, and protected by, the bony ribcage. The airways terminate in millions of balloonlike sacs known as alveoli (see *alveolus, pulmonary*), where gas exchange with the tiny surrounding blood vessels takes place. These small blood vessels feed into larger pulmonary vessels for transport to and from the heart (see *Respiration* box, left).

Air is inhaled and exhaled (see *breathing*) by the action of the dome-shaped diaphragm and the abdominal and chest muscles, including the intercostal muscles located between the ribs. Respiration is controlled by the respiratory centre in the *brainstem*.

DISORDERS

Some disorders of the respiratory system can affect the air passages, causing obstruction of the air flow into or out of the lungs; other disorders can affect the lung tissues, resulting in a poor exchange of oxygen and carbon dioxide. The functioning of the respiratory system may also be impaired by certain disorders (such as *poliomyelitis*) that have an adverse effect on the chest muscles and diaphragm, thereby impeding the inflation of the lungs. (See also *respiratory tract infection*).

ANATOMY OF THE RESPIRATORY SYSTEM

The system includes the upper air passages, lungs, and the muscles that control breathing (not shown).

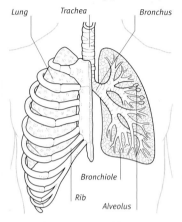

Lung   Trachea   Bronchus

Bronchiole

Rib

Alveolus

respiratory tract infection

Infection of the breathing passages, which extend from the nose to the alveoli (the tiny, balloonlike sacs in the lungs; see *alveolus, pulmonary*). This type of infection is divided into upper and lower respiratory tract infections.

Upper respiratory tract infections affect the nose, *pharynx* (throat), *sinuses*, and larynx (voicebox). Examples of such infections include the common cold, (see *cold, common*) and inflammatory conditions such as *pharyngitis*, *tonsillitis*, *sinusitis*, *laryngitis*, and *croup*.

Lower respiratory tract infections, which involve inflammation of the *trachea* (windpipe), *bronchi*, and *lungs*, include acute *bronchitis*, acute *bronchiolitis*, and *pneumonia*.

restless legs

A syndrome characterized by unpleasant tickling, burning, prickling, or aching sensations in the leg muscles.

Symptoms of restless legs tend to come on at night in bed and can interrupt sleep; they may also be triggered by prolonged sitting. The condition tends to run in families and is most common in middle-aged women, people with *rheumatoid arthritis* or *diabetes mellitus*, smokers, and pregnant women.

The cause of restless legs is unknown and there is no single cure: some patients benefit from cooling the legs; others from warming them. Relief may be obtained through movement, such

R

as walking. Treatment with *levodopa*, *benzodiazepine drugs* (such as clonazepam), or certain *anticonvulsant drugs* (such as carbamazepine) may help to improve the condition.

restoration, dental

The reconstruction of part of a damaged tooth. Restoration also refers to the material or substitute part used to rebuild the tooth.

Small repairs are usually made by filling the tooth (see *filling, dental*). For more extensive repairs, an inlay (see *inlay, dental*) or a crown (see *crown, dental*) may be fitted. Chipped front teeth may be repaired by bonding (see *bonding, dental*), in which the surface of the tooth is etched with an acidic solution and plastic or porcelain material is attached to the roughened surface.

restricted growth

See *short stature*.

resuscitation

See *cardiopulmonary resuscitation*; *rescue breathing*.

retardation

The slowing up of a process. The term mental retardation was once commonly used to refer to impaired intellectual development (see *learning difficulties*).

retching

Repeated unsuccessful, usually involuntary, attempts to vomit (see *vomiting*).

reticular formation

A network of *nerve* cells that are scattered throughout the *brainstem* (the stalk of nerve tissue that links the brain to the spinal cord).

reticulocyte

The medical term for a newly formed *red blood cell*. Reticulocytes are made in the bone marrow from *stem cells*. They remain in the bone marrow for between one and two days and then pass into the bloodstream, where they eventually mature into red blood cells.

reticulosarcoma

See *lymphoma, non-Hodgkin's*.

retina

The light-sensitive membrane that lines the back inner surface of the *eye*, and on which images are cast by the *cornea* (the transparent dome that forms the front of the eyeball) and the *lens* (the part of the eye responsible for fine focusing). The retina contains specialized nerve cells (rods and cones) that convert light into nerve impulses. The impulses travel from the rods and cones through other cells in the retina and along the *optic nerve* to the *brain*.

The rods are extremely sensitive and respond to very dim light; the cones are responsible for *colour vision*, producing impulses that vary in strength depending on the colour of the light striking them. Near the centre of the retina is the fovea, the area of the eye that is responsible for detailed vision because it contains the highest concentration of light-sensitive cells. (See also *Disorders of the retina* box, opposite.)

retinal artery occlusion

Blockage of an artery supplying blood to the *retina* (the light-sensitive inner layer at the back of the eye), most commonly due to *thrombosis* (abnormal blood clot formation) or *embolism* (in which a blood clot or fatty deposit is carried in the bloodstream to lodge in another area). Retinal artery occlusion may affect either the main retinal artery or one of its branches.

The disorder can result in sudden blindness or loss of part of the visual field, which is painless and can be permanent. The extent of visual loss depends on the artery affected and how quickly the condition can be treated. (See also *retinal vein occlusion*.)

LOCATION OF THE RETINA

The retina covers the back inner surface of the eye. It contains light-sensitive rod and cone cells, which send impulses along the optic nerve.

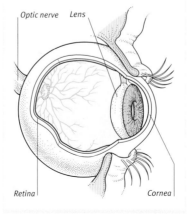

Optic nerve Lens

Retina Cornea

retinal detachment

Separation of the *retina* (the light-sensitive inner layer at the back of the *eye*) from the outer layers at the back of the eye. Retinal detachment may follow an eye injury but usually occurs spontaneously. It is usually preceded by a *retinal tear* (a split in the retina), and is more common in highly myopic (shortsighted) people, people who have had *cataract surgery*, and people with a family history of the condition.

SYMPTOMS

Retinal detachment is painless. The first indication may be the appearance of bright flashes of light caused by stimulation of the light-sensitive cells as the tear occurs. This may be accompanied by *floaters* (fragments perceived to be floating in the field of vision) that result from the release of blood or pigment into the vitreous humour (the gel-like substance that fills the rear compartment of the eye). Alternatively, the appearance of a black "drape" that gradually obscures vision may be the first sign of retinal detachment.

TREATMENT

Urgent treatment is required to prevent detachment of the macula (the site of central vision) and usually involves surgical repair of the underlying tear. A soft silicone rubber sponge may be sewn onto the outside of the *sclera* (the outer layer of the eye) overlying the detachment. The sponge indents the sclera and results in the absorption of the fluid under the retina, causing the retina to settle back into place. The retina is then fixed in place by cryopexy (the application of extreme cold), or by *laser treatment*. If the macula has not been detached, the results can be excellent.

retinal haemorrhage

Bleeding into the *retina* (the light-sensitive inner layer at the back of the eye) from one or more blood vessels. It may be due to *diabetes mellitus*, *hypertension* (high blood pressure), or *retinal vein occlusion* (blockage of a vein that drains blood from the retina).

When the macula (the site of central vision) is involved, vision is severely impaired. Peripheral haemorrhages may be detected only when the eye is examined using an *ophthalmoscope*.

retinal tear

The development of a split in the *retina* (the light-sensitive inner layer situated at the back of the eye), usually caused

R

DISORDERS OF THE **RETINA**

Despite its small size, the retina is subject to a wide variety of disorders, many of which seriously affect vision and, in some cases, result in blindness.

Congenital and genetic disorders

Colour blindness (see *colour vision deficiency*), an abnormality of retinal cones (colour receptors in the retina), usually has a genetic basis. Hereditary degenerative disorders of the macula may appear at any age, leading to serious impairment of central vision. Other degenerative disorders of the retina with a genetic basis include *Tay-Sachs disease* and *retinitis pigmentosa*.

Retrolental fibroplasia may result from exposure of a premature baby to excessive oxygen concentration (needed to treat lung immaturity), which causes abnormalities in the retinal vessels.

Infection

Toxoplasmosis is an infection of the retina that is acquired before birth and recurs later in life, causing progressive damage to the retina.

Toxocara canis is a parasitic worm whose larvae may lodge in the retina and cause severe retinal destruction, producing a white mass resembling a tumour (see *toxocariasis*). *Onchocerciasis*, an infestation by a tropical worm, may cause severe retinal damage.

Bacterial and fungal infections elsewhere in the body can be carried in the blood to the retina. People whose immune systems are impaired are more susceptible to infections that can involve the retina.

Tumours

Retinoblastoma is a cancerous tumour that usually appears in the first three years of life. There may be visual loss in the affected eye and a visible whiteness

in the pupil; *squint* often develops. The tendency to this cancer can be inherited.

Secondary cancerous tumours, spreading to the eye from primary tumours elsewhere in the body, can also occur. Malignant melanoma (see *melanoma, malignant*) can arise from the choroid (the layer beneath the retina). A variety of noncancerous tumours may also occur in the retina.

Injury

The retina may be torn or detached due to severe penetrating or blunt (non-penetrating) injury (see *retinal detachment*; *retinal tear*). Permanent damage may be caused by a retinal burn, which is sometimes caused by looking directly at the sun (even during an eclipse).

Metabolic disorders

Diabetes mellitus may cause *retinopathy*, with fluid leakage and haemorrhage into the retina (see *retinal haemorrhage*) and with the growth of new, fragile blood vessels on the retinal surface, which bleed readily. Vitreous haemorrhage (bleeding into the vitreous humour, the gel-like substance that fills the rear compartment of the eye) may occur from blood vessels, and fibrous tissue can grow forwards on to the vitreous humour in cases of "proliferative" retinopathy. This is a major cause of permanent loss of vision.

Impaired blood supply

Retinal vein occlusion (or *retinal artery occlusion*), a common cause of blindness, results from blockage of the central vein (or artery) of the retina. Hypertensive retinopathy is damage to the retina caused by high blood pressure, which leads to narrowing and *atherosclerosis* (fat deposits on the artery walls) of the retinal arteries, both of which may lead to retinal damage.

Poisons

A combination of heavy tobacco-smoking, heavy alcohol intake, and poor nutrition may lead to visual loss. Vitamin deficiency in combination with lead poisoning may cause visual loss. *Methanol* causes widespread and permanent destruction of certain retinal tissues, leading to blindness.

Drugs

Many drugs can damage the retina. Examples are *chloroquine*, used in large doses over a long period for the treatment of conditions such as rheumatoid arthritis.

Other disorders

Age-related *macular degeneration*, causing progressive loss of vision, is a common condition in older people. Detachment of the retina often occurs in the absence of any injury, and it may be more common in individuals who suffer from severe *myopia* (shortsightedness).

INVESTIGATION

Retinal disorders are investigated by checking the visual acuity and the visual fields (see *vision tests*; *retinoscopy*). After dilating the pupils with drops, the retinas are inspected by means of a direct or indirect ophthalmoscope (an instrument used to examine the eye). Fluorescein can be injected into an arm, where it is carried by the blood to outline the retinal vessels and to detect leaks. Electrophysiological tests can also be carried out to study certain ocular diseases. Ultrasound scanning can be used to study tumours in or under the retina.

by degeneration. A retinal tear is more likely to occur in people who have severe *myopia* (shortsightedness) but the condition may also be caused by a severe eye injury. *Retinal detachment* usually follows a retinal tear.

If a retinal tear is diagnosed at a stage before detachment has occurred, the hole may be sealed by means of *laser treatment* or cryopexy (the application of extreme cold).

retinal vein occlusion

Blockage of a vein carrying blood from the *retina* (the light-sensitive layer at the back of the eye). It usually results from *thrombosis* (abnormal blood clot formation) in the affected vein and is more common in people who have *glaucoma* (a condition in which the pressure of fluid in the eye is abnormally high). Retinal vein occlusion may affect either the main retinal vein or one of its branches.

Retinal vein occlusion may cause visual disturbances, glaucoma, and can result in blindness, depending on which vein is affected and how quickly the condition can be treated. (See also *retinal artery occlusion*.)

retinitis

Inflammation affecting the *retina* (the light-sensitive inner layer at the back of the eye). (See also *retinopathy*.)

retinitis pigmentosa

An inherited condition in which there is degeneration of the rods and cones of the *retina* (the light-sensitive inner layer at the back of the eye) in both eyes.

The first symptoms of retinitis pigmentosa usually appear during or after adolescence and include night blindness (the inability to see well in dim light). Tests show a ring-shaped area of blindness which, over some years, extends to destroy an increasing area of the *visual field*, although central vision is often retained for many years.

Ophthalmoscopy (examination of the retina) reveals several masses of black pigment corresponding to the areas of visual loss. Affected individuals and their parents should seek *genetic counselling*.

retinoblastoma

A cancer of the *retina* (the light-sensitive inner layer at the back of the eye) that affects infants and children. The first indications of this disorder may be a *squint*, caused by blindness in the affected eye, or a visible whiteness in the pupil. Without early treatment, retinoblastoma can spread to the orbit and along the *optic nerve* to the brain.

In some cases, the underlying cause of retinoblastoma is an inherited abnormal gene; this form of the disease may affect one or both eyes. Newborn infants from affected families are given regular eye examinations; prospective parents in affected families should seek genetic counselling. There is also a non-inherited form of the condition, which usually affects only one eye; the cause of this form is unknown.

Treatment depends on the size and position of the tumour. In general, small tumours are treated by *cryotherapy* (freezing), laser therapy, or *brachytherapy* (a type of *radiotherapy*) to destroy the tumour; in addition, *chemotherapy* may also be used. Larger tumours may be treated by chemotherapy or radiotherapy; in some cases, it may be necessary to remove the affected eye. If both eyes are involved, the one worse affected may be removed and the other given radiotherapy.

retinoids

A group of drugs derived from *vitamin A*, of which *tretinoin* is an example.

retinol

The principal form of *vitamin A* found in the body.

retinopathy

Disease affecting the *retina* (the light-sensitive inner layer at the back of the eye), which is usually caused by *diabetes mellitus* or persistent *hypertension* (high blood pressure).

In diabetic retinopathy, the capillaries (tiny blood vessels) within the retina are affected by *aneurysms* (balloonlike swellings). They also leak fluid and haemorrhage (bleed) into the retina. Abnormal capillaries then grow on the retinal surface and, as these are fragile, vitreous haemorrhage (bleeding into the *vitreous humour*, the gel-like substance that fills the rear compartment of the eye) may occur. Fibrous tissue may also grow into the vitreous humour. *Laser treatment* can often halt the progress of the condition.

In hypertensive retinopathy, the retinal arteries become narrowed. Areas of retina may be destroyed and bleeding and white deposits may occur in the retina. (See also *retrolental fibroplasia*.)

retinoscopy

A type of *vision test* in which a beam of light is shone from an instrument called a retinoscope into each eye in turn. The effect of different lenses on the beam of light determines whether glasses are needed to correct refractive errors such as *hypermetropia* (longsightedness), *myopia* (shortsightedness), or *astigmatism*. Retinoscopy is particularly useful for assessing the sight of babies and young children.

retractor

A surgical instrument used to hold an incision open or to hold back surrounding tissue so that the *surgeon* has free access to the area being operated on.

retrobulbar neuritis

A form of *optic neuritis* in which the *optic nerve* becomes inflamed behind the eyeball.

retrograde

Moving backwards or in the opposite direction to normal. In retrograde ejaculation, for example, semen is forced into the bladder rather than out through the tip of the penis (see *ejaculation, disorders of*).

retrolental fibroplasia

A condition, also called *retinopathy* of prematurity, that mainly affects the eyes of premature infants. The usual cause of retrolental fibroplasia is high concentrations of *oxygen* being given to premature infants as part of the treatment for *respiratory distress syndrome* (an acute lung disorder that makes breathing difficult).

Excess oxygen causes the tissues at the margin of the *retina* (the light-sensitive layer at the back of the eye) to shut down their blood vessels. When oxygen concentrations return to normal, the affected tissues may send strands of new blood vessels and fibrous scar tissue into the vitreous humour (the gel-like substance in the rear compartment of the eye), which may interfere with vision and cause *retinal detachment*.

Retrolental fibroplasia may be successfully treated by *laser treatment*.

retroperitoneal fibrosis

Inflammation and scarring of tissues at the back of the abdominal cavity. Retroperitoneal fibrosis often blocks the *ureters*, preventing urine flow from the kidneys to the bladder. In severe cases, this results in *kidney failure*.

Retroperitoneal fibrosis usually occurs in middle-aged men and is of unknown cause; it may be an *autoimmune disorder*. The condition may be associated with long-term treatment with drugs such as *methysergide* or *bromocriptine*. Treatment may involve *corticosteroid drugs*, insertion of a stent (a rigid tube) to relieve obstruction of the ureters, and surgery.

retrosternal pain

Pain in the central region of the chest, behind the sternum (breastbone). Causes include irritation of the *oesophagus*, *angina pectoris* (chest pain due to impaired blood supply to the heart muscle), or *myocardial infarction* (heart attack). (See also *chest pain*.)

retrovirus

A type of *virus* whose genetic material is *RNA*, rather than *DNA*, and that uses an *enzyme* called reverse transcriptase to produce DNA from the RNA template. The DNA can then be incorporated into its host cells. One notable example of a retrovirus is *HIV*.

Rett's syndrome

A *brain* disorder, thought to be a *genetic disorder*, that affects only girls. Symptoms usually first appear when the child is between 12 and 18 months old. Acquired skills, such as walking and communication skills, disappear and the affected girl becomes progressively handicapped, sometimes with signs of

R

autism. Repetitive writhing movements of the hands and limbs and inappropriate outbursts of crying or laughter are characteristics of the condition.

There is no cure for Rett's syndrome and sufferers need constant care and attention. Parents of an affected child should receive *genetic counselling* if they are thinking of having another child.

reverse transcriptase inhibitors

A class of drugs used in the treatment of certain infectious diseases, including *HIV* infection and hepatitis B infection. The drugs affect the ability of the virus to reproduce by blocking reverse transcriptase, a key *enzyme*. Examples of reverse transcriptase inhibitors are *lamivudine*, *zidovudine* (AZT), efavirenz, and stavudine.

reversible monoamine oxidase inhibitors (RIMAs)

A reversible type of *monoamine oxidase inhibitor* (MAOI), which is a type of *antidepressant drug*. Reversible monoamine oxidase inhibitors are reported to have fewer adverse interactions with other drugs and with foods such as cheese and red wine than other MAOIs. *Moclobemide* is currently the only RIMA available.

Reye's syndrome

A rare disorder in which brain and liver damage follow a viral *infection*. People over the age of 16 are rarely affected. The cause is unknown, but taking *aspirin* seems to be a predisposing factor; aspirin should therefore not be taken by children under the age of 16 nor by women who are breast-feeding, except on the advice of a doctor.

SYMPTOMS AND SIGNS
The disorder starts as the child recovers from the infection. Symptoms include uncontrollable vomiting, lethargy, memory loss, and disorientation. Swelling of the brain may cause seizures, disturbances in heart rhythm, *coma*, and cessation of breathing.

TREATMENT AND OUTLOOK
Brain swelling may be controlled by *corticosteroid drugs* and by *intravenous infusion* of mannitol. *Dialysis* or *blood transfusions* may be needed to correct changes in blood chemistry caused by damage to the liver. If breathing stops, the patient is placed on a *ventilator*.

The death rate in Reye's syndrome is at least ten per cent, and higher for those who have seizures, lapse into deep coma, and stop breathing. Patients who survive a serious attack may suffer permanent brain damage.

rhabdomyolysis

Destruction of *muscle* tissue accompanied by the release of *myoglobin* (the oxygen-carrying muscle pigment) into the blood. The most common cause is a severe, crushing muscle injury (see *crush syndrome*). Other causes of the condition include *polymyositis* (a viral infection of muscle), some *statins*, and, rarely, excessive exercise.

There is usually temporary *paralysis* or weakness of the affected muscle. Except in cases of severe injury, the condition usually clears up without treatment.

rhabdomyosarcoma

A very rare cancerous *muscle* tumour. Rhabdomyosarcoma may develop during infancy, usually affecting the throat, bladder, prostate gland, or vagina; it may also occur in old age when it may affect a large muscle in the arm or leg. The tumour grows rapidly and quickly spreads to other tissues. Treatment involves surgical removal, *radiotherapy*, and *anticancer drugs*.

rhesus immunoglobulin

See *anti-D(Rh₀) immunoglobulin*.

rhesus incompatibility

A mismatch between the blood group of a rhesus (Rh)-negative pregnant woman and that of her baby. In certain circumstances, this mismatch may lead to *haemolytic disease of the newborn*.

CAUSES
The Rh system is based on the presence or absence in the blood of several factors, the most important of which is a substance called D *antigen* (a substance that can trigger an immune response). Rh-positive blood contains D antigen, whereas Rh-negative blood does not. Blood type is determined by *genes*.

A common way in which rhesus incompatibility results is if a Rh-negative woman is exposed to the blood of her Rh-positive baby during the birth. There are usually no problems during the first pregnancy with a Rh-positive baby but the woman may produce *antibodies* against the D antigen; in a subsequent pregnancy with a Rh-positive baby, these antibodies may cross the placenta and attack the red blood cells of the fetus.

A Rh-negative woman can also be sensitized to Rh-positive blood if she has had a *miscarriage, abortion*, or *amniocentesis* in which the fetus's Rh-positive blood enters her circulation. A *placental abruption* (separation of part or all of the placenta from the wall of the uterus) may also cause a transfer of blood between the mother and the fetus.

TREATMENT
Rhesus incompatibility is now uncommon because injections of *anti-D(Rh₀) immunoglobulin* are given routinely to Rh-negative women during pregnancy and at delivery. This substance destroys any of the baby's blood cells that have entered the mother's system before she is able to become sensitized to them.

Anti-D(Rh₀) immunoglobulin is also given to Rh-negative women after miscarriage, abortion, amniocentesis, or following any other procedure that might result in exposure of the mother to fetal blood cells.

R

HOW **RHESUS (Rh) INCOMPATIBILITY** OCCURS

Without preventive treatment, an Rh-negative woman who is exposed to Rh-positive blood during pregnancy may develop antibodies that will attack the red blood cells of any future Rh-positive babies.

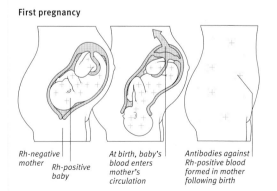

First pregnancy

Subsequent pregnancies

Rh-negative mother
Rh-positive baby

At birth, baby's blood enters mother's circulation

Antibodies against Rh-positive blood formed in mother following birth

Antibodies cross placenta and destroy red blood cells of subsequent Rh-positive babies

rhesus isoimmunization

The development of *antibodies* (proteins that are manufactured by the immune system) against rhesus (Rh)-positive blood in a person who has blood that is Rh-negative (see *haemolytic disease of the newborn*; *rhesus incompatibility*).

rheumatic fever

A disease that causes inflammation throughout the body, especially in the *joints*. Now rare in developed countries, it is an important cause of heart disease in developing countries and is most common in children aged five to 15 years.

CAUSE

Rheumatic fever is believed to be an *autoimmune disorder* (in which the body's immune system attacks its own tissues) induced by certain strains of streptococcal bacteria. Rheumatic fever always follows a throat infection. The development of rheumatic fever can usually be prevented by treatment with *antibiotic drugs*.

SYMPTOMS AND SIGNS

Rheumatic fever causes fever with pain, inflammation, and swelling of one or more of the larger joints. The *heart valves* may be scarred, leading to *mitral stenosis* (narrowing of the mitral valve) or *mitral incompetence* (leaking of the mitral valve). If the *nervous system* is involved, *Sydenham's chorea* may occur, in which there are irregular, uncontrollable, jerky movements.

DIAGNOSIS AND TREATMENT

Rheumatic fever may be suspected whenever *arthritis* (joint inflammation) moves from joint to joint, but may be discovered only after development of heart failure or a heart murmur.

Treatment is with *penicillin drugs* to eradicate streptococci; with *aspirin* or other salicylate drugs to control joint pain and inflammation and to minimize heart damage; and, in some cases, with *corticosteroid drugs*. If damage to the heart valves occurs, *heart valve surgery* may be required.

rheumatism

A popular term for any disorder that causes pain and stiffness in *muscles* and *joints*. The term is used to refer both to minor aches and twinges as well as to disorders such as *rheumatoid arthritis*, *osteoarthritis*, and *polymyalgia rheumatica*.

rheumatoid arthritis

A type of *arthritis* (joint inflammation) in which the joints in the limbs, and sometimes in other parts of the body, become painful, swollen, stiff, and, in severe cases, deformed. Tissues that are outside the joints, for example the heart, can also be affected.

CAUSES AND INCIDENCE

Rheumatoid arthritis is an *autoimmune disorder* (in which the body's immune system attacks its own tissues) that usually starts in early adulthood or middle age but can also develop in children (see *juvenile chronic arthritis*) or elderly people. Women are affected more commonly than men. There are usually recurrent attacks.

SYMPTOMS AND SIGNS

Early symptoms of rheumatoid arthritis include mild fever and aches followed by swelling, redness, pain, and stiffness in the joints, particularly in the morning. *Ligaments*, *tendons*, and *muscles* around the affected joint may also be involved. *Raynaud's phenomenon* (a condition in which the fingers turn white on exposure to cold) may occur and there may also be *rheumatoid nodules* (small lumps under the skin) over pressure points, such as the elbows or finger joints. Swelling of the wrist may cause *carpal tunnel syndrome* (tingling and pain in the fingers due to pressure on the median nerve) and also *tenosynovitis* (inflamed, painful tendon sheaths).

Complications of severe rheumatoid arthritis may include *anaemia* (a reduced level of the oxygen-carrying pigment haemoglobin in the blood), *pericarditis* (inflammation of the membranous heart covering), *ulcers* on the hands and feet, *pleural effusion* (accumulation of fluid around the lungs), *pulmonary fibrosis* (scarring and thickening of lung tissue), and *Sjögren's syndrome* (in which the eyes and mouth become excessively dry).

DIAGNOSIS AND TREATMENT

A diagnosis can be confirmed through *X-rays* of the affected joints and *blood tests* (including a check for specific antibodies known as *rheumatoid factor*).

Once the diagnosis has been confirmed, treatment with *disease-modifying antirheumatic drugs* (DMARDs) is started as soon as possible to slow down pro-

RHEUMATOID ARTHRITIS

One of the most serious forms of joint disease, rheumatoid arthritis may occur as a single episode or a succession of progressively severe attacks. It results from a disturbance in the body's immune system, causing the body to attack its own tissues. The joints are usually the worst affected, but other tissues such as the heart and lungs may also be involved.

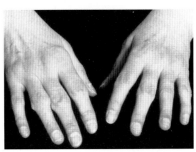

The hands in rheumatoid arthritis
This condition commonly affects the fingers. In this photograph, there is pronounced swelling around the knuckles, particularly of the right hand.

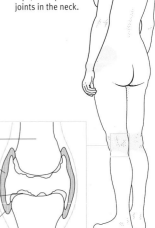

Affected joints
Rheumatoid arthritis can affect virtually any joint, but especially the fingers, wrists, shoulders, knees, hips, and spinal joints in the neck.

Disease progression
The synovium (membrane lining the capsule of an affected joint) becomes inflamed and thickened (right). Later, inflammation may spread to the cartilage and bone.

Bone

Inflamed synovium

Cartilage

Capsule

R

gression of the disease and help prevent further joint damage. These drugs take several weeks to start working and during this period *nonsteroidal anti-inflammatory drugs* (NSAIDs) or, less commonly, *corticosteroid drugs* may be used to relieve symptoms.

Once the DMARDs have started working, it may be necessary to continue with lower-dose NSAIDs to provide adequate symptom relief. Corticosteroids may also sometimes be used to treat flare-ups of symptoms.

If DMARDs are ineffective or unsuitable, drugs called *cytokine inhibitors* may sometimes be used instead. These drugs also slow down progression of the disease and help prevent joint damage.

Physiotherapy is needed to prevent or limit deformity and to help relieve symptoms and maintain mobility. People who are disabled by arthritis can be helped to cope with everyday tasks through *occupational therapy*.

In severe cases, surgery may be performed to replace damaged joints with artificial ones (see *arthroplasty*). Hip and knee replacements are the most common operations of this type.

Most sufferers must continue drug treatment for life, but many can achieve a near-normal level of activity with effective control of their symptoms.

rheumatoid factor

A specific autoantibody (a protein manufactured by the *immune system* that acts against the body's own cells) that attaches itself to naturally occurring *immunoglobulin* G (another type of antibody that, in this case, has actually triggered the immune response). This combination of immunoglobulin and autoantibody is a type of *immune complex*; it can settle in joints, causing *rheumatoid arthritis*. Most people with rheumatoid arthritis have rheumatoid factor in their blood. (See also *autoimmune disorders*; *hypersensitivity*.)

rheumatoid nodules

Small lumps that may develop under the skin in people who are suffering from *rheumatoid arthritis*. Rheumatoid nodules are *granulomas* (clumps of a type of cell that is associated with chronic inflammation); they are found particularly in areas of the body that are often under pressure, such as the elbows. Rheumatoid nodules may also develop in the lungs and can be identified on a chest X-ray.

rheumatoid spondylitis

See *ankylosing spondylitis*.

rheumatology

The branch of medicine that is concerned with the causes, development, diagnosis, and treatment of diseases and disorcers that affect the *joints, muscles,* and *connective tissue*.

rhinitis

Inflammation affecting the *mucous membrane* that lines the nose, which may lead to a feeling of stuffiness, with nasal discharge and sneezing.

TYPES

Viral rhinitis is a feature of the common cold (see *cold, common*), and may sometimes lead to *sinusitis*.

Rhinitis due to allergy (see *rhinitis, allergic*) may be seasonal (usually caused by pollens) or occur throughout the year (due to house dust, moulds, or pets). Allergic rhinitis commonly occurs with vasomotor rhinitis.

Vasomotor rhinitis may be intermittent or continual. The nose becomes over-responsive to stimuli such as pollutants, changes or extremes in temperature or humidity, certain foods or medicines, or certain emotions. Vasomotor rhinitis is common in pregnancy and in those taking combined *oral contraceptives* or other *oestrogen drugs*.

Hypertrophic rhinitis, which is characterized by thickening of the mucous membrane in the nose and chronic congestion of the nasal veins, can result from repeated nasal infections. The condition results in constant stuffiness and sometimes impairment of the sense of smell. In severe cases, treatment may involve surgical removal or shrinkage of part of the swollen tissue.

Atrophic rhinitis is characterized by wasting of the mucous membrane in the nose and can result from aging, chronic bacterial infections, or extensive nasal surgery. Features include persistent nasal infection, a nasal discharge, loss of smell, and an unpleasant odour. Treatment may include *antibiotic drugs* and nose drops.

rhinitis, allergic

A common condition that is characterized by inflammation of the *mucous membrane* lining the nose due to *allergy* to pollen, dust, or other airborne substances. Allergic rhinitis causes sneezing, a runny nose, nasal congestion, and, in most cases, watering eyes. The eyes, soft palate, and ears may also itch. The eyes may also be affected by *conjunctivitis*, making them red and sore.

CAUSES

In some people, the inhalation of particles of certain harmless substances, known as allergens, provokes an exaggerated response by the *immune system*, which forms *antibodies* against them. These allergens also trigger the release of *histamine* and other chemicals that cause inflammation and fluid production in the linings of the nose and nasal *sinuses* (air cavities around the nose). Allergens that cause allergic rhinitis include tree, grass, and weed pollens; moulds; animal skin scales, hair, or feathers; house dust; and *house dust mites*.

Seasonal allergic rhinitis is pollen-induced and is commonly known as hay fever. Tree pollens are most prevalent in spring, grass pollens in summer, and weed pollens in summer and autumn. Sufferers are worst affected during hot and windy weather, especially in heavily vegetated, low-lying areas. People affected by household allergens, such as dust, tend to have less severe symptoms but are affected throughout the year, a condition that is known as perennial rhinitis.

PREVENTION AND TREATMENT

Oral *antihistamine drugs* are often effective at relieving symptoms. Nasal symptoms may also be helped by inhaled antihistamines or nasal *corticosteroid drugs*, and eye symptoms may be alleviated by antihistamine or *sodium cromoglicate* eye-drops.

rhinophyma

A bulbous deformity and redness of the *nose* that occurs almost exclusively in elderly men. Rhinophyma is a complication of severe *rosacea* (a skin disorder of the nose and cheeks). The tissue of the nose thickens, small blood vessels enlarge, and the *sebaceous glands* become overactive, which results in making the nose excessively oily.

An operation to cut away the swollen tissue, performed under general anaesthetic (see *anaesthesia, general*), can restore the nose to a satisfactory shape.

rhinoplasty

A surgical operation to alter the structure of the *nose* in order to improve its appearance or correct a deformity.

Under either a local or general anaesthetic (see *anaesthesia*), incisions are made within the nose to avoid visible

R

scars. The *septum* (the vertical wall of cartilage and bone that divides the nose) may be altered if breathing passages are blocked; the cartilage and bone are then reshaped. The nose is finally splinted in position for about ten days.

Rhinoplasty usually causes considerable bruising and swelling and the results may not be clearly visible for a number of weeks or months.

rhinorrhoea

The discharge of watery mucus from the nose, usually due to *rhinitis*. Rarely, the discharge consists of *cerebrospinal fluid* and is the result of a head injury. (See also *nasal discharge*.)

rhinovirus

Any one of a group of *RNA*-containing viruses that cause infections of the upper respiratory tract, typically the common cold (see *cold, common*).

rhythm method

See *contraception, natural methods of*.

rib

Any of the flat, curved bones that form a framework for the chest and a protective cage around the heart, lungs, and other underlying organs.

There are 12 pairs of ribs, each joined at the back of the ribcage to a vertebra in the spine (see *Anatomy of the ribs*, right). The upper seven pairs, known as "true ribs", link directly to the *sternum* (breastbone) at the front of the body by flexible costal cartilage (connective tissue formed of collagen). The next two or three pairs of "false ribs" connect indirectly to the sternum by way of cartilage attached to the cartilage of the ribs above. The lowest two pairs of ribs are not attached to the sternum at the front and, therefore, they are known as "floating ribs". Between and attached to the ribs are thin sheets of muscle (called intercostal muscles) that expand and relax the chest during *breathing*. The spaces between the ribs also contain nerves and blood vessels.

DISORDERS

The ribs can easily be fractured by a fall or blow (see *rib, fracture of*). A rib is also a common site for a noncancerous *bone tumour* or for a *metastasis* (a secondary cancerous tumour that has spread from elsewhere in the body). *Tietze's syndrome* is a condition in which chest pain is caused by inflammation of one or more areas of rib cartilage.

In rare cases a person is born with one or more extra ribs, known as *cervical ribs*, above the uppermost normal rib. Cervical ribs may cause a variety of problems, such as putting pressure on nerves supplying the arm.

ribavirin

An *antiviral drug*, also called tribavirin, used to treat children with severe *bronchiolitis* caused by respiratory syncytial virus. It is also used in combination with other drugs in the treatment of chronic *hepatitis C*.

rib, fracture of

A crack or break in one or more of the *rib* bones. Such a fracture may be caused by a fall or blow or by stress on the ribcage, such as that produced by prolonged coughing.

The fracture of a rib causes severe pain, which worsens during periods of deep breathing, as well as tenderness and swelling of the overlying tissue. Pain may be relieved by *analgesic drugs* (painkillers) or by an injection of a local anaesthetic (see *anaesthesia, local*). *X-rays* may be used to confirm a diagnosis.

Most rib fractures are undisplaced (the bone ends remain in alignment) and usually heal without specific treatment. Strapping is rarely used because it hinders chest expansion and thereby increases the risk of *pneumonia*. Instead, the patient is encouraged to take deep breaths while holding the injured side.

A fracture that is displaced or splintered may pierce a lung, thereby causing lung collapse (see *pneumothorax*). Multiple rib fractures can result in *flail chest* (a chest injury in which part of the chest wall moves in the direction opposite to normal during breathing).

riboflavin

The chemical name of vitamin B_2 (see *vitamin B complex*).

ribonucleic acid

See *RNA*.

rickets

A disease caused by nutritional deficiency that results in *bone* deformities in childhood. Bones become deformed because inadequate amounts of *calcium* and *phosphate* are incorporated into

ANATOMY OF THE RIBS

There are seven true ribs attached to the sternum; three false ribs, each attached to a rib above; and two floating ribs, attached only to the spine, on each side. Every rib is attached to the spine at the back. The intercostal muscles (between the ribs) pull the ribs up, expanding the chest and drawing air into the lungs. The front ends of the true ribs are linked to the sternum by cartilages.

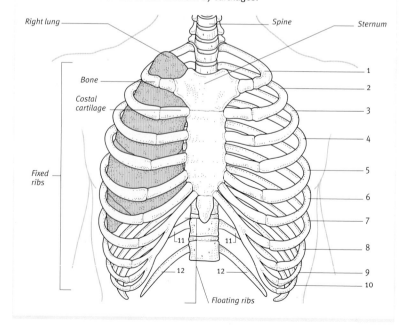

them as they grow. A similar deficiency of calcium and phosphate in adults results in *osteomalacia*.

CAUSES
The most common cause of rickets is deficiency of *vitamin D*, which is vital for the absorption of calcium from the intestines into the blood and for its incorporation into bone. Vitamin D is found in fat-containing animal foods, such as oily fish, butter, egg yolk, and liver. There are also small amounts in human and animal milk. Vitamin D is also made in the body through the action of sunlight on the skin.

Rickets occasionally develops as a complication of a digestive disorder that causes *malabsorption* (failure to absorb nutrients from the intestine). It may also occur in certain rare forms of kidney and liver disease.

SYMPTOMS AND SIGNS
The principal feature of advanced rickets is deformity of the bones, especially of the legs and spine. Typically, there is bowing of the legs and, in infants, flattening of the head as a result of softness of the skull. Infants with rickets often sleep poorly and show delay in crawling and walking. Other features that occur in rickets include *kyphoscoliosis* (spinal curvature), a tendency to *fractures*, and enlargement of the wrists, ankles, and ends of the ribs. There may also be pelvic pain and muscle weakness.

DIAGNOSIS AND TREATMENT
Diagnosis is based on the child's physical appearance, *X-rays*, and *blood tests*.

Rickets due to dietary deficiency is treated with vitamin D supplements, which can restore normal bone growth. Deformities usually disappear as the child grows. The type of rickets that occurs as a complication of another disorder is treated according to the cause.

rickettsia

A type of parasitic microorganism. Rickettsiae resemble small *bacteria* but, much like viruses, they can multiply only by invading other living cells. Rickettsiae are primarily parasites of arthropods, such as ticks, lice, fleas, and mites, but can be transmitted to the blood of larger animals via insect bites. Human rickettsial diseases include *Q fever*, *Rocky Mountain spotted fever*, and *typhus*.

rifabutin

A drug used in the treatment of *tuberculosis* and in the prevention of other *mycobacterial infections*.

rifampicin

An *antibacterial drug* used principally in the treatment of *tuberculosis*, but also *Hansen's disease* (leprosy) and *legionnaires' disease*. It may also be used to prevent meningococcal *meningitis* in people who are in close contact with the disease. Rifampicin is usually prescribed in combination with other antibacterials because some strains of bacteria develop resistance to it if it is used alone.

Side effects include harmless, orange-red discoloration of the urine, saliva, and other body secretions; muscle pain; nausea and vomiting; diarrhoea; *jaundice*; flulike symptoms; rash; and itching. Rifampicin also interferes with the action of *oral contraceptives*.

Rift Valley fever

A viral disease found in East Africa and South Africa that is transmitted from animals to humans by mosquitoes. The symptoms of Rift Valley fever resemble those of *dengue* or *influenza*, although in some cases the condition may be symptomless. In extremely severe and rare cases, Rift Valley fever may lead to *retinitis* (inflammation of the retina), *encephalitis* (inflammation of the brain), haemorrhage (bleeding), and even death.

right bundle branch block

See *heart block*.

rigidity

Increased tone in one or more *muscles*, causing them to feel tight; as a result, the affected part of the body becomes stiff and inflexible.

Causes of rigidity include muscle injury, *arthritis* in a nearby joint, a neurological disorder (such as *Parkinson's disease*), *stroke*, or *cerebral palsy* (a movement disorder caused by damage to the brain). Rigidity of the abdominal muscles is a sign of *peritonitis* (inflammation of the membranous lining of the abdominal cavity). (See also *spasticity*.)

rigor

A violent attack of shivering, which is often associated with a fever. Rigor may also refer to stiffness or rigidity of body tissues, as in *rigor mortis*.

rigor mortis

The stiffening of *muscles* that starts three to four hours after death. Rigor mortis is usually complete after about 12 hours; the stiffness then disappears over the next 48 to 60 hours.

The greater the physical exertion before death, the sooner rigor mortis begins. Similarly, the sooner rigor mortis begins, the quicker it passes. These facts are used to help assess the time of death.

Riley–Day syndrome

A *genetic disorder* that affects the function of nerves in many parts of the body. The condition may begin in infancy.

SYMPTOMS
Children with Riley-Day syndrome often have diminished sensitivity to pain and may not notice when they hurt themselves. Problems with swallowing are common, and affected infants may develop pneumonia as a result of inhaling food into their airways (see *aspiration pneumonia*). Vomiting may also occur. The children may also suffer from lack of tears, increased sweating, poor coordination, problems with speech, and an unsteady gait. Puberty may be delayed (see *delayed puberty*).

INVESTIGATION AND TREATMENT
Genetic testing may be arranged to look for the specific gene abnormality. Any additional tests performed depend on the symptoms. For example, if the child is unwell with a cough, a *chest X-ray* may be arranged and may show evidence of pneumonia.

Treatment is aimed at relieving specific problems as they arise, such as giving *antibiotic drugs* for pneumonia.

People with a family history of Riley–Day syndrome who are considering having children can obtain *genetic counselling*, and prenatal diagnostic testing can identify an affected fetus.

RIMAs

The abbreviation for *reversible monoamine oxidase inhibitors*.

rimonabant

An *appetite suppressant* drug.

ringing in the ears

See *tinnitus*.

ring pessary

A plastic, ring-shaped device inserted into the vagina to hold a prolapsed uterus (see *uterus, prolapse of*) in position.

ringworm

A popular name for certain fungal skin infections commonly found on the feet, groin, scalp, nails, or trunk. Ringworm causes ring-shaped, reddened, scaly, or blistery skin patches. (See also *tinea*.)

R

Rinne's test

A type of *hearing test* that is used to determine whether *deafness* is conductive (due to the faulty conduction of sound from the outer ear to the inner ear) or sensorineural (due to problems of the inner ear, the nerves, or the auditory area of the brain).

A vibrating tuning fork is placed against the mastoid process (the bone behind the ear) and then held close to the ear. A positive result, when the sound conducted by the air is heard more clearly than that conducted by the bone, indicates sensorineural deafness. A negative result, when the sound conducted by bone is heard more loudly, indicates conductive deafness. Rinne's test is used in conjunction with other hearing tests.

risk factor

Any feature or attribute that predisposes a person to an increased risk of developing an illness. For example, tobacco *smoking*, working with asbestos (see *asbestos-related diseases*), or having a family history of a condition are all considered to be risk factors.

risperidone

An *antipsychotic drug* that is used in the treatment of psychoses such as *schizophrenia* and *mania*. Possible side effects include weight gain, agitation, and dizziness. Risperidone is also associated with an increased risk of *stroke* in elderly people who have *dementia*.

ritodrine

A drug used to prevent or delay premature labour (see *prematurity*) by relaxing the muscles of the uterus (womb). Possible side effects of ritodrine include tremor, chest pain, *palpitations*, nausea, vomiting, and hot flushes.

rivalry, sibling

See *sibling rivalry*.

rivastigmine

An *acetylcholinesterase inhibitor* drug used to treat mild to moderate dementia in *Alzheimer's disease* and *Parkinson's disease*. It slows the progression of dementia and loss of mental abilities. Possible side effects include nausea, vomiting, dizziness, headaches, agitation, and difficulty in passing urine.

river blindness

See *onchocerciasis*.

RNA

The abbreviation for ribonucleic acid. RNA and *DNA* (deoxyribonucleic acid) carry the inherited, coded genetic instructions in cells. In all animal and plant cells, DNA carries the instructions and RNA helps to decode them, but, in some *viruses*, the instructions are held by RNA. (See also *nucleic acids; protein synthesis*).

RNI

See *reference nutrient intake*.

Rocky Mountain spotted fever

A rare, infectious disease causing fever and a rash with spots that spread over the body, darken, enlarge, and bleed. The disease occurs in North and South America and is caused by a microorganism called a *rickettsia* that is transmitted from small mammals to humans by tick bites (see *ticks and disease*). Treatment is with *chloramphenicol* or *tetracycline*.

rod

One of the two specialized types of nerve cell in the *retina* (the light-sensitive inner layer at the back of the eye) that convert light into nerve impulses. The rods are very sensitive and can respond to very dim light. (See also *cone*.)

rodent ulcer

A common name for *basal cell carcinoma*.

role-playing

The acting of a role (a pattern of behaviour expected in a given situation). The phrase "sick role" describes the type of passive behaviour expected and allowed of a patient; people with social or emotional problems may unconsciously adopt this role to gain sympathy.

root-canal treatment

A dental procedure performed to save a tooth in which the pulp (the living tissue in the tooth) has died or become untreatably diseased, usually due to extensive dental *caries*.

Root-canal treatment may be performed under a local anaesthetic (see *anaesthesia, local*). *X-rays* are first taken in order to establish the length of the root canal. The main stages of treatment are shown in the illustrations (right).

A hole is drilled into the crown to remove all material from the pulp chamber. The root canals are then enlarged slightly and shaped with fine-tipped instruments, and their length is measured. The procedure is sometimes monitored by X-rays. The cavity is washed out, and antibiotic paste and a temporary filling are packed into it. Some days later, the filling is removed and the canals are checked for sterility. If no infection is detected, the cavity is filled with a sealing paste and/or tapering solid "points" made of gutta-percha resin mixed with zinc and bismuth oxides. The roots are then sealed with cement. If the cavity is not filled completely, bacteria may enter, leading to *periodontitis* (inflammation of the tissues surrounding the teeth).

Treated teeth may turn grey but their appearance can be restored by the use of bonding techniques (see *bonding*,

ROOT-CANAL TREATMENT

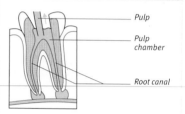

1 The pulp is removed from the pulp cavity through a hole drilled in the crown. The root canals are enlarged and shaped with fine-tipped instruments. Sometimes, X-rays may be used to monitor the procedure.

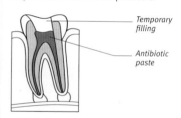

2 An antibiotic paste and a temporary filling are packed into the pulp chamber. A few days later, the filling is removed and the root canals are checked to ensure that no infection is present.

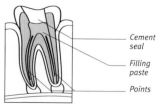

3 If no infection can be detected, the cavity is filled and the roots are sealed with cement and/or tapering solid "points" made of gutta-percha. The cavity is filled completely in order to avoid the risk of bacteria entering.

R

dental), by fitting an artificial crown (see *crown, dental*) or veneer, or by bleaching (see *bleaching, dental*).

rooting reflex

An automatic reflex action seen in newborn infants (see *reflex, primitive*). The rooting reflex, which can be evoked by touching the baby's cheek with the fingertip, enables the baby to find the mother's nipple to suckle.

root pain

Pain that occurs as a result of damage to, pressure on, or disease of the roots of a *sensory nerve*. Root pain is felt in areas of skin supplied by the affected sensory nerve roots.

Rorschach test

A psychological test based on a person's responses to a set of ink-blot pictures. The Rorschach test was intended to reveal an individual's attitudes, conflicts, and emotions, but is now rarely used. (See also *personality tests*.)

rosacea

A chronic skin disorder in which the nose and cheeks are abnormally red. In most cases the cause is unknown but the condition may be associated with the use of corticosteroid creams; other triggers include spicy foods, alcohol, caffeine, and stress. The disorder is most common in middle-aged women.

Rosacea usually begins with temporary flushes, but may develop into permanent redness of the skin, sometimes accompanied by acne-like pustules. In elderly men, it may lead to *rhinophyma* (bulbous swelling of the nose).

Treatment is with topical (applied to the skin) *metronidazole* or, if this is ineffective oral *tetracycline*. There is no cure for rosacea but treatment can alleviate the symptoms. The symptoms may recur after stopping treatment.

roseola infantum

A common infectious disease, caused by a type of *herpes* virus, that mainly affects children between the ages of six months and two years.

Roseola infantum is characterized by an abrupt onset of irritability and fever. The child's temperature drops to normal after four or five days and, at about the same time, a rash appears on the trunk, often spreading to the neck, face, and limbs. The rash usually clears up within two days. Other symptoms may include a sore throat and enlargement of the *lymph nodes* in the neck. Convulsions (see *convulsion, febrile*) may occur during the fever, but there are usually no serious effects.

The only treatment for roseola infantum is to keep the child cool and give *paracetamol* to reduce the fever.

rose spots

A rash of pink or red spots that erupts on the skin of the chest, the abdomen, and sometimes the thighs in the second week of *typhoid fever*. Rose spots last a few days.

rosiglitazone

An oral hypoglycaemic drug (see *hypoglycaemics, oral*) used alone or in combination with other oral hypoglycaemics (either *metformin* or a sulphonylurea) in the treatment of type 2 *diabetes mellitus*. Rosiglitazone acts by reducing peripheral *insulin* resistance. Side effects of rosiglitazone may include gastrointestinal disturbances, weight gain, and *anaemia* (a reduced level of haemoglobin in the blood).

rotator cuff

A reinforcing structure around the shoulder *joint*, composed of four muscle tendons that merge with the fibrous capsule enclosing the joint. The rotator cuff may be torn as the result of a fall. A partial tear may cause *painful arc syndrome* (pain when the arm is lifted away from the body in a particular arc). A complete tear seriously limits the person's ability to raise the arm and, in cases of severe disability, may require surgical repair.

rotavirus

A type of *virus* that is a common cause of *gastroenteritis*; rotavirus particularly affects young children.

roughage

See *fibre, dietary*.

roundworms

A class of elongated, cylindrical worms, also known as nematodes. Some types of roundworm are human *parasites* (the table below summarizes the main ones). The adult worms usually inhabit the human intestines, often without causing symptoms. Sometimes worm larvae pass through other parts of the body, which may cause symptoms.

The only common roundworm disease in the UK is *threadworm infestation*, which mainly affects children; occasionally, *ascariasis, whipworm infestation*, and *toxocariasis* occur. Some people return from abroad with *hookworm infestation*.

DISEASES CAUSED BY **ROUNDWORMS** (NEMATODES)

Disease	Adult length	Distribution	How acquired
Ascariasis (common roundworm)	15–38 cm	Worldwide	By swallowing worm eggs that have contaminated food or fingers
Enterobiasis (threadworm)	0.2–1.5 cm	Worldwide	By swallowing worm eggs that have contaminated fingers
Trichuriasis (whipworm)	2.5–5 cm	Worldwide	By swallowing worm eggs that have contaminated food or fingers
Ancylostomiasis (hookworm)	1.5 cm	Tropics	By penetration of skin of feet by worm larvae in soil
Strongyloidiasis	0.2 cm	Tropics	By penetration of skin of feet by worm larvae in soil
Toxocariasis	Several cm	Worldwide	By swallowing worm eggs from dirt or dog faeces
Trichinosis (porkworm)	0.1 cm	Worldwide	By eating undercooked pork containing encysted worm larvae
Filariasis	2–50 cm	Tropics	By mosquito and other insect bites

R

In tropical countries, roundworm diseases are much more common; they include those mentioned above as well as *strongyloidiasis*, *guinea worm disease*, and various types of *filariasis*.

For most roundworm infestations, treatment is with *anthelmintic drugs*.

Roussy–Levy disease

A rare *genetic disorder* affecting nerves and muscles; symptoms usually begin in early childhood. Roussy–Levy disease resembles *peroneal muscular atrophy* and results from degeneration of the nerves supplying the lower legs and forearms.

Features include weakness, muscle wasting, and poor coordination of the legs; *claw-foot*; and tremors of the hands. There may also be abnormal curvature of the spine (see *kyphoscoliosis*). Roussy–Levy disease displays an autosomal dominant pattern of inheritance.

RSI

The abbreviation used for *repetitive strain injury*, a type of overuse injury.

rubber dam

A rubber sheet used to isolate one or more teeth during certain dental procedures. The dam acts as a barrier against saliva and prevents the inhalation of debris. To fit a dam, the dentist punches small holes in a rubber sheet, through which the teeth protrude. The sheet is then secured in place with clamps and a frame.

rubefacient

A substance that causes redness of the skin by increasing blood flow to it. Rubefacients are sometimes included in ointments used to relieve muscular aches and pains and they work by producing counter-irritation: they stimulate nerve endings to create a superficial feeling of heat or cold and distract the brain from the deeper muscular pain. Examples of rubefacients include methyl salicylate and menthol.

rubella

A viral infection, also known as German measles. Rubella is serious only if it affects a nonimmune woman in the early months of pregnancy, when there is a risk that the *virus* will cause severe *birth defects* (known as congenital rubella syndrome) in the fetus.

TRANSMISSION AND SYMPTOMS

The rubella virus is spread through mother-to-baby transmission and from person to person in airborne droplets; it has an *incubation period* (the time between infection and the onset of symptoms) of two to three weeks. Infection usually occurs in children between the ages of six and 12 and is almost invariably mild.

The first symptoms may be a slight fever, malaise, and enlarged *lymph nodes* at the back of the neck. A rash then appears on the face, spreads to the trunk and limbs, and disappears within about three days. In adolescents and adults the symptoms may be more marked, such as a headache before the rash appears and a more pronounced fever.

The virus may be transmitted from about a week before the rash appears until a few days after its onset. An unborn baby is at risk if the mother is infected during the first four months of pregnancy. The earlier the infection occurs, the more likely the infant is to be affected and the more serious the resulting abnormalities tend to be. The most common abnormalities are *deafness*, congenital *heart disease*, *learning difficulties*, *cataract*, *purpura*, *cerebral palsy*, and bone abnormalities. About one in five affected babies dies in early infancy.

DIAGNOSIS AND TREATMENT

Rubella is easily confused with other viral infections, *scarlet fever*, and drug reactions, which may produce similar symptoms. Rubella can be positively diagnosed only by laboratory isolation of the virus, for example from a throat *swab* or by tests to look for *antibodies* (proteins manufactured by the immune system) to the virus in the blood.

There is no specific treatment. *Paracetamol* can be given to reduce fever. Treatment of congenital rubella syndrome depends on the defects present.

PREVENTION

Rubella vaccine provides immunity to the disease; it is now given in the MMR vaccine (see *MMR vaccination*) to babies at around the age of 13 months, with a booster at three years four months to five years of age. Rubella infection also confers immunity.

Any woman who is planning a pregnancy should have her rubella status checked. If she is not immune, she should be vaccinated immediately and she should then avoid becoming pregnant for a month afterwards. If a nonimmune pregnant woman comes into contact with a person who has rubella, passive immunization by *immunoglobulin injection* may help to prevent infection of the fetus.

rubeola

Another name for *measles*.

running injuries

Disorders resulting from the effects of jogging or running. Running injuries are common but most can be avoided by taking some simple precautions, such as wearing the correct footwear.

TYPES

Common types of running injury include *tendinitis* (inflammation of a tendon, particularly the *Achilles tendon*); *stress fractures* of bones in the leg and foot; plantar *fasciitis* (inflammation of tissue in the sole of the foot); torn *hamstring muscles* at the back of the thigh; back pain due to jarring of the spine; tibial *compartment syndrome* (painful cramp in the lower leg due to muscle compression); knee pain; ligament injuries in the ankle; and *shin splints* (pain along the tibia or shin).

PREVENTION

Shoes should fit snugly to provide stability but they should not cramp the foot; insoles help to cushion the jarring force on the legs and spine. Shoes that have become worn down should not be used because this can cause abnormal positioning of the foot during running, leading to foot strain.

Before running, warming-up exercises should be performed to reduce the risk of injury. Beginners should run only short distances at first and experienced runners should keep within sensible bounds. Runners should maintain an upright posture, with trunk, neck, and arms relaxed. Long periods of running uphill, downhill, or along the side of a slope should be avoided as they increase stress on the ankles and knees.

Following diagnosis of a running injury, assessment by a sports physiotherapist may be required in order to help prevent a recurrence of the injury.

rupture

A common term for a *hernia*. The term also refers to a complete break in a structure, as in rupture of a *tendon*.

Rynacrom

A brand name for *sodium cromoglicate*, an antiallergy drug. Rynacrom is used specifically in the prevention of allergic rhinitis (see *rhinitis, allergic*).

R

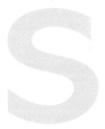

S

sac

A baglike organ or body structure.

saccharin

An *artificial sweetener*.

sacralgia

Pain in the *sacrum* (the triangular spinal bone below the lumbar *vertebrae*) that is caused by pressure on a spinal nerve. Sacralgia is usually the result of a *disc prolapse*. Rarely, it may be due to *bone cancer*. (See also *back pain*.)

sacralization

Fusion of the fifth (lowest) lumbar *vertebra* with the upper *sacrum* (the triangular spinal bone that is positioned below the lumbar vertebrae). Sacralization may be present at birth, in which case there are usually no symptoms. Sacralization may also be produced deliberately by a surgical procedure for the treatment of a *disc prolapse* or *spondylolisthesis*. (See also *spinal fusion*.)

sacroiliac joint

One of a pair of rigid *joints* on each side of the body that form an interface between the *sacrum* (the triangular spinal bone below the lumbar *vertebrae*) and the *ilium* (hip bone). The bony surfaces within the joint are lined with cartilage and have a small amount of synovial fluid between them. Strong ligaments positioned between the sacrum and ilium allow only minimal movement at the joint.

The sacroiliac joint can be strained, usually by childbirth or overstriding when running. Such an injury causes pain in the lower back and buttocks. The sacroiliac joint can also become inflamed (see *sacroiliitis*).

sacroiliitis

Inflammation of a *sacroiliac joint*, one of a pair of joints situated between each side of the *sacrum* (the triangular spinal bone below the lumbar vertebrae) and each *ilium* (hip bone).

Sacroiliitis can be due to various disorders, such as *ankylosing spondylitis*, *Reiter's syndrome*, *rheumatoid arthritis*, or arthritis associated with *psoriasis*. The main symptom is pain in the lower back, buttocks, groin, and back of the thigh. Treatment is with *nonsteroidal anti-inflammatory drugs*.

sacrum

The large triangular bone in the lower *spine*. The sacrum lies in the centre back of the *pelvis*. Its broad upper part articulates with the fifth (lowest) lumbar *vertebra*, and its narrow lower part with the *coccyx*. The sides are connected by the *sacroiliac joints* to each *ilium* (hip bone). Disorders affecting the sacrum include *sacralgia*, *spondylolisthesis*, and *sacralization*. (See also *spine, disorders of*.)

SAD

The abbreviation for *seasonal affective disorder*.

sadism

The tendency or practice of deriving pleasure, particularly sexual pleasure, from inflicting pain or suffering on others. (See also *sadomasochism*.)

sadomasochism

The tendency or practice of deriving sexual pleasure by inflicting pain (see *sadism*) and receiving abuse (see *masochism*); one

STRUCTURE OF THE SACROILIAC JOINT

The joint forms an interface between the sacrum at the back of the pelvis and the ilium (hip bone) on each side of the body.

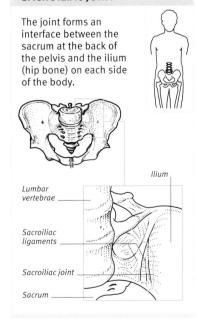

Ilium

Lumbar vertebrae

Sacroiliac ligaments

Sacroiliac joint

Sacrum

STRUCTURE OF THE **SACRUM**

The sacrum consists of five vertebrae (spinal bones) that are fused together to form a single solid structure.

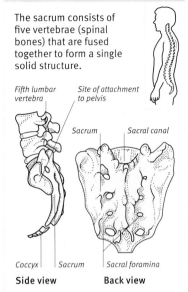

Fifth lumbar vertebra

Site of attachment to pelvis

Sacrum

Sacral canal

Coccyx

Sacrum

Sacral foramina

Side view

Back view

trait usually predominates. It also describes a sexual relationship in which one partner is very dominant and one is submissive.

safe period

See *contraception, natural methods of*.

safer sex

Preventive measures that are undertaken to reduce the risk of *sexually transmitted infections*. These include taking simple precautions such as maintaining a monogamous sexual relationship with someone who is free of infection; avoiding casual sex or sex with multiple partners; avoiding activities that can damage the skin or mucous membranes, or that involve contact with body fluids; and using a *condom*.

salbutamol

A *bronchodilator drug* that is used in the treatment of *asthma*, chronic *bronchitis*, and *emphysema*. It is also occasionally used to help prevent premature labour (see *prematurity*).

salicylic acid

A *keratolytic drug* that is used to treat skin disorders such as *dermatitis*, *eczema*, *psoriasis*, *dandruff*, *ichthyosis*, *acne*, *warts*, (including verrucas) and callosities (see *callus, skin*). Salicylic acid is also sometimes used to treat *fungal infections*. Side effects are few; they may include irritation and dryness of the skin.

S

SAFER SEX: HOW TO USE A CONDOM

Using a condom is not a guarantee against transmission of HIV (the AIDS virus) or other sexually transmitted infections, but it does reduce the risks substantially. Condoms that are prelubricated with a spermicide offer extra protection against pregnancy. Hypoallergenic condoms are available for people who are sensitive to rubber. In addition, condoms are available that are made from a thicker type of rubber and these should be used during anal intercourse.

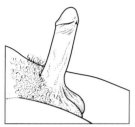

1 The penis should be fully erect before the condom is put on. The condom should be in place before any vaginal or anal penetration by the penis and before oral sex.

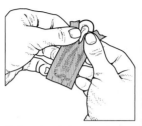

2 Use a brand of condom that conforms to British Standards. Do not use one that has no teat, is beyond its "use by" date or appears to be defective. Open the condom carefully to avoid tearing it.

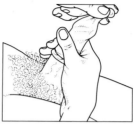

3 The teat-end should be squeezed so it is free of air and the condom unrolled fully over the penis. Do not stretch the condom tightly because a tight condom is more likely to burst.

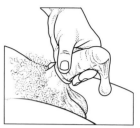

4 The penis should be withdrawn soon after ejaculation. During withdrawal, the base of the condom should be held in order to prevent the semen from spilling out of the condom.

saline

A solution of salt (sodium chloride). Solutions with the same concentration of salt as body fluids are known as normal, or physiological, saline. Saline is used in contact lens solutions and may be given by *intravenous infusion* to replace fluids lost in severe dehydration.

saliva

The slightly alkaline fluid secreted into the mouth by the *salivary glands* and the *mucous membranes* lining the mouth. Saliva contains the digestive enzyme amylase, which helps to break down carbohydrates in food. In addition, saliva keeps the mouth moist, lubricates food to aid swallowing, and helps the tongue and mouth to register *taste*.

salivary glands

Three pairs of glands that secrete *saliva*, via ducts, into the mouth.

The largest, the *parotid glands*, lie on each side of the jaw, just below and in front of the ears; the ducts of these glands run forwards and inwards to open inside the cheeks. The sublingual glands lie on the floor of the front of the mouth, where they form a low ridge on each side of the frenulum (the band of tissue that attaches the underside of the tongue to the floor of the mouth). This ridge has a row of small openings through which saliva is excreted. The submandibular glands lie towards the back of the mouth, close to the sides of the jaw. Their ducts run forwards and open under the tongue at two small swellings, one on each side of the frenulum.

DISORDERS

The parotid glands can be infected with the *mumps* virus, and stones (calculi) can form in a salivary gland or duct. A stone in a duct causes a swelling that enlarges during eating because saliva flow is blocked; it may also cause pain. Surgical removal of a stone from a duct

ANATOMY OF THE SALIVARY GLANDS

Each gland consists of thousands of saliva-secreting sacs. Tiny ducts carry the saliva into the main ducts leading to the mouth.

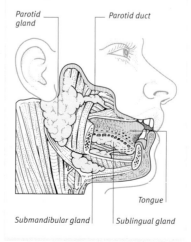

Parotid gland
Parotid duct
Tongue
Submandibular gland
Sublingual gland

is usually straightforward, but if the stone is within the gland, the entire gland may have to be removed.

Poor *oral hygiene* may allow bacterial infection in a gland, sometimes leading to an abscess. Tumours may develop; however, they are rare, except for a type of parotid tumour that is slow-growing, noncancerous, and painless.

Insufficient salivation causes a dry mouth (see *mouth, dry*). This problem may be due to *dehydration* or *Sjögren's syndrome*, or it may occur as a side effect of certain drugs.

salivation, excessive

The production of too much *saliva*. Excess salivation sometimes occurs during pregnancy and prior to vomiting. Other causes include mouth problems such as irritation of the mouth lining, *gingivitis* (gum inflammation), or *mouth ulcers*; digestive tract disorders such as *peptic ulcers* and *oesophagitis*; and nervous system disorders such as *Parkinson's disease*. In some cases, it may be reduced by *anticholinergic drugs*.

salmeterol

A *bronchodilator drug* used as a preventer in the treatment of *asthma*. It is also used in the treatment of chronic obstructive pulmonary disease (see *pulmonary disease, chronic obstructive*). Salmeterol is administered by inhalation. Side effects of the drug may include slight tremor, agitation, insomnia, and, rarely, a rapid heartbeat.

S

salmonella infections

Infections caused by any of the salmonella group of bacteria. One type of salmonella causes *typhoid fever*; another causes *paratyphoid fever*, others commonly result in bacterial *food poisoning*. Infants, elderly people, and those who are debilitated are most susceptible.

In many cases, the source of salmonella poisoning has been traced to poultry products, and particularly to hens' eggs and chicken meat. The infection of eggs can originate in the hen's ovaries or may occur as a result of faecal contamination via the egg shell.

SYMPTOMS
Symptoms of salmonella food poisoning usually appear suddenly 12–24 hours after infection and include headache, nausea, abdominal pain, diarrhoea, and sometimes fever. They usually last for only two or three days, but in severe cases *dehydration* or *septicaemia* (blood poisoning) may develop, especially in the very young and old.

TREATMENT
Treatment is by *rehydration therapy* to replace lost fluids. In severe cases, fluid may need to be replaced by means of *intravenous infusion* and *antibiotic drugs* may be required.

PREVENTION
In general, it is advisable to avoid foods that contain raw egg (such as homemade mayonnaise). The risk of infection is reduced in very fresh eggs. Salmonella bacteria are not killed by light cooking, and eggs given to children or the frail or elderly should be well cooked.

salmon patch

See *stork mark*.

salpingectomy

Surgical removal of one or both *fallopian tubes*. Salpingectomy may be performed if the tube is infected (see *salpingitis*) or to treat *ectopic pregnancy*. (See also *salpingo-oophorectomy*.)

salpingitis

Inflammation of a *fallopian tube*. Salpingitis is commonly caused by infection (usually a sexually transmitted infection, such as *gonorrhoea* or *chlamydial infection*) spreading up from the vagina, cervix, or uterus. Salpingitis is also a feature of *pelvic inflammatory disease*.

Symptoms include abdominal pain and fever, which may be severe. Pus may collect in the fallopian tube, and a pelvic *abscess* may develop.

Diagnosis is by examination of vaginal and cervical discharge, to identify the infectious organism, or *laparoscopy* to view the abdominal cavity. Blood tests may be carried out if *septicaemia* is suspected and the woman is very unwell. Treatment of the condition is with *antibiotics*. Surgery may be needed if an abscess has formed.

If the infection has damaged the inside of the fallopian tubes, *infertility* or an increased risk of an *ectopic pregnancy* may result. In some cases, damage to a tube can be corrected surgically.

salpingo-oophorectomy

Removal of one or both *fallopian tubes* and *ovaries*. This operation may be performed to treat some types of *ovarian cyst*. It may also be performed together with a *hysterectomy* to treat cancer of the ovary (see *ovary, cancer of*) or the uterus (see *uterus, cancer of*).

salt

A substance formed when an acid and a base react. The word is commonly used to refer to sodium chloride (table salt).

salve

A healing, soothing ointment.

sandfly bites

Bites from sandflies, which are found in many warm climates and can pass disease to humans. In tropical and subtropical areas they transmit *leishmaniasis*. In parts of Asia and the Mediterranean, they transmit sandfly fever, an illness like influenza. In the western Andes, they transmit bartonellosis, different forms of which cause either joint pain and fever or a rash. The risk of bites can be minimized by wearing clothing with long arms and legs that fits closely at the wrists and ankles, and using insect repellent, especially after dusk (when the flies are most active).

sanitary protection

A variety of articles, including pads and tampons, that are used to absorb blood and protect the clothing during *menstruation*. Most are disposable.

saphenous vein

A major vein that runs the length of the leg just under the skin (see *circulatory system*). The saphenous vein is sometimes removed and used to bypass blockages in blood vessels supplying the heart (see *coronary artery bypass*).

sarcoidosis

A rare disease of unknown cause in which there is inflammation of tissues throughout the body, especially the lymph nodes, lungs, skin, eyes, and liver. It occurs mainly in young adults.

Symptoms do not always occur. When they do, they include fever, generalized aches, painful joints, and eye problems such as conjunctivitis and uveitis (painful, bloodshot eyes). Sarcoidosis may also cause enlargement of the lymph nodes, breathlessness, *erythema nodosum* (purplish swellings on the legs), a purplish facial rash, and areas of numbness. Possible complications of sarcoidosis include *hypercalcaemia* (excess calcium in the blood), which may damage the kidneys, and *pulmonary fibrosis* (scarring of lung tissue).

Treatment is not always needed. Most people recover fully within two years, with or without treatment, but some develop a persistent, chronic form of the disease. *Corticosteroid drugs* are given to treat persistent fever or erythema nodosum, to prevent blindness in an affected eye, and to reduce the risk of permanent lung damage.

sarcoma

A cancer of *connective tissue* (which holds body structures together). Types include *osteosarcoma*, *Kaposi's sarcoma*, *chondrosarcoma*, and *fibrosarcoma*.

SARS

The abbreviation for severe acute respiratory syndrome, a potentially serious viral infection that may cause *pneumonia*. SARS is caused by a new strain of coronavirus and, in most cases, is spread by close personal contact.

Symptoms appear two to seven days after infection and include acute fever (sometimes with chills), aching muscles, and headache. After a further three to seven days, a dry (nonproductive) cough (accompanied by shortness of breath that may become severe) may develop, which may indicate pneumonia.

Various tests may be performed to confirm the diagnosis and exclude other possible causes of pneumonia. These may include a blood test to check for antibodies associated with the virus, a viral culture, and a genetic test to look for viral *DNA* in the blood, faeces, or nasal secretions.

Treatment includes oxygen therapy, (with artificial ventilation if necessary) and, in some cases, antibiotic and/or

S

antiviral drugs. There is no vaccine or curative treatment available at present, and therefore control of the disease depends on physical measures, including the use of face masks, hand washing, and isolation of infected individuals. Most people recover from SARS, including those who develop pneumonia, although in some cases the illness is fatal.

saturated fats

See *fats and oils*; *nutrition*.

scab

A crust that forms on the skin or on a mucous membrane at the site of a healing wound or infected area. (See also *blood clotting*.)

scabies

A skin infestation caused by the mite *SARCOPTES SCABIEI*, which burrows into the skin to lay eggs. Scabies is highly contagious by close physical contact. It is most common in infants, children, and young adults.

The mite's burrows may appear on the skin as grey, scaly swellings, usually between the fingers, on the wrists and genitals, and in the armpits. Later, small papules may appear on the limbs and trunk. The infestation causes intense itching, particularly at night, and scabs may form on the papules.

Treatment is with an insecticide lotion that is usually applied to all of the skin including the head. All occupants of the person's household, and any sexual partners, should be treated at the same time.

scald

A *burn* due to hot liquid or steam.

scalded skin syndrome

A rare skin disease that causes redness followed by peeling of large areas of skin. It is caused by certain toxins from the bacterium *STAPHYLOCOCCUS AUREUS*. Children are particularly susceptible. Treatment is with intravenous injection or infusion of antibiotics.

scaling, dental

Removal of hard deposits from the teeth (see *calculus, dental*) to prevent or treat *periodontal disease* in the tissues supporting the teeth.

scalp

The skin of the head and its underlying tissue layers. The scalp is normally covered with hair. The skin of the scalp is tougher than other skin and overlies a sheet of muscle that extends from the eyebrows, over the top of the head, to the nape of the neck.

The scalp may suffer injuries such as cuts and tears; it is richly supplied with blood vessels, so such wounds bleed profusely. Disorders affecting the scalp include *dandruff*; *alopecia* (hair loss); *sebaceous cysts*; *psoriasis*; fungal infections such as *tinea* (ringworm); and parasitic infestations such as *lice*. *Cradle cap* is common in infants.

scalpel

A surgical knife for cutting tissue.

scan

An image produced by one of several *scanning techniques*.

scanning techniques

Methods of producing images of organ structure (or sometimes function) using sound waves, radio waves, *X-rays*, or other forms of radiation directed through body tissues.

Ultrasound scanning is a widely used technique in which inaudible, ultra-high-frequency sound waves are passed into the body. These sound waves are reflected by various body structures in a pattern that is detected by one or more transducers and displayed on a screen.

CT scanning uses X-rays to measure variations in the density of an organ. The method compiles an image or picture by computer analysis.

Radionuclide scanning, which is also known as scintigraphy, involves injection into the body of radioactive substances, which are taken up in different amounts by different organs. Radioactive iodine, for example, becomes concentrated in the thyroid gland. A detector is positioned in close proximity to the organ being examined and the pattern of radiation being emitted is recorded and displayed on a screen.

MRI (magnetic resonance imaging) uses a powerful electromagnet to align the nuclei of atoms of hydrogen in the body. The nuclei are then knocked out of position by radio waves; in realigning themselves with the magnetic field, the nuclei produce a radio signal that can be detected and transformed into a computer-generated image.

PET scanning (positron emission tomography) is based on the detection of positively charged particles that are emitted by radioactively marked sub-stances introduced into the body. A computer is used to build up an image that reflects the chemical activity of the tissue that is being studied.

scaphoid

One of the eight *wrist* bones. It is the outermost bone on the thumb side of the hand, in the row of wrist bones nearest the elbow.

A fracture of the scaphoid is a common wrist injury usually caused by a fall on an outstretched hand. A characteristic symptom is tenderness in the anatomical snuffbox (the space between the tendons at the base of the thumb on the back of the hand). Treatment is by immobilizing the wrist in a *cast*.

scapula

The anatomical term for the shoulder-blade. The two scapulae are flat, triangular bones situated in the upper back. On the rear surface of each one is a prominent spine (which can be felt under the skin) that runs diagonally upwards and outwards to a bony prominence (the acromion) at the shoulder tip. The acromion articulates with the end of the *clavicle* (collarbone) to form the *acromioclavicular joint*. Just below the acromion is a socket (the glenoid cavity) into which the head of the humerus (upper-arm bone) fits to form the shoulder joint.

The scapula serves as an attachment for some of the muscles and tendons of the arm, neck, chest, and back and aids movements of the arm and shoulder.

LOCATION OF THE **SCAPULAE**

The two scapulae are the prominent wing-shaped bones in the upper back. They form a major part of the shoulder joint.

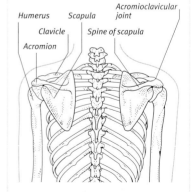

scar

A mark left where damaged tissue has healed. Scar tissue forms not only on the skin but on all internal wounds, such as at the site of a muscle tear or where surgery has been performed.

The body repairs a wound or other lesion by increasing production of the tough, fibrous protein *collagen* at the site of the damage. This helps to form new *connective tissue* around the lesion. If the edges of a lesion are brought together during healing, a narrow, pale scar forms; if they are left apart, more extensive scarring occurs.

ABNORMAL SCARS

A hypertrophic scar is a large, unsightly scar that may develop at the site of an infected wound. Some people have a family tendency to develop such scars.

A *keloid* is a large, irregularly shaped scar that continues to grow in size as the body continues to produce extra collagen after a wound has healed. This type of scar is more common in black people than in white.

Adhesions are areas of scar tissue that form between unconnected parts of internal organs. They are a potential complication of intestinal surgery.

scarlatina

Another name for *scarlet fever*.

scarlet fever

An uncommon infectious disease, more often seen in childhood, that is caused by a strain of streptococcal bacteria and spread by exhaled breath or coughing. Symptoms appear four to seven days after infection; they include a severe sore throat, high fever, vomiting, and a rapidly spreading rash of tiny red spots on the neck and upper trunk. The face is flushed, except around the mouth. A white coating with red spots may develop on the tongue ("strawberry tongue"), which then comes off after a few days to reveal a bright red colour. After this event, the fever soon subsides, the rash fades, and the skin may peel. *Glomerulonephritis* (inflammation in the kidney) or *rheumatic fever* may, rarely, develop some weeks later. *Antibiotics* prevent this and promote a rapid recovery.

Scheie syndrome

A *mucopolysaccharidosis* (an inherited metabolic disorder) causing clouding of the cornea (surface of the eye), deformed hands, and aortic disease, but normal motor development.

Scheuermann's disease

A form of *osteochondritis juvenilis*, a bone disorder affecting children and adolescents. It causes degeneration of the thoracic *vertebrae* (the spinal bones that support the ribcage), leading to *kyphosis* (a forward bend in the spine).

Schilling test

A test used to measure intestinal absorption of vitamin B_{12}, in order to detect disorders such as *pernicious anaemia* (failure to absorb vitamin B_{12}). A person is given a radioactive dose of the vitamin by mouth, then the urine is tested over 24 hours to see how much of the radioactive substance is excreted.

schistosome

A fluke that causes *schistosomiasis*.

schistosomiasis

A parasitic tropical disease, also called bilharzia, that is caused by flukes (parasitic flatworms) called schistosomes, and acquired from infested lakes, rivers, or other waters. The larvae penetrate the skin and develop in the body into adult flukes, which settle in the veins of the bladder and intestines. Their eggs cause inflammatory reactions; there may be bleeding and ulceration in the bladder and intestinal walls, and the liver may be affected.

The first symptom of infestation is usually tingling and an itchy rash where the flukes have entered the skin. An influenza-like illness may develop many weeks later, when the adult flukes produce eggs. Subsequent symptoms include blood in the urine or faeces, abdominal or lower back pain, and enlargement of the liver or spleen. Complications of long-term infestation include liver *cirrhosis*, *bladder tumours*, and *kidney failure*.

Treatment is with the drug *praziquantel*. No vaccine is available, so people visiting infested areas should avoid bathing or wading in fresh water.

CYCLE OF **SCHISTOSOMIASIS**

The disease affects a large proportion of the population in some parts of the world, such as the Nile valley in Egypt. Many methods have been tried to break the cycle of the disease in affected areas, with varying success. Methods used have included strict sanitary regulations and measures to eradicate freshwater snails.

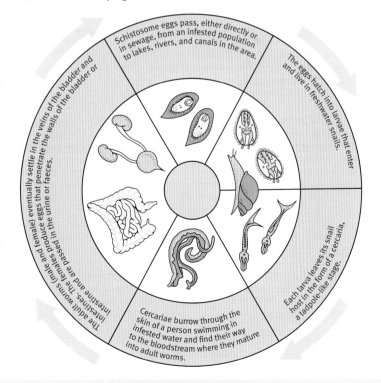

Schistosome eggs pass, either directly or in sewage, from an infested population to lakes, rivers, and canals in the area.

The eggs hatch into larvae that enter and live in freshwater snails.

Each larva leaves its snail host in the form of a cercaria, a tadpole-like stage.

Cercariae burrow through the skin of a person swimming in infested water and find their way to the bloodstream where they mature into adult worms.

The adult worms (male and female) eventually settle in the veins of the bladder and intestines. The females produce eggs that penetrate the walls of the bladder or intestine and are passed in the urine or faeces.

S

schizoid personality disorder

An inability to relate socially to other people. Individuals who have this trait, which is apparent from childhood, are often described as "loners" and make few, if any, friends. They are eccentric, seem to lack concern for others, and are apparently detached from normal day-to-day activities.

schizophrenia

A general term for a group of psychotic illnesses (disorders in which a person loses contact with reality) that are characterized by disturbances in thinking, emotional reaction, and behaviour. Schizophrenia is a disabling illness with a prolonged course that almost always results in chronic ill health and some degree of personality change.

Onset can be at any age but is most common in late adolescence and the early 20s. No causes have been identified, but many have been implicated. It is likely that inheritance plays a role, and various trigger factors may be involved, including life events such as bereavement and the use of drugs such as cannabis. Disruption of the activity of some neurotransmitters (chemicals that transmit signals between nerve cells) in the brain is a possible mechanism. Brain imaging has revealed abnormalities of structure and function in affected people.

SYMPTOMS AND SIGNS

Schizophrenia may begin insidiously, with the person becoming slowly more withdrawn and losing motivation. In other cases, it comes on suddenly, often in response to external stress. The main signs are delusions (fixed, irrational ideas) such as those of persecution (which are typical of paranoid schizophrenia); *hallucinations* (perceptions that occur without any external stimulus), and thought disorder. Hallucinations are usually auditory (in which the person hears voices talking about him or her), but may also be visual or tactile. Thought disorder leads to impaired concentration and thought processes; it is often reflected in muddled and disjointed speech and bizarre responses to questions. The person may believe that his or her thoughts are being controlled by outside forces or broadcast to others.

As the illness progresses, the person's emotions become blunted; he or she also becomes detached from others and loses interest in usual occupations. Behaviour is eccentric, and self-neglect common. In a rare form of schizophrenia,

catatonia may occur. In this condition, rigid postures are adopted for prolonged periods, or there are outbursts of repeated movement.

DIAGNOSIS AND TREATMENT

Diagnosis may take some time, and in some cases, it may be difficult to make a diagnosis at all. Treatment, which is usually through a community mental health team, is mainly with *antipsychotic drugs*, such as *phenothiazine drugs*, and antipsychotic drugs such as risperidone. In some cases, the drugs are usually given as monthly depot injections. Once the symptoms are controlled, community care, vocational opportunities, and family counselling can help to prevent a relapse.

Some people may make a complete recovery; however, most sufferers have relapses punctuated with partial or full recovery. A small proportion of people have a severe lifelong disability.

sciatica

Pain that radiates along the *sciatic nerve*. The pain usually affects the buttock and thigh, sometimes extending down the leg to the foot. In severe cases, the pain may be accompanied by numbness and/or weakness in the affected area.

The most common cause is a ruptured intervertebral disc pressing on the nerve root (see *disc prolapse*). Other causes include a muscle spasm, sitting awkwardly for long periods, or, less commonly, pressure on the nerve from a tumour. Sometimes the cause is unknown.

Treatment of sciatica is with *analgesic drugs* (painkillers) and *nonsteroidal anti-inflammatory drugs*. If the pain is severe, a short period of bed rest may be helpful, although prolonged rest may cause the sciatica to worsen. *Physiotherapy* may help in some cases, but neurosurgery may be needed if other treatments are ineffective or if there is nerve root compression. It is important to try and maintain a healthy posture and weight.

sciatic nerve

The main *nerve* in each leg and the largest nerve in the body. It is formed from roots in the spinal cord. The sciatic nerve supplies the hip joint, some of the thigh muscles, and the back of the thigh. Lower down it branches to form the nerves that supply the lower leg and the foot.

SCID

The abbreviation for *severe combined immune deficiency*.

scintigraphy

A less common alternative name for *radionuclide scanning*. Renal scintigraphy is also known as *renography*.

scirrhous

A term meaning "hard and fibrous". It is usually applied to cancerous tumours containing dense, fibrous tissue.

sclera

The white, fibrous, tough coating that protects the *eye*. The sclera may be injured by sharp objects. Disorders of the sclera include *scleritis* (inflammation) and *osteogenesis imperfecta* (a condition in which the sclera is abnormally thin and may appear blue).

scleritis

Inflammation of the *sclera*. It usually accompanies a *collagen disease* such as *rheumatoid arthritis*, but also occurs in *herpes zoster* ophthalmicus and *Wegener's granulomatosis*. Scleritis may cause some parts of the sclera to become thin and perforated. It is usually persistent but often responds to *corticosteroid* eye-drops.

LOCATION OF THE SCIATIC NERVE

The diagram below shows the sciatic nerve in the back of the right thigh and knee. Branches of the nerve extend down the leg to the sole of the foot.

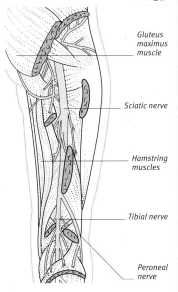

Gluteus maximus muscle

Sciatic nerve

Hamstring muscles

Tibial nerve

Peroneal nerve

S

S

LOCATION OF THE **SCLERA**

The sclera is the white tissue at the front of the eye. It is about 0.5 mm thick and is continuous with the cornea. It is extremely tough and protects the eye's inner structures.

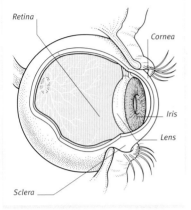

Retina

Cornea

Iris

Lens

Sclera

scleroderma

A slowly progressive condition characterized by hardening and thickening of the skin. With progression, internal organs are affected (see *systemic sclerosis*).

scleromalacia

Softening of the *sclera* (the white outer coat of the eye). It is a common complication of *scleritis*, especially when associated with *rheumatoid arthritis*.

sclerosing cholangitis

A rare condition in which many of the bile ducts are narrowed, causing progressive liver damage for which the only treatment may be a *liver transplant*. In many cases, it is related to *inflammatory bowel disease*. (See also *cholangitis*.)

sclerosis

Hardening of a body tissue. The term is usually used to refer to hardening of blood vessels (as in *arteriosclerosis*) or nerve tissue (as in *multiple sclerosis*).

sclerotherapy

A method of treating *varicose veins*, especially those in the legs; *haemorrhoids*; and *oesophageal varices*. The affected vein is injected with an irritant solution, which causes scar tissue formation and obliteration of the vein.

scoliosis

A deformity in which the *spine* is curved to one side. The thoracic (chest) or lumbar (lower back) regions are most commonly affected. Scoliosis usually starts in childhood or adolescence and becomes progressively more marked until growth stops. In many cases, another part of the spine curves to compensate, resulting in an S-shaped spine. Scoliosis may also be associated with *kyphoscoliosis*. The condition may be very mild and cause no symptoms, or it may be noticed by a doctor during investigation of back pain.

The cause of juvenile scoliosis is not known. Rarely, the condition is due to a congenital abnormality of the vertebrae (bones forming the spine). Sometimes it may occur temporarily as a result of a spinal injury.

If an underlying cause is found, it will be treated. In some cases, *physiotherapy* may be sufficient to control scoliosis of unknown cause. Progressive or severe scoliosis may require immobilization of the spine in a brace, followed by surgery (see *spinal fusion*) to straighten it.

scorpion stings

Many species of scorpions are not dangerous, but some in North Africa, the southern US, South America, the Caribbean, and India are highly venomous. Some stings may cause only mild pain and tingling; but in more venomous species severe pain, restlessness, sweating, diarrhoea, and vomiting can occur. They are rarely fatal in adults, but pose a greater risk to children and elderly people.

Scorpion stings require prompt attention. If pain is the only symptom, *analgesics* and a cold compress may be enough. In severe cases, treatment with *antivenom* may be needed.

scotoma

An area of abnormal vision occurring within the *visual field*.

screening

The testing of people with the aim of detecting disease at an early stage when it is still treatable.

Women routinely undergo various screening tests during pregnancy to check both the woman's health and that of the fetus (see *antenatal care*). After the birth, the newborn baby is also screened for certain disorders, such as *phenylketonuria*, congenital *hypothyroidism*, and *sickle cell anaemia*. Newborn babies are also given a physical examination and hearing tests (see *newborn screening tests*). Women are also routinely screened for breast cancer (see *mammography*) and cervical cancer (see *cervical smear test*).

People at high risk of developing certain conditions may also be given specific screening tests, such as screening for colon cancer (see *colon, cancer of*), *glaucoma*, and *hyperlipidaemia* (high blood lipid levels). People with a family history of some inherited conditions, such as *cystic fibrosis*, may be offered genetic tests to assess the likelihood of their children being affected. (See also *cancer screening*; *familial screening*.)

scrofula

Tuberculosis of the lymph nodes in the neck, often those just beneath the angle of the jaw. Scrofula is rare in developed countries. Antituberculous drugs clear up the condition in most cases.

scrofuloderma

A type of *tuberculosis* in which the infection spreads from inside the body, most commonly from the lymph nodes in the neck (see *scrofula*), to the skin. It causes painless swellings under the skin that develop into *abscesses* or *ulcers*.

ANATOMY OF THE **SCROTUM**

The scrotum has oil-secreting glands and thinly scattered hairs on its surface. Internally it is divided by a membrane into two halves, each containing a testis.

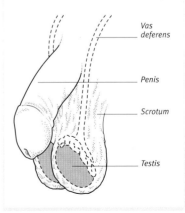

Vas deferens

Penis

Scrotum

Testis

scrotum

The pouch that hangs behind the penis and contains the *testes*. It consists of an outer layer of thin, wrinkled skin over a layer of muscular tissue. Swelling of the scrotum may have a number of causes including *inguinal hernia*, a swollen testis, *hydrocele*, *varicocele*, or fluid accumulation due to *heart failure* or injury.

scuba-diving medicine

A medical speciality concerned with the hazards of diving with self-contained underwater breathing apparatus (SCUBA). Most hazards stem from the increased pressure: at a depth of 10 m, the total pressure is twice the surface pressure; at 30 m, it is four times the surface pressure.

MECHANICAL EFFECTS OF PRESSURE

During descent, divers must introduce gas into their middle-ear cavities and facial sinuses to prevent damage as the pressure increases. This increasing pressure is also what airline passengers experience during descent and repressurization (see *barotrauma*). Whatever depth they attain, divers must be supplied with breathing mixtures at a pressure equal to the external water pressure. During ascent, gas in the lungs expands and can rupture lung tissues if the diver panics and inadvertently holds his or her breath. This is a serious condition, which is known as pulmonary barotrauma (burst lung). Symptoms may include coughing up blood, inability to pass urine, breathing difficulties, and unconsciousness.

TOXIC EFFECTS OF GASES

Amateur divers breathe compressed air, which consists mainly of nitrogen and oxygen. These gases are harmless at surface pressures but become toxic at high pressure. Nitrogen impairs the nervous system when air is breathed at depth, causing slowed mental functioning and other symptoms that mimic alcohol intoxication (a condition known as nitrogen narcosis). Oxygen becomes toxic when air is breathed at increased pressure, and in such situations it can cause convulsions or lung damage.

To attain greater depths without risking nitrogen and oxygen poisoning, professional divers use gas mixtures other than air. A typical mixture consists of helium, with the addition of only small amounts of oxygen and nitrogen.

THE BENDS

At depth, divers accumulate in their tissues excessive quantities of any inert gas they are breathing (nitrogen, if air is being breathed). If the diver ascends too quickly and if a large amount of gas has accumulated because the diver remained at depth for too long, this gas may form bubbles in tissues and blood, causing *decompression sickness*.

OTHER HAZARDS

Additional hazards include *hypothermia* due to immersion in cold water, and bites or stings from marine animals (see *bites, animal*; *venomous bites and stings*). In addition, there is a risk of drowning.

ACCIDENT PREVENTION AND TREATMENT

Anyone who is thinking of taking up scuba diving should first have a medical checkup and undergo training at a recognized diving school.

Pressure-related accidents, such as burst lung and decompression sickness, are treated by recompression of the diver in a special pressure chamber. This allows any bubbles or gas in the blood or tissues to be reabsorbed. The following stage is slow release of the pressure.

scurvy

A disease, now rare in developed countries, caused by inadequate *vitamin C* intake. Scurvy disturbs the production of *collagen*. The collagen is unstable, causing weakness of small blood vessels and poor wound healing. Haemorrhages (bleeding) may occur anywhere in the body, including the brain. If it occurs in the skin, the bleeding appears as bruising. Bleeding into the gums and loosening of teeth are common. Bleeding into the muscles and joints causes pain.

Scurvy is treated with large doses of vitamin C. Bleeding stops in 24 hours, healing resumes, and muscle and bone pain quickly disappear.

seafood poisoning

Bacterial or viral infections caused by eating shellfish that has been badly stored or cooked, or has been in water contaminated by human faeces. Symptoms include vomiting, diarrhoea, and abdominal pain. They may be relieved with plenty of fluids and salts (see *rehydration therapy*), but severe cases may need hospital treatment.

sealants, dental

Plastic coatings that are applied to crevices in the chewing surfaces of the back *teeth* to help prevent decay.

seasickness

A type of *motion sickness*.

seasonal affective disorder

A form of *depression* in which mood changes occur with the seasons. People with seasonal affective disorder, or SAD, tend to become depressed in winter, when natural light decreases, and feel better in spring. In some people, exposure to bright light for two to four hours each morning seems to prevent it.

sebaceous cyst

A harmless, smooth nodule under the skin, most commonly on the scalp, face, ear, or genitals. The cyst contains a yellow, cheesy material and may become very large and infected by bacteria, making it painful. Large or infected cysts can be surgically removed.

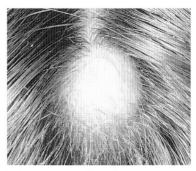

Sebaceous cyst on the scalp
These smooth nodules under the surface of the skin are filled with a cheeselike substance known as sebum. Those cysts that grow very large or become infected need to be removed surgically.

sebaceous glands

Glands in the *skin* that secrete a lubricating substance called *sebum*. Sebaceous glands either open into hair follicles or discharge directly on to the surface of the skin. These glands are most numerous on the scalp, face, and anus, but do not exist on the palms or the soles of the feet. Disorders of the glands may lead to *seborrhoea* or *acne* vulgaris.

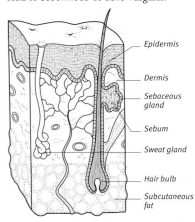

Cross-section of skin with sebaceous gland
These glands occur in the skin and are most numerous on the scalp. They secrete a lubricating substance called sebum, which discharges directly on to the surface of the skin or into hair follicles.

seborrhoea

Excessive secretion of *sebum*, causing oiliness of the face and a greasy scalp. The cause is unclear, but *androgen hormones* play a part. Seborrhoea is most common in adolescent boys; those affected are more likely to develop seborrhoeic *dermatitis* and *acne* vulgaris. The condition usually improves in adulthood without any treatment.

seborrhoeic dermatitis

See *dermatitis*.

seborrhoeic wart

Also called a seborrhoeic *keratosis*, a small, harmless, brown or black skin growth with a rough, greasy surface.

sebum

The oily secretion that is produced by the *sebaceous glands*. Sebum has several functions: it lubricates the skin, keeps it supple, and protects it from becoming waterlogged or dried out and cracked. Sebum also protects against bacteria and fungi. Production of sebum is partly controlled by *androgen hormones*. Oversecretion (see *seborrhoea*) of sebum causes greasy skin and may lead to seborrhoeic *dermatitis* or *acne*.

secondary

A term applied to a disease or disorder that results from or follows another disease (the *primary* disease). It also refers to a malignant tumour that has spread from a primary cancer elsewhere in the body (see *metastasis*).

secondary haemorrhage

Bleeding that results from an injury or surgical procedure but that occurs at a later time, rather than immediately. Secondary haemorrhage may be the result of infection.

secondary infection

An infection that results from or follows a pre-existing infection. One example is a bacterial respiratory infection that follows a viral infection. (See also *superinfection*).

secretin

A hormone produced by the *duodenum* (the first part of the small intestine) when acidic food enters it from the stomach. Secretin stimulates the release of pancreatic juice, which contains sodium bicarbonate to neutralize the acid, and bile from the liver.

secretion

The manufacture and release by a cell, gland, or organ of substances (such as *enzymes*) needed for metabolic processes elsewhere in the body.

secretory otitis media

An alternative name for *glue ear*.

sectioning

A commonly used term for the implementation of a section of the *Mental Health Act* to detain a mentally ill person against his or her will.

security object

A significant item, such as a favourite blanket, garment, or soft toy, that provides comfort and reassurance to a young child. These items are sometimes referred to as transitional objects. The child may become deeply attached to the object and show great distress if it is lost or if any attempt is made to take it away from him or her.

Security objects are often important during the toddler stage and may be used for several years. However, most children grow out of the need for such an item by the time they are about seven or eight years old.

sedation

The use of a drug to calm a person. Sedation is used to reduce excessive *anxiety* and control dangerously aggressive behaviour. It may also be used as part of *premedication* (drugs given to prepare a person for surgery). *Sleeping drugs* are used for night sedation.

Location of electrodes

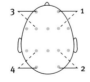

Each numbered trace shows changes in electrical potential between two points on the skull surface.

Normal traces **Abnormal traces during seizure**

EEG changes during a seizure
The traces are recordings of electrical activity in a patient's brain, obtained from electrodes placed at various locations on the scalp and linked to an EEG machine. They show the change in activity at the onset of a seizure.

sedative drugs

A group of drugs used to produce *sedation*. Sedatives include *sleeping drugs*, *antianxiety drugs*, *antipsychotic drugs*, and some *antidepressant drugs*.

sedimentation rate

See *ESR*.

seizure

A sudden episode of abnormal electrical activity in the *brain*. Recurrent seizures occur in *epilepsy*.

Seizures may be partial or generalized. In a partial seizure, the abnormal activity is confined to one area of the brain. Symptoms include tingling or twitching of a small area of the body, *hallucinations*, fear, or *déjà vu*. In a generalized seizure, the abnormal activity spreads through the brain, causing loss of consciousness.

Causes of seizures include *head injury*, *stroke*, *brain tumour*, infection, metabolic disturbances, withdrawal in *alcohol dependence*, or hereditary alcohol intolerance. In children, high fever may cause seizures (see *convulsion, febrile*). *Anticonvulsant drugs* can control seizures or reduce their frequency.

selective serotonin reuptake inhibitors (SSRIs)

A group of drugs that are mainly used to treat *depression* but may also be used in the treatment of *panic disorder*, *bulimia*, *obsessive–compulsive disorder post-traumatic stress disorder*, and certain *anxiety* disorders. SSRIs block the reabsorption of *serotonin* following its release in the brain; the increased serotonin levels that result are associated with improved mood. Common SSRIs include fluoxetine, *paroxetine*, and *sertraline*. The drugs are usually taken orally once a day; beneficial effects may not be felt for up to three weeks. SSRIs usually produce fewer side effects than other types of antidepressant but may cause diarrhoea, nausea, restlessness, and anxiety. Stopping SSRIs suddenly can cause withdrawal symptoms. Most SSRIs are not recommended for treating depression in those under 18 years old.

selegiline

A drug that is used in the treatment of *Parkinson's disease*, either alone (in the disease's early stage) or in combination with *levodopa*. Side effects may include nausea, vomiting, diarrhoea or constipation, dry mouth, and sore throat.

S

selenium

A *trace element* that may help to preserve the elasticity of body tissues. The richest dietary sources are meat, fish, whole grains, and dairy products.

self-help organizations

Charity or voluntary organizations that provide people affected by particular conditions with information, support, and, sometimes, financial aid.

self-image

A person's view of his or her own personality and abilities. Some neurotic disorders stem from an incongruity between self-image and how others see one. *Psychotherapy* aims to treat neurosis by changing a person's self-image.

self-injury

The act of deliberately injuring oneself, for example by cutting the wrists or burning the skin. It most often occurs in young adults, and is three times more common in women. In some cases, it is a way of dealing with stress, such as that caused by *child abuse*. It may also occur as a feature of *autism*. There are more unusual forms of self-harm, for example genital mutilation, and these are usually due to *psychosis*. Self-destructive biting features in Lesch–Nyhan syndrome, a rare *metabolic disorder*.

semen

Fluid discharged from the penis on *ejaculation*. Semen comprises fluid from the *seminal vesicles*, fluid from the *prostate* and Cowper's glands, and *sperm*. (See also *reproductive system, male*.)

semen analysis

Analysis of sperm concentration, shape, and motility (ability to move) to investigate male *infertility*. It is also performed about 12 weeks after *vasectomy* to ensure that semen no longer contains sperm.

semen, blood in the

The appearance of a small amount of blood in the semen is usually harmless, and many cases are assumed to have been caused by minor trauma to the testes or genital tract. It may also occur after a prostate *biopsy*. However, occasionally there is a more serious underlying cause (such as infection, prostate cancer, or various disorders of the urethra), particularly if blood persistently appears in the semen, and therefore all cases need medical assessment.

semicircular canal

A structure in the inner *ear* that plays a role in *balance*. There are three semicircular canals in each ear, at right angles to each other, and connected via a chamber called the vestibule. The fluid-filled canals contain small hairs that detect movement and acceleration and transmit information to the brain via the vestibular nerve.

seminal vesicle

One of a pair of sacs behind the bladder in the male that produce seminal fluid, which is mixed with sperm to make semen (see *reproductive system, male*).

seminoma

See *testis, cancer of.*

senile dementia

See *dementia*.

senile purpura

A skin condition in which some areas become purple or red-brown. It occurs in middle to old age and is more common in women. It is caused by bleeding from small blood vessels under the skin.

senility

Old age or, more commonly, the decline in mental ability that may occur with age.

senna

A *laxative drug* from leaves and pods of the Arabian shrubs CASSIA ACUTIFOLIA and CASSIA ANGUSTIFOLIA. It stimulates bowel contractions and may darken the urine.

PRINCIPAL **SENSORY PATHWAYS** INTO THE BRAIN

Some information entering the brain passes via the brainstem and/or thalamus to the cerebral cortex (outer surface of the brain), where sensations are perceived. Other information does not lead to conscious sensation. This includes certain data about body posture, processed in the cerebellum, and about internal body functioning, processed in the brainstem.

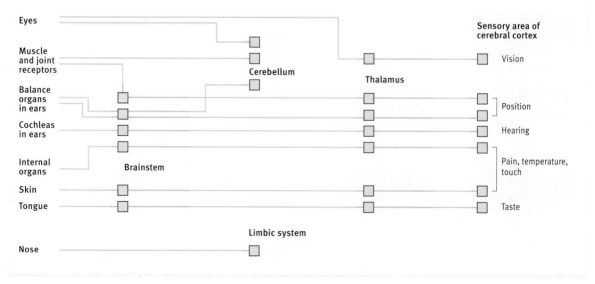

S

sensate-focus technique

A method taught to couples who are experiencing sexual difficulties caused by psychological rather than physiological factors. The technique's aim is to make people more aware of their own and their partner's pleasurable bodily sensations, and to reduce anxiety about performance. It is particularly effective in treating loss of sexual desire (see *sexual desire, inhibited*), or inability to achieve orgasm (see *orgasm, lack of*), and in helping men to overcome *erectile dysfunction* or premature ejaculation (see *ejaculation, disorders of*).

sensation

A feeling or impression (such as a sound, smell, touch, or hunger) that has entered consciousness. The senses convey information about the external environment and the body's internal state to the *central nervous system* (the *brain* and *spinal cord*).

SENSORY RECEPTORS

Information is collected by millions of *receptors* (specialized nerve structures) found throughout the body in the skin, muscles, and joints, in the internal organs, in the walls of blood vessels, and in special sense organs such as the *eye* and inner *ear*.

Receptors are attuned to a particular stimulus, such as light of a certain wavelength, chemical molecules of a particular shape, vibration, or temperature. Each receptor "fires" (sends an electrical signal) when stimulated.

Some receptors are the terminals (free nerve cell fibres) of long nerve cell fibres, others are specialized cells that connect to such fibres. When a receptor fires, a signal passes along the appropriate nerve fibre to the spinal cord and/or brain. A proportion of this information reaches the *sensory cortex* of the brain and is consciously perceived.

SPECIAL SENSES

The special senses include *vision*, *hearing*, *taste*, and *smell*. The receptor cells for these senses are collected into special organs: the retina in the eye, the auditory apparatus in the ear, the tastebuds in the *tongue*, and the organ for smell in the *nose*. Information from these organs passes directly to the brain via the *cranial nerves*. Much of the collected information passes to the cerebral cortex, although some goes to other areas of the brain (for example, from the eyes to the cerebellum, where it is used to help maintain balance).

NEUROLOGICAL SENSORY TESTING

When examining a patient's nervous system, a doctor usually includes several standard tests of touch, position, pain, and vibration senses, such as those below.

Light touch
With the patient's eyes closed, a wisp of cotton wool is brushed lightly across the face.

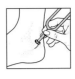

Vibration
A vibrating tuning fork is held against a prominent bone, such as the ankle bone or mastoid bone.

Pinprick
The prick tests pain sensation and may be repeated at different locations on the patient's body.

Position sense
The patient, with eyes closed, tells in which direction his or her finger is moved.

Pain pinch
Pain sense may be further tested by pinching the Achilles tendon at the back of the heel.

Two-point discrimination
Measures the ability to distinguish two pinpricks from a single prick.

INTERNAL AND TOUCH SENSES

These senses include pain, temperature, pressure, and proprioception (position), sensations. Proprioception relies on receptors in the muscles and joints to provide information on the position in space of parts of the body. Pain is one of the most primitive senses; its role is to warn of harmful stimuli through receptors that occur both at the surface of the skin and internally.

Many types of receptors are found in the skin. Some are sensitive to pressure, others to the movement of hairs or to temperature changes. Skin receptors are made up of the terminals of nerve fibres, which are wrapped around the roots of hairs, formed into discs, or surrounded by a series of membranes to form onionlike structures called pacinian corpuscles. Different patterns of stimulation of these receptors produce such sensations as pain, tickling, firm or light pressure, heat or cold. Certain skin areas (lips, palms of the hands, and genitals) have a particularly high concentration of receptors.

Most of the signals from these receptors pass, through the cranial or *spinal nerves* and tracts in the brain or spinal cord, to the *thalamus* and then to two regions of the sensory cortex called the somatosensory cortices. Sensations that are perceived at certain points within these regions correspond to the parts of the body from which the signals originated. Much larger areas of cortex are devoted to sensations originating from the highly receptive hands and lips than from less sensitive parts.

sensation, abnormal

Dulled, unpleasant, or otherwise altered *sensations* in the absence of an obvious stimulus. Abnormal sensation is also known as paraesthesia.

TYPES

Numbness and *pins-and-needles* are common abnormal sensations, which are sometimes combined with pain or feelings of coldness or burning. *Neuralgia* is characterized by pain with a brief stabbing, repetitive quality.

More examples of unusual abnormal sensations include a feeling that fluid is trickling down the skin, tight constriction in part of the body, and the feeling that insects are crawling over the skin (known as formication).

The special senses can also be impaired or altered as a result of damage to the relevant sensory mechanism or nerve tracts (see *deafness*; *smell*; *tinnitus*; *vision, disorders of*).

CAUSES

Neuropathy (peripheral nerve damage) from thiamine (vitamin B_{12}) deficiency in alcoholics, *diabetes mellitus*, or certain types of poisons (such as lead) is a common cause of abnormal sensation. The sufferer may complain of tingling or a feeling of walking on cotton wool. The peripheral nerves may also be damaged or irritated by infections such as *herpes zoster* (shingles) or by a tumour pressing on a nerve, which often causes severe pain. *Spinal injury*, *head injury*, *stroke*, and *multiple sclerosis* are other causes of disruption to nerve pathways in the *brain* or *spinal cord*.

Damage to the *thalamus* (a relay station for sensory pathways in the brain) can produce particularly unpleasant results, such as a spreading sensation like an electric shock that occurs after a simple pinprick. Damage that affects the parietal lobe in the brain can lead to loss of the ability to locate or recognize objects by touch.

DIAGNOSIS AND TREATMENT
Various tests may be needed to find the cause of abnormal sensation. These include simple neurological sensory testing; testing of *reflexes*; tests on blood and urine; and *CT scanning* and *MRI*.

Pressure on or damage to nerves can sometimes be relieved by surgery or other treatments for the cause. In other cases, distressing abnormal sensation can be relieved by drugs or by cutting the relevant nerve fibres or giving injections to block the transmission of signals.

senses
See *sensation*. (See also *hearing*; *taste*; *touch*; *smell*; *vision*.)

sensitization
The initial exposure of a person to an allergen or other substance recognized as being foreign by the *immune system*, which leads to an immune response. On subsequent exposures to the same substance, there is a much stronger and faster immune reaction. This response forms the basis of *allergy* and other types of *hypersensitivity* reaction.

sensorineural deafness
A type of *deafness* that occurs as a result of problems either relating to the inner ear itself, or to the nerves connecting the inner ear to the brain, or to the auditory area of the brain.

sensory cortex
A region of the outer *cerebrum* of the *brain* in which sensory information comes to consciousness.

Pressure, pain, and temperature sensations are perceived in the parietal lobes of the cerebrum, as is taste. Visual sensations are perceived in the occipital lobes, at the back of the cerebrum; sound is perceived in the temporal lobes, at the sides.

sensory deprivation
The removal of normal external stimuli, such as sight and sound, from a person's environment. Prolonged sensory deprivation can produce feelings of unreality, difficulty in thinking, and *hallucinations* (perceptions occurring without any external stimulus).

sensory nerve
A type of *nerve* fibre that carries information from a *receptor* or sense organ towards the brain.

separation anxiety
The feelings of distress experienced by a young child parted from his or her parents or home. Signs include crying and clinging to a parent. This is a normal aspect of infant behaviour and usually diminishes by the age of three or four.

In separation anxiety disorder, the reaction to separation is greater than that expected for the child's age and maturity. The anxiety may manifest as physical symptoms such as headaches, nausea, and difficulty in sleeping. Separation anxiety disorder may sometimes be a feature of *depression*.

sepsis
Bacterial infection of a wound or body tissue that leads to the formation of *pus* or to the multiplication of the bacteria in the blood. (See also *bacteraemia*; *septicaemia*; *septic shock*.)

septal defect
A congenital *heart* abnormality in which there is a hole in the septum (partition) between the left and right sides of the heart. The hole can be between either the atrial (upper) or the ventricular (lower) chambers. Commonly known as a hole in the heart, septal defect varies in its effects according to its type and size. Usually, the cause is unknown.

TYPES
When the hole is in the septum separating the two ventricles, the abnormality is known as a ventricular septal defect; when it is in the septum between the two atria, it is called an atrial septal defect. In both types, the hole allows some of the freshly oxygenated blood in the left half of the heart (which supplies tissues throughout the body) to flow into the right half, mix with deoxygenated blood and recirculate through the lungs.

Some children are born with both types of defect. Either type may be accompanied by one or more additional heart abnormalities and/or some other congenital defects.

SYMPTOMS AND SIGNS
A small defect has little or no effect. A large ventricular hole may cause *heart failure* six to eight weeks after birth, causing breathlessness, feeding difficulties, pallor, and sweating. A large atrial defect may cause heart failure to develop around the age of 30 or there may be no heart failure at all, but fatigue may occur on exertion. *Pulmonary hypertension* (high blood pressure in the arteries supplying the lungs) may develop in both types of defect but is especially likely if there is a large ventricular defect.

With a ventricular defect there is also a slight risk of *endocarditis* (inflammation of the lining of the heart); in atrial septal defect, *atrial fibrillation* (rapid, irregular beating of the atria) may occur after the age of 30.

DIAGNOSIS AND TREATMENT
Diagnosis may be aided by a *chest X-ray*, *ECG*, or *echocardiography*. Atrial holes are repaired surgically if they cause symptoms or if complications develop. Small ventricular holes often become smaller, or even close up, on their own as the child grows. A ventricular defect that

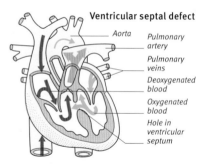

Ventricular septal defect

Aorta

Pulmonary artery

Pulmonary veins

Deoxygenated blood

Oxygenated blood

Hole in ventricular septum

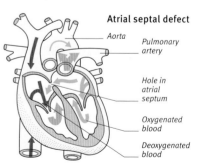

Atrial septal defect

Aorta

Pulmonary artery

Hole in atrial septum

Oxygenated blood

Deoxygenated blood

Two types of septal defect
In both cases (atrial and ventricular), oxygenated blood is forced from the left to the right side of the heart through the hole in the septum. Too much blood passes to the lungs (via the pulmonary artery) and too little to the body tissues (via the aorta).

S

is causing heart failure is treated with drugs such as *diuretics*. If the hole does not close spontaneously, it may be repaired by *open heart surgery*, usually before the child reaches school age. The operation has a very high success rate and most children go on to lead normal lives.

septate uterus

A defect in which the interior of the uterus (womb) is divided by a septum (wall of tissue). A septate uterus may result in *miscarriages*; however, it can be corrected surgically, and most women have successful pregnancies after treatment.

septic abortion

A complication of *miscarriage* or abortion (see *abortion, induced*) in which the uterus and any tissue retained from the fetus and the placenta become infected. Symptoms include fever, abdominal pain, and a vaginal discharge that may contain blood. Hospital treatment is needed to prevent *septic shock*. (See also *septicaemia*.)

septicaemia

A serious or even life-threatening condition, also called blood poisoning, in which bacteria multiply rapidly in the bloodstream and bacterial *toxins* are present in the blood.

Septicaemia is usually due to bacteria that have escaped from a site of infection, such as an *abscess*. The condition is more likely to occur in people whose resistance to infection is lowered by an *immunodeficiency disorder* or *immunosuppressant drugs*. Those with *cancer* or *diabetes mellitus*, and drug addicts who inject, are also at higher risk.

Signs include a high fever, chills, rapid breathing, headache, and clouding of consciousness. The sufferer may go into life-threatening *septic shock*.

Glucose and/or saline are administered by *intravenous infusion*, and *antibiotics* given by injection or infusion. Tests are performed to identify the bacteria and, if necessary, the site of infection. Surgery may be needed to remove tissue at the site. If treatment is given before septic shock develops, the outlook is good.

septic arthritis

A type of *arthritis* caused by a bacterial infection entering a joint via an open wound or from the bloodstream. Symptoms of septic arthritis appear suddenly and may include swelling, tenderness, and fever. If pus builds up, the joint may be permanently damaged.

Fluid is taken from the joint and is analysed to determine the presence of infection (see *aspiration*), and pus may be drained to help relieve pain. Initially, treatment is with intravenous *antibiotic drugs*, followed by oral antibiotics for several weeks or months after that.

septic shock

A life-threatening condition in which there is tissue damage (especially affecting the kidneys, heart, and lungs) and a dramatic drop in blood pressure as a result of *septicaemia* (multiplication of bacteria and the presence of bacterial toxins in the blood).

In many cases, the main danger comes from the toxins because they can damage cells and tissues, promote blood clotting in the smallest blood vessels, and seriously interfere with the normal circulation of the blood. Toxins may also cause fluid leakage from blood vessels and reduced ability of the vessels to constrict. This leads to a drop in blood pressure and may also lead to a further problem, *disseminated intravascular coagulation* (a clotting disorder).

CAUSES
Septic shock is most common in people who have debilitating disorders, such as *diabetes mellitus*, *cancer*, or liver *cirrhosis*, who also have an infection (often in the intestines and urinary tract) that has led to septicaemia. Septic shock is particularly likely to occur in people with an *immunodeficiency disorder*, and in individuals taking *immunosuppressant drugs*. Newborn babies are also particularly susceptible.

SYMPTOMS AND SIGNS
The symptoms vary with the extent and site of major tissue damage but they are broadly the same as those that occur in septicaemia. Additionally, however, there may be cold hands and feet, often with cyanosis (blue coloration) due to slowed blood flow, a weak, rapid pulse, and much reduced blood pressure. There may be vomiting and diarrhoea. Heart failure, abnormal bleeding, and damage to the kidneys, leading to kidney failure, may also develop.

TREATMENT
Septic shock requires immediate treatment with *antibiotic drugs*, and sometimes surgery to remove the focus of infection. Rapid fluid replacement to prevent kidney failure occurring is an essential aspect of treatment. Measures are also taken to raise blood pressure and promote better blood supply to the tissues.

Septrin

A brand name for the antibacterial drug *co-trimoxazole*.

septum

A thin dividing wall that occurs within or between parts of the body; an example is the nasal septum, the partition between the nostrils.

sequela

A condition that results from or follows a disease, disorder, or injury. The term is usually used in the plural (sequelae) to refer to complications of a disease.

sequestration

Separation of a sequestrum (a piece of dead bone) from healthy living bone. Sequestration also refers to loss of blood or other fluid into body spaces, removing it from the circulation and causing *hypotension*. Sequestration crises, in which blood pools in the spleen and liver, occur in *sickle cell anaemia*.

seroconversion

The development, in the blood *serum*, of *antibodies* (proteins made to combat a specific infection) that can be detected by testing (see *serology*).

serology

A branch of laboratory medicine concerned with analysis of blood *serum*. Applications of serological techniques include the diagnosis of infectious diseases by the identification of *antibodies*, the development of *antiserum* preparations for passive *immunization*, and the determination of *blood groups* in *paternity testing* and forensic investigations.

seronegative

A term that is used to describe blood *serum* that has undergone testing for an infection (see *serology*) and is found to have no antibodies to the infectious organism under investigation. The term also refers to the absence of an autoantibody (one that reacts against the body's own cells) in a specific condition. An example of this usage is the lack of rheumatoid factor that occurs in seronegative rheumatoid arthritis.

seropositive

A term that is used to describe blood *serum* that has undergone testing for a certain infection (see *serology*) and is found to contain antibodies to the infectious organism.

S

serotonin

Also known as 5-hydroxytryptamine (5HT), a substance found in many tissues, particularly in blood platelets, digestive tract lining, and brain. Serotonin is released from platelets at sites of bleeding, where its function is to constrict small blood vessels, thereby reducing blood loss. In the digestive tract, serotonin inhibits gastric secretion and stimulates smooth muscle in the intestine wall. In the brain, it acts as a *neurotransmitter* (a chemical that passes signals between nerve cells). Serotonin levels in the brain are reduced in people who are depressed, but certain *antidepressant drugs* raise the level. *Serotonin agonists* are used in the treatment of acute migraine attacks.

serotonin agonists

A group of drugs, also known as $5HT_1$ agonists, used to treat acute attacks of *migraine*, in which the headache is caused by dilation of blood vessels in the brain. Serotonin agonists act on the same receptors in the brain as *serotonin* (a chemical messenger), returning the dilated vessels to their normal size and thereby relieving the symptoms of the migraine attack.

Common serotonin agonists include *naratriptan* and *sumatriptan*. These drugs can cause chest pain, particularly in people with heart disease. They should be used with caution in those at increased risk of coronary artery disease. Other side effects include flushing, tingling, and nausea.

serotonin antagonists

A group of drugs, also known as $5HT_3$ antagonists, used to treat nausea and vomiting that is caused by *radiotherapy* and *anticancer drugs* or following general anaesthesia given for surgery. In these cases, the symptoms occur when *serotonin* stimulates the vomiting centre in the brain; the drugs prevent them by inhibiting the action of serotonin. Common serotonin antagonists include granisetron and *ondansetron*.

serous

A word that refers to blood *serum* or clear, watery body fluid. It is also used of body structures containing or producing these substances.

Seroxat

The brand name for *paroxetine*, an SSRI antidepressant drug.

Sertoli cell tumour

A tumour arising from the Sertoli cells (which support and nourish the developing sperm) within the testis. Some Sertoli cell tumours are malignant (see *testis, cancer of*).

sertraline

A *selective serotonin reuptake inhibitor* drug used in the treatment of *depression* and *obsessive–compulsive disorder*.

serum

The clear fluid that separates from *blood* when it clots. It contains salts, glucose, and proteins, including *antibodies*. Serum from the blood of a person who has had an infection usually contains antibodies to the infectious organism; if injected into other people, it can protect them from that disease. The serum preparation is called an *antiserum*; its use forms the basis of passive *immunization*. (see also *plasma*).

serum sickness

A type of *hypersensitivity* reaction that may develop about 10 days after injection with an *antiserum* of animal origin or after taking certain drugs, such as *penicillins*. Symptoms may include an itchy rash, joint pain, fever, and enlarged lymph nodes. In severe cases, a state that is similar to *shock* develops. Symptoms of serum sickness usually clear up in a few days; *antihistamine drugs* may hasten recovery. In severe cases, a *corticosteroid drug* may be prescribed.

severe acute respiratory syndrome (SARS)

See *SARS*.

severe combined immunodeficiency (SCID)

A rare *congenital* (present from birth) disorder in which the immune system functions inefficiently, or not at all. Babies born with severe combined immunodeficiency (SCID) are highly susceptible to infections. They may fail to thrive and have many severe infections (such as those of the respiratory and gastrointestinal tracts), skin rashes, recurrent oral thrush (see *candidiasis*), and *pneumonia*.

Early diagnosis of SCID is vital; the disorder is confirmed by blood tests to check levels of *lymphocytes* (a type of white blood cell). A *stem cell* or *bone marrow transplant* offers the best chance of a cure, provided it is performed in the first few months of life. Many children with SCID are treated successfully and are able to lead normal lives thereafter.

sex

Another term for gender; also a commonly used term for *sexual intercourse*.

sex change

Radical surgical procedures, usually combined with hormone therapy, that alter a person's anatomical gender. Sex-change operations are performed on transsexuals (see *transsexualism*) and on infants whose external sex organs are neither completely male nor completely female (see *genitalia, ambiguous*). The procedures are carried out in order to give a person the physical appearance that coincides with his or her psychological *gender identity*, or to provide a more defined sexual identity.

PROCEDURES

For transsexuals, sex-change procedures involve a series of major operations on the genitourinary tract, which are carried out after courses of hormone therapy and extensive counselling. The male-to-female sex change operation is the one more commonly performed and the results are more satisfactory than the female-to-male procedure.

Babies with ambiguous genitalia are assigned a gender as soon as possible after birth, and given appropriate surgical and hormonal treatment.

OUTLOOK

Hormone therapy may need to be continued for life to maintain secondary sexual characteristics, such as body shape and hair distribution. Female transsexuals can have intercourse but cannot conceive; males cannot ejaculate, and achieve an erection only with mechanical aids.

sex chromosomes

The pair of *chromosomes* that determines a person's sex. All the cells in the human body (except for egg or sperm cells) contain a pair of sex chromosomes together with 22 other pairs of chromosomes known as autosomes. In women, the sex chromosomes are of similar appearance and are called X chromosomes. In men, one sex chromosome is an X and the other, smaller, one is a Y. The normal sex chromosome complement for women is XX, and for men, XY.

FUNCTION

Like all chromosomes, the X and Y chromosomes exert their effects in the body through the activities of their constituent *genes*. These genes contain the coded instructions for chemical processes within cells and for aspects of growth and development within the whole body.

The X and Y chromosomes differ in one way: genes on the Y chromosome are concerned solely with *sex determination*. Their presence ensures a male: their absence a female. The X chromosome, occurring in both sexes, contains many genes vital to general development and functioning. Absence of the X chromosome is incompatible with life.

The presence of a single X chromosome and 22 pairs of autosomes in the nuclei of ordinary body cells appears to provide the blueprint for general body functioning and development, which seems to have an underlying female pattern. This can be seen in people with *Turner's syndrome*, who have only one sex chromosome, an X. Although full female sexual characteristics never develop, these people are unmistakably female in appearance and identity. The full complement of female sexual characteristics will develop only in the presence of a second X chromosome. It is the addition of a Y chromosome that is responsible for converting the female to the male pattern.

sex determination

The factors that determine biological sex. The underlying determinants are the *sex chromosomes* in a person's cells: two X chromosomes in females and one X and one Y chromosome in males. Early in embryonic development, these chromosomes cause the development of different gonads (the testes in males and the ovaries in females). In males, the testes then produce hormones that cause the development of a male reproductive tract, including a penis. In females, absence of these male hormones leads to a different pattern of development, with the formation of fallopian tubes, uterus, and vagina. At *puberty*, another surge of hormones from the gonads leads to the appearance of secondary *sexual characteristics*, such as facial hair in males, breasts in females, and pubic hair in both sexes.

Defects sometimes occur in the process of sex determination, and may result in ambiguous sex (see *genitalia, ambiguous*). Some people acquire an abnormal complement of sex chromosomes (see *chromosomal abnormalities*) and all the characteristics of one sex do not develop.

True *hermaphroditism* (the presence of both ovaries and testes in the body) is a very rare occurrence.

sex hormones

Hormones that control the development of primary and secondary *sexual characteristics* and that regulate sex-related functions, such as the menstrual cycle. There are three main types: *androgen hormones*, *oestrogen hormones*, and *progesterone hormone*.

sex-linked inheritance

The passing on to the next generation of a trait or disorder that is determined by the *sex chromosomes*, or by the *genes* that are carried on them.

Disorders due to an abnormal number of sex chromosomes include *Turner's syndrome* and *Klinefelter's syndrome*. Most other sex-linked traits or disorders are caused by *recessive* genes on the X chromosome (see *X-linked disorders*).

sex therapy

Counselling for, and treatment of, sexual difficulties not due to a physical cause. Sex therapy (also called psychosexual therapy) may involve changing the partners' attitudes towards sex, increasing their understanding of sexual needs, and teaching techniques, such as the *sensate-focus technique* or *pelvic floor exercises*, for specific problems. Sex therapy is particularly successful in treating certain disorders including *vaginismus*, premature ejaculation (see *ejaculation, disorders of*), lack of orgasm (see *orgasm, lack of*), and *erectile dysfunction*.

sexual abuse

Subjection of a person to sexual activity that has caused, or is likely to cause, physical or psychological harm. (See also *child abuse*; *incest*; *rape*.)

sexual characteristics, primary

Physical features, which are present from birth, that show a person's sex, such as a penis and testes in a male or a vagina and vulva in a female.

sexual characteristics, secondary

Physical features appearing at *puberty* that indicate the onset of adult reproductive life. In girls, breast enlargement is the first sign. Shortly afterwards, pubic and underarm hair appears, and body fat increases around the hips, stomach, and thighs to produce the

female body shape. In boys, the first sign is enlargement of the testes, followed by thinning of the scrotal skin and enlargement of the penis. Pubic, facial, underarm, and other body hair appears, the voice deepens, and muscle bulk and bone size increase.

sexual desire, inhibited

Lack of sexual desire (libido) or of the ability to become physically aroused during sexual activity. Either condition may be physical or psychological.

LACK OF DESIRE

A high proportion of women and some men experience loss of sexual desire at some time in the their lives. Common physical causes include fatigue, ill health, and discomfort after childbirth. Certain drugs, including sleeping pills, antidepressants, antihypertensives, oral contraceptives, and alcohol, can also reduce sexual desire. Psychological factors include *depression*, anxiety, stress, unsatisfactory relationships, fear of pregnancy, or a traumatic sexual experience.

LACK OF PHYSICAL AROUSAL

It is rare for anyone of either sex to be incapable of some degree of physical sexual arousal. A common reason for failure is the partner's poor or insensitive sexual technique, although guilt about the sex act or anxiety about sexual inadequacy may contribute to the problem.

TREATMENT

Sex therapy or *relationship counselling* may be helpful in resolving problems with a psychological basis. Sexual problems with a physical or chemical cause often improve once the underlying condition is resolved.

sexual deviation

See *deviation, sexual*.

sexual dysfunction

See *psychosexual dysfunction*.

sexual intercourse

A term sometimes used to describe a variety of sexual activities, but which specifically refers to the insertion of a man's penis into a woman's vagina. Sexual intercourse is the usual means of achieving *fertilization*. It is also a means of achieving *orgasm* for one or both partners.

sexuality

A term describing the capacity for sexual feelings and behaviour, or a person's sexual orientation or preference. *Heterosexuality* is sexuality directed towards

S

SEXUAL INTERCOURSE

The term sexual intercourse usually refers to the act during which the male's penis is inserted into the female's vagina. However, some people use the term more broadly to refer to a much wider range of sexual activity. Physiologically, intercourse falls into four main stages – arousal (which generally includes a period of foreplay), a plateau (during which penetration usually occurs), orgasm, and resolution. The duration of each stage of intercourse varies.

Arousal in men
Sexual thoughts, the sight and feel of his partner's body, and foreplay may sexually arouse a man. Blood enters the penis so that it becomes firm and erect.

Plateau phase in men
Vaginal penetration usually takes place during this phase and thrusting movements begin. The penis reaches maximum size and the testes elevate.

Orgasm in men
Muscular contractions in the ducts connecting the testes, prostate, and penis force semen out of the penis, accompanied by intensely pleasurable sensations.

Resolution in men
The penis returns to half its fully erect size and the testes descend.

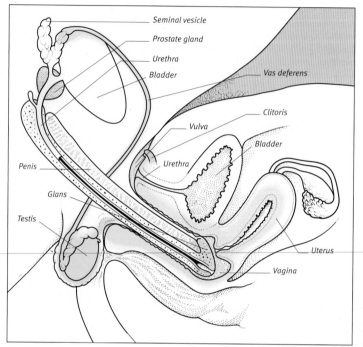

Arousal in women
Similar factors lead to arousal in women as in men, though foreplay may be more important. The clitoris lengthens, the vagina enlarges, and its walls secrete a lubricating fluid.

Plateau phase in women
Muscular contractions in the walls of the vagina help grip the penis. The uterus rises, and the clitoris may pull back beneath its hood of skin.

Orgasm in women
The walls of the outer part of the vagina contract rhythmically and strongly several times and an intense sensual feeling spreads from the clitoris and throughout the body.

Resolution in women
The clitoris subsides and, more gradually, the vagina relaxes and the uterus falls.

the opposite sex; *homosexuality* is attraction to the same sex; and *bisexuality* is attraction to both sexes.

sexually transmitted infection

An infection transmitted primarily (but not exclusively) by sexual intercourse. Common sexually transmitted infections (STIs) include *genital herpes*, *chlamydial infections*, *pubic lice*, *genital warts*, *trichomoniasis*, *syphilis*, *gonorrhoea*, and *HIV* infection. Certain sexual activities carry a high risk of infection with STIs. They include casual sex or having multiple partners (particularly if partners are not known to be free of disease); activities that involve contact with sperm or other body fluids; and activities that may damage the skin or mucous membranes. Practising *safer sex* can minimize these risks and help prevent STIs.

Antibiotics can be used to treat most bacterial STIs. Confidential tracing and treatment of an affected person's partners is essential in the management of STIs (see *contact tracing*).

sexual problems

Any difficulty associated with sexual performance or behaviour. Sexual problems are often psychological in origin; *sex therapy* may help such problems. They may also be due to physical disease, such as a disorder affecting blood flow; a hormonal dysfunction; or a disorder of the genitals. Such problems are addressed by treating the cause, where possible. See also *ejaculation, disorders of*; *erectile dysfunction*; *orgasm, lack of*; *sexual desire, inhibited*; *vaginismus*.

Sézary syndrome

A rare condition in which there is an abnormal overgrowth of *lymphocytes* (white blood cells active in the immune system) in the skin, liver, spleen, and lymph nodes. It mainly affects middle-aged and elderly people. The first symptom is the appearance of red, scaly patches on the skin that spread to form an itchy, flaking rash. There may also be an accumulation of fluid under the skin; baldness; and distorted nail growth.

Sézary syndrome is sometimes associated with *leukaemia*. Treatment includes *anticancer drugs* and *radiotherapy*.

shared care

Management of a pregnant woman's care by her general practitioner and the community midwives (see *primary care*), in combination with a hospital antenatal team. The term shared care also refers increasingly to the management of certain chronic conditions, for example asthma and diabetes.

Sheehan's syndrome

A form of hypopituitarism (underactivity of the pituitary gland) in women who have just given birth. The disorder occurs when cells in the pituitary die as a result of heavy bleeding or *shock* during the delivery. The treatment for Sheehan's syndrome involves replacement of the deficient hormones.

shellfish poisoning

See *seafood poisoning*.

S

shell shock

See *post-traumatic stress disorder*.

shigellosis

An acute infection of the intestine by SHIGELLA bacteria; also called bacillary dysentery. The bacteria exist in faeces and are spread by poor hygiene. *Endemic* in some countries, shigellosis occurs in isolated outbreaks in the UK.

The disease usually starts suddenly, with bloody diarrhoea, abdominal pain, nausea, vomiting, generalized aches, and fever. Persistent diarrhoea may cause *dehydration*, especially in certain groups such as babies and elderly people. Occasionally, *toxaemia* (presence of bacterial toxins in the blood) develops.

Shigellosis usually subsides after a week or so, but hospital treatment may be needed for severe cases. Dehydration is treated by *rehydration therapy*. *Antibiotics* may be given.

shingles

See *herpes zoster*.

shin splints

Pain in the front and sides of the lower leg that develops or worsens during exercise. There may also be tenderness and swelling in the area. Shin splints is a common problem in runners. Possible causes include inflammation of a tendon or muscle or *periostitis* (inflammation of the outer layer of a bone). (See also *compartment syndrome*.)

In most cases, the pain in the shins disappears within two months of rest. *Nonsteroidal anti-inflammatory drugs* may help alleviate the pain. In rare cases, surgery is performed in order to alleviate excessive pressure in a muscle. Some people benefit from *physiotherapy*.

shivering

Involuntary trembling of the entire body caused by rapid contraction and relaxation of muscles. Shivering is the body's normal automatic response to cold; it also occurs in fever.

When the body becomes cold, temperature-sensitive nerve cells in the hypothalamus (part of the brain) act as a thermostat, initiating the shivering reflex. This causes muscles to contract, generating heat. Shivering caused by cold usually disappears as soon as the body is warmed to a near-normal temperature.

Shivering during fever is caused by the release of certain substances by the white blood cells. The trigger for this release is usually an infection. These substances effectively "reset" the thermostat at a higher point, causing the body to shiver when it needs to lose, rather than retain, heat.

shock

A dangerous reduction of blood flow throughout the body tissues, which may occur with severe injury or illness. Shock in this sense is a physiological reaction, as distinct from the mental distress that may follow a traumatic experience.

In most cases, reduced blood pressure is a major factor in causing shock and it is also one of its main features. Shock may develop in any situation in which blood volume is reduced, blood vessels are abnormally widened, the heart's action is weak, blood flow is obstructed, or there is a combination of a few of these factors. Causes of shock include severe bleeding or burns, persistent vomiting or diarrhoea, *myocardial infarction* (heart attack), *pulmonary embolism* (a blood clot in the lung), *peritonitis* (inflammation of the abdominal lining) and some types of *poisoning*.

Signs include rapid, shallow breathing; cold, clammy skin; a rapid, weak pulse; dizziness; weakness; and fainting. If left untreated, shock can impair the oxygen supply to vital organs, such as the brain, which will eventually lead to collapse, coma, and death.

Emergency treatment is needed. This involves an *intravenous infusion* of fluid, a blood transfusion, *oxygen therapy*, and, if pain relief is necessary, *morphine* or similar powerful *analgesic drugs* (painkillers). Any further treatment that is given depends on the underlying cause. (See also *anaphylactic shock*; *hypovolaemia*; *septic shock*; *toxic shock syndrome*.)

shock, electric

The sensation that is caused by an electric current passing through the body, and its effects. A current of sufficient size and duration can cause loss of consciousness, cardiac arrest, respiratory arrest, burns, and tissue damage. (See also *electrical injury*.)

shock therapy

See *ECT*.

shock wave lithotripsy

See *lithotripsy*.

shortsightedness

See *myopia*.

short sight, operations for

See *LASIK*; *photorefractive keratectomy*.

short stature

A height that is significantly below the normal range for a person's age. Short stature in children is often due to hereditary factors or to slow bone growth. In most cases, growth eventually speeds up, resulting in normal adult height. Less commonly, it is due to a disorder that interferes with bone growth, such as bone disease (as in untreated *rickets* or *achondroplasia*), or hormonal disorders including *growth hormone* deficiency and *hypothyroidism* (underactivity of the thyroid gland). *Emotional deprivation*, *malabsortion*, and chronic malnutrition, can also limit growth.

Certain chromosomal disorders cause short stature: restricted growth occurs in *Down's syndrome*, and the normal pubertal growth spurt is absent in girls with *Turner's syndrome*. Other causes of restricted growth in children include prolonged use of *corticosteroid drugs* and *anticancer drugs*. Severe untreated respiratory disease or congenital heart disease can also cause short stature by restricting the supply of oxygen to growing tissues.

When assessing a child, the doctor will take into account the parents' heights, and will look for signs of any underlying disease. An affected child's growth rate is monitored by regular measurement of his or her height. *X-rays* and *blood tests* may help to identify an underlying cause, which will then be treated. Growth hormone is given for any hormone deficiency, and also as treatment for short stature due to disorders such as Turner's syndrome. (See also *growth, childhood*.)

short wave diathermy

The application of a high-frequency electric current to the body to relieve pain. The current produces an electromagnetic field that generates deep heat in the tissues.

Short-wave diathermy may be used to treat certain soft-tissue injuries, such as *sprains* and *strains*; joint disorders such as *osteoarthritis*; and inflammatory disorders such as *sinusitis* and chronic *pelvic inflammatory disease*. It may also be used to help speed wound healing. It must not be used, however, on any individuals who have metal implants or other non-removable prostheses, or on people who are fitted with *pacemakers*.

S

shoulder

The area of the body where the arm attaches to the trunk. The rounded bony surface at the front of the shoulder is the upper part of the *humerus* (upper-arm bone); the bony surfaces that form the top and back of the shoulder are parts of the *scapula* (shoulderblade). The *clavicle* (collarbone) articulates with the acromion (the bony prominence at the outer top part of the scapula) at the *acromioclavicular joint* and extends across the top of the chest to the *sternum* (breastbone), to which it is attached at the sternoclavicular joint.

Just below the acromion, on the outer wall of the scapula, is a socket (called the glenoid cavity) into which the head of the humerus fits to form the shoulder joint. A bursa (fluid-filled sac) under the acromion reduces friction at the joint. The shoulder joint is a ball-and-socket joint with the widest range of movement of all joints; movement is produced by part of the *biceps muscle*, several small muscles that make up the *rotator cuff*, various muscles in the chest wall, and the *deltoid* muscle at the top of the upper arm and shoulder.

DISORDERS
Shoulder injuries are relatively common, including dislocation of the shoulder joint (see *shoulder, dislocation of*) or of the acromioclavicular joint, and *fractures* of the clavicle or of the upper part of the humerus. Fractures of the scapula are less common.

STRUCTURE OF THE **SHOULDER**

Three bones meet at the shoulder – the scapula (shoulderblade), clavicle (collarbone), and humerus (upper-arm bone). The shoulder is an example of a ball-and-socket joint.

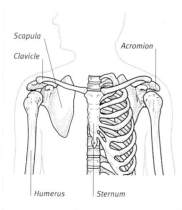

Scapula
Clavicle
Acromion
Humerus
Sternum

The shoulder joint may be affected by any joint disorder, including *arthritis* and *bursitis* (inflammation of a bursa). In severe cases, a joint disorder may lead to *frozen shoulder* (a condition in which movements at the joint are severely restricted). Movement of the shoulder may also be painful and/or restricted because of *tendinitis* (inflammation of a tendon). Tendinitis or bursitis can cause *painful arc syndrome*, in which raising the arm to the side causes pain.

shoulderblade

The common name for the *scapula*.

shoulder, dislocation of

Displacement of the head of the *humerus* (upper-arm bone) out of the shoulder joint. The main symptom is pain in the shoulder and upper arm that is made worse by movement. A forward dislocation often produces obvious deformity; however, a backward dislocation usually does not.

Diagnosis is by *X-rays*. The head of the humerus is repositioned in the joint socket, and the shoulder is immobilized in a sling for about three weeks. In cases of recurrent shoulder dislocation, surgery may be required.

Complications of shoulder dislocation include damage to nerves, causing temporary weakness and numbness in the shoulder; damage to an artery in the upper arm, causing pain and discoloration of the arm and hand; and damage to the muscles that support the shoulder.

shoulder–hand syndrome

Pain and stiffness of one shoulder and the hand on that side; the hand may also become hot, sweaty, and swollen. Arm muscles may waste through lack of use.

The cause of shoulder–hand syndrome is not known, but the condition may sometimes occur as a complication of *myocardial infarction* (heart attack), *stroke*, *herpes zoster* (shingles), or shoulder injury. Recovery usually occurs in about two years. However, this period may be shortened by *physiotherapy* and *corticosteroid drugs*. In rare cases, a cervical *sympathectomy* is performed.

shunt

An abnormal passage between two normally unconnected body parts (as in a *septal defect* of the heart). The term also refers to a passage created surgically between unconnected areas for purposes such as draining excess fluid.

Shy–Drager syndrome

A rare degenerative disorder of unknown cause that progressively damages the *autonomic nervous system*. It begins gradually between the ages of 60 and 70 and is more common in men. Symptoms include dizziness and fainting due to postural *hypotension*; urinary incontinence; *erectile dysfunction*; reduced ability to sweat; and *parkinsonism*. The condition eventually leads to disability and sometimes premature death. There is no cure or means of slowing degeneration, but many symptoms are relieved by drugs.

SIADH

The abbreviation for "syndrome of inappropriate antidiuretic hormone (secretion)", in which oversecretion of antidiuretic hormone (ADH) results in water retention and a low sodium level in the body. SIADH is associated with certain lung disorders such as COPD (see *pulmonary disease, chronic obstructive*) or *pneumonia*. Other conditions, for example brain disorders such as *encephalitis* or *brain haemorrhage*, and some cancers including small cell carcinoma (see *lung cancer*) and cancer of the pancreas (see *pancreas, cancer of*), may also be associated with SIADH.

Siamese twins

See *twins, conjoined*.

sibling rivalry

A term that describes the intense competition that sometimes occurs between siblings.

sibutramine

A centrally acting *appetite suppressant* drug that is used to treat obesity in people who have not responded to other methods of weight loss, such as dieting and exercise. Common side effects include constipation, dry mouth, and *hypertension*. People taking this drug should have regular follow-ups with their blood pressure and pulse monitored.

sicca syndrome

Occurring in *Sjögren's syndrome*, dryness of the eyes, mouth, and other mucous membranes (such as the lining of the vagina) due to destruction of exocrine (such as tear, salivary, or sweat) glands.

sick building syndrome

A collection of symptoms reported by some workers in office buildings. Symptoms include loss of energy, fatigue,

S

poor concentration, headaches, and dry, itchy eyes, nose, and throat. Although the exact cause is unknown, various factors may be involved, including air conditioning, lack of natural light and ventilation, and psychological stress.

sickle cell anaemia

An inherited *genetic disorder* in which the red blood cells contain an abnormal type of *haemoglobin* (oxygen-carrying pigment) called haemoglobin S. When red cells enter capillaries (tiny blood vessels) under conditions of low oxygen (due to the atmosphere or infection or dehydration, for example), haemoglobin S crystallizes. The cells become sickle-shaped and fragile, leading to haemolytic *anaemia*. Also, because the abnormal cells are unable to pass easily through capillaries, they intermittently block the blood supply to organs. The result is a sickle cell crisis, which may also occur for no apparent reason.

CAUSE
Sickle cell anaemia occurs mainly in black African people, and the defective gene is inherited from both parents. (If the gene is passed on from only one parent, the result is sickle cell trait, in which carriers are at risk of passing the gene to their children.)

SYMPTOMS AND SIGNS
Symptoms usually appear after six months of age and often begin with painful swelling of the hands and feet. Chronic haemolytic anaemia causes fatigue, headaches, shortness of breath on exertion, pallor, and *jaundice*. Sickle cell crises start suddenly; there may be pains (especially in the bones), blood in the urine (from kidney damage) or damage to the lungs or intestines. If the brain is affected, *seizures*, a *stroke*, or unconsciousness may result.

In some affected children, the *spleen* becomes enlarged and traps red cells at a very high rate, which causes a life-threatening form of anaemia. After adolescence, the spleen usually stops functioning, thereby increasing the risk of infection in those affected.

People who have sickle cell trait generally have no disability, and may be protected from falciparum *malaria*, but they may experience similar blood-vessel blocking events if oxygen levels are low.

DIAGNOSIS AND TREATMENT
Diagnosis is made from examination of a blood smear and *electrophoresis* to detect haemoglobin S. Babies may be screened for the condition shortly after birth.

Supportive treatment may include supplements of *folic acid*, and *antibiotics* and immunization to protect against infection. The treatment of life-threatening crises involves the use of *intravenous infusions* of fluids, *oxygen therapy*, antibiotics, and *analgesic drugs*. If the crisis still does not respond, an exchange *blood transfusion* may be performed. This may be done regularly for people who suffer from frequent severe crises.

sick sinus syndrome

Abnormal function of the heart's *sinoatrial node* (its natural "pacemaker") that leads to episodes of *bradycardia* (slow heart rate), alternating bradycardia and *tachycardia* (fast heart rate), or very short episodes of *cardiac arrest*.

The cause of sick sinus syndrome is usually *coronary artery disease*; alternatively, it may be a *cardiomyopathy* (a condition that leads to weakened heart muscle contractions). Symptoms may include lightheadedness, fainting, and palpitations. The diagnosis is confirmed by a 24-hour *ECG* recording. Sick sinus syndrome is usually treated with *antiarrhythmic drugs* and the fitting of an artificial *pacemaker*.

side effect

A reaction or consequence of medication or therapy that occurs in addition to the desired effect. The term is usually used with reference to an unwanted or adverse effect usually following a normal dose, rather than the toxic effects resulting from a *drug overdose*.

siderosis

Any condition in which there is too much iron in the body, including *pneumoconiosis*, when it is caused by inhalation of iron particles. (See also *haemosiderosis*.)

SIDS

An abbreviation for *sudden infant death syndrome*.

sievert

A unit for measuring doses of ionizing *radiation*. (See *radiation units*.)

sight

See *vision*.

sight, partial

Loss of vision short of total *blindness*. Partial sight may involve loss of *visual acuity* and/or *visual field*.

sigmoid colon

The S-shaped part of the *colon* in the lower abdomen, extending from the brim of the pelvis, usually down to the third segment of the *sacrum*. It is connected to the descending colon above and the *rectum* below.

sigmoidoscopy

Endoscopy (examination with a viewing instrument) of the *rectum* and *sigmoid colon* (parts of the large intestine). Sigmoidoscopy is used to investigate symptoms relating to the lower gastrointestinal tract, such as bleeding from the rectum or lower colon, and to look for evidence of disorders, such as polyps (small noncancerous growths), *ulcerative colitis*, or cancer (see *colon, cancer of*). Attachments on the end of the sigmoidoscope allow a *biopsy* (removal of a tissue sample for analysis) to be performed.

sign

An objective indication of a disease or disorder (for example, jaundice) that is observed or detected by a doctor, as opposed to a *symptom* (for example, pain), which is noticed by the patient.

sign, vital

See *vital sign*.

sildenafil

Commonly known by its brand name Viagra, a drug used in the treatment of *erectile dysfunction*. It is also sometimes used to treat *pulmonary hypertension* (high blood pressure in the arteries supplying the lungs). Possible side effects include indigestion, nausea, vomiting, headaches, flushing, dizziness, visual disturbances, and nasal congestion, and *priapism*. Sildenafil should not be used by people who have had a recent *myocardial infarction* (heart attack) or *stroke*, or those with certain eye disorders. It should also not be used by people taking *nitrate drugs* because of a possible serious interaction.

silent myocardial infarct

A heart attack (see *myocardial infarction*) that occurs without the usual signs and symptoms (such as sudden chest pain).

silicone

A long-chain, carbon-containing compound of silicon and oxygen. Synthetic silicone implants are sometimes used in *cosmetic surgery*, notably breast enlargement. Leakage from silicone implants

S

LOCATION AND FUNCTION OF THE **SINOATRIAL NODE**

The sinoatrial (SA) node is a small mass of specialized muscle cells in the right atrium of the heart. It sends out impulses at an inherent rate of about 100 impulses per minute. External control by the vagus nerve reduces the rate to about 70 per minute. Other mechanisms also affect the rate.

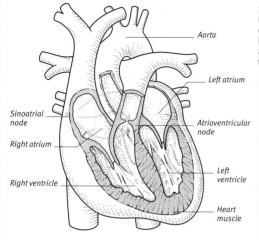

Aorta

Left atrium

Sinoatrial node

Atrioventricular node

Right atrium

Left ventricle

Right ventricle

Heart muscle

Spread of the impulse
From the SA node, the waves of contraction spread over both atria and then to the atrioventricular node serving the ventricles.

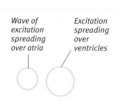

Wave of excitation spreading over atria

Excitation spreading over ventricles

Electrocardiogram
The spread of excitation over the two atria is fairly slow; the spread over the ventricles is rapid.

can occur and may cause autoimmune disorders (in which the immune system attacks the body's own tissues).

silicosis

A lung disease caused by the inhalation of dust containing silica from rock or sand. (See also *pneumoconiosis*.)

silver sulfadiazine

An *antibacterial drug* applied as a cream to prevent infection after skin grafts or in burns, leg ulcers, and pressure sores. Side effects may include permanent grey skin discoloration, rashes, or itching.

simian crease

A single deep, horizontal crease on the palm of the hand. This feature is associated with chromosomal disorders such as *Down's syndrome*.

simple linctus

See *linctus*.

simvastatin

A *lipid-lowering drug* that acts on the liver enzymes that produce *cholesterol*. Simvastatin may cause bowel upsets, headaches, and muscle pains. It may also raise liver enzyme levels, which must be monitored.

sinew

A nonmedical term for a *tendon*.

singer's nodes

Small, greyish-white nodules that develop on the vocal cords. Singer's nodes are the result of constant voice strain, causing hoarseness or loss of voice.

A *biopsy* (removal of a sample of tissue for microscopic examination) may be carried out to exclude the possibility of a malignant tumour (see *larynx, cancer of*) being present. Treatment of acute

cases of singer's nodes consists of resting the voice. In chronic cases, surgical removal of the nodes may be necessary.

sinoatrial node

The natural pacemaker of the *heart*. The sinoatrial node consists of a cluster of specialized muscle cells in the right atrial wall. These cells emit rapid electrical impulses that initiate the heart's contractions (beats). Various hormones and nervous system activities may alter the rate at which the node emits impulses. (See also *heart rate*.)

sinus

A cavity in a bone; in particular, one of the air-filled spaces in the bones surrounding the nose (see *sinus, facial*).

The term "sinus" also refers to any wide channel that contains blood, or to an abnormal, often infected, tract.

sinus arrhythmia

A normal variation in the heart rate that occurs with breathing and is particularly found in children and young adults. During inspiration (breathing in), the heart rate is increased; during expiration (breathing out) it decreases.

sinus bradycardia

A slow, but regular, heart rate (fewer than 60 beats per minute) that is the result of reduced electrical activity in the *sinoatrial node*. The symptom of sinus bradycardia is normal in athletes

LOCATION AND FUNCTION OF THE **SINUSES**

The air spaces, or sinuses, in the skull bones lighten the skull and improve the resonance of the voice. The sinuses surround the nose and are lined with mucous membrane. Mucus produced by this membrane drains into the nasal cavity via narrow channels.

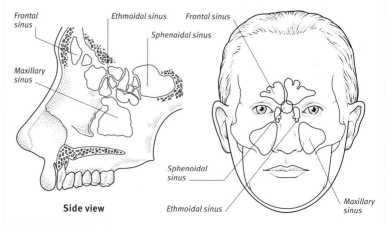

Frontal sinus

Ethmoidal sinus

Frontal sinus

Sphenoidal sinus

Maxillary sinus

Sphenoidal sinus

Side view

Ethmoidal sinus

Maxillary sinus

S

and people who are fit, but in others it may be caused by *hypothyroidism*, a *myocardial infarction*, or drugs such as *beta-blockers* or *digoxin*.

sinus, facial

Also referred to as a paranasal sinus, any of the air-filled cavities in the bones surrounding the nose. Facial sinuses include two frontal sinuses that are situated in the lower forehead; two ethmoidal sinuses between the eyes; two maxillary sinuses in the cheekbones; and the sphenoidal sinuses in the skull behind the nose. The sinuses decrease the weight of the skull and alter voice resonance. Each sinus is lined with mucous membrane; and mucus drains along a channel that opens into the nose.

sinusitis

Inflammation of the membrane that lines the facial sinuses (see *sinus, facial*). Sinusitis is most often due to infection, usually spread from the nose. The maxillary and ethmoidal sinuses are most commonly affected.

Sinusitis may cause pressure, headache, facial pain, and a feeling of fullness in the affected area; there may also be fever, a stuffy nose, and loss of the sense of smell. A common complication is the formation of pus, causing pain and nasal discharge.

Treatment of sinusitis is usually by *steam inhalations* and a *decongestant*, but in some cases antibiotics may be needed. If sinusitis persists despite treatment, surgical drainage of the affected sinuses may be performed.

sinus tachycardia

A fast but regular heart rate (more than 100 beats per minute) due to increased electrical activity in the *sinoatrial node*. Such a heartbeat is normal in sudden stressful moments or during exercise. Persistent sinus tachycardia at rest may be caused by fever or *hyperthyroidism*.

situs inversus

An unusual condition in which the internal organs are situated in a mirror image of their normal positions. No treatment is needed provided that all the organs are functioning normally.

Sjögren's syndrome

A condition, mostly affecting middle-aged women, in which the eyes and mouth are excessively dry. Other areas including the nasal cavity, throat, and

BONES OF THE **SKELETON**

There are two main parts to the skeleton, called the axial and appendicular skeletons (shown below). Some parts, such as the skull and pelvis, consist of several fused or associated bones. The skeleton is not merely an inert framework that supports and protects organs and makes movement possible; the bones are active living structures that are constantly producing blood cells and interchanging minerals with the blood.

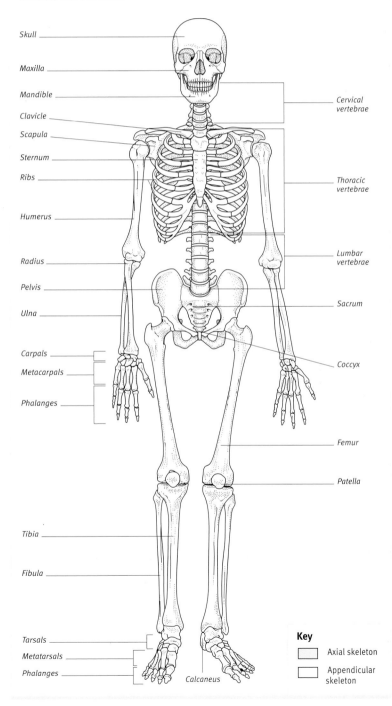

Skull
Maxilla
Mandible
Clavicle
Scapula
Sternum
Ribs
Humerus
Radius
Pelvis
Ulna
Carpals
Metacarpals
Phalanges
Tibia
Fibula
Tarsals
Metatarsals
Phalanges
Calcaneus

Cervical vertebrae
Thoracic vertebrae
Lumbar vertebrae
Sacrum
Coccyx
Femur
Patella

Key
Axial skeleton
Appendicular skeleton

S

vagina may also be affected. Sjögren's syndrome tends to occur with certain *autoimmune disorders* (in which the immune system attacks the body's own tissues), such as *rheumatoid arthritis* and systemic *lupus erythematosus*. The dryness is due to destruction by the immune system of the lubricant-producing exocrine glands.

skeletal muscle

See *muscle*.

skeleton

The framework of bones that gives the body its shape and provides attachment points for the muscles and underlying soft tissues. The average human adult skeleton has 213 *bones* (counting each of the nine fused vertebrae of the sacrum and coccyx as individual bones). The bones are linked to each other with *ligaments* (which are slightly elastic) at the *joints* and are joined to muscles by *tendons* (which are inelastic).

STRUCTURE

The skeleton consists of two main parts: the axial and appendicular skeletons.

The axial skeleton comprises the *skull*, *spine*, *ribs*, and *sternum* (breastbone). Together, these make up a total of 87 bones: 29 in the skull (including the *hyoid* bone in the upper part of the neck and three pairs of auditory *ossicles* in the inner ear); 33 in the spine (seven cervical, 12 thoracic, and five lumbar vertebrae, the five fused vertebrae of the

DISORDERS AFFECTING THE **SKIN**

The skin is the largest and most vulnerable organ of the body. Skin conditions are seldom life-threatening, but many can be severely debilitating and can cause psychological problems.

Congenital disorders

A *birthmark* is a type of *naevus* (pigmented skin blemish) present from birth. Naevi include moles, freckles, and *haemangiomas*, such as port-wine stains and strawberry marks.

Infection and inflammation

Viral infections of the skin include *cold sores*, *warts*, and *molluscum contagiosum*. Systemic infections such as *chickenpox* and *herpes zoster* (shingles) also affect the skin. Bacterial infections include *boils*, *cellulitis*, *erysipelas*, and *impetigo*. Fungal infections, such as *tinea*, cause *athlete's foot* and ringworm.

Inflammation of the skin occurs in *dermatitis* and *eczema*; it may be caused by an allergic reaction to a substance (such as nickel), a detergent, a plant, or a drug. *Psoriasis* is a common and persistent skin disease of unknown cause that consists of large, red patches with silvery, scaly surfaces. *Prickly heat* is an irritating rash caused by blockage of the sweat glands.

Tumours

Benign (noncancerous) skin tumours are extremely common. These include seborrhoeic *keratoses* and most types of naevi. *Bowen's disease* is a skin disorder that may slowly become cancerous. Three common forms of skin cancer are *basal cell carcinoma*, *squamous cell carcinoma*, and malignant melanoma (see *melanoma, malignant*). Less common skin cancers include *Paget's disease of the nipple*, *mycosis fungoides*, and *Kaposi's sarcoma*.

Injury

The skin is vulnerable to many minor injuries, including cuts and bites (see *bites, animal*; *insect bites*) as well as more serious *wounds*. *Burns* can be among the most serious of all skin injuries and may cause extensive scarring or death.

Hormonal disorders

Acne is partly related to the action of androgens (male sex hormones) on the sebaceous glands; it is particularly common among adolescents.

Nutritional disorders

Deficiency of vitamins A, B, and C can cause *rashes* and other problems.

Impaired blood supply

Leg ulcers, which are particularly common in the elderly, may be caused by poor blood flow to the skin as a result of *atherosclerosis*, by poor drainage of blood through *varicose veins*, or by the leg swelling associated with heart failure.

Drugs

Many drugs, including antibiotics, barbiturates, and sulphonamides, may cause a rash. Some cause *urticaria* (hives), others cause *eczema* or a measles-like rash, and some cause *photosensitivity*.

Radiation

All forms of radiation are potentially damaging to the skin. Overexposure to sunlight (ultraviolet radiation) causes premature aging of the skin and increases the risk of skin cancer (see *sunlight, adverse effects of*). High doses of other forms of radiation, such as X-rays, may cause severe injury to the skin and may lead to cancer.

Autoimmune disorders

Many autoimmune disorders are systemic but have manifestations in the skin. They include *lupus erythematosus*, which may affect the skin alone or the skin and other organs; *vitiligo*, which is characterized by unpigmented patches and caused by destruction of the skin's pigment cells; *dermatomyositis*, which is characterized by a specific skin rash and muscle weakness; *morphoea* and *systemic sclerosis*, in which there is progressive hardening of the skin and other tissues; and *pemphigoid* and *pemphigus*, in which large blisters develop on the skin.

Other disorders

A *keloid* is an abnormally large and protruding scar caused by the continuing production of scar tissue long after healing would usually be complete. *Striae* (stretch-marks) often develop during pregnancy and may also develop as a side effect of *corticosteroid drugs*.

Erythema simply means redness and has many possible causes. Purpura is a condition in which blood leaks into tissues, giving rise to petechiae (tiny pinpoints of blood) or larger bruises. *Xanthelasma* are fatty yellowish patches that tend to occur on the eyelids; they are associated with raised levels of cholesterol in the blood.

INVESTIGATION

Most skin disorders can be diagnosed from their physical characteristics. A swab or skin scraping may be taken if infection is suspected. A *biopsy* (taking a tissue sample for microscopic analysis) may also be performed, usually to confirm the diagnosis of a skin problem or to exclude skin cancer.

S

sacrum, and the four fused vertebrae of the coccyx); and 25 in the chest (the 12 pairs of ribs and the sternum).

The appendicular skeleton consists of the limb girdles (the *shoulder* and the *pelvis*) and their attached limb bones. Altogether there are 126 bones: 64 in the shoulders and upper limbs and 62 in the pelvis and lower limbs. There are two bones in each shoulder: the *clavicle* (collarbone) and *scapula* (shoulderblade); three in each arm: the *humerus* (upper-arm bone) and *radius* and *ulna* (forearm bones); eight carpals in each *wrist*; five *metacarpals* in each palm; and 14 *phalanges* in the digits of each hand (two in each thumb and three in each finger).

The pelvic girdle is made up of two hip bones. There are 30 bones in each of the lower limbs: a *femur* (thighbone), *patella* (kneecap), and *tibia* and *fibula* (lower-leg bones) in each leg; seven tarsals in the *ankle*, heel (see *calcaneus*), and the back part of the foot; five *metatarsals* in the middle section of each foot; and 14 phalanges in the toes (two of which are in each big toe and three in each of the other toes).

There are minor differences between the skeletons of men and women. In general, men's bones tend to be larger and heavier, but the female pelvic cavity is wider to facilitate childbirth.

FUNCTION

The skeleton plays an indispensable role in movement by providing a strong, stable, but mobile framework on which muscles can act to move the body. It also supports and protects internal body organs, notably the brain and spinal cord, which are encased in the skull and spine, and the heart and lungs, which are protected by the ribs.

However, the skeleton is not an inert frame. It is an active organ that produces blood cells (formed in bone marrow) and acts as a reservoir for minerals such as calcium, which can be drawn on, if required, by other parts of the body.

skin

The outermost covering of body tissue, and the largest organ of the body. Skin has two layers: the epidermis (outer layer) and dermis (inner layer), beneath which is the fatty subcutaneous tissue.

EPIDERMIS

The epidermis comprises sheets of flat cells, which resemble paving stones when viewed under the microscope. It varies in thickness, being thickest on the soles and palms and thinnest on the eyelids.

The outermost part of the epidermis is composed of dead cells, which form a tough, horny, protective coating. As these dead cells are worn away, they are replaced by new ones that are produced by the rapidly dividing living cells in the innermost part of the epidermis. Between the outer and inner parts is a transitional region that consists of both living and dead cells.

Most of the cells produce the protein *keratin*, a tough substance that is the main constituent of the outermost part. Some of the cells make the pigment *melanin*, which protects the body from *ultraviolet light* in sunlight and determines skin colour.

DERMIS

The dermis is composed of *connective tissue* that is interspersed with *hair* follicles, *sweat glands*, *sebaceous glands*, blood and lymph vessels, and sensory receptors (specialized nerve structures) that are capable of detecting pressure, temperature, and pain.

FUNCTION

The skin's most important function is a protective one. It acts as the main barrier between the environment and the internal organs of the body, shielding them from injury, the harmful rays of sunlight, and infection with microorganisms such as bacteria.

The skin is a sensory organ containing many cells that are sensitive to touch, temperature, pain, pressure, and itching. The skin also plays a role in keeping body temperature constant. When the body is hot, the sweat glands cool it by producing perspiration and the blood vessels in the dermis dilate (widen) to dissipate heat; if the body gets cold, blood vessels in the skin constrict (narrow), to conserve the body's heat.

The epidermis contains a fatty substance that waterproofs the skin and stops it soaking up moisture like a sponge. The outer epidermis also has an effective water-holding capacity, which contributes to its elasticity and helps maintain the body's balance of fluid and electrolytes. If the water content drops below a certain level, the skin becomes cracked and its barrier effect less efficient.

skin allergy

Irritation of the skin following contact with an allergen (a substance that provokes an inappropriate reaction from the *immune system*).

There are two main types of allergic skin reaction. In contact allergic *dermatitis*, red, itchy patches develop a few hours to two days after skin contact. Trigger substances include adhesives in plasters, nickel in jewellery, and cosmetics.

STRUCTURE OF **SKIN**

The skin consists essentially of two distinct layers – the dermis (true skin), which contains most of the living elements, and the epidermis, which is a tough protective covering that has an outer layer of dead cells.

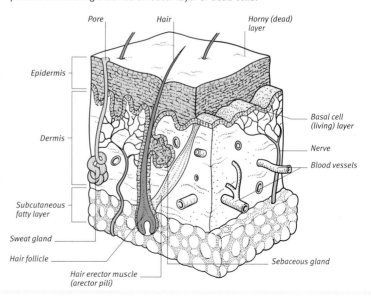

Pore   Hair   Horny (dead) layer

Epidermis

Basal cell (living) layer

Dermis

Nerve

Blood vessels

Subcutaneous fatty layer

Sweat gland

Hair follicle

Sebaceous gland

Hair erector muscle (arector pili)

S

In contact *urticaria*, red, raised areas appear a few minutes after skin contact. Possible causes include certain chemicals, plants, and insect bites.

If possible, contact with the trigger substance should be kept to a minimum. In many cases the trigger is obvious, but sometimes *skin tests* are needed to identify the allergen. (See also *atopic eczema*.)

skin biopsy

Removal of a portion of skin for laboratory analysis to diagnose a skin disorder.

skin cancer

A malignant skin tumour. *Basal cell carcinoma*, *squamous cell carcinoma*, and malignant melanoma (see *melanoma, malignant*) are forms associated with exposure to sun. *Bowen's disease*, a rare disorder that can become cancerous, may also be related to sun exposure. Less common types include *Paget's disease of the nipple* and *mycosis fungoides*.

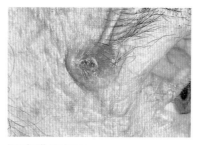

Basal cell carcinoma
This is the most common form of skin cancer. Also called a rodent ulcer, a basal cell carcinoma develops most commonly on the face.

Kaposi's sarcoma is a type usually found in *AIDS* patients. Most skin cancers are curable if treated early.

skin flap

A surgical technique in which a section of *skin* and underlying tissue, sometimes including muscle, is moved to cover an area from which skin and tissue have been lost or damaged by injury, disease, or surgery. Unlike a *skin graft*, a skin flap retains its blood supply. Therefore, skin flaps can be either attached (in which they remain attached to their donor site) or free (in which they are reattached to blood vessels at the recipient site by *microsurgery*). Skin flaps adhere well, even where there is extensive loss of deep tissue. For this reason, they may be used to cover areas that have lost their blood supply.

skin graft

A technique that is carried out in order to repair areas of lost or damaged *skin* that are too large to heal naturally, that are slow to heal, or that would otherwise leave tightening or unsightly scars. A skin graft is often used in the treatment of burns or sometimes for ulcers that are not healing.

A piece of healthy skin is detached from one part of the body and transferred to the affected area. New skin cells grow from the graft and cover the damaged area. In a meshed graft, donor skin is removed and made into a mesh by cutting. The mesh is stretched to fit the recipient site; new skin cells grow to fill the spaces in the mesh. In a pinch graft, multiple small areas of skin are pinched up and removed from the donor site. Placed on the recipient site, the new skin cells gradually expand to form a new sheet of healthy skin. (See also *skin flap*.)

skin patch

See *transdermal patch*.

skin peeling, chemical

A cosmetic procedure to remove acne scars, freckles, delicate wrinkles, or other skin blemishes. The procedure involves application of a caustic paste to peel away the outer layers of skin.

skin tag

A harmless, small, brown or flesh-coloured flap of skin that is often found on the neck, under the breasts, or in skin folds. A skin tag may appear spontaneously, or it may result from poor healing of a wound.

skin tests

Procedures to determine how the body reacts to various substances by applying them to the skin (usually on patches) or by injecting a small quantity of a substance under the skin. *Patch tests* are used in the diagnosis of contact allergic

TECHNIQUE FOR A FREE **SKIN AND MUSCLE FLAP**

A flap of skin and underlying tissue can be moved to a new site to replace lost tissue; if its blood supply is reconnected, the flap will heal in place. Microsurgery to rejoin blood vessels facilitates the technique.

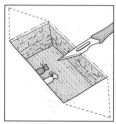

1 The donor area needs a good blood supply if muscle is also to be taken.

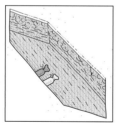

2 The ends of the donor area need to be tapered to allow satisfactory closure.

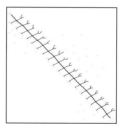

3 The skin may have to be undercut and freed before the wound is closed.

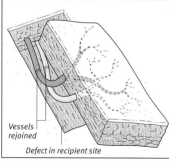

Vessels rejoined

Defect in recipient site

4 At the recipient site, an artery and a vein of suitable size must be available to be joined to blood vessels in the flap.

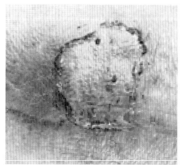

Skin flaps are particularly useful where there has been an extensive loss of deep tissue. The results are usually excellent.

S

TYPES OF **SKIN GRAFT**

The two main types of skin graft are split-thickness (in which less than the full thickness of skin is removed from the donor site) and full-thickness (in which a deeper thickness is removed). There are advantages to each of these types.

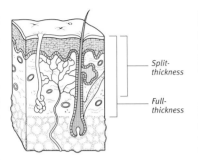

Split-thickness

Full-thickness

Split-thickness graft
When large areas need to be covered, such as after burns, split-thickness grafts are used and the donor sites are left to regenerate, which they do in a few days. Such sites can be repeatedly harvested.

Full-thickness graft
Full-thickness skin grafts are usually preferred for the face because they more closely match the appearance of normal skin. However, donor sites are limited and must be sutured (stitched).

HOW A FULL-THICKNESS GRAFT IS DONE

Most skin grafts are performed under general anaesthesia. Full-thickness grafts can be obtained easily with a scalpel. Subcutaneous fat is avoided and any bleeding at the recipient site prevented.

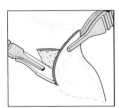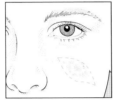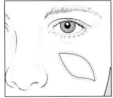

1 Skin for a full-thickness graft is often taken from behind the ear.

2 The graft must be slightly larger than the area to be covered, to allow for shrinkage.

3 Precise fitting and firm pressure are needed to ensure there is a satisfactory "take".

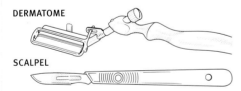

DERMATOME

SCALPEL

Instruments
Split-skin grafts are cut, usually from the abdomen or thigh, with an instrument called a dermatome. If necessary, the skin can be expanded into a trellis-like mesh on the donor site.

dermatitis; allergens will cause patches of reddened or blistered skin. Injections may sometimes be used to help identify substances that are causing allergic illnesses such as *asthma*. They may also be used to test immunity to certain infectious diseases (as in the *tuberculin test* for tuberculosis).

skin tumour

A growth developing on or in the *skin* that may be cancerous (see *skin cancer*) or noncancerous. *Keratoses* and squamous *papillomas* are common types of

noncancerous tumour; other types include *sebaceous cysts*, cutaneous *horns*, *keratoacanthomas*, and *haemangiomas*.

skull

The bony skeleton of the head, which protects the brain; houses the special sense organs (eyes, ears, tongue, and nose); provides attachment points for face, scalp, and neck muscles; and forms part of the respiratory and digestive tracts.

All the skull bones, except the mandible (lower jaw) are fixed to one another by immovable sutures; the skull bones

do not fuse until about 18 months of age (see *fontanelle*). The cranial cavity houses the brain; other skull structures include the nasal cavity and eye orbits.

Several of the skull bones, especially those around the nasal area, contain *sinuses* (air spaces). In the cranium, there are many holes for the passage of nerves and blood vessels. The largest of the holes, called the foramen magnum, is situated in the occipital bone (which forms part of the base and back of the cranium); this hole allows the *brainstem* to enter the spinal canal, where it continues as the spinal cord.

The skull rests on the atlas (the first cervical vertebra), which is a ring-shaped bone that articulates with the occipital bone and permits nodding movement of the head. Turning the head is a function of the joint between the atlas and the second cervical vertebrae, which is called the axis. The occipital bone, atlas, and axis are connected together by numerous small muscles.

DISORDERS
The skull may be affected by any disorder that involves the skeleton, such as *Paget's disease*, but the most common disorder is injury. A blow to the head may cause a fracture (see *skull, fracture of*), possibly leading to brain damage. (See also *head injury*.)

skull, fracture of

A break occurring in one or more of the *skull* bones as a result of a *head injury*. In most skull fractures, there are no complications. In a severe injury, however, the broken bones may be displaced. If this happens, bone fragments may rupture blood vessels in the *meninges* (the membranes covering the brain) or, rarely, tear the meninges, resulting in bleeding and, in some cases, damage to the brain.

S

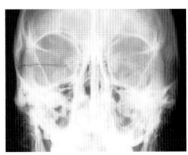

Skull fracture
In this X-ray image, a fracture of the back of the skull is visible as a long, dark, horizontal line across the orbit of the right eye (left on the image).

An uncomplicated skull fracture usually heals by itself. However, if there is damage to brain structures, neurosurgery is often required. (See also *depressed skull fracture*; *extradural haemorrhage*; *subarachnoid haemorrhage*; *subdural haemorrhage*).

skull X-ray

A technique for providing images of the *skull*. The X-rays are taken after some cases of *head injury* to look for a fracture or foreign body, or to evaluate disorders affecting the skull bones.

slapped cheek syndrome

Another name for *fifth disease*.

SLE

The abbreviation for the disorder systemic *lupus erythematosus*.

sleep

A natural state of lowered consciousness and reduced *metabolism*. Sleep takes up about one third of an average life.

PHYSIOLOGY

EEG recordings of the electrical impulses produced by the brain during sleep show that there are two distinct types of sleep: REM (rapid eye movement) and NREM (nonrapid eye movement). These types alternate in cycles lasting approximately 90 minutes throughout the sleep period. NREM sleep, which accounts for the major part of sleep, starts with drowsiness; brain waves become increasingly deeper and slower until brain activity and metabolism fall to their lowest level. Dreams are infrequent.

In REM sleep, the brain suddenly becomes more active and its temperature and blood flow increase. The eyes move rapidly and *dreaming* occurs. REM sleep, also known as paradoxical sleep, periodically interrupts NREM sleep. The first REM period usually takes place 90 to 100 minutes after the onset of sleep and lasts about five to 10 minutes. REM sleep periods increase in length as sleep continues; the last of a night's four or five REM sleep periods may last about an hour.

FUNCTIONS OF SLEEP

Sleep is a fundamental human need, as is shown by the detrimental effects of *sleep deprivation*. The way in which sleep is beneficial is not understood, however.

SLEEP REQUIREMENTS

The need for sleep decreases with age. A one-year-old infant needs about 14 hours of sleep a night, a five-year-old child about 12 hours, and adults seven or eight hours on average. (Some adults, however, need more than 10 hours' sleep, while others can manage on five hours or less.) Elderly people tend to sleep less than young adults at night, but doze during the day.

SLEEP DISORDERS

Sleep disorders are divided into four main categories: difficulty in falling or remaining asleep (see *insomnia*); difficulty in staying awake (see *narcolepsy*); disruption of the sleep/wake cycle, for example, by working shifts or travelling across time zones (see *jet-lag*); and other miscellaneous problems such as *bedwetting*, *night terrors*, or *sleepwalking*. (See also *sleep apnoea*.)

sleep apnoea

A disorder in which there are episodes of temporary breathing stoppage (lasting 10 seconds or longer) during sleep.

TYPES

Obstructive sleep apnoea (OSA) is the most common type and may affect anyone, but more often middle-aged men, especially those who are overweight. The most common cause is over-relaxation of the muscles of the soft palate, which obstructs air flow. Obstruction may also be caused by enlarged *tonsils* or *adenoids*. The obstruction causes snoring. If complete blockage occurs, breathing stops. This triggers the brain

---

STRUCTURE OF THE **SKULL**

The skull consists of the cranium, surrounding the brain, and the facial skeleton. The cranium is formed by the frontal bone, two temporal bones, two parietal bones, the occipital bone at the back, the ethmoid bone behind the nose, and the sphenoid. The face consists of 14 bones, including nasal, cheek, and jaw bones.

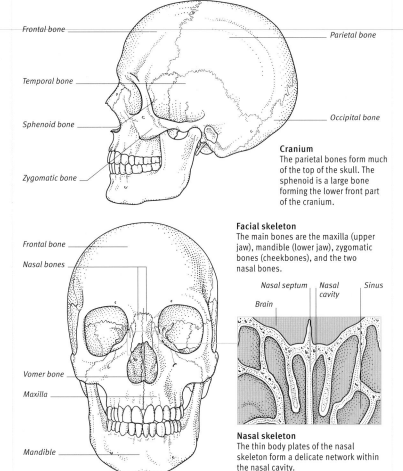

Frontal bone
Temporal bone
Sphenoid bone
Zygomatic bone

Parietal bone
Occipital bone

Cranium
The parietal bones form much of the top of the skull. The sphenoid is a large bone forming the lower front part of the cranium.

Frontal bone
Nasal bones
Vomer bone
Maxilla
Mandible

Facial skeleton
The main bones are the maxilla (upper jaw), mandible (lower jaw), zygomatic bones (cheekbones), and the two nasal bones.

Nasal septum · Nasal cavity · Sinus
Brain

Nasal skeleton
The thin body plates of the nasal skeleton form a delicate network within the nasal cavity.

S

to restart breathing, and the person may gasp and wake briefly. People with OSA may not be aware of any problem at night but they may be sleepy during the day, with poor memory and concentration. They are also at increased risk of an accident due to tiredness. In addition, OSA may increase the risk of *hypertension* (high blood pressure), *myocardial infarction*, (heart attack), or *stroke*.

People who are overweight may find losing weight helps. Alcohol and sleeping drugs aggravate OSA. The condition may be treated by continuous positive airways pressure (CPAP), in which air at higher than normal pressure is breathed through a mask. *Tonsillectomy*, *adenoidectomy*, or surgery to shorten or stiffen the soft palate may be performed.

In central sleep apnoea (CSA), breathing stops because the chest and diaphragm muscles temporarily cease to work. It is usually due to disturbance in the nervous system's control of breathing, which may result from various causes, such as a disorder of the *brainstem* or *encephalitis*. CSA may also occur in people with certain neuromuscular disorders or *heart failure*. Treatment of CSA depends on the underlying cause.

sleep deprivation

Insufficient *sleep*. Irritability and a shortened attention span may occur after a short night's sleep. Longer sleepless periods leave a person less able to concentrate or perform normal tasks. Three or more sleepless nights may lead to *hallucinations* and, sometimes, to *paranoia*.

sleeping drugs

COMMON DRUGS

BENZODIAZEPINE DRUGS •Flurazepam •Loprazolam •Lormetazepam •Nitrazepam •Temazepam

OTHERS •Clomethiazole •Chloral hydrate •Promethazine •Zolpidem •Zopiclone

A group of drugs that are used for the treatment of *insomnia*. Sleeping drugs include *benzodiazepine drugs*; *antihistamine drugs*, which are often available over-the-counter; *antidepressant drugs*; and chloral hydrate. These drugs promote sleep by reducing the activity of nerve cells in the brain.

Sleeping drugs should always be taken in the smallest effective dose for the shortest period of time. In general, they should be used for no more than three weeks, and preferably for no more than one week and not every night.

SLEEP PATTERNS

The brain does not rest when a person is sleeping, but there is some reorganization of activity within it. EEGs (electroencephalograms) and other recordings reveal cyclical patterns to this activity.

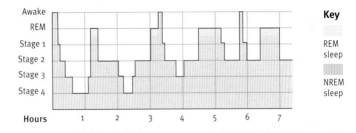

Key

REM sleep

NREM sleep

Phases of sleep
There are two types of sleep, REM (rapid eye movement) and NREM (nonrapid eye movement). They can be distinguished by the presence of absence of REMs and by EEGs or other recordings. The chart shows how a sleeper passes in cycles between the four stages of NREM sleep during the night, with bursts of REM sleep.

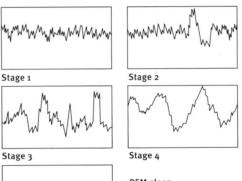

Stage 1

Stage 2

Stage 3

Stage 4

REM sleep

NREM sleep
This is sometimes called orthodox sleep; in adults it makes up about 80 per cent of the sleeping pattern. It has four stages of progressively greater "depth" of sleep, characterized by EEG waves (left) of increasingly larger voltage (amplitude) and lower frequency (number of waves per second). People awakened during NREM sleep often report they were "thinking" about everyday matters but rarely report dreams.

REM sleep
The EEG (left) shows high-frequency, low-voltage waves. People awakened during REM sleep often report dreams.

Sleeping drugs do not treat the underlying cause of the insomnia, which needs to be investigated.

ADVERSE EFFECTS
Sleeping drugs may cause drowsiness, unsteadiness, and impaired concentration on waking. They can be especially hazardous to anyone driving or operating machinery. Long-term use may induce *tolerance* and *dependence*.

sleeping sickness

A serious infectious disease of tropical Africa caused by the protozoan parasite TRYPANOSOMA BRUCEI, which is transmitted to humans by the bite of a tsetse fly.

One form of the disease, which occurs in West and Central Africa, takes a slow course, with bouts of fever and lymph node enlargement. After months

or years, the disease spreads to the brain, causing headaches, confusion, and, eventually, severe lassitude. Without treatment, coma and death follow. The other, East African, form runs a faster course. Fever develops after a few weeks of infection, and the heart may suffer fatal effects before the disease has reached the brain.

Drugs may effect a cure, but there may be residual brain damage if the infection has already spread to the brain. People in infested areas should wear long clothing fastened at the wrists and ankles to help prevent tsetse fly bites.

sleep paralysis

The sensation of being unable to move at the moment of going to sleep or waking up. It usually lasts only a few

S

LIFE-CYCLE OF TRYPANOSOMES IN **SLEEPING SICKNESS**

The life-cycle of the trypanosomes that cause sleeping sickness is shown. They multiply in a person's blood and lymph vessels and may spread to the brain or heart with serious effects.

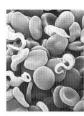

Trypanosomes
The parasites (pale, irregular shapes) are shown here in blood.

A tsetse fly ingests some parasites when it bites an infested person or animal.

Within the fly, the parasites reproduce by simple division and mature in the fly's gut.

A person contracts sleeping sickness from the bite of a fly with parasites in its saliva.

The parasites then move to the salivary glands of the fly; here the parasites become infective.

---

seconds, and may be accompanied by *hallucinations*. Sleep paralysis most often occurs in people with *narcolepsy*.

sleep terror

See *night terror*.

sleepwalking

Walking while asleep, also known as somnambulism. It occurs during NREM (nonrapid eye movement) *sleep*, or during arousal from this type of sleep, and does not represent the acting out of dreams. Some people regularly sleepwalk.

Usually a sleepwalker gets out of bed, wanders around aimlessly, and then goes back to bed. Sometimes, however, sleepwalking occurs with *night terror*, in which case the person may show distress or cry out. Waking a sleepwalker and is not necessary; he or she should simply be steered gently back to bed.

In children, sleepwalking is not normally a cause for concern and tends to disappear with age. In adults, it may be related to anxiety or the use of sleeping drugs, especially in the elderly.

slimming

See *weight reduction*.

sling

A triangular bandage used to immobilize, support, or elevate an injured arm. The arm may be supported horizontally or held elevated, depending on the injury.

slipped disc

See *disc prolapse*.

slipped femoral epiphysis

See *femoral epiphysis, slipped*.

slit-lamp

An illuminated type of microscope used to examine internal structures of the front of the eye. A slit-lamp may also be used to view the retina at the back of the eye. (See also *eye, examination of*.)

slough

Dead tissue that has been shed from its original site; for example, dead cells from the skin's surface. Sloughing is also part of the healing process.

small cell carcinoma

The most rapidly spreading and dangerous form of *lung cancer*.

small intestine

The section of the digestive tract (see *digestive system*) that lies between the stomach and large intestine. The small intestine, which consists of the *duodenum*, *jejunum*, and *ileum*, is the area in which nutrients are extracted from food and absorbed into the body.

smallpox

A highly infectious disease, caused by the variola virus, that was eradicated in 1980 after a global vaccination campaign.

Smallpox was transmitted from person to person. It caused an illness resembling influenza and was characterized by a rash that spread over the body and eventually developed into pus-filled blisters. The blisters became crusted and sometimes left pitted scars. Complications included blindness, pneumonia, and kidney damage. There was no effective treatment for the disease, which killed up to 40 per cent of its victims.

Eradication of smallpox was achieved through cooperative international use of a highly effective vaccine. Routine vaccination has now been discontinued throughout the world.

smear

A specimen for microscopic examination prepared by spreading a thin film of cells on to a glass slide. Common types of smear include blood cells for a *blood film* and cells from the neck of the uterus for a *cervical smear test*. Less commonly, cells may be collected from the inside of the cheek (known as a buccal smear) for *DNA* or *chromosome analysis* or *genetic fingerprinting*.

smegma

An accumulation of sebaceous gland secretions under the foreskin in an uncircumcised male, usually due to poor hygiene. Fungal or bacterial infection of smegma may cause *balanitis* (inflammation of the foreskin and the head of the penis).

smell

One of the five senses. In the nose, hair-like projections from smell receptor cells lie in the mucous membrane. When the receptors are stimulated by certain molecules, they transmit impulses along the olfactory nerves to the smell centres in the *limbic system* and the temporal and frontal lobes of the brain, where smell is perceived.

Loss of sense of smell may result from inflammation of the nasal membrane, as in a common *cold*; cigarette *smoking*; hypertrophic *rhinitis*, in which a thickened nasal membrane obscures olfactory nerve endings; atrophic rhinitis, in which the nerves waste away; head injury that tears the nerves; or a tumour of the *meninges* (membranes covering the brain) or nasopharynx (upper part of the throat).

The perception of illusory, unpleasant odours may be a feature of *depression*, *schizophrenia*, some forms of *epilepsy*, or alcohol withdrawal.

S

THE SENSE OF **SMELL**

The smell receptors are specialized nerve cell endings that are situated in a small patch of mucous membrane lining the roof of the nose. The axons (fibres) of these sensory cells pass up through tiny perforations in the overlying bone to enter the two elongated olfactory bulb lying on top of the bone. These bulbs are swellings at the ends of the olfactory nerves; the nerves contain millions of nerve fibres and enter the brain on its lower surface. The olfactory nerves carry sensory information to smell centres (parts of the limbic system and frontal lobes) situated within the brain.

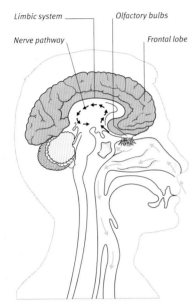

Physiological basis of smell
The receptor cell bodies that are situated in the nasal cavity are swollen at their lower ends; each one has several cilia that extend down to the surface of the mucous membrane. The cilia contain the receptor sites at which stimulation by the molecules of odorous substances gives rise to nerve impulses. These nerve impulses pass from the olfactory bulb along the olfactory nerve to smell centres in the brain (which include parts of the limbic system and frontal lobes). Although we know that we are able to distinguish between as many as several thousand different odours, the exact basis of this high degree of specificity is uncertain. No microscopic difference in structure can be detected among the different receptors.

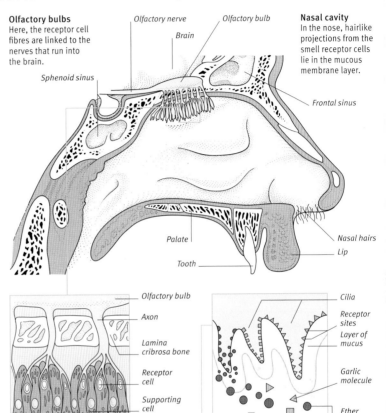

Olfactory bulbs
Here, the receptor cell fibres are linked to the nerves that run into the brain.

Nasal cavity
In the nose, hairlike projections from the smell receptor cells lie in the mucous membrane layer.

Probable mechanism of smell
The smell process is probably based on a physical "fit" between the odour molecules and the receptor sites. For example, the receptors on some cells may fit only with ether molecules, others with molecules of bleach. The molecules must dissolve in the mucus before they can stimulate the receptors. The sensitivity of the system is remarkable; as few as four molecules can give a recognizable smell.

S

Smith's fracture

A break in the lower part of the radius (the shorter of the two bones of the forearm, on the thumb side of the arm) in which the fragment underneath the fracture is displaced forwards.

smoking

Inhalation of tobacco smoke from cigarettes, cigars, or pipes. More than 110,000 deaths per year in the UK are attributed to smoking, and it is the greatest avoidable cause of premature death in the UK.

EFFECTS OF SMOKING

Smoking increases the heart rate and blood pressure, and levels of the *neurotransmitters* dopamine and noradrenaline (norepinephrine) in the brain, the effects of which are to elevate mood, increase alertness, and improve concentration. These effects are caused mainly by the nicotine in tobacco smoke. Nicotine is highly addictive, and can also cause a dangerous rise in blood pressure in some people who suffer from *hypertension*.

In addition to nicotine, tobacco smoke contains many other substances, such as tar, carbon monoxide, and oxidant gases, that can cause a wide range of serious diseases, including *lung cancer*, *bronchitis*, *emphysema*, chronic obstructive pulmonary disease (see *pulmonary disease, chronic obstructive*), *coronary artery disease*, *stroke*, and *peripheral vascular disease*. Smoking also increases the risk of developing *mouth cancer*, *lip cancer*, throat cancer (see *pharynx, cancer of*), oesophageal cancer (see *oesophagus, cancer of*), bladder cancer (see *bladder tumours*), cervical cancer (see *cervix, cancer of*), *kidney cancer*, stom-

EFFECTS OF **SMOKING**

About 20 per cent of all deaths in the UK are attributed to smoking. The main harmful effects of smoking are respiratory diseases (lung cancer and COPD) and cardiovascular diseases (coronary artery disease and peripheral vascular disease). Smoking also causes a range of other cancers, including cancer of the bladder, cervix, tongue, larynx, and stomach. Smoking kills around half of all smokers.

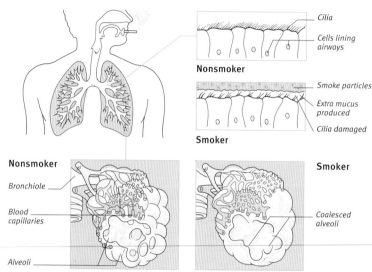

Nonsmoker — Cilia / Cells lining airways

Smoker — Smoke particles / Extra mucus produced / Cilia damaged

Nonsmoker — Bronchiole / Blood capillaries / Alveoli

Smoker — Coalesced alveoli

How smoking damages the lungs
Smoke particles irritate the lungs' airways, causing excess mucus production (top right). The smoke particles also indirectly destroy the walls of the lungs' alveoli, which merge together (above right), resulting in a smaller area overall for oxygen absorption. Both factors reduce lung efficiency. In addition, tar in tobacco smoke has a direct cancer-causing action.

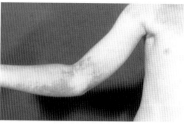

Snake bite
Following an adder bite, this boy's arm has become bruised and swollen, and the lymph nodes in his armpit have become enlarged.

ach cancer, and pancreatic cancer (see *pancreas, cancer of*). It also increases the risk of respiratory tract infections (such as *pneumonia*), *macular degeneration*, *peptic ulcers*, *osteoporosis*, *erectile dysfunction*, and *infertility*, and may make some pre-existing conditions (such as *asthma* and diabetic *retinopathy*) worse or more prolonged.

There is also evidence that passive smokers are at increased risk of smoking-related disorders, especially lung cancer and heart disease, Also, passive smokers suffer immediate discomfort when breathing in smoke, such as coughing, and sore eyes. Babies exposed to tobacco smoke are at increased risk of *sudden infant death syndrome* (SIDS), and children with parents who smoke are more likely to suffer from asthma or other respiratory diseases.

Smoking is extremely harmful during pregnancy. It increases the risk of *miscarriage*, premature birth (see *prematurity*), and *stillbirth*. Babies of women who smoke are smaller and may grow more slowly than babies of nonsmokers.

STOPPING SMOKING

Most people are aware of the benefits of stopping smoking in terms of significantly improving the health and reducing the chance of premature death of themselves and those around them. However, many people find it diffcult to stop smoking because they are addicted to nicotine. It is the physiological effects of this addiction that cause the craving that gradually builds up between cigarettes and the withdrawal symptoms (such as depressed mood, agitation, irritability, increased appetite, dizziness, and difficulty sleeping) that occur after a longer period without smoking.

Various aids are available to help smokers quit. These include smoking help lines, personal support at home, and support groups run by specialist advisers. There are different types of *nicotine replacement therapy* (such as nicotine gum and patches) available over the counter to help reduce tobacco cravings and withdrawal symptoms. In addition, drugs such as *amfebutamone* (bupropion) or *varenicline* may be

prescribed by a doctor as an aid to stopping, in conjunction with self-help measures. Some people also find alternative therapies, such as *hypnotherapy* and *acupuncture*, helpful.

snail track ulcer

A shallow, greyish mouth ulcer. Snail track ulcers are a characteristic symptom that occur during the secondary stage of *syphilis*.

snake bites

Every year, hundreds of thousands of people all over the world are bitten by snakes, but the chance of death or serious injury following a bite is relatively small. Most bites are by nonvenomous species of snake; furthermore, medical treatment of poisonous bites is usually effective, provided the victim can be taken to hospital quickly. Even the most powerful snake venom takes hours or days to kill a human being.

VENOMOUS SPECIES

Venomous snakes are found mainly in the tropics; the only poisonous species native to the UK is the adder, a member of the Viperidae (viper family). Round the world, this group of snakes includes lance-headed vipers, water moccasins (cottonmouths), American rattle-snakes, and the saw-scaled or carpet viper.

Another group of venomous snakes, Elapidae, includes cobras, coral snakes, kraits, and mambas. Venomous bites are caused by other snakes including Atractaspididae (burrowing asps), Hydrophiidae (sea snakes), and a relatively small number of the Colubridae family.

EFFECTS OF A BITE

The effects of a venomous bite depend on the species and size of the snake, the amount of venom injected, and the age and health of the victim.

A bite from a viper such as a rattle-snake is characterized by two distinct puncture wounds. Typically, there is an immediate burning pain and swelling at the site, followed by dizziness and nausea. The blood pressure drops and heart rate increases. A pins-and-needles sensation, thirst, and headache are other common symptoms. The venom may prevent the blood from clotting, causing bleeding from the wound and bruising under the skin. There may also be internal bleeding from the urinary tract, mouth, rectum, or vagina.

Elapidae also make puncture wounds but may chew the skin. Their venom primarily affects the nervous system. Serious symptoms develop from 10 minutes to eight hours after the bite and may include drooping eyelids, slurred speech, and double vision. The victim becomes drowsy or delirious and may have convulsions. Without treatment, respiratory paralysis eventually leads to death.

TREATMENT
Snakebite victims need medical help as quickly as possible. *Antibiotic drugs* and *tetanus* antitoxin injections are given for all bites, venomous or not, to prevent infection and tetanus. For a venomous bite, an injection of *antivenom* (a serum that contains antibodies against the poison) is given. Most victims recover completely with prompt treatment.

Snellen chart

A method of measuring *visual acuity* used during *vision tests*. The Snellen chart has several rows of letters, of standard sizes, with each row smaller than the one above. The patient is positioned at a set distance from the chart, then each eye in turn is covered and the patient is asked to read down the chart as far as possible with the open eye.

snoring

Noisy breathing through the open mouth produced by vibrations of the soft palate during sleep. Snoring is often caused by a condition that hinders breathing through the nose, such as a *cold*, allergic *rhinitis*, or enlarged *adenoids*. It is also a feature of *sleep apnoea*. Snoring is more common in people sleeping on their backs. If the underlying cause can be treated, it may stop.

snow-blindness

A common name for actinic *keratopathy*.

snuff

A preparation of powdered *tobacco* (often with other substances) for inhalation. Snuff is addictive because it contains *nicotine*; it also irritates the nasal lining and increases the risk of cancer of the nose and throat.

snuffles

A general term that is used to describe nasal obstruction, especially that occurring in infants suffering from an upper *respiratory tract infection*.

social and communication disorders

A collective term for disorders such as *Asperger's syndrome* and *autism*, which are marked by difficulties in social interaction and obsessive behaviour. Problems begin in childhood and tend to persist throughout life.

social skills training

A type of behaviour modification in which individuals are encouraged to improve their ability to communicate. It is an important part of *rehabilitation* for people with *learning difficulties* or those with chronic psychological disorders, such as *schizophrenia*. *Role-playing* is a commonly used technique in which social situations are simulated to improve a person's confidence and performance.

sociopathy

An outdated term for *antisocial personality disorder*.

sodium

A *mineral* that helps to regulate the body's water balance and maintain normal heart rhythm. It is also involved in conduction of nerve impulses and contraction of muscles. The level of sodium in the blood is controlled by the kidneys, which eliminate any excess in the urine.

Almost all foods contain sodium naturally or as an ingredient added during processing or cooking; the main forms are sodium chloride (salt) and sodium bicarbonate. Consequently, deficiency is rare and usually results from excessive loss of sodium through persistent diarrhoea or vomiting or profuse sweating. Signs include weakness, dizziness, and muscle cramps. In severe cases, there may be a drop in blood pressure, leading to confusion, fainting, and palpitations. Treatment is with supplements, which, in hot climates, may help to prevent *heat disorders* by compensating for sodium lost through heavy sweating.

Excessive intake of sodium is thought to be a contributory factor in *hypertension* (high blood pressure). Another adverse effect is fluid retention, which may cause dizziness and swelling of the legs in severe cases.

sodium aurothiomalate

A *disease-modifying antirheumatic drug* (DMARD) used to treat active, progressive *rheumatoid arthritis*. A preparation of gold, sodium aurothiomalate is given by injection. It may have serious side effects, including gastrointestinal bleeding, and lung, liver, and kidney damage.

sodium bicarbonate

An alkali used to neutralize acid in *cystitis* and severe *acidosis* (blood acidity) in kidney failure. It is also an ingredient in over-the-counter *antacid drugs* for *indigestion*, *heartburn*, and *peptic ulcer*. Sodium bicarbonate often causes symptoms such as belching and abdominal discomfort. Long-term use can cause swollen ankles, muscle cramps, tiredness, and nausea.

sodium citrate

A drug used to relieve discomfort in urinary infections such as *cystitis*, by making the urine less acidic.

sodium cromoglicate

A drug given by inhaler to prevent *asthma* attacks. It is also used as a nasal spray to treat allergic *rhinitis*, in eye-drops for allergic *conjunctivitis*, and orally (in conjunction with dietary restrictions) for *food allergy*. Side effects include coughing and throat irritation on inhalation.

sodium picosulfate

A stimulant *laxative* drug used to treat *constipation* and to empty the bowel prior to procedures such as X-ray, *endoscopy*, and intestinal surgery. Side effects may include abdominal cramps and diarrhoea. The drug should be avoided in cases of intestinal obstruction.

sodium valproate

An *anticonvulsant drug* used to treat *epilepsy* and *mania*. Possible side effects include drowsiness, abdominal discomfort, temporary hair loss, weight gain, and rash. Sodium valproate may rarely cause liver damage and blood tests may sometimes be carried out while taking the drug to monitor liver function.

soft-tissue injury

Damage to the tissues (such as *ligaments*, *tendons*, or *muscles*) that surround bones and joints. (See also *sports injuries*.)

soiling

Inappropriate passing of *faeces* that, in children, occurs after the age at which bowel control is achieved (usually at about two or two and a half years). It can also occur in elderly people and those with physical or mental disability.

Causes include slow development of bowel control, longstanding *constipation* (in which faecal liquid leaks around hard faeces blocking the large intestine), poor *toilet-training*, and emotional stress (caused, for example, by starting school). Soiling due to constipation is usually resolved with treatment. If no physical cause can be found, a course of *psychotherapy* may help.

Encopresis is a type of soiling in which children deliberately pass faeces in inappropriate places, such as behind furniture. Such children have no specific physical problem, but often refuse to use a potty or toilet. Encopresis usually improves with time and is rare after the age of 10.

solar keratosis

A crumbly yellow-white crust occurring on the skin in older people as a result of repeated overexposure to sunlight. The skin growth is also known as an actinic *keratosis*.

solar lentigo

Also known as a liver spot, a flat, brown frecklelike patch that appears on exposed skin. Solar lentigos occur in older white people. (See also *lentigo*.)

solar plexus

The largest network of autonomic nerves in the body, located behind the stomach between the adrenal glands. The solar plexus incorporates branches of the *vagus nerve* and the splanchnic (visceral) nerves, and sends branches into the stomach, intestines, and other abdominal organs.

Solpadeine

A brand-name *analgesic drug* (painkiller) containing *paracetamol* and *codeine*.

solvent abuse

The practice of inhaling the intoxicating fumes given off by certain volatile liquids. Glue-sniffing is the most common form of solvent abuse. The usual method of inhalation is from a plastic bag containing the solvent, but sometimes aerosols are sprayed into the nose or mouth. Solvent abuse is usually a group activity, especially among boys.

Inhalation of solvent fumes produces a feeling of intoxication similar to that produced by alcohol. Solvent abuse can cause headache, vomiting, confusion, and coma. Death may occur due to a variety of reasons including a direct toxic effect on the heart, a fall, choking on vomit, or asphyxiation by a clinging plastic bag. The effects of repeated solvent abuse include erosion of the lining of the nose and throat, and damage to the kidneys, liver, and nervous system.

The signs of solvent abuse include intoxicated behaviour, a flushed face, ulcers around the mouth, a smell of solvent, and personality changes, such as moodiness and nervousness. Acute symptoms such as vomiting or coma require urgent medical attention. In the longer term, counselling may be helpful in discouraging the behaviour.

somatic

A term meaning "related to the body" (soma), as opposed to the mind (psyche), or "related to body cells", as opposed to germ cells (eggs and sperm). It also refers to the body wall, in contrast to "visceral" (of the internal organs).

somatization disorder

A condition in which a person complains over a period of several years of various physical problems for which no organic cause can be found. The disorder, previously classified as *hysteria*, usually begins before age 30 and leads to numerous tests by many doctors. Unnecessary surgery and other treatments may result.

The symptoms that are most commonly complained of are neurological (such as double vision, seizures, weakness), gynaecological (painful menstruation, pain on intercourse), and gastrointestinal (abdominal pain, nausea). The condition is often associated with *anxiety*, *depression*, or substance abuse.

The physical symptoms in somatization disorder are caused by underlying emotional conflicts, anxiety, and depression that the person is unable to confront and unconsciously displaces on to the body. (See also *conversion disorder*; *hypochondriasis*.)

somatostatin analogues

Synthetic versions of somatostatin, a hormone that acts on the *pituitary gland* controlling the release of growth hormone. The drugs are used to treat *acromegaly* and symptoms associated with some other hormone-secreting tumours (particularly in *carcinoid syndrome*). *Octreotide* is one of the more commonly used somatostatin analogues.

somatotype

A person's physical build.

somatropin

A synthetic *growth hormone* given to children to treat *short stature* as a result of growth-hormone deficiency.

somnambulism

See *sleepwalking*.

sorbitol

A carbohydrate used as a substitute for cane sugar in foods manufactured for diabetics. It is also used in disorders of carbohydrate metabolism and in drip feeding. (See also *artificial sweeteners*.)

sore

A term that is used to describe any disrupted area of the skin or mucous membranes. The word is also used as a description of an unpleasant feeling of pain or tenderness.

sore throat

A rough or raw feeling in the back of the throat that causes discomfort, especially when swallowing.

Sore throat is a common symptom, usually caused by *pharyngitis* and occasionally by *tonsillitis*. It is often the first symptom of the common *cold*, *influenza*, *laryngitis*, *infectious mononucleosis*, and many childhood viral illnesses, such as *chickenpox*, *measles*, and *mumps*.

A sore throat may be relieved by gargling with salt water. Sore throats that are due to bacterial infection are usually treated with *antibiotic drugs*. (See also *strep throat*.)

space medicine

A medical speciality that is concerned with the physiological effects of space flight. Examples are the effects of acceleration or *motion sickness* that are caused by weightlessness.

spacer device

A plastic device that is used to aid the delivery of drugs from metered-dose *inhalers* as part of the treatment of *asthma* and other lung conditions. The mouthpiece of the inhaler is slotted in to one end of the spacer and the user's mouth is positioned tightly over the other end. During administration of a dose, the inhaler is compressed so that the drug enters the air in the spacer, then the user slowly breathes in and out, drawing the drug particles into the lungs. A valve prevents the gas from escaping out of the spacer except during the time it is being inhaled through the mouthpiece. Spacers are particularly helpful for children and older people who have difficulty coordinating their breathing with activating an inhaler.

spasm

An involuntary contraction of a *muscle*. Spasms are not necessarily painful. Examples of spasm include cramps (often affecting the calf muscles), *hiccups* (in which the diaphragm goes into spasm) and *tics* (which frequently affect the facial muscles).

Less commonly, a spasm may be caused by an abnormality in the central nervous system (brain and spinal cord) or a symptom of a muscle disorder. Spasms caused by disease of the nervous system include *myoclonus* and *chorea*. Other disorders that are characterized by spasm include *trigeminal neuralgia* (affecting the muscles of the face and head), *tetany* (spasm caused by a drop in blood calcium level), and *tetanus* (a serious bacterial infection). *Bronchospasm* is a contraction of muscles in the small airways of the lungs that occurs in asthma. In *vasospasm* (which is one of the symptoms of *Raynaud's disease*) there is a tightening of the muscles in the walls of blood vessels.

spasm, clonic

A type of spasm in which the affected muscle undergoes rapid contractions and relaxations. (See also *clonus*.)

spasm, facial

See *tic*.

spasm, infantile

A severe condition that affects infants and is associated with deterioration of brain function. The spasms involve forward flexion of the head, neck, and trunk and extension or flexion of the arms and legs.

spasm, tonic

A prolonged, involuntary muscular contraction. (See also *tetany*; *tetanus*; *tonic–clonic seizure*.)

spastic diplegia

Also called spastic paraplegia, a condition in which the lower body muscles are paralysed and abnormally rigid.

spasticity

Increased rigidity in a group of *muscles*, causing stiffness and restricted movement. Spasticity is a feature of disorders such as *Parkinson's disease*, *multiple sclerosis*, *cerebral palsy*, and *tetanus*.

spastic paralysis

Inability to move a part of the body, accompanied by rigidity of the muscles. Causes of spastic paralysis include *stroke*, *cerebral palsy*, and *multiple sclerosis*. (See also *paralysis*.)

specific gravity

The ratio of the *density* of a substance to that of water. The specific gravity of urine, for example, indicates whether the urine has a large amount of material dissolved in it (near 1.030) or whether it is almost water (near 1.010).

specific learning disability

Difficulty in one or more areas of learning in a child of average or above average intelligence. Specific learning disabilities include *dyslexia*, in which the child cannot recognize letters, and dyscalculia, in which the child has a problem with mathematics.

specimen

A sample of tissue, fluids, waste products, or an infective organism taken from the body for analysis, identification, and/or diagnosis.

SPECT

The abbreviation for single photon emission computed tomography, a type of *radionuclide scanning*.

spectacles

See *glasses*.

speculum

A device for holding open an orifice (body opening) to enable a doctor to perform an examination. For example, a speculum is used to perform a cervical smear or gynaecological swab.

speech

A system of sounds by which humans communicate. Speech involves the muscles that are used in breathing and the larynx (voicebox), tongue, palate, lips, jaw, and face.

SPEECH PRODUCTION

The production of speech sounds originates in two regions of the cerebral cortex, on each side of the *brain*, that

SPEECH DEVELOPMENT IN CHILDHOOD	
3 months	Period of babbling begins. The child produces strings of sounds for pleasure. Babbling is important in building sequences of muscle movements that will be used later to produce meaningful speech sounds.
9 months	The child echoes the speech of others, but words are not yet used with meaning. By listening to and copying adults, the child learns that clusters of sounds refer to specific objects, people, or situations.
12 to 18 months	The child beings to utter simple words with meaning, often accompanied by gestures. Examples include "bye-bye", "dog", "hot", and "daddy". Single words are used, with vocabulary gradually increasing from two or three words initially.
18 to 24 months	The child begins to combine concepts to form two-word sentences (e.g. "Hello John" or "That hot!"). By the age of two years, the child may be using 100 or more different words.
2 to 3 years	The child's sentences become longer (e.g. "I like cake" or "Peter hit Mary"). He or she also begins to incorporate adjectives and adverbs into sentences (e.g. "That's daddy's old coat" or "I want lunch now"). By the age of three years, the average sentence length is four words. Most sounds have developed, with the possible exceptions of "the", "r", "j", "ch", and "sh".
3 years and older	More elaborate sentences with several nouns, verbs in past and future tenses, and linked phrases begin to be used (e.g. "We went to Amy's and we had milk and biscuits" or "I think mummy went downstairs"). However, mistakes are often made (e.g. "What did you played?"), reflecting the child's linguistic immaturity. Language skills continue to develop throughout childhood.

S

are linked to the centre for language expression (Broca's area) in the dominant hemisphere of the brain. The areas send signals down nerve pathways to muscles controlling the larynx, tongue, and other parts involved in speech; the cerebellum, at the back of the brain, plays a part in coordinating movements of these parts. Air from the lungs is vibrated through the vocal cords in the larynx. The vibration produces a noise that is amplified in the cavities of the throat, nose, and sinuses. The vibrated air is shaped by movements of the tongue, mouth, and lips in order to produce speech sounds.

Children learn speech by listening to and imitating the speech of others. Normal speech development occurs in several stages (see *Speech development in childhood*, previous page). It depends on maturation of the child's nervous system and muscles, normal hearing, and the child's interaction with other people and the environment.

speech disorders

Defects or disturbances in *speech* that lead to inability to communicate effectively. Some of these disorders are more accurately described as disturbances of language rather than speech, as they are caused by impaired ability to understand or to form words in the language centres of the brain, rather than any fault of the apparatus of speech production. Most people who have speech disorders can be helped with the use of *speech therapy*.

DISORDERS OF LANGUAGE
Damage to the language centres of the brain (usually due to a *stroke*, *head injury*, or *brain tumour*) leads to *dysphasia* (difficulty with, or disorder of, language skills). The ability to speak and write and/or to comprehend written or spoken words is impaired to a varying degree, depending on the site and extent of the damage.

Delayed development of language in a child is characterized by slowness to understand speech and/or slow growth in vocabulary and sentence structure. Delayed development has many causes, including hearing loss (see *deafness*), lack of stimulation, or emotional disturbance (see *developmental delay*).

DISORDERS OF ARTICULATION
Articulation is the ability to make speech sounds. A defect of articulation is sometimes referred to as *dysarthria*. Damage to nerves passing from the brain to muscles in the larynx (voicebox), mouth, or

lips can make speech slurred, indistinct, slow, or nasal. The causes of the damage are similar to those that cause aphasia or dysphasia (including stroke, head injury, *multiple sclerosis*, or *Parkinson's disease*), although they affect different regions of the brain. A structural abnormality of the mouth, such as a *cleft lip and palate*, can also be a cause of poor articulation.

DISORDERS OF VOICE PRODUCTION
Disorders of voice production include hoarseness, inappropriate pitch or loudness, and abnormal nasal resonance. In many cases, the cause is a disorder affecting closure of the vocal cords (see *larynx, disorders of*). A voice that is too high or low or too loud or soft may be caused by a hormonal or psychiatric disturbance or by hearing loss.

Abnormal nasal resonance is caused by too much air (hypernasality) or too little air (hyponasality) flowing through the nose during speech. Hypernasality may result from damage to the nerves supplying the palate (roof of the mouth) or from cleft palate, and causes deterioration in the intelligibility of speech. Hyponasality is caused by blockage of the nasal airways which may be a result of congestion or excess mucus.

DISORDERS OF FLUENCY
Disorders of fluency include *stuttering*, which is marked by hesitant speech and sound repetition. The underlying cause of such problems is not understood.

speech therapy

A form of treatment for people who suffer from a *speech disorder*. A speech therapist tests speech and *hearing* and devises exercises to improve the deficient aspect of speech.

sperm

The male sex cell, also called a spermatozoon (spermatozoa in the plural), which is responsible for *fertilization* of the female cell (ovum). Each sperm is about 0.05 mm long and consists of a

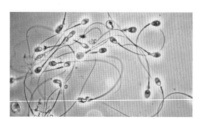

Human sperm magnified 350 times
Each sperm consists of a head that contains the hereditary material (DNA) and a long, whiplike tail that propels it along.

head, which contains genetic material, and a tail, which propels the sperm through the woman's reproductive tract after *ejaculation*. The top of the sperm's head contains enzymes that enable it to penetrate the ovum's outer covering.

Sperm production starts at *puberty*. Sperm are formed in the seminiferous tubules of the *testes* and mature in the *epididymis*, just behind each testis. This process depends on *testosterone* and *gonadotrophin hormones* secreted by the *pituitary gland*. Oligospermia (low sperm count) or azoospermia (absence of sperm) can be causes of *infertility*. (See also *reproductive system, male*; *semen analysis*.)

spermatic cord

The structure, in males, that runs from the abdomen to the scrotum and contains the *vas deferens* (a tube that conveys *sperm*). (See also *reproductive system, male*.)

spermatocele

A harmless cyst of the *epididymis* (the tube that conveys sperm from the testis) containing fluid and sperm. A very large or uncomfortable spermatocele is usually removed surgically.

spermatozoa

See *sperm*.

spermicides

Contraceptive preparations in the form of creams, gels, foams, and pessaries that kill *sperm*. They are usually recommended for use with a barrier device such as a condom or diaphragm.

SPF

The abbreviation for *sun protection factor*.

sphenoid bone

A bone at the base of the *cranium* (the part of the skull holding the brain). The sphenoid bone contains the sphenoidal

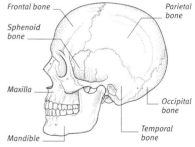

Location of the sphenoid bone
The sphenoid bone is a bat-shaped bone that lies in front of the temporal bones at the base of the skull.

S

sinuses (see *sinuses, facial*); channels for the *optic nerve* and other nerves; and a space for the *pituitary gland*.

spherocytosis, hereditary

An inherited disorder in which there are a large number of unusually small, round red blood cells (spherocytes) in the circulation. These abnormal cells are fragile and easily broken up when blood passes through the *spleen*. At times, the rate of red blood cell destruction (*haemolysis*) exceeds the rate at which new cells can be made in the bone marrow, leading to *anaemia*.

SYMPTOMS

The characteristic symptoms of anaemia, such as tiredness, shortness of breath, and pallor, may develop. Other symptoms include *jaundice* (yellowing of the skin and whites of the eyes) and enlargement of the spleen. Occasionally, crises occur (usually triggered by infection) in which all of the symptoms worsen. *Gallstones* are a frequent complication of hereditary spherocytosis.

DIAGNOSIS AND TREATMENT

The diagnosis of spherocytosis is made by blood tests. *Splenectomy* (removal of the spleen) usually leads to permanent improvement.

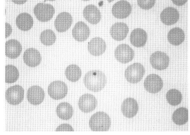

Spherocytes in blood
A person with hereditary spherocytosis has a large number of these unusually small, round, fragile, red cells in the blood.

sphincter

A ring of muscle around a natural body opening or passage that regulates inflow or outflow, such as the anal sphincter.

sphincter, artificial

A surgically created valve or other device used to treat or prevent urinary or faecal *incontinence*.

sphincterotomy

A surgical procedure that involves cutting a *sphincter* muscle that closes a body opening or constricts the opening between body passages.

TYPES OF **SPINA BIFIDA**

There are different forms of spina bifida. In one type (spina bifida occulta), the only defect is a failure of the fusion of the bony arches behind the spinal cord. When the bone defect is more extensive, there may be a meningocele, with protrusion of the meninges (the membranes surrounding the cord) or, more seriously, a myelocele, with malformation of the spinal cord itself.

MENINGOCELE

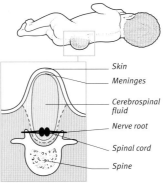

Skin
Meninges
Cerebrospinal fluid
Nerve root
Spinal cord
Spine

Meningocele
In this type, of spina bifida, the nerve tissue of the spinal cord is usually intact; there is skin over the bulging sac and therefore there may be no functional problems. However, repairs are necessary early in life.

MYELOCELE

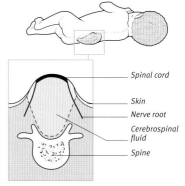

Spinal cord
Skin
Nerve root
Cerebrospinal fluid
Spine

Myelocele
In this type of the condition, the baby is born with a raw swelling over the spine. It consists of malformed spinal cord, which may or may not be contained in a membranous sac. The child is likely to be disabled.

---

sphygmomanometer

An instrument for measuring *blood pressure*. In the traditional type of sphygmomanometer, a cuff attached to the device is wrapped around a person's arm and inflated until it compresses the main artery in the arm; it is then deflated while the user listens to the blood flow with a stethoscope. The blood pressure is read off a graduated dial or, occasionally, a mercury-filled glass column. In more modern instruments, the cuff is attached to an electronic measuring device, which displays the readings on a digital display; such devices may also measure the pulse rate.

spider bites

Almost all spiders produce venom, which they use to kill their prey. Only a few species, such as the black widow in North America, are harmful to humans. *Antivenoms* are available as an antidote for many of the potentially fatal spider bites.

spider naevus

A red, raised pinhead-sized dot, from which a number of small blood vessels radiate. A spider naevus is formed by a dilated minor artery and its connecting capillaries. Small numbers of spider

naevi are common in children and pregnant women, but larger numbers may indicate liver disease.

spina bifida

A *congenital* defect in which one or more of the *vertebrae* fails to develop completely in a fetus. As a result, when the baby is born a portion of the *spinal cord* is left exposed. Spina bifida is a type of *neural tube defect*.

The risk of spina bifida can be substantially reduced by the mother taking the recommended dose of *folic acid* supplements before conception and during the first 12 weeks of pregnancy. Spina bifida can also be detected before birth by blood tests and *ultrasound scanning*.

spinal anaesthesia

Injection of an anaesthetic into the cerebrospinal fluid in the spinal canal to block *pain* sensations before they reach the *central nervous system*. Spinal anaesthesia is used mainly during surgical procedures on the lower abdomen and legs and in obstetrics. (See also *epidural anaesthesia*.)

spinal canal decompression

see *decompression, spinal canal*.

S

LOCATION OF THE **SPINAL CORD**

The cord runs about 45 cm downwards from the brain via a canal in the spine, tapering at its lower end. It is covered by meninges, which are continuous with the covering of the brain.

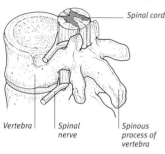

Spinal cord

Vertebra | Spinal nerve | Spinous process of vertebra

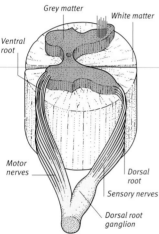

Grey matter — White matter

Ventral root

Motor nerves — Dorsal root — Sensory nerves — Dorsal root ganglion

Structure of the spinal cord
The grey matter contains nerve cell bodies, whereas the white matter consists of tracts of nerve fibres. Spinal nerves join the cord at regular intervals.

ANATOMY OF THE **SPINAL NERVES**

The 31 pairs of nerves are divided into groups – cervical, thoracic, lumbar, and sacral – according to the section of spine from which they emerge. Those emerging from the middle of the spinal cord encircle the body, branching to supply a fairly distinct segment of trunk. Those emerging from the top and bottom of the spine join to form networks, called plexuses, from which branches arise to supply the arms and legs.

Nerve twig

Spinal nerve

Ventral root

Dorsal root
Spinal cord

Spinous process of vertebra

Spinal nerve
Nerve bundle
Nerve axon
Vertebra
Intervertebral discs

Brain
Cervical nerves
Thoracic nerves
Spinal cord
Lumbar nerves
Sacral nerves
Cauda equina

Distribution
The branches of each nerve divide as they travel further from the spinal cord. As a result, all parts of the trunk, arms, and legs are supplied with a network of nerve twigs.

Structure
Each nerve consists of bundles of the axons, or fibres, of individual nerve cells that have their cell bodies in or close to the spinal cord.

S

spinal cord

A cylinder of *nerve* tissue, about 45 cm long and about the width of a finger, that runs from the *brain* down the central canal in the *spine* to the first lumbar vertebra. Below that point, the lowest nerve roots continue within the spinal canal as the *cauda equina*. The spinal cord is a major component of the *central nervous system*.

STRUCTURE
At the core of the spinal cord is grey matter, which contains the cell bodies of nerve cells, along with various supporting cells. Some of the nerve cells are motor neurons from which long pro-

jecting fibres (called axons) pass out of the spinal cord in bundles with the *spinal nerves* and extend to glands or muscles in the trunk and limbs. Surrounding the grey matter are areas of white matter, which consist of bundles of nerve cell axons running lengthwise through the cord.

Sprouting from each side at regular intervals are the sensory and motor spinal nerve roots. These combine to form the spinal nerves, which link the cord to all areas of the trunk and limbs. The cord is bathed in *cerebrospinal fluid* and surrounded by three protective membranes known as the *meninges*.

FUNCTION
The nerve tracts in the white matter act mainly as highways for sensory information passing up to the brain or motor signals passing down; however, the cord processes some sensory information, and provides motor responses, without any involvement of the brain. Many automatic reflex actions are controlled in this way.

DISORDERS
The spinal cord may be injured by trauma to the spine (see *spinal injury*). Severing of nerve tracts interrupts communication between the brain and parts of the body served from the section of

STRUCTURE OF THE **SPINE**

The spine is made up of a column of 33 roughly cylindrical bones called vertebrae. Running through the centre of this bony structure is the spinal cord.

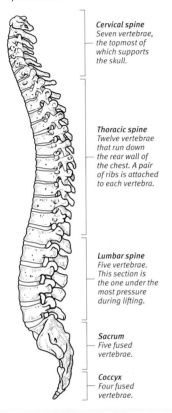

Cervical spine
Seven vertebrae, the topmost of which supports the skull.

Thoracic spine
Twelve vertebrae that run down the rear wall of the chest. A pair of ribs is attached to each vertebra.

Lumbar spine
Five vertebrae. This section is the one under the most pressure during lifting.

Sacrum
Five fused vertebrae.

Coccyx
Four fused vertebrae.

the cord below the injury. This can lead to various types of paralysis and/or loss of sensation, which are usually permanent because nerve cells and fibres in the cord cannot regenerate. However, reflexes that are controlled by the spinal cord are usually maintained. Pressure on the cord, which may be due to a blood clot or a tumour, for example, can also affect movement and sensation but can sometimes be relieved by surgery.

Infections of the spinal cord are rare but can cause serious damage. An example of such an infection is *poliomyelitis*. In the degenerative disease *multiple sclerosis* there is patchy loss of the insulating sheaths around nerve fibres.

spinal fusion

Major surgery in which two or more adjacent *vertebrae* are joined together. It is performed if there is abnormal move-

DISORDERS OF THE **SPINE**

Many disorders of the spine, despite their different causes, result in just one symptom: *back pain*.

Congenital disorders

Some children are born with a gap in the vertebrae because part of one or more vertebrae has failed to develop completely. This leaves part of the spinal cord exposed. The condition, known as *spina bifida*, may cause paralysis of the lower limbs and incontinence.

Infection

Osteomyelitis (infection of bone and bone marrow) may in rare cases affect a vertebra, destroying both bone and disc. The most common cause of osteomyelitis is the spread of an infection, such as *tuberculosis*, from elsewhere in the body.

Inflammation

In *ankylosing spondylitis*, and in some cases of *rheumatoid arthritis*, the joints in the spine become inflamed and eventually fuse, causing permanent stiffness. *Osteochondritis juvenilis* (inflammation of the growing area of bone in children and adolescents) can affect the vertebrae, when the disease may cause deformity of the spine.

Injuries

Lifting heavy objects, twisting suddenly, or adopting bad posture can cause any of the following spinal injuries: sprained ligament, torn muscle, *spondylolisthesis* (dislocated vertebra), dislocated facet joint, or *disc prolapse* (rupture of the tough outer layer of the disc).

ment between adjacent vertebrae that causes severe back pain or risks damaging the spinal cord.

spinal injury

Damage to the *spine* and sometimes to the *spinal cord*, most often due to falling from a height or a road traffic accident.

Damage to the *vertebrae* and their *ligaments* usually causes severe pain and swelling of the affected area. Damage to the spinal cord results in *paralysis* and/or loss of sensation below the site of injury. *X-rays* and/or *MRI* or *CT scanning* of the spine are carried out to determine the extent of damage. If the

A direct blow, a fall from a height, or sudden twisting can result in fracture of one or more vertebrae.

Tumours

Tumours of the bones of the spine are usually malignant; in most cases, they have spread from cancer elsewhere in the body (see *bone cancer*).

Degeneration

Osteoarthritis (degeneration of joint cartilage due to wear and tear) affects the spine joints of virtually everyone over 60, particularly people who do heavy manual work or those whose spines have already been affected by disease or injury.

Osteoporosis (thinning and softening of bone), which is most common in postmenopausal women, can weaken the vertebrae. Vertebrae may fracture and collapse, under the weight of the trunk.

Other disorders

In some people, the spine is abnormally curved. Excessive curvature may be inwards in the lower back (see *lordosis*), outwards in the upper back (see *kyphosis*), or to one side (see *scoliosis*). Causes include infection, osteoporosis, and congenital and muscle disorders.

INVESTIGATION

Spinal disorders are investigated by *X-rays*, *CT scanning*, and *MRI*. Other bone imaging techniques, such as *radionuclide scanning*, may also be performed.

S

bones are dislocated, surgery is needed to manipulate them back into position. Surgery may also be needed to remove pressure on the cord, but damaged nerve tracts cannot be repaired. *Physiotherapy* may stop joints locking and muscles contracting due to paralysis.

If there is no spinal cord damage, recovery is usually complete. In cases of spinal cord damage, some improvement may occur for up to 12 months.

spinal nerves

A set of 31 pairs of *nerves* that connect to the *spinal cord*. The nerves emerge in two rows from either side of the spinal cord and leave the spine through gaps between adjacent vertebrae. They then branch out to supply all parts of the trunk, arms, and legs with sensory and motor nerve fibres.

Disc prolapse may lead to pressure on a spinal nerve, which causes pain. Nerve injury may result in loss of sensation or movement in the specific area that is supplied by the nerve.

spinal tap

See *lumbar puncture*.

spine

The column of bones and cartilage that extends from the base of the skull to the pelvis, enclosing the *spinal cord* and supporting the trunk and head.

STRUCTURE AND FUNCTION

The spine is made up of 33 roughly cylindrical bones called *vertebrae*. Each pair of adjacent vertebrae is connected by a facet *joint*, which helps both to stabilize the spine and allow movement in it. Between the vertebrae lie pads of tough fibrous cartilage with a jellylike core, called intervertebral discs (see *disc, intervertebral*). These pads act as shock-absorbers during such movements as running and jumping.

In a normal spine, the topmost section, consisting of seven vertebrae and known as the cervical spine, curves forwards; the thoracic spine, made up of the 12 vertebrae at the rear of the chest, curves backwards; the lumbar (lower back) section curves forwards, particularly in women; and the pelvic section (consisting of the sacrum and coccyx) curves backwards.

The spine encloses the *spinal cord*, a column of nerve tracts running from the brain. *Spinal nerves* branch off from the spinal cord, at the nerve roots, to form the peripheral nerves (see *peripheral nervous system*), the roots of which pass between the vertebrae to supply every part of the body.

The vertebrae are bound together by two long, thick *ligaments* running the length of the spine and by smaller ligaments between the individual bones. Attached to the spine are several groups of *muscles*, which control its movement and help to support it. See *Structure of the spine* box and *Disorders of the spine* box, previous page.

spiral fracture

A type of *fracture* in which the bone is broken by severe twisting.

SPIROMETRY

A spirometer is used to measure the volume of air (in litres) that you can inhale and exhale over a period of time. The results of spirometry show whether or not the airways are narrowed as a result of lung disorders such as asthma. The procedure can also be used to monitor the effectiveness of certain treatments for lung disorders, such as bronchodilator drugs, which widen the airways.

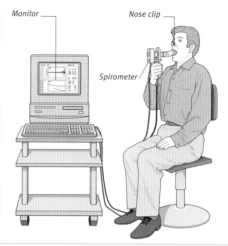

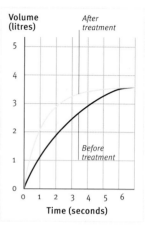

Using the spirometer
The patient is asked to inhale and exhale fully through a mouthpiece several times. The volume of air inhaled and exhaled is displayed on the monitor.

Spirometry graph
This graphs shows the effect of drug treatment to widen the air passages in a person with asthma. The volume of air that is exhaled in 1 second rises from about 1 litre to 2 litres soon after the drugs have been taken.

---

spirochaete

Any of a group of spiral-shaped bacteria that cause various infections, including *syphilis*, *leptospirosis*, *relapsing fever*, and *Lyme disease*.

spirometry

A *pulmonary function test* used to diagnose or assess a *lung* disorder or to monitor treatment. It records the rate at which a person exhales air from the lungs and the total volume exhaled.

Spirometry may be used to assess conditions in which the airways are narrowed, such as *asthma*, or those in which lung expansion is restricted, such as *interstitial pulmonary fibrosis*.

spironolactone

A potassium-sparing *diuretic drug* used to treat *heart failure*, *oedema*, and *ascites* (fluid buildup in the peritoneal cavity of the abdomen). Possible side effects include numbness, weakness, and nausea; less commonly, the drug may cause diarrhoea, lethargy, *erectile dysfunction*, rash, and irregular menstruation. High doses may cause *gynaecomastia* (abnormal breast enlargement) in men.

spleen

A fist-sized, dark red spongy organ in the upper left of the abdomen behind the lower ribs. The spleen removes worn-out and defective red blood cells from the circulation and helps to fight infection by producing some of the *antibodies* (proteins) and *lymphocytes* and *phagocytes* (types of white blood cell) that destroy invading microorganisms.

The spleen enlarges in many diseases, including infections such as *malaria* and *infectious mononucleosis*; blood disorders such as *leukaemia*, *thalassaemia*, and *sickle cell anaemia*; and tumours such as *lymphomas*. Enlargement may be accompanied by *hypersplenism* (overactivity of the spleen). The organ may be ruptured by a severe blow to the abdomen; this may cause potentially fatal haemorrhage, needing an emergency *splenectomy* (removal of the spleen).

splenectomy

Surgical removal of the *spleen*. Splenectomy is performed after the spleen has been seriously injured, or to treat *hypersplenism* or certain forms of *anaemia*. The absence of the spleen does not normally cause any problems because its function is largely taken over by other parts of the *lymphatic system* and the *liver*. People who have had a splenectomy are more susceptible to certain infections and are given pneumococcal, meningococcal, Hib, and influenza vaccines and long-term *antibiotics*.

splint

A device used to immobilize a part of the body. Splints are usually made of firm or rigid material and sometimes they are padded. An uninjured part of a person's own body may also be used as a splint.

splinter haemorrhage

Bleeding under the fingernails, visible as tiny, splinter-like marks. Splinter haemorrhage is usually due to trauma but can also be a sign of infective *endocarditis*.

splinting

The application of a *splint*, most often to immobilize fracture.

splinting, dental

The mechanical joining of several teeth to hold them in place while an injury heals or while *periodontal disease* is treated.

split personality

A common term for *multiple personality*. It is also used, incorrectly, to describe *schizophrenia*.

spondylitis

Inflammation of the joints between the vertebrae in the *spine*. Spondylitis is usually caused by *osteoarthritis*, *rheumatoid arthritis*, or *ankylosing spondylitis*.

spondylolisthesis

The slipping of a *vertebra* over the one below it. In most cases, the fifth (lowest) lumbar vertebra slips; in other cases, it is

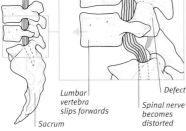

Normal spine   **Spondylolisthesis**

Lumbar: Defect
vertebra
slips forwards
Sacrum   *Spinal nerve*
                 becomes
                 distorted

Lumbar spondylolisthesis
If the lowest lumbar vertebra slips forwards over the sacrum, it may distort or press on a spinal nerve, causing symptoms such as backache or sciatica.

the fourth lumbar vertebra or a cervical (neck) vertebra. The displaced bone may press on nearby spinal nerves.

Lumbar spondylolisthesis may be due to bone weakness caused by *spondylolysis* or *osteoarthritis*, and may result in *back pain* and *sciatica*. Cervical spondylolisthesis may be due to neck injury, spinal abnormality, or *rheumatoid arthritis*; it leads to neck pain and stiffness and, in severe cases, pain, numbness, and weakness in the hands or arms.

Treatment may include *traction*, immobilizing the area in a plaster corset or with an orthopaedic collar, and *physiotherapy*. If there is nerve damage or severe back pain, *spinal fusion* may be needed to fuse the affected vertebrae.

spondylolysis

A disorder of the *spine* in which the arch of the fifth (or, rarely, the fourth) lumbar vertebra consists of soft fibrous tissue instead of normal bone. As a result, the arch is weak and prone to damage under stress, which may produce *spondylolisthesis*. Otherwise, the condition is usually symptomless.

spongiform encephalopathy

A brain disorder in which the brain tissue shrinks and spaces develop in it, producing severe signs such as paralysis and dementia. (See also *Creutzfeldt–Jakob disease*; *encephalopathy*; *kuru*; *prion*.)

spontaneous abortion

See *miscarriage*.

sporotrichosis

A chronic infection caused by the fungus SPOROTHRIX SCHENCKII, which grows on plants. The infection is most often contracted through a skin wound; gardeners are particularly vulnerable. An ulcer develops at the site of the wound; nodules then form in lymph channels around the site. Potassium iodide solution taken orally usually clears up the infection. Rarely, in people with reduced immunity, sporotrichosis spreads to other parts of the body and requires treatment with amphotericin, an *antifungal drug*.

sports, drugs and

The use of drugs to improve athletic performance has been condemned by authorities because it endangers the health of users and gives them an unfair advantage. Random drug tests on urine (and sometimes other body fluids) are performed in most sports during competitions and sometimes also in training. Many drugs affect the performance of athletes who are taking them. Some are medications that have been prescribed to treat specific medical conditions but are abused by athletes who want to benefit from the body-building and performance-enhancing effects of these drugs. Others are everyday nonprescription substances, such as caffeine and nicotine, which have a relatively minor effect on performance. However, even these substances can cause drug levels in the body to rise to unacceptable levels if they are taken in excess.

PROHIBITED DRUGS

Various classes of drugs are prohibited in international sports and their use may lead to an athlete being banned from competitions, sometimes for life. The regulations concerning drug use in sports are complex, with some drugs being banned at all times and others banned only during competition. However, the International Olympic Committee completely prohibits five classes of drugs at all times, in and out of competition. These are anabolic agents, such as anabolic steroids (see *steroids, anabolic*); hormones and related substances, such as erythropoietin and *growth hormone*; *beta-blockers*; hormone antagonists and modulators, such as anti-oestrogens; and *diuretics* and other masking agents. Many other drugs, such as stimulants, narcotics, cannabinoids, glucocorticosteroids, and alcohol, are banned during competitions. Caffeine, which is in tea, coffee, and many soft drinks, is prohibited only in high doses.

In addition to drugs, certain performance-enhancing methods are prohibited, such as blood doping, gene doping, and any intravenous infusion.

LEGITIMATE DRUG USE

Certain prescribed medications can legitimately be used by athletes for some medical disorders, such as *asthma* or *epilepsy*. However, the use of prescribed medications must be declared in writing to the appropriate authority before any competition. Other prescribed drugs, such as antibiotics, may not noticeably affect athletic performance but the underlying disorder for which the drugs are being taken may make strenuous activity inadvisable. Athletes also need to be careful when using over-the-counter medications because they may contain low doses of prohibited substances. In general, athletes should obtain medical advice

S

before taking drugs of any kind to avoid inadvertently taking a prohibited substance or endangering their health.

sports injuries

Any injury that arises during participation in sports. Typical sports injuries include *fractures, head injury* (including *concussion*), muscle *strain* or *compartment syndrome, tendinitis* or tendon rupture, ligament *sprain*, and joint *dislocation* or *subluxation*. Some "sports" injuries, such as *tennis elbow*, are in fact a type of *overuse injury*. (See also *running injuries*.)

sports medicine

A medical speciality concerned with the assessment and improvement of *fitness* and the treatment and prevention of injuries and disorders related to sports.

spot

A general term for a small lump, mark, or inflamed area on the skin.

spotting

See *breakthrough bleeding*.

sprain

Tearing or stretching, due to a sudden pull, of *ligaments* that hold the bone ends together in a joint. A sprain causes painful swelling, and the joint cannot be moved without increasing the pain. There may also be spasm of surrounding muscles.

Treatment consists of applying an *icepack*, wrapping the joint in a bandage, resting it in a raised position, and taking *analgesic drugs*. In severe cases, surgical repair may be necessary.

sprue

An intestinal disorder that prevents the small intestine absorbing sufficient nutrients from food. There are two forms: tropical sprue (see *sprue, tropical*), and *coeliac disease*, which is more common and is caused by sensitivity to gluten.

sprue, tropical

A disease of the small intestine that interferes with the absorption of nutrients. Occurring mainly in India, the Far East, and the Caribbean, sprue may be due to intestinal infection. Symptoms include loss of appetite and weight, an inflamed mouth, and fatty diarrhoea. Sprue leads to *malnutrition* and megaloblastic *anaemia*.

Diagnosis is confirmed by *jejunal biopsy*. The condition responds well to *antibiotic drug* treatment and vitamin and mineral supplements.

sputum

Also called phlegm, mucous fluid that is produced by cells lining the airways in the lungs. Sputum production may be increased by *respiratory tract infection*, an allergic reaction, or inhalation of irritants.

squamous cell carcinoma

Also known as SCC, a cancer that arises in epithelial cells, which line most hollow structures within the body and cover the body's surface. SCC can occur in many body organs, including the mouth (see *mouth cancer*) and lungs (see *lung cancer*). SCC of the skin is one of the most common types of *skin cancer* and is linked to long-term exposure to sunlight; it is most common in fair-skinned people over 60.

SCC of the skin starts as a small, painless lump or patch, usually on the lip, ear, or back of the hand. It enlarges fairly rapidly, often resembling a wart or ulcer. It can also arise from a pre-existing solar keratosis (a patch of rough or thickened skin). Left untreated, the cancer may spread to other parts of the body and prove fatal.

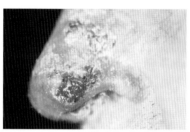

Squamous cell carcinoma
The tumour has spread to cover much of the area around the side of this patient's nose. It can be treated with radiotherapy. Squamous cell carcinoma is the second most common form of cancer.

Diagnosis is based on a *skin biopsy*. The tumour is removed surgically or destroyed by *radiotherapy*. (See also *basal cell carcinoma*; *melanoma, malignant*.)

squint

Known medically as strabismus, a deviation of one eye in relation to the other. A squint can be either convergent (in which the eye turns inwards) or divergent (in which it turns outwards).

Many babies have a squint because the mechanism for aligning the eyes has not yet developed. A squint that starts later in childhood is usually due to breakdown of the alignment mechanism; longsightedness is a common contributory factor. In some cases, there

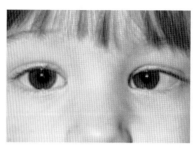

Squint
This child has a convergent squint of the left eye (right in image), in which the eye is directed too far inwards, towards the nose. Left untreated, a squint can lead to permanent loss of sight in one eye.

is an additional problem in that the brain suppresses the image from the deviating eye, leading to *amblyopia* (reduced sharpness of vision).

In adults, squint may be a symptom of *stroke, diabetes mellitus, multiple sclerosis, hyperthyroidism*, or a tumour. A squint in adults causes double vision.

Squint in children should be treated as soon as possible to prevent potential visual impairment. Treatment may include covering the normal eye with a patch, which forces the child to use the weak eye; alternatively, deviation of the squinting eye may be controlled by glasses. In a few cases, it may be possible to treat a squint with special eye exercise or eye-drops. If none of these treatments is effective, surgery may be required. The sudden onset of a squint in adults may have a serious underlying cause and must be investigated promptly.

SSRIs

See *selective serotonin reuptake inhibitors*.

stable

A term used in medicine to describe a patient's condition that is neither deteriorating nor improving; a personality that is not susceptible to mental illness; or a chemical substance that is resistant to changes in its composition or physical state, or is not radioactive.

stage

A phase in the course of a disease; the term is used particularly to describe the progression of *cancer*. Staging is a method of assessing cancer according to the size of the main tumour, the degree to which it has invaded surrounding tissues, and the extent to which it has spread elsewhere in the body. Treatment and outlook of diseases depend on the stage, hence the importance of staging.

S

staghorn calculus

A large kidney stone, with several branches, that forms in the renal pelvis (the central area of the kidney, where urine collects before leaving the organ). (See *calculus, urinary tract*.)

staining

The process of dyeing specimens of cells, tissues, or microorganisms to make them clearly visible or easily identifiable under a *microscope*.

stammering

See *stuttering*.

Stanford–Binet test

A type of *intelligence test*.

stanozolol

A type of anabolic steroid drug (see *steroids, anabolic*).

stapedectomy

An operation on the *ear* to replace the *stapes* (the innermost of the three bones in the middle ear) with a device that takes over the bone's function. It is used to treat *deafness* due to *otosclerosis*.

stapes

The innermost of the three tiny, sound-conducting bones in the middle *ear*. The stapes is the smallest bone in the body. Its head articulates with the *incus* and its base fits into the oval window in the wall of the inner ear.

In *otosclerosis*, the stapes becomes fixed and cannot transmit sound to the inner ear. The resultant hearing loss can be treated by *stapedectomy*.

staphylococcal infections

Infections caused by *bacteria* of the genus STAPHYLOCOCCUS. Different species of staphylococci are responsible for a range of disorders, including skin infections such as *pustules*, *abscesses*, and *boils*, and a rash in newborn babies (see *necrolysis, toxic epidermal*); *pneumonia*; *toxic shock syndrome* in menstruating women; *urinary tract infection*; and *food poisoning*. If the bacteria enter the circulation, they may cause *septicaemia* or *septic shock*, infectious *arthritis*, *osteomyelitis*, or bacterial *endocarditis*. (See also *Staphylococcus aureus*.)

Staphylococcus aureus

A species of STAPHYLOCOCCUS bacterium that produces toxins, causing a range of *staphylococcal infections*. Some strains of the bacterium have developed resistance to methicillin and many other antibiotics; these strains are known as *MRSA* (methicillin-resistant STAPHYLOCOCCUS AUREUS).

stapling

A surgical procedure to treat severe *obesity*, in which the *stomach* is partitioned using surgical staples, to leave only a small volume for digestion and food storage. Staples are also used for *suturing*.

starch

See *carbohydrates*.

startle reflex

A reflex action seen in newborn babies that is similar to the *Moro reflex*.

starvation

A condition that results from lack of food over a long period and results in weight loss, changes in *metabolism* (the body's chemical processes) and extreme hunger. (See also *anorexia nervosa*; *fasting*; *nutritional disorders*.)

stasis

Slowing down or cessation of flow.

stasis ulcer

An open sore that develops on the lower leg (see *leg ulcer*) as a result of poor blood flow in that area.

statins

A group of *lipid-lowering drugs* used to treat high blood levels of *cholesterol*. They are also used to lower blood lipid (fat) levels in people with *coronary artery disease* or those at risk of developing it, such as people with a family history of the disease, smokers, and those with *diabetes mellitus*. Possible side effects of statins include headache, abdominal discomfort, vomiting, constipation, and diarrhoea. Rarely, *myositis* (muscle inflammation) and liver damage may occur. People taking statins may have blood tests to monitor the effectiveness of the drugs and possible side effects.

statistics, medical

The collection and analysis of numerical data that relates to medicine, such as information on the *incidence* and *prevalence* of various conditions.

status asthmaticus

A severe and prolonged *asthma* attack. This condition is potentially life-threatening and needs urgent treatment.

status epilepticus

Prolonged or repeated epileptic seizures in which there is no recovery of consciousness between attacks. It is a medical emergency, which may be fatal if it is not treated promptly. It is more likely to occur in people with *epilepsy* if *anticonvulsant drugs* are taken erratically or are withdrawn suddenly.

STDs

The abbreviation for sexually transmitted diseases; another name for *sexually transmitted infections*.

steatorrhoea

Excessive fat in the faeces, causing bulky, loose, pale-coloured, greasy, and offensive-smelling faeces that float in the toilet. It may occur in *pancreatitis* and *coeliac disease* (which interfere with the breakdown of fat from food) and after the removal of substantial segments of small intestine. It is also a side effect of *orlistat* and some *lipid-lowering drugs*.

Stein–Leventhal syndrome

See *ovary, polycystic*.

stem cell

A basic cell in the body from which more specialized cells are formed. Stem cells in the *bone marrow* produce *blood cells* through a series of maturation steps. Stem cells are also found in the blood itself, and in the blood in a baby's umbilical cord.

The terms "stem cell transplant" and "bone marrow transplant" are often used interchangeably, and their therapeutic uses are the same. Strictly, however, a bone marrow transplant utilizes stem cells obtained only from the bone marrow whereas a stem cell transplant may utilize stem cells from any source.

Stem cells for transplantation can be obtained from the patient him- or herself (autologous transplantation), with the cells harvested and stored to be reinfused later after treatment has damaged the patient's bone marrow. Alternatively, stem cells can be obtained from a donor sibling or a matched but unrelated donor, or from stored umbilical blood (allogeneic transplantation). Allogeneic transplantation carries the risk of rejection (known as *graft-versus-host disease*); autologous transplantation does not.

stenosis

Narrowing of a duct, canal, passage, or tubular organ. (See also *pyloric stenosis*.)

S

FEMALE **STERILIZATION**

Laparoscopic sterilization (below) is the most common method. Both fallopian tubes must be cut, sealed, or obstructed so that eggs and sperm cannot meet for fertilization. Sterilization is usually permanent.

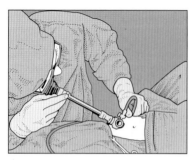

Laparoscopic sterilization
An endoscope (viewing tube) and an operating instrument are passed through separate small incisions in the abdomen.

Cutting
A small loop of the fallopian tube may be drawn up, secured by a tight ligature, and then cut off.

Constriction
A loop of the fallopian tube may be constricted at the base by a tight band, preventing eggs from passing through.

Clipping
A plastic or metal clip may be applied to the fallopian tube, sealing it so that eggs cannot pass through.

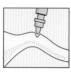

Cautery
Electrocoagulation (diathermy) can be used to burn through, and thus seal, the fallopian tube.

Instruments
The trocar is a sharp-pointed inner stylus surrounded by a close-fitting tube, the cannula. The instrument can be passed through the abdominal wall. After insertion, the trocar is removed, leaving the hollow cannula in place. Other instruments are passed through the hollow cannula.

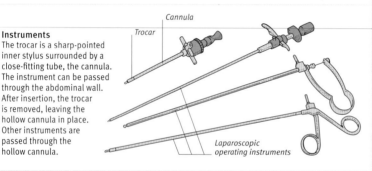

Cannula

Trocar

Laparoscopic operating instruments

stent

A rigid tube that is surgically inserted to open up, or keep open, any body canal that has become narrowed or closed up due to disease. Stents are used to open narrowed *coronary arteries* in heart disease. Some arterial stents are coated with slow-release drugs to reduce the risk of arterial renarrowing. Stents are also used to relieve blockages caused by a tumour, for example in the oesophagus or pancreas.

sterculia

A bulk-forming *laxative* used to treat constipation. It is especially useful when stools are small and hard. It should be used only if fibre intake cannot be increased. During its use, intake of fluids must be sufficient to avoid intestinal obstruction. Side effects may include flatulence, bloating, and gastrointestinal obstruction or impaction.

stereotaxic surgery

Brain operations carried out by inserting delicate instruments through a surgically created hole in the skull and guiding them, with the aid of *CT scanning*, to a specific area of the brain. Stereotaxic procedures can be used to treat *pituitary tumours*; for a brain *biopsy*; or to destroy small areas of the brain as treatment for some disabling neurological disorders.

sterility

The state either of being germ-free or of permanent *infertility*.

sterilization

Complete destruction or removal of living microorganisms, which is usually carried out to prevent the spread of infection. The term also refers to a procedure that renders a person infertile. (See also *sterilization, female*; *vasectomy*.)

sterilization, female

A method of *contraception* in which the fallopian tubes are sealed to prevent sperm from reaching the ova. Female sterilization is usually performed by *laparoscopy*, which involves two small incisions in the abdomen. Sometimes it is performed by minilaparotomy, in which a single incision is made in the pubic area. The fallopian tubes are sealed using clips or by cutting and tying. The operations have a low failure rate, although if failure does occur, there is a risk of *ectopic pregnancy*. After the operation, women should therefore seek medical advice if they have vaginal bleeding, abdominal pain, or think they might be pregnant. Although sterilization is usually permanent, fertility can sometimes be restored by *microsurgery*.

sterilization, male

See *vasectomy*.

sternum

The long, narrow, flat plate of bone at the front of the chest. The sternum consists of the manubrium (uppermost part); the body (long middle part); and

LOCATION OF THE **STERNUM**

The sternum, or breastbone, is joined to the ribs and clavicles by flexible couplings that allow the chest to move while breathing in and out.

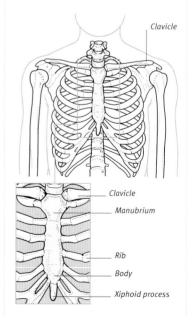

Clavicle

Clavicle

Manubrium

Rib

Body

Xiphoid process

S

the xiphoid process, or xiphisternum (a small, leaf-shaped projection). The top of the sternum articulates with the inner ends of the *clavicles* (collarbones). The *ribs* are attached to the sides by cartilage. Between the manubrium and the body is a *symphysis* that joins the two parts firmly but allows the sternum to move slightly during breathing.

Great force is required to fracture the sternum, the main danger of which is the possibility of the broken bone being driven inwards and damaging the heart, which lies behind the sternum.

steroid

A term used to describe either a naturally occurring hormone or a steroid drug. Steroid hormones include the *sex hormones* and hormones produced by the adrenal glands (see *corticosteroid hormones*). Steroid drugs include *corticosteroid drugs* and anabolic steroids (see *steroids, anabolic*).

steroids, anabolic

COMMON DRUG
• Nandrolone

Drugs that have an anabolic (protein-building) effect similar to *testosterone*. They build tissue, promote muscle recovery after an injury, and strengthen bones. They are used medically to treat some types of *anaemia*. The drugs may, however, be abused by athletes (see *sports, drugs and*). Possible adverse effects include acne, *oedema*, liver damage, *infertility*, *erectile dysfunction* in men, and *virilization* in women.

stethoscope

An instrument used for listening to sounds within the body, particularly those made by the heart or lungs (see *auscultation*). A stethoscope has ear-

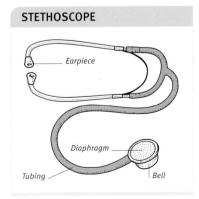

STETHOSCOPE

Earpiece

Diaphragm

Tubing

Bell

pieces; a diaphragm, which picks up high-pitched sounds; and a bell-shaped piece, which picks up low sounds.

Stevens–Johnson syndrome

A rare, life-threatening type of *erythema multiforme* that is characterized by severe blistering and sometimes bleeding in the mucous membranes of the eyes, mouth, nose, and genitals.

sticky eye

A sign of the eye condition *conjunctivitis* in which the eyelids become stuck together with discharge.

stiff neck

A common symptom, which is usually due to muscle spasm at the side or back of the neck. In most cases, it occurs suddenly and for no apparent reason. It may result from a neck injury, such as a ligament *sprain*, *disc prolapse*, or *whiplash injury*. A rare cause is *meningitis*.

Mild stiffness may be relieved by massage and warming. Severe or persistent stiffness requires medical attention. (See also *torticollis*.)

stiffness

A term for difficulty in moving a joint or stretching a muscle. Morning joint stiffness is characteristic of conditions such as *rheumatoid arthritis*. In degenerative conditions, such as *osteoarthritis*, pain and stiffness may be worse at the end of the day. *Cramp* and *spasticity* (muscle rigidity) may cause stiffness.

stilbestrol

See *diethylstilbestrol*.

stillbirth

Delivery of a dead fetus after the 24th week of *pregnancy*.

CAUSES

The cause of stillbirth is often unknown. Some stillborn babies have severe malformations, such as *anencephaly*, *spina bifida*, or *hydrocephalus*. Other possible causes include a maternal disorder that damages the placenta (the organ supplying nutrients to the baby), such as *antepartum haemorrhage* or *hypertension*; *diabetes*; *kidney disease*; or severe *rhesus incompatibility* (in which the mother's *antibodies* attack the baby's red blood cells).

Infectious diseases, such as *rubella*, *chickenpox*, *influenza*, *toxoplasmosis*, *cytomegalovirus*, and *herpes simplex*, may harm the fetus if contracted in pregnancy, increasing the risk of stillbirth.

PSYCHOLOGICAL EFFECTS

After a stillbirth, the parents usually experience a sense of loss as intense as if any other loved one had died. Often, they experience feelings of depression, guilt, anger, and inadequacy. Emotional support from friends, relatives, and self-help groups is useful; some people are helped by professional counselling.

Still's disease

See *juvenile chronic arthritis*.

stimulant drugs

COMMON DRUGS

CENTRAL NERVOUS SYSTEM STIMULANTS
• Caffeine • Dexamfetamine
• Methylphenidate
RESPIRATORY STIMULANTS • Doxapram

Drugs that increase *brain* activity by initiating the release of *noradrenaline* (norepinephrine). There are two types of stimulant drug: central nervous system stimulants (such as *amphetamines*), which are used in the treatment of *narcolepsy* and *ADHD*; and respiratory stimulants (see *analeptic drugs*).

stings

Sharp structures, on plants or animals, that discharge venom or irritants. Stinging animals include scorpions, some insects, jellyfish, and some fish (see *venomous bites and stings*). Stinging plants may cause an allergic skin reaction. (See also *poisonous plants*.)

STIs

See *sexually transmitted infections*.

stitch

A temporary, sudden, sharp pain in the abdomen or side that occurs during severe or unaccustomed exercise. A stitch is also the common name for a suture (see *suturing*) to close a wound.

St John's wort

A herbal remedy derived from the plant HYPERICUM PERFORATUM. Tablets, capsules, or infusions taken orally are effective in treating mild depression. St John's wort is also used in creams for burns, wounds, and joint problems. However, it interacts with a wide variety of other medications (including the contraceptive pill) so St John's wort preparations should not be used unless a doctor or pharmacist has been consulted beforehand. Its safety during pregnancy and breast-feeding has not been established.

S

Stokes–Adams attacks

Recurrent episodes of temporary loss of consciousness as a result of insufficient blood flow from the heart to the brain. Stokes–Adams attacks may be caused by an irregular heartbeat (see *arrhythmia, cardiac*), which prevents the heart from pumping properly, or by complete *heart block*, which causes the heart to stop beating briefly. Most affected people are fitted with a *pacemaker* to prevent attacks.

stoma

A term with the literal meaning mouth or orifice. A common use of the term is to describe the stoma that can be created surgically in the abdominal wall (see *colostomy*; *ileostomy*) to allow the intestine to empty into a bag or pouch on the surface of the skin.

stomach

A hollow, baglike organ of the *digestive system* located in the left side of the abdomen under the diaphragm. At its upper end, the stomach is connected to the *oesophagus* (gullet), and at the lower end it joins the *duodenum* (the first part of the small intestine).

ANATOMY OF THE **STOMACH**

Food enters the stomach from the oesophagus and exits into the duodenum. The stomach lining secretes gastric juice and protective mucus.

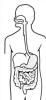

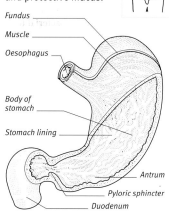

Fundus
Muscle
Oesophagus

Body of stomach

Stomach lining

Antrum
Pyloric sphincter
Duodenum

Parts of the stomach
The fundus, the body of the stomach, and the antrum are the three main parts; the lower oesophageal segment and pyloric sphincters control entry and exit of food.

STRUCTURE AND FUNCTION

The stomach is flexible and in the average adult can expand to hold around 1.5 litres of food. Its wall consists of layers of longitudinal and circular muscle, lined by special glandular cells that secrete gastric juice, and supplied by blood vessels

DISORDERS OF THE **STOMACH**

Disorders of the stomach have a variety of causes. Because the stomach is a reservoir, disorders of the emptying of stomach contents occur. Other problems relate to the stomach's role in the preparation of ingested food for digestion.

Infection

The large amount of hydrochloric acid secreted by the stomach protects it from some infections by destroying many of the bacteria, viruses, and fungi that are taken in with food and drink. When the protective power is insufficient, a variety of gastrointestinal infections may occur.

Tumours

Stomach cancer is one of the commonest forms of cancer. Early symptoms are often mistaken for *indigestion*, and diagnosis is often delayed until it is too late for a cure. Any change in the customary functioning of the digestive system is important, especially after the age of 50. A persistent feeling of fullness, or pain before or after meals, should never be ignored. Unexplained loss of appetite or frequent nausea should always be reported to a doctor. A tumour in the upper part of the stomach, near the opening of the oesophagus, can cause obstruction and difficulty in swallowing. Sometimes a stomach tumour remains "silent" and the first signs are due to the appearance of secondary growths elsewhere in the body. Benign (noncancerous) *polyps* can also develop in the stomach.

Ulceration

The acid and other digestive juices secreted by the stomach sometimes attack the stomach lining. The healthy stomach is prevented from digesting itself mainly by the protective layer of mucus secreted by the lining and by the speed with which damaged surface cells are replaced by the deeper layers. Many influences can upset this delicate balance. One of the most important is

and nerves. A strong muscle at the lower end of the stomach forms a ring called the pyloric sphincter that can close the outlet leading to the duodenum.

The main function of the stomach is to contribute to the breakdown of food that is started in the mouth and com-

excessive acid secretion. The resulting *peptic ulcers* are probably the most common serious stomach disorder. Peptic ulcers are most often caused by HELICOBACTER PYLORI infection, but are sometimes caused by stress, severe injury such as major burns, or after surgery and serious infections; often they occur for no apparent reason. The stomach lining can be damaged by large amounts of aspirin or alcohol, sometimes causing *gastritis* (inflammation of the stomach lining. This may eventually lead to ulceration.

Autoimmune disorders

Pernicious anaemia (see *anaemia, pernicious*) is caused by the failure of the stomach lining to produce intrinsic factor, a substance that facilitates the absorption of vitamin B_{12} (necessary for red blood cell formation). Failure to produce intrinsic factor occurs if there is atrophy of the stomach lining, which also causes failure of acid production. Tests that determine a person's ability to absorb vitamin B_{12} are important in the investigation of this condition. Pernicious anaemia is usually due to an *autoimmune disorder*.

Other disorders

Enlargement of the stomach may be caused when scarring from a chronic peptic ulcer occurs at the stomach outlet. It may also be a complication of *pyloric stenosis*, a rare but serious condition in which there is narrowing of the stomach outlet. Rarely, the stomach may become twisted and obstructed, a condition called volvulus.

INVESTIGATION

Stomach disorders are investigated primarily by *gastroscopy* and/or *barium X-ray examinations*. Occasionally, a *biopsy* (removal of a tissue sample for microscopic analysis) is performed.

S

pleted in the small intestine. However, it also acts as a storage organ; if storage were not possible, food would have to be eaten about every 20 minutes.

The sight and smell of food, and its arrival in the stomach, stimulate the stomach lining to secrete gastric juice. This fluid contains pepsin, an enzyme that breaks down protein; hydrochloric acid, which kills bacteria and creates the optimum *pH* for pepsin activity; and intrinsic factor, which is essential for absorption of vitamin B$_{12}$ in the small intestine. The lining also secretes mucus to stop the stomach from digesting itself.

The layers of muscle in the stomach wall produce rhythmic contractions about every 20 seconds that churn the food and gastric juice. This process converts semi-solid food into a creamy fluid (chyme). At regular intervals, the stomach muscles contract, as the pyloric sphincter relaxes, propelling partly digested food into the duodenum.

stomachache

Discomfort in the upper abdomen. (See also *indigestion*.)

stomach cancer

A malignant tumour that arises from the lining of the *stomach*. The exact cause is unknown, but Helicobacter pylori infection is linked to increased risk. Other risk factors include smoking and drinking alcohol. Diet may also play a part, particularly eating large amounts of salted or pickled foods. Pernicious *anaemia*, partial *gastrectomy*, and belonging to blood group A also seem to increase the risk. Stomach cancer rarely affects people under the age of 40 and is more common in men, especially Japanese men.

Symptoms may start with loss of appetite, weight loss, and difficulty swallowing; they may also be indistinguishable from those of *peptic ulcer* and may include burning abdominal pain, nausea, and vomiting.

Diagnosis is usually made by *gastroscopy* and *biopsy*, or by *barium X-ray examination*. Partial gastectomy may be performed if the tumour is detected early; otherwise, the only effective treatment is gastrectomy (removal of the stomach). In advanced cases, in which the tumour has spread, *anticancer drugs* may prolong life.

stomach imaging

See *barium X-ray examinations*.

stomach pump

See *lavage, gastric*.

stomach ulcer

Also known as a gastric ulcer, a type of *peptic ulcer*.

stomatitis

Any type of inflammation or ulceration of the mouth.

stones

Small, hard collections of solid material within the body. (See also *calculus, urinary tract*; *gallstones*.)

stool

Another word for *faeces*; in particular, a quantity of faeces passed in one bowel movement.

stork mark

A harmless small, flat, pinkish-red, skin blemish found in many newborn babies, usually around the eyes or at the nape of the neck. Stork marks, a type of *haemangioma*, may be only temporary.

strabismus

A medical term for a *squint*.

straight leg raising

A neurological test carried out during investigation of lower-back or leg pain to test for nerve root irritation, such as occurs with a *disc prolapse*. The test involves lying down and raising the leg to see if and where pain is felt.

strain

Tearing or stretching of *muscle* fibres as a result of suddenly pulling them too far. There is bleeding into the damaged area of muscle, causing pain, swelling, muscle spasm, and bruising.

Treatment may include resting the affected part (in a raised position if possible) and applying an *ice-pack* to reduce pain and swelling; taking *analgesic drugs*; and *physiotherapy*. (See also *sprain*.)

strangulation

Constriction (usually by twisting or compression) of a tube or passage in the body, blocking blood flow and interfering with the function of the affected organ. Strangulation may occur with a *hernia*, for example.

Strangulation of the neck is a life-threatening accidental or deliberate injury involving compression of the *jugular veins*, preventing blood from flowing out of the brain, and compression of the windpipe, which restricts breathing. The victim loses consciousness; brain damage and death caused by lack of oxygen follow.

strangury

A painful and frequent urge to empty the bladder, although only a few drops of urine can be passed. Causes include inflammation (see *cystitis*; *prostatitis*), bladder stones (see *calculus, urinary tract*), and bladder cancer (see *bladder tumours*).

strapping

The application of adhesive tape to part of the body to exert pressure and thus reduce pain and swelling, or to support a weakened area.

strawberry naevus

A bright red, raised spot appearing in early infancy. Strawberry naevi are a type of *haemangioma*. Treatment is not usually needed unless they occur near the eye, where they might interfere with visual development.

strawberry tongue

A white coating with red spots that develops on the tongue in a person with *scarlet fever*.

strep throat

A *streptococcal infection* of the *throat* that is most common in children. The bacteria are spread in droplets coughed or breathed into the air.

In some people, the bacteria cause no symptoms. In others, sore throat, fever, and enlarged lymph nodes in the neck occur. In some cases, the bacterial toxins produce a rash (see *scarlet fever*).

Treatment is usually with *penicillin* or *erythromycin*. Very rarely untreated strep throat may lead to *glomerulonephritis* or *rheumatic fever*.

streptococcal infections

Infections caused by *bacteria* of the Streptococcus genus. Streptococci are spherical bacteria that grow in lines, like beads on a string. They are among the most common disease-causing bacteria in humans.

Certain types of streptococci are present harmlessly in the mouth and throat of most people. If the bacteria enter the bloodstream (which may happen after dental treatment), they are usually destroyed. However, in some people with heart-valve defects, bacteria

S

can settle in the heart to cause bacterial *endocarditis*. Another type of streptococcus is normally present harmlessly in the intestines but can spread to cause a *urinary tract infection*.

Haemolytic streptococci can cause *tonsillitis*, *strep throat*, *scarlet fever*, *otitis media* (middle-ear infection), *pneumonia*, *erysipelas*, and wound infections.

Streptococcus pneumoniae

Also called *pneumococcus*, a type of STREPTOCOCCUS bacterium that can cause *pneumonia* and other serious disorders such as *meningitis* and *septicaemia*.

streptokinase

A *thrombolytic drug* that is used to dissolve blood clots following a *myocardial infarction* (heart attack), *pulmonary embolism* (a clot that blocks a blood vessel in a lung), or deep-vein thrombosis (see *thrombosis, deep-vein*).

Streptokinase is given under strict supervision because of the side effect of excessive bleeding; other adverse effects of the drug include nausea, rash, and cardiac *arrhythmias*.

streptomycin

An *antibiotic drug* that, usually in combination with other drugs, is used to treat certain uncommon infections, including *tuberculosis* and *brucellosis*. It may damage nerves in the inner ear, disturbing balance and causing dizziness, *tinnitus* (noises in the ears), or deafness. Other side effects of streptomycin include facial numbness, tingling in the hands, and headache.

stress

Any disturbance of a person's mental and physical wellbeing. Stress may be felt in response to a range of physical and emotional stimuli.

In stressful situations, the body responds by increasing production of the hormones *adrenaline* (epinephrine) and *hydrocortisone*. These hormones increase the heart rate and blood pressure and affect the metabolism to improve performance. Above a certain level, however, they impair a person's ability to cope. Continued exposure to stress often leads to mental and physical symptoms such as *anxiety* and *depression*, *indigestion*, palpitations, and muscular aches and pains. *Post-traumatic stress disorder* is a severe response to a specific stressful event. (See also *relaxation techniques*; *stress ulcer*.)

STRESS AND HEART RATE

The graph shows how a person's heart rate varies over a typical day. Exercise and stress both activate the body's "fight-or-flight" system and increase heart rate, but repeated alerting of the system without accompanying physical activity is probably harmful. Although the home and workplace both present stress, for many city workers the most stressful parts of the day are those spent commuting.

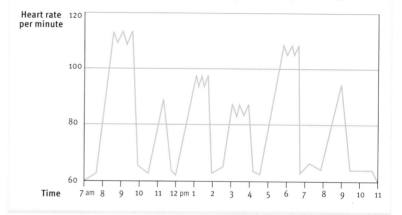

stress fracture

A *fracture* that results from repetitive jarring of a bone. Common sites include the metatarsal bones in the foot (see *march fracture*), the *tibia* and *fibula* (lower leg bones), the neck of the femur (thigh bone), and the lumbar spine (lower back). The main symptoms are pain and tenderness at the fracture site. Diagnosis is by *bone imaging*. Treatment consists of resting the affected area for four to six weeks, depending on the site; the fracture may be immobilized in a *cast*.

stress ulcer

An acute (of sudden onset) *peptic ulcer* that develops after *shock*, a severe burn or injury, or during a major illness. Stress ulcers are usually multiple and most commonly occur in the stomach. The exact cause is unknown. Severely ill hospital patients are often given drugs to prevent stress ulcers from developing.

stretcher

A horizontal frame used to carry seriously ill or injured people in order to minimize the risk of further injury or disturbance to the body.

stretch-mark

See *stria*.

stria

Also called a stretch-mark, a line on the *skin* caused by thinning and loss of elasticity in the dermis. Striae initially appear as red, raised lines, then turn purple and eventually fade to form shiny, silvery streaks. They often develop, during the adolescent growth spurt, on the shoulders in boys and on the hips and thighs in athletic girls. They are a common feature of pregnancy, occurring on the breasts, thighs, and lower abdomen. Purple striae are a characteristic feature of *Cushing's syndrome*.

Striae are thought to be caused by an excess of *corticosteroid hormones*, which decreases the level of *collagen* in the skin. There is no means of prevention.

stricture

Narrowing of a passage in the body. Stricture may be due to inflammation, development of scar tissue, or a growth such as a tumour. In some cases, it may be *congenital* (present at birth).

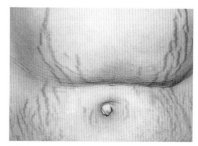

Striae
Commonly known as stretch-marks, striae often develop on the abdomen, thighs, and breasts of pregnant women. The striae shown here result from obesity associated with Cushing's syndrome.

stridor

An abnormal sound, on breathing, that is due to narrowing or obstruction of the *larynx* or *trachea*. Stridor is most common in young children and usually occurs in *croup*. Other causes include *epiglottitis*, an inhaled *foreign body*, *hypocalcaemia*, and some larynx disorders.

stroke

Damage to part of the *brain* due to interruption to its blood supply. The most common cause is blockage of a cerebral artery by a blood clot, which may have formed in the artery (see *thrombosis*) or may have been carried in the circulation from another part of the body (see *embolism*). Stroke may also result from localized haemorrhage due to a ruptured blood vessel (including an *aneurysm*) or *bleeding disorder* in or near the brain.

The incidence of stroke rises with age and is higher in men. Certain factors increase the risk; the most important are *hypertension* and *atherosclerosis*, which damage artery walls. *Smoking* increases the risk of stroke by increasing the risk of all these disorders; and the risk of atherosclerosis is increased with *diabetes*. *Atrial fibrillation* (irregular, very rapid heartbeats), a damaged *heart valve*, or a recent *myocardial infarction* (heart attack) can cause clots in the heart that may migrate to the brain.

SYMPTOMS AND SIGNS

Symptoms usually develop abruptly and depend on the site, cause, and extent of the brain damage. The movement, function, or sensation controlled by the damaged area of the brain is impaired (see *Types and causes of stroke* box, overleaf). The possible complications of a major stroke include *pneumonia* and blood clots in the legs (see *thrombosis, deep vein*), which could lead to pulmonary embolism. Roughly one third of major strokes are fatal, a third result in some disability, and the final one third have no lasting ill effects (see *transient ischaemic attack*).

DIAGNOSIS AND TREATMENT

A range of techniques may be used to investigate the cause and extent of brain damage. These include *ECG*, *CT scanning*, *chest X-rays*, *blood tests* (which may include clotting tests), *angiography*, *MRI*, and *carotid doppler scanning* (to assess narrowing of the carotid artery).

In some cases of stroke, urgent treatment may improve the chances of recovery. If a scan shows that the stroke is due to thrombosis, *thrombolytic drugs* may be given to dissolve the clot. *Anticoagulants* may be given if there is an obvious source of an embolism, such as atrial fibrillation. Antiplatelet agents such as *aspirin* may be used in order to help prevent further clotting.

Attention to hydration and pressure areas, and good nursing care, are important influences on the outcome. *Physiotherapy* may restore lost movement or sensation; *speech therapy* may help language disturbances. To reduce the risk of recurrence, any underlying risk factors, such as hypertension, diabetes, and high blood cholesterol, should be treated, and it is also important to stop smoking.

stroma

The tissue that forms an organ's framework, as distinct from functional tissue (the *parenchyma*) and the fibrous outer layer that holds the organ together.

strongyloidiasis

An infestation of the intestines by the parasitic worm STRONGYLOIDES STERCORALIS. Strongyloidiasis is widespread in the tropics. It is contracted by walking barefoot on soil that is contaminated with faeces. Larvae penetrate the soles and migrate via the lungs and throat to the small intestine, where they develop into adults and produce larvae. Most of the larvae are passed out in the faeces, but some enter the skin around the anus to begin a new cycle. An individual may be infested for more than 40 years.

The larvae cause itching and red weals where they enter the skin. In the lungs they may cause *asthma* or *pneumonia*. Heavy intestinal infestation may cause symptoms such as swelling of the abdomen and diarrhoea. Occasionally, an infected person with reduced immunity dies of complications, such as *septicaemia* or *meningitis*.

Treatment with an *anthelmintic drug*, usually tiabendazole or albendazole, kills the worms.

strontium

A metallic element occurring in various compounds in certain minerals, seawater, and marine plants. A compound of strontium, strontium ranalate, is used in the treatment of *osteoporosis* in postmenopausal women.

A radioactive variety of strontium, strontium 90, is produced during nuclear reactions and may be present in nuclear fallout. Strontium 90 accumulates in bone, where the *radiation* it emits may cause *leukaemia* and/or *bone tumours*. Other forms of radioactive strontium have been used to diagnose and treat bone tumours.

Strümpell–Marie disease

Another name for *ankylosing spondylitis*.

strychnine poisoning

Strychnine is a poisonous chemical found in the seeds of STRYCHNOS species (a group of tropical trees and shrubs). Its main use is in some rodent poisons; most cases of strychnine poisoning occur in children who accidentally ingest such poisons.

The symptoms, which begin soon after ingestion, include restlessness, stiffness of the face and neck, increased sensitivity of hearing, taste, and smell, and *photosensitivity*, followed by alternating episodes of seizures and floppiness. Death may occur from *respiratory arrest*.

Strychnine poisoning requires emergency medical treatment. There is no specific antidote for strychnine and treatment of poisoning involves controlling symptoms (for example, with drugs to control seizures) plus, if necessary, supportive measures such as artificial ventilation.

stuffy nose

See *nasal congestion*.

stump

The end part of a limb that remains after *amputation*.

stupor

A state of almost complete *unconsciousness* from which a person can be aroused only briefly and by vigorous external stimulation. (See also *coma*.)

Sturge–Weber syndrome

A rare, *congenital* condition affecting the skin and the brain in which there is abnormal distribution of blood vessels. Typically, a large, purple birthmark (port wine stain) extends over one side of the face, including the eye. Malformation of cerebral blood vessels may cause weakness on one side of the body, progressive *learning difficulties*, and *epilepsy*. *Glaucoma* may develop in the affected eye, leading to loss of vision.

Seizures can usually be controlled with *anticonvulsant drugs*. However, in severe cases, brain surgery may be necessary.

S

TYPES AND CAUSES OF **STROKE**

Stroke may be caused by any of three mechanisms (below): cerebral thrombosis, cerebral embolism, or haemorrhage . Thrombosis and embolism both lead to cessation of the blood supply to part of the brain and thus to infarction (tissue death). Rupture of a blood vessel in or near the brain may cause an intracerebral haemorrhage or a subarachnoid haemorrhage. Any part of the brain may be affected by a stroke; accordingly the symptoms vary considerably.

CEREBRAL THROMBOSIS

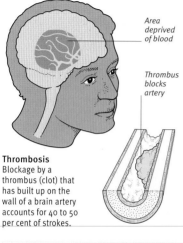

Area deprived of blood

Thrombus blocks artery

Thrombosis
Blockage by a thrombus (clot) that has built up on the wall of a brain artery accounts for 40 to 50 per cent of strokes.

CEREBRAL EMBOLISM

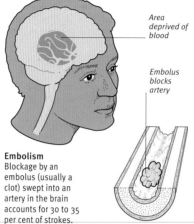

Area deprived of blood

Embolus blocks artery

Embolism
Blockage by an embolus (usually a clot) swept into an artery in the brain accounts for 30 to 35 per cent of strokes.

HAEMORRHAGE

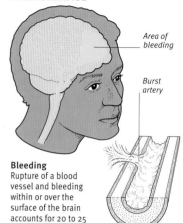

Area of bleeding

Burst artery

Bleeding
Rupture of a blood vessel and bleeding within or over the surface of the brain accounts for 20 to 25 per cent of strokes.

Key
● Cerebral infarction
○ Intracerebral haemorrhage
● Subarachnoid haemorrhage

Estimated incidence per 1,000 population

Age <45 45–54 55–64 65–74 75–84 >84

Incidence with age
Strokes are rare under age 45. Incidence of cerebral infarction increases with age, but incidence of intracerebral haemorrhage and subarachnoid haemorrhage falls after age 75.

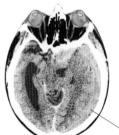

Cerebral haemorrhage
This CT (computed tomography) scan shows a subdural haematoma. The left side of the brain (right on image) is filled with blood, which has clotted to form a solid mass.

Haematoma

SYMPTOMS

The symptoms of a stroke usually develop abruptly over minutes or hours, but occasionally over several days. Depending on the size, site, cause, and extent of damage, any or all of the symptoms shown on the right may be present, in any degree of severity. A serious stroke may lead to rapid loss of consciousness, coma, and death. Up to 30 per cent of people are dependent on others after stroke, but some strokes cause barely noticeable symptoms.

Hemiplegia
Weakness, paralysis, or loss of sensation on one side of the body are the more common efects of a serious stroke.

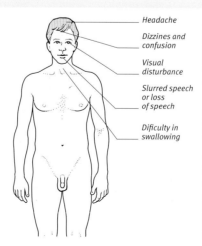

Headache

Dizzines and confusion

Visual disturbance

Slurred speech or loss of speech

Dificulty in swallowing

RISK FACTORS

● Age
● High blood pressure
● Atherosclerosis (narrowing of arteries by fatty deposits)
● Heart disease
● Diabetes mellitus
● Smoking
● Polycythaemia
● Hyperlipidaemia
● Obesity

S

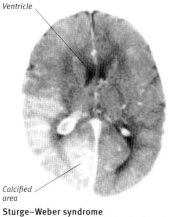

Sturge–Weber syndrome
Sturge–Weber syndrome is evident in this MRI of the brain. The black areas are the fluid-filled ventricles, and the white section (bottom left of the image) is part of the brain that has calcified.

stuttering

A speech disorder in which there is repeated hesitation and delay in uttering words, unusual prolongation of sounds, and repetition of word elements. Stuttering usually starts before the age of eight and may continue into adult life. It is more common in males, twins, and left-handed people, and may occur with *tics* or *tremors*. The severity may be related to social circumstances. The exact cause is unknown, although it tends to run in families. *Speech therapy* often helps.

St Vitus' dance

See *Sydenham's chorea*.

stye

Also called a hordeolum, a small, pus-filled *abscess* at the base of an eyelash that is caused by bacterial infection.

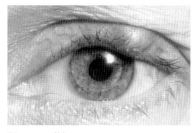

Stye on eyelid
Caused by infection at the base of an eyelash, a stye most often forms near the inner corner of the eye. This stye has formed in the centre, resulting in swelling and inflammation of the upper eyelid.

subacromial bursitis

Inflammation of the fluid-filled sac that cushions the acromion, part of the *scapula* (shoulderblade). The con-dition occurs if the bursa becomes trapped in the shoulder joint after a fall or overuse of the arm (for example, in sports involving throwing). It causes pain and restricted movement of the shoulder, particularly when lifting the arm sideways.

Treatment of subacromial bursitis usually includes rest, *analgesic drugs* and *nonsteroidal anti-inflammatory drugs*; *physiotherapy* may be given to help maintain mobility in the joint. For persistent cases, a corticosteroid injection into the joint may be needed.

subacute

A term that is used to describe a disease that runs a course between *acute* (of sudden onset and/or short duration) and *chronic* (long-term).

subacute bacterial endocarditis

See *endocarditis*.

subacute combined degeneration of the spinal cord

Progressive damage to columns of nerves running through the spinal cord due to vitamin B$_{12}$ deficiency. Subacute combined degeneration of the spinal cord may occur as a complication of *pernicious anaemia*. Symptoms may include tingling and numbness of the limbs. Weakness and *dementia* (deterioration in brain function) may eventually develop. If left untreated, the disease may be fatal after around five years. Treatment is with vitamin B$_{12}$ injections.

subacute sclerosing panencephalitis

A rare and fatal type of *encephalitis* in children and young adults that is caused by the *measles* virus. Subacute sclerosing panencephalitis, which may not begin until several years after initial infection, causes progressive deterioration in brain function over several weeks or months, and results in *seizures*, *spasticity*, *personality change*, *coma*, and, eventually, death.

subarachnoid haemorrhage

A type of *brain haemorrhage* in which a blood vessel ruptures and blood leaks into the space between the middle and inner meninges (the membranes lining the brain). Subarachnoid haemorrhage is most common in individuals between the ages of 35 and 60. Bleeding usually occurs spontaneously but may follow unaccustomed exercise; the most com-mon source of the bleeding is a burst *berry aneurysm* (a swollen, weakened area of artery wall).

An attack may cause loss of consciousness, sometimes preceded by a sudden, violent headache at the back of the head. If the person remains conscious, *photophobia* (abnormal sensitivity to light), drowsiness, nausea, vomiting. and a stiff neck may develop. Both conscious and unconscious patients can recover, but it is common to have further attacks, which are often fatal.

Diagnosis of a subarachnoid haemorrhage is by *CT scanning*, *lumbar puncture*, and *angiography*. Treatment includes life-support procedures and control of blood pressure to prevent recurrence. Burst or leaking aneurysms are usually treated by surgery. Ninety per cent of people who survive for a month survive for at least a year; some of these make a complete recovery, and some may have a residual disability such as paralysis.

subclavian steal syndrome

Recurrent attacks of blurred or double vision, loss of coordination, or dizziness when one arm (usually the left) is moved. The cause of subcalvian steal syndrome is narrowing of the arteries that supply the arms, usually due to *atherosclerosis*. The blood supply is sufficient while the arm is at rest, but during movement extra blood is diverted from the base of the brain in order to supply the arm. Treatment of the syndrome is by *arterial reconstructive surgery*.

subclinical

A term for a disorder that produces no symptoms or signs, being either mild or in the early stages of development.

subconjunctival haemorrhage

S

Bleeding under the *conjunctiva* (the clear membrane covering the white of the eye), due to rupture of tiny, fragile

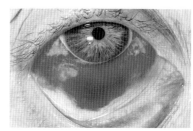

Subconjunctival haemorrhage
The bleeding causes a bright red area to appear in the white of the eye. A subconjunctival haemorrhage may look alarming but is usually harmless.

blood vessels. A subconjunctival haemorrhage is usually harmless and disappears in a few days without any treatment.

subconscious

A term used to describe various mental events (such as thoughts) of which one is temporarily unaware but that can be recalled under the right circumstances.

subcutaneous

A term meaning "beneath the skin".

subdural haemorrhage

Bleeding into the space between the outer and middle *meninges* (the membranes surrounding the brain), usually following *head injury*. The trapped blood forms a large clot within the skull that presses on brain tissue.

Signs and symptoms tend to fluctuate and may include headache, confusion, drowsiness, and one-sided weakness or *paralysis*. Bleeding occurs slowly; the interval between the injury and start of symptoms varies from days to months.

Diagnosis is by *CT scanning* or *MRI* to locate the clot. If a skull fracture is suspected, an X-ray may also be taken. In many cases, surgery is needed. This involves drilling burr holes in the skull (see *craniotomy*) to drain the blood and repair damaged blood vessels. If treatment is carried out at an early enough stage, the person usually makes a full recovery. A small subdural haemorrhage that produces few symptoms may not require treatment. The affected person is usually monitored with regular scans, and the clot may clear up on its own. (See also *extradural haemorrhage*.)

sublimation

In *psychoanalytic theory*, the unconscious process by which primitive, unacceptable impulses are redirected into socially acceptable forms of behaviour.

sublingual

A term meaning "under the tongue". Drugs taken sublingually are rapidly absorbed through the lining of the mouth into the blood. For example, nitrate drugs are given sublingually to provide rapid relief of an angina attack.

subluxated tooth

A tooth displaced in its socket following an accident. The upper front teeth are the most vulnerable. A subluxated tooth can usually be manipulated back into position before being immobilized (see

splinting, dental). If the blood vessels of the tooth are torn in the accident, *root-canal treatment* is required.

subluxation

Incomplete *dislocation* of a *joint*, in which the bone surfaces are displaced but remain in partial contact.

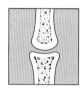

Normal
The diagram on the left shows the normal position of the bony surfaces in a simple joint, such as the joint in the middle of a finger.

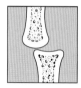

Subluxation
In a subluxation, the surfaces of the bones are slightly displaced from their normal positions relative to each other but are still in contact.

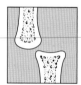

Dislocation
Here, there is almost complete loss of contact between the bone surfaces and, in most cases, considerable damage to surrounding tissues.

submucous resection

Also called septoplasty, surgery to correct a deviated *nasal septum* (deformed partition between the nostrils).

subphrenic abscess

An *abscess* under the diaphragm (the sheet of muscle dividing the chest from the abdomen).

substance abuse

The use of drugs or other substances for a purpose other than the recommended one, usually to cause intoxication or alter mood. Stimulant drugs, solvents, and glue are all commonly abused. Problems may arise as a result of the adverse effects of the substance or from its habit-forming potential. (See also *drug abuse*.)

substrate

A substance on which an *enzyme* acts.

sucking chest wound

An open wound in the chest wall through which air passes, causing the lung on that side of the body to collapse. Severe breathlessness and a life-threatening lack of oxygen result. (See also *pneumothorax*.)

suckling reflex

See *rooting reflex*.

sucralfate

An *ulcer-healing drug* used to treat *peptic ulcer*. Possible side effects are constipation and abdominal pain.

sucrose

The chemical name for culinary sugar, which is obtained from sugar cane and sugar beet (see *carbohydrates*.)

suction

The removal of unwanted fluid or semi-fluid material from the body with a syringe and a hollow needle or an intestinal tube and a mechanical pump.

suction lipectomy

See *body contour surgery*.

Sudafed

The brand name for the *decongestant drug* pseudoephedrine.

sudden death

See *death, sudden*.

sudden infant death syndrome (SIDS)

The sudden, unexpected death of an infant that cannot be explained. Possible risk factors include laying the baby face-down to sleep; overheating; parental smoking before and after the birth; *prematurity* and low birth weight; and the baby sleeping in the parent's bed.

Preventive measures include ensuring the baby sleeps on his or her back at the foot of the cot; making sure the baby does not overheat; not sharing a bed with the baby but keeping the baby's cot in the parent's room for the first six months; and stopping smoking. If a baby is unconscious, unresponsive, and/or not breathing, emergency medical help should be sought.

Sudeck's atrophy

Swelling and loss of use of a hand or foot after a *fracture* or other injury. Treatment includes elevation of the affected hand or foot, gentle exercise, and *heat treatment*. Full recovery is usual within about four months.

suffocation

A condition in which there is a lack of oxygen due to obstruction to the passage of air into the lungs. (See also *asphyxia*; *choking*; *strangulation*.)

S

sugar

See *carbohydrates*.

suicide

The act of intentionally killing oneself. Suicide results from a person's reaction to a perceivedly overwhelming problem, for example, social isolation, a stressful event such as death of a loved one, serious physical illness, or financial problems. It is often associated with a psychiatric illness, such as severe *depression* or *schizophrenia*, or dependency on drugs or alcohol.

Suicide is most common among young men. More men than women commit suicide, although women attempt it more often (see *suicide, attempted*). The most common methods among men are hanging and suffocation; drug overdose is the most common method among women.

suicide, attempted

A deliberate act of self-harm that is or is believed to be life-threatening but proves to be nonfatal.

Many more people attempt suicide than actually succeed. It is more common in women than men, and is most common in the 15–25 age group. The rate is highest in people who have personality disorders and in those who live in deprived urban areas or have alcohol or drug problems. Trigger factors for attempted suicide include the death of a loved one, breakdown of a relationship, financial worries, or any severe loss that results in *depression*. One of the most common methods is drug overdose.

A person who has attempted suicide needs urgent medical help to treat the self-inflicted physical trauma, such as treatment for *drug poisoning*. Longer-term support and therapy is also often needed for underlying psychological problems, such as depression.

sulfasalazine

An *immunosuppressant drug* that is used to relieve inflammation in *Crohn's disease* and *ulcerative colitis*. It is also a *disease-modifying antirheumatic drug* used to treat *rheumatoid arthritis* and psoriatic arthritis (see *psoriasis*). Possible side effects of sulfasalazine include nausea, headache, fever, and loss of appetite.

sulfinpyrazone

A drug used to reduce the frequency of attacks of *gout*. Possible side effects include nausea and abdominal pain.

sulindac

A *nonsteroidal anti-inflammatory drug* (NSAID) that is used to relieve joint pain and stiffness in *arthritis* and acute *gout*. Side effects of sulindac are the same as for other NSAIDs and include indigestion and sometimes bleeding or ulcers in the stomach.

sulphasalazine

See *sulfasalazine*.

sulphinpyrazone

See *sulfinpyrazone*.

sulphonamide drugs

COMMON DRUGS
- Sulfadiazine • Sulfamethoxazole

A group of *antibacterial drugs*. They have largely been superseded by more effective and less toxic alternatives.

sulphonylurea drugs

A type of oral hypoglycaemic drug (see *hypoglycaemics, oral*) used to treat type 2 *diabetes mellitus*.

sulphur

A mineral that is a constituent of vitamin B_1 (see *vitamin B complex*) and several essential *amino acids*. In the body, sulphur is needed to make *collagen*, which is found in bones, tendons, and skin, and is a constituent of *keratin* (the protein in skin, hair, and nails). Sulphur is also used as a cream in the treatment of *acne*.

sulpiride

An *antipsychotic drug* used in the treatment of *schizophrenia*.

sumatriptan

A *serotonin agonist* drug that is used to relieve acute attacks of *migraine*, especially those that have not responded to *analgesic drugs*; it is particularly effective in treating cluster headaches. Sumatriptan may cause chest pain and tightness, tingling, flushing, dizziness, and weakness. It should not be used by people who have ischaemic heart disease (see *heart disease, ischaemic*).

sunbed

A bedlike device that encloses both sides of the body and exposes the skin to *ultraviolet light* to give a fast suntan. Because of various health risks associated with sunbeds (in particular, the risk of *skin cancer)* their use is not advised.

sunburn

Inflammation of the *skin* caused by overexposure to the sun. The *ultraviolet light* in sunlight may destroy cells in the outer layer of the skin and damage tiny blood vessels beneath. Severe sunburn in childhood increases the risk of *skin cancer* in later life.

Fair-skinned people are most susceptible. The affected skin becomes red and tender and may blister. The dead skin cells are later shed by peeling.

Calamine lotion soothes burnt skin. *Analgesic drugs* can relieve discomfort. Avoiding exposure to the midday sun, wearing protective clothing, and applying a high protection factor *sunscreen* help to prevent sunburn.

sunlight, adverse effects of

Problems resulting from overexposure to the sun and in particular from the effects of the *ultraviolet light* in sunlight. Fair-skinned people are most susceptible. Short-term overexposure causes *sunburn* and, in intense heat, can lead to *heat exhaustion* or *heatstroke*. Repeated overexposure over a long period can cause premature aging of the skin and solar *keratoses*, and increases the risk of *skin cancer*. Protecting the skin with *sunscreens* helps to prevent sun damage.

Other adverse effects of sunlight include *photosensitivity* (an abnormal sensitivity to sunlight), resulting in a rash. Exposure to sunlight can also affect the eyes, causing irritation of the conjunctiva, actinic *keratopathy*, or *pterygium*. Good quality sunglasses help to prevent eye problems.

sun protection factor (SPF)

A measure of the amount of UVB radiation that a *sunscreen* absorbs and thus the degree of protection that it provides against sunburn. It is given as a number (SPF number); the higher the SPF number, the greater the protection. The number refers to how many times longer an individual can stay out in the sun without burning.

sunscreens

Also called sunblocks, preparations that help to protect the skin from the harmful effects of sunlight. To remain effective, however, sunscreens must be reapplied on a regular basis.

WARNING
Some suntanning preparations do not contain a sunscreen and therefore provide no protection against sunburn.

S

sunstroke

A common form of *heatstroke*.

suntan

Darkening of the *skin* after exposure to sunlight. Specialized cells in the epidermis (the outer skin layer) respond to *ultraviolet light* by producing the protective pigment *melanin*. However, even if a suntan develops, the skin may still suffer damage from overexposure to the sun. (See also *sunburn; sunlight, adverse effects of*.)

superego

The part of the personality, as described in *psychoanalytic theory*, that is thought to be responsible for maintaining a person's standards of behaviour. Popularly termed the "conscience", the superego arises as a result of a child incorporating the moral views of those in authority (usually parents).

superficial

Situated near the surface.

superinfection

A second *infection* that occurs during the course of an existing infection. The term usually refers to an infection by a microorganism that is resistant to drugs being used against the original infection. One example is candidiasis (thrush) caused by treatment with antibiotic drugs. The antibiotic destroys the body's normal flora (microorganisms that are present in the body but do not produce any ill effects), which usually keep the candida yeast under control, preventing it from proliferating.

superiority complex

An individual's exaggerated and unrealistic belief that he or she is better than other people. In modern *psychoanalytic theory*, a superiority complex is considered to be a compensation for unconscious feelings of inadequacy or low self-esteem.

superior vena cava obstruction

A condition in which blood flow through the superior vena cava (the major vein that returns blood to the heart from the upper body) is restricted, often by pressure in the chest. The restriction is most commonly the result of a tumour, particularly *lung cancer* or *lymphoma*. Pressure may build up in the blood vessels behind the obstruction, causing swelling of the face, neck, and arm.

supernumerary

A term meaning "more than the normal number". Supernumerary teeth can also occur; they are usually extracted.

supernumerary nipple

One or more nipples in excess of the usual number.

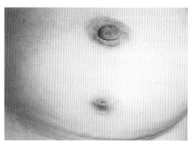

Supernumerary (extra) nipple
Additional nipples can develop along a line that extends from the armpit to the groin; the extra nipples are not usually associated with underlying glandular tissue.

supination

The act that involves turning the body to a supine position (lying on the back with the face upwards) or of turning the hand to a position in which the palm faces forwards. The opposite position to supination is *pronation*.

suppository

A solid medical preparation, of cone or bullet shape, designed to be placed in the rectum to dissolve. Suppositories are used to treat rectal disorders such as *haemorrhoids* or *proctitis*, or to soften faeces and stimulate defaecation. They may also be used to administer drugs into the general circulation via blood vessels in the rectum, if vomiting is likely to prevent absorption after oral administration or if the drug would cause irritation of the stomach.

suppressor T-cell

A type of white blood cell, also known as a suppressor T-lymphocyte (see *lymphocyte*) that is involved in the *immune system*. These cells act to prevent the immune response.

suppuration

The formation or discharge of *pus*.

suprarenal glands

Another name for the *adrenal glands*.

suprasellar cyst

See *craniopharyngioma*.

supraspinatus syndrome

Inflammation of the supraspinatus tendon, which is in the shoulder, causing *painful arc syndrome*.

supraventricular tachycardia

An abnormally fast but regular heart rate that occurs in episodes that vary in duration from several hours to a number of days. Supraventricular tachycardia occurs when abnormal electrical impulses that arise in the atria (upper chambers) of the *heart* take control of the heartbeat from the *sinoatrial node* (the cluster of cells that stimulates heartbeats). Symptoms include palpitations, breathlessness, chest pain, or fainting (see *Stokes–Adams syndrome*).

Diagnosis is by an *ECG*. An attack can sometimes be stopped by *Valsalva's manoeuvre* or by drinking cold water. Recurrent attacks are treated with *antiarrhythmic drugs*. Occasionally, supraventricular tachycardia may require *cardioversion* (application of an electric shock to the heart).

surfactant

A substance that reduces surface tension in a liquid. Pulmonary surfactant is secreted by the alveoli in the lungs, preventing them from collapsing during exhalation. Because surfactant is absent in significantly premature babies, breathing difficulties can occur that can lead to *respiratory distress syndrome*. In such cases, *artificial ventilation* and an artificial surfactant need to be given.

surfer's nodules

Multiple bony outgrowths on the foot bones and on the bony prominence just below the knee.

surgery

Treatment of injury or other disorders by direct physical intervention, often with instruments. The word is also used for aspects of medicine that deal with the study, diagnosis, and management of disorders treated surgically.

surgical emphysema

The presence of gas trapped under the skin tissues following an injury or surgical procedure.

surgical spirit

A liquid, consisting mainly of ethyl alcohol, that has a soothing and hardening effect when applied to the skin. It may be used before injections as an *antiseptic*.

S

surrogacy

The agreement by a woman to become pregnant and give birth to a child with the understanding that she will surrender the child after birth to the contractual parents. Pregnancy may be achieved either by *artificial insemination* or by *in vitro fertilization*.

susceptibility

Total or partial vulnerability to an infection or disorder.

Sustac

A brand name for *glyceryl trinitrate*, a drug used to prevent attacks of *angina pectoris* (chest pain due to insufficient oxygen reaching the heart).

Sustanon

A brand name for the male sex hormone *testosterone*, given as a treatment to males whose bodies produce too little testosterone.

suture

A type of *joint*, found only between the bones of the skull, in which the adjacent bones are mobile during birth but then become so closely and firmly joined by a layer of connective tissue that movement between them is impossible.

The term "suture" is also used to refer to a surgical stitch (see *suturing*).

suturing

The closing of a surgical incision or a wound by sutures (stitches) to promote healing. Suturing may be carried out by means of a single continuous stitch under the skin (subcuticular) or by using individual stitches (interrupted). Some materials used in suturing, such as catgut, eventually dissolve in the body and may therefore not need to be removed; skin sutures made of other, nonsoluble materials are removed about one to two weeks after insertion, depending on the site in the body.

swab

A wad of absorbent material used to apply antiseptics or soak up body fluids during surgery or to obtain a sample of bacteria from an infected patient.

A surgical swab is commonly a folded piece of cotton gauze held in the hand or in a clamp. It is used to apply cleansing and antiseptic solutions to the skin before an incision is made and to soak up blood and other fluids during an operation. The swab often contains

METHODS OF **SUTURING**

Suturing is carried out under either a general or a local anaesthetic. The type of stitch used depends on the nature of the wound or incision (two types are shown below). In all cases the surgeon sews the wound edges together to produce minimal distortion of tissue.

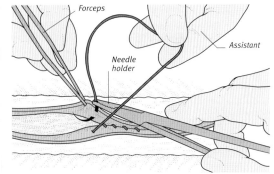

Technique
The surgeon grasps the edge of the wound with forceps held in one hand and inserts the needle through the skin using the other hand. In this illustration, the surgeon is using a needle holder, which gives greater control for very fine stitches. In other cases, the needle may be held in the hand. Suturing sometimes requires assistance.

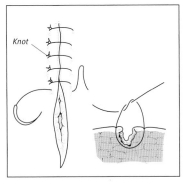

Standard interrupted sutures
The needle is passed into one skin edge, through the full depth of the wound, and out of the other skin edge. Each stitch is then knotted at the side.

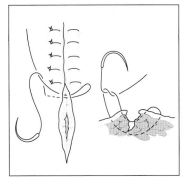

Mattress sutures
For deeper wounds, the needle is passed through the wound twice: first shallowly, close to the skin edges, and then more deeply, farther from the edges.

OTHER METHODS OF CLOSURE

Alternatives to suturing include removable staples and clips (staples are also used internally), adhesive tape, and tissue glue.

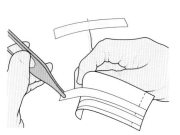

Adhesive tape
When the wound is shallow, tape may be applied directly. For deeper wounds, absorbable stitches are first inserted just beneath the skin.

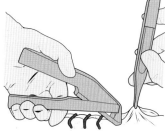

Inserting staples
The wound edges are held up with forceps and staples, which are spaced out at equal intervals, are inserted using an automatic stapling device.

S

material opaque to X-rays to enable it to be detected if it is accidentally left in the body after an operation.

A microbiological swab consists of a twist of cotton wool at the end of a thin stick, supplied in a sterile container. The swab is applied to an infected area of the body to absorb pus, mucus, or any other discharge or exudate for microscopic examination.

swallowing

The process by which food or liquid is sent from the mouth to the stomach via the oesophagus.

In the mouth, food is chewed and mixed with saliva to form a soft mass called a bolus; the tongue then pushes the bolus to the back of the mouth and voluntary muscles in the palate push it into the throat.

The rest of the swallowing process occurs by a series of *reflexes*. Entry of food into the throat causes the epiglottis to tilt down to seal the trachea (windpipe) to prevent inhalation of food and choking, and the soft palate to move back to close off the nasal cavity. The throat muscles push the food into the oesophagus (gullet). Waves of contractions (peristalsis) along the oesophagus propel the food towards the stomach.

swallowing difficulty

Known medically as dysphagia, a common symptom with various possible causes. These include a foreign object in the throat; insufficient production of saliva (see *mouth, dry*); a disorder of the oesophagus, such as *oesophageal stricture*; pressure on the oesophagus, for example from a *goitre* or tumour (see *oesophagus, cancer of*); a nervous system disorder such as *myasthenia gravis* or *stroke*; or a psychological problem such as *globus hystericus*.

Investigations of swallowing difficulty may include barium swallow (see *barium X-ray examinations*) or *oesophagoscopy*. Treatment depends on the cause.

swamp fever

Another name for *leptospirosis*, a disorder caused by contact with water contaminated by rats' urine. The term is also sometimes applied to *malaria*.

sweat glands

Structures deep within the *skin* that produce sweat, which is composed mainly of water but also contains other substances, including sodium chloride

(salt) and urea (a nitrogen-containing compound). There are two types of sweat gland, known as eccrine and apocrine glands. Eccrine glands are the most numerous, and they open directly on to the skin's surface. Apocrine glands open into a hair follicle. Developing at puberty, the apocrine glands occur only in hairy areas of skin, particularly in the armpits, in the pubic region, and around the anus.

The sweat glands are controlled by the *autonomic nervous system*. The glands usually produce sweat in order to keep the body cool, but they may also release sweat in response to anxiety or fear. Sweat is odourless until bacteria act on it, producing *body odour*.

Disorders of the sweat glands include *hyperhidrosis* (excessive sweating); and *hypohidrosis* (insufficient sweating); and hidradenitis suppurativa (a disorder of the apocrine glands in which painful resistant papules, nodules, and scars occur in the armpit and groin).

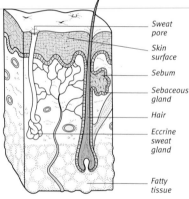

Cross-section of skin showing sweat gland
Sweat produced by the numerous eccrine sweat glands is carried up through the sweat duct and directly on to the skin's surface. Apocrine sweat glands open on to a hair follicle.

Labels on figure:
- Sweat pore
- Skin surface
- Sebum
- Sebaceous gland
- Hair
- Eccrine sweat gland
- Fatty tissue

sweating

The process by which the body cools itself. (See also *hyperhidrosis*, *hypohydrosis*; *sweat glands*.)

sweeteners, artificial

See *artificial sweeteners*.

swimmer's ear

A common name for *otitis externa*.

swimmer's itch

A skin rash that occurs after swimming in fresh water contaminated with a form of *fluke* that infests snails and wildfowl. The itching is caused by fluke

larvae burrowing through the skin. Swimmer's itch may be a manifestation of *schistosomiasis*.

sycosis barbae

Inflammation of the beard area due to infection of the hair follicles, usually with STAPHYLOCOCCUS AUREUS bacteria from razors or towels. Pus-filled blisters appear around the follicles. Treatment is usually with *antibiotic drugs*.

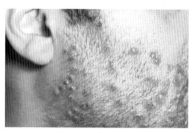

Sycosis barbae
Caused by infection and inflammation of the hair follicles in the beard area, sycosis barbae tends to affect men with greasy skin, and may be persistent.

Sydenham's chorea

Formerly called St Vitus' Dance, a rare childhood disorder of the *central nervous system*. The condition, which usually follows *rheumatic fever*, causes involuntary jerky movements of the head, face, limbs, and fingers; voluntary movements are clumsy, and the limbs become floppy.

Sydenham's chorea usually clears up after two to six months and has no long-term adverse effects.

Symmetrel

A brand name for the antiviral drug *amantadine*.

sympathectomy

An operation in which the ganglia (nerve terminals) of certain sympathetic nerves are destroyed to interrupt the nerve pathway.

WHY IT IS DONE

The sympathetic nerves form part of the *autonomic nervous system* and control involuntary (automatic) activities in the body, including widening and narrowing of blood vessels. In *peripheral vascular disease* (a disorder in which the blood vessels in the legs, and sometimes the arms, become narrowed), stimulation from the sympathetic nerves produces spasms in the blood vessels and worsens the narrowing. Sympathectomy prevents these spasms from occurring and may improve the blood supply flowing to the affected area.

S

The sympathetic nerves also play an important part in producing the sensation of *pain*. In some cases of *causalgia* (persistent severe pain usually caused by nerve injury), only sympathectomy can provide relief.

sympathetic nervous system

One of the two divisions of the *autonomic nervous system*, which, along with the parasympathetic nervous system, controls many of the involuntary activities in the body. The sympathetic nervous system increases body activities (it quickens the heartbeat and widens blood vessels in muscles, for example) in preparation for coping with stress (see *fight-or-flight response*).

sympathomimetic drugs

Drugs that stimulate the *sympathetic nervous system* by mimicking the effects of natural chemicals that control functions such as heart rate, blood flow, and digestion. Sympathomimetic drugs include *decongestant drugs*, which work by constricting blood vessels in the nasal membranes, and *bronchodilator drugs*, which work by widening the small airways of the lungs.

symphysis

A type of *joint* in which two bones are firmly joined by tough cartilage. Such joints occur in various parts of the body: between the *vertebrae*; between the pubic bones, at the front of the *pelvis*; and between the upper and middle parts of the *sternum* (breastbone).

symptom

An indication of a disease or disorder that is noticed by the sufferer him- or herself – pain, for example. By contrast, the indications that a doctor notes are called signs.

symptoms, first rank

Certain features of mental illness, the presence of which indicate a likely diagnosis of *schizophrenia*. They include auditory *hallucinations* (the person hears voices having a conversation or commenting on him or her); thought broadcasting (the belief that one's thoughts are being broadcast to the outside world); thought insertion (the belief that thoughts are being put into one's head); thought withdrawal (thoughts are being removed from one's head); and passivity (thoughts and actions are being controlled from an

external source). Such symptoms may be caused by other conditions, such as psychiatric problems related to the toxic effects of certain illegal drugs (see *drug psychosis*), and these other problems must be ruled out before the diagnosis of schizophrenia can be confirmed.

symptothermal method

See *contraception, natural methods of*.

Synacthen

A brand name for *tetracosactide*, a drug that is used to assess the function of the adrenal glands.

synaesthesia

A condition in which stimulation of one of the senses produces an unusual response in addition to the normal perception that is associated with the particular stimulus; for example, when a sound causes a person to see a colour as well as hear the noise.

synapse

A junction between two *neurons* (nerve cells) across which a signal can pass. At a synapse, the two neurons do not come directly into contact but are separated by a gap called the synaptic cleft. When an electrical signal passing along a neuron reaches a synapse, it causes the release of a chemical called a *neurotransmitter*. The neurotransmitter crosses the synaptic cleft to the next neuron, where it stimulates an electrical signal in that neuron. Signals can cross a synapse in one direction only.

Most drugs affecting the nervous system work as a result of their effects on synapses. Such drugs may affect the release of neurotransmitters, or they may modify their effects.

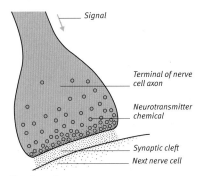

Structure of a synapse
When a signal arrives at the terminal of a nerve cell axon, it causes the release of a neurotransmitter; this chemical crosses the synaptic cleft and has an effect on the next cell.

syncope

The medical term for *fainting*.

syncope, micturition

See *micturition syncope*.

syndactyly

A *congenital* defect in which two or more fingers or, more commonly, toes are joined. Syndactyly is often inherited and is more common in males. In mild cases, adjacent digits (fingers or toes) are joined by only a web of skin; in more serious cases, the bones are fused. Surgery to separate the digits may be performed in early childhood.

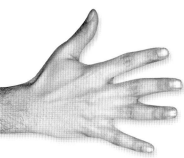

Syndactyly
The congenital fusion of digits, syndactyly may range in severity from a slight degree of webbing between fingers, as shown here, to almost complete fusion.

Syndol

A brand-name *analgesic drug* (painkiller) containing *paracetamol*, *caffeine*, *codeine*, and doxylamine.

syndrome

A group of symptoms and/or signs that, when they occur together, constitutes a particular disorder. An example is *irritable bowel syndrome*, which includes a range of symptoms including abdominal pain, wind and bloating, and irregular bowel movements.

syndrome of inappropriate antidiuretic hormone (secretion)

See *SIADH*.

syndrome X

A term that is used to describe two types of cardiovascular problem. The first, which is also called cardiac syndrome X, is a condition in which there are symptoms of *angina pectoris* (chest pain), and *exercise ECGs* show changes suggesting *ischaemic heart disease*, but the coronary arteries appear normal when viewed by *angiography*.

S

The term "syndrome X" is also used for a group of factors that are often found in people with ischaemic heart disease, and whose presence is associated with an increased risk. These risk factors include excessive fat around the abdomen (central obesity), *hyperlipidaemia* (high levels of fats in the blood), *hypertension* (high blood pressure), and *insulin resistance*.

synergistic drug

A drug that interacts with another to produce a combined effect that is greater than the effects produced by either of the drugs given separately. Drug synergy may be useful by allowing lower doses of certain drugs to be given. However, many combinations of drugs produce dangerous synergistic effects, as do some drugs and foods, notably *monoamine oxidase inhibitors* and foods containing tyramine, which may interact to produce a dangerous rise in blood pressure.

synergistic muscles

Muscles that work together to produce a particular movement.

synovectomy

Surgical removal of the membrane lining a joint capsule to treat recurrent or persistent *synovitis*, usually in cases of severe *rheumatoid arthritis*.

synovitis

Inflammation of the membrane lining the capsule of a movable *joint*. The condition may be *acute*, in which case it is usually caused by an attack of *arthritis*, injury, or infection; or *chronic*, due to a disorder such as *rheumatoid arthritis*. The joint becomes swollen, painful, and often warm and red.

To find the cause of synovitis, joint aspiration (taking a sample of the joint's lubricating fluid) or *biopsy* of the synovium (taking a sample of the membrane) may be needed.

The symptoms of synovitis are relieved by rest, supporting the affected joint with a splint or a cast, *analgesic drugs*, *nonsteroidal anti-inflammatory drugs*, and, occasionally, a *corticosteroid* injection. Chronic synovitis may be treated by *synovectomy* (surgical removal of the synovium).

synovium

The membrane lining the capsule around a movable *joint*. The synovium also forms a sheath for certain tendons of the hands and feet. It secretes synovial fluid, which lubricates the joint or tendon. The synovium can become inflamed; in a joint this problem is known as *synovitis*, while in a tendon sheath it is known as *tenosynovitis*.

syphilis

An infection caused by TREPONEMA PALLIDUM bacteria. Syphilis is spread by sexual intercourse or other intimate body contact; the organism enters the body through broken skin or *mucous membranes*, then spreads rapidly via the bloodstream and lymphatic system. Syphilis can also be spread by nonsexual means, such as through broken skin or saliva, although these nonsexual methods of transmission occur mainly in the Middle East and Africa. Rarely, syphilis may be transmitted from a mother to her fetus during pregnancy (congenital syphilis).

SIGNS AND SYMPTOMS

In sexual infection, the first sign is a painless ulcer (chancre) that develops on the genitals, anus, rectum, lips, throat, or fingers. The chancre may develop any time from 10 days to three weeks after infection and it heals in four

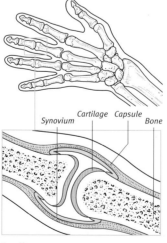

LOCATION OF **SYNOVIUM**

Every movable joint is enclosed within a fibrous capsule. The inner lining of the capsule is known as the synovium.

Synovium Cartilage Capsule *Bone*

Function
The membrane secretes a thick fluid, called synovial fluid, that lubricates the joint. If the joint is injured, excess fluid may accumulate and cause pain.

to eight weeks. A rash then develops, which may be transient or recurrent, or may last for months. Other possible signs include lymph node enlargement, headache, bone pain, loss of appetite, fever, and fatigue. Thickened, grey or pink patches may develop on moist areas of skin and are highly infectious. *Meningitis* may also develop.

Following this symptomatic phase, the disease becomes latent (hidden) for a few years, or sometimes indefinitely. A few untreated cases proceed, eventually, to a final stage characterized by widespread tissue destruction. Other serious effects include cardiovascular syphilis, which affects the aorta and leads to *aneurysm* and heart valve disease; *neurosyphilis*, with progressive brain damage and paralysis; and *tabes dorsalis*, a disorder that affects part of the spinal cord.

Signs of congenital syphilis include a rash, persistent snuffles, bone abnormalities, jaundice, and enlargement of the liver and spleen. *Keratitis* (inflammation of the cornea), a characteristic flat face, peg-shaped teeth, arthritis, and learning difficulties may appear later in childhood.

DIAGNOSIS AND TREATMENT

Diagnosis is by examination of chancre serum and by blood tests. All forms of syphilis are treated with *antibacterial drugs*. Organ damage already caused by the disease cannot be reversed.

Pregnant women are given a blood test for syphilis infection early in pregnancy. If the test is positive, antibacterial drugs are given, which also treat the unborn baby. The baby will be given antibacterial drugs again after birth to ensure that the infection is completely eradicated.

PREVENTION

Practising *safer sex* can help to prevent syphilis infection but does not entirely eliminate the risk. People with syphilis are infectious in the early stages and sometimes in the early latent stage but not in the final stage.

syringe

A hollow, cylindrical instrument that is commonly used with a needle to inject fluid into, or withdraw fluid from, a body cavity, blood vessel, or tissue.

syringe driver

A portable device comprising a syringe of medication attached to a small pump. It is used to provide continuous pain

S

relief in conditions such as cancer. The syringe driver delivers a certain amount of an *analgesic* (painkiller), over a set period of time, through a needle inserted into the skin.

syringe, oral

A form of syringe with no needle that is used to give medicines by mouth, especially to young children. To use an oral syringe, a small, accurately measured dose of a drug is drawn up into the syringe, then the tip of the device is placed inside the child's mouth and the drug is directed against the inside of the child's cheek.

EAR SYRINGING

This procedure should be carried out by a doctor or nurse; amateur attempts can damage the eardrum.

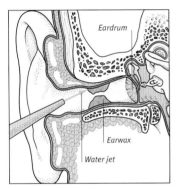

Syringing the ear
After softening with sodium bicarbonate, a jet of warm water is directed (avoiding the eardrum) along the upper wall of the ear canal to dislodge earwax or a foreign body.

syringing of ears

The flushing of excess *earwax* or a foreign body from the outer ear canal by introducing water from a syringe into the ear canal.

syringomyelia

A rare, progressive condition in which a cavity forms in the *brainstem* (the lowest part of the brain) or in the *spinal cord* at the neck or thoracic level. The cavity gradually expands, filling with *cerebrospinal fluid* and compressing nearby nerve fibres.

Syringomyelia is usually congenital (present at birth) and may be associated with congenital deformity of the brain. It may also occur after spinal cord injury.

Signs usually appear in early adulthood and include lack of temperature or pain sensation; muscle wasting in the neck, shoulders, arms, and hands; and some loss of the sense of touch. Later, there is difficulty in moving the legs and controlling the bladder and bowel, and the joints may become deformed.

There is no drug treatment. Surgery can relieve pressure in the central cavity to prevent further enlargement, relieve pressure on the distended spinal cord (see *decompression, spinal canal*), or slow the deterioration.

syrinx

An abnormal cavity in the brainstem or spinal cord; a feature of *syringomyelia*.

system

A group of interconnected or interdependent organs with a common function, as in the *digestive system*.

systemic

A term applied to something that affects the whole body rather than a specific part of it. For example, fever is a systemic symptom, whereas swelling is a localized symptom. The term "systemic" is also applied to the part of the blood circulation that supplies all parts of the body except the lungs.

systemic lupus erythematosus

See *lupus erythematosus*.

systemic sclerosis

A progressive form of scleroderma, systemic scleroderma is a rare *autoimmune disorder* (in which the immune system attacks the body's own tissues). The condition can affect many organs and tissues, particularly the skin, arteries, kidneys, lungs, heart, gastrointestinal tract, and joints. Systemic sclerosis is three times as common in women as in men and is most likely to appear between the ages of 30 and 50.

The disease varies in severity. It often begins with the symptoms of *Raynaud's phenomenon*, a disorder in which the fingers and toes become white, numb, and painful when exposed to cold. This is followed some years later by thickening and tightness of the skin of the face, hands, forearms, and feet. In more severe cases, the internal organs are affected. Symptoms may include heartburn or difficulty swallowing due to damage to the oesophagus. *Pulmonary hypertension* (high blood pressure in

the arteries that supply the lungs) may develop, sometimes up to 15 years after the onset of the disease.

Systemic sclerosis often progresses rapidly in the first few years and then slows down or even stops. In a minority of people, degeneration is rapid, and leads to death from *heart failure, respiratory failure,* or *kidney failure*. There is no cure for systemic sclerosis, but many of the symptoms can be relieved by drug treatment or *physiotherapy*.

systole

Muscular contraction of a chamber of the *heart* that alternates with a resting period (*diastole*). There are two stages of systole, namely atrial and ventricular. With each *heartbeat*, the atria (upper chambers) contract, squeezing blood into the ventricles (lower chambers). This action is followed by ventricular systole, in which the ventricles squeeze blood into the arteries.

The first of the two heartbeat sounds is associated with systole and represents the closing of the valves between the atria and ventricles; this action prevents blood from flowing back into the atria. The second sound relates to the diastole and signifies the closing of the aortic and pulmonary valves at the exits of the ventricle. (See also *heart sounds; pulse.*)

systolic murmur

A heart murmur (a sound, made by the heart, that can be detected by a doctor) that occurs during *systole*, the phase of the heartbeat during which the heart muscle contracts.

A systolic murmur is usually caused by backflow of blood through the mitral or tricuspid *heart valves* between the upper and lower heart chambers. It can also be due to a type of *hypertrophic cardiomyopathy* called hypertrophic obstructive cardiomyopathy (narrowing of the outflow passage from the left ventricle). Heart valve problems such as hardening (sclerosis) or narrowing (stenosis) of the aorta (see *aortic stenosis*) or pulmonary valve (see *pulmonary stenosis*) are also possible causes.

S

T

tabes dorsalis

A rare complication of untreated *syphilis* that appears years after infection. The condition affects the spinal cord and causes abnormalities of sensation, sharp pains, incoordination, and incontinence.

tablet

A type of drug preparation in the form of a compressed plug. As well as the drug itself, a tablet contains other ingredients, such as disintegrating agents (to help the tablet dissolve), binding agents, and lubricants, and may have a sugar or membrane coating.

tachycardia

An adult heart rate of over 100 beats per minute. The average heart rate is 72–78 beats per minute. Tachycardia occurs in healthy people during exercise. At rest, tachycardia may be due to *fever*, *anxiety*, *hyperthyroidism* (overactivity of the thyroid gland), *coronary artery disease*, high *caffeine* intake, or treatment involving *anticholinergic drugs*.

There are various types of tachycardia, which originate in different areas of the heart; these include *atrial fibrillation*, *sinus tachycardia*, *supraventricular tachycardia*, and *ventricular tachycardia*.

The symptoms of tachycardia may include palpitations, breathlessness, and lightheadedness.

tachypnoea

An abnormally fast rate of breathing, which may be caused by exercise, anxiety, or lung or cardiac disorders.

tadalafil

A drug used in the treatment of *erectile dysfunction*. It is similar to *sildenafil* but is longer-acting. Possible side effects include indigestion, nausea, vomiting, headaches, flushing, dizziness, visual disturbances, and nasal congestion, and *priapism*. It should not be used by people who have had a recent *myocardial infarction* (heart attack) or stroke, or those with certain eye disorders. It

should also not be used by people who are taking *nitrate drugs* because of a possible serious interaction.

Taenia

A genus of tapeworms (see *tapeworm infestation*), some species of which can infest humans. These include TAENIA SOLIUM, which is passed on through contaminated pork, and TAENIA SAGINATA, whose larvae develop in beef.

Tagamet

A brand name for *cimetidine*, an *ulcer-healing drug*.

T'ai chi

A Chinese exercise system based on a series of over 100 postures between which slow, continuous movements are made. The aim is to exercise the muscles and integrate mind and body.

Takayasu's syndrome

A disorder, also known as Takayasu's arteritis, in which the arteries branching from the *aorta* become inflamed and progressively blocked. The cause is unknown. Takayasu's syndrome is rarely diagnosed outside Asian countries such as Japan. Absence of a pulse in the arms or neck is a characteristic feature, and blood pressure is increased. Symptoms such as paralysis of facial muscles and episodes of unconsciousness may occur as a result of minor *strokes*.

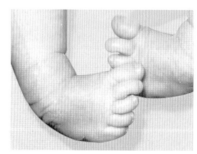

Talipes equinovarus
This birth defect, commonly known as club-foot, affects about one baby in 900. Treatment is by gentle manipulation, repeated several times a day.

talipes

A *birth defect* (commonly called club-foot) in which the foot is twisted out of shape or position. Most cases are thought to be due to pressure on the baby's feet from the mother's uterus in late pregnancy. A genetic factor is also sometimes present. The most common form of talipes is an equinovarus deformity,

in which the heel turns inwards and the rest of the foot bends down and inwards. Also, the tibia (shinbone) may be twisted inwards and the lower-leg muscles may be underdeveloped. Both feet may be affected. This defect is twice as common in boys as in girls.

TREATMENT
Talipes equinovarus is treated by repeated manipulation of the foot and ankle, starting soon after birth. A plaster *cast*, *splint*, or *strapping* may be used to hold the foot in position. If these measures are not successful by the time the baby is three to six months of age, surgery may be performed.

talus

The square-shaped foot bone that forms the ankle joint together with the *tibia* and *fibula* bones of the lower leg.

tamoxifen

An *anticancer drug* used to treat certain forms of *breast cancer* and some types of *infertility*. It may cause nausea, vomiting, hot flushes, swollen ankles, and irregular vaginal bleeding. Use of the drug is associated with a slight increased risk of endometrial cancer (see *uterus, cancer of*) and deep vein thrombosis (see *thrombosis, deep vein*).

tampon

A plug of absorbent material inserted into a wound or body opening to soak up blood or other secretions. The term commonly refers to a vaginal tampon, used to absorb menstrual blood.

tamponade

Compression of the heart by fluid within the *pericardium* (the membrane surrounding the heart), which may cause breathlessness and collapse. Causes include *pericarditis* (inflammation of the pericardium), complications after heart surgery, or a chest injury.

A diagnosis is made by *echocardiography*. Treatment of tamponade involves removing the fluid.

tamsulosin

An *alpha-blocker drug* used to treat urinary symptoms due to enlargement of the prostate gland (see *prostate, enlarged*). Side effects include low blood pressure, drowsiness, dry mouth, and gastrointestinal disturbances.

tan

See *suntan*.

tannin

Also known as tannic acid, a chemical that occurs in many plants, particularly tea. It may cause constipation, and large amounts cause liver damage.

tantrum

An outburst of bad behaviour, common in toddlers, usually indicating frustration and anger. During a tantrum, the child may scream, cry, yell, kick, bang the feet and fists, roll on the floor, go red in the face, spit, and bite. Some toddlers hold their breath, turning blue and, in rare cases, momentarily losing consciousness (see *breath-holding attacks*).

CAUSES

Tantrums occur at the age when a child starts to gain independence and becomes frustrated by restraints imposed by others, but is not yet able to express feelings verbally. Outbursts are more likely when a child is tired or when normal routine is disrupted, for example, by the birth of another baby. Occasional tantrums are considered normal; frequent outbursts may indicate an underlying *behavioural problem* or communication difficulty.

TREATMENT

Firm and consistent handling of the child is essential. Tantrums should be ignored as much as possible; a child's attention can often be diverted to a game or project. Most children grow out of tantrums when they develop the ability to express their feelings.

tapeworm infestation

Ribbon-shaped worms that infest the intestines of humans and animals. Tapeworms (cestodes) are usually acquired by eating undercooked meat or fish. An adult tapeworm has a flat, segmented body and suckers or hooks on its head, by which it attaches itself to the intestinal wall.

TYPES

Three large species of tapeworms are acquired by eating undercooked, infected beef, pork, and fish. The adults may grow up to 6 to 9 m long. Typically, tapeworms such as this have life-cycles that usually involve another animal host (see illustrated box). Tapeworms occur worldwide but infestations are largely prevented in countries that have adequate measures for inspecting meat and disposing of sewage.

The much smaller dwarf tapeworm, which is only 2.5 cm long, can be acquired through accidental transfer of worm eggs in human faeces to fingers and then to mouth. This worm is most common in the tropics and primarily affects children.

Humans may also act as intermediate hosts to the larvae of a tapeworm for which dogs are the main host.

SYMPTOMS

Despite their size, tapeworms from beef, pork, and fish usually only cause mild abdominal discomfort or diarrhoea. However, if eggs of pork worms are ingested, the hatched larvae form cysts in body tissues. This leads to cysticerosis, the symptoms of which are muscle pain and convulsions. Rarely, fish tapeworms cause anaemia. Tapeworm larvae acquired from dogs grow and develop into cysts in the liver and lungs, a condition called *hydatid disease*.

DIAGNOSIS AND TREATMENT

A diagnosis is made from the presence of worm segments or eggs in the faeces. Treatment with *anthelmintic drugs* is usually effective.

tar

A dark, sticky substance distilled from organic materials such as peat, coal, or wood. Coal tar is used as an ingredient in some skin preparations for the treatment of *psoriasis* and *eczema*, and in some soaps and shampoos. Tar residue in cigarette smoke collects as deposits in smokers' lungs.

tardive dyskinesia

Abnormal, uncontrolled movements, mainly of the face, tongue, mouth, and neck. Tardive dyskinesia may be caused by prolonged use of *antipsychotic drugs*, and is distinct from the movement disorder *parkinsonism*.

tarsal

A term denoting or relating to any of the seven bones that make up the *tarsus*.

tarsalgia

Pain in the rear part of the foot, usually associated with *flat-feet*.

tarsal tunnel syndrome

An uncommon disorder arising from abnormal pressure on the tibial nerve in the foot. Where this nerve curves round the inside of the ankle, it passes through the tarsal tunnel, a space formed between the bones of the ankle joint and bands of supporting fibrous tissue. If this space becomes constricted, the nerve is trapped and compressed.

Tarsal tunnel syndrome sometimes occurs when injury, or stress from over-activity, damages foot structures. It is also more common in people with flat feet. The usual symptoms are pain and a burning or tingling sensation on the sole of the foot.

Rest and *anti-inflammatory drugs* may be all that is needed. Persistent cases may be treated by *physiotherapy*, injections of *corticosteroid drugs* or, possibly, surgery to open up the tarsal tunnel.

LIFE-CYCLE OF TAPEWORM

Many tapeworms have life-cycles in which the adult and larval worms infest different hosts. In the cycle on the right, the adult worms infest humans and the larvae infest cattle (called the intermediate hosts). Pigs and fish may also act as intermediate hosts to human tapeworms, and humans may act as intermediate hosts to dog and pig tapeworms.

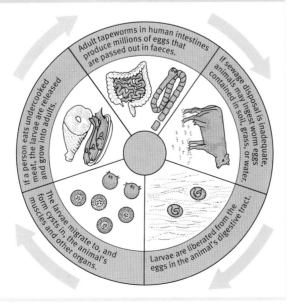

Adult tapeworms in human intestines produce millions of eggs that are passed out in faeces.

If sewage disposal is inadequate, animals may ingest worm eggs contained in soil, grass, or water.

Larvae are liberated from the eggs in the animal's digestive tract.

The larvae migrate to, and form cysts in, the animal's muscles and other organs.

If a person eats undercooked meat, the larvae are released and grow into adults.

tarsorrhaphy

Surgery in which the upper and lower eyelids are partially or completely sewn together. Tarsorrhaphy may be used as part of the treatment of corneal ulcer, or to protect the corneas of people who cannot close their eyes or those with *exophthalmos* (bulging eyes). The eyelids are later cut apart and allowed to open.

tarsus

The seven bones that make up the back of the foot and the ankle.

tartar

See *calculus, dental.*

tartrazine

A yellow dye that is commonly used as a food colouring in soft drinks, confectionery, and ready-prepared meals. (See also *food additives.*)

taste

One of the five senses. There are generally thought to be five basic tastes: sweet, salty, sour, bitter, and umami (a savoury taste), although in combination with the sense of *smell*, many different flavours can be distinguished. Tastes are detected by *taste buds*, most of which are on the tongue although there are also some on the palate and at the back of the throat.

taste bud

One of 10,000 specialized structures located mainly on the *tongue*, with some at the back of the throat and on the palate. Each bud contains about 50 sensory receptor cells, with tiny taste hairs that respond to food and drink. Taste buds on different parts of the tongue sense the five basic *tastes*: bitter, sour, salty, sweet, and umami.

taste, loss of

Loss of the sense of *taste*, usually as a result of loss of the sense of *smell*. The most common cause is inflammation of the nasal passages. Other causes include

THE SENSE OF **TASTE**

Tastes are detected by special structures, which are called taste buds. Every person has some 10,000 taste buds, mainly situated on the tongue, with a few at the back of the throat and on the palate. These taste buds surround pores within papillae (protuberances) on the tongue surface and elsewhere. There are five types of taste buds (sensitive to sweet, salty, sour, bitter, and umami chemicals). All tastes are formed from a mixture of these five elements.

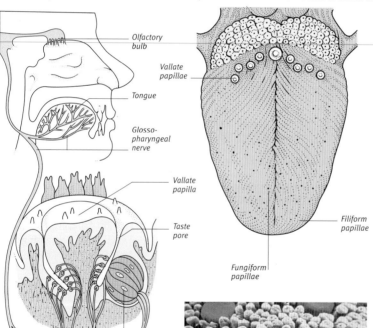

How a substance is tasted
Chemicals in food or drink dissolve in saliva and enter pores in the papillae on the tongue. Around these pores are groups of taste receptor cells – the taste buds. The chemicals stimulate hairs projecting from the receptor cells, causing signals to be sent from the cells along nerves to taste centres in the brain.

Magnified photograph of tongue surface
This photograph shows large (fungiform) and small (filiform) papillae. Taste buds are arranged around pores in the surface of the papillae.

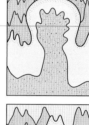

Fungiform papillae
These mushroom-shaped papillae occur in small numbers at random over the tongue surface, mainly at the tip and sides.

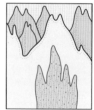

Filiform papillae
These smaller peak-shaped protuberances occur in large numbers over all except the back of the tongue's upper surface, and on the palate.

TASTE CENTRES

Taste buds sensitive to sweet, salty, sour, or bitter are grouped in particular areas on the surface of the tongue. The areas sensitive to umami are not yet known.

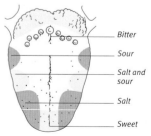

Bitter
Sour
Salt and sour
Salt
Sweet

any condition that causes a dry mouth (see *mouth, dry*); natural degeneration of the *taste buds* with age; damage to the taste buds from *stomatitis* (inflammation of the mouth), *mouth cancer*, or *radiotherapy* to the mouth; or damage to nerves that carry taste sensations.

tattooing

The introduction of permanent colours under the skin. Tattooing is used to create a picture on the skin for decorative purposes or may be carried out therapeutically (for example to "draw" on a nipple after breast surgery). Tattooing, even by professionals, is potentially dangerous. Unless strict sterile procedures are followed, there is a risk of infection (including with the viruses that cause *hepatitis* and *AIDS*) from the tattooist's needles. There is also a risk of scarring and allergic reactions to the dyes.

Complete tattoo removal is usually difficult. *Laser treatment* is the most common method, although sometimes *dermabrasion* or surgical excision may be used.

taxanes

A group of *anticancer drugs* used to treat certain cancers, such as ovarian cancer (see *ovary, cancer of*) and *breast cancer*. They work by preventing the growth of cancer cells. Common taxane drugs include *paclitaxel* and docetaxel.

Tay–Sachs disease

A serious inherited metabolic disorder (see *metabolism, inborn errors of*) that causes premature death. The cause is deficiency of the enzyme hexosaminidase A, which results in a buildup in the brain of a harmful substance. Symptoms usually appear after the age of six months and include blindness, paralysis, and seizures, leading to death by age three to five years.

Diagnosis is made by analysis of the enzymes of white blood cells. There is no treatment for the disorder but it is now largely prevented by screening and *genetic counselling* of high-risk groups, such as Ashkenazi Jews.

TB

An abbreviation for *tuberculosis*.

T-cell

A class of *lymphocyte*.

Td/IPV

A combined vaccine that provides immunity against *tetanus*, *diphtheria*, and *poliomyelitis*. It is given as a booster to young people between 13 and 18 years old as part of the childhood immunization programme. (See *Typical childhood immunization schedule*, p.414.)

tear duct

One of the channels, also known as a nasolacrimal duct, through which tears drain into the nose. (See also *lacrimal apparatus*.)

tear gas

See *CS spray*.

tears

The watery, salty secretion produced by the lacrimal glands, which are part of the *lacrimal apparatus* of the *eye*. Tears keep the *cornea* and *conjunctiva* moist to maintain transparency of the cornea and prevent ulcers; to aid blinking; and to wash away any foreign particles in the eye. Tear production increases in response to eye irritation and emotion. (See also *artificial tears*.)

technetium

A radioactive element used in *radionuclide scanning*.

teeth

Hard, bonelike projections set in the jaws and surrounded by the gums. The teeth are used for *mastication* (chewing), help to form speech, and give shape to the face. At the centre of each tooth is the pulp, which contains blood vessels and nerves and is surrounded by hard dentine. The crown, the part of the tooth above the gum, is covered by enamel, the hardest substance in the body. The roots of the tooth, which fit into the jawbone, are covered by bonelike cementum. (See *Structure and arrangement of teeth* box, overleaf.)

Adult humans have 32 *permanent teeth*, which erupt after the *primary teeth* are lost, starting from about the age of six. These permanent teeth comprise eight chisel-shaped, biting incisors; four sharp, pointed canines; eight grinding premolars; and 12 large, grinding molars. (See also *anodontia*.)

teeth, care of

See *oral hygiene*.

teething

The period when a baby cuts his or her *primary teeth* (see *eruption of teeth*). Usually, the first signs of teething occur at about six months of age.

While teething, a baby may be irritable, fretful, clingy, may have difficulty sleeping, and may cry more than usual. Extra saliva may be produced, resulting in dribbling, and the baby tends to chew on anything that comes to hand.

Before a tooth emerges, the gum may become red and swollen. When molars erupt, the cheek may feel warm and look red on the affected side.

Symptoms may be relieved by the use of painkilling gels that are rubbed on the gums, or liquid preparations.

teichopsia

A visual disturbance in which shimmering, jagged patterns of light appear in front of the eyes. Teichopsia is sometimes experienced just before the onset of a *migraine* attack.

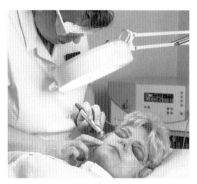

Cosmetic laser surgery for telangiectasia
A hand-held laser is used to remove the broken veins. Although often referred to as "broken", the blood vessels are, in fact, simply larger than usual.

telangiectasia

An increase in the size of small blood vessels beneath the skin, causing redness and a "broken veins" appearance. It most commonly occurs on the nose and cheeks. There may be no obvious cause for telangiectasia, or it may be due to many years of excessive alcohol consumption, the skin condition *rosacea*, overexposure to sunlight, or a connective tissue disease such as *dermatomyositis*.

Telangiectasia is not a cause for concern, but if very unsightly the veins can be removed in some cases by electro-desiccation (electrical destruction of the upper layers of the skin) or by *laser treatment*. (See also *spider naevus*.)

telecardiography

The recording of an *ECG* by transmission of impulses (such as via a telephone line) to a site that is remote from the patient. (See also *Holter monitor*.)

T

STRUCTURE AND ARRANGEMENT OF **TEETH**

At the heart of each tooth is the living pulp, which contains blood vessels and nerves. A hard substance called dentine surrounds the pulp. The part of the tooth above the gum, the crown, is covered by enamel. The roots of the tooth, which fit into sockets in the jawbone, are covered by a sensitive, bonelike material, the cementum. The periodontal ligament connects the cementum to the gums and to the jaw. It acts as a shock absorber and prevents jarring of the teeth and skull when food is being chewed.

Cross-section

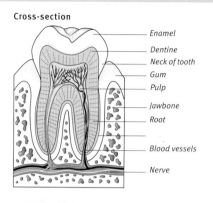

- Enamel
- Dentine
- Neck of tooth
- Gum
- Pulp
- Jawbone
- Root
- Blood vessels
- Nerve

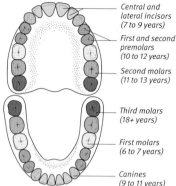

- Central and lateral incisors (7 to 9 years)
- First and second premolars (10 to 12 years)
- Second molars (11 to 13 years)
- Third molars (18+ years)
- First molars (6 to 7 years)
- Canines (9 to 11 years)

The permanent teeth
The illustration above shows the arrangement in the jaw of the permanent teeth – eight incisors, four canines, eight premolars, and 12 molars. The ages when these teeth erupt are indicated.

X-ray of teeth
The panoramic X-ray on the left shows all the teeth (there are no wisdom teeth) of the upper and lower jaw and their surrounding structures. The tooth roots, buried in jawbones, can be clearly seen; several teeth have been filled.

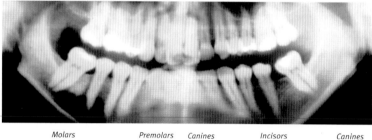

| Molars | | | Premolars | Canines | Incisors | Canines | Premolars | Molars |
| Third | Second | First | | | | | | |

Molars
The molars are large, strong teeth, efficient at grinding food. The third molars, or wisdom teeth, are the last to erupt; in some people, the wisdom teeth never appear.

Premolars
Also known as bicuspids, because of their two distinct edges, the premolars are concerned with grinding food. There are no premolars among the primary (milk) teeth.

Incisors
These teeth have a chisel-shaped, sharp cutting edge that is ideal for biting. The upper incisors overlap the lower incisors slightly when the jaws are closed.

Canines
These are sharp, pointed teeth, ideal for tearing food. They are larger and stronger than the incisors, with very long roots. The upper canines are often known as eye teeth.

temazepam

A *benzodiazepine drug* that is used to treat *insomnia*. It is also a drug of abuse.

temperature

In the human body, temperature must be maintained at around 37°C for optimum functioning. This varies slightly, not only among individuals but also in the same person, as temperature is affected by such factors as exercise, sleep, eating and drinking, time of day, and, in women, the stage of the menstrual cycle.

Body temperature is maintained by the *hypothalamus*, an area in the brain, which monitors blood temperature and automatically compensates for changes. When body temperature falls, the hypothalamus sends nerve impulses to stimulate *shivering*, which creates heat by muscle activity, and to constrict blood vessels in the skin, which minimizes heat loss. When body temperature rises, the hypothalamus stimulates *sweating* and dilates blood vessels in the skin to increase heat loss. Many factors (such as infections or extremes of heat and cold) may disrupt the heat-regulating system, making temperature too high or too low. (See also *fever*; *heatstroke*; *hypothermia*.)

T

TEMPORAL ARTERITIS

In this disorder, the temporal artery and other arteries in the head are inflamed. Early treatment of temporal arteritis is vital, because if the condition is left untreated, there is a risk of sudden blindness.

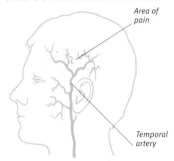

Telltale symptoms
If the temporal artery is inflamed, it is usually prominent and there is a persistent severe headache and scalp tenderness in the area of the head shown above.

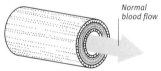

Normal artery
In a normal artery, there is a smooth lining, and the blood flow through it is sufficient to meet the needs of the tissues it supplies.

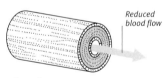

Inflamed artery
In arteritis, the walls of the artery become disrupted and thickened, and blood flow through it is therefore markedly reduced.

temporal

Of or near the temples or a temple.

temporal arteritis

An uncommon disease of older people in which the walls of the arteries in the scalp over the temples become inflamed. Other arteries in the head and neck may also be affected, as may the *aorta* and its main branches. The inflamed vessels become narrowed, reducing blood flow through them.

CAUSES
The cause of temporal arteritis is unknown, but it may be associated with *polymyalgia rheumatica*.

SYMPTOMS
The most common symptom is a severe headache on one or both sides of the head. The temporal artery (located at the side of the head above the earlobe) may be prominent and the scalp may be tender, especially over the artery. In about half of the cases, the ophthalmic arteries supplying the eyes are affected, which may cause sudden blindness if untreated. Other symptoms include fever and poor appetite.

DIAGNOSIS AND TREATMENT
Early reporting of symptoms is essential due to the risk of blindness. The diagnosis of temporal arteritis is made by *blood tests*, notably the *ESR* (erythrocyte sedimentation rate), which is elevated in temporal arteritis. In some cases a *biopsy* (taking a tissue sample for analysis) of the artery may also be done.

Treatment with a *corticosteroid drug* usually produces a rapid alleviation of symptoms and prevents visual loss. Initially, a high dose is used and then the dose is gradually reduced to the minimum necessary to control inflammation, as assessed by ESR tests. Corticosteroid treatment needs to be continued until the condition clears up completely, which usually occurs within two years.

temporal lobe epilepsy

A form of *epilepsy* in which abnormal electrical discharges occur in the temporal lobe (most of the lower side of each half of the *cerebrum*) in the *brain*.

LOCATION OF THE TEMPORAL LOBE

The temporal lobe forms much of the lower side of each half of the cerebrum (main mass of the brain).

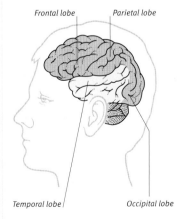

Frontal lobe   *Parietal lobe*

Temporal lobe   *Occipital lobe*

The usual cause of this type of epilepsy is damage to the temporal lobe, which may be due to a *birth injury*, *head injury*, *brain tumour*, *brain abscess*, or *stroke*.

SYMPTOMS
Attacks of this form of epilepsy cause dreamlike states, unpleasant *hallucinations* of smell or taste, the perception of an illusory scene, or *déja vu*. There may also be grimacing, rotation of the head and eyes, and sucking and chewing movements. The affected person may have no memory of activities during an attack, which can last for minutes or hours. Sometimes, the seizure develops into a *grand mal* seizure.

DIAGNOSIS AND TREATMENT
Diagnosis and drug treatment is the same as for other forms of epilepsy.

LOCATION OF THE TEMPOROMANDIBULAR JOINT

The head of the mandible (jawbone) fits neatly into a hollow situated on the underside of the temporal bone of the skull at the joint.

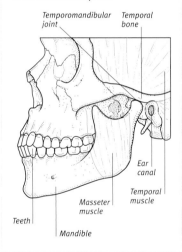

Temporomandibular joint   *Temporal bone*

Ear canal

Temporal muscle

Masseter muscle

Teeth

Mandible

temporomandibular joint

The joint between the mandible (lower jaw bone) and the *skull*.

temporomandibular joint dysfunction

Pain and other symptoms affecting the head, jaw, and face that are thought to occur when the *temporomandibular joints* and the muscles and ligaments attached to them do not work together correctly.

A common cause of temporomandibular joint dysfunction is spasm of the chewing muscles, which is often

T

caused by clenching or grinding the teeth as a result of emotional tension. *Malocclusion* (an incorrect bite) may be a contributing factor because it places additional stress on the muscles. Temporomandibular joint problems may also be caused by jaw, head, or neck injuries. In rare cases, *osteoarthritis* may be the cause.

SYMPTOMS

Common symptoms include headaches, tenderness of the jaw muscles, and an aching facial pain, especially in or around the ear. There may also be difficulty in opening the mouth, locking of the jaws, clicking noises as the mouth is closed or opened, or pain caused by opening the mouth wide or chewing.

TREATMENT

In many cases, the condition clears up without treatment. If treatment is necessary, it may include drugs such as *analgesics, nonsteroidal anti-inflammatory drugs, muscle relaxants,* or *antidepressants*. These may be used alone or in combination with other treatments, such as jaw exercises, biofeedback, and the use of bite guards. Some people also find self-help measures beneficial, including eating only soft foods, avoiding overuse of the jaw, massaging and applying heat to the affected muscles; and relaxation techniques. In severe, persistent cases, injections of *corticosteroid drugs* into the joint or surgery may be necessary.

tendinitis

Inflammation of a tendon, usually due to injury or overuse. Symptoms of tendinitis include restricted movement, pain, and tenderness. Treatment is with *nonsteroidal anti-inflammatory drugs*, *ultrasound treatment*, or injection of a *corticosteroid drug* around the tendon.

tendolysis

An operation performed to free a *tendon* from *adhesions* (fibrous bands) that limit its movement.

tendon

A fibrous cord that joins muscle to bone. Tendons are strong and flexible, but inelastic. They are made up principally of bundles of collagen (a white, fibrous protein) and contain some blood vessels. The tendons in the hands, wrists, and feet are enclosed in synovial sheaths (fibrous capsules) that secrete a lubricating fluid, which allows movement without excessive friction.

FINGER TENDONS

Tendons on the top and underside of the finger control bending and extension; the tendons originate from forearm muscles.

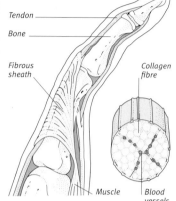

Tendon
Bone
Fibrous sheath
Collagen fibre
Muscle
Blood vessels

Internal structure
A cross-section of a tendon (above right) shows that it consists of numerous parallel bundles of collagen fibres together with some blood vessels.

DISORDERS

Tendinitis (inflammation of a tendon) may follow an injury. *Tenosynovitis* (inflammation of the inner lining of a tendon sheath) usually affects tendons in the hands and wrists and results from overuse. *Tenovaginitis* (inflammation of the outer wall of a tendon sheath), may restrict movement of the tendon through the sheath.

Injury may cause a *tendon rupture*. The *Achilles tendon* in the heel can rupture during vigorous sprinting and jumping. In many cases, however, because tendons are strong, severe stress results in pulling off a piece of bone where the tendon is attached, rather than tearing of the tendon itself.

tendon repair

Surgery to join the cut or torn ends of, or to replace, a damaged *tendon*.

tendon rupture

A complete tear in a *tendon*. A tendon may rupture when the muscle to which it is attached contracts suddenly and powerfully, such as during vigorous exercise. Rupture may also be the result of an injury or a joint disorder such as *rheumatoid arthritis*.

Symptoms include a snapping sensation, impaired movement, pain, and

---

swelling. Diagnosis is usually obvious from the symptoms alone. Surgery to repair the tendon may be needed. In some cases, the tendon may heal if immobilized in a plaster *cast*.

tendon transfer

Surgery to reposition a *tendon* so that the tendon makes a muscle perform a different function. The tendon is cut from its original point of attachment on the muscle and reattached elsewhere, making the muscle lie in a different position. The procedure may be used to treat *talipes* (club-foot) or permanent muscle injury or paralysis.

tenecteplase

A *thrombolytic drug* that is used in the treatment of *myocardial infarction* (heart attack). Tenecteplase is administered by intravenous injection.

tenesmus

A feeling of incomplete emptying of the bowel in which the urge to pass *faeces* accompanies ineffective straining. Tenesmus may be a symptom of inflammation of the bowel or a tumour (see *colon, cancer of*).

tennis elbow

Pain and tenderness on the outside of the elbow and in the back of the forearm. Also called lateral epicondylitis, tennis elbow is caused by inflammation of the *tendon* that attaches the muscles that straighten the fingers and wrist to the *humerus* (upper-arm bone).

Treatment of tennis elbow consists of resting the arm, applying *ice-packs*, and taking *analgesic drugs* (painkillers) or *nonsteroidal anti-inflammatory drugs*. In some cases, *ultrasound treatment*, injection of a *corticosteroid drug*, or surgery may be necessary.

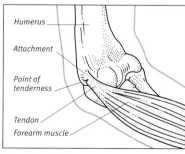

Humerus
Attachment
Point of tenderness
Tendon
Forearm muscle

Site of tennis elbow
Pulling of the forearm muscles at the point where they attach to the humerus causes tenderness on the outer side of the elbow.

T

tenosynovitis

Inflammation of the lining of the sheath that surrounds a *tendon*. The usual cause is excessive friction caused by repetitive movements; bacterial infection is a rare cause. The hands and wrists are most often affected in tenosynovitis. Symptoms include pain, tenderness, and swelling over the tendon.

Treatment is with *nonsteroidal anti-inflammatory drugs* (NSAIDs) or a local injection of a *corticosteroid drug*. However, if infection is the cause, *antibiotics* are prescribed. A *splint* to immobilize the joint, or surgery, may also be needed.

tenovaginitis

Inflammation or thickening of the fibrous wall of the sheath that surrounds a *tendon*. Tenovaginitis affecting the sheath of one of the tendons that bends a finger results in *trigger finger*.

TENS

Abbreviation for transcutaneous electrical nerve stimulation, a method of pain relief. Minute electrical impulses, which block pain messages to the brain, are relayed from an impulse generator to electrodes attached to the skin in the area of the pain. TENS can help relieve chronic pain not controlled by *analgesic drugs* and may be used in *childbirth*.

tension

A feeling of mental and physical strain associated with *anxiety*. Muscle tension may cause headaches and stiffness. Persistent tension is related to generalized anxiety disorder. (See also *stress*.)

teratogen

A physical, chemical, or biological agent, such as radiation, the drug *thalidomide*, or the *rubella* virus, that causes abnormalities in a developing *embryo* or *fetus*.

teratoma

A primary *tumour*, which may be cancerous or noncancerous, consisting of cells totally unlike those normally found in that part of the body. For example, teratomas in the ovary may form cysts containing skin, hair, teeth, or bone.

terbinafine

An *antifungal drug* that may be used orally or topically to treat fungal infections of the skin and nails, particularly *tinea* (ringworm). Topical preparations may also be used to treat candida skin infections (see *candidiasis*).

Side effects are rare with topical use of terbinafine. Those that occur are generally mild and transient and may include local irritation. Taken orally, the drug may cause nausea, abdominal pain, a rash, or, rarely, liver problems.

terbutaline

A *bronchodilator drug* that is used to treat *asthma* and chronic obstructive *pulmonary disease*. Terbutaline is also used to prevent premature labour. Possible adverse effects of the drug include nervousness, restlessness, tremor, and nausea. These effects may be reduced with an adjustment in dosage, however. Palpitations and headache may also occur, but they are rare.

terminal care

See *dying, care of the*.

termination of pregnancy

See *abortion, induced*.

testicular feminization syndrome

A rare inherited condition in which an individual who is genetically male with internal *testes* has the external appearance of a female. The syndrome is a form of *intersex* and is the most common type of male *pseudohermaphroditism*.

CAUSE

The cause is a defective response of the body tissues to the male sex hormone *testosterone*. The causative genes are carried on the X chromosome, and so females can be carriers and pass on the genes to their sons.

SYMPTOMS

Those affected seem to be girls throughout childhood. Most develop normal female secondary *sexual characteristics* at *puberty* but *menstruation* does not occur because there is no uterus and the vagina is short and blind-ending. People with the syndrome tend to be tall, and are of normal health.

DIAGNOSIS AND TREATMENT

Testicular feminization syndrome may be diagnosed before puberty if a girl is found to have an inguinal *hernia* or a swelling in the labia that turns out to be a testis. Otherwise, the diagnosis is usually made during investigations at puberty to find the cause of *amenorrhoea* (failure to menstruate). This is confirmed by *chromosome analysis*, which shows the presence of male chromosomes, and blood tests, which show male levels of testosterone.

Treatment of testicular feminization syndrome involves surgical removal of the testes, to prevent cancerous change in later life, and therapy with *oestrogen drugs*. An affected person is not fertile but can live a normal life as a woman.

testicular self-examination

Regular, manual self-examination of the testes to detect any unusual lumps, swellings, or other abnormalities that could indicate an underlying problem, particularly testicular cancer (see *testis, cancer of*).

When the testes are relaxed (after a hot shower or bath, for example), the man should gently roll each testis between fingers and thumb to feel for unusual lumps and swellings or changes in skin texture. Anything that feels different from normal – particularly any new lump or swelling – should be reported to a doctor as soon as possible. Testicular tumours are usually firm but not tender or painful. A painful lump may be due to infection, and the man should therefore not have sex until he has seen a doctor. Most testicular abnormalities are not due to cancer, and even testicular cancer can be cured in the majority of cases if it is detected early.

SELF-EXAMINATION OF THE TESTIS

Most lumps are not cancerous but should be considered potentially malignant until medical tests prove otherwise. Cancers tend to be firm to the touch and are usually not tender or painful when pressed.

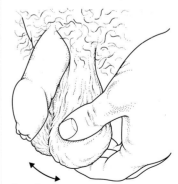

Procedure
After a hot shower or bath, gently roll the testis between the fingers and thumb to feel for any unusual hard lumps that were not present before. The entire surface of each testis should be felt, and each testis should be examined in turn.

T

LOCATION OF THE **TESTIS**

Each testis is suspended in the scrotum by a spermatic cord, which contains the vas deferens, and the arteries, veins and nerves that supply the testis.

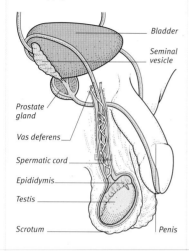

Bladder

Seminal vesicle

Prostate gland

Vas deferens

Spermatic cord

Epididymis

Testis

Scrotum

Penis

testis

One of the two male sexual organs, also called testicles, that produce *sperm* and the male sex hormone *testosterone*.

The testes form within the abdomen early in fetal development. In response to hormones produced by both the mother and the fetus, the testes gradually descend. At birth, or within the next few months, they have usually reached the surface of the body and hang suspended in the pouch of skin called the *scrotum*.

STRUCTURE

Within each testis are the seminiferous tubules, delicate coiled tubes that produce sperm. These tubules lead via the vasa efferentia (small ducts) to the *epididymis*, a structure lying behind the testis in which the newly formed sperm mature. Cells between the seminiferous tubules produce testosterone, which passes into small blood vessels in the testis and from there into the general blood circulation.

Each testis is protected by a tough, fibrous capsule (called the tunica albuginea) and is suspended from the body by the *spermatic cord*. This cord is composed of the *vas deferens* (the tube that transports sperm from the epididymis to the urethra), and a number of blood vessels and nerves. (See also *testis, undescended*.)

testis, cancer of

A cancerous tumour of the *testis*. Testicular cancer occurs most commonly in young to middle-aged men, and the risk increases in individuals who have a history of undescended testis (see *testis, undescended*).

TYPES

The most common types of testicular cancer are seminomas, which are made up of only one type of cell, and *teratomas*, which are made up of cells that do not resemble other cells in the testis. Other cancers affecting the testis are extremely rare and develop from testicular tissue or from lymphatic tissue within the testis (see *lymphoma*).

SYMPTOMS

The cancer usually appears as a firm, painless swelling of one testis. In some cases, there may be pain and inflammation.

DIAGNOSIS

Men are recommended to examine their testes regularly to check for unusual changes (see *testicular self-examination*). If a lump is found, the doctor will perform tests, such as *ultrasound scanning*, to exclude other causes of testicular swelling (see *testis, swollen*).

TREATMENT

Biopsy, followed by *orchidectomy* (surgical removal of the testis) is the usual course of action for testicular cancer, and may be combined with *chemotherapy*. If detected at an early stage, a tumour usually responds well to treatment. Provided the other testis is healthy, treatment generally does not destroy its fertility.

testis, ectopic

A *testis* that is absent from the *scrotum* because it has descended into an abnormal position, usually in the groin or at the base of the penis. The condition is most often discovered soon after birth during a routine physical examination. It is treated by *orchidopexy*, an operation to place the testis in the scrotum. (See also *testis, undescended*.)

testis, pain in the

Pain in a *testis* may have a number of causes, including mild injury, a tear in the wall of the testis due to a direct blow, *orchitis* (inflammation of the testis), *epididymo-orchitis* (inflammation of the testis and the epididymis), and torsion of the testis (see *testis, torsion of*).

Sometimes, no cause is found and the pain disappears without treatment. If the wall of the testis is torn, an operation to repair it may be needed.

testis, retractile

A *testis* that is drawn up high into the groin by a pronounced muscle reflex in response to cold or touch. A retractile testis is normal in young children, but it usually disappears by *puberty*.

testis, swollen

Harmless, painless swellings include *epididymal cysts*, *hydroceles*, *varicoceles*, and *spermatoceles*. Cancer of the testis (see *testis, cancer of*) is a rare cause of usually painless swelling. Painful testicular swelling may be due to a direct blow, torsion of the testis (see *testis, torsion of*), *orchitis* (inflammation of the testis), or *epididymo-orchitis* (inflammation of the testis and epididymis). Any swelling of the testes should be assessed promptly by a doctor. An *ultrasound* scan may be done to aid diagnosis.

testis, torsion of

Twisting of the *spermatic cord* that causes severe pain and swelling of the *testis*. The pain develops rapidly and is sometimes accompanied by abdominal pain and nausea. The testis becomes swollen and very tender, and the skin of the *scrotum* becomes discoloured. Unless the torsion

TORSION OF THE **TESTIS**

If a testis rotates, veins in the spermatic cord become obstructed, causing severe swelling and pain. The condition is most common around puberty but can occur at any age.

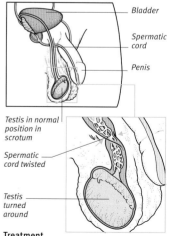

Bladder

Spermatic cord

Penis

Testis in normal position in scrotum

Spermatic cord twisted

Testis turned around

Treatment
Torsion must be treated by surgery within a few hours, otherwise the testis will have to be removed. In surgery, both testes are secured in the scrotum to prevent recurrence.

T

is treated within a few hours, permanent damage to the testis results. The condition is most common around puberty. It is more likely to occur if the testis is unusually mobile within the scrotum.

Diagnosis is by physical examination. Surgery is performed to untwist the testis and anchor it in the scrotum to prevent recurrence. If the damage is irreversible, *orchidectomy* (removal of the testis) is performed. In either case, the other testis is anchored to the scrotum to prevent torsion on that side.

testis, undescended

A testis that has failed to descend from the abdomen to the *scrotum*. The condition usually affects only one testis. An undescended testis often descends within months of birth and has usually descended within the first year but rarely descends after this time. The condition is more common in premature babies.

An undescended testis does not develop normally, cannot produce normal sperm, and is at increased risk of testicular cancer (see *testis, cancer of*). If both testes are undescended, *infertility* results.

CAUSES
The final descent of the testis into the scrotum is controlled by hormones produced by the mother and by the testis itself. If these do not have an effect, the spermatic cord fails to lengthen sufficiently to allow full descent. Less commonly, a normal testis is prevented from reaching the scrotum because of fibres blocking its route.

DIAGNOSIS AND TREATMENT
A diagnosis is made during a physical examination after birth or later in infancy. Treatment is by *orchidopexy*, an operation to place the testis in the scrotum, which usually reduces the risk of later infertility or testicular cancer. A poorly developed undescended testis may be removed if the other is normal.

test meal

A procedure to measure the output of acid by the *stomach*. A *nasogastric tube* is passed into the stomach after an overnight fast, and a sample of gastric fluid is sucked up through the tube. An injection of a drug that stimulates gastric secretion is given and further samples of stomach fluid are taken and analysed for hydrochloric acid content. The test is used for people thought to have *Zollinger–Ellison syndrome*, and to confirm the absence of stomach acid in people with pernicious anaemia (see *anaemia, pernicious*).

testosterone

The main *androgen hormone* (male sex hormone). It stimulates bone and muscle growth and sexual development. It is produced by the *testes* and, in small amounts, the *ovaries*. Synthetic or animal testosterone is used to stimulate delayed *puberty* or treat some forms of male *infertility*.

tests, medical

Tests may be performed to investigate the cause of symptoms and establish a diagnosis, to monitor the course of a disease, or to assess response to treatment. Testing carried out on people who are apparently in good health to find disease at an early stage is known as *screening*.

TYPES OF MEDICAL TESTS

The table below lists some commonly performed medical tests, classified by the body system they are used to study, although any of the tests may be done as part of the investigation for any system. Each test listed in the table has its own entry. Only some of the most important imaging techniques for each body organ have been included; a complete list appears in the appropriate imaging article.

System	Test	
Brain and nervous system	• EEG • Evoked responses • Hearing tests • Vision tests • Lumbar puncture • Intelligence tests	• Myelography • Brain imaging • CT scanning • MRI • PET scanning
Skin, bones, and muscles	• EMG • Biopsy	• Bone imaging • X-rays
Endocrine system and metabolism	• Thyroid-function tests • Thyroid scanning	• Blood tests • Urinalysis
Blood and immune system	• Blood tests • Lymphangiography	• Skin tests • Bone marrow biopsy
Heart and circulation	• Heart imaging • Chest X-ray • Angiography • Echocardiography • Venography	• ECG (plus exercise and 24-hour ECG) • Catheterization, cardiac • Cardiac stress test • Thallium scan
Lungs	• Pulmonary function tests • Blood gases/oxygen saturation • Peak-flow meter • Spirometry	• Chest X-ray • Bronchoscopy • Sputum analysis
Biliary system	• Liver-function tests • Liver imaging • Ultrasound scanning • Cholangiography	• Cholecystography • ERCP • Liver biopsy
Gastrointestinal tract	• Endoscopy • Colonoscopy • Gastroscopy • Sigmoidoscopy	• Barium X-ray examinations • Jejunal biopsy • Occult blood, faecal • Microbiology/parasitology
Urinary tract	• Kidney imaging • Urography (IVU) • Ultrasound scanning	• Urinalysis • Kidney-function tests • Cystoscopy
Reproductive system	• Pregnancy test • Hysterosalpingography • Mammography • Ultrasound scanning • Laparoscopy	• Amniocentesis • Cervical smear test • Chorionic villus sampling • Chromosome analysis • Seminal fluid analysis

T

The accuracy of a test is based on its sensitivity (ability to correctly identify diseased subjects), specificity (ability to correctly identify healthy subjects), and predictive value. The predictive value is determined by a mathematical formula that involves the number of accurate test results and the total number of tests performed. The best tests have both high specificity and high sensitivity, and therefore high predictive value. (See also *Medical tests* box, previous page.)

test-tube baby

The colloquial term for a baby born following *in vitro fertilization*, in which an egg (ovum) is taken from a woman's ovary, fertilized outside the body, and then implanted in the uterus.

tetanus

A serious, sometimes fatal, disease of the *central nervous system* (brain and spinal cord) caused by infection of a wound with spores of the bacterium CLOSTRIDIUM TETANI.

CAUSE
The spores live mainly in soil and manure but are also found elsewhere, including in the human intestine. When the spores infect poorly oxygenated tissues they multiply and produce a *toxin* that acts on the nerves responsible for controlling muscle activity.

SYMPTOMS
The most common symptom is *trismus* (stiffness of the jaw, commonly known as lockjaw). Other symptoms include stiffness and aching of the abdominal and back muscles, and contraction of facial muscles, producing a fixed grimace. There may also be a fast pulse, mild fever, and profuse sweating. Painful muscle spasms then develop, and may result in *asphyxia* if they affect the *larynx* or chest wall. The spasms usually subside after 10 to 14 days.

DIAGNOSIS AND TREATMENT
The diagnosis is made from the symptoms and signs, and a course of tetanus *antitoxin* injections is started. Artificial ventilation may be needed. Most people recover completely if treated promptly.

PREVENTION
In the UK tetanus is prevented by routine immunization, with three doses during the first year (at two, three, and four months of age), a booster at three years four months to five years, and another booster at 13 to 18 years. Generally, five doses of vaccine provide lifelong immunity, although further boosters may be required after a dirty wound or if travelling in an area with poor medical services.

tetany

Spasms and twitching of the muscles, most commonly in the hands and feet, although the muscles of the face, *larynx* (voicebox), or spine may also be affected. The spasms are caused by a biochemical disturbance and are painless at first; if the condition persists, the spasms tend to become increasingly painful.

Muscle damage may result if the cause is not treated. The most common underlying cause is *hypocalcaemia* (a low level of calcium in the blood). Other causes include *hypokalaemia* (a low level of potassium), *hyperventilation* during a panic attack, or, more rarely, *hypoparathyroidism* (underactivity of the parathyroid glands).

tetracosactide

A drug used to test the functioning of the *adrenal glands*. Tetracosactide is a chemical analogue (imitation) of the natural hormone corticotrophin (*ACTH*). ACTH stimulates the cortices of the adrenal glands to secrete hormones such as *cortisol*. To diagnose a disorder of the adrenal glands, a tetracosactide injection is given and the blood cortisol level measured. Failure of the level to rise indicates an abnormality.

tetracosactrin

The former name for *tetracosactide*.

tetracycline drugs

COMMON DRUGS
- Doxycycline • Minocycline • Oxytetracycline
- Tetracycline

A group of *antibiotic drugs* that are commonly used as a treatment for certain infections including *chlamydial infections*, flare-ups of chronic *bronchitis*, *Lyme disease*, *leptospirosis*, and certain types of *pneumonia*. They are also used to treat some cases of *acne*. It should be noted that if taken with milk or *antacid drugs*, tetracyclines are not absorbed effectively in the intestines.

Possible side effects of tetracyclines include nausea, vomiting, diarrhoea, headache, and worsening of kidney disorders and liver function. Tetracyclines may discolour developing teeth and are therefore not usually prescribed for children under the age of 12 or women who are pregnant or breast-feeding.

tetralogy of Fallot

A form of congenital *heart disease* in which the heart has four coexisting anomalies: displacement of the aorta, narrowing of the pulmonary valve, a hole in the ventricular septum, and thickening of the right ventricle wall. Because of these defects, blood pumped from the heart to the body is insufficiently oxygenated, resulting in *cyanosis* (bluish coloration) and breathlessness.

SYMPTOMS AND SIGNS
Affected infants appear normal at birth, although disturbed blood flow in the heart may be heard as *murmurs* through a stethoscope. Severely affected infants may become cyanosed and breathless early in life, and may be prone to fainting. Those less severely affected develop these symptoms gradually. Other symptoms include failure to gain weight and poor development.

DIAGNOSIS AND TREATMENT
An *ECG*, echocardiogram (see *echocardiography*), and sometimes cardiac *catheterization* are performed to confirm the diagnosis and also to assess the severity of the condition.

Tetralogy of Fallot is corrected by *open heart surgery*. Carrying out the repair

Normal heart

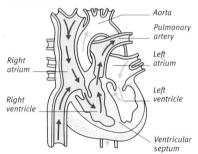

Aorta

Pulmonary artery

Right atrium

Left atrium

Right ventricle

Left ventricle

Ventricular septum

Tetralogy of Fallot

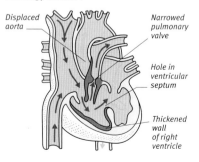

Displaced aorta

Narrowed pulmonary valve

Hole in ventricular septum

Thickened wall of right ventricle

Defects of tetralogy of Fallot
The four defects are shown above. Insufficient blood passes to the pulmonary artery and lungs to be oxygenated, and the blood pumped to the body via the aorta is therefore lacking in oxygen.

T

before the child reaches school age provides the best chance of success and normal future development.

tetraplegia

An alternative term for the condition *quadriplegia*.

thalamus

One of a pair of structures in the *brain*, the thalamus is a walnut-sized mass of nerve tissue. The thalami sit at the top of the *brainstem* and are connected to all parts of the brain.

Each thalamus relays sensory information flowing into the brain. Some basic sensations, such as pain, may reach consciousness within the thalamus. Other types of sensory information are processed and relayed to parts of the cerebral cortex (the outer layer of the brain), where sensations are perceived.

The thalamus acts as a filter by selecting only information that is of particular importance. Certain centres in the thalamus are also thought to play a part in long-term memory.

LOCATION OF THE **THALAMUS**

The two thalami are situated deep within the brain, at a position just above the brainstem.

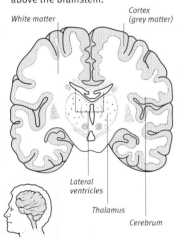

White matter
Cortex (grey matter)
Lateral ventricles
Thalamus
Cerebrum

thalassaemia

A group of inherited *blood* disorders in which there is a fault in the production of the oxygen-carrying pigment *haemoglobin*. This pigment is normally made in the *bone marrow* for incorporation into red *blood cells*. Many of the red blood cells become fragile and haemolyse (break up), leading to anaemia (see *anaemia, haemolytic*). Thalassaemia is prevalent in the Mediterranean, the Middle East, and Southeast Asia, and in families originating from these areas.

CAUSES AND TYPES

Normal adult haemoglobin contains two pairs of globins (protein chains), known as alpha and beta. In thalassaemia, a recessive defective gene results in reduced synthesis of one of the chains. Usually beta-chain production is disturbed (beta-thalassaemia). Beta-thalassaemia minor (thalassaemia trait), which is never severe, is caused by a single defective gene. The presence of two defective genes causes beta-thalassaemia major (Cooley's anaemia). The rare disorder alpha-thalassaemia varies in severity, but alpha-thalassaemia major usually results in fetal death.

SYMPTOMS

Symptoms of beta-thalassaemia major appear three to six months after birth and include shortness of breath, *jaundice*, and an enlarged *spleen*. If the condition is untreated, bone marrow cavities expand, leading to characteristic enlargement of the skull and facial bones; normal body growth is arrested and death is likely to occur in early childhood.

DIAGNOSIS AND TREATMENT

Beta-thalassaemia major is diagnosed by microscopic examination of the blood and other *blood tests*. Treatment is with *blood transfusions* and, sometimes, *splenectomy* (removal of the spleen). However, successive *blood transfusions* cause a buildup of iron in the body (see *haemosiderosis*). *Chelating agents* are given by mouth or by infusion to help the body excrete the excess iron. A *stem cell* or *bone marrow transplant* offers a cure.

PREVENTION

Genetic counselling is advised for parents or other close relatives of a child with thalassaemia, and also for any person with thalassaemia trait.

thalidomide

A drug that was withdrawn in the UK in 1961 after it was found to cause limb deformities in many babies born to women given the drug during pregnancy. Although thalidomide is not generally available, it may still be used in specific cases to treat *Hansen's disease* (leprosy) and certain types of cancer.

thallium

A rare metallic element that is present as compounds in some zinc and lead ores. Poisoning over a prolonged period causes loss of hair, disorders of the nerves in the limbs, and disturbance of the stomach and intestines. Thallium-201 (an artificial radioactive isotope) is sometimes used during *radionuclide scanning* of the heart.

THC

The abbreviation for tetrahydrocannabinol, the active ingredient in *marijuana*.

theca

A sheath of tissue covering a body part. An example is the *pericardium*, the membrane that encloses the heart.

thenar

The medical name for the palm of the hand. The term thenar is also used to refer specifically to the fleshy part of the palm at the base of the thumb.

theobromine

A substance that is chemically similar to caffeine and occurs naturally in coffee, tea, and cocoa. Theobromine has a weak diuretic effect and also dilates the blood vessels.

theophylline

A *bronchodilator drug* sometimes used to treat severe *asthma* in cases that have failed to respond to other treatments. Theophylline is given orally, but it is sometimes mixed with another drug in a preparation called *aminophylline* so that it can be given intravenously as emergency treatment.

Possible side effects of theophylline include nausea, vomiting, dizziness, diarrhoea, *palpitations*, and *seizures*.

therapeutic

A term meaning related to treatment. The therapeutic dose of a drug is the amount required to have the greatest beneficial effect.

therapeutic community

A method of treating *drug dependence*, *alcohol dependence*, and some *personality disorders* that involves patients living together as a group in a nonhospital environment, usually under supervision. (See also *social skills training*.)

therapy

The treatment of any disease or abnormal physical or mental condition.

therapy, aversion

See *aversion therapy*.

T

therapy, cognitive

See *cognitive–behavioural therapy*.

therapy, family

See *family therapy*.

therapy, occupational

See *occupational therapy*.

thermography

A technique by which the variations in temperature of different areas of skin are recorded. Thermography provides clues to the presence of diseases and abnormalities that alter the temperature of the skin, such as problems of the circulation, inflammation, and tumours. There are two types of thermography. In one, a camera or scanner picks up infrared radiation naturally emitted from the skin. In the other, sheets of temperature-sensitive liquid crystals are applied to the skin; they change colour in response to changes in temperature.

thermometer

An instrument that is used to measure *temperature*. A traditional clinical thermometer consists of a glass capillary tube (a tube with a very fine bore), which is sealed at one end and has a mercury-filled bulb at the other.

Mercury thermometers are being phased out and modern versions of the clinical thermometer include an electronic probe that is connected to a digital display, and an aural thermometer, which measures the temperature of the *eardrum*. Both of these versions give an almost instant reading. There are also disposable skin thermometers, which employ heat-sensitive chemicals that change colour at specific temperatures. These are not as reliable, however, as standard thermometers.

Clinical thermometers may be calibrated in degrees Celsius (sometimes referred to as centigrade), degrees Fahrenheit, or sometimes both.

thermoregulation

The body's internal, automatic temperature-regulating mechanism, which is controlled by the *hypothalamus* in the brain. (See also *temperature*; *heat disorders*; *hyperthermia*; *hypothermia*.)

thiamine

See *vitamin B complex*.

thiazides

A type of *diuretic drug*.

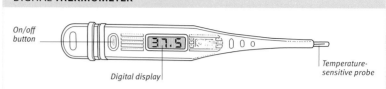

DIGITAL **THERMOMETER**

On/off button

Digital display

Temperature-sensitive probe

thiazolidinediones

Sometimes referred to as glitazones, a group of oral hypoglycaemic drugs (see *hypoglycaemics, oral*) that are used in the treatment of type 2 *diabetes mellitus*. Thiazolidinediones work by reducing the resistance of the body cells to *insulin* and are often used in combination with other oral hypoglycaemics, such as *metformin* or a sulphonylurea drug. The two main thiazolidinediones are *pioglitazone* and *rosiglitazone*.

thiopental

A *barbiturate drug* that is widely used as a general anaesthetic (see *anaesthesia, general*). Thiopental is given by intravenous injection.

thirst

The desire to drink. Thirst is one means by which the amount of water in the body is controlled (the other is the volume of urine excreted).

Thirst is stimulated by an increased concentration of salt, sugar, or certain other substances in the blood. As the blood passes through the *hypothalamus* in the brain, special nerve receptors are stimulated, inducing the sensation of thirst. Thirst is also stimulated if blood volume decreases as a result of sweating, vomiting, diarrhoea, severe bleeding, or extensive burns. Thirst may also be caused by a dry mouth.

thirst, excessive

A strong and persistent need to drink, most commonly due to *dehydration*. Other possible causes include untreated *diabetes mellitus* and *diabetes insipidus*, kidney failure, treatment with certain drugs such as *phenothiazine drugs*, and severe blood loss. Abnormal thirst may also be due to a psychological condition known as psychogenic polydipsia.

Thomsen's disease

A rare inherited disorder, also called myotonia congenita, in which myotonia (a condition in which muscles contract and then cannot relax again) begins in early childhood and persists throughout life. The myotonia is usually mild. An affected person may experience stiffness and cramps at rest, but symptoms usually subside on exercise. The disorder is inherited in an autosomal dominant manner (see *genetic disorders*).

thoracic outlet syndrome

A condition in which pressure on the *brachial plexus* (the nerve roots that pass into the arms from the neck) causes pain in the arms and shoulders, pins-and-needles sensation in the fingers, and weakness of grip and other hand movements. Severe symptoms are usually caused by a *cervical rib*, which is an extra rib located above the first rib. Thoracic outlet syndrome may also be caused by drooping of the shoulders, an enlarged scalenus muscle in the neck, or a tumour. The condition is made worse by lifting and carrying heavy loads or increases in body weight.

Treatment of thoracic outlet syndrome usually consists of exercises to improve posture, which may sometimes be combined with *nonsteroidal anti-inflammatory drugs*. Severe cases may be treated by surgical removal of the first rib.

thoracic surgery

A surgical speciality that is concerned with operations on organs within the chest cavity. Sometimes, thoracic surgery is combined with heart surgery, in which case it is known as cardio-thoracic surgery.

thoracotomy

An operation in which the chest is opened to provide access to organs in the chest (thoracid) cavity.

There are two types of thoracotomy: lateral and anterior. In a lateral thoracotomy the chest is opened between two ribs to provide access to the *lungs*, major blood vessels, and the *oesophagus*. In an anterior thoracotomy, an incision down the length of the sternum (breastbone) provides access to the *heart* and the *coronary arteries*.

T

thorax

The medical name for the chest. The thorax extends from the base of the neck to the *diaphragm muscle*.

thought

The complex mental activity that enables humans to reason, form judgments, and solve problems. The essential features of thought processes include the substitution of symbols (in the form of words, numbers, or images) for objects, the formation of symbols into ideas, and the arrangement of ideas into a certain order in the mind. (See also *thought disorders*.)

thought disorders

Abnormalities in the structure or content of *thought*, as reflected in a person's speech, writing, or behaviour. *Schizophrenia* causes several types of thought disorder, including the loss of logical connections between associations, the invention of new words (*neologisms*), thought blocking (sudden interruption in the train of thought), the feeling that thoughts are being inserted into or withdrawn from the mind, and *hallucinations*, usually of an auditory form.

Incoherent thoughts occur in all types of *confusion*, including *dementia* and delirium. Rapidly jumping from one idea to another occurs in *hypomania* and *mania*. In *depression*, thinking becomes slow, and there is a lack of association and a tendency to dwell in great detail on trivial subjects. In *obsessive–compulsive disorder*, recurrent ideas seem to come into a person's mind involuntarily. *Delusions*, which occur in schizophrenia and other psychotic illnesses, may be an expression of distorted thinking.

threadworm infestation

A common infestation with a small worm, ENTEROBIUS VERMICULARIS (also called pinworm), that lives in the intestines. Threadworms mainly affect children.

Female adult threadworms are white and about 1 cm long (large enough to see). They lay eggs in the skin around the anus, and their movements cause itching in the anal region, often at night. Eggs are transferred from the fingers to the mouth to cause reinfestation or are carried on toys or blankets to other children. Swallowed eggs hatch in the intestine and the worms reach maturity after a period of two to six weeks. For further information see *Cycle of threadworm infestation* box, overleaf.

DIAGNOSIS AND TREATMENT
Adult worms can sometimes be seen in the faeces or on the buttocks. The worms and their eggs can be collected by applying a piece of sticky tape to the anal area. Treatment is with an *anthelmintic drug*, which usually clears up the problem. Doctors recommend that all members of a family be treated at the same time to prevent reinfection.

threatened miscarriage

Warning signs that a pregnancy may be about to end before full term (see *miscarriage*). There is bleeding from the vagina, although the cervix remains closed and the fetus stays in the uterus. An *ultrasound* scan may help confirm whether the fetus is alive.

thrill

A vibrating sensation felt when the flat of the hand is held against an area of the body. Thrill is caused by turbulent blood flow in an *artery* or the *heart*. The term is also used to describe the feeling produced by fluid within the abdominal cavity in *ascites*.

throat

A popular term for the *pharynx*. The term is also sometimes used to refer to the front of the neck.

throat cancer

See *pharynx, cancer of*; *larynx, cancer of*.

thrombectomy

The removal of a *thrombus* (blood clot) that is blocking a blood vessel. It is performed as an emergency procedure if a major artery is blocked, or as a precautionary measure if there is a risk of an *embolus* (fragment) breaking off. Before surgery, the site of the thrombus is established by *angiography* and the patient may be given *anticoagulant drugs*.

thromboangiitis obliterans

Another name for *Buerger's disease*.

thrombocyte

An alternative name for a *platelet* (the smallest type of blood cell).

thrombocytopenia

A reduction in the number of *platelets* (the smallest type of blood cell) in the blood. Because platelets play a vital role in the blood-clotting process, thrombo-

---

ANATOMY OF THE **THORAX**

The heart, lungs, and large blood vessels (such as the aorta) occupy almost all of the thoracic cavity; a section of the oesophagus and the trachea are also in the thorax. The thoracic contents are protected and supported by a framework composed of the ribs, sternum (breastbone), and vertebrae.

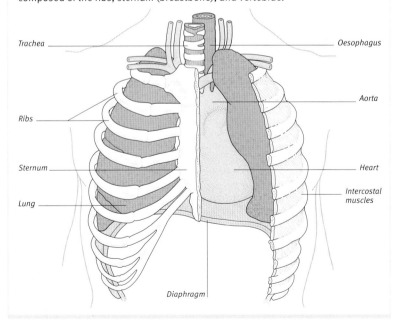

Trachea — Oesophagus — Aorta — Ribs — Sternum — Heart — Intercostal muscles — Lung — Diaphragm

T

CYCLE OF **THREADWORM INFESTATION**

The adult worms live in the large intestine, from where the females migrate to lay eggs around the anal region. Eggs may be transferred to the mouth (via fingers, sheets, or toys), are swallowed, and hatch to start a new infestation. Occasionally, in a girl, worms can affect the vagina, causing discharge.

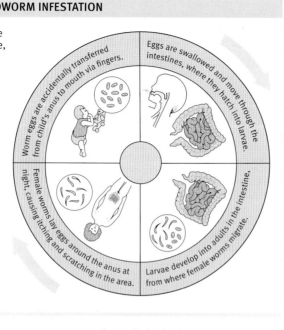

Worm eggs are accidentally transferred from child's anus to mouth via fingers.

Eggs are swallowed and move through the intestines, where they hatch into larvae.

Female worms lay eggs around the anus at night, causing itching and scratching in the area.

Larvae develop into adults in the intestine, from where female worms migrate.

symptoms. Women with thrombophilia are advised not to use *oral contraceptives* or *hormone replacement therapy*.

thrombophlebitis

Inflammation of a section of vein, usually just under the skin, with clot formation in the affected part. This can occur after minor injury to the vein or as a complication of *varicose veins* or *Buerger's disease*. The affected blood vessel is swollen, red, and tender, and feels hard. Fever and malaise may occur. In some cases, there may be an underlying deep vein thrombosis (see *thrombosis, deep vein*), and an *ultrasound scan* may be performed to check for this possibility.

If there is an underlying deep vein thrombosis, treatment is for this cause. Otherwise, treatment includes support with a bandage, *nonsteroidal anti-inflammatory drugs*, and sometimes antibiotic drugs. The condition usually clears up in 10–14 days.

cytopenia causes a tendency to bleed, especially from smaller vessels. Thrombocytopenic *purpura* (abnormal bleeding into the skin) sometimes develops.

CAUSES

The cause of thrombocytopenia may be a reduced rate of platelet production or a fast rate of platelet destruction. The disorder can be a feature of certain diseases, including *leukaemia*, *lymphoma*, systemic *lupus erythematosus*, *HIV* infection, megaloblastic *anaemia*, and *hypersplenism*. It can also be caused by excessive alcohol intake, a viral illness, exposure to *radiation*, or an adverse reaction to a drug such as a thiazide *diuretic*. Idiopathic *thrombocytopenic purpura* (ITP) is an *autoimmune disorder*.

DIAGNOSIS AND TREATMENT

Thrombocytopenia is confirmed by a *blood count*; a bone marrow test may also be performed. Any underlying disease is treated, if possible. Children with ITP may not need treatment but adults are usually given *corticosteroid drugs*. In some cases of severe, acute bleeding, a transfusion of platelets may be given. Persistent thrombocytopenia may be treated with a *splenectomy* (removal of the spleen).

thromboembolism

Blockage of a blood vessel by a piece of a blood clot (embolus) that has broken off from a *thrombus* elsewhere in the circulation. (See also *thrombosis*; *embolism*.)

thrombolytic drugs

COMMON DRUGS
• Alteplase • Reteplase • Streptokinase
• Tenecteplase

Sometimes called fibrinolytic drugs, this group of drugs is used to treat acute *myocardial infarction* (heart attack), *thrombosis* and *embolism* in which a blood vessel is blocked by a blood clot, and some cases of acute *stroke*. Thrombolytic drugs act within blood vessels to dissolve clots. They are administered intravenously and must be given promptly to be effective. Possible side effects include abnormal bleeding and allergic reaction.

thrombophilia

A tendency for blood to clot too readily, which leads to an increased risk of disorders, such as deep vein thrombosis (see *thrombosis, deep vein*) and *stroke*, due to blockage of blood vessels by clots (called *thrombosis*). This tendency may be due to an inherited deficiency or abnormality in proteins such as *factor V* that are involved in clotting. Thrombophilia may also be caused by the immune disorder antiphospholipid syndrome, which is associated with an increased risk of miscarriage as well as of circulatory disorders due to thrombosis.

Thrombophilia may go unrecognized until conditions, such as air travel or injury, that increase the risk of clots cause

thrombosis

The formation of a *thrombus* (blood clot) in an undamaged blood vessel. Clotting is a normal response when a blood vessel wall is injured, but abnormal when a vessel has not been punctured.

A thrombus that forms within an artery supplying the heart muscle (coronary thrombosis) is the usual cause of *myocardial infarction* (heart attack). A thrombus in an artery of the brain (cerebral thrombosis) is a common cause of *stroke*.

Thrombi may block arteries supplying blood to the legs, kidneys, retinas, intestines, and other organs, sometimes causing severe damage and symptoms such as pain and loss of function. Another danger is that an embolus (fragment of a thrombus) may break off and be carried by the blood to block an important blood vessel in another area (see *embolism*).

Thrombi can also form in veins, either just beneath the skin or in deeper veins (see *thrombosis, deep vein*).

CAUSES

In the blood there is a fine balance between the mechanisms that encourage and discourage clotting, so there is neither a tendency to bleed nor to form clots too readily (see *blood clotting*). Thrombosis can occur if this mechanism is disturbed in favour of clotting. (See *thrombophilia*.)

In arteries, thrombus formation is encouraged by *atherosclerosis* (a buildup of fatty deposits on the walls of

T

arteries), smoking, *hypertension* (high blood pressure), and damage to blood vessel walls from inflammation in *arteritis* and *phlebitis*. An increased clotting tendency may occur in *pregnancy*, with the use of *oral contraceptives or hormone replacement therapy (HRT)*, or through prolonged immobility.

SYMPTOMS

An arterial thrombosis may cause no symptoms until the blood flow is impaired. When this occurs, it leads to reduced function in the tissue supplied by the affected artery, and sometimes severe pain. Venous thrombosis may cause pain and swelling.

DIAGNOSIS AND TREATMENT

Diagnosis of thrombosis is by Doppler *ultrasound*. In some cases, *angiography* or *venography* may also be used. Treatment may include *anticoagulant*

drugs* or *thrombolytic drugs*, *nonsteroidal anti-inflammatory drugs*, and, in some cases, *antibiotic drugs*. In life-threatening cases, *thrombectomy* (surgical removal of the blood clot) may be needed.

thrombosis, deep vein

The formation of a *thrombus* (blood clot) within deep-lying veins in the leg.

CAUSES

The cause is usually a combination of slow blood flow through one part of the body (such as when sitting for long periods or when tissues are compressed, as occurs in long-haul aircraft flights) and an increase in the blood's clotting tendency, which occurs in dehydration, after surgery or injury, in pregnancy, in some inherited conditions (see *thrombophilia*), and in women taking *oral contraceptives or hormone replacement*

therapy (HRT). Deep vein thrombosis may also be due to *polycythaemia* (increased numbers of red cells in the blood).

Deep vein thrombosis is common in people with *heart failure*; those who have had a *stroke*; and those who have been bedridden. People who are obese and/or smoke are at increased risk of developing the condition.

SYMPTOMS

Clots in the leg veins may cause pain, tenderness, swelling, discoloration, and ulceration of the skin, but they can be symptomless. A deep vein thrombosis is not necessarily serious in itself, but part of the clot may break off and travel in the bloodstream to the lungs. This is known as a *pulmonary embolism*.

DIAGNOSIS AND TREATMENT

A diagnosis is made by Doppler *ultrasound scanning* or *venography*. A special

DEEP VEIN THROMBOSIS

Thrombi, or clots, tend to form when blood flow is sluggish or if there is a rise in the level of coagulation factors in the blood. Once a clot has formed, it may provide a site for further clotting, so that a long, snaky clot may grow along the length of a vein. There is a risk that the end of such a clot may break off into the circulation. Thrombi form most commonly in the leg veins and may interfere with the drainage of blood from a leg (below right), causing signs and symptoms of varying severity.

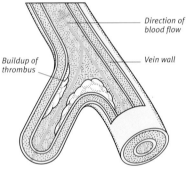

Direction of blood flow

Buildup of thrombus

Vein wall

Partly blocked vein **Healthy vein**

Normal and obstructed vein
Thrombi tend to form at points where a vein lining is damaged and may then grow to obstruct blood flow. The main danger is that a piece of clot will detach and be carried to the heart and lungs to cause a potentially fatal obstruction.

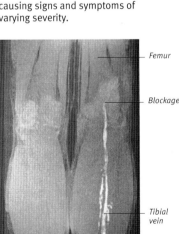

Femur

Blockage

Tibial vein

Example of deep vein thrombosis
This MRI of the leg of a patient with deep vein thrombosis shows the vein blocked by a thrombus (blood clot).

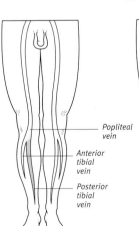

Popliteal vein

Anterior tibial vein

Posterior tibial vein

Calf vein thrombosis
When clots are localized in the lower-leg veins, there is usually some pain in the calf but there may be little swelling.

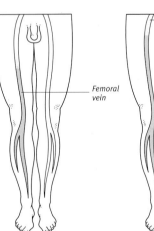

Femoral vein

Femoral vein thrombosis
If clots are present in the femoral and the lower-leg veins, there is usually pain and swelling up to the region above the knee.

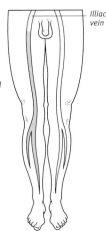

Illiac vein

Iliac vein thrombosis
Clots in the iliac vein may affect drainage of blood from the whole leg, causing severe pain and swelling in the leg.

T

blood test (called the D-dimer test) may also be carried out to check the coagulability of the blood.

Treatment is usually with *anticoagulant drugs* to prevent further clotting. In some cases, *thrombolytic drugs* may be used to dissolve clots. If there is a high risk of pulmonary embolism, *thrombectomy* (surgical removal of the clot) may be performed. Subsequently, the risk of recurrence can be reduced by wearing compression stockings, and in some cases long-term use of anticoagulant drugs may be recommended.

PREVENTION

The risk of deep vein thrombosis during long-haul flights can be reduced by wearing compression stockings, moving the legs and feet frequently, and drinking plenty of nonalcoholic fluids. For people who are overweight and/or smoke, losing the excess weight and stopping smoking can reduce the risk.

thrombus

A blood clot that has formed inside an intact blood vessel. A thrombus is life-threatening if it obstructs the blood supply to an organ such as the heart or brain. A thrombus may also lead to *gangrene* (tissue death) in an organ or extremity, or to *embolism*, in which a fragment of the thrombus breaks off and is carried to obstruct the blood circulation elsewhere in the body. (See also *blood clotting*; *thrombosis*.)

thrush

A common name for the fungal infection *candidiasis*.

thumb-sucking

A common habit in young children, which provides comfort, oral gratification, and reassurance. Thumb-sucking tends to decrease after age three, and most children grow out of it by age seven. In most cases it is not harmful but *malocclusion* (incorrect alignment) of the permanent teeth may develop if the habit continues past seven years of age. This problem is usually temporary, but if the thumb-sucking persists, an *orthodontic appliance* may be needed.

thymoma

A rare *tumour* of the *thymus gland*. The tumour can arise from any of the cell types in the thymus gland and can be cancerous or noncancerous. Thymoma is associated with the autoimmune disorder *myasthenia gravis*.

thymoxamine

See *moxisylyte*.

thymus gland

A gland that forms part of the *immune system*. It lies behind the *sternum* (breastbone) and consists of two lobes that join in front of the *trachea* (windpipe). Each lobe is made of lymphoid tissue consisting of *lymphocytes* (white blood cells), *epithelium* (lining cells), and fat.

The thymus conditions lymphocytes to become *T-cells*. It plays a part in the immune response until *puberty*, gradually enlarging during this time. After puberty, it shrinks, but some glandular tissue remains until middle-age.

thyroglossal disorders

A set of congenital defects caused by failure of the thyroglossal duct to close before birth. In *embryos*, the duct runs from the base of the tongue to the *thyroid gland*. Abnormal development may cause the duct to persist in its entirety or partly as a cyst. A cyst may become infected and swollen, which may lead to formation of a *fistula* (abnormal passage) between the cyst and surface of the neck. The cyst and any remnants of the duct are removed.

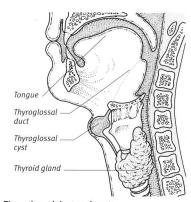

Thyroglossal duct and cyst
The thyroglossal duct, lying between the tongue and the thyroid, sometimes persists after fetal life, and a cyst may form at any point along the duct.

thyroid cancer

Rare *tumours* of the *thyroid gland*. In most cases the cause is unknown, although exposure to radioactive fallout increases the risk of the condition.

TYPES AND SYMPTOMS

There are several types, depending on the cells involved. In all types, the first sign is a firm nodule in the neck, which may grow slowly or rapidly (however, a nodule does not necessarily indicate cancer: about 10 per cent of thyroid

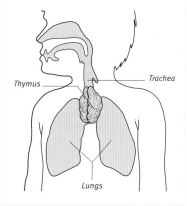
tumours are found to be cancerous). In many cases, the cancer is painless and symptoms such as difficulty swallowing, and hoarseness or loss of voice, only develop when the tumour presses on other structures.

DIAGNOSIS AND TREATMENT

A diagnosis is made by *thyroid scanning* and *needle aspiration* or a *biopsy*. A *thyroidectomy* (surgical removal of thyroid tissue) is usually followed by treatment with radioactive *iodine* to destroy any residual cancer. Cure rates depend on the cell type and on the size and spread of the tumour when it is diagnosed. Patients need to take the thyroid hormone *thyroxine* for the rest of their lives.

thyroidectomy

Surgical removal of all or part of the *thyroid gland*, which is performed as a treatment for *thyroid cancer*, some cases of *hyperthyroidism* (overactivity of the thyroid) and of *goitre* (enlargement of the thyroid), or a noncancerous tumour of the thyroid gland.

thyroid-function tests

A group of blood tests used to evaluate the function of the *thyroid gland* and to diagnose under- or overactivity of the gland. Tests may include measurement of levels of the thyroid hormones T_3 and T_4, as well as thyroid-stimulating hormone (TSH), the *pituitary gland* hormone that stimulates the thyroid gland.

thyroid gland

One of the main *endocrine glands*, which helps to regulate the rate of all the body's internal processes. The thyroid is situated in the front of the neck, just below the *larynx* (voicebox). It consists of two lobes, one on each side of the *trachea* (windpipe), joined by a piece of tissue called the isthmus.

STRUCTURE AND FUNCTION

Thyroid tissue is composed of follicular cells, which secrete the iodine-containing hormones triiodothyronine (T_3) and thyroxine (T_4), and parafollicular cells (C cells), which secrete the hormone *calcitonin*. T_3 and T_4 are important in controlling metabolism. Calcitonin helps to regulate calcium balance in the body. (See also *thyroid hormones*; *Disorders of the thyroid gland* box.)

LOCATION OF THE THYROID GLAND

This major gland lies at the base of the neck just in front of the trachea (windpipe).

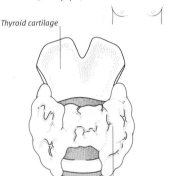

Thyroid cartilage

Trachea

Thyroid gland

---

thyroid hormones

The three hormones produced by the *thyroid gland* are thyroxine (T_4) and triiodothyronine (T_3), which regulate metabolism, and *calcitonin*, which helps regulate calcium levels. See *Control of thyroid hormone production* box, overleaf.

thyroiditis

Inflammation of the *thyroid gland*; it occurs in several different forms. The most common is *Hashimoto's thyroiditis*, an *autoimmune disorder* that causes *hypothyroidism*. Less commonly, thy-

---

DISORDERS OF THE **THYROID GLAND**

The function of the thyroid gland is controlled by both the pituitary gland and the hypothalamus, so thyroid disorders may be due not only to defects in the gland itself, but also to disruption of the hypothalamic-pituitary hormonal control system. Disorders of the thyroid gland may cause overproduction of thyroid hormones (*hyperthyroidism*), underproduction of these hormones (*hypothyroidism*), or enlargement or distortion of the gland. *Myxoedema*, *Graves' disease*, and *Hashimoto's thyroiditis* are common disorders. *Goitre* (enlargement of the thyroid gland) may sometimes occur with no accompanying abnormality of thyroid function.

Congenital disorders

In rare cases, the thyroid gland is absent at birth, producing *cretinism*. However, congenital thyroid deficiency more often takes the form of underdevelopment or maldevelopment, in which there is some thyroid tissue but not enough to secrete normal amounts of hormones. A blood test is performed on newborns to screen for hypothyroidism. Sometimes the thyroid develops in an abnormal position in the neck, causing, rarely, difficulty swallowing or breathing.

Genetic disorders

Rarely, genetic disorder may impair the thyroid's ability to make hormones. The low blood level of thyroid hormones results in greatly increased secretion by the pituitary gland of thyroid-stimulating hormone (TSH), which, in turn, causes the thyroid to enlarge.

Infection

Thyroid infection is uncommon; it leads to *thyroiditis* (inflammation of the thyroid gland). Viral infection can cause an extremely painful gland and temporary hyperthyroidism.

Tumours

Thyroid tumours may be either cancerous or noncancerous. Thyroid *adenomas* are noncancerous tumours that may secrete thyroid hormone,

sometimes in large enough amounts to cause hyperthyroidism. *Thyroid cancers* are relatively rare. They may be suspected if a single firm or hard lump can be felt in the gland.

Autoimmune disorders

Graves' disease is a form of thyroid overactivity thought to be due to the body's immune system producing antibodies that attack the thyroid gland. In Hashimoto's thyroiditis, antibodies damage glandular cells.

Myxoedema

Deficiency of thyroid hormone, which may occur for a variety of reasons, causes a condition known as myxoedema, in which the skin becomes dry and thickened and facial features become coarse. Constipation, cold intolerance, and fatigue are other common symptoms.

Hormonal disorders

Hormonal changes during puberty or pregnancy may cause a degree of goitre temporarily. Hyperthyroidism due to excessive production of TSH by the pituitary gland is rare but it may result from a *pituitary tumour*.

Iodine deficiency

Because iodine is necessary for the production of thyroid hormone, its deficiency may lead to goitre, but it is uncommon in developed countries. severe iodine deficiency in children may cause myxoedema.

INVESTIGATION

Blood samples may be taken for *thyroid-function tests*, in which the levels of thyroid or pituitary hormones are measured. The thyroid gland itself may be imaged by various *thyroid scanning* techniques or ultrasound. In some cases, such as a suspected tumour, a *biopsy* may be carried out to obtain a sample of thyroid tissue for microscopic examination.

T

CONTROL OF **THYROID** HORMONE PRODUCTION

The blood levels of the hormones T3 (triiodothyronine) and T4 (thyroxine) produced by the thyroid must be kept within narrow limits, otherwise hyperthyroidism or hypothyroidism may result. The control systems below exist to achieve this balance but certain disorders may interfere with the system.

Raised blood levels of thyroid hormones

Bloodstream
If blood levels of the thyroid hormones T3 and T4 rise, they decrease the sensitivity of the pituitary to thyrotrophin-releasing hormone (TRH), secreted by the hypothalamus.

Hypothalamus
Secretes TRH.

Pituitary gland
The pituitary becomes less sensitive to TRH, so it secretes less thyroid-stimulating hormone (TSH).

Thyroid gland
In response to lowered TSH stimulation, the thyroid reduces its production of the hormones T3 and T4.

Bloodstream
The blood levels of T3 and T4 thus gradually fall back to normal.

Reduced blood levels of thyroid hormones

Bloodstream
If blood levels of the thyroid hormones T3 and T4 fall, the hypothalamus is stimulated to produce more TRH.

Hypothalamus
Increases secretion of TRH.

Pituitary gland
In response to stimulation by TRH, the pituitary increases production of TSH.

Thyroid gland
In response to increased TSH stimulation, the thyroid increases its production of T3 and T4.

Bloodstream
The blood levels of T3 and T4 thus gradually rise back to normal.

---

roiditis is associated with a viral infection, or it may occur temporarily in women after childbirth.

thyroid scanning

Techniques, such as *radionuclide scanning* and *ultrasound scanning*, that are able to

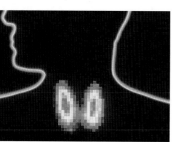

Thyroid scanning
This is a gamma scan (scintigram) of a healthy thyroid gland. An injected radioactive tracer substance shows areas of activity within the gland.

give information on the location, anatomy, and function of the *thyroid gland* and detect tumours.

thyroid-stimulating hormone

A hormone that is produced in the *pituitary gland*, which is located at the base of the brain. Thyroid-stimulating hormone (TSH) travels in the bloodstream to the *thyroid glands*, which are then stimulated by TSH to release other hormones (known as T$_3$ and T$_4$) that are involved in the body's use of energy. (See also *thyroid hormones*.)

thyrotoxicosis

Overactivity of the thyroid gland, also called *hyperthyroidism*.

thyroxine

Represented by the symbol T$_4$, the most important *thyroid hormone*. For thera-

peutic use in the treatment of *hypothyroidism* (underactivity of the thyroid gland), a synthetic form of thyroxine (called *levothyroxine*) is given orally.

TIA

The abbreviation for *transient ischaemic attack*, a brief interruption of the blood supply to part of the brain. Sometimes called a mini stroke, a TIA causes temporary impairment of vision, speech, sensation, or movement. Symptoms disappear completely within 24 hours.

tibia

Also called the shin, the inner and thicker of the two long bones in the lower leg. The tibia is the supporting bone of the lower leg. It runs parallel to the *fibula*, the narrower bone to which it is attached by *ligaments*. The upper end articulates with the *femur* (thigh bone) to form the *knee* joint; the lower end articulates with the *talus* to form part of the *ankle* joint. On the inside of the ankle, the tibia is widened and protrudes to form a bony prominence known as the medial malleolus.

FRACTURE

One of the most commonly fractured bones, the tibia may break across the shaft or at the upper end from a blow to the outside of the leg below the knee. Prolonged walking or running on hard ground may cause a *stress fracture*.

LOCATION OF THE **TIBIA**

Also called the shin, the tibia can easily be felt beneath the skin of the lower leg.

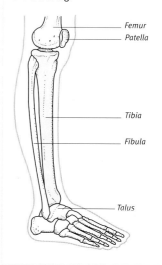

Femur
Patella
Tibia
Fibula
Talus

tibolone

A drug used in the short-term treatment of menopausal symptoms (see *hormone replacement therapy*), although it is not suitable for use during the perimenopausal period nor within a year of the last menstrual period. Tibolone is also used to protect against *osteoporosis* (although it is not usually recommended as a first-line treatment). It is given continuously and combines the effects of *oestrogen* and *progestogen drugs*.

Possible adverse effects are irregular vaginal bleeding, changes in weight, ankle *oedema* (fluid swelling), dizziness, skin reactions, headache, and facial hair growth. Tibolone also increases the risk of *breast cancer*, but to a lesser extent than combined HRT.

tic

A repeated, uncontrolled, purposeless contraction of a *muscle* or group of muscles, most commonly in the face, shoulders, or arms. Typical tics include blinking, mouth twitching, and shrugging. Often, the cause is unknown, although a tic may be a sign of a minor psychological problem. Tics usually develop in childhood; most stop within about a year of onset, although in some cases they may persist into adult life. (See also *Gilles de la Tourette's syndrome*.)

tic douloureux

Another name for *trigeminal neuralgia*.

ticks and disease

Ticks are small, eight-legged animals that feed on blood and sometimes transmit diseases to humans via their bites. They are about 3 mm long before feeding and become larger when full of blood. Ticks may be picked up in long grass, scrub, woodland, or caves.

In the UK, the only disease known to be transmitted to humans by ticks is *Lyme disease*. In other parts of the world tick-borne diseases include *relapsing fever*, *Rocky Mountain spotted fever*, *Q fever*, *tularaemia*, tick typhus, and certain types of viral *encephalitis*. The prolonged bite of certain female ticks can cause tick paralysis, in which a toxin in the tick saliva affects nerves that control movement; in extreme cases, this can prove fatal.

Tietze's syndrome

Chest pain localized to an area on the front of the chest wall, usually made worse by movement of the arms or trunk or by pressure on the chest wall. The syndrome, also called costochondritis, is caused by inflammation of one or several rib cartilages and symptoms may persist for months. Treatment is with *analgesics*, *nonsteroidal anti-inflammatory drugs*, or, if symptoms persist, a local injection of *corticosteroid drugs* into the cartilage.

Tildiem

A brand name for diltiazem, a *calcium channel blocker* used to treat *hypertension* (high blood pressure) and *angina*.

timolol

A *beta-blocker drug* used to treat *hypertension* (high blood pressure) and *angina pectoris* (chest pain due to inadequate blood supply to the heart). Timolol may be given after a *myocardial infarction* (heart attack) and may also be used to prevent *migraine* attacks. Timolol is used as eye-drops in the treatment of *glaucoma* (raised pressure in the eye).

Possible side effects, such as cold hands and feet, are typical of other betablockers. The eye-drops may cause irritation, blurred vision, and headache.

tinea

Any of a group of common *fungal infections* of the skin, hair, or nails. Most are caused by fungi called dermatophytes. The infections, often called ringworm, may be acquired from other people, animals, soil, shower floors, or household objects, such as chairs or carpets.

TYPES AND SYMPTOMS

The most common type of tinea infection is tinea pedis (*athlete's foot*). Tinea corporis (ringworm of the body) causes itchy, usually circular, patches with a prominent edge. Tinea cruris (which is commonly called jock itch) produces a reddened, itchy area spreading from the genitals over the inside thighs. This form of tinea is more common in males. Tinea capitis (scalp ringworm) causes round, itchy, patches of hair loss on the scalp; it occurs mainly in children. Ringworm of the nails (tinea unguium) is often accompanied by scaling of the soles or palms. The nails become thick and turn white or yellow.

DIAGNOSIS AND TREATMENT

Most types of tinea are easily recognizable by appearance, but the diagnosis may be confirmed by culturing the organisms in a laboratory. Treatment is usually with topical *antifungal drugs* in the form of skin creams or ointments. However, for widespread infections or those affecting the hair or nails, oral drug treatment may be necessary.

tinea versicolor

An alternative name for *pityriasis versicolor*, a common skin disorder caused by a fungus.

tingling

See *pins-and-needles*.

tinidazole

An *antibacterial* drug that is particularly useful in treating *anaerobic* infections. Tinidazole is also used with other drugs to eradicate infection with the HELICOBACTER PYLORI bacterium. Possible adverse effects of tinidazole include nausea, vomiting, gastrointestinal disturbances, headache, and dizziness. Alcohol should be avoided during treatment.

tinnitus

A ringing, buzzing, whistling, hissing, or other noise heard one or both ears in the absence of external noise.

CAUSES

In tinnitus, the *acoustic nerve* transmits impulses to the brain, not as the result of vibrations produced by external sound waves, but, for reasons that are not fully understood, as the result of stimuli originating inside the head or within the ear itself. Tinnitus is almost always associated with hearing loss, particularly that due to *presbyacusis* (age-related loss of hearing) and exposure to loud noise. The condition can also occur as a symptom of ear disorders such as *labyrinthitis*, *Ménière's disease*, *otitis media*, *otosclerosis*, *ototoxicity*, and blockage of the ear canal with earwax. It may also be caused by certain drugs, such as *aspirin* or *quinine*, or may follow a *head injury*.

SYMPTOMS

The noise in the ear can sometimes change in nature or intensity. In most cases, however, it is present continuously, although the affected individual may not be aware of its presence all the time. Tolerance of tinnitus varies from one person to another. Many people learn to live with the condition, while other people find it almost intolerable.

TREATMENT

Any underlying disorder is treated if possible. Many sufferers of tinnitus make use of various means, such as a radio, television, cassette player, or headphones, to block out the noise in

T

their ears. A tinnitus masker, a hearing-aid type device that plays white noise (a random mixture of sounds at a wide range of frequencies), may be effective.

tinzaparin

A type of low molecular weight *heparin* (anticoagulant drug) that may be injected once daily in the treatment of deep vein thrombosis (see *thrombosis, deep vein*)or *pulmonary embolism*. It may also be used to prevent *thromboembolism* in patients undergoing some times of surgery.

tiotropium

A drug used in the treatment of chronic obstructive pulmonary disease (see *pulmonary disease, chronic obstructive*). Tiotropium, which is taken by inhalation (see *inhaler*), can help to relieve shortness of breath.

tiredness

A common complaint that is usually the result of overwork or poor quality or insufficient sleep. Persistent tiredness may be caused by a number of conditions, including *depression*, *anxiety*, *anaemia*, and *diabetes mellitus*.

tissue

A collection of *cells* specialized to perform a particular function. Examples include muscle tissue, which consists of cells specialized to contract (shorten); epithelial tissue, which forms the *skin* and *mucous membranes* that line the respiratory and other tracts; nerve tissue, comprising cells specialized to conduct electrochemical nerve impulses; and *connective tissue*, which includes *adipose tissue* (fat), and the various fibrous and elastic tissues (such as tendons and cartilage) that hold the body together.

tissue fluid

The watery liquid present in the tiny gaps between body cells, also known as interstitial fluid. Tissue fluid is one component of extracellular fluid (any body fluid outside the cells, including blood and lymph).

To reach the body's cells, oxygen and nutrients must pass from the blood vessels and into the tissue fluid. Similarly, there is a reverse movement of carbon dioxide and other waste products from the cells into the tissue fluid, and then into the bloodstream.

In addition to nutrients and wastes, tissue fluid also contains *ions*. This fluid contains a much higher level of sodium ions, and a much lower level of potassium ions, than intracellular fluid. It is this difference in ion levels that helps to control the movement of water into and out of cells by osmosis; ion levels also play a role in the transmission of electrical impulses through nerves and muscles.

Tissue fluid is formed by the filtration of liquid out through the walls of the first part of blood capillaries (that is, the part nearest an arteriole), where it is forced out by the high blood pressure. In the last part of capillaries (nearest to a venule), blood pressure is much lower, and tissue fluid passes back into the capillaries; some tissue fluid is also drained away into the lymphatic vessels. Thus, there is a continual flow that keeps the amount of tissue fluid constant. Various disorders, for example, congestive *heart failure*, disrupt the balance between formation and drainage of tissue fluid, leading to the accumulation of excess fluid in the tissues, a condition called *oedema*.

tissue-plasminogen activator

Also called TPA, a substance produced by the inner lining of blood vessels that helps dissolve blood clots. TPA can be prepared artificially for use as a *thrombolytic drug*, which is called alteplase. This is used to treat acute *myocardial infarction* (heart attack), *pulmonary embolism* (blockage of the artery supplying the lungs), and acute *stroke*. Possible side effects of TPA include nausea and vomiting, bleeding or the formation of a *haematoma* (collection of blood) at the injection site, and an allergic reaction. (See also *fibrinolysis*.)

tissue-typing

The classification of certain characteristics of the *tissues* of prospective organ donors and recipients (see *transplant surgery*). This minimizes the risk of rejection of a donor organ by the recipient's *immune system* after transplantation.

A person's tissue type is classified in terms of his or her *histocompatibility antigens*, the most important of which are human leukocyte antigens (HLAs), on the surface of cells. A person's set of HLAs is inherited and unique (except for identical twins, who have the same set). Nevertheless, close relatives often have closely matching HLA types.

HOW IT IS DONE

A person's tissue-type is established by laboratory tests on cells from a blood sample. In one method, an antiserum containing *antibodies* to a particular HLA is added to the test specimen. If the HLA is present, it is detected by an observable colour or other change.

titanium dental implants

See *implants, dental*.

titubation

Tremor or a nodding movement of the head and/or a stumbling gait, seen in some disorders of the *central nervous system* (brain and spinal cord).

T-lymphocyte

A type of *white blood cell*, also known as a T-cell, that plays a role in the *immune system*. (See also *helper T-cell*; *killer T-cell*; *memory T-cell*; *suppressor T-cell*.)

TMJ dysfunction

See *temporomandibular joint dysfunction*.

toadstool poisoning

See *mushroom poisoning*.

tobacco

The dried leaf of the plant NICOTIANA TAB-ACUM. Tobacco is used for smoking, chewing, or as snuff by billions of people. It contains a variable percentage of *nicotine*, and several carcinogenic substances. There is a direct relationship between the amount of tobacco used, the period over which it is used, and the likelihood of *cancer*. All tobacco users have an increased risk of cancers of the oral cavity (see *mouth cancer*), pharynx (see *pharynx, cancer of*), larynx (see *larynx, cancer of*) and oesophagus (see *oesophagus, cancer of*). Smokers are also at increased risk of developing a wide range of other disorders, as are passive smokers. For more information about the risks, see *smoking*.

tobacco-smoking

See *smoking*.

tobramycin

An *antibiotic drug* that is used to treat serious infections such as *septicaemia*, *meningitis*, and severe infections of the bile ducts, kidneys, prostate gland, and lining of the heart. Tobramycin is sometimes used in the form of eye-drops to treat eye inflammation. High doses of injected preparations of the drug may result in kidney damage, deafness, nausea, vomiting, and headache. Any preparation of tobramycin may cause rash and itching.

tocography

An obstetric procedure that is used to record muscular contractions of the uterus during *childbirth*. It is usually combined with *fetal heart monitoring* (see *cardiotocography*).

tocopherol

A constituent of *vitamin E*. Together, four tocopherols (alpha, beta, gamma, and delta) and several tocopherol derivatives make up the vitamin.

toddler's diarrhoea

A common condition affecting some children for a period after the introduction of an adult diet. It occurs because the child is unable to digest food properly, perhaps because of inadequate chewing. The diarrhoea is no cause for concern, and no treatment is needed.

Todd's paralysis

Weakness in part of the body following some types of epileptic seizure (see *epilepsy*). The weakness may last for minutes, hours, or even days, but there is no lasting effect. The cause is thought to be temporary damage to the motor cortex (the area of the *brain* that controls movement).

toe

One of the digits of the foot. Each toe has three *phalanges* (bones), except for the *hallux* (big toe), which has two. The phalanges join at hinge joints, which are moved by tendons that flex (bend) or extend (straighten) the toe. An artery, vein, and nerve run down each side of the toe, and the whole structure is enclosed in skin with a nail at the top. The main function of the toes is to maintain balance during walking.

DISORDERS

Congenital disorders include toes missing at birth, *polydactyly* (extra toes), *syndactyly* (fused toes), or *webbing* (skin flaps between the toes).

Injuries to the toes, including fractures, are fairly common. Inflammation of the joints, with pain, stiffness, and swelling, may be caused by *osteoarthritis*, *rheumatoid arthritis*, or *gout*.

A common deformity of the big toe is *hallux valgus*, in which the toe turns inwards to the others. This often leads to the development of a *bunion* over the joint at the base of the toe. Abnormality of a tendon in one of the toes may also cause distortion (see *hammer toe*).

toenail, ingrowing

A painful condition of a toe (usually the big toe) in which one or both edges of the nail press into the adjacent skin, leading to infection and inflammation. The cause is usually incorrect cutting of the nail or wearing tight-fitting shoes.

Pain relief can be obtained by bathing the foot once or twice daily in a strong, warm, salt solution, then covering the nail with a dry gauze dressing. *Antibiotics* may be prescribed. In some cases, the edge of the nail is removed and the nail bed obliterated to prevent recurrence.

toilet-training

The process of teaching a young child to acquire complete bowel and bladder control. A child is unlikely to be completely toilet-trained before age three and may normally take much longer to remain dry at night (see *enuresis*).

WHEN TO START

Up to about 18 months, emptying of the bladder or bowel is a totally automatic reaction. The child is not yet able to connect the actions of defaecation and urination with their results, and cannot control these actions at will.

At around 18 months, a child can usually indicate that he or she has passed urine or a bowel movement, but is not yet aware when he or she is about to do so. At this stage, the child is not quite ready to use a potty, but can practise sitting on it. By the age of two, a child is aware when he or she is about to pass urine or a bowel movement and says so. At this stage, the child is ready to start using the potty.

METHODS

Toilet-training should be approached in a relaxed, unhurried manner. A child should never be forced to sit on a potty. Boys initially urinate sitting down but soon learn how to manage standing up. Once a child uses the potty confidently, he or she can gradually progress to using the toilet.

When reasonable control has been achieved, the child can be taken out of nappies during the day. Nappies should be worn at night until the child is usually dry on waking.

Toilet accidents, particularly wetting, are common up to the age of five, because a young child can delay urination for only a few minutes. Some children revert to soiling or wetting when anxious or under stress. (See also *encopresis*; *enuresis*; *soiling*.)

tolbutamide

An oral hypoglycaemic drug (see *hypoglycaemics, oral*) used in the treatment of type 2 *diabetes mellitus*.

tolerance

The need to take ever higher doses of a *drug* to obtain the same physical or mental effect. It develops after taking a drug over a period of time, and usually results from the liver becoming more efficient at breaking the drug down or from tissues becoming less sensitive to it.

tolnaftate

An *antifungal drug* applied to the skin to treat, and sometimes prevent, recurrent *tinea* infections, including *athlete's foot*. In rare cases, tolnaftate may cause skin irritation or a rash.

tomography

An *imaging technique* that produces a cross-sectional image ("slice") of an organ or part. Most tomography is performed using *CT scanning* or *MRI*.

-tomy

A suffix denoting the operation of cutting or making an incision.

tone, muscle

The natural tension in *muscle* fibres. At rest, all muscle fibres are kept in a state of partial contraction by nerve impulses from the spinal cord. Abnormally high muscle tone causes increased resistance to movement, *spasticity*, and rigidity. Abnormally low muscle tone causes floppiness (see *hypotonia*).

ANATOMY OF THE TOES

Each hallux, or big toe, has two bones called phalanges, which are connected by hinge joints. All the other toes have three phalanges.

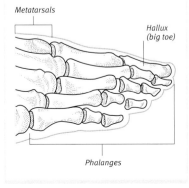

Metatarsals

Hallux (big toe)

Phalanges

T

tongue

A muscular, flexible organ in the floor of the *mouth*.

STRUCTURE AND FUNCTION

The tongue is composed of a mass of muscles covered by a *mucous membrane*. The muscles are attached to the *mandible* (lower jaw) and *hyoid* bone above the *larynx* (voicebox). The tongue is supplied by four *cranial nerves*.

Tiny nodules called papillae stick out from the tongue's upper surface, giving it a rough texture. On the papillae at the sides and base of the tongue are *taste buds*. The tongue plays an essential part in *mastication* (chewing), *swallowing*, and *speech*.

DISORDERS

A large tongue is a feature of *Down's syndrome*, *cretinism*, and *acromegaly*. Temporary enlargement of the tongue as a result of swelling and inflammation may occur in *glossitis*.

Cracks on the surface of the tongue are common and usually cause no problems. However, they are occasionally deep enough to trap food particles, causing discomfort. Unnatural smoothness of the tongue that is accompanied by redness and soreness (glossitis) is a feature of certain types of anaemia (see *anaemia, iron-deficiency*; *anaemia megaloblastic*). Dryness or excessive furring

of the tongue may be an indication of *dehydration* or may be symptoms of *Sjögren's syndrome* or, in infants, *candidiasis*.

In rare cases, for unknown reasons, the papillae become elongated and turn black or brown, a condition known as black tongue. This is harmless but unsightly and persistent. The discoloration can be removed by cleaning the tongue twice a day with a soft toothbrush dipped in antiseptic mouthwash.

The tongue can be a site for *mouth ulcers* and *leukoplakia* (thickened white or grey patches), a condition that occasionally becomes cancerous (see *tongue cancer*). Any ulcer developing on the tongue that does not disappear within about three weeks should be reported to a doctor without delay.

tongue cancer

The most serious type of *mouth cancer* due to its rapid spread. It mainly affects people over 40 and is associated with *smoking*, heavy alcohol consumption, and poor oral hygiene. The edge of the tongue is most commonly affected. The first sign may be a small ulcer with a raised margin, a white patch of thickened tissue called a *leukoplakia*, a fissure, or a raised, hard mass.

Diagnosis of tongue cancer is made by a *biopsy* (tissue sampling). Small tumours, especially those at the tip of the tongue, are removed surgically. Larger tumours or those that have spread often require *radiotherapy*.

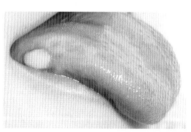

Appearance of tongue cancer
The cancer often starts at the edge of the tongue. It may appear as a raised mass (as here), as a fissure, or as an ulcer.

tongue depressor

A flat instrument used to hold the tongue on the floor of the mouth to allow examination of the throat.

tongue-tie

A minor *mouth* defect, also known as ankyloglossia, in which the frenulum (band of tissue attaching the underside of the tongue to the floor of the mouth)

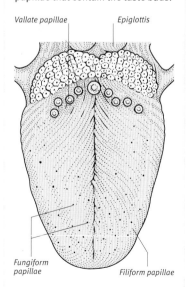
LOCATION OF THE TONSILS

The tonsils can be easily seen on either side of the back of the throat. They reach their maximum size at about the age of seven years and then shrink.

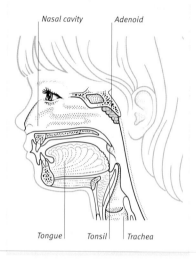

Nasal cavity *Adenoid*

Tongue *Tonsil* *Trachea*

is too short and extends forwards to the tip of the tongue. There are usually no symptoms apart from limited movement of the tongue. Rarely, the condition causes a speech defect, and minor surgery is required to divide the frenulum.

tonic

One of a group of remedies intended to relieve symptoms such as malaise, lethargy, and appetite loss. Evidence suggests that tonics mainly have a *placebo* effect. The term is also used adjectivally to relate to muscle tone (see *tone, muscle*), as in tonic neck reflex, one of the primitive *reflexes* found in newborn infants.

tonic–clonic seizure

Formerly called grand mal, a type of seizure in which consciousness is lost and there is muscle stiffness followed by uncontrolled jerking movements. The seizure normally lasts only a few minutes; prolonged tonic–clonic seizures can be life-threatening. (See *epilepsy*.)

tonometry

The procedure for measuring the pressure of the fluid within the *eye*, usually performed by an ophthalmologist or optician during an eye examination (see *eye, examination of*). Tonometry is useful in diagnosing *glaucoma* (increased pressure within the eyeball).

T

tonsil

One of a pair of oval tissue masses at the back of the throat on either side. The tonsils are made up of lymphoid tissue and form part of the *lymphatic system*. Along with the *adenoids*, the tonsils protect against upper respiratory tract infections. The tonsils gradually enlarge from birth until age seven, after which time they shrink substantially. *Tonsillitis* is a common childhood infection.

tonsillectomy

Surgical removal of the *tonsils*, which is now performed only if the patient suffers from frequent, recurrent attacks of severe *tonsillitis*. The operation is also carried out as a treatment for *quinsy* (an abscess around the tonsil).

PROCEDURE FOR TONSILLECTOMY

A tonsillectomy may be performed if the tonsils are very enlarged, after an abscess on the tonsil, or if tonsil infections are frequent and severe.

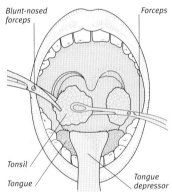

Blunt-nosed forceps
Forceps
Tonsil
Tongue
Tongue depressor

Standard technique
With the patient under a general anaesthetic, the tongue is depressed downwards and the tonsils prised from the back of the throat so that they can then be cut away.

tonsillitis

Inflammation of the *tonsils* as a result of infection. Tonsillitis mainly occurs in children under age nine. Sometimes the tonsils become repeatedly infected by the microorganisms they are supposed to protect against.

SYMPTOMS

The main symptoms are a sore throat and difficulty in swallowing. The throat is visibly inflamed. Other common symptoms are fever, headache, earache, enlarged and tender *lymph nodes* in the neck, and bad breath. Occasionally, there may be additional problems, such as temporary deafness or *quinsy* (an abscess around the tonsil).

TREATMENT

Tonsillitis is treated with plenty of fluids and an *analgesic drug* (painkiller) such as paracetamol; in some cases *antibiotic drugs* may also be prescribed.

tooth

See *teeth*.

tooth abscess

See *abscess, dental*.

toothache

Pain in one or more *teeth* and sometimes the *gums*.

CAUSES

Early dental *caries* (decay) may cause mild toothache when very hot, cold, or sweet food is eaten. More advanced decay or a fractured tooth (see *fracture, dental*), or a deep, unlined filling (see *filling, dental*) may lead to pulpitis (pulp inflammation). This usually causes a sharp, stabbing pain, which is often worse when the person is lying down.

If the inflammation spreads, the supporting tissues round the root of the tooth may be affected (a disorder known as periapical *periodontitis*). This causes localized pain brought on mainly by biting and chewing. A dental abscess (see *abscess, dental*) may also occur. In this case, pain is severe and often continuous, the gum surrounding the affected tooth is tender and swollen, and there may be swelling of the face and neck accompanied by fever.

Sometimes, toothache is caused by *sinusitis* (inflammation of the membrane lining the facial air cavities), when pain is referred to the upper molar and premolar teeth (see *referred pain*).

TREATMENT

Analgesic drugs may provide temporary pain relief. A visit to the dentist should be arranged as early as possible.

tooth avulsion

See *avulsed tooth*.

toothbrushing

Cleaning of the *teeth* with a brush in order to remove *plaque* and food particles from the tooth surfaces and to stimulate the gums. Brushing the teeth should be carried out twice a day using a *dentifrice* (usually toothpaste) that contains fluoride.

tooth decay

See *caries, dental*.

tooth extraction

See *extraction, dental*.

toothpaste

See *dentifrice*.

tophus

A collection of *uric acid* crystals that is deposited in certain tissues, especially those around the joints, but occasionally in other places such as the ear. Tophus is a sign of *hyperuricaemia*, a condition that accompanies *gout*.

topical

A term describing a *drug* that is applied to the surface of the body, not swallowed or injected.

toric lens

A type of *contact lens* specially shaped to correct *astigmatism*.

torsion

A term that means twisting, often applied to the intestine or *testis*.

torticollis

Twisting of the neck, causing the head to be tilted and fixed in an abnormal position (wry neck). There is often neck pain and stiffness. The cause is usually a minor neck injury that irritates cervical nerves, leading to *muscle spasm*. Other causes are sleeping in an awkward position, a neck-muscle injury at birth, and a burn or injury that has caused heavy scarring.

Torticollis due to muscle spasm may be treated with *nonsteroidal anti-inflammatory drugs*, *heat treatment*, *ultrasound treatment*, or *physiotherapy*, In severe cases, torticollis may be treated with

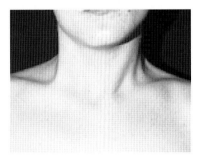

Woman with torticollis
The muscles on the left side of the neck have gone into spasm, causing the head to be pulled over to that side and causing pain.

THE SENSE OF **TOUCH**

The skin contains many thousands of specialized cells that respond to a variety of external stimuli, such as touch, heat, cold, and pressure. These cells (receptors) are divided into two different types. One type of receptor consists only of a thin nerve fibre, which may wrap around an individual hair and respond to its movement. The other type of receptor has a specialized structure, which is known as an end organ, that surrounds the nerve ending. Some skin receptors consist of several layers of cells that are attached to one nerve fibre. Others contain several nerve fibres that are arranged in a loop or coil. It is probable that several varieties of receptors play a part in each of the different types of touch modality.

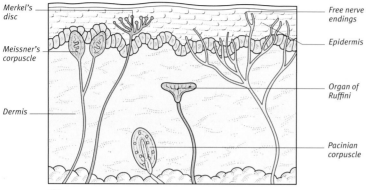

Merkel's disc

Meissner's corpuscle

Dermis

Free nerve endings

Epidermis

Organ of Ruffini

Pacinian corpuscle

Skin receptors
These receptors vary from free nerve endings to corpuscular or bulb-like structures. Individual receptors do not seem to be associated exclusively with any one skin sensation (e.g. cold or pain).

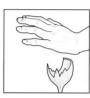

Delicate touch
The ability to detect light contact between an object and the skin. Areas with more receptors are more sensitive.

Pain
Pain warns the brain about possible injury from an external stimulus and can trigger a reflex withdrawal.

Heat
Some free nerve endings respond to heat. The inner wrist is good for testing temperature. Extreme heat stimulates pain receptors.

Cold
Cold on the skin is detected by specialized end organs. Extreme cold also stimulates pain receptors.

Pressure
A change in pressure on the skin is detected by specialized end organs called pacinian corpuscles.

TOUCH PERCEPTION

General sensations that emanate from various parts of the body are perceived at specific points within the brain's cerebral cortex. Some of the more highly sensitive body parts, such as the lips and hands, are represented in the brain by correspondingly large regions within the cortex.

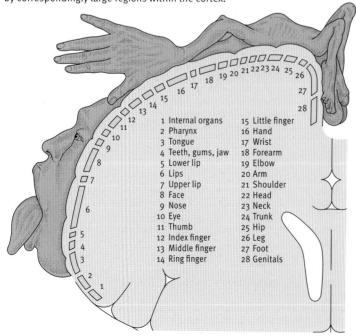

1 Internal organs	15 Little finger
2 Pharynx	16 Hand
3 Tongue	17 Wrist
4 Teeth, gums, jaw	18 Forearm
5 Lower lip	19 Elbow
6 Lips	20 Arm
7 Upper lip	21 Shoulder
8 Face	22 Head
9 Nose	23 Neck
10 Eye	24 Trunk
11 Thumb	25 Hip
12 Index finger	26 Leg
13 Middle finger	27 Foot
14 Ring finger	28 Genitals

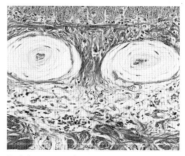

Pacinian corpuscle
These receptors are 1 mm to 4 mm long and occur in hairless areas of skin, especially the fingers.

T

injections of *botulinum toxin*. When the cause of torticollis is an injury arising from birth, the muscle is gently stretched several times each day; occasionally, an operation is necessary.

touch

The sense by which certain characteristics of objects, such as their shape, size, temperature, and surface texture, can be ascertained by physical contact.

The skin has many types of touch *receptors*, including Meissner's corpuscles and Merkel's discs to detect light touch, and Pacinian corpuscles to sense deep pressure and vibration. Signals from these receptors pass via sensory nerves to the spinal cord, then to the *thalamus* in the brain, and on to the *sensory cortex*, where touch sensations are perceived and interpreted.

The various parts of the body differ markedly in their sensitivity to touch discrimination. For example, the fingertips are considerably more sensitive to the sense of touch than the trunk. (See also *sensation*.)

Tourette's syndrome

See *Gilles de la Tourette's syndrome*.

tourniquet

A device that is placed around a limb in order to compress blood vessels. A tourniquet may be used to locate a vein for the purposes of an intravenous injection or the withdrawal of blood. An inflatable tourniquet, called an *Esmarch's bandage*, is used to control blood flow in some limb operations. The use of a tourniquet as a first-aid measure to stop severe bleeding can cause *gangrene* (tissue death); first-aid courses now teach use of pressure to control bleeding in preference to a tourniquet.

toxaemia

Presence in the bloodstream of *toxins*, commonly produced by *bacteria*. (See also *pre-eclampsia*; *toxic shock syndrome*.)

toxaemia of pregnancy

See *pre-eclampsia*.

toxicity

The property of being toxic (poisonous). The term also refers to the severity of adverse effects or illness produced by a *toxin*, a *poison*, or a drug overdose.

toxicology

The study of *poisons*.

toxic shock syndrome

An uncommon, severe illness caused by a *toxin* produced by the bacterium STAPHYLOCOCCUS AUREUS.

CAUSES

The condition occurs mostly in women who use highly absorbent vaginal tampons. Other cases have been linked to use of a contraceptive cap, diaphragm, or sponge (see *contraception*), or to skin wounds or staphylococcus infections elsewhere in the body.

SYMPTOMS AND COMPLICATIONS

A high fever, vomiting, diarrhoea, headache, muscle aches and pains, dizziness, and disorientation develop suddenly. A widespread skin rash that resembles sunburn and also affects the palms and soles, develops. Blood pressure may fall dangerously low, and *shock* may develop. Other complications include *kidney failure* and *liver failure*.

TREATMENT

Antibiotics and treatment in an intensive care unit may be needed.

toxin

A poisonous protein produced by pathogenic (disease-causing) bacteria, various animals, or some plants. Bacterial toxins are sometimes subdivided into three categories: *endotoxins*, which are released from dead bacteria; *exotoxins*, which are released from live bacteria; and *enterotoxins*, which inflame the intestine. (See also *poison*; *poisoning*; *toxaemia*.)

toxocariasis

An infestation of humans, usually children, with the larvae of TOXOCARA CANIS: a small, threadlike worm that lives in the intestines of dogs.

CAUSE

Children who play with an infested dog or soil contaminated with dog faeces, and who then put their fingers in their mouths, may swallow worm eggs. The eggs hatch in the intestines and release larvae, which then migrate to organs such as the liver, lungs, brain, and eyes.

SYMPTOMS

Usually, infestation causes only mild fever and *malaise*, which soon clear up. However, heavy infestation may lead to *asthma*, *pneumonia*, and *seizures*. Vision may be lost if worm larvae enter the eye and die there.

DIAGNOSIS AND TREATMENT

A diagnosis of toxocariasis is made from sputum analysis, and by a *liver biopsy*. Severe cases require treatment in hospital with an *anthelmintic drug*.

toxoid

An inactivated bacterial *toxin*. Certain toxoids are used to immunize against specific diseases, such as *tetanus*.

toxoplasmosis

Infection with the *protozoan* TOXOPLASMA GONDII, often caused by eating undercooked meat from infected animals, or by handling faeces from infected cats.

SYMPTOMS AND COMPLICATIONS

In most cases, there are no symptoms, but there may be a feverish illness that resembles infectious *mononucleosis* (glandular fever). Eye problems, such as retinitis (inflammation of the retina) and *choroiditis* (inflammation of the choroid) may also develop. In people who are *immunocompromised*, such as those with *AIDS* or patients undergoing chemotherapy, toxoplasmosis can be very serious, causing problems such as heart and lung damage and severe *encephalitis* (brain inflammation).

Toxoplasmosis that is contracted by a pregnant woman may be transmitted to the fetus. The infection may result in *miscarriage* or *stillbirth*, or the infant may have an enlarged liver and spleen, blindness, *hydrocephalus* (fluid around the brain), learning difficulties, seizures, or may die during infancy. Infection in late pregnancy usually has no ill effects.

DIAGNOSIS AND TREATMENT

The diagnosis is made from blood tests. Treatment (with antibiotics) may not be necessary except in certain people, such as those with severe symptoms, those who are immunocompromised, and those who have developed retinitis or choroiditis. If toxoplasmosis is acquired in pregnancy, antibiotics will be given, although a termination may be offered in some cases.

TPA

See *tissue-plasminogen activator*.

trabecula

A band of fibrous tissue that divides the inner part of an organ, for example the penis, into different sections. The term trabecula (plural trabeculae) is also used to describe the bony struts that make up the meshlike structure inside spongy *bone*.

trabeculectomy

A surgical procedure used to control *glaucoma* (raised pressure in the eye). It enables the fluid that accumulates in the front chamber of the eye to drain out under the conjunctiva.

T

trace elements

Minerals necessary in minute amounts in the diet to maintain health. Examples are *chromium*, *copper*, *zinc*, and *selenium*. (See also *nutrition*.)

tracer

A radioactive substance introduced into the body so that its distribution, processing, and elimination from the body can be monitored.

trachea

The air passage, also called the windpipe, that runs from just below the *larynx* (voicebox) to behind the upper part of the *sternum* (breastbone), where it divides to form the *bronchi*.

STRUCTURE

The trachea is made up of fibrous and elastic tissue and also smooth muscle. It also contains about 20 rings of *cartilage*, which help to keep it open. The trachea lining has specialized cells (goblet cells) that secrete mucus and cells with *cilia* (hairlike structures), which beat the mucus upwards to help keep the lungs and airways clear.

LOCATION OF THE **TRACHEA**

The trachea extends down from the larynx (voicebox) for about 10 cm to the point where it divides into the two bronchi.

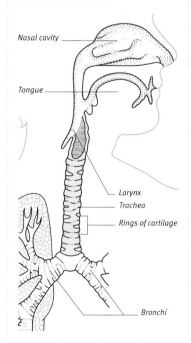

Nasal cavity

Tongue

Larynx

Trachea

Rings of cartilage

Bronchi

DISORDERS

One of the most common disorders of the trachea is *tracheitis* (inflammation of the trachea lining), which is usually caused by an infection (especially by a virus) and is often associated with *bronchitis* or *laryngitis*. Obstruction of the trachea by an inhaled object is rare because the narrowest part of the upper respiratory tract is the larynx, and any objects that pass through there usually also continue through the trachea. However, the trachea may become obstructed by a tumour or narrowed as a result of scarring from a *tracheostomy* tube inserted to create an artificial airway through the front of the neck.

Rarely, a congenital malformation occurs in which an abnormal channel forms between the trachea and the oesophagus immediately behind it (see *tracheoesophageal fistula*).

tracheitis

Inflammation of the *trachea* (windpipe). Tracheitis is usually caused by a viral infection and is aggravated by inhaled fumes and especially by tobacco smoke. Tracheitis often occurs with *laryngitis* and *bronchitis* in a condition known as laryngotracheobronchitis.

Symptoms include a painful dry cough and hoarseness. In most cases, no treatment is needed.

tracheoesophageal fistula

A rare *birth defect* in which an abnormal passage connects the *trachea* (windpipe) with the *oesophagus* (gullet). In the most common form of this type of fistula, the lower end of the oesophagus connects with the trachea, and the upper end of the oesophagus is underdeveloped, forming a blind-ended pouch.

SYMPTOMS AND SIGNS

The affected baby cannot swallow saliva and drools constantly. During feeding, food is regurgitated and enters the lungs, causing the baby to choke, cough, and sometimes to turn blue due to lack of oxygen. The abdomen swells because inhaled air passes into the stomach through the fistula. The acidic fluid in the stomach passes up into the lungs through the fistula, leading to *pneumonia* and *atelectasis* (lung collapse).

DIAGNOSIS AND TREATMENT

The condition is often discovered soon after birth, although mild forms may not be detected until childhood or even adult life, usually after recurrent attacks of pneumonia. The diagnosis may be confirmed by *X-rays*. Treatment of tracheoesophageal fistula consists of an operation that closes the fistula and connects the trachea and oesophagus together correctly.

tracheostomy

A surgical procedure in which an opening is made in the *trachea* (windpipe) and a tube is inserted in order to maintain an effective airway. A tracheostomy is used for the emergency treatment of various airway problems involving the *larynx* (voicebox).

A planned tracheostomy is most commonly performed on a person who has lost the ability to breathe naturally and is undergoing long-term *ventilation* or is unable to keep saliva and other secretions out of the trachea. Permanent tracheostomy is needed after a *laryngectomy* (removal of the larynx).

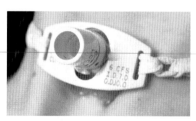

Tracheostomy tube
The tube readily becomes blocked by secretions; it has a metal inner lining that can be removed for cleaning.

tracheotomy

Cutting of the *trachea* (windpipe). (See also *tracheostomy*.)

trachoma

A persistent infectious disease of the *cornea* and *conjunctiva* of the eye. Trachoma is caused by the bacteria CHLAMYDIA TRACHOMATIS and is spread by direct contact and possibly by flies (see *chlamydial infections*). Trachoma is uncommon in the UK, but worldwide it is the most common cause of blindness. Treatment is with *antibiotic drugs*.

tract

Any one of a group of organs that form a common pathway with the purpose of performing a particular function. The term also refers to a bundle of nerve fibres with a common function.

traction

A procedure in which part of the body is placed under tension to correct the alignment of two adjoining structures

T

TRACTION FOR FEMORAL FRACTURE

The thigh muscles have a tendency to go into spasm, because of their immense power, and fractures of the femur (thigh-bone) tend to override this force. Without traction to prevent this, the bone would heal with overlapping ends, with the result that the leg would be permanently shortened.

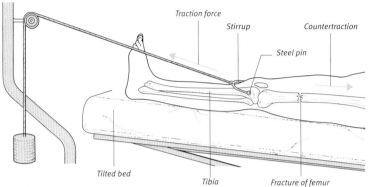

Traction force

Stirrup

Countertraction

Steel pin

Tilted bed

Tibia

Fracture of femur

Procedure
Traction is usually performed by means of a narrow steel pin that is pushed through the upper end of the tibia (shin); a steel stirrup is attached to this in order that a cord and weight can be used to apply the force. The other end of the femur must be immobilized (or counter-traction applied) in order that the fractured bone ends are kept in alignment.

or to hold them in place. Traction is most commonly used to treat a *fracture* in which muscles around the bone ends are pulling the bones out of alignment.

tragus

The small projection of cartilage in front of the opening of the ear canal.

training

A programme of exercises that is undertaken to prepare for a particular sport. Training may be concentrated on improving skills or on improving physical *fitness*. Fitness training should include both *aerobic* and anaerobic exercises, which together build up strength, flexibility, and endurance. Interval training is a type of fitness programme in which a particular exercise is repeated several times with a rest period between. Circuit training consists of performing a set number of different exercises.

trait

Any characteristic or condition that is inherited (which means that is determined by one or more *genes*). Blue or brown eye colour, dark or light skin, and nose shape are examples of genetic traits. The term trait is also sometimes used to describe a mild form of a recessive *genetic disorder*, for example *thalassaemia* trait.

tramadol

An *opioid drug* that is used to relieve severe pain following a heart attack, surgery, or serious illness. Tramadol is less likely to cause dependence with long-term use than most opioids. Possible side effects include nausea, vomiting, drowsiness, confusion, and impaired consciousness.

trance

A sleeplike state in which consciousness is reduced, voluntary actions lessened or absent, and body functions diminished. Trances are claimed to be induced by *hypnosis* and have been reported as part of a group experience. Trances may be a feature of *catalepsy*, *automatism*, and petit mal *epilepsy*.

tranexamic acid

An antifibrinolytic drug that promotes *blood clotting*. Tranexamic acid is particularly useful in treating *menorrhagia* (heavy menstrual periods). Side effects of the drug may include diarrhoea, nausea, and vomiting.

tranquillizer drugs

Drugs that have a sedative effect. Tranquillizers are divided into two types: major tranquillizers (see *antipsychotic drugs*) and minor tranquillizers (see *antianxiety drugs*).

transcutaneous electrical nerve stimulation

See *TENS*.

transdermal patch

A method of administering medication through the skin, using a drug-impregnated, adhesive patch. The drug is released from the patch over a period of time and is absorbed by the skin.

transference

The unconscious displacement of emotions from people who were important during one's childhood, such as parents, to other people during adulthood. For example, during psychotherapy, anger that the analysand feels towards his or her father may be transferred to the therapist. (See also *psychoanalysis*.)

transfusion

See *blood transfusion*.

transfusion, autologous

See *blood transfusion, autologous*.

transient ischaemic attack (TIA)

A brief interruption of the blood supply to part of the brain, which causes temporary impairment of vision, speech, sensation, or movement. The episode typically lasts from several minutes to a few hours, but symptoms disappear completely within 24 hours with no permanent after-effects. TIAs are sometimes described as mini strokes, and can be the prelude to a *stroke*. A stroke occurs within a year in up to 10 per cent of people who have had a TIA. Having had a TIA is also a risk factor for a subsequent *myocardial infarction* (heart attack).

CAUSES
TIAs may be caused by a blood clot (see *embolism*) that temporarily blocks an artery supplying the brain, or by narrowing of an artery as a result of *atherosclerosis* (buildup of fatty deposits in the artery wall).

INVESTIGATION
After a TIA, tests such as *CT scanning*, *blood tests*, and *angiography* or Doppler *ultrasound scanning* of the carotid artery in the neck may be needed to find a cause. In some cases, the heart is studied as a possible source of blood clots.

TREATMENT
Treatment, which is aimed at preventing a stroke, includes *anticoagulant drugs* or *aspirin*. *Endarterectomy* (an operation to remove the lining of an artery affected by atherosclerosis) may also sometimes

T

be advised. It is also important to treat any risk factors, such as *hypertension* (high blood pressure) and high blood cholesterol. Stopping smoking is vital.

transillumination

A procedure that is sometimes carried out during the physical examination of a lump or swelling. Light that comes from a small torch is shone onto one side of the lump; if the light can be seen on the other side, the lump contains clear fluid.

transitional cell carcinoma

A type of cancerous tumour that can develop in the bladder or kidney. In the bladder, transitional cell carcinomas develop within the bladder lining (see *bladder tumours*). In the kidney (see *kidney cancer*), this type of tumour develops in the lining of the renal pelvis (the urine-collecting chamber at the centre of the kidney).

translocation

A rearrangement of the *chromosomes* inside a person's cells; it is a type of *mutation*. Sections of chromosomes may be exchanged or the main parts of two chromosomes may be joined. A translocation may be inherited or acquired as the result of a new mutation.

Often a translocation has no obvious effect and causes no apparent abnormality. However, it sometimes means that some of the affected person's sperm or egg cells carry too much or too little chromosomal material, which may cause a *chromosomal abnormality*, such as *Down's syndrome*, in the person's children.

transmissible

Capable of being passed from one person, or one organism, to another.

transplant surgery

Replacement of a diseased organ or tissue with a healthy, living substitute. The organ is usually taken from a person who has just died. Some kidneys are transplanted from a patient's living relatives (see *organ donation*). The results of surgery have been improved by testing for *histocompatibility antigens* and *tissue-typing*. However, rejection remains a major problem and every patient who has to undergo an organ transplant operation must be given *immunosuppressant drugs* for an indefinite period. (See also *heart–lung transplant*; *heart transplant*; *kidney transplant*; *liver transplant*.)

EFFECT OF CHROMOSOMAL **TRANSLOCATION**

A translocation is a rearrangement of the chromosomes in body cells. A person carrying a translocation may show no abnormality but there is a risk of his or her child having a chromosomal abnormality.

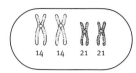

Normal cell
A body cell normally contains 22 paired chromosomes (called autosomes) plus two sex chromosomes (XX in women and XY in men). Just two pairs of autosomes – numbers 14 and 21 – are shown here.

Example of translocation
In a typical translocation, a large part of one of the chromosomes is joined to a large part of another. In this particular example, most of chromosome number 21 and chromosome number 14 are joined together.

Balanced translocation (parent)
The remaining bits of chromosomes 21 and 14 disappear. If, as is illustrated here, the translocation is balanced – that is, the total amount of chromosomal material is normal or very close to the normal situation – no outward abnormality is seen.

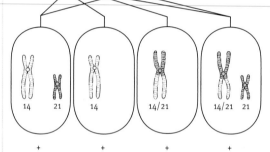

Eggs or sperm produced
A parent with the above translocation makes four types of egg or sperm. They are (from left) – normal, missing a chromosome 21, carrying joined chromosomes 14 and 21, and the same with an extra chromosome 21.

Normal egg or sperm
An egg or sperm from the parent with the translocation combines with one from the other parent, which has one number 21 and one number 14 chromosome. Any of the four outcomes below may result.

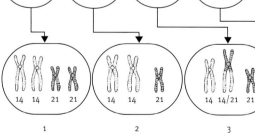

The effect in the child
The child may have any of the following: (1) normal chromosomes, (2) a missing chromosome 21 (incompatible with life), (3) a balanced translocation (like the parent), and (4) effectively, an extra chromosome 21, leading to Down's syndrome. In the last case, the parents of the affected child may benefit from genetic counselling.

T

transposition of the great vessels

A serious form of congenital *heart disease* in which the two major vessels that carry blood away from the heart (the *aorta* and the pulmonary artery) are transposed. This means that insufficient oxygenated blood is supplied to the body's tissues. *Cyanosis* (blueness of the skin) usually develops and the baby becomes increasingly short of breath and feeds poorly. *Open heart surgery* is needed in order to correct the defect.

transsexualism

A rare condition in which an individual wishes to live as a member of the opposite sex. Transsexuals commonly seek hormonal or surgical treatment in order to bring about a physical *sex change*. A psychiatric evaluation and a physical examination are necessary before such treatment is undertaken.

transverse colon

One of the four major sections of the *colon*, or large intestine. The transverse colon lies across the abdomen.

transverse fracture

A *fracture* in which there is a straight break across the bone.

transverse myelitis

See *myelitis*.

transvestism

A persistent desire by a man to dress in women's clothing, also known as cross-dressing. Transvestism ranges from the occasional wearing of female underclothes to dressing in female clothes in public and involvement in transvestite subculture. Most transvestites are heterosexual and many have a sexual relationship with a female partner who is aware of the cross-dressing and can accept it as a special need.

tranylcypromine

An *antidepressant drug* that belongs to the *monoamine-oxidase inhibitor* (MAOI) group and is used mainly in patients with severe depression.

trapezius muscle

A large, diamond-shaped *muscle* that extends from the back of the skull to the lower part of the spine in the chest and across the width of the shoulders. The trapezius muscle is attached to the top and back of the shoulderblade and

LOCATION OF THE TRAPEZIUS MUSCLE

The trapezius is a large, diamond-shaped muscle in the upper part of the back. The trapezius muscle helps to support the neck and head and is also involved in raising the arms.

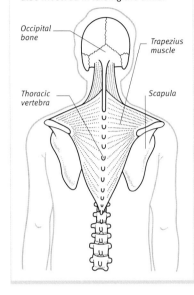

to the outermost part of the collarbone. It helps to support the neck and spine and is also involved in moving the arm.

trapped nerve

See *nerve, trapped*.

trastuzumab

More commonly known by its brand name Herceptin, a monoclonal antibody (see *antibody, monoclonal*) used to treat some cases of advanced *breast cancer* in which the cancer has metastasized (spread to other parts of the body). It may be used alone or in combination with *chemotherapy*. Trastuzumab may also be used as follow-on treatment in some cases of early breast cancer after initial treatment with surgery, chemotherapy, and *radiotherapy*. Possible adverse effects include headache, diarrhoea, gastrointestinal disturbances, breathing problems, rash, and heart damage.

trauma

Any serious physical injury or severe emotional shock. (See also *post-traumatic stress disorder*.)

traumatic amputation

See *amputation, traumatic*.

traumatology

Emergency treatment of patients suffering from acute trauma (such as severe and/or multiple injuries).

travel immunization

Anyone planning to travel abroad may need immunizations. Although few are compulsory for international travel, some are recommended for the protection of the traveller and to prevent the spread of diseases. (See *Guidelines for travel immunization* box, overleaf). Wherever the travel destination, everybody should be immunized against *diphtheria*, *tetanus*, and *polio*, and should have had any necessary boosters.

Advice on travel immunizations may change from time to time and travellers should consult a doctor, travel nurse, pharmacist, or travel clinic for the most up-to-date information about their individual needs. Some vaccines must be given in several doses, with an interval between each dose. Therefore, medical advice should be sought at least two to three months before departure. Children under one year of age, pregnant women, and people who have a compromised immune system or a serious illness may not be able to have some vaccinations, such as that for yellow fever.

traveller's diarrhoea

People visiting foreign countries may suffer episodes of diarrhoea, which range in severity and are usually due to *gastroenteritis*. Attention to hygiene, drinking bottled water, avoiding ice in drinks, and eating peelable fruit can prevent a large proportion of episodes.

travel sickness

See *motion sickness*.

trazodone

An *antidepressant drug* with a strong sedative effect that is used to treat *depression* accompanied by *anxiety* or *insomnia*. Possible side effects of trazodone include drowsiness, constipation, a dry mouth, dizziness, and, rarely, *priapism*.

treadmill test

A test that involves exercise at varying degrees of inclination on a treadmill while the heart function is monitored (see *exercise ECG*).

treatment

A measure taken to prevent or cure a disease or disorder or to relieve symptoms.

GUIDELINES FOR **TRAVEL IMMUNIZATION**

Immunization	Who should be immunized	Period of protection
Cholera	People travelling to areas where cholera is endemic or epidemic. Immunization does not provide complete protection; travellers to these areas should pay scrupulous attention to food, water, and personal hygiene.	Up to 2 years.
Hepatitis A	Frequent travellers to the Mediterranean or developing countries, particularly countries where sanitation is poor.	Up to 20 years.
Hepatitis B	People travelling to countries in which hepatitis B is prevalent; those who might need medical or dental treatment while in a developing country; and people likely to have unprotected sex.	Up to 5 years.
Japanese B encephalitis	People staying in rural areas of certain countries in Southeast Asia and the Far East, particularly those doing outdoor activities.	Up to 3 years.
Meningitis A, C, W135, and Y	People travelling to sub-Saharan Africa and parts of Saudi Arabia. Immunization certificate needed if travelling to Saudi Arabia for the Hajj or Umrah pilgrimages.	Up to 5 years.
Rabies	People travelling to areas where rabies is endemic, particularly those at high risk (such as veterinary surgeons) and/or are travelling to areas with limited medical facilities. The vaccine may also be given after exposure to rabies.	Up to 3 years.
Typhoid	People travelling to areas with poor sanitation, although it is also important to pay scrupulous attention to personal hygiene.	Up to 3 years.
Yellow fever	Compulsory for entry to some countries and advisable for visits to others within yellow fever zones in Africa and South America. May also be needed when travelling from yellow fever zones to some Asian countries. A vaccination certificate is provided.	At least 10 years.

trematode

The scientific name for any *fluke* or *schistosome*.

trembling

See *tremor*.

tremor

An involuntary, rhythmic, oscillating movement in the *muscles* of part of the body; the most commonly affected muscles are those of the hands, feet, jaw, tongue, or head. Tremor is the result of rapidly alternating muscle contraction and relaxation. Occasional tremors are experienced by the majority of people and are due to increased production of the hormone *adrenaline* (epinephrine). A slight, persistent tremor is common in elderly people.

Essential tremor, a type that runs in families, is a fine-to-moderate tremor (about six to ten movements per second) that may be temporarily relieved by consuming a small amount of alcohol or by taking *beta-blocker drugs*.

Coarse tremor (about four to five movements per second) is present at rest but reduced during movement, and is often a sign of the movement disorder *Parkinson's disease*. An intention tremor (tremor that is worse on movement of the affected part) may be a sign of *cerebellar ataxia*.

Tremor may also be caused by *multiple sclerosis*, *Wilson's disease*, *mercury poisoning*, *thyrotoxicosis*, or hepatic *encephalopathy*; drugs, such as *amphetamines* and *caffeine*; and withdrawal from drugs, including *alcohol*.

trench fever

An infectious disease that is now rare or unknown in most parts of the world. The disease is caused by *rickettsiae* (microorganisms that are similar to bacteria) spread by body *lice*. Symptoms include headache, muscle pains, and fever, which may occur in bouts. Treatment is with *antibiotic drugs*.

trench foot

See *immersion foot*.

trench mouth

See *gingivitis, acute ulcerative*.

Trendelenburg's test

A test that is used to assess the function of each hip in turn. It involves standing on one leg and lifting the other leg while keeping the spine straight. Normally, as the leg is raised the pelvis on the same side should lift. Drooping of the pelvis on the side of the raised leg indicates that there may be a problem, such as a hip dislocation or weakness of the buttock muscles.

trephine

A hollow, cylindrical instrument with a saw-toothed edge used for cutting a circular hole, usually in bone.

Treponema pallidum

The species of bacteria responsible for causing *syphilis*.

tretinoin

A *topical* drug that is chemically related to *vitamin A* and is mainly used to treat *acne*. Tretinoin may aggravate acne at the start of treatment but usually improves the condition within three to four months. Possible side effects include irritation, peeling, and skin discoloration. Exposing the skin to sunlight while using tretinoin may aggravate irritation and can lead to *sunburn*. Because of possible adverse effects on a fetus, tretinoin is not prescribed to women who are pregnant. Women of child-bearing age must use effective contraception for at least a month before starting the drug, during treatment, and for at least a month after stopping.

triage

A classification system for establishing priority for treatment among a group of patients. Triage is used in hospital accident and emergency departments to sort patients into categories according to the nature of their injuries and their need for emergency treatment. It is intended to give the best chance of survival to the greatest number of people.

trial, clinical

A test on human volunteers of the effectiveness and safety of a drug. A clinical trial can also involve systematic comparison of alternative forms of medical or surgical treatment for a particular disorder. Patients involved in clinical trials have to give their consent, and the trials are approved and supervised by an ethics committee.

triamcinolone

A *corticosteroid drug* that is used to treat inflammation of the mouth, gums, skin, and joints; *asthma*; and allergic rhinitis (see *rhinitis, allergic*).

triamterene

A *diuretic drug* that is used to treat *hypertension* (high blood pressure) and *oedema* (accumulation of fluid in tissues). Possible adverse effects include nausea, vomiting, weakness, and rash.

tribavirin

see *ribavirin*.

triceps muscle

The *muscle* at the back of the upper arm. At the upper end of the triceps are three "heads"; one is attached to the outer edge of the *scapula* (shoulderblade), and the other two to either side of the *humerus* (upper-arm bone). The lower part of the triceps is attached to the olecranon process of the ulna (the bony prominence on the elbow). Contraction of the muscle straightens the arm. (See also *biceps muscle*.)

trichiasis

An alteration in the direction of eyelash growth, in which the lashes grow inwards towards the eyeball. They can rub against the eye, causing severe discomfort and sometimes damage to the *cornea*. *Trachoma* is a possible cause.

trichinosis

An infestation with the larvae of the TRICHINELLA SPIRALIS worm, which is usually acquired by eating undercooked pork. Trichinosis is rare in the UK. The thorough cooking of pork products, and freezing meat to a temperature below -18°C for 24 hours, helps to avoid infection.

LOCATION OF THE TRICEPS MUSCLE

This muscle at the back of the upper arm functions to straighten the elbow joint, thus opposing the action of the biceps at the front of the upper arm.

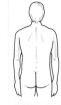
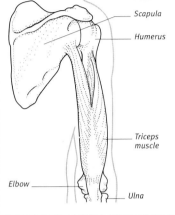

Scapula

Humerus

Triceps muscle

Elbow

Ulna

SYMPTOMS
Slight infestation usually causes no symptoms. However, heavy infestation may cause diarrhoea and vomiting within a day or two of eating the infected meat; gastointestinal symptoms are followed by fever; swelling around the eyelids; severe muscle pains, which may last for several weeks; and inflammation of the heart muscle (*myocarditis*).
DIAGNOSIS AND TREATMENT
Trichinosis may be suspected from the symptoms, and the diagnosis is confirmed by *blood tests*, or by a muscle *biopsy* (tissue sample). Treatment of the infestation is with an *anthelmintic drug*.

trichology

The study of hair, including its structure, patterns of growth, and diseases.

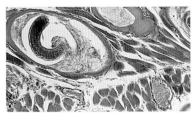

Biopsy specimen showing trichinosis
This light micrograph of a section of a patient's muscle shows a cyst formed by a *Trichinella spiralis* larva.

---

trichomoniasis

An infection caused by the *protozoan* (single-celled microorganism) TRICHOMONAS VAGINALIS. Trichomoniasis is one of the common causes of *vaginitis* (inflammation of the vagina) in women. The infection is usually sexually transmitted. Trichomoniasis is less common in men, in whom it affects the urethra.
CAUSES
In women, the causative organism may inhabit the vagina for many years without causing symptoms. However, if symptoms do occur, they include painful inflammation of the vagina and *vulva*, and a greenish, frothy, offensive-smelling discharge. Sexual intercourse may be painful. Men usually have no symptoms, but some may have discomfort on passing urine.
DIAGNOSIS AND TREATMENT
The diagnosis is made from examination of a sample of the discharge. However, diagnosis is usually difficult to confirm in men.

Treatment is usually with *metronidazole*. The sexual partner or partners of an infected person should be treated at the same time to prevent reinfection.

Trichophyton

A genus of fungi that can cause diseases of the hair, skin, and nails in humans (see *fungal infections*). *Athlete's foot* and ringworm of the scalp (see *tinea*) are among common disorders caused by TRICHOPHYTON species.

trichotillomania

The habit of constantly pulling out one's own hair. It can be associated with severe *learning difficulties* or with a psychotic illness. Trichotillomania may also occur in psychologically disturbed children. The trichotillomania sufferer will typically pull, twist, and break off chunks of hair from his or her scalp, leaving visible bald patches. Occasionally, the pubic hair is pulled out in addition to or instead of hair on the head.

Children sometimes eat the removed hair, which may form a hairball in the stomach, known medically as a trichobezoar (see *bezoar*).

Treatment depends on the cause of the problem, and it may consist of *psychotherapy* or *antipsychotic drugs*.

trichuriasis

A parasitic infestation with the mainly tropical worm TRICHURIS TRICHURIA (whipworm). Children are most commonly

T

affected. Infestation occurs when eggs are ingested and then develop into adult worms in the intestines. Severe infestation may cause bloody diarrhoea, abdominal pain, and weight loss. Treatment of trichuriasis is with *anthelmintic drugs*.

triclosan

An *antiseptic* used for disinfecting the skin. For example, triclosan may be used by doctors and other hospital staff for cleansing the hands before carrying out surgical procedures.

tricuspid incompetence

Failure of the heart's *tricuspid valve* to close fully, allowing blood to leak back into the right atrium (upper chamber) when the right ventricle (lower chamber) contracts. Tricuspid incompetence, also known as tricuspid insufficiency, reduces the heart's pumping efficiency.

CAUSES

The usual cause is *pulmonary hypertension* (high pressure in the blood supply to the lungs). More rarely, it follows *rheumatic fever*, or, in intravenous drug users, bacterial infection of the heart.

SYMPTOMS

Tricuspid incompetence results in symptoms of right-sided *heart failure*, notably *oedema* (fluid swelling) of the ankles and abdomen. The liver is swollen and tender, and veins in the neck are distended.

DIAGNOSIS AND TREATMENT

A diagnosis is made from the symptoms, from hearing a heart *murmur* through a stethoscope, and by tests that may include an *ECG*, *chest X-rays*, *echocardiography*, and cardiac *catheterization*. Treatment with *diuretic drugs* and *ACE inhibitors* often relieves the symptoms. In severe cases, surgery may be recommended.

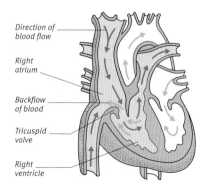

Defect in tricuspid incompetence
The tricuspid valve lies between the atrium and ventricle in the right side of the heart. Incompetence means that when the right ventricle contracts, some blood escapes back into the right atrium.

Labels on diagram:
Direction of blood flow
Right atrium
Backflow of blood
Tricuspid valve
Right ventricle

tricuspid stenosis

Narrowing of the opening of the *tricuspid valve* of the heart (the valve between the right upper chamber and right lower chamber of the heart), usually caused by a previous attack of *rheumatic fever*. Tricuspid stenosis is uncommon and often occurs with another heart-valve disorder. For example, *tricuspid incompetence* may also occur in intravenous drug users who have a bacterial infection of the heart. Tricuspid stenosis causes enlargement of the right atrium (upper heart chamber).

The symptoms and diagnosis of tricuspid stenosis are similar to those of tricuspid incompetence. Treatment is with *diuretic drugs*, and *heart-valve surgery* is sometimes needed.

tricuspid valve

One of the valves in the *heart* that consists of three flaps that lies between the right atrium (upper chamber) and the right ventricle (lower chamber). Its function is to ensure that that blood flow from the atrium to the ventricle occurs in one direction only.

tricyclic antidepressants

A type of *antidepressant drug*. Tricyclic antidepressants work by preventing *neurotransmitters* (chemicals released from nerve endings) in the brain from being reabsorbed, thereby increasing their level. Examples include *amitriptyline*, *clomipramine*, and *imipramine*.

trifluoperazine

An *antipsychotic drug* that is used in the treatment of *schizophrenia*. It is also used to treat severe nausea and vomiting.

trigeminal nerve

The fifth *cranial nerve*. The trigeminal nerves, one on each side of the face, arise from the *brainstem*. Both nerves divide into three branches that supply sensation to the face, scalp, nose, teeth, lining of the mouth, upper eyelid, *sinuses*, and the front portion of the tongue. They also stimulate contraction of the *jaw* muscles for chewing.

trigeminal neuralgia

A disorder of the *trigeminal nerve* in which brief episodes of severe, stabbing pain affect the cheek, lips, gums, or chin on one side of the face. The disorder usually occurs in people over the age of 50. Pain may come in bouts that last for weeks at a time. The cause is uncertain, and pain is often brought on by touching the face, eating, drinking, or talking.

Treatment of trigeminal neuralgia is usually with the anticonvulsant drugs *carbamazepine* or gabapentin. If drug treatment is ineffective, surgery may be recommended in some cases.

trigger finger

Locking of one or several fingers in a bent position due to inflammation of the sheath enclosing the *tendon* of the affected finger. The finger is usually ten-

LOCATION OF THE **TRIGEMINAL NERVE**

The trigeminal nerve splits into three main branches. The ophthalmic nerve supplies most of the scalp, the upper eyelid, and the cornea; the maxillary nerve supplies the upper jaw; and the mandibular nerve supplies the tongue, lower jaw, and jaw muscles.

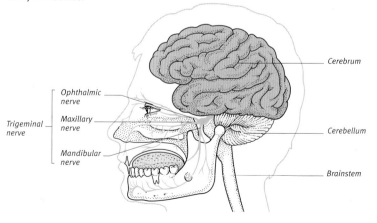

Labels on diagram:
Ophthalmic nerve
Maxillary nerve
Mandibular nerve
Trigeminal nerve
Cerebrum
Cerebellum
Brainstem

T

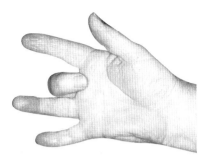

Appearance of trigger finger
The disorder is caused by inflammation of the sheath of one of the tendons involved in controlling the finger's movements.

der at the base and slightly swollen over the tendon. Treatment involves local injection of a *corticosteroid drug* or, if this is unsuccessful, surgery.

trigger point

A localized area of the body that is painful to the touch or to pressure.

triglyceride

A type of simple fat (see *fats and oils*) made up of a molecule of *glycerol* and three molecules of fatty acids. Triglycerides are the main type of fat found in stores of body fat.

trimeprazine

A former name for *alimemazine*, an *antihistamine drug*.

trimester

A period of three months; the term is used particularly with reference to human *pregnancy*, which is conventionally divided into three trimesters.

trimethoprim

An *antibacterial drug* that is used to treat a range of infections, most commonly those of the urinary and respiratory tracts. It is also used in combination with another antibacterial drug, sulfamethoxazole, in a preparation known as *co-trimoxazole*, which is used mainly to treat *pneumocystis pneumonia*, *toxoplasmosis*, and *nocardiosis*.

Possible side effects of trimethoprim include rash, itching, nausea, vomiting, diarrhoea, and a sore tongue.

trimipramine

A tricyclic *antidepressant drug* that is used to treat *depression* accompanied by *anxiety* or *insomnia*. Possible side effects include dry mouth, blurred vision, dizziness, constipation, and nausea.

triplets

Three offspring resulting from one pregnancy (see *pregnancy, multiple*).

triple X syndrome

A group of features that may occur in females due to inheriting three female sex chromosomes (XXX) rather than the usual two (see *chromosomes*). The defect results from errors in the division of one parent's egg or sperm cells.

The features of triple X syndrome can vary greatly. In some cases there are no obvious signs. More severely affected females may show delays in developing speech and motor skills, an IQ that may be lower than that of any siblings, and behavioural problems such as tantrums or shyness. Adult women may be taller than average, but show normal sexual development and are fertile.

trismus

Involuntary contraction of the jaw muscles, which causes the mouth to become tightly closed; commonly known as lockjaw. Trismus may develop as a symptom of *tetanus*, *tonsillitis*, *mumps*, or acute ulcerative *gingivitis* (gum disease), or of other dental problems that affect the back teeth. Treatment is for the underlying cause.

trisomy

Any condition in which there is an extra *chromosome* within a person's cells, making three of a particular chromosome instead of the usual two.

CAUSE

A fault during *meiosis* (cell division) to form egg or sperm cells can sometimes leave an egg or sperm with an extra chromosome. When the egg or sperm takes part in fertilization, the resulting embryo inherits an extra chromosome in each of its cells.

TYPES AND SYMPTOMS

The most common type of trisomy is of chromosome 21 (*Down's syndrome*). Trisomy 18 (Edwards' syndrome) and trisomy 13 (Patau's syndrome) are less common; trisomy 8 and trisomy 22 are very rare. Partial trisomy, with only part of a chromosome reproduced in triplicate, also occurs.

Full trisomies cause abnormalities such as skeletal and heart defects and learning difficulties. Except in Down's syndrome, babies usually die in early infancy. The effects of partial trisomies depend on the amount of extra chromosomal material present.

DIAGNOSIS AND PREVENTION

Diagnosis is made by *chromosome analysis* of cells, which may be obtained from the fetus by *amniocentesis* or after the birth. There is no specific treatment. Parents of an affected child may wish to have *genetic counselling*.

trisomy 21 syndrome

Another name for *Down's syndrome*.

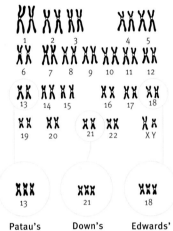

Types of trisomy
In all trisomies a child is born with three chromosomes, instead of the usual complement of two, of a particular number. Down's syndrome is by far the most common trisomy.

trochanteric bursitis

Inflammation of the bursa (fluid-filled sac) located towards the upper end of the femur (thigh-bone). Trochanteric bursitis may be due to repeated strain on the hip joint in activities such as running, or may result from sudden injury (for example, in a fall or during contact sports). It may also occur after surgery on the hip, or develop in a person whose legs are of different lengths. In some cases, there is no apparent cause. The main symptom is pain at the side of the hip; the pain may also spread down the side of the thigh.

Treatment often includes rest, application of ice-packs (or heat treatment), and the use of *nonsteroidal anti-inflammatory drugs* (NSAIDs) for pain relief. A *corticosteroid* injection may be given into the bursa, often providing a rapid relief from the symptoms. *Physiotherapy* may also be helpful.

trochlear nerve

The fourth *cranial nerve*. There are two trochlear nerves, which arise in the brainstem, one on each side of the midbrain (the uppermost of the brainstem's three main parts). They enter the eye sockets through gaps in the skull bones. Each trochlear nerve controls one of the two superior oblique muscles, which are responsible for rotation of the eyes downwards and outwards.

trophic

A term that means relating to nutrition. It is also used of a hormone or its effects to indicate stimulation of another hormone-producing gland.

trophic ulcer

An *ulcer* that develops when nerves in the skin are damaged or destroyed by disease or injury. Trophic ulcers most

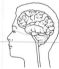

LOCATION OF THE TROCHLEAR NERVE

This nerve emerges from the brain and supplies a muscle that rotates the eye down and outwards.

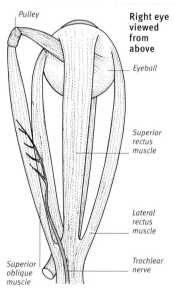

Pulley

Right eye viewed from above

Eyeball

Superior rectus muscle

Lateral rectus muscle

Superior oblique muscle

Trochlear nerve

commonly appear on the feet and can be a complication of disorders such as *diabetes mellitus* and *Hansen's disease*.

trophoblastic tumour

A growth arising from the tissues that develop into the *placenta*. The most common type is a *hydatidiform mole*. (See also *choriocarcinoma*.)

tropical diseases

Many diseases prevalent in the tropics are primarily caused by overcrowded living conditions and inadequate diet. *Malnutrition* is one of the major causes of illness in the tropics. Apart from resulting in nutritional deficiency disorders, a poor diet weakens the body's ability to fight infectious diseases such as *measles*, *diphtheria*, and *tuberculosis*.

Lack of sanitary facilities, which encourages the contamination of water and soil with human excrement, causes a number of diseases, including *typhoid fever*, *shigellosis*, *cholera*, *amoebiasis*, and *nemotode* and *tapeworm infestations*.

Diseases that are spread through the tropics by insects include *malaria*, *yellow fever*, *sleeping sickness*, and *leishmaniasis*. Exposure to strong tropical sunlight causes an increased tendency to *skin cancer* among people with fair skin; sunlight may also damage the outer tissues of the eye, leading to such disorders as *pinguecula* and *pterygium*.

tropical sprue

See *sprue, tropical*.

tropical ulcer

An area of persistent skin and tissue loss caused by infection with one or more organisms. The condition is most common in malnourished people living in the tropics. Treatment is cleaning and dressing of the ulcer, a course of *antibiotic drugs*, and a high protein diet. The ulcer usually heals but may scar.

tropicamide

A drug used to dilate the *pupil* before an eye examination. Adverse effects of the drug include blurred vision, increased sensitivity to light, stinging, and, rarely, dry mouth, flushing, and *glaucoma*.

trunk

The centre of the body, comprising the chest and abdomen. It also refers to any large blood vessel or nerve, from which smaller vessels or nerves branch off.

truss

An elastic, canvas, or padded appliance used to hold an abdominal *hernia* in place. Trusses are used only when corrective surgery cannot be undertaken.

trypanosomiasis

A tropical disease that is caused by Trypanosoma parasites. (See also *Chagas' disease*; *sleeping sickness*.)

trypsin

A type of *enzyme*, secreted by the pancreas, that plays an important role in the process of digestion by breaking down proteins.

tryptophan

An essential *amino acid* (a building block of proteins). Tryptophan, which is necessary for normal growth, is not manufactured within the body but must be obtained from the diet.

tsetse fly bites

The bites of tsetse flies, which are found in Africa, can be very painful. The flies, resembling brown houseflies, spread *sleeping sickness*.

TSH

The abbreviation for *thyroid-stimulating hormone*.

T-tube cholangiography

An *imaging technique* that is performed in order to check that there are no *gallstones* left in the bile duct following a *cholecystectomy* (surgical removal of the gallbladder). A T-shaped rubber tube is inserted into the bile duct during the surgery and is left in place. After about a week, *contrast medium* is inserted into the tube and *X-rays* are taken. If there are no stones, the tube is pulled out. If there are, they may be removed by *ERCP* or by a stone-dissolving solvent administered through the tube.

tubal ligation

See *sterilization, female*.

tubal pregnancy

See *ectopic pregnancy*.

tubercle

A grey, nodular mass that is found in tissues affected by *tuberculosis*. The term also refers to a small rounded protrusion that sometimes occurs on the surface of a bone.

tuberculin tests

Skin tests used to determine whether or not an a person has been exposed to the bacterium that causes *tuberculosis*, and whether or not they require *BCG vaccination*. A small amount of tuberculin (purified protein from the bacteria) is injected into the skin. A few days later, the skin reaction, if any, is noted. A reaction indicates previous exposure, by infection or vaccination. Tuberculin tests are carried out only on people considered to be at higher than normal risk of tuberculosis infection due to their being in contact with people who are infected.

tuberculosis

A notifiable infectious disease, commonly called TB, caused in humans by the bacterium *MYCOBACTERIUM TUBERCULOSIS*.

CAUSES AND TYPES

TB is usually transmitted in airborne droplets expelled when an infected person coughs or sneezes. Inhaled droplets enter the lungs and the bacteria multiply.

The immune system usually seals off the infection at this point, but in some cases the infection spreads to the *lymph nodes*. It may also spread to other organs, which may lead to miliary tuberculosis, a potentially fatal form of the disease, or to *meningitis* (inflammation of the membranes around the brain and spinal cord), bone infection, genitourinary infection, or *pericarditis* (inflammation of the membranes around the heart).

In other cases, bacteria held in a dormant state by the immune system become reactivated months, or even years, later; this may occur when old age, poor health, or reduced immunity increase susceptibility to the infection. The infection may then progressively damage the lungs.

SYMPTOMS

The primary infection is usually without symptoms. Progressive infection in the lungs causes coughing (sometimes bringing up blood), chest pain, shortness of breath, fever and sweating, poor appetite, and weight loss. *Pleural effusion* (collection of fluid between the lung and chest wall) or *pneumonia* may develop. The lung damage may be fatal.

DIAGNOSIS

A diagnosis is made from the symptoms and signs, from a *chest X-ray*, and from

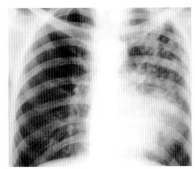

Chest X-ray showing tuberculosis
The right lung (left) appears normal, but the left lung shows dense opacities (white areas) adjoining the heart shadow, indicating tuberculosis.

tests on the sputum. Alternatively, a *bronchoscopy* may also be carried out to obtain samples for culture.

TREATMENT

Treatment usually starts with a course of four drugs (*isoniazid*, *rifampicin*, *pyrazinamide*, and *ethambutol*), which are taken daily for two months. Treatment is then continued for a further four months with daily doses of isoniazid and rifampicin. If the full course of drugs is taken, most patients recover. However, drug-resistant forms of TB are an increasing problem and alternative drugs may be required in these cases.

Tuberculosis is a notifiable disease and any contacts of an infected person are traced and, if infected, treated to reduce the risk of the infection spreading.

PREVENTION

Tuberculosis can be prevented by *BCG vaccination*, which is offered to people at risk of contracting the disease and for whom a *tuberculin test* is negative. At-risk infants (those who are considered to be at higher than normal risk of infection due to having been in contact with infected people or having come from an area or population with a high incidence of tuberculosis) are immunized without having a tuberculin test.

tuberosity

A prominent area on a *bone* to which *tendons* are attached.

tuberous sclerosis

An inherited disorder that affects the skin and *nervous system*. Symptoms may include a condition of the face that is similar to acne, *epilepsy*, and *learning difficulties*. In addition, noncancerous tumours of the brain, kidney, retina, and heart may also develop.

There is no cure for tuberous sclerosis, and treatment consists of measures to relieve symptoms. In severe cases, tuberous sclerosis is fatal before the age of 30. *Genetic counselling* is recommended for affected families.

tuboplasty

Surgery in which a damaged *fallopian tube* is repaired to treat *infertility*. It may be performed by *microsurgery*.

tularaemia

A bacterial infection that affects wild animals which is sometimes transmitted to humans. Tularaemia does not occur in the UK but is seen in North America. It may result from contact with an

infected animal or carcass, or a tick, flea, fly, or louse bite. Diagnosis is by blood tests. Treatment of the infection is with *antibiotic drugs*.

tumbu fly

A tropical fly found in Africa whose larvae infest the skin and cause *myiasis*.

tumour

A term that describes any swelling but which is generally used to refer to an abnormal mass of tissue that forms when cells in a specific area reproduce at an increased rate. Tumours can be *cancerous* or *noncancerous*.

Cancerous tumours invade surrounding tissues and may spread through the bloodstream or lymphatic system to form a secondary growth (a *metastasis)* elsewhere in the body. A cancerous tumour that arises from epithelial tissues (such as the skin) is known as a carcinoma; one that arises from connective tissue (such as muscle, bone, or fibrous tissue) is called a sarcoma.

Noncancerous tumours usually grow slowly and do not metastasize. They tend to stay confined within a fibrous capsule, which makes surgical removal relatively straightforward. Noncancerous tumours sometimes grow large enough to press on nearby structures, which can be dangerous in confined spaces such as the skull.

tumour marker

A substance produced by a *tumour* that can be detected in the bloodstream. Tests for the presence of markers can assist in the diagnosis and treatment of tumours. Markers are often substances that occur normally in the body, but are produced in larger amounts when a particular kind of tumour is present. For example, *alpha-fetoprotein*, which is produced in normal pregnancy, is present at elevated levels in a certain type of primary liver cancer.

tuning fork tests

Hearing tests that are carried out in order to differentiate between conductive *deafness* and sensorineural deafness. In the Weber test, a vibrating tuning fork is held against the forehead. If there is conductive hearing loss, the sound seems louder in the affected ear. In the Rinne test, a vibrating tuning fork is held first near the ear, then against the bone behind it. If it sounds louder when against the bone, there is conductive hearing loss.

T

tunnel vision

Loss of the peripheral *visual field* to the extent that only objects straight ahead can be seen clearly. Tunnel vision is most often caused by chronic *glaucoma* (raised pressure within the eyeball). *Retinitis pigmentosa* (degeneration of the retina) is another possible cause.

turbinate

One of the three shell-shaped bony projections in the side of the nasal cavity.

Turner's syndrome

A disorder caused by a *chromosomal abnormality* that only affects females.

CAUSES

The abnormality may arise in one of three ways: affected females may possess only one X *chromosome* instead of the normal two; they may possess one normal and one defective X chromosome; or they may possess a mixture of cells (see *mosaicism*), in which some of the cells are missing an X chromosome, some have extra chromosomes, and others have the normal complement of chromosomes.

SYMPTOMS

The characteristics of Turner's syndrome are short stature; webbing of the skin of the neck; absence or retarded development of sexual characteristics; *amenorrhea* (failure to menstruate), *coarctation of the aorta*, and abnormalities of the eyes and bones.

TREATMENT

Treatment with *growth hormone* from infancy helps girls with Turner's syndrome to achieve near normal height. Coarctation of the aorta is treated surgically. Treatment with *oestrogen drugs* induces menstruation, but it does not make affected girls fertile.

TURP

The abbreviation for transurethral resection of the prostate. A type of *prostatectomy*, TURP is a surgical procedure in which part of an enlarged *prostate gland* is removed (see *prostate, enlarged*). A viewing instrument called a resectoscope is passed along the *urethra* until it reaches the prostate. A heated wire loop, or sometimes a cutting edge, is inserted through the resectoscope and used to cut away excess prostate tissue.

twins

Two offspring resulting from one pregnancy. Twins may develop from a single ovum (egg) or from two ova.

Monozygotic, or identical, twins develop when a single fertilized egg divides at an early stage of development. Incomplete division of the egg results in conjoined twins (see *twins, conjoined*). Monozygotic twins share the same *placenta*. Although one is often much bigger than the other at birth, they are always of the same sex and look remarkably alike.

Dizygotic, or fraternal, twins develop when two eggs are fertilized at the same time. The ova they develop from may be released by the same or different ovaries; fertilization occurs simultaneously. They each have a placenta and may be of different sexes and look quite different.

Twins occur in about one in 80 pregnancies. (See also *pregnancy, multiple*.)

twins, conjoined

Identical *twins* physically joined due to a failure to separate during development from a single fertilized egg. Conjoined twins are also called Siamese twins.

twitch

See *fasciculation*; *tic*.

TWO TYPES OF **TWINS**

During each menstrual cycle, either one ovum or a small number of ova are released. if one ovum is fertilized and the two cells formed from its first division develop independently, the result is identical twins. if two ova are fertilized and mature normally, nonidentical twins result.

IDENTICAL TWINS

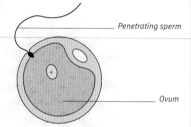

Penetrating sperm

Ovum

Fertilization of a single ovum
Identical twins come from a single fertilized ovum. When the ovum splits, the two cells formed develop independently.

NONIDENTICAL TWINS

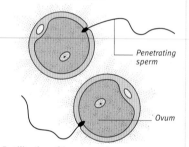

Penetrating sperm

Ovum

Fertilization of two separate ova
Nonidentical twins are the result of two separate ova that have been fertilized by two separate sperm.

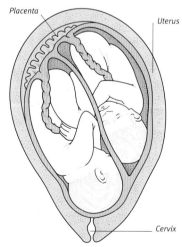

Placenta

Uterus

Cervix

Identical twins in the uterus
The result is a pair of genetically identical twins sharing the same placenta. They are also known as monozygotic, or monovular, twins.

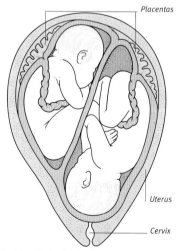

Placentas

Uterus

Cervix

Nonidentical twins in the uterus
The resulting individuals are genetically distinct and have separate placentas. They are also known as dizygotic, or binovular, twins.

T

tympanic cavity

The medical term for the middle *ear*.

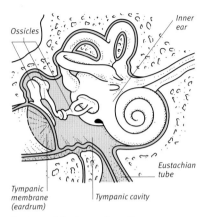

Anatomy of the tympanic cavity
The tympanic cavity contains three movable bones (the malleus, incus, and stapes), which transmit sound from the tympanic membrane (the eardrum) to the inner ear.

tympanic membrane

The medical term for the *eardrum*.

tympanometry

A type of *hearing test* that is used to establish the cause of conductive *deafness*. During the test, a probe that contains a tone generator, a microphone, and an air pump is introduced into the outer-ear canal. The air pressure in the ear is varied and tones are played into it. The tone pattern reflected from the *eardrum* and received by the microphone shows if the eardrum is moving normally.

Tympanometry is a particularly useful technique for use in children because it does not rely on a response from the person being tested.

tympanoplasty

An operation on the *ear* to treat conductive *deafness* by repairing a hole in the eardrum (see *myringoplasty*) or by repositioning or reconstructing the diseased *ossicles* (tiny bones in the middle ear that conduct sound).

tympanum

A term referring either to the middle-*ear* cavity (tympanic cavity) or to the *eardrum* (tympanic membrane).

type 1 diabetes

See *diabetes mellitus*.

type 2 diabetes

See *diabetes mellitus*.

typhoid fever

An infectious disease, also known as enteric fever, contracted by eating food or drinking water contaminated with the bacterium *SALMONELLA TYPHI*. An almost identical disease, *paratyphoid fever*, is caused by related bacteria.

CAUSES

The infection is contracted from the faeces of a person who has the disease or who is a symptomless carrier of the bacteria. Typhoid fever is commonly spread by drinking water contaminated with sewage, by flies carrying the bacteria from faeces to food, or by infected people handling food.

The bacteria pass from the intestines into the blood, then to the spleen and liver, where they multiply. The organisms are excreted from the liver, accumulate in the gallbladder, and are released in large numbers into the intestine. Carriers, after recovering from the condition, may continue to harbour typhoid bacteria in the gallbladder and shed them in faeces for many years.

SYMPTOMS

Typhoid has an incubation period of seven to 21 days. The first symptom is usually a severe headache followed by fever, loss of appetite, *malaise*, abdominal pain, constipation, and often delirium. Diarrhoea soon develops. In the second week of illness, small, raised pink spots develop on the chest and abdomen, and the liver and *spleen* become enlarged.

The illness usually clears up within four weeks. However, potentially fatal complications may develop, including intestinal bleeding, perforation of the intestine leading to *peritonitis*, *osteomyelitis*, *pyelonephritis*, and *kidney failure*.

DIAGNOSIS, TREATMENT, AND PREVENTION

Diagnosis of typhoid is confirmed by a *blood test* or by obtaining a *culture* of typhoid bacteria from blood, faeces, or urine. Treatment with *antibiotic drugs* usually brings the disease under control within a few days.

Immunization against typhoid is recommended for travellers to areas with poor sanitation. It is also important to pay scrupulous attention to personal hygiene to reduce the risk of infection.

typhus

Any of a group of infectious diseases with similar symptoms that are caused by *rickettsiae* (microorganisms similar to bacteria) and are spread by insects or similar animals.

TYPES

Of the various types, epidemic typhus, which is spread between humans by body lice, is historically the most important. This disease formerly killed hundreds of thousands of people in times of war, famine, or other natural disasters. Except in some highland areas of tropical Africa and South America, epidemic typhus is rare today.

Endemic typhus, also called murine typhus, is a disease of *rats* that is occasionally spread to humans by fleas; sporadic cases occur in North and Central America. Scrub typhus is spread by *mites* and occurs in India and Southeast Asia.

SYMPTOMS

The symptoms and complications of all types of typhus are similar. Symptoms include severe headache, back and limb pain, coughing, constipation, high fever, a measles-type rash that may develop into *purpura*, confusion, and exhaustion. If typhus is left untreated, the condition may be fatal, especially in elderly or debilitated people.

DIAGNOSIS AND TREATMENT

Diagnosis is made by *blood tests*, and the infection is treated with *antibiotic drugs* and supportive treatment.

typing

A general term for procedures by which blood or tissues are classified (see *blood groups*; *tissue-typing*).

tyramine

An *amino acid* present in various foods, including cheese, chocolate, red wine, and beer. Tyramine has a stimulating effect on the body. The substance interacts with certain drugs (*monoamine oxidase inhibitors*) used to treat depression; taking both together can cause adverse reactions such as headache and a dangerous rise in blood pressure.

tyrosine

A nonessential *amino acid* (a building-block of proteins). Tyrosine plays a role in the healthy functioning of the nervous and endocrine systems.

T

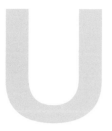

ulcer

An open sore appearing on the skin or on a *mucous membrane* that results from the destruction of surface tissue. Ulcers may be shallow, or deep and crater-shaped, and they are usually inflamed and painful. An indolent ulcer is one that is slow to heal but is not painful.

SKIN ULCERS

Skin ulcers most commonly occur on the leg (see *leg ulcer*), usually as the result of inadequate blood supply to, or drainage from, the limb. In some cases skin cancers, particularly *basal cell carcinomas* or *squamous cell carcinomas*, may be ulcerated. Rarely, a cancer may develop in the skin at the edge of a longstanding ulcer.

DIGESTIVE TRACT ULCERS

Ulcers of the mucous membranes most commonly develop within the digestive tract. The ulcers include *mouth ulcers* (see also *ulcer, aphthous*), *peptic ulcers* (affecting the stomach or duodenum), and the ulcers that occur in *ulcerative colitis*, an inflammatory disorder of the colon or rectum.

GENITAL ULCERS

Ulcers may also affect the skin or mucous membranes of the genitalia (see *genital ulcer*). Most genital ulcers are caused by sexually transmitted infections. Examples of this type of ulcer are hard chancres (see *chancre, hard*), which develop during the first stage of *syphilis*, and soft chancres (see *chancroid*).

EYE ULCERS

Ulcers may also develop on the cornea, the transparent covering at the front of the eyeball (see *corneal ulcers*).

SOLITARY RECTAL ULCER

A break in the lining of the lower part of the large intestine that fails to heal. Symptoms may include bleeding or mucus discharge from the anus, tenesmus (a feeling that the rectum has not been completely emptied), and pain. There may also be diarrhoea or constipation; and rectal prolapse (in which part of the rectum protrudes outside the anus) is often present.

Diagnosis may be made by *sigmoidoscopy* (endoscopic examination of the rectum) and biopsy (taking a tissue sample). Treatment may include laxatives and a high-fibre diet. Surgery may be recommended to excise the ulcer.

ulcer, aphthous

A small, painful *ulcer* that occurs, alone or in a group, on the inside of the cheek or lip or underneath the tongue.

Aphthous ulcers are most common in people between the ages of 10 and 40 and affect more women than men. The most severely affected people have continually recurring ulcers; others have just one or two ulcers each year.

CAUSES

The ulcer, which usually lasts for one to two weeks, may be a hypersensitive reaction to haemolytic streptococcus *bacteria*. Other factors commonly associated with the occurrence of these ulcers are minor injuries (such as at an injection site or from a toothbrush), acute stress, or allergies. In women, aphthous ulcers are most common during the premenstrual period. They may also be more likely to occur if other family members suffer from recurrent ulcerative conditions such as *Crohn's disease*.

SYMPTOMS

Each ulcer is usually small and oval, with a grey centre and a surrounding red, inflamed halo. The ulcers usually last for one to two weeks.

TREATMENT

Analgesic mouth gels or mouthwashes may ease the pain of an aphthous ulcer. Some ointments form a waterproof covering that protects the ulcer while it is healing. Ulcers heal by themselves, but a doctor may prescribe a paste or lozenge containing a *corticosteroid drug* or a mouthwash containing an antiseptic to speed up the healing process.

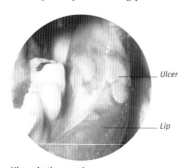

Ulcers in the mouth
Aphthous ulcers are common, painful, and they typically last for one or two weeks. Most aphthous ulcers heal well without leaving scars.

ulceration

The formation or presence of one or more *ulcers*.

ulcerative colitis

Chronic inflammation and ulceration of the lining of the *colon* and *rectum*, or, especially at the start of the condition, of the rectum alone. The cause of ulcerative colitis is not known, but the condition is most common in young and middle-aged adults.

SYMPTOMS

The main symptom of ulcerative colitis is bloody diarrhoea; the faeces may also contain mucus. In severe cases, the diarrhoea and bleeding are extensive, and there may be abdominal pain, fever, weight loss, and general malaise. The incidence of attacks varies considerably from person to person. Most commonly, the attacks occur at intervals of a few months. However, in some cases, there may be only a single episode.

COMPLICATIONS

Ulcerative colitis may lead to *anaemia*, due to blood loss. Other complications include a toxic form of *megacolon* (an abnormally enlarged colon), which may become life-threatening; rashes; *mouth ulcers*; arthritis; *conjunctivitis* (inflammation of the membrane covering the eyeball); and *uveitis* (inflammation of the iris or choroid of the eye). In addition, people whose entire colon has been affected for more than 10 years are at increased risk of developing cancer of the colon (see *colon, cancer of*).

DIAGNOSIS

Diagnosis is based on examination of the rectum and the lower colon (see *sigmoidoscopy*) or of the entire colon (see *colonoscopy*), or is made by a barium enema (see *barium X-ray examination*). During sigmoidoscopy or colonoscopy, a *biopsy* (removal of a tissue sample) may be performed. Samples of faeces may be taken for analysis in a laboratory to exclude the possibility of infection by bacteria or parasites. *Blood tests* may also be necessary.

People who have suffered from ulcerative colitis for a number of years need periodic colonoscopy and biopsy to check for the development of cancer.

TREATMENT

In most cases, treatment with drugs effectively controls the disease by relieving the symptoms and preventing complications from occurring. For ulcerative colitis occurring in the last part of the colon or the rectum, the

U

drugs may be administered locally, as suppositories for example. If the condition occurs higher up in the intestine or is diffuse (affecting several areas of the colon and/or rectum), the drugs are taken orally.

In mild to moderate ulcerative colitis, acute attacks are treated with *sulfasalazine*, *mesalazine*, or *corticosteroid drugs*. In severe cases or those that do not respond to treatment with these drugs, treatment may be with intravenous corticosteroids and, in some cases, the immunosuppressant drugs *ciclosporin* or *infliximab*. Once the disease is under control, sulfasalazine, mesalazine, and *azathioprine* or infliximab may be used to prevent relapses.

Colectomy (surgical removal of the colon) may be required for a severe attack that fails to respond to other treatments, for those with complications such as toxic megacolon, or to avoid colon cancer in those people who are at high risk of developing this type of cancer. This operation usually produces a dramatic improvement in health, although the person is usually left with an *ileostomy* (an opening in the surface of the abdomen through which faeces are passed).

ulcer-healing drugs

COMMON DRUGS

H₂-RECEPTOR ANTAGONISTS •Cimetidine •Famotidine •Nizatidine •Ranitidine

PROTON PUMP INHIBITORS •Lansoprazole •Omeprazole •Pantoprazole •Rabeprazole

OTHER DRUGS •Antacids •Antibiotics •Bismuth •Misoprostol •Sucralfate

A group of drugs used to treat or to prevent ulcers of the stomach or duodenum (see *peptic ulcers*). The ulcers occur when some of the mucus covering these areas is eroded and irritants attack the tissues, causing a sore to develop. Causes of peptic ulcers include infection with the bacterium HELICOBACTER PYLORI; external irritants, such as tobacco smoke, alcohol, or nonsteroidal anti-inflammatory drugs (NSAIDS); or excessive production of stomach acid.

HOW THEY WORK

Ulcer-healing drugs work in several ways. They may either reduce or neutralize stomach acid or protect the ulcerated area, thus allowing the damaged tissue to heal.

Taking *antacid drugs* regularly may be effective in healing duodenal ulcers

because the drugs neutralize excess stomach acid; however, the rate of healing may be slow.

H2-receptor antagonists function by blocking the effects of histamine, a chemical that normally stimulates the release of acid into the stomach. Drugs such as *omeprazole* are called proton pump inhibitors. They work by blocking an enzyme system called the proton pump, which stimulates the secretion of acid; as a result, they stop acid production until the body can make new supplies of the enzymes. Other drugs, such as misoprostol, also work by reducing acid secretion.

Other ulcer-healing drugs, such as *sucralfate*, are believed to work by forming a protective barrier over the ulcer, allowing healing of the underlying tissues to take place.

CHOICE OF DRUG

Antacids may be all that is needed for the relief of occasional symptoms. If HELICOBACTER PYLORI is confirmed as the cause of a peptic ulcer, treatment is with a proton pump inhibitor to reduce stomach acid secretion and an antibiotic to eradicate the infection. In other cases of peptic ulcer, including those that may have been caused by NSAIDS, H₂-receptor antagonists or proton pump inhibitors may be used.

POSSIBLE ADVERSE EFFECTS

Ulcer-healing drugs do not usually produce adverse side effects. Those that do occur may include diarrhoea, constipation, skin rashes, or dizziness. H₂-receptor antagonists may cause confusion in elderly people. Misoprostol can induce miscarriage or may cause fetal abnormalities, so this drug should not be taken by any woman who is (or may be) pregnant.

ulcer, trophic

See *trophic ulcer*.

ulna

The longer of the two bones of the forearm; the other is the *radius*. The ulna is the bone running down the forearm on the side of the little finger.

The upper end of the ulna articulates with the radius and extends into a rounded projection (which is known as the *olecranon* process) that fits around the lower end of the humerus to form part of the *elbow* joint. The lower end of the ulna articulates with the carpals (*wrist* bones) and the lower part of the radius.

The ulna hinges at the elbow on the inner side of the lower end of the humerus (upper-arm bone). It is less mobile than the radius.

Right arm

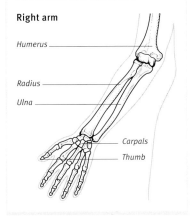

Humerus

Radius

Ulna

Carpals

Thumb

ulna, fracture of

A fracture of the *ulna*, one of the two bones of the forearm. Ulnar fractures typically occur across the shaft or at the *olecranon* process (the rounded projection at the tip of the elbow).

A fracture to the shaft usually results from a blow to the forearm or a fall onto the hand. Sometimes the radius (the other bone in the forearm) is fractured at the same time (see *radius, fracture of*). Surgery is usually needed to reposition the broken bone ends and fix them together using either a plate and screws or a long nail down the centre of the bone. The arm is immobilized in a *cast*, with the elbow at a right-angle, until the fracture heals.

A fracture of the olecranon process is usually the result of a fall onto the *elbow*. If the bone ends have not been displaced, the arm is immobilized in a cast that holds the elbow at a right-angle. If the bone ends are displaced, however, they are fitted together and fixed with a metal screw.

ulnar nerve

One of the principal *nerves* of the arm. The ulnar nerve, which is a branch of the *brachial plexus*, runs down the full length of the arm and into the hand. The ulnar nerve controls muscles that move the thumb and fingers. It also conveys sensation from the fifth finger, part of the fourth finger, and the area of the palm that is closest to these fingers.

U

DISORDERS

A blow to the *olecranon* process (the rounded projection at the tip of the elbow), over which the ulnar nerve passes, causes a pins-and-needles sensation and pain in the forearm and fourth and fifth fingers. Repeated leaning on the elbow can have a similar effect.

Persistent numbness and weakness in areas controlled by the ulnar nerve may be caused by an abnormal bony outgrowth from the *humerus* (upper-arm bone), which may be due to *osteoarthritis* or to a fracture of the humerus. Surgery is needed to relieve the pressure on the nerve. If the condition is left untreated, it may cause permanent damage to the ulnar nerve, which can result in *claw-hand*.

ultrasonography, Doppler

See *Doppler ultrasonography*.

ultrasound

Sound with a frequency that is greater than the human ear's upper limit of perception: that is, higher than 20,000 hertz (cycles per second). Ultrasound is used in medicine to produce images of body structures and thus aid diagnosis (see *ultrasound scanning*), or in treatment to aid healing or to destroy abnormalities such as kidney stones (see *ultrasound treatment*; *lithotripsy*). Ultrasound that is used for these purposes is typically in the range of 1–15 million hertz.

ultrasound scanning

A diagnostic technique in which very high frequency sound waves are passed into the body and the reflected echoes analysed to build a picture of the internal organs or of a fetus in the uterus. Unlike most other imaging techniques, ultrasound scanning can produce moving images. The procedure is painless and is considered safe.

WHY IT IS DONE

The ability of ultrasound scanning to show soft tissues makes the procedure useful for examining fluid-filled or soft structures within the body. Ultrasound waves cannot, however, pass through bone or gas; therefore, they are of limited use for viewing any areas that are surrounded by bone (such as the brain in adults) or those that are filled with gas (such as the lungs or the intestines).

Obstetric and neonatal uses One of the most common uses of ultrasound is to view the uterus and fetus, at any time during *pregnancy*.

HOW **ULTRASOUND SCANNING** WORKS

Ultrasound waves are emitted by a transducer, a device placed on the skin over the area to be viewed. Gel is used to ensure good contact between the transducer and the skin. The transducer contains a crystal that converts an electric current into sound waves. The waves have frequencies in the range of 1 to 15 million hertz. At these high frequencies, they can be focused into a fine parallel beam, which passes through a "slice" of the body if the transducer crystal is oscillated back and forth. Some of the waves are reflected at tissue boundaries, so a series of echoes is returned. The transducer also acts as a receiver, converting these echoes into electrical signals, which are processed and displayed on a screen as two-dimensional images of the scanned body slice. By moving the transducer, different slices can be seen.

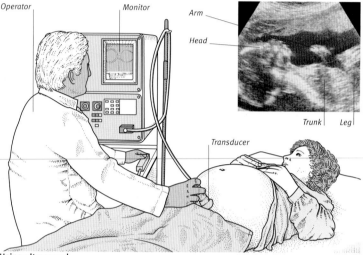

Using ultrasound
Ultrasound has wide applications in medicine and is especially useful in obstetrics. It has no known risk to the baby. By movement of the transducer across the outer wall of the abdomen, views of the growing fetus are obtained from various angles, so it is possible to screen for abnormalities.

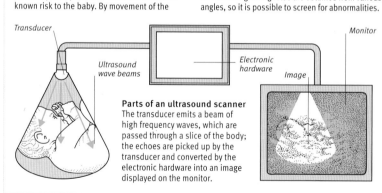

Parts of an ultrasound scanner
The transducer emits a beam of high frequency waves, which are passed through a slice of the body; the echoes are picked up by the transducer and converted by the electronic hardware into an image displayed on the monitor.

The age, size, and growth rate of the fetus can be determined by means of ultrasound. If the date of conception is known, the scan shows whether the fetus is of the expected size for its age; conversely, the size of the fetus can help to establish the accurate date of conception and therefore help doctors and midwives to predict the expected date of delivery.

Ultrasound scans will show if there is more than one fetus (see *pregnancy, multiple*). They also aid the detection of certain problems in the fetus, such as *neural tube defects* or congenital heart disease, so that an affected infant can receive treatment as soon as possible after birth. In addition, the scans show the position of the placenta (the organ through which the fetus receives oxy-

U

gen and nutrients). If the placenta is in a position that could obstruct normal delivery (see *placenta praevia*), delivery by *caesarean section* may be necessary.

The first scan is usually done early in pregnancy (typically before 15 weeks) to accurately date the pregnancy, check for *ectopic pregnancy* (the presence of an embryo outside the uterus), check for major fetal abnormalities, and check for multiple pregnancy. At 18–20 weeks another scan (known as an anomaly scan) is done to check in more detail for any fetal abnormalities, check the fetus is growing properly, and to check the position of the placenta.

Scanning is also a vital part of procedures such as *amniocentesis* (removal of amniotic fluid for analysis) and *chorionic villus sampling* (removal of tissue from the placenta); it shows the position of the fetus and placenta, and helps in guiding the needle into the uterus. Scans may be performed later in pregnancy if the growth rate of the fetus seems slow, if fetal movements cease or become excessive, or if the mother has vaginal bleeding. For high-risk or overdue pregnancies, a scan may be carried out just before delivery to check on fetal size, development, and position in the uterus, assess the amount of amniotic fluid, and to recheck the position of the placenta.

Non-obstetric uses The liver can be clearly viewed by ultrasound; scans can be used to diagnose liver disorders such as *cirrhosis*, cysts, abscesses, or tumours. Ultrasound shows the presence of *gallstones* in the gallbladder or bile ducts. In a patient with *jaundice*, a scan can help to establish whether the jaundice is due to obstruction of the bile ducts or to liver disease. The pancreas can be scanned for cysts, tumours, or for *pancreatitis*, and the kidneys for congenital defects, cysts, tumours, and *hydronephrosis* (swelling due to obstruction preventing the outflow of urine). Other organs that may be scanned by ultrasound (primarily for the purpose of looking for cysts, solid tumours, or foreign bodies) include the thyroid gland, breasts, bladder, testes, uterus, fallopian tubes, ovaries, spleen, and eyes.

Ultrasound can also be used to assess the risk of fracture in suspected *osteoporosis*; to screen for abdominal aortic *aneurysm* (ballooning of the aorta, the body's main artery); and to assess the size of the prostate gland and any changes in the gland.

Echocardiography is an ultrasound technique that is used to look at the heart. This technique is particularly useful for investigating heart *murmurs*, congenital heart disease, heart failure, and disorders of the heart valves.

Ultrasound scanning is also used during needle *biopsy* (insertion of a very thin hollow needle into an organ to remove cells, tissue, or fluid for examination) to help guide the needle accurately to a specific spot.

Doppler ultrasound scanning This technique is a modified form of ultrasound scanning that uses the *Doppler effect* (the change in pitch that occurs when a sound source is moving relative to the detector) for the purposes of investigating moving objects. Doppler ultrasound scanning can be used to examine the fetal heartbeat and to obtain information about the rate of blood flow in blood vessels, for example through the fetus's umbilical cord.

HOW IT IS DONE
The patient removes all clothing that is covering the area to be viewed. A gel is then smeared over the skin to ensure that there is good contact between the skin and the transducer (the device that emits and receives ultrasonic waves). The transducer is placed on the skin over the part of the body that is to be viewed and is moved back and forth. At the boundaries, or edges, of tissues, echoes are bounced back to the transducer. The device converts the sound echoes into electrical signals and sends these to a computer, which converts the data into an image. For scans in early pregnancy or for gynaecological purposes, a transducer may instead be inserted into the vagina (which is known as transvaginal ultrasound).

For a scan in early pregnancy, the woman is usually asked not to pass urine for a few hours beforehand; a full bladder helps to improve the view of the uterus by displacing nearby loops of intestine. For a liver or gallbladder scan, the patient is usually asked to fast for several hours beforehand.

ultrasound treatment

The use of high-frequency sound waves in order to treat soft-tissue injuries (such as injuries to ligaments, muscles, and tendons). Ultrasound treatment reduces inflammation and speeds up the healing process. It is thought to work by improving blood flow in tissues under the skin.

ELECTROMAGNETIC SPECTRUM

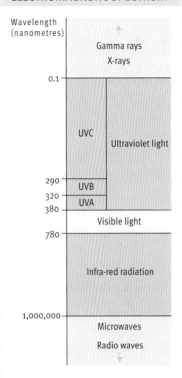

Ultraviolet light in the spectrum
Different types of electromagnetic radiation are defined according to their wavelengths. The diagram shows the different types (which together make up the electromagnetic spectrum) and their wavelength limits in nanometres (one nanometre equals one thousand-millionth of a metre). Ultraviolet light is the part of the electromagnetic spectrum between visible light and X-rays.

ultraviolet light

Invisible light from the part of the electromagnetic spectrum immediately beyond the violet end of the visible light spectrum (see *colour vision*). Long-wavelength ultraviolet light is termed UVA, intermediate UVB, and short-wavelength UVC.

Ultraviolet light occurs in sunlight, but much of it is absorbed by the *ozone* layer of the atmosphere. The ultraviolet light (mainly UVA) that reaches the Earth's surface causes the tanning effects of sunlight and the production of *vitamin D* in the skin. It can also have harmful effects, such as *skin cancer* (see *sunlight, adverse effects of*).

This form of light is generated by tanning beds to produce a suntan. Tanning beds are designed to emit only UVA rays; in practice they also give off a small amount of UVB (which is more

U

likely to cause burning than UVA). Tanning beds may also cause skin cancer. Ultraviolet light is also produced by certain other types of equipment, such as welding torches, carbon arcs, and lasers. Special precautions, such as the use of goggles, should always be taken when using such equipment.

MEDICAL USES
Ultraviolet light is sometimes used in *phototherapy* to treat certain skin disorders, such as psoriasis and eczema, and jaundice in newborn babies. A mercury-vapour lamp (Wood's light) can be used to produce ultraviolet light artificially. This device is used to diagnose skin conditions such as *tinea* because it causes the infected area to fluoresce.

umbilical cord

The ropelike structure connecting the *fetus* to the *placenta*. The umbilical cord supplies the fetus with oxygen and nutrients from the mother's circulation. It is usually 40–60 cm long. It consists of a jellylike substance that contains two arteries and a vein.

After delivery, the umbilical cord is clamped and then cut about 2.5 cm from the baby's abdomen. The stump falls off within a couple of weeks, leaving a scar called the umbilicus (navel).

DISORDERS
In rare cases, the umbilical cord protrudes down through the mother's cervix during labour. This situation is dangerous, because the cord can be squeezed between the mother's pelvis and the baby's body, causing the baby's oxygen supply to be cut off. Prompt delivery, by caesarean section or forceps, is necessary. Another problem that may occur during delivery is the cord wrapping around the baby's neck, causing strangulation. This problem can usually be remedied by someone slipping the cord over the baby's head.

Rarely, there is only one artery in the umbilical cord. This condition may be associated with birth defects.

umbilical hernia

A soft swelling at the *umbilicus* (navel) caused by the protrusion of the abdominal contents through a weak area of abdominal wall. Umbilical hernias, which are common in newborn babies, occur twice as often in boys as in girls. The swelling increases in size when the baby cries, and may cause discomfort. Umbilical hernias usually disappear without treatment by the age of two. If

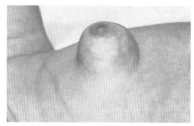

Umbilical hernia
This condition, which is present from birth, is caused by a localized weakness in the abdominal wall. It usually disappears without treatment.

a hernia is still present after this age, surgery may be needed.

Umbilical hernias sometimes develop in adults, especially in women after *childbirth*. Surgery may be needed for a large, persistent, or disfiguring hernia.

umbilicus

The scar on the abdomen that marks the site of attachment of the *umbilical cord* to the *fetus*. It is commonly called the navel or belly button.

DISORDERS
Various umbilical disorders may occur in newborns. Occasionally, problems may occur in adults.

Problems in newborns The baby's umbilical stump sometimes becomes infected and may ooze pus. Called omphalitis, this condition generally begins during the first week of life. Treatment involves gently wiping the umbilicus with sterile cotton wool and water. Treatment with *antibiotic drugs* may also be necessary. Another common problem is the development of an *umbilical hernia*.

Quite commonly, a fleshy protuberance called a granuloma grows on the umbilical stump, sometimes as a result of chronic infection. Umbilical granulomas may be destroyed by topical application of silver nitrate. Another form of growth is an umbilical polyp (also called umbilical adenoma): a shiny, bright red, raspberry-like growth. Such polyps may require surgical removal.

Problems in adults Adults occasionally develop umbilical hernias. Other problems are rare.

One possible problem is a discharge from the umbilicus, which may be due to an infection or to an abnormal connection between the umbilicus and the urinary, biliary, or intestinal tracts. Such structural abnormalities may result from a birth defect, *cancer*, or *tuberculosis*. It may be possible to correct them surgically. Occasionally,

secondary cancerous tumours may develop in the umbilicus as a result of cancers in the breast, colon, ovary, or stomach. In rare cases, women develop *endometriosis* in the umbilicus, causing it to bleed during *menstruation*.

unconscious

A specific part of the mind in which ideas, memories, perceptions, or feelings that a person is not currently aware of are stored and processed. The contents of the unconscious mind are not easily retrieved, in contrast to those of the *subconscious*. (See also *Freudian theory*; *Jungian theory*.)

unconsciousness

An abnormal loss of awareness of self and one's surroundings due to a reduced level of activity in the reticular formation of the *brainstem*. An unconscious person can be roused only with difficulty or not at all. Unconsciousness may be brief and light, as in *fainting* or *concussion*, or deep and prolonged (see *coma*).

underbite

See *prognathism*.

undescended testis

See *testis, undescended*.

undulant fever

Another name for *brucellosis*.

unit of alcohol

See *alcohol, unit of*.

unsaturated fats

See *fats and oils*.

unstable angina

A form of *angina pectoris* (chest pain due to impaired blood supply to the heart) that develops during sleep or without provocation (pain is usually provoked by exercise in angina). The term may also refer to angina that is becoming more frequent or more severe. Unstable angina is a medical emergency because there is a high risk of *myocardial infarction* (heart attack). Drugs are given and *angioplasty* may be necessary.

unstable bladder

Another name for *irritable bladder*.

uraemia

The presence of excess *urea* and other chemical waste products in the blood, caused by *kidney failure*.

U

uranium

A radioactive metallic element that does not occur naturally in its pure form but is widely found in ores such as pitchblende, carnotite, and uraninite. Radioactive decay of uranium causes *radiation* to be emitted and yields a series of radioactive products, including *radium* and *radon*, which may cause tissue damage or cancer (see *radiation hazards*; *radiation sickness*). Uranium is also chemically poisonous and can cause damage to the urinary system.

urea

A waste product from the breakdown of proteins. Proteins in food are digested to form *amino acids*. In the liver, excess amino acids are converted into urea, which is carried by the bloodstream to the kidneys and excreted in the urine (a small amount of urea is also excreted by the sweat glands). A high-protein diet increases the amount of urea produced.

The kidneys are usually highly efficient at eliminating urea from the body. Healthy kidneys can cope with increased urea production, but *kidney failure* lessens this ability and leads to uraemia (abnormally high blood levels of urea). For this reason, the measurement of urea levels in the blood may be one of the routine *kidney-function tests*.

Urea is also formed in the body from the breakdown of cell proteins. If there is a large increase in urea from this source (due, for example, to severe tissue damage), the kidneys are sometimes unable to cope and uraemia results.

Certain conditions (such as liver damage) may lead to a decrease in the blood level of urea. Blood levels of urea also fall during pregnancy, when the blood is more dilute than usual.

MEDICAL USES

Urea is used in various creams and ointments to moisturize and soften the skin in disorders such as *psoriasis*, atopic *dermatitis*, *ichthyosis*, and other conditions in which the skin is dry and scaly.

ureter

One of the two tubes that carry urine from the *kidneys* to the *bladder*. Urine flows down the ureters, partly by gravity, but mainly by *peristalsis* (rhythmic contractions of the muscular ureter walls).

Each ureter is 25–30 cm long. The walls of the ureters have three layers: a fibrous outer layer; a muscular middle layer; and an inner watertight layer. The ureters are supplied by blood vessels

and nerves. They join the bladder via a tunnel in the bladder wall, which is angled to prevent reflux (backflow) of urine, into the ureters when the bladder muscle contracts.

DISORDERS

Some people are born with duplex (double) ureters, on one or both sides of the body, usually in association with partial *duplex kidney* on an affected side. Double ureters may be separate along their entire length, or they may join to form a Y shape. In many cases, the condition causes no problems, but if duplicated ureters enter the bladder separately there may be *vesicoureteric reflux* (backflow of urine into the ureter). There may also be problems, such as *incontinence* or infection, if a ureter enters the urethra or the vagina instead of the bladder. Corrective surgery can be performed if necessary.

Spasms of the ureter may occur if a stone (see *calculus, urinary tract*) passes down or becomes stuck in a ureter. This extremely painful condition is commonly known as *renal colic*.

Ureteritis is an inflammatory condition that may occur if the ureter is blocked by a stone, or be caused by the spread of infection from the bladder.

ANATOMY OF THE **URETER**

The ureters are tubes that carry urine from the kidneys to the bladder. They enter the back of the bladder at an angle.

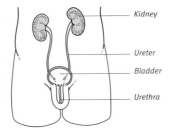

Kidney
Ureter
Bladder
Urethra

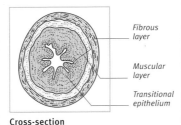

Fibrous layer
Muscular layer
Transitional epithelium

Cross-section
Each ureter has three layers: a fibrous layer, muscular middle layer, and inner transitional epithelial layer, which is the same tissue that lines the bladder.

---

ureteric colic

See *renal colic*.

ureterolithotomy

The surgical removal of a stone (see *calculus, urinary tract*) from a *ureter* (tube that carries urine from a kidney to the bladder). Ureterolithotomy is not often used because *lithotripsy* and *cystoscopy* can deal with stones.

urethra

The tube through which *urine* is excreted from the *bladder*. In females, the urethra is short and opens to the outside of the body in front of the *vagina*. In males, the urethra is much longer; it is surrounded by the *prostate gland* at its upper end, and it forms a channel through length of the penis, with its outlet in the *glans*. (see *Location of the urethra*, overleaf).

DISORDERS

Urethral infections, scarring, and congenital abnormalities occur in both sexes, but these are much more common and serious in males than in females.

Inflammation of the urethra, called *urethritis*, may be due to an infection such as chlamydia or gonorrhoea, irritation, or minor surgery. It may lead to *urethral stricture* (narrowing of a section of the urethra) in men. In addition, the male urethra is easily damaged in accidents involving pelvic injury and may require surgical repair.

Male infants sometimes have a urethral valve, which is a flap that grows from the lining of the urethra. The valve impedes the flow of urine and causes back pressure on the kidneys as urine overfills the bladder, ureters, and collecting ducts of the kidneys. Permanent and severe damage to the kidneys can occur if the urethral valve is not removed surgically.

urethral dilatation

The procedure in which a *urethral stricture* (a narrowed section of the urethra) in a male is widened by the insertion of a slim, round-tipped instrument through the opening of the urethra at the tip of the *penis*.

urethral discharge

A fluid, distinct from urine, that flows from the *urethra* in some cases of *urethritis* (urethral inflammation) caused by infection. In some infections, the discharge is clear whereas in others, such as *gonorrhoea* and sometimes *chlamydial infections*, it is cloudy.

U

LOCATION OF THE **URETHRA**

The urethra is the tube through which urine is passed from the bladder. There is no voluntary muscle in the urethra. The flow of urine is controlled by muscles in the wall and outlet of the bladder.

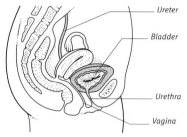

Ureter
Bladder
Urethra
Vagina

Urethra in a woman
The female urethra is short (about 4 cm long) and runs down to open to the exterior just in front of the vagina.

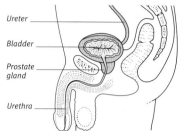

Ureter
Bladder
Prostate gland
Urethra

Urethra in a man
The male urethra is about 18–20 cm long. It passes through the prostate gland and along the full length of the penis.

urethral stricture

A rare condition in which the male *urethra* becomes narrowed and sometimes shortened due to shrinkage of scar tissue in its walls. Scar tissue may form after injury to the urethra or persistent *urethritis* (inflammation of the urethra).

A stricture may make passing urine or ejaculation difficult or painful, and it may cause some deformation of the penis when erect. It may also encourage the development of *urinary tract infection* due to a buildup of stagnant urine. In some cases, trapped urine puts back-pressure on the kidneys and may result in kidney damage.

Treatment is usually by *urethral dilatation* (surgical widening of the urethra). If this operation fails, a surgeon may cut through the scar tissue or, in some cases, the stricture may be completely removed and the urethra is reconstructed by *plastic surgery*.

urethral syndrome, acute

A set of symptoms, usually affecting women, that are very similar to *cystitis* but which occur without the presence of any infection. The symptoms consist of pain and discomfort in the lower abdomen, a frequent urge to pass urine, and, in women, pain around the *vulva*. Middle-aged women are the most commonly affected by this syndrome.

In most cases, kidney function and urinary tract anatomy are normal. The symptoms often occur after sexual intercourse. In women who have gone through the *menopause*, the symptoms may be due to inflammation of the vulva associated with thinning of tissues (see *vulvitis*). Emotional and psychological factors may contribute.

Treatment may be difficult. Cases due to vulvitis may be relieved by creams containing *oestrogen drugs*. Antiseptic creams and strong soaps should be avoided because they may worsen the symptoms. Good personal hygiene and a high fluid intake are usually recommended. Changing sex positions, for example, with the woman on top, may be helpful, as may passing urine before and after sex.

urethritis

Inflammation of the *urethra*. Urethritis may be caused by various infectious organisms, including chlamydia and the bacterium that causes *gonorrhoea*. *Non-gonococcal urethritis* may be caused by any of a large number of different types of microorganism. Urethritis may also be caused by damage from an accident or from a *catheter* or *cystoscope*. Other possible causes include irritant chemicals, such as some spermicides.

SYMPTOMS AND TREATMENT

Urethritis causes a burning sensation and intense pain when passing urine. The urine may be bloodstained and, particularly if gonorrhoea is the cause, may contain a pus-filled discharge.

The inflammation may lead to *urethral stricture* (narrowing), which can make it difficult for the person to pass urine.

The cause of urethritis is identified by analysis of a urine sample or swabs taken from the urethra. Infections are treated with *antibiotic drugs*.

urethrocele

An anatomical abnormality in females caused by a weakness in the tissues in the front wall of the *vagina*. The urethra bulges backwards and downwards into the vagina. A urethrocele may be congenital, but more commonly develops after *childbirth*. It is usually treated by surgery to tighten the vaginal tissues.

-uria

A suffix relating to *urine*. For example, haematuria means blood in the urine.

uric acid

A waste product of the breakdown of *nucleic acids* in body cells. A small amount is also produced by the digestion of foods rich in nucleic acids, such as liver, kidney, and other offal. Most uric acid produced in the body passes to the kidneys, which excrete it in the *urine*, but some goes into the intestine, where it is broken down into chemicals excreted in the *faeces*.

When uric acid metabolism and/or excretion is disrupted, it may result in *hyperuricaemia* (abnormally high levels of uric acid in the blood), which may in turn lead to *gout* and kidney stones (see *calculi, urinary tract*).

urinal

A container for *urine*, useful for bedridden men (women use a *bedpan*).

urinalysis

Tests that are carried out on *urine*, including measurements of its physical characteristics (such as colour, cloudiness, and concentration); microscopic examination to identify abnormalities such as blood or uric acid crystals; a urine *culture* to detect infectious organisms; and chemical testing such as dipstick urinalysis.

Dipstick urinalysis involves dipping a test stick into a urine sample; chem-

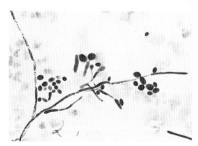

Candida in urine
This infection can be diagnosed using urinalysis. In this light micrograph, the hyphae (strands) and blastospores of the fungus are clearly visible.

ically impregnated squares on the stick change colour in the presence of test substances. The intensity of the colour change shows the amount of the substance present in the urine.

Urinalysis can be used to check kidney function and to diagnose urinary tract infections and disorders such as *diabetes mellitus*. Urinalysis is also used in *pregnancy tests*.

urinary diversion

Any surgical procedure (temporary or permanent) that enables urine to flow when the outlet of the *urinary tract*, via the bladder and urethra, is obstructed or cannot be used, or the bladder has been surgically removed.

TEMPORARY DIVERSION

Temporary urinary diversion may be necessary when the passage of urine is blocked by *prostate gland* enlargement or by *urethral stricture* (narrowing of the urethra). A tube is passed into the bladder through an opening in the abdomen (see *catheterization, urinary*). Temporary diversion is also required after some urinary tract operations; a tube is introduced into the kidney and brought to the abdominal surface.

PERMANENT DIVERSION

Permanent urinary diversion is needed when the bladder has been surgically removed; when neurological bladder control is severely disturbed, such as after severe spinal injury; or if there is an irreparable *fistula* (an abnormal opening) between a woman's bladder or urethra and her vagina.

A section of the *ileum* (the lower part of the small intestine) is removed to create a substitute bladder, into one end of which the surgeon implants the ureters. The other end of the substitute bladder is then brought out through an incision in the abdominal wall. The patient wears a bag attached to the skin to collect urine.

urinary incontinence

See *incontinence, urinary*.

urinary retention

Inability to empty the *bladder* or difficulty in doing so. Urinary retention may be complete (in which urine cannot be passed voluntarily at all) or incomplete (in which the bladder fails to empty completely).

CAUSES

In males, causes of urinary retention include *phimosis* (tight foreskin), *urethral stricture* (narrowing of the urethra), *prostatitis* (inflammation of the prostate gland), a stone in the bladder (see *calculus, urinary tract*), and enlargement or tumour of the prostate (see *prostate, enlarged*; *prostate, cancer of*). In females, causes include pressure on the urethra from uterine *fibroids* or from a growing *fetus* in the uterus. In either sex, the cause may be a bladder tumour.

Urinary retention may also be caused by a defective functioning of the nerve pathways that supply the bladder as a result of general or spinal *anaesthesia*, of drugs affecting the bladder, of surgery, of injury to the nerves, or of disease of the spinal cord.

SYMPTOMS

Complete urinary retention causes discomfort and lower abdominal pain (except when the nerve pathways are defective). The full bladder can be felt above the pubic bone. Chronic or partial urinary retention, however, may not cause problems, and the affected individual may be unaware of the condition. Urinary retention can lead to kidney damage and, often, a urinary tract infection.

TREATMENT

The condition is treated by catheterization (see *catheterization, urinary*). The cause is then investigated. Obstruction can usually be treated; if nerve damage is the cause, permanent or intermittent catheterization is sometimes necessary.

URINARY DIVERSION USING ILEAL CONDUIT

This is one of the standard operations that can be performed when the bladder has to be removed. A midline incision in the abdomen is used; before making the incision, the surgeon creates an opening through the abdominal wall in a good position for later attachment of the collecting bag.

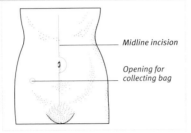

Midline incision

Opening for collecting bag

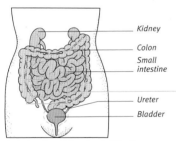

Kidney
Colon
Small intestine
Ureter
Bladder

1 A short length is cut out of the ileum (the lower part of the small intestine), retaining the mesentery (supporting folds of tissue) and the essential blood vessels that supply the freed section.

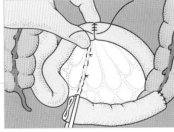

2 The cut ends of the intestine are rejoined. One end of the freed length of intestine is closed, and the other end is temporarily clamped. The bladder is removed.

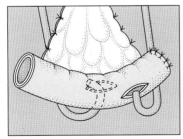

3 The ureters are now implanted into the isolated length of ileum. The open end of this segment is brought through the abdominal wall and stitched in place.

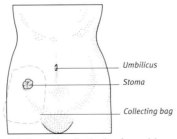

Umbilicus
Stoma
Collecting bag

4 A disposable collecting bag for receiving the patient's urine is attached with adhesive around the new stoma (opening) in the wall of the abdomen.

U

urinary system

See *urinary tract*.

urinary tract

The part of the body concerned with the formation and excretion of *urine*. The urinary tract consists of the *kidneys* (with their blood and nerve supplies), the renal pelvises (funnel-shaped ducts that channel urine from the kidneys), the *ureters*, the *bladder*, and the *urethra*.

The kidneys make urine by filtering blood. The urine collects in the renal pelvises and is then passed down the ureters into the bladder by the actions of gravity and *peristalsis* (wavelike contractions of the muscular ureter walls). Urine is stored in the bladder until there is a sufficient amount present to stimulate *micturition* (passage of urine). When the bladder contracts, the urine is expelled through the urethra. (See also *urinary tract infection*.)

urinary tract infection

An infection anywhere in the *urinary tract*. These often cause inflammation of the urethra (see *urethritis*), bladder (see *cystitis*), or kidneys (see *pyelonephritis*). The symptoms depend on the area affected.

CAUSES AND INCIDENCE

Urethritis is often due to a *sexually transmitted infection*, such as gonorrhoea, but may have other causes. Cystitis and pyelonephritis are almost always the result of a bacterial infection that has travelled up the urinary tract from the urethra; the causative organisms are often bacteria from the rectum that have entered the urethra. Backflow of urine into the ureters from the bladder (see *vesicoureteric reflux*) causes recurrent urinary infection in children that often results in acute pyelonephritis. Infectious organisms may also be carried to the urinary tract in the bloodstream.

Infections of the urethra are more common in men. Infections further up the urinary tract are more common in women, and are more likely to occur during pregnancy. However, an enlarged prostate gland (see *prostate, enlarged*) is often a predisposing factor to bladder or kidney infection in men.

In both sexes, causes of urinary tract infections include stones (see *calculus, urinary tract*), *bladder tumours*, *congenital* abnormalities of the urinary tract, or defective bladder emptying as a result of *spina bifida* or a *spinal injury*.

The risk of a urinary tract infection can be reduced by taking care over personal hygiene, regularly emptying the bladder, and drinking plenty of fluids.

TYPES AND SYMPTOMS

Urethritis causes a burning sensation when urine is passed. Cystitis causes a frequent urge to pass urine, lower abdominal discomfort or pain, *haematuria* (blood in the urine), and, often, general malaise with a mild fever. Pyelonephritis causes fever, pain in the back under the ribs, and sometimes also violent shivering, nausea, and vomiting.

COMPLICATIONS

Urethritis can lead to the formation of a *urethral stricture* (narrowing of a section of the urethra). Cystitis does not usually cause complications unless the infection spreads to the *kidneys*. Pyelonephritis, if left untreated, can lead to permanent kidney damage, *septicaemia* (blood poisoning), and *septic shock*.

DIAGNOSIS AND TREATMENT

Urinary tract infection is diagnosed by examination of a urine *culture*. Further investigations using *intravenous urography* or *ultrasound scanning* may be necessary. Most urinary tract infections are treated with *antibiotic drugs*. Increasing fluid intake and taking preparations such as potassium citrate that make the urine less acidic can relieve the symptoms.

urination, excessive

The production by an individual of more *urine* than is usual for them. In an adult, an output of about 3 litres a day would be considered abnormal, a condition known medically as polyuria.

CAUSES

Various diseases may cause abnormal amounts of certain substances to be excreted in the urine; these substances draw water with them, thus increasing the urine volume. The most important disease in this group is *diabetes mellitus*, in which excess glucose passes from the blood into the urine. Certain kidney diseases, called salt-losing states, lead to excessive salt loss in the urine, with an accompanying increase in volume.

Excessive urination may also be due to *diabetes insipidus*. In central diabetes insipidus, the production of *ADH* (antidiuretic hormone) by the pituitary gland is reduced. ADH normally acts on the kidneys to concentrate the urine, so low levels of this hormone cause a marked increase in urine volume. In nephrogenic diabetes insipidus, which may result from various kidney disorders, normal amounts of ADH are produced but the kidneys fail to respond to it.

Excessive urination is sometimes due to psychiatric problems, which may cause a person to drink compulsively. This leads inevitably to a high urine output.

Alcoholic drinks and drinks containing caffeine have a *diuretic* effect, which temporarily increases urine output.

DIAGNOSIS

Any person who starts to pass larger quantities of urine than is usual for them should consult a doctor.

One simple diagnostic test involves restricting the patient's fluid intake. In a compulsive drinker, urine volume soon drops if water intake is restricted, but if a person has diabetes insipidus, urine production will remain excessive. If diabetes insipidus is suspected, synthetic ADH may be given to establish the type; central diabetes insipidus improves after administration of ADH, but the nephrogenic form does not.

Chemical tests on urine (see *urinalysis*) may also aid diagnosis. In patients with diabetes mellitus, the glucose level in the blood and urine is high; in salt-losing patients, an excessive amount of sodium is detectable in the urine.

TREATMENT

Treatment of excessive urination varies according to the underlying cause. (See also *urination, frequent*.)

urination, frequent

Also known as urinary frequency, passing of urine more often than the average of four to six times daily.

Causes of frequent urination include excessive production of urine (see *urination, excessive*), *cystitis* (inflammation of the bladder), *anxiety*, stones in the bladder (see *calculus, urinary tract*), enlargement of the prostate gland (see *prostate, enlarged*) in men, and, rarely, a *bladder tumour*. In addition, some people who are suffering from *kidney failure* pass urine more frequently, especially during the night. A temporary increase in frequency can result from consuming alcoholic or caffeinated drinks.

Treatment of frequent urination is always aimed at the underlying cause.

urination, painful

Pain or discomfort that occurs when urine is being passed. Painful urination is known medically as dysuria. The pain is often described as burning; sometimes it is preceded by difficulty in starting urine flow. Pain after the flow has ceased, with a strong desire to continue, is called strangury.

U

THE **URINARY TRACT**

Also known as the urinary system, the urinary tract consists of the kidneys, in which urine is formed to carry away waste materials from the blood; the ureters, which transport the urine from the kidneys; the bladder, where the urine is stored until it can be conveniently disposed of; and the urethra, through which the bladder is emptied to the outside. The kidneys require a large blood supply and are connected close to the body's main artery, the aorta. More than a litre of blood passes through the kidneys every minute.

X-ray showing urinary tract
The X-ray on the left, taken using the technique of intravenous urography, shows (as lighter areas) the calyces and pelvis of each kidney, the ureters and bladder, as well as the bones of the lower spine and pelvic girdle.

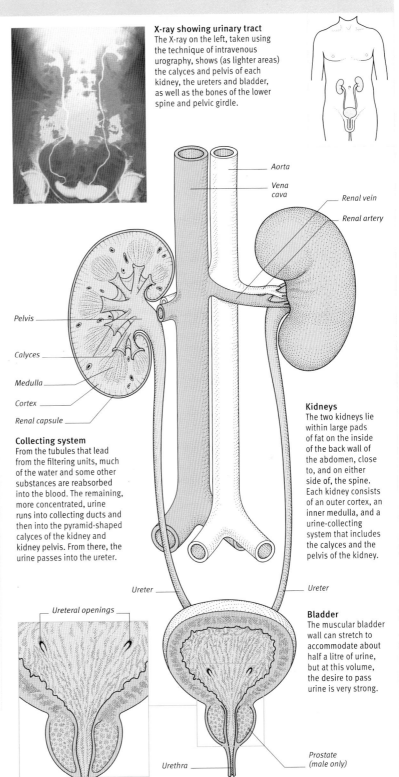

Aorta

Vena cava

Renal vein

Renal artery

Pelvis

Calyces

Medulla

Cortex

Renal capsule

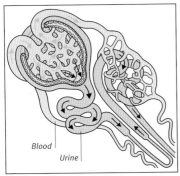

The filtering units
Each kidney has about one million of these units, which form dilute urine by filtering the blood.

Blood

Urine

COMPOSITION OF URINE

Urine consists almost entirely of water, with only small amounts of urea (the main waste product), other waste products (e.g. creatinine and uric acid), and sodium chloride (salt).

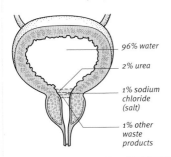

96% water

2% urea

1% sodium chloride (salt)

1% other waste products

Interior of bladder
The two ureteral openings, shown on the right, and the urethral orifice form a triangle at the base of the bladder. In males, the urethra runs through the body of the prostate gland situated below the bladder.

Collecting system
From the tubules that lead from the filtering units, much of the water and some other substances are reabsorbed into the blood. The remaining, more concentrated, urine runs into collecting ducts and then into the pyramid-shaped calyces of the kidney and kidney pelvis. From there, the urine passes into the ureter.

Kidneys
The two kidneys lie within large pads of fat on the inside of the back wall of the abdomen, close to, and on either side of, the spine. Each kidney consists of an outer cortex, an inner medulla, and a urine-collecting system that includes the calyces and the pelvis of the kidney.

Ureter

Ureter

Ureteral openings

Bladder
The muscular bladder wall can stretch to accommodate about half a litre of urine, but at this volume, the desire to pass urine is very strong.

Prostate (male only)

Urethra

U

The most common cause of strangury, especially in women, is *cystitis* (inflammation of the bladder). Other causes include a *bladder tumour*, bladder stone (see *calculus, urinary tract*), and *urethritis* (inflammation of the urethra). In men, possible causes include *balanitis* (inflammation of the head of the penis) and *prostatitis* (inflammation of the prostate gland). Vaginal *candidiasis* (thrush) may be a cause in women.

Strangury is usually caused by spasm of an inflamed bladder wall, but it may be due to bladder stones. Mild discomfort when passing urine may be caused by highly concentrated urine.

Dysuria may be investigated by means of a physical examination, *urinalysis*, *intravenous urography*, or *cystoscopy*. Treatment is of the cause. (See also *urethral syndrome, acute*.)

urine

The pale yellow fluid produced by the *kidneys* and excreted from the body via the *ureters*, *bladder*, and *urethra*. Urine is normally sterile when passed and has only a faint odour. Stale urine has an unpleasant smell, however, because of the action of bacteria, which causes the release of ammonia.

URINE PRODUCTION
Urine is produced when blood is filtered through the *kidneys* to remove waste products and excess water or chemical substances.

A healthy adult produces 0.5–2 litres of urine per day. The minimum volume needed to remove all waste products is about 0.5 litres. A high fluid intake increases the amount of urine produced. High fluid loss from sweating, vomiting, or diarrhoea leads to reduced production.

COMPOSITION
After water, the main component of urine is *urea*. The other substances that are normally excreted in urine are shown in the diagram on p.775.

The volume, acidity, and salt concentration of urine are carefully regulated by hormones such as *ADH* (antidiuretic hormone), *atrial natriuretic peptide*, and *aldosterone*. These hormones act on the kidneys to ensure that the body's levels of water and salt, and the *acid–base balance* (the acidity or alkalinity of the blood and tissue fluids), are kept within narrow limits.

Measurements of the composition of urine are useful in the diagnosis of numerous conditions, from kidney disease and diabetes mellitus to pregnancy.

urine, abnormal

Urine may be produced in abnormal amounts or have an abnormal appearance or composition.

ABNORMAL VOLUME
Certain conditions may cause excess urine to be passed (see *urination, excessive*): in adults, more than about 3 litres of urine per day. In contrast, abnormally low urine production (see *oliguria*), of less than about 0.4 litres per day, may occur in severe *dehydration* or acute *kidney failure*. If severely damaged, the kidneys may fail to produce any urine (see *anuria*). Obstruction of the urinary tract by a stone, for example, may also cause the cessation of urine flow.

ABNORMAL APPEARANCE
Cloudy urine may be due to a *urinary tract infection*, a stone (see *calculus, urinary tract*), or the presence of salts. Haematuria (blood in the urine) may be due to bleeding in the urinary tract. Urine may become discoloured due to ingestion of certain foods or drugs. An excess of protein may cause urine to become frothy.

ABNORMAL COMPOSITION
Certain disorders cause abnormal substances to be excreted in the urine. In *diabetes mellitus*, glucose enters the urine. *Glomerulonephritis* (inflammation of the filtering units of the kidneys) or *nephrotic syndrome* cause protein to leak into the urine. Some disorders cause abnormal levels of normal waste products, or other chemical imbalances. *Kidney failure* reduces the total amounts of waste products such as urea. Other kidney disorders, such as *Fanconi's syndrome* and *renal tubular acidosis*, may make the urine too acid or alkaline, or may cause it to contain excess amino acids, phosphates, salts, or water.

urine tests

See *urinalysis*.

urodynamics

A group of tests carried out to investigate problems with *bladder* control, such as *incontinence*. These studies range from simple measurement of urine flow rate to more invasive procedures to assess bladder function.

HOW THEY ARE DONE
Urine flow rate measurement is a straightforward procedure in which the volume of urine in a given time is measured, usually with an external electronic device. The more complex studies may include cystometry to measure pressure in the bladder and assessments

of bladder function and shape. These studies involve the insertion of probes and catheters into the bladder and into the rectum or vagina to monitor pressure changes while the bladder is filled and emptied. The procedures are carried out under X-ray monitoring in order to produce a visual record of changes in bladder shape.

urography

See *intravenous urography*.

urology

A branch of medicine concerned with the structure, functioning, and disorders of the *urinary tract* in males and females, and of the *reproductive system* in males. Investigative techniques that are used in urology include *intravenous urography*, *cystoscopy*, *ultrasound scanning*, *cystometry*, and *urinalysis*.

ursodeoxycholic acid

A drug used to dissolve *gallstones*. Ursodeoxycholic acid is suitable only if the stones are made exclusively of *cholesterol* and only if the gallbladder is functioning normally.

Side effects of ursodeoxycholic acid are rare but can include diarrhoea, indigestion, and a rash. Drug treatment is less commonly used since the introduction of *minimally invasive surgery*.

urticaria

A skin condition, also known as nettle rash or hives, characterized by the development of itchy weals, usually on the limbs and trunk. Large weals may merge to form irregular, raised patches.

SYMPTOMS
Urticaria is generally harmless and lasts only a few hours, but sometimes a persistent or recurrent form develops. The condition is sometimes accompanied by *angioedema* (an allergic condition in which swelling occurs in various parts of the body). *Dermographism* is a less common form of urticaria in which weals form after the skin is stroked. The symptoms of urticaria can be exacerbated by stress.

CAUSES
The cause is often unknown. The most common known cause is an allergic reaction (see *allergy*), often to a food or drug. Urticaria may also follow exposure to heat, cold, or sunlight. Less commonly, it may be associated with another disorder, such as *vasculitis*, systemic *lupus erythematosus*, or *cancer*.

U

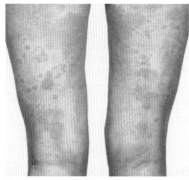

Appearance of urticaria
This skin condition is characterized by itchy weals with a white or yellow centre and an outer area of inflammation.

TREATMENT

Itching can be relieved by the application of *calamine lotion* or by taking *antihistamine drugs*. Severe cases of urticaria may require *corticosteroid drugs*. Identifying and avoiding trigger factors can help prevent future reactions. A tendency to urticaria often disappears in time without treatment.

urticaria, neonatal

A very common, harmless skin condition, also called erythema neonatorum or toxic erythema, that affects newborn infants. The cause is unknown. Neonatal urticaria produces a blotchy rash, in which raised white or yellow lumps are surrounded by ill-defined red areas of inflammation. The rash mainly affects the face, chest, arms, and thighs. It usually clears up without treatment.

uterine muscle relaxants

Drugs that are used to delay premature delivery of a *fetus*. Beta$_2$-adrenoceptor stimulants, such as *salbutamol* and *ritodrine*, may be used in at-risk pregnancies of 24–33 weeks' gestation; these drugs relax the muscles of the *uterus* and may postpone labour for days or weeks. Delaying of premature labour for up to 48 hours allows time for *corticosteroid drugs* to be given to the mother, to help the fetus's lungs to mature.

uterovaginal prolapse

See *uterus, prolapse of.*

uterus

The hollow, muscular organ of the female reproductive system in which the fertilized *ovum* (egg) normally becomes embedded and in which the unborn baby (see *embryo*; *fetus*) develops.

The uterus, which is commonly known as the womb, is situated within the pelvic cavity, behind the *bladder* and in front of the intestines.

STRUCTURE

In a nonpregnant woman, the uterus is 7.5–10 cm long and weighs 60–90 g. The lower part of the uterus opens into the *vagina* at the *cervix*; the upper part opens into the *fallopian tubes*.

The inside of the uterus is lined with *endometrium*. During the menstrual cycle, the endometrium thickens to prepare for the possible implantation of a fertilized egg. If conception and fertilization do not occur, hormone levels fall, causing the endometrium to be expelled from the uterus (see *menstruation*). After the *menopause* (when egg production and menstruation cease), the endometrium atrophies (becomes thinner) and muscle and connective tissue are reduced.

The uterus expands in pregnancy to accommodate the growing baby. At full term, the uterine muscles expel the baby via the birth canal (see *childbirth*).

DISORDERS

Conditions that affect the uterus include *congenital* disorders such as malformation or absence of the uterus, *duplex uterus*, or *septate uterus*; tumours, including *polyps*, *fibroids*, and cancer of the endometrium (see *uterus, cancer of*); infections, causing inflammation of the lining of the uterus (see *endometritis*); and hormonal disorders. (See also *uterus, prolapse of*; *uterus, retroverted*.)

ANATOMY OF THE **UTERUS**

The nonpregnant uterus lies deep in the pelvis immediately behind and above the urinary bladder and in front of the rectum. It is usually tilted forwards at an angle to the vagina, and is curved downwards slightly. When the bladder is full, the uterus is pushed up and back.

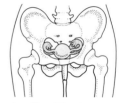
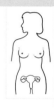

Location of the uterus

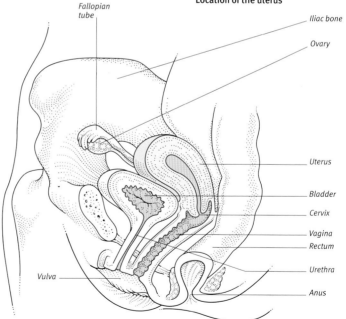

Fallopian tube

Iliac bone

Ovary

Uterus

Bladder

Cervix

Vagina

Rectum

Urethra

Anus

Vulva

The uterus
This thick-walled organ consists mainly of muscle. The fallopian tubes enter on both sides of the uterus just below its uppermost point. The small uterine cavity is lined with a mucous membrane called the endometrium, which undergoes changes during the different phases of the menstrual cycle. The vaginal surface of the cervix is lined with a flatter mucous membrane, which is identical to that of the vagina.

U

uterus, cancer of

A malignant growth in the tissues of the *uterus*. Cancer of the uterus mainly affects the cervix (see *cervix, cancer of*) and *endometrium* (the lining of the uterus). Rarely, the uterine muscle is affected by a type of cancer called a leiomyosarcoma. The term "uterine cancer" is usually used to refer to cancer of the endometrium.

CAUSES

Risk factors for endometrial cancer include anything that may raise levels of the female sex hormone oestrogen in the body, such as *obesity*, a history of failure to ovulate, or taking *oestrogen hormones* long term if these are not balanced with *progestogen drugs*. The drug *tamoxifen*, used to treat breast cancer, increases the risk of uterine cancer. The cancer is more common in women who have had no children, and most cases occur after the menopause.

SYMPTOMS

Before the *menopause*, the first symptom of cancer of the uterus may be *menorrhagia* (heavy periods), or bleeding between periods or after sexual intercourse. After the menopause, the first symptom is usually a bloodstained vaginal discharge.

DIAGNOSIS AND TREATMENT

Diagnosis is made by transvaginal *ultrasound* and *hysteroscopy* (examination of the inside of the uterus using a viewing instrument), with a *biopsy* (taking a tissue sample for microscopic analysis).

Very early endometrial cancer is usually treated by *hysterectomy* (surgical removal of the uterus) and removal of the fallopian tubes and ovaries. If the cancer has spread beyond the uterus, *radiotherapy* and *anticancer drugs* may also be used.

uterus, prolapse of

A condition in which the *uterus* descends from its normal position into the *vagina*. The degree of prolapse varies from first-degree prolapse, in which there is only slight displacement of the uterus, to third-degree prolapse (procidentia), in which the uterus can be seen outside the *vulva*.

The condition may sometimes be associated with defects of the vagina that include *cystocele*, in which the bladder bulges into the front wall of the vagina; *urethrocele*, in which the urethra bulges into the front wall of the vagina; and *rectocele*, in which the rectal wall bulges into the back wall of the vagina.

CAUSES

Stretching of the ligaments that support the uterus is the most common cause of prolapse. Prolapse of the uterus is also aggravated by obesity.

SYMPTOMS AND DIAGNOSIS

There are often no symptoms, but there is sometimes a dragging feeling in the pelvis. In severe cases, part or all of the uterus may be visible. An accompanying cystocele, urethrocele, or rectocele may cause leakage of urine or difficulty in passing urine or faeces. Diagnosis is made by examination.

PREVENTION AND TREATMENT

Pelvic floor exercises strengthen the muscles of the vagina and can therefore reduce the risk of a prolapse, especially following childbirth. Often, surgery is necessary to repair structures that support the uterus.

For a severe prolapse, treatment usually involves *hysterectomy* (removal of the uterus) and tightening of the ligaments. Rarely, if surgery is not advised, a plastic, ring-shaped pessary may be inserted into the vagina to hold the uterus in position. (See also *cystocele*; *rectocele*; *urethrocele*.)

uterus, retroverted

A harmless variation in the position of the uterus, which is normally retroverted in infancy, tilting forwards at puberty; a

---

PROLAPSE OF THE **UTERUS**

This condition is caused by weakening and slackness of the various ligaments, muscles and connective tissues that help to keep the uterus in position in the pelvis. Prolapse of the uterus, which is more common in women who have had children, may occur in conjunction with a rectocele or cystocele. There are three degrees of uterine prolapse, as shown below.

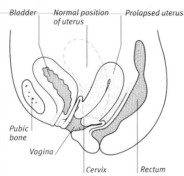

First degree prolapse
In this, the least severe degree of prolapse, strain causes the cervix (neck) of the uterus to move farther down in the vagina; however, it remains well within the vagina.

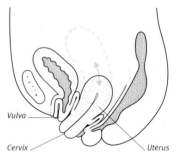

Second degree prolapse
The cervix protrudes beyond the vulva during straining, but retracts on relaxation. The vagina is partly everted (turned inside out).

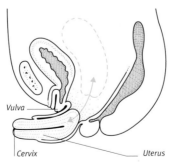

Third degree prolapse
The whole uterus projects outside the vulva. The surface of the cervix and the everted vaginal wall eventually dry out and are replaced by thick white tissue.

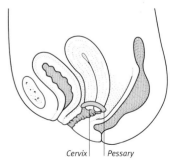

Treatment of prolapse
Surgery to repair the prolapse or, if necessary, to perform a hysterectomy, is the usual treatment. The uterus may be held in position by a plastic pessary inserted into the vagina.

U

RETROVERTED **UTERUS**

In about 80 per cent of women, the uterus is anteverted (tilted forwards). In addition, the body of the organ is anteflexed (bent forwards). In simple retroversion, the organ is tilted back, but not bent back. A retroverted uterus may also be retroflexed (bent back). Retroversion is a normal variant and does not cause symptoms.

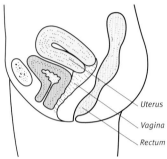

Anteflexion (most common position)
The illustration shows the usual position of the uterus, lying bent and tilted forwards, at right angles to the vagina.

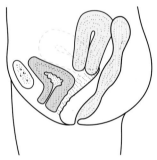

Simple retroversion
A retroverted uterus that can easily be anteverted by manipulation seldom causes any symptoms.

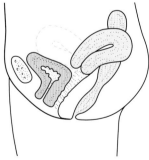

Retroversion and retroflexion
The retroversion and retroflexion may be the result of disease such as endometriosis. There may be symptoms including painful intercourse.

retroverted uterus inclines backwards. About 1 in 5 females has a retroverted uterus. In some cases, the uterus has failed to incline forwards during the normal process of maturation. Other cases are due to changes in position after childbirth. Less commonly, retroversion is caused by a disease, such as a tumour; scarring caused by *endometriosis*; or *pelvic inflammatory disease*.

A retroverted uterus rarely causes problems. If it is associated with underlying disease, however, it may cause symptoms such as *dysmenorrhoea* (painful periods), pain during intercourse (see *intercourse, painful*), and *infertility*. Rarely, a retroverted uterus may fail to lift out of the pelvis after about 12 weeks of pregnancy, as is usual, which may lead to urinary retention needing catheterization.

Diagnosis of a retroverted uterus is by means of physical examination (see *pelvic examination*). *Laparoscopy* (examination of the abdominal cavity with a viewing instrument) may be performed if an underlying disease is suspected. Treatment of the condition is not necessary unless the retroversion is causing symptoms, in which case the underlying cause is treated or the uterus may be manipulated back into position or surgically repositioned.

uvea

Part of the *eye*, comprising the *iris* (the pigmented area around the pupil), the *ciliary body* and its muscle, which focuses the *lens*, and the *choroid* (the blood-rich layer just under the *retina*).

The uvea is well supplied with blood vessels. Those in the iris supply the muscles that control dilation (widening) and constriction (narrowing) of the pupil. The vessels in the choroid supply oxygen and nutrients to the retina.

Pigment cells, which are concentrated in the back of the iris and scattered throughout the choroid, give the eye its colour and improve optical efficiency.

uveitis

Inflammation of the *uvea*. It may affect any part of the uvea, including the *iris* (when it is known as iritis), the *ciliary body* (when it is called cyclitis), or the *choroid* (when it is called choroiditis).

CAUSES

Uveitis may occur as a result of a wide range of underlying causes, including *autoimmune disorders* (in which the immune system attacks the body's own

LOCATION OF THE **UVEA**

The uvea consists of the iris, ciliary body, and choroid.

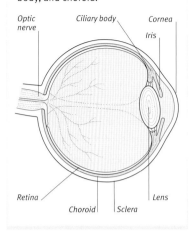

tissues), infections, cancer, eye injury, impaired circulation to the eye, certain medications, and some inherited disorders. In some cases, uveitis occurs without any identifiable cause.

SYMPTOMS

The symptoms can vary, depending on which part of the uvea is affected. They may include painful, red eye, blurred vision, photophobia (excessive sensitivity to light), and gradual loss of vision. One or both eyes may be affected. However, in some cases symptoms may not be noticeable.

TREATMENT

Early treatment is vital to prevent irreversible loss of vision. When an underlying cause can be identified, this will be treated. Treatment of the uveitis itself may include cycloplegic drugs drugs such as cyclopentolate or *atropine* and *corticosteroid drugs*.

uvula

The small, fleshy protuberance that hangs from the middle of the lower edge of the soft *palate*. It is composed of muscle and connective tissue, with a covering of mucous membrane.

U

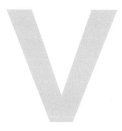

vaccination

A form of *immunization* in which a *vaccine*, in the form of weakened or killed *microorganisms* or inactivated bacterial *toxins*, is introduced into the body. A vaccine is given, usually in the form of an injection, in order to sensitize the *immune system*. If disease-causing organisms or toxins of the same type enter the body in the future, the sensitized immune system rapidly produces *antibodies* that destroy them.

vaccine

A preparation that is given to induce *immunity* against an infectious disease. Most vaccines contain the organisms (or parts of the organisms) against which protection is sought.

Vaccines are usually given by injection into the upper arm. Some vaccines require several doses that are spaced some weeks apart; others require only one dose. (See also *immunization*.)

vacuum extraction

An obstetric procedure that is undertaken to facilitate the delivery of a baby. Vacuum extraction may be used if the second stage of labour (see *childbirth*) is

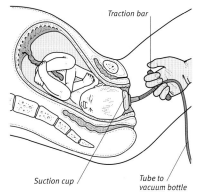

Technique of vacuum extraction
Once the suction cup is attached to the baby's head, the obstetrician pulls on the traction bar during each contraction, and the baby is drawn out through the vagina.

STRUCTURE OF THE **VAGINA**

The vagina has highly elastic muscular walls to allow intercourse and childbirth; it has a ribbed inner lining that secretes a lubricating fluid during sexual arousal and intercourse. It has no glands itself but is kept moist by cervical and uterine glands.

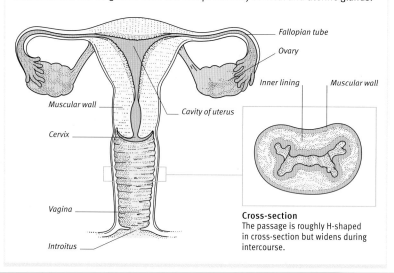

Cross-section
The passage is roughly H-shaped in cross-section but widens during intercourse.

prolonged, if the mother becomes exhausted, or if the baby begins to show signs of *fetal distress*.

The vacuum extraction instrument consists of a suction cup connected to a vacuum bottle. The suction cup is placed on the baby's head in the birth canal, and the vacuum machine sucks the baby's scalp into the cup. The obstetrician draws the baby out of the mother's vagina by gently pulling on the cup with each uterine contraction.

The baby is born with a swelling on the scalp, but this disappears after a few days, usually without treatment.

vagina

The muscular passage, forming part of the female *reproductive system*, occurring between the *cervix* (the neck of the uterus) and the external genitalia. The vagina has highly elastic muscular walls to enable *sexual intercourse* and *childbirth* to take place and are richly supplied with blood vessels.

vaginal bleeding

Bleeding, via the *vagina*, that may originate in the *uterus*, the *cervix* (neck of uterus), or in the vagina itself.

BLEEDING FROM THE UTERUS
The uterus is the most common source of vaginal bleeding and the most likely cause is *menstruation*. From puberty to the menopause, menstrual bleeding

usually occurs at regular intervals. However, problems may occur with either the character or the timing of the bleeding (see *menstruation, disorders of*).

Nonmenstrual bleeding from the uterus may have a variety of causes. Hormonal drugs, such as *oral contraceptives*, can cause spotting. *Endometritis* (infection of the uterine lining) and endometrial cancer (see *uterus, cancer of*) are other possible causes. Bleeding in early pregnancy may be a sign of threatened *miscarriage*. Later in pregnancy, it may indicate *placenta praevia* (implantation of the placenta in the lower part of the uterus) or *placental abruption* (separation of all or part of the placenta from the uterus wall).

BLEEDING FROM THE CERVIX
Bleeding from the cervix may be due to *cervical erosion*, in which case it may occur after intercourse. *Cervicitis* (infection of the cervix) and cervical *polyps* may also cause bleeding. More seriously, bleeding may be a sign of cervical cancer (see *cervix, cancer of*).

BLEEDING FROM THE VAGINA
A possible cause of bleeding from the vagina is injury during intercourse, especially following the menopause, when the walls of the vagina become thinner and more fragile. Occasionally, severe *vaginitis* (inflammation of the vagina) leads to bleeding. Rarely, vaginal bleeding is caused by cancer of the vagina.

V

vaginal discharge

The emission of secretions from the *vagina*. Some mucous secretion from the vaginal walls and the cervix is normal during the reproductive years; its amount and nature vary from woman to woman and at different times in the menstrual cycle (see *menstruation*). *Oral contraceptives* can increase or decrease this discharge. Vaginal secretions tend to be greater during pregnancy. Sexual stimulation also produces increased vaginal discharge.

ABNORMAL DISCHARGE

Discharge may be abnormal if it is excessive, offensive-smelling, yellow or green, or if it causes itching. Abnormal discharge may accompany *vaginitis* (inflammation of the vagina), which may be the result of infection, such as *candidiasis* (thrush) or *trichomoniasis*, or may be due to a foreign body, such as a forgotten tampon, in the vagina.

vaginal itching

Irritation in the *vagina*, often associated with *vulval itching*. Itching is, in many cases, a symptom of *vaginitis* (inflammation of the vagina), which may be due to infection or by an allergic reaction to chemicals in hygiene or spermicidal products. Vaginal itching is common after the *menopause*, when it may be caused by low oestrogen levels. Treatment depends on the cause; it may involve topical *oestrogen drugs*.

vaginal repair

An operation to correct prolapse (displacement) of the vaginal wall. This may be accompanied by a vaginal *hysterectomy* (surgical removal of the uterus and vagina) if the uterus is also prolapsed (see *uterus, prolapse of*).

vaginismus

Painful, involuntary spasm of the muscles surrounding the entrance to the *vagina*. Vaginismus interferes with *sexual intercourse*. It can sometimes also interfere with medical vaginal examinations. The cause of the condition is usually psychological. (See also *intercourse, painful*; *psychosexual dysfunction*.)

vaginitis

Inflammation of the *vagina*. It may be caused by infection, commonly with the fungus CANDIDA ALBICANS (see *candidiasis*), the parasite TRICHOMONAS VAGINALIS (see *trichomoniasis*), or bacteria. There is also a form of the condition called

atrophic vaginitis that occurs after the *menopause* and is due to a reduction in the production of *oestrogen hormones*. The reduced level of hormones causes the vaginal lining to become fragile and prone to inflammation.

Infections are treated with *antibiotic drugs* or *antifungal drugs*. In cases of allergy, irritants should be avoided. Any foreign bodies, including tampons that may have been left in, are removed. Atrophic vaginitis is treated with *oestrogen drugs*. (See also *vulvitis*; *vulvovaginitis*.)

vagotomy

An operation in which the *vagus nerve*, which controls production of digestive acid by the stomach wall, is cut. Once widely used to treat some cases of *peptic ulcer*, vagotomy has now largely been replaced by drug treatment.

vagus nerve

The tenth *cranial nerve* and the principal component of the parasympathetic division of the *autonomic nervous system*.

COURSE OF THE **VAGUS NERVE**

There are two vagus nerves: right and left. The right vagus nerve supplies the rear portion of the stomach, and the left (shown here) supplies the front portion of the stomach.

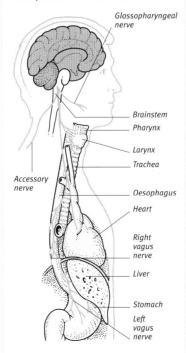

Glossopharyngeal nerve

Brainstem
Pharynx
Larynx
Trachea
Accessory nerve
Oesophagus
Heart
Right vagus nerve
Liver
Stomach
Left vagus nerve

The vagus nerve passes from the medulla oblongata (in the *brainstem*) through the neck and chest to the abdomen and has branches to most of the major organs, including the larynx (voicebox), pharynx (throat), trachea (windpipe), lungs, heart, and digestive system.

valgus

The medical term for outward displacement of a part of the body.

Valium

A former brand name for diazepam, a *benzodiazepine* antianxiety drug, *muscle relaxant*, and *anticonvulsant drug*.

valproate

See *sodium valproate*.

Valsalva's manoeuvre

A forcible attempt to breathe out when the airway is closed. The manoeuvre occurs naturally when an attempt is made to breathe out while holding the *vocal cords* tightly together. This happens, for example, at the beginning of a sneeze. When performed deliberately by pinching the nose and holding the mouth closed, the manoeuvre can prevent pressure damage to the eardrums (see *barotrauma*).

valve

A structure that allows fluid or semifluid material to flow through a tube or passageway in one direction but which closes to prevent reflux (backflow) in the opposite direction.

The valves at the exits from the heart chambers (see *heart valve*) and in the *veins* are essential components of the *circulatory system*. There are also small valves in the lymphatic vessels that make up the *lymphatic system*.

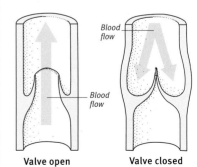

Blood flow
Blood flow

Valve open   **Valve closed**

Valves in the circulatory system
The valves are flaps that open to allow blood to flow in one direction but close to prevent blood flow in the opposite direction.

V

valve replacement

A surgical operation to replace a defective or diseased heart valve. (See also *heart-valve surgery*.)

valvotomy

An operation that is performed to correct a narrowed *heart valve*. Cuts are made, or pressure is applied, to separate the flaps of the valve where they have joined, reducing the degree of narrowing. Valvotomy is performed either by opening the heart up (see *heart-valve surgery*) or by balloon *valvuloplasty*.

valvular heart disease

A defect that occurs in one or more of the *heart valves*.

valvuloplasty

Reconstructive or repair surgery on a defective heart valve (see *heart-valve surgery*). Valvuloplasty may be performed as *open heart surgery*. However, the technique of balloon valvuloplasty makes it possible to treat a narrowed valve without opening the chest. A *balloon catheter* is passed into a blood vessel and from there to the heart. Inflation of the balloon via the catheter then separates the flaps of a narrowed valve.

vancomycin

A glycopeptide *antibiotic drug* given by injection to treat serious bacterial infections, such as *endocarditis* and *MRSA*. Given by mouth, it may be used to treat a form of *colitis* induced by antibiotic drugs. Possible side effects of vancomycin include rash, nausea, kidney damage, and hearing damage.

vardenafil

A drug similar to *sildenafil* used in the treatment of *erectile dysfunction*. Possible side effects of vardenafil include indigestion, nausea, vomiting, headaches, flushing, dizziness, visual disturbances, nasal congestion, and *priapism*. It should not be used by people who have had a recent *myocardial infarction* (heart attack) or *stroke*, or those with certain eye disorders. It should also not be used by people taking *nitrate drugs* because of a possible serious interaction.

varenicline

A drug used, along with self-help measures, as an aid to stopping *smoking*. Varenicline works by partially stimulating the same nerve receptor sites that are stimulated by nicotine. Possible side

effects of varenicline include gastrointestinal disturbances, a dry mouth, taste disturbances, headache, drowsiness, dizziness, and sleep problems.

variant angina

A form of *angina pectoris* (chest pain as a result of insufficient blood supply to the heart muscle), also known as Prinzmetal's angina, in which chest pain occurs when at rest, often during sleep. The pain may be accompanied by breathlessness and *palpitations*. Variant

---

VARICOSE VEINS

When a vein's valves work correctly, the weight of the blood column is well distributed. When they fail, the back pressure is from a much larger column of blood; some veins become engorged with blood and swell.

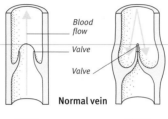

> Blood flow
> Valve
> Valve

Normal vein

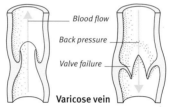

> Blood flow
> Back pressure
> Valve failure

Varicose vein

How varicosities are caused
In a normal vein, valves stop blood from draining down due to gravity. If valves fail, blood is able to pool downwards.

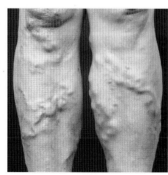

Appearance of varicose veins
This varicosity of the saphenous vein on the front of the lower legs shows the typical tortuous, swollen appearance.

---

angina is thought to be due to narrowing of the *coronary arteries* by muscular spasm in their walls. Treatment with *calcium channel blockers* or *nitrate drugs* is usually effective.

variant CJD

One form of *Creutzfeldt–Jakob disease*.

varicella

Another name for *chickenpox*.

varicella–zoster

The virus that is responsible for *chickenpox* and *shingles*.

varices

Enlarged, tortuous, or twisted sections of vessels, usually veins. Varices is the plural of varix. A vein affected by varices is called a *varicose vein*.

varicocele

Varicose veins surrounding a *testis*. Varicocele is a common condition. It almost exclusively affects the left testis and is usually harmless, although there may be aching in the *scrotum* or an abnormally low sperm count (see *infertility*). Aching may be relieved by supportive underwear. Surgery to divide and tie off the swollen veins may be performed if the sperm count is low.

varicose veins

Enlarged, tortuous *veins* just beneath the surface of the skin. Varicose veins most commonly occur in the legs but can also occur in the anus (see *haemorrhoids*), oesophagus (see *oesophageal varices*), and scrotum (see *varicocele*).
CAUSES
A defect of the *valves* in the leg's perforating veins (which lie between the superficial veins (those near the skin's surface) and the deeplying veins) causes blood to pool in the superficial veins. The buildup of pressure in these veins causes them to become varicose. Factors that contribute to varicose veins include *obesity*, hormonal changes and pressure on the pelvic veins during *pregnancy*, hormonal changes occurring at the *menopause*, and standing for long periods of time. Varicose veins are common, tend to run in families, and affect more women than men.
SYMPTOMS
Varicose veins may not cause any problems, but they may ache severely and the feet and ankles may be swollen; persistent itching can also occur. These

V

symptoms may worsen during the day and may be relieved by sitting with the legs raised. In women, symptoms are often worse just before menstruation. In severe cases, *leg ulcers* may develop. *Thrombophlebitis* (inflammation and clotting of blood in the veins) may be associated with varicose veins.

TREATMENT

In some cases. the symptoms can be adequately controlled by wearing compression stockings, regular walking, and sitting with the feet up as much as possible. However, these measures do not treat the varicose veins themselves and, if they are ineffective, surgery to remove or seal off the varicose veins may be recommended.

Various surgical techniques may be used, including avulsion, in which individual varicosed sections of vein are removed; stripping or powered phlebectomy, two methods of removing entire veins; and *radiofrequency ablation* or *laser therapy*, which seal off veins. *Sclerotherapy*, in which an irritant chemical is injected into a vein to seal it, may also sometimes be used. Varicose veins have a tendency to recur, and repeat treatment may be required.

variola

Another name for *smallpox*.

varus

The medical term for an inward displacement of part of the body.

LOCATION OF THE **VAS DEFERENS**

The vas deferens passes from the epididymis, up and around the bladder, before entering the prostate, where it connects to a tube from the seminal vesicle to form the ejaculatory duct.

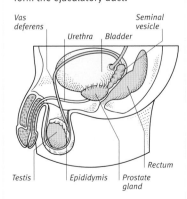

HOW **VASECTOMY** IS PERFORMED

This operation blocks the passage of sperm from the testes but does not prevent the prostate and other glands from secreting the fluids that form most of the semen. Hence it has little effect on the volume of the ejaculate and no effect no orgasm.

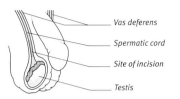

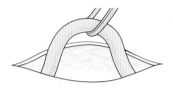

1 Under a local anaesthetic, incisions are made on both sides of the scrotum; the vas deferens is then cut free of the spermatic cord.

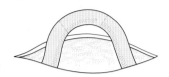

2 A loop of the vas deferens is freed and brought out through the incision. There are now several possibilities; usually, a length of the vas deferens is cut out.

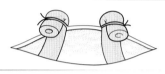

3 In order to prevent the cut ends from rejoining, they are often bent back and tightly closed with ligatures. They are then pushed back into the spermatic cord.

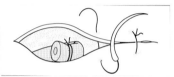

4 The skin incision is now closed with three or four dissolvable or tape sutures. When the local anaesthetic wears off, there is usually a mild, dull, aching pain for a few days.

---

vasculitis

Inflammation of blood vessels. Vasculitis usually leads to damage to the lining of blood vessels, with narrowing or blockage that restricts or stops blood flow. As a result, the body tissues supplied by affected vessels are damaged, or they are destroyed by *ischaemia*.

Vasculitis is thought to be caused in most cases by the presence of minute bodies, called immune complexes, in the blood. Immune complexes (*antigens* bound to *antibodies*) are normally destroyed by white blood cells, but sometimes adhere to the walls of blood vessels, where they cause inflammation. In some cases, the antigens are *viruses*.

Vasculitis is a disease process that occurs in various disorders, such as *polyarteritis nodosa*, *erythema nodosum*, *Henoch–Schönlein purpura*, *serum sickness*, *temporal arteritis*, and *Buerger's disease*.

vas deferens

Either of a pair of tubes that convey *sperm* from each *testis* to the *urethra* (the tube that carries sperm and urine through the penis to be expelled). The plural form is vasa deferentia.

vasectomy

The operation of male sterilization. Vasectomy is a minor surgical procedure, performed under a local anaesthetic (see *anaesthesia, local*), that consists of cutting out a short length of each *vas deferens* (a duct that carries sperm from a testis to the urethra). For more information about how the procedure is performed, see *How vasectomy is performed* box, above.

After vasectomy, the man continues to achieve orgasm and ejaculate as normal, but the *semen* no longer contains *sperm*, which are reabsorbed in the testes. However, sterility does not occur immediately after the operation and contraception should be used until a semen analysis indicates that there are no sperm present in the semen.

Male sterilization is a safe and effective method of *contraception*. Rarely, the severed ends of a vas deferens reunite, and sperm appear in the ejaculate. If this occurs, the man can safely undergo another vasectomy. Some operations to restore fertility after vasectomy are successful, but the process should be regarded as irreversible.

V

vasodilator drugs

A group of drugs that widen blood vessels. They include *ACE inhibitor drugs*, *alpha-blocker drugs*, *calcium channel blockers*, and *nitrate drugs*. Some vasodilators are used to treat disorders in which abnormal narrowing of blood vessels reduces blood flow through tissues. Such disorders include *angina pectoris peripheral vascular disease*, and *Raynaud's disease*. Vasodilators are also used to treat *hypertension* (high blood pressure) and *heart failure* (reduced pumping efficiency). Vasodilator drugs may cause flushing, headaches, dizziness, fainting, and swollen ankles. (See also *antihypertensive drugs*.)

vasopressin

Another name for *ADH*.

vasovagal attack

Temporary loss of consciousness as a result of sudden slowing of the heartbeat, usually brought on by severe pain, stress, shock, or fear. A vasovagal attack, a common cause of *fainting* in healthy people, results from overstimulation of the *vagus nerve*.

vector

An animal that transmits a particular *infectious disease*. A vector picks up disease-causing organisms from a source of infection (such as the blood or faeces of an infected person or animal), carries them in or on its body, and then deposits them, where they go on to infect a new host. Part of the disease-causing organism's life-cycle must usually take place in the body of a vector. Mosquitoes, fleas, lice, ticks, and flies are the most important vectors of disease to humans.

veganism

Eating a diet that excludes all meat and fish and all animal products, including milk and eggs. A vegan diet is likely to result in deficiency of *vitamin B₁₂* because this vitamin occurs naturally only in foods of animal origin; vegans should therefore take B₁₂ supplements or eat fortified foods, such as yeast extract. Supplements of B₁₂ are essential during pregnancy, and dietary advice should be sought before putting a baby or child on a vegan diet.

vegetarianism

Eating a diet that excludes meat and fish, and sometimes other animal products. It is not essential to eat meat or animal

STRUCTURE OF **VEIN AND ARTERY**

Like arteries, the walls of veins have a smooth inner layer, a muscular middle layer, and a fibrous outer layer. However, the walls are thinner and less muscular than those of arteries.

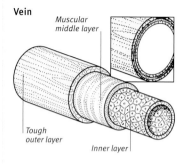

Vein

Muscular middle layer

Tough outer layer

Inner layer

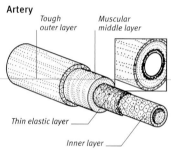

Artery

Tough outer layer

Muscular middle layer

Thin elastic layer

Inner layer

products as long as the plant foods provide a balanced diet (see *nutrition*). However, people who exclude all animal products (vegans) need to plan their diet carefully or take supplements to avoid deficiency of *vitamin B₁₂* or *calcium*.

Vegetarian diets are relatively rich in *fibre*, which may help to protect against *diverticular disease* and intestinal cancer (see *colon, cancer of*; *rectum, cancer of*). Vegetarian diets tend to be lower in *fats*, especially saturated fats (which may contribute to *coronary artery disease* and possibly some forms of cancer). These diets are also likely to contain much less *sodium* and more *potassium*, and vegetarians tend to have lower blood pressure than people who eat meat.

vegetative state, persistent

See *persistent vegetative state*.

vein

A blood vessel that returns blood towards the *heart* from the organs and tissues. The walls of veins, like those of arteries, consist of a smooth inner lining, a muscular middle layer, and a fibrous outer covering. However, blood pressure in the veins is lower than in the arteries. In addition, the walls of veins are thinner, less elastic, less muscular, and weaker than those of arteries. The linings of many veins contain folds,

LOCATION OF THE **VENAE CAVAE**

All the circulating blood, after being pumped to the body, returns to the heart via the venae cavae. The superior vena cava collects blood from the whole of the upper trunk, head, neck, and arms. The inferior vena cava drains blood from all parts of the body below the chest.

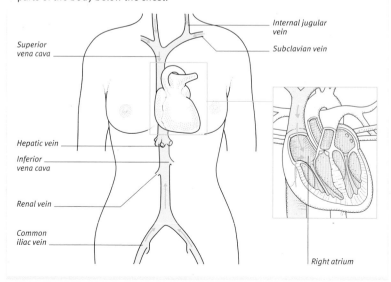

Superior vena cava

Internal jugular vein

Subclavian vein

Hepatic vein

Inferior vena cava

Renal vein

Common iliac vein

Right atrium

which act as valves, ensuring that the blood flows only towards the heart. Blood is helped on its way through the veins by pressure on the vessel walls from the contraction of surrounding muscles. (See also *circulatory system*.)

veins, disorders of

Common disorders that affect the *veins* include *varicose veins*, in which the affected vein becomes enlarged, tortuous, or twisted; deep vein thrombosis (see *thrombosis, deep vein*), in which a blood clot forms in a deep-lying vein of the leg; and *thrombophlebitis*, which involves inflammation of and blood clotting in a vein.

vena cava

Either of two large *veins* into which all circulating deoxygenated blood drains. The venae cavae (superior and inferior) deliver blood to the right atrium (the upper chamber) of the *heart* for pumping to the lungs.

SUPERIOR VENA CAVA

The superior vena cava starts at the top of the chest, near the *sternum* (breastbone), and passes down through the *pericardium* (outer lining of the heart) before connecting to the right atrium. It collects blood from the upper trunk, head, neck, and arms.

INFERIOR VENA CAVA

The inferior vena cava starts in the lower abdomen and travels upwards in front of the spine, behind the liver, and through the *diaphragm* before joining the right atrium. It collects blood from the legs, pelvic organs, liver, and kidneys.

venepuncture

A common procedure in which a *vein*, usually in the forearm, is pierced with a needle to inject fluid or withdraw blood. A tourniquet is used to swell the veins, and a sterile needle is inserted. A syringe is attached to the needle if blood is to be taken or medication injected. For *intravenous infusion*, a cannula (tube) is inserted via the needle.

venereal diseases

See *sexually transmitted infections*.

venesection

Withdrawing blood from a *vein* for *blood donation* or therapeutic bloodletting. Regular bloodletting is performed to treat *polycythaemia* (in which the blood is too thick) and *haemochromatosis* (in which iron accumulates in the body).

venlafaxine

A serotonin and noradrenaline reuptake inhibitor (SNRI) drug that is used in the treatment of *depression*. Venlafaxine combines the effects of *selective serotonin reuptake inhibitors* and *tricyclic antidepressants*. The drug produces fewer side effects than other tricyclic antidepressants. Possible side effects of venlafaxine may include nausea, dry mouth, and constipation.

venography

A diagnostic procedure that enables *veins* to be seen on an *X-ray* film after they have been injected with a radiopaque dye (a substance that is opaque to X-rays). Venography is used to detect abnormalities or diseases of the veins, such as narrowing or blockage from *thrombosis* (formation of blood clots).

venomous bites and stings

The injection of venom by certain animals via their mouthparts (bites) or other injecting apparatus (stings). Venoms are often carried to discourage predators, and are sometimes used to kill or immobilize prey. It is rare for a venomous animal to attack a person unless it has been provoked or disturbed. Specific *antivenoms* are available to treat many, although not all, types of animal venom. (See also *insect stings*; *jellyfish stings*; *scorpion stings*; *snake bites*; *spider bites*.)

ventilation

The use of a machine called a *ventilator* to take over or assist *breathing*. Arrested or severely impaired breathing may occur as a result of various conditions, including *head injury*, brain disease, an overdose of *opioid drugs*, chest injury, respiratory disease, a nerve or muscle disorder, or major chest or abdominal surgery.

Ventilation may be needed if a muscle relaxant has been given, as part of general *anaesthesia*, during an operation. Premature babies with *respiratory distress syndrome* may also need ventilation until their lungs have developed sufficiently. Positive pressure ventilation (continuous pumping of air under high pressure) may be used in the home to treat *sleep apnoea* (the temporary cessation of breathing during sleep).

ventilator

A device used for the artificial *ventilation* of a person who is unable to breathe naturally. A ventilator is an electrical pump connected to an air supply that works like bellows. Air is directed through a tube passed down the windpipe to inflate the lungs. The air is then expelled by the natural elasticity of the lungs and ribcage. A valve on the ventilator prevents the expelled air from re-entering the lungs.

ventilatory failure

See *respiratory failure*.

TECHNIQUE OF **ARTIFICIAL VENTILATION**

Machine-assisted breathing may be needed when a person has lost the ability to breathe naturally (often following a severe head injury, narcotic drug overdose, or in various other medical emergencies). It may also be needed when a muscle relaxant has been given during an operation as part of a general anaesthetic.

Procedure
The air is delivered to the patient's lungs via a tube inserted into the windpipe. After each inflation, the air is expelled by the natural elasticity of the lungs. Fluids and drugs must be given to the patient by intravenous infusion.

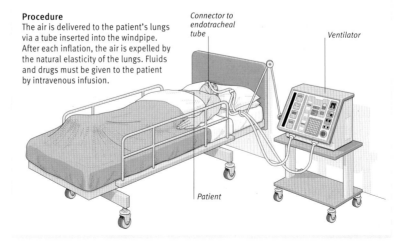

Connector to endotracheal tube

Ventilator

Patient

V

LOCATION OF THE VENTRICLES

The location of the ventricles in the brain (seen from above) and in the heart are shown below. Of the heart ventricles, the right ventricle pumps blood to the lungs, the left pumps blood to the rest of the body.

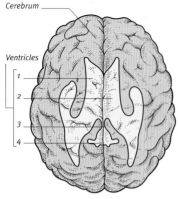

Ventricles in the brain
Together, these four irregularly shaped cavities contain approximately 25 ml of cerebrospinal fluid.

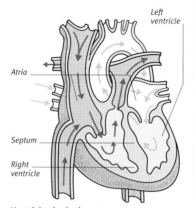

Ventricles in the heart
The ventricles of the heart are the large lower chambers that are separated by a muscular wall, the septum.

ventouse

See *vacuum extraction*.

ventral

Relating to the front of the body, or describing the lowermost part of a body structure when a person is lying face-down. The opposite is *dorsal*.

ventricle

A cavity or chamber. Both the *heart* and *brain* have anatomical parts that are known as ventricles.

The brain has four ventricles: one in each of the two cerebral hemispheres; a third at the centre of the brain, above the brainstem; and a fourth between the brainstem and cerebellum. These cavities are filled with *cerebrospinal fluid*.

The ventricles of the heart are its two lower chambers. The ventricles receive blood from each *atrium* (upper chamber) and pump it to the lungs and to the rest of the body.

ventricular aneurysm

A balloonlike bulge in the wall of the left ventricle of the *heart* (the chamber that pumps oxygen-rich blood around the body). Commonly developing as a result of a *myocardial infarction* (heart attack), ventricular aneurysm may, in turn, cause *heart failure* (reduced pumping efficiency) or *arrhythmias* (abnormal heart rhythms). Another possible com-plication is that a blood clot may form within the bulge, and fragments may become dislodged and travel around the circulation to block blood vessels elsewhere in the body (see *embolism*).

Diagnosis is by *echocardiography* (an ultrasound heart scan). Treatment involves drugs to treat heart failure or arrhythmias, as well as *anticoagulant drugs*. Surgical removal of the aneurysm may be needed in some cases.

ventricular ectopic beat

A type of cardiac *arrhythmia* in which abnormal heartbeats are initiated from electrical impulses within the *ventricles* (the lower chambers) of the *heart*. In a normal heart, beats are initiated by the *sinoatrial node* in the right atrium.

Ventricular ectopic beats may be detected on an *ECG*. For frequent abnormal heartbeats that are causing symptoms, or beats that arise from more than one site in the ventricles, an *antiarrhythmic drug* may be required.

ventricular fibrillation

One of the two life-threatening cardiac *arrhythmias* (the other is asystole, absence of a heartbeat) that occur in *cardiac arrest*. The *heart* has rapid, unco-ordinated, ineffective contractions and does not pump blood. The problem is due to abnormal heartbeats initiated by electrical activity in the *ventricles* (lower heart chambers). It is a common com-plication of *myocardial infarction* (heart attack) and may also be caused by electrocution or drowning.

The diagnosis is confirmed by *ECG*. Emergency treatment is with *defibrillation* (administration of an electric shock to the heart) and *antiarrhythmic drugs*.

ventricular septal defect

A hole between the lower two chambers of the heart. The abnormality is present from birth and in many cases is small and closes without treatment. Surgery may be performed for larger defects, usually with good results.

ventricular tachycardia

A serious cardiac *arrhythmia* in which each heartbeat is initiated from electrical activity in the *ventricles* (the lower heart chambers) rather than from the *sinoatrial node* in the right atrium (upper heart chamber).

It is an abnormally fast heart rate due to serious heart disease, such as *myocardial infarction* (heart attack) or *cardiomyopathy* (disease of the heart muscle). It may last for a few seconds or for several days.

Diagnosis is confirmed by *ECG*. Emergency treatment is with *defibrillation* (administration of an electric shock to the heart) and an *antiarrhythmic drug*.

verapamil

A drug that acts as a *calcium channel blocker* to treat *hypertension* (high blood pressure), *angina pectoris* (chest pain due to inadequate blood supply to the heart), and certain *arrhythmias* (abnormalities of the heartbeat). Possible side effects include headache, flushing, dizziness, and ankle swelling.

vernix

The white, cheeselike substance covering a newborn baby. Vernix comprises fatty secretions and dead cells. It protects the skin, insulates against heat loss before birth, and lubricates the baby's passage down the birth canal.

verruca

The Latin name for a *wart*, commonly applied to warts on the soles of the feet.

version

A change in the direction in which a *fetus* lies so that a *malpresentation*, most commonly a breech (bottom-down) presentation, replaces the normal head-down presentation.

V

vertebra

Any of the 33 roughly cylindrical bones that form the *spine*. There are seven vertebrae in the cervical spine; 12 in the thoracic; five in the lumbar; five (fused) in the *sacrum*; and four (fused) in the *coccyx*. The top 24 vertebrae are separated by discs of cartilage (see *disc, intervertebral*). Each vertebra has a hole in the centre through which the *spinal cord* runs, and processes to which muscles are attached. (See also *Location and structure of the vertebrae* box, p.789.)

vertebrobasilar insufficiency

Intermittent episodes of dizziness, weakness, double vision, and difficulty in speaking caused by reduced blood flow to parts of the *brain*. The condition is usually a result of *atherosclerosis* (narrowing due to accumulation of fatty deposits) of the basilar and vertebral arteries and other arteries in the base of the brain. Vertebrobasilar insufficiency sometimes precedes a *stroke*.

vertigo

An illusion that an individual or his or her surroundings are spinning. Vertigo is usually the result of a disturbance of the *semicircular canals* in the inner ear or the nerve tracts leading from them. The condition may also be caused by certain *brain* disorders affecting the brainstem, the cerebellum, or the cerebral cortex. Sudden-onset vertigo is treated with rest and *antihistamine drugs*, which, in some cases, are also given to prevent recurrent attacks.

vesicle

A small *blister*, usually filled with clear fluid, that forms at a site of skin damage. The term is also used to refer to any small saclike structure in the body.

vesicoureteric reflux

Backflow of urine from the bladder into the ureters (tubes that carry urine from the kidneys to the bladder). Vesicoureteric reflux causes recurrent urinary infection in children that often results in acute *pyelonephritis* and scarring of the kidneys. The condition, which is caused by a faulty valve mechanism, is diagnosed using voiding cystourethrography (see *cystourethrography, voiding*). *Antibiotic drugs* may be given to prevent infection, but corrective surgery may also be needed.

vestibule

A chamber. The vestibule in the inner ear is a hollow chamber that connects the three *semicircular canals*.

vestibulitis

Inflammation of the nasal vestibule (the part of the nasal cavity just inside the nostril) or of the area between the labia minora in the vulva, usually as a result of bacterial infection.

vestibulocochlear nerve

The eighth *cranial nerve*. The vestibulocochlear nerve consists of two branches: the vestibular nerve (which is concerned with balance) and the cochlear nerve (which is concerned with hearing). Each vestibulocochlear nerve (one on each side) carries sensory impulses from the inner *ear* to the *brain*, which it enters between the pons and medulla oblongata (in the *brainstem*).

DISORDERS
A tumour of the cells that surround the vestibulocochlear nerve (see *acoustic neuroma*) may result in loss of balance, *tinnitus* (ringing in the ear), and *deafness*. Deafness may also be the result of damage to the vestibulocochlear nerve,

---

TYPES OF **VENTRICULAR ARRHYTHMIA**

The ventricles (lower chambers) of the heart usually beat regularly in response to excitatory waves that spread from the upper chambers. Any disturbances to that rhythm (arrhythmia) may be associated with heart disease. The different types of ventricular arrhythmia can be seen on these electrocardiograph (ECG) recordings.

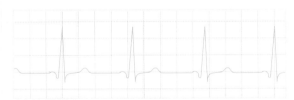

Normal heartbeat
This is the normal ECG appearance of the heartbeat. The regular spikes coincide with beats of the ventricles (lower heart chambers). The small rises before each spike coincide with contractions of the atria (upper chambers).

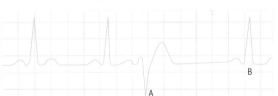

Ventricular ectopic beat
Here there is an abnormal beat, which has a broad, bizarre-looking waveform on the ECG; it occurs just before the expected normal beat. To the patient, the heart may seem to stop at time A and restart with a thump at time B.

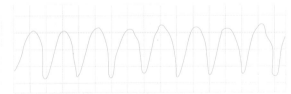

Ventricular tachycardia
Here, there is a rapid succession of abnormal beats, caused by an abnormal focus of electrical activity in a ventricle. It usually indicates serious underlying heart disease. The rate of beating may be very high – up to 220 beats per minute.

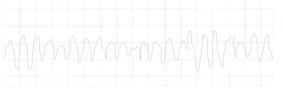

Ventricular fibrillation
This pattern is seen only when the heart is in a state of virtual arrest, usually after a heart attack, with the ventricles twitching in a rapid and totally irregular manner. Unless a normal rhythm can be restored, the condition is rapidly fatal.

V

LOCATION OF THE VESTIBULOCOCHLEAR NERVE

This nerve originates in the brainstem. It conducts sensory impulses concerned with hearing and balance from different parts of the inner ear to the brain.

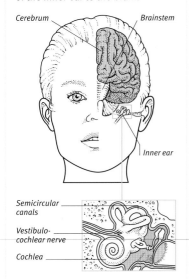

which may be caused by an infection, such as *meningitis* or *encephalitis*, or to a reaction to a drug such as *streptomycin*.

Viagra

The brand name for *sildenafil*, a drug used to treat *erectile dysfunction*.

vibration white finger

See *hand–arm vibration syndrome*.

villus

A minute fingerlike projection from a membranous surface. Millions of villi are present on the mucous lining of the small *intestine*. Each intestinal villus

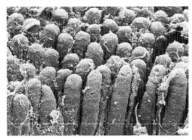

Microvilli in the intestine
This scanning electron micrograph shows numerous microvilli projecting from a single cell in the lining of the small intestine.

contains a small *lymph* vessel and a network of *capillaries* (tiny blood vessels). Its surface is covered with hundreds of hairlike structures (microvilli). The villi and microvilli provide a large surface area for the absorption of food molecules from the intestine into the blood and the lymphatic system.

vinca alkaloids

A group of substances derived from the periwinkle plant (*VINCA ROSEA*) that are used to treat *leukaemias* (cancers of the blood), *lymphomas* (cancers of lymphoid tissue), and some solid tumours, such as *breast cancer* and *lung cancer*.

All vinca alkaloids can cause neurological toxicity, which appears as *neuropathy* (nerve damage). Other side effects may include abdominal pain, constipation, and reversible *alopecia* (hair loss). Common vinca alkaloids include vinblastine, vindesine, and *vincristine*.

Vincent's disease

A severe form of gingivitis (gum disease) in which bacterial infection causes painful ulceration of the gums. (See also *gingivitis, acute ulcerative*.)

vincristine

A *vinca alkaloid* used to treat certain cancers. One particular side effect of vincristine is peripheral or autonomic *neuropathy* (nerve damage); but, unlike the other vinca alkaloids, it causes very little reduction in blood-cell production by the bone marrow. Other side effects may include abdominal pain, constipation, and reversible *alopecia* (hair loss).

viraemia

The presence of *virus* particles in the blood. Viraemia can occur at certain stages in various viral infections. Some viruses, such as those responsible for viral *hepatitis*, *yellow fever*, and *poliomyelitis*, are transported in the bloodstream to their target tissue or organ, for example the liver, where they multiply. Others, such as the *rubella* virus and *HIV*, multiply in, and spread via, certain white blood cells. If viraemia is a feature of a viral infection, there may be a risk that the infection will be transmitted to other people in blood or blood products, or by insects that feed on blood.

viral haemorrhagic fever

Diseases that are prevalent in Africa and cause severe bleeding. There are several types, including Ebola fever, Lassa fever,

Hantavirus, and Marburg fever. The diseases are fatal in a large percentage of cases, but Lassa fever may respond to *antiviral drugs* if given in the first week.

virginity

The physical state of not having experienced sexual intercourse.

virilism

The presence in a woman of masculine characteristics, caused by excessive levels of *androgen hormones*. Androgens are male sex hormones which, in women, are normally secreted in small amounts by the adrenal glands and ovaries.

Raised levels induce various changes in women, including *hirsutism* (excessive hairiness); male-pattern baldness (see *alopecia*); disruption or cessation of *menstruation*; enlargement of the *clitoris*; loss of normal fat deposits around the hips; development of the arm and shoulder muscles; and deepening of the voice (see *virilization*).

virility

A term used to describe the quality of maleness, especially in sexual characteristics and performance.

virilization

The development in a woman of male characteristics as a result of overproduction of *androgen hormones* by the adrenal glands and/or ovaries. This may be due to various conditions such as certain *adrenal tumours*, polycystic ovary (see *ovary, polycystic*) and some other *ovarian cysts*, or congenital *adrenal hyperplasia* (a rare genetic disorder).

virion

A single, complete, *virus* particle.

virology

The study of *viruses* and the *epidemiology* and treatment of diseases caused by viruses. In a more restricted sense, virology also refers to the isolation and identification of viruses to diagnose specific viral infections. Depending on the type of virus, this may involve growing viruses in cultures of human or animal cells, *staining* or microscopic examination of specimens containing viruses, or *immunoassay* techniques.

virulence

The ability of a microorganism to cause disease. This can be assessed by measuring what proportion of the population exposed to the microorganism develops symptoms of disease, how rapidly the infection spreads through the body, or the mortality from the infection.

viruses

One of the smallest known types of infectious agent. It is debatable whether viruses are truly living organisms or just collections of molecules capable of self-replication under specific conditions. Their sole activity is to invade the cells of other organisms, which they then take over to make copies of themselves. Outside living cells, viruses are inert.

STRUCTURE

A single virus particle (virion) consists of an inner core of *nucleic acid*, which may be either *DNA* or *RNA*, surrounded by one or two protective protein shells (capsids). Surrounding the outer capsid may be another layer, the viral envelope, which consists mainly of protein. The nucleic acid consists of a string of *genes* that contain coded instructions for making copies of the virus (see *Viruses and disease* box, overleaf).

VIRAL DISEASES

Common viral conditions include the common cold (see *cold, common*), *influenza*, *chickenpox*, *cold sores*, and *warts*. *AIDS* is caused by the human immunodeficiency virus (see *HIV*).

viscera

A collective term used to describe the internal organs.

viscosity

The resistance to flow of a fluid; its "stickiness". The viscosity of blood affects its ability to flow through small vessels. An increased blood viscosity increases the risk of *thrombosis* (abnormal blood clotting).

vision

The faculty of sight. When light-rays reach the *eye*, most of the focusing is done by the *cornea*, but the eye also has *accommodation*, an automatic fine-focusing facility that operates by altering the curvature of the *lens*. Together, these systems form an image on the *retina*. The light-sensitive rod and cone cells in the retina convert the elements of this image into nerve impulses that pass into the visual cortex of the *brain* via the *optic nerves*. The rods, which are more concentrated at the periphery of the retina, are highly sensitive to light but not to colour. The colour-sensitive cones are concentrated more at the centre of the retina (see *colour vision*).

The brain coordinates the motor nerve impulses to the six tiny muscles that move each eye to achieve alignment of the eyes. Accurate alignment allows the brain to fuse the images from each eye, but because each eye has a slightly different view of a given object, the brain obtains information that is interpreted as solidity or depth. This stereoscopic vision is important in judging distance. (See also *Types of vision test* box, p.791; *The sense of vision* box, p.792.)

vision, disorders of

The most common visual disorders are refractive errors, such as *astigmatism* (the abnormal curvature of the front of the eye), *myopia* (shortsightedness), and

---

LOCATION AND STRUCTURE OF THE **VERTEBRAE**

The 33 vertebrae are arranged as shown. Apart from the top two, all have a similar structure. The top cervical vertebra (atlas) has no body. The second (the axis) forms a pivot on which the atlas can rotate, allowing the head to be turned in all directions.

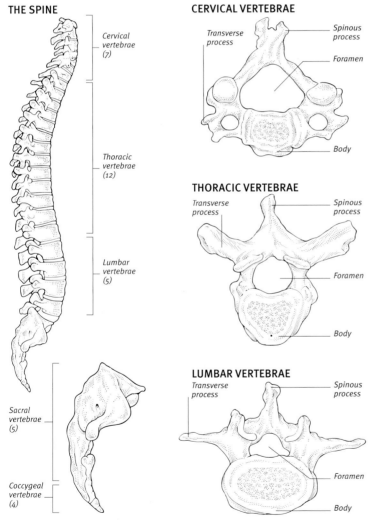

THE SPINE

Cervical vertebrae (7)

Thoracic vertebrae (12)

Lumbar vertebrae (5)

Sacral vertebrae (5)

Coccygeal vertebrae (4)

CERVICAL VERTEBRAE

Transverse process

Spinous process

Foramen

Body

THORACIC VERTEBRAE

Transverse process

Spinous process

Foramen

Body

LUMBAR VERTEBRAE

Transverse process

Spinous process

Foramen

Body

Arrangement
The vertebrae fall into five groups – cervical, thoracic, lumbar, sacral, and coccygeal. The top 24 are separated by discs of cartilage.

Structure
Three typical vertebrae are shown above. The foramen in each is the channel through which the spinal cord runs. The processes serve as muscle attachments.

V

VIRUSES AND DISEASE

All viruses have the same basic structure (right), but they come in various shapes and sizes. Examples from the main families are shown below (some in cross-section). All are tiny – from about 15 to 300 nanometres in diameter (one nanometre equals one thousand-millionth of a metre); most are so small that they can be seen only with an electron microscope. All types of viruses can multiply only within cells of their host (far right).

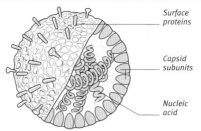

Structure of typical virus particle
Nucleic acid in the centre is surrounded by one or more capsids made of protein subunits.

VIRAL REPLICATION

The sequence below shows how a virus multiplies. The signs and symptoms of viral infection are caused by the virus interfering with or destroying the host's cells.

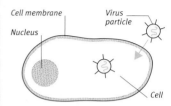

1 The virus particle first attaches itself to and then injects itself into the host cell.

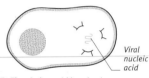

2 The viral capsid breaks down and the viral nucleic acid (DNA or RNA) contained inside is released.

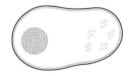

3 The viral nucleic acid replicates itself; the new copies are made from raw materials in the host cell.

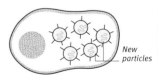

4 Each of the new copies of the viral nucleic acid now directs the manufacture of a capsid for itself.

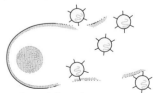

5 The newly formed virus particles are released in large numbers, and the host cell may be destroyed.

TYPES OF VIRUS

Papova-viruses	Adeno-viruses	Herpes-viruses	Pox-viruses	Picorna-viruses	Toga-viruses
Orthomyxo-viruses	Paramyxo-viruses	Corona-viruses	Arena-viruses	Rhabdo-viruses	Retro-viruses

Family	Examples of conditions or diseases
Papovaviruses	Warts, cervical cancers, anal cancers
Adenoviruses	Respiratory and eye infections
Herpesviruses	Cold sores, genital herpes, chickenpox, herpes zoster (shingles), glandular fever, cytomegalovirus (CMV)
Poxviruses	Cowpox, smallpox (eradicated), molluscum contagiosum
Picornaviruses	Poliomyelitis, viral hepatitis type A, respiratory infections, myocarditis
Togaviruses	Rubella, yellow fever, dengue, encephalitis
Orthomyxoviruses	Influenza
Paramyxoviruses	Mumps, measles, respiratory syncytial virus (RSV)
Coronaviruses	Common cold
Arenaviruses	Lassa fever
Rhabdoviruses	Rabies
Retroviruses	AIDS, some leukaemias

V

hypermetropia (longsightedness), which can almost always be corrected by *glasses* or *contact lenses*. Other disorders of vision include *amblyopia* (lazy eye); *double vision*; and disorders of the *eye* or *optic nerve*, of the nerve pathways connecting the optic nerves to the *brain*, and of the brain itself.

CAUSES IN THE EYE

The eye may lose its transparency through corneal opacities, *cataract*, or *vitreous haemorrhage* (bleeding into the gel of the eye behind the lens). Defects near the centre of the retina cause loss of the corresponding parts of the *visual field* (see *macular degeneration*). *Floaters*, which are usually insignificant, may indicate a *retinal tear* or haemorrhage, or they may herald a *retinal detachment*. *Optic neuritis* (inflammation of the optic nerve) can cause a blind spot in the centre of the visual field.

CAUSES IN THE BRAIN

Damage to the brain (for example, from a *stroke*) may cause visual impairment such as *hemianopia* (loss of half the visual field), *agnosia* (failure to recognize objects), visual perseveration (in which a scene continues to be perceived after the direction of gaze has shifted), and visual hallucinations.

vision, loss of

The inability to see. Loss of vision may develop slowly or suddenly, and it may be temporary or permanent, depending on the cause. Loss of vision may affect one eye or both of the eyes. It can cause complete *blindness* or may affect only peripheral or central vision.

SLOW VISION LOSS

Progressive loss of visual clarity is common with increasing age and may be cause by any of a number of disorders (see *vision, disorders of*).

SUDDEN VISION LOSS

Sudden loss of vision may be caused by disorders such as *hyphaema* (bleeding into the aqueous humour), severe *uveitis* (inflammation of the iris or the choroid), *vitreous haemorrhage* (bleeding into the gel within the eye), or *retinal haemorrhage*. *Optic neuritis* (inflammation of the optic nerve) can reduce vision in one eye.

Damage to the nerve connections between the eyes and brain, or to the visual area of the brain, can cause loss of peripheral vision. This nerve damage may be caused by a number of disorders such as an *embolism*, *ischaemia*, tumour, inflammation, or injury.

vision tests

The part of an *eye examination* that determines reduction in the ability to see.

VISUAL ACUITY TESTS

Tests of *visual acuity* (sharpness of central vision) include a *Snellen chart*, which is used to test a patient's distance vision, and close-reading test cards, which may be used to assess his or her near vision.

REFRACTION TESTS

Refraction tests assess the ability of the eye to focus light clearly on the retina via the cornea and lens. They can be used to detect *hypermetropia* (longsightedness), *myopia* (shortsightedness), and *astigmatism* (abnormal curvature of the front of the eye). By observing the effect of different lenses on movement

---

TYPES OF VISION TESTS

These tests are performed to measure a number of variables: the acuity of a patient's distance vision and the power of the lenses he or she may need (visual acuity and refraction test), the extent of peripheral vision (visual field test), and the ability to focus on near objects (accommodation tests).

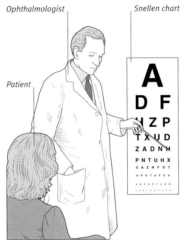

Visual acuity test
These tests use the familiar Snellen chart. Visual acuity is measured according to how far down the chart the patient can read accurately.

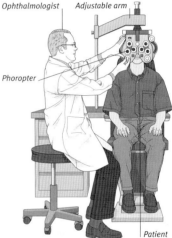

Refraction test
Lenses in the phoropter are changed until the letters near the bottom of the Snellen chart can be read. This allows the optician to make a prescription for appropriate lenses.

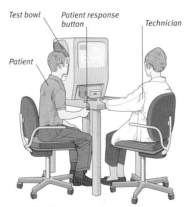

Visual field test
One eye is covered and the other is fixed on a central target inside the test bowl. A response button is pressed when the patient sees lights flashing in different parts of the visual field.

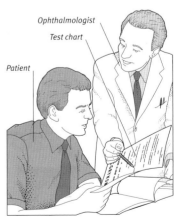

Accommodation test
After any distance-focusing ability has been corrected with glasses, the ability to read small print close-up is measured to test accommodation.

V

THE SENSE OF **VISION**

Vision starts in the retina, the membrane at the back of the eye that contains the light-sensitive rod and cone cells. Much of the rest of the eye is concerned with focusing light, in the right quantities, on to the retina. Huge amounts of data are sent from the retina, through the optic nerves, to the brain for analysis.

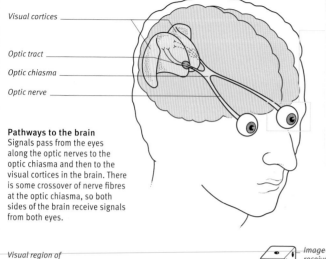

Visual cortices

Optic tract

Optic chiasma

Optic nerve

Pathways to the brain
Signals pass from the eyes along the optic nerves to the optic chiasma and then to the visual cortices in the brain. There is some crossover of nerve fibres at the optic chiasma, so both sides of the brain receive signals from both eyes.

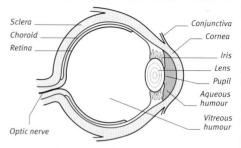

Sclera
Choroid
Retina

Conjunctiva
Cornea
Iris
Lens
Pupil
Aqueous humour
Vitreous humour

Optic nerve

Cross-section through the eye

IMAGE RECEPTION

The light-rays from an object stimulate a group of receptors in the retina within an area that has the same shape as the object but is upside down. The brain automatically interprets the image the right way up.

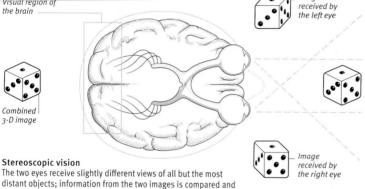

Visual region of the brain

Image received by the left eye

Combined 3-D image

Image received by the right eye

Stereoscopic vision
The two eyes receive slightly different views of all but the most distant objects; information from the two images is compared and processed in the brain to give a single 3-D interpretation of the object.

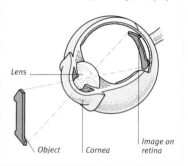

Lens

Object   Cornea   Image on retina

EYEBALL MOVEMENTS

In order to maintain the image of any moving object on the centre of the retina, precise eyeball movements, which are achieved by the six muscles shown below, are necessary.

The muscles act to swivel the eyeball (here, the right) in the directions indicated. The muscles always act in groups to achieve movement.

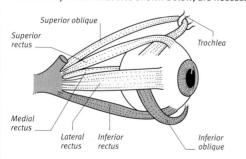

Superior oblique
Superior rectus
Trochlea
Medial rectus
Lateral rectus
Inferior rectus
Inferior oblique

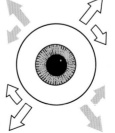

Inferior oblique
Upwards, outwards and anticlockwise rotation

Lateral rectus
Outwards

Superior oblique
Downwards, outwards, and clockwise rotation

Superior rectus
Upwards, inwards, and clockwise rotation

Medial rectus
Inwards

Inferior rectus
Downwards, inwards, and anticlockwise rotation

V

of light reflected from the eye, the strength and type of *glasses* or *contact lenses* needed to correct the visual defect can be assessed objectively. Visual acuity tests are then used to check that the patient can see clearly using the new lenses. Further minor adjustments to the lenses may be required.

VISUAL FIELD TESTS

Tests of the *visual field* may be performed to assess disorders of the eye, such as *glaucoma* (increased pressure of fluid within the eyeball), or disorders of the nervous system, such as a *stroke*.

visual acuity

Sharpness of central *vision*. Refractive errors, such as *myopia* (shortsightedness), *hypermetropia* (longsightedness), and *astigmatism* (abnormal curvature of the front of the eye), are the most common causes of poor visual acuity. Poor visual acuity for near objects occurs in the condition *presbyopia* (age-related deterioration in focusing power).

visual field

The total area in which visual perception is possible while a person is looking straight ahead. The visual fields normally extend outwards over an angle of about 90 degrees on either side of the midline of the face, but are more restricted above and below, especially if the eyes are deep-set or the eyebrows are prominent. The visual fields of the two eyes overlap to a large extent, giving binocular vision (see the illustrated box). Partial loss of the visual field may occur in *glaucoma* (raised pressure within the eyeball) or *stroke*.

vital sign

An indication that a person is still alive. Vital signs include chest movements that are caused by breathing, the presence of a pulse, and the constriction of the *pupil* of the eye when it is exposed to a bright light.

vitamin

Any of a group of complex organic substances essential, in small amounts, for the normal functioning of the body. There are 13 vitamins: A, C, D, E, K, B_{12}, and seven grouped under the *vitamin B complex*. Apart from vitamin D, which the body can synthesize itself, vitamins must be obtained from the diet. For most healthy people, a balanced diet contains adequate amounts of all the vitamins and supplements are not necessary; in fact,

certain vitamins may be harmful if taken in excess. However, specific vitamin supplements may be recommended for certain groups, such as women who are planning a pregnancy or are pregnant and people who are taking drugs that interfere with vitamin function.

TYPES

Vitamins can be categorized as fat-soluble or water-soluble.

Fat-soluble vitamins (A, D, E, and K) are absorbed with fats from the intestine into the bloodstream and are then stored in fatty tissue (mainly in the liver). Because body reserves of some of these vitamins last for several years, a daily intake is not usually necessary. Deficiency of a fat-soluble vitamin is usually the result of a disorder in which

intestinal absorption of fats is impaired (see *malabsorption*) or is due to having a poor diet for a prolonged period.

Vitamins C, B_{12}, and those of the B complex are water-soluble. Vitamin C and B complex vitamins can be stored in the body in only limited amounts and are excreted in the urine if taken in greater amounts than needed. A regular intake is therefore essential to prevent deficiency. However, vitamin B_{12} is stored in the liver; these stores may last for years.

FUNCTION IN THE BODY

The role of all the vitamins is not fully understood. Most have several important actions on one or more body systems, and many are involved in the activities of *enzymes*. (See also individual vitamin entries; *Reference Nutrient Intake*, overleaf.)

THE **VISUAL FIELDS**

The field of vision of each eye (with the head and eyes immobile) extends through an angle of 130 degrees and is divided into an area that overlaps with the visual field of the other eye (binocular vision) and an area that can be seen only by one eye.

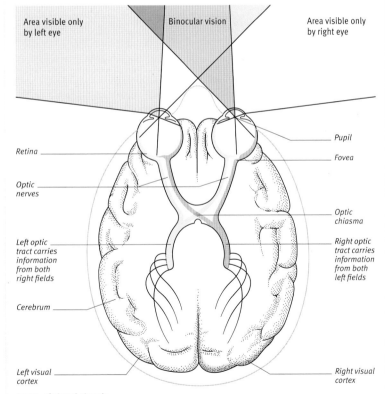

Area visible only by left eye

Binocular vision

Area visible only by right eye

Retina

Optic nerves

Left optic tract carries information from both right fields

Cerebrum

Left visual cortex

Pupil

Fovea

Optic chiasma

Right optic tract carries information from both left fields

Right visual cortex

Route of visual signals
Note that all light from the fields left of the centre of both eyes (grey) falls on the right sides of the two retinas; and information about these fields goes to the right visual cortex. Information about the right fields of vision (coloured) goes to the left cortex. Data about the area of binocular vision (visible to both eyes) go to both left and right visual cortices.

V

vitamin A

A fat-soluble *vitamin* vital for growth, for bone and teeth formation, for cell structure, for night vision, and for protecting the linings of the respiratory, digestive, and urinary tracts against infection.

Vitamin A is absorbed by the body in the form of retinol. This is found in liver, fish-liver oils, egg yolk, dairy produce, and is added to margarines. *Carotene*, which the body converts into retinol, is found in various vegetables and fruits.

DEFICIENCY

Vitamin A deficiency is rare in developed countries. In most cases, it is due to *malabsorption*. Vitamin A deficiency may also result from long-term treatment with certain *lipid-lowering drugs*. Deficiency is common in some developing countries due to poor diet. The first symptom of deficiency is night blindness, followed by dryness and eye inflammation (see *xerophthalmia*), *kerato-malacia* (damage to the cornea), and eventually blindness. Deficiency also causes reduced resistance to infection, dry skin, and, in children, stunted growth.

EXCESS

Prolonged excessive intake of vitamin A can cause headache, nausea, loss of appetite, skin peeling, hair loss, and irregular menstruation. In severe cases, the liver and spleen become enlarged. Excess vitamin A, especially in the form of retinol, has been linked with an increased risk of bone fractures. Excessive intake during pregnancy may cause birth defects, and women who are pregnant or planning a pregnancy should not take vitamin A supplements except on the advice of a doctor; they should also avoid eating liver products. In infants, excessive intake of vitamin A may cause skull deformities, which disappear if the diet is corrected.

MEDICAL USES

The drug *tretinoin* (a derivative of vitamin A) is used to treat severe *acne*.

vitamin B

See *vitamin B₁₂*; *vitamin B complex*.

REFERENCE NUTRIENT INTAKE (RNI) FOR SELECTED VITAMINS

The table gives the reference nutrient intake (RNI) of vitamins for which amounts have been established; when different, the RNI for males and females is denoted by M and F. The figures are for healthy individuals; they are not applicable for babies or people with medical conditions or special nutritional requirements.

Vitamin	1–3 years	4–6 years	7–10 years	11–14 years	15–18 years	19–50 years	51+ years	Extra needed: Pregnancy	Extra needed: Breast-feeding
Folic acid (mcg/day)	70	100	150	200	200	200	200	+400*	+60
Niacin (mg/day)	8	11	12	M 15 F 12	M 18 F 14	M 17 F 13	M 16 F 12	0	+2
Vitamin B6 (mg/day)	0.7	0.9	1.0	M 1.2 F 1.0	M 1.5 F 1.2	M 1.4 F 1.2	M 1.4 F 1.2	0	0
Riboflavin (mg/day)	0.6	0.8	1.0	M 1.2 F 1.1	M 1.3 F 1.1	M 1.3 F 1.1	M 1.3 F 1.1	+0.3	+0.5
Thiamine (mg/day)	0.5	0.7	0.7	M 0.9 F 0.7	M 1.1 F 0.8	M 1.0 F 0.8	M 0.9 F 0.8	+0.1**	+0.2
Vitamin A (mcg/day)	400	400	500	M 300 F 600	M 700 F 600	M 700 F 600	M 700 F 600	+10	+350
Vitamin B12 (mcg/day)	0.5	0.8	1.0	1.2	1.5	1.5	1.5	0	+0.5
Vitamin C (mg/day)	30	30	30	35	40	40	40	+10	+30
Vitamin D (mcg/day)***	7	0	0	0	0	0	10†	+10	+10

Vitamin E
There is no recommended intake for vitamin E. The amount needed depends on the amount of polyunsaturated fatty acids in the diet.

Units

mg = milligrams (thousandths of a gram)

mcg = micrograms (millionths of a gram)

* Most women are advised to take a supplementary daily dose of 400mcg before conception through to week 12 of pregnancy. If there is a high risk of the fetus having a neural tube defect, the recommended daily supplementary dose is 5mg.

** For last trimester only

*** Vitamin D is synthesized in the body using sunlight. Certain individuals or at-risk groups may require dietary vitamin D.

† For people aged 65 years or older only

V

vitamin B₁₂

A water-soluble *vitamin* that plays a vital role in the activities of several *enzymes* in the body. Vitamin B₁₂ is important in the production of the genetic material of cells (and thus in growth and development), in the production of red blood cells in bone marrow, in the utilization of folic acid in the diet, and in the functioning of the nervous system. Only foods of animal origin naturally contain vitamin B₁₂; foods that are rich in this vitamin include liver, kidney, chicken, beef, pork, fish, eggs, and dairy products.

DEFICIENCY

Deficiency is almost always due to inability of the intestine to absorb vitamin B₁₂, usually because of pernicious anaemia (see *anaemia, megaloblastic*). Less commonly, deficiency may result from *gastrectomy* (removal of all or part of the stomach), *malabsorption*, or *veganism*.

The effects of deficiency are megaloblastic anaemia, sore mouth and tongue, and symptoms resulting from damage to the *spinal cord*, such as numbness and tingling in the limbs. There may also be depression and loss of memory.

EXCESS

A high intake of vitamin B₁₂ has no known harmful effects.

vitamin B complex

A group of water-soluble *vitamins* that comprise thiamine (vitamin B₁), riboflavin (vitamin B₂), niacin, pantothenic acid, pyridoxine (vitamin B₆), biotin (vitamin H), and folic acid. *Vitamin B₁₂* is discussed above.

THIAMINE

Thiamine plays a role in the activities of various *enzymes* involved in the utilization of *carbohydrates* and thus in the functioning of nerves, muscles, and the heart. Sources include wholegrain cereals, wholemeal bread, brown rice, liver, kidney, pork, fish, beans, nuts, and eggs.

Those who are susceptible to deficiency include elderly people on a poor diet, and people with *hyperthyroidism* (overactivity of the thyroid gland), *malabsorption*, or severe *alcohol dependence*. Deficiency may also occur as a result of severe illness, surgery, or injury.

Mild deficiency of the vitamins may cause tiredness, irritability, and loss of appetite. Severe deficiency may cause abdominal pain, constipation, depression, memory impairment, and *beriberi*; in alcoholics, it may cause *Wernicke–Korsakoff syndrome*.

RIBOFLAVIN

Riboflavin is necessary for the activities of various enzymes that are involved in the breakdown and utilization of carbohydrates, fats, and proteins; production energy in cells; utilization of other B vitamins; and hormone production by the adrenal glands. Liver, whole grains, milk, eggs, and brewer's yeast are good sources of these vitamins.

People who are susceptible to riboflavin deficiency include those taking phenothiazine *antipsychotic drugs*, tricyclic *antidepressant drugs*, or oestrogen-containing *oral contraceptives*, and those with malabsorption or severe alcohol dependence. Deficiency may also occur through serious illness, surgery, or injury.

Prolonged deficiency may cause soreness of the tongue and the corners of the mouth, and eye disorders such as *amblyopia* and *photophobia*.

NIACIN

Niacin plays an essential role in the activities of various enzymes involved in the metabolism of carbohydrates and fats, the functioning of the nervous and digestive systems, the manufacture of sex hormones, and the maintenance of healthy skin. The main dietary sources are liver, lean meat, fish, nuts, and dried beans. Niacin can be made in the body from tryptophan (an *amino acid*).

Most cases of deficiency are due to malabsorption disorders or to severe alcohol dependence. Prolonged deficiency causes *pellagra*, the main symptoms of which are soreness and cracking of the skin, inflammation of the mouth and tongue, and mental disturbances.

PANTOTHENIC ACID

Pantothenic acid is essential for the activities of various enzymes that are involved in carbohydrate and fat metabolism, manufacture of *corticosteroids* and *sex hormones*, utilization of other vitamins, the functioning of the nervous system and *adrenal glands*, and growth and development. It is present in almost all vegetables, cereals, and animal foods.

Deficiency of pantothenic acid usually occurs as a result of malabsorption or alcoholism, but may also occur after severe illness, surgery, or injury. The effects include fatigue, headache, nausea, abdominal pain, numbness and tingling, muscle cramps, and susceptibility to respiratory infections.

PYRIDOXINE

Pyridoxine aids the activities of various enzymes and hormones involved in the utilization of carbohydrates, fats, and proteins, the manufacture of red blood cells and antibodies, the functioning of the digestive and nervous systems, and the maintenance of healthy skin. Dietary sources are liver, chicken, pork, fish, whole grains, wheat-germ, bananas, potatoes, and dried beans. Pyridoxine is also manufactured by intestinal bacteria.

People susceptible to pyridoxine deficiency include those with malabsorption or severe alcohol dependence, those taking certain drugs (including *penicillamine* and *isoniazid*), and elderly people who have a poor diet. Deficiency may cause weakness, irritability, depression, skin disorders, inflammation of the mouth and tongue, *anaemia*, and, in infants, *seizures*. Long-term use of high-dose pyridoxine supplements has been associated with nerve damage.

BIOTIN

Biotin is essential for the activities of various enzymes involved in the breakdown of fatty acids and carbohydrates and for the excretion of the waste products of protein breakdown. It is present in many foods, especially liver, peanuts, dried beans, egg yolk, mushrooms, bananas, grapefruit, and watermelon. Biotin is also manufactured by bacteria in the intestines.

Deficiency of biotin may occur during prolonged treatment with *antibiotics* or *sulphonamide drugs*. Symptoms are weakness, tiredness, poor appetite, hair loss, depression, inflammation of the tongue, and eczema.

FOLIC ACID

Folic acid is vital for various enzymes involved in the manufacture of *nucleic acids* and consequently for growth and reproduction, the production of red blood cells, and the functioning of the nervous system. Sources of folic acid include green vegetables, mushrooms, liver, nuts, dried beans, peas, egg yolk, and wholemeal bread.

Mild folic acid deficiency is common, but it can usually be corrected by increasing dietary intake. More severe deficiency may occur during pregnancy or breast-feeding, in premature or low-birthweight infants, in people on *dialysis*, in people with certain blood disorders, the skin disorder *psoriasis*, malabsorption, or alcohol dependence, and in people taking certain drugs.

The main effects include anaemia, sores around the mouth, and, in children, poor growth. The recommended dose of folic acid supplements, taken before conception and during the first

V

12 weeks of pregnancy, has been shown to reduce the risk of a *neural tube defect* in the baby; a higher dose may be recommended if there is a family history.

vitamin C

A water-soluble *vitamin* that plays an essential role in the activities of various *enzymes*. Vitamin C is important for the growth and maintenance of healthy bones, teeth, gums, blood vessels, and ligaments; in the production of certain *neurotransmitters* (chemicals that transmit nerve impulses) and adrenal gland hormones; in the response of the *immune system* to infection; in wound healing; and in the absorption of *iron*. However, there is no evidence that vitamin C supplements can protect against the common cold.

The main dietary sources are fruits and vegetables. Considerable amounts of the vitamin are lost when foods are processed, cooked, or kept warm.

DEFICIENCY
Mild deficiency of vitamin C may result from a serious injury or severe burn. It may also occur from use of *oral contraceptives* or continual inhalation of carbon monoxide (from traffic fumes or tobacco smoke), or after major surgery or a fever. It may cause weakness, general aches, swollen gums, and *nosebleeds*. More serious deficiency is usually due to a very restricted diet. Severe deficiency leads to *scurvy* and *anaemia*.

EXCESS
High doses of vitamin C are not usually toxic for healthy adults. However, very high doses may sometimes cause nausea, stomach cramps, and diarrhoea.

VITAMINS AND MAIN FOOD SOURCES

A varied diet usually provides all the body's vitamin needs. For vegans (who eat no fish or animal products, including dairy products), vitamin B$_{12}$ and vitamin D may be lacking; these vitamins can be obtained from supplements or, in the case of vitamin D, through adequate exposure to sunlight.

Fat-soluble	Good sources
Vitamin A	Liver, fish-liver oils; egg yolk, milk and dairy products; margarine, various fruits and vegetables (such as oranges and carrots)
Vitamin D	Cod-liver oil, oily fish (such as sardines, herring, salmon, and tuna); liver; egg yolk; margarine
Vitamin E	Vegetable oils (such as corn, soya bean, olive and sunflower oils); nuts; meat; green, leafy vegetables; cereals; wheat-germ; egg yolk
Vitamin K	Green, leafy vegetables (especially cabbage, broccoli, and turnip greens); vegetable oils; egg yolk; cheese; pork liver

Water-soluble	Good sources
Thiamine (vitamin B1)	Wheat-germ; bran; whole-grain or enriched cereals; wholemeal bread; brown rice; pasta; liver; kidney; pork; fish; beans; nuts; eggs
Riboflavin (vitamin B2)	Brewer's yeast; liver; kidney; milk; cheese; eggs; whole grains; enriched cereals; wheat-germ
Niacin	Liver; lean meat; poultry; fish; nuts; dried beans; enriched cereals; bread; wheat-germ; potatoes
Pantothenic acid	Liver; heart; kidney; fish; egg yolk; wheat-germ; most vegetables; most cereals
Pyridoxine (vitamin B6)	Liver; chicken; pork; fish; whole grains; wheat-germ; bananas; potatoes; dried beans
Biotin (vitamin H)	Liver; peanuts; dried beans; egg yolk; mushrooms; bananas; grapefruit; watermelons
Folic acid	Green, leafy vegetables; mushrooms; liver; nuts; dried beans; peas; egg yolk; wholemeal bread
Vitamin B12 (cyanocobalamin)	Liver; kidney; chicken; beef; pork; fish; eggs; milk; cheese; enriched cereals
Vitamin C	Citrus fruits; tomatoes; green leafy vegetables; potatoes; green peppers; strawberries; blackcurrants

vitamin D

The collective term for a group of substances that help to regulate the balance of *phosphate* and *calcium* in the body, aid calcium absorption in the intestine, and promote strong bones and teeth.

Good sources of vitamin D include oily fish, liver, and egg yolk; the vitamin is also added to margarines. In the body, vitamin D is synthesized by the action of ultraviolet light on a particular chemical in the skin.

DEFICIENCY
Deficiency of vitamin D may occur in individuals with a poor diet, in premature infants, and in those who are deprived of sunlight. It can also result from *malabsorption*. Other causes include liver or kidney disorders and some genetic defects. Prolonged use of certain drugs, such as the anticonvulsant *phenytoin*, may also lead to deficiency. Deficiency in young children causes the bone disorder *rickets*; long-term deficiency in adults leads to *osteomalacia*.

EXCESS
Excessive intake of vitamin D may lead to *hypercalcaemia* (an abnormally high level of calcium in the blood) and abnormal calcium deposits in the soft tissues, kidneys, and blood vessel walls. In children, it may cause growth retardation.

vitamin E

The collective term for a group of substances that are essential for normal cell structure, for maintenance of the activities of certain *enzymes*, and for the formation of red blood cells. Vitamin E

V

also protects the lungs and other tissues from damage by pollutants and is believed to slow aging of cells. Sources include vegetable oils, nuts, meat, green vegetables, cereals, and egg yolk.

DEFICIENCY

Dietary deficiency of vitamin E is rare; deficiency is most common in people with *malabsorption*, certain liver disorders, and in premature infants. It leads to the destruction of red blood cells, which eventually leads to *anaemia*. In infants, it causes irritability and *oedema* (accumulation of fluid in tissues).

EXCESS

Prolonged excessive intake of vitamin E may cause abdominal pain, nausea, and diarrhoea. It may also reduce intestinal absorption of vitamins A, D, and K.

vitamin K

A fat-soluble *vitamin* that is essential for the formation in the liver of substances that promote blood clotting. Green vegetables, vegetable oils, egg yolk, cheese, pork, and liver are good sources of vitamin K, which is also manufactured by bacteria in the intestine.

DEFICIENCY

Dietary deficiency of vitamin K rarely occurs. Deficiency may develop in people with *malabsorption*, certain liver disorders, or chronic diarrhoea. It may also result from prolonged treatment with *antibiotic drugs*. Vitamin K deficiency may cause nosebleeds and bleeding from the gums, intestine, and urinary tract.

Newborn babies lack the intestinal bacteria that produce vitamin K and are routinely given supplements to prevent deficiency. Without supplements, there is a risk of *brain haemorrhage*, which may be life-threatening.

vitamin supplements

A group of dietary preparations containing one or more *vitamins*. Some multivitamin preparations also contain *minerals*, such as iron and calcium. A healthy person with a balanced diet should not need to take supplements (see *nutrition*). Excessive doses of certain vitamins (especially vitamins A, B₆, and D) may actually be harmful.

Vitamin supplements may be given in order to prevent vitamin deficiency in susceptible people, including those with increased requirements (such as women who are pregnant or breast-feeding); infants (see *feeding, infant*); people who follow a restricted diet (such as *veganism*); those who have severe *alcohol*

dependence; and people suffering from disorders that may cause vitamin deficiencies, such as *malabsorption* and some liver and kidney disorders.

Vitamin supplements are also used in the treatment of certain disorders, including diagnosed vitamin deficiency. For example, vitamin D is used to treat the bone condition *osteomalacia* and vitamin A derivatives may be given in the treatment of severe *acne*. Supplementary vitamins may be given orally or may be injected.

vitiligo

A common disorder of *skin* pigmentation in which patches of skin, most commonly on the face, hands, armpits, and groin, lose their colour. Vitiligo is thought to be an *autoimmune disorder* (in which the body's immune system attacks its own tissues). The condition may occur at any age, but it usually develops in early adulthood.

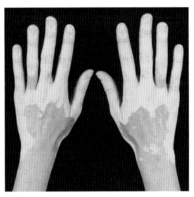

Vitiligo affecting the hands
Loss of pigment is the only skin change that occurs. The usual remedy for the condition is to mask the white patches with cosmetics.

Spontaneous repigmentation occurs in some cases. A course of *phototherapy* using *PUVA* can also induce repigmentation of the skin, and creams containing *corticosteroid drugs* may help.

vitreous haemorrhage

Bleeding into the *vitreous humour*, the gel-like substance that fills the main cavity of the eye. A common cause of a vitreous haemorrhage is diabetic *retinopathy*, in which new, fragile blood capillaries form on the retina.

Vitreous haemorrhage often affects vision; a major haemorrhage causes poor vision until the blood is reabsorbed, which may not be for several months, and may not occur at all.

vitreous humour

The transparent, gel-like body that fills the rear compartment of the *eye* between the crystalline lens and the retina. The vitreous humour is composed almost entirely of water.

vivisection

The performance of a surgical operation on a live animal, particularly for the purposes of research. (See also *animal experimentation*.)

vocal cords

Two fibrous sheets of tissue in the *larynx* (voicebox) that are responsible for voice production. The vocal cords are attached at the front to the thyroid cartilage and at the rear to the arytenoid cartilages (see *Location of the vocal cords* box, overleaf).

In order to produce sound, the vocal cords (which normally form a V-shaped opening) close and vibrate as air that is expelled from the lungs passes between them. Alterations in cord tension produce sounds of different pitch, which are modified by the tongue, mouth, and lips to form speech.

voicebox

See *larynx*.

voice, loss of

Inability to speak normally. Temporary partial loss of voice commonly results from straining of the muscles of the *larynx* (voicebox) through overuse of the voice or from inflammation of the *vocal cords* in *laryngitis*.

Persistent or recurrent loss of voice may be the result of *polyps* on the vocal cords, thickening of the vocal cords in *hypothyroidism* (underactivity of the thyroid gland), or interference with the nerve supply to the larynx muscles as a result of cancer of the larynx, *thyroid gland*, or *oesophagus*. Total loss of the voice is rare and is usually of psychological origin. (See also *hoarseness*; *larynx, disorders of*).

Volkmann's contracture

A disorder of the wrist and fingers in which they become permanently fixed in a bent position.

CAUSE

Volkmann's contracture occurs because of an inadequate blood supply to the forearm muscles that control the wrist and fingers. This is most likely to be the result of an injury.

V

LOCATION OF THE **VOCAL CORDS**

The vocal cords are located at the top of the larynx (voicebox). Their top edges stretch between the thyroid cartilage at the front and the arytenoid cartilages at the back. If they are brought close together, the vocal cords vibrate and emit sounds as air passes between them.

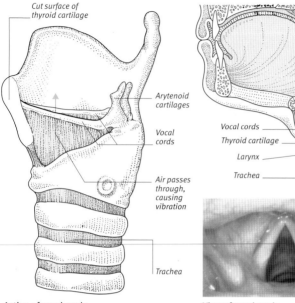

Cut surface of thyroid cartilage

Arytenoid cartilages

Vocal cords

Air passes through, causing vibration

Trachea

Action of vocal cords
For voice production, the cords are brought close together by muscles that act on the arytenoid cartilages.

Vocal cords
Thyroid cartilage
Larynx
Trachea

View of vocal cords
This photograph shows the two vocal cords in their position at rest: spaced apart to form a V-shaped opening.

SYMPTOMS
Initially, the fingers become cold, numb, and white or blue. Finger movements are weak and painful, and there is no pulse at the wrist. Unless treatment is started within a few hours, wrist and finger deformity develops.

TREATMENT
Treatment of the condition is by manipulation back into position of displaced bones, followed, if necessary, by surgical restoration of blood flow in the forearm. If there is permanent deformity, *physiotherapy* may help to restore function of the affected parts.

volvulus

Twisting of a loop of *intestine* or, in rare cases, of the *stomach*. Volvulus is a serious condition that causes obstruction of the passage of intestinal contents (see *intestine, obstruction of*) and a risk of *strangulation*. If strangulation occurs, blockage of blood flow to the affected area leads to potentially fatal *gangrene* (death of tissues in the area).

The symptoms of volvulus are severe episodes of abdominal pain followed by vomiting. Volvulus may be present from birth or may be a result of *adhesions* (areas of scar tissue binding loops of intestine). It requires emergency treatment, usually by surgery.

vomiting

The involuntary forcible expulsion of stomach contents through the mouth. Vomiting may be preceded by nausea, pallor, sweating, excessive salivation, and a slowed heart rate.

MECHANISM
It occurs when the vomiting centre in the *brainstem* is activated by signals from one of three places in the body: the digestive tract; the balancing mechanism of the inner *ear*; or the brain, either due to thoughts and emotions or via the part of the brain that responds to poisons in the body.

The vomiting centre sends messages to both the *diaphragm*, which presses down on the stomach, and the abdominal wall, which presses inwards; the combined effect of these actions is to expel the stomach contents upwards through the *oesophagus*.

CAUSES
Vomiting may be the result of overindulgence in food or alcohol. It is also a common side effect of many drugs, and it may follow general *anaesthesia*.

Vomiting is also common in gastro-intestinal disorders such as *peptic ulcer*, acute *appendicitis*, *gastroenteritis*, and *food poisoning*. Less commonly, it is due to intestinal obstruction (for example, due to *pyloric stenosis* or *intussusception*) or a tumour of the digestive tract. It may also be due to inflammation of associated digestive-tract organs (see *hepatitis*; *pancreatitis*; *cholecystitis*).

Other possible causes of vomiting are pressure within the skull (see *encephalitis*; *hydrocephalus*; a *brain tumour*; a *head injury*), *migraine*, conditions that affect the ear's balancing mechanism (see *Ménière's disease*; *labyrinthitis*; *motion sickness*), and hormonal disorders such as *Addison's disease*.

Vomiting may be a symptom of keto-acidosis in poorly controlled *diabetes mellitus*. It may also be a symptom of an emotional problem or be part of the disorders *anorexia nervosa* or *bulimia*.

TREATMENT
Persistent vomiting requires medical investigation. Treatment depends on the cause. *Antiemetics* may be given. (See also *vomiting blood*; *vomiting in pregnancy*.)

vomiting blood

A symptom of bleeding from within the digestive tract. The vomiting of blood may be the result of a tear in the lower oesophagus (see *Mallory–Weiss syndrome*), bleeding from *oesophageal varices* (enlarged veins in the oesophagus), erosive *gastritis* (inflammation of the stomach lining), a *peptic ulcer*, or, rarely, *stomach cancer*. A person can also vomit blood if the blood is swallowed during a nosebleed.

Vomited blood may be dark red, brown, black, or it may resemble coffee grounds. Vomiting of blood is often accompanied by the passing of black, tarry faeces.

The cause of vomiting blood is investigated by *endoscopy* (examination using a viewing instrument) of the oesophagus and stomach, or by *barium X-ray examinations*. If blood loss is severe, a *blood transfusion*, and possibly surgery to stop the bleeding, may be required.

V

vomiting in pregnancy

Nausea and vomiting in early *pregnancy* are common and are most likely to be caused by changes in hormone levels. Vomiting occurs most frequently in the morning, but it may occur at any time. It is sometimes precipitated by stress, travelling, or food.

In rare cases, the vomiting becomes severe and prolonged. This condition, known as hyperemesis gravidarum (see *hyperemesis*), can cause dehydration, nutritional deficiency, alterations in blood acidity, and weight loss. Hyper-emesis gravidarum requires immediate hospital admission to replace lost fluids and chemicals by *intravenous infusion*, to rule out any serious underlying disorder, and to control the vomiting.

von Recklinghausen's disease

Another name for *neurofibromatosis*.

von Willebrand's disease

An inherited lifelong *bleeding disorder* similar to *haemophilia*. People with the condition have a reduced concentration in their blood of a substance called von Willebrand factor, which helps *platelets* to plug injured blood vessel walls and forms part of *factor VIII* (a substance that is vital to blood coagulation).

SYMPTOMS

Symptoms include excessive bleeding from the gums and from nosebleeds and cuts. Women may have heavy menstrual bleeding. In severe cases, bleeding into joints and muscles may occur.

DIAGNOSIS AND TREATMENT

The condition is diagnosed by *blood-clotting tests* and measurement of blood levels of von Willebrand factor. Bleeding episodes can be prevented or controlled by desmopressin (a substance that is similar to *ADH*). Factor VIII or concentrated von Willebrand factor may also be used to treat bleeding.

voyeurism

The observation, on a regular basis, of unsuspecting individuals who may be naked, undressing, or engaged in sexual activity, in order to achieve sexual arousal.

VSD

The abbreviation for *ventricular septal defect*.

vulva

The external part of the female genitalia, comprising the *clitoris* and two pairs of skin folds called *labia*.

Conditions that affect the vulva include *vulval itching*; inflammation (see *vulvitis* and *vulvovaginitis*); skin conditions, such as *dermatitis* and *lichen sclerosus et atrophicus*; genital warts (see *warts, genital*); genital herpes (see *herpes, genital*); *leukoplakia* (raised white patches due to tissue thickening); and cancer (see *vulva, cancer of*).

vulva, cancer of

A malignant tumour of the vulva (the external part of the female genitalia), a rare disorder that most commonly affects postmenopausal women. Cancer of the vulva may be preceded by a phase of vulval cell changes that cause itching, but, in many cases, the first symptom of the condition is a lump or painful ulcer on the vulva.

Diagnosis is confirmed using *biopsy* (removal of a sample of tissue for analysis). Treatment is by surgical removal of the affected tissue, sometimes together with *radiotherapy* and *chemotherapy*. The outlook depends on how early treatment is commenced.

vulval itching

Irritation of the vulva (the external part of the female genitalia), known medically as pruritus vulvae. Vulval itching

ANATOMY OF THE **VULVA**

The outer skin folds (labia majora) are usually in contact. If parted, they reveal the clitoris and the inner folds (labia minora), which enclose the urethral and vaginal openings.

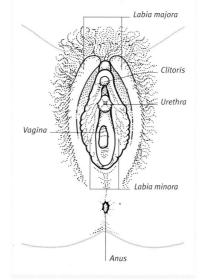

may be caused by localized conditions, including infections (such as *candidiasis*), infestations (such as with *pubic lice*), or abnormal changes in the vulval skin (due, for example, to *leukoplakia* or *cancer*). It may also be caused by any condition leading to generalized itching or by skin conditions, such as *dermatitis* and *psoriasis*. Itching may also result from an *allergy* to chemicals in spermi-cidal or hygiene products. Treatment of vulval itching depends on the cause.

vulvitis

Inflammation of the vulva (the external part of the female genitalia). Infections that may lead to vulvitis include *candidiasis* (thrush) and genital herpes (see *herpes, genital*). Infestations with *pubic lice* or *scabies* are other possible causes. Vulvitis may also occur as a result of changes in the vulval skin, which tend to affect women after the *menopause*. Such changes may take the form of red or white patches and/or thickened or thinned areas that may be inflamed (see *lichen sclerosus et atrophicus*; *leukoplakia*). Other possible causes of vulvitis include allergic reactions to hygiene products, excessive vaginal discharge, or urinary incontinence (see *incontinence, urinary*).

Treatment depends on the cause, but may involve the topical application of a combination of drugs; good hygiene is usually recommended. If there are skin changes, a *biopsy* (tissue sample) may be taken to exclude the possibility of vulval cancer. (See also *vaginitis*; *vulvovaginitis*.)

vulvovaginitis

Inflammation of the vulva (see *vulvitis*) and vagina (see *vaginitis*). Vulvovaginitis is often caused by infections such as *candidiasis* (thrush) or *trichomoniasis*.

V

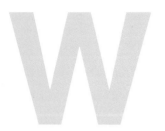

walking

Movement of the body by lifting the feet alternately, bringing one foot into contact with the ground before the other starts to leave it. A person's gait (style of walking) is determined by body shape, size, and posture. The age at which children first walk varies enormously.

Walking is controlled by nerve signals to the muscles. The signals travel to the muscles, via the spinal cord, from the motor cortex of the brain (see *cerebrum*), *basal ganglia*, and *cerebellum*.

DISORDERS

Abnormal gait may be caused by joint stiffness, muscle weakness (sometimes due to conditions such as *poliomyelitis* or *muscular dystrophy*), skeletal abnormalities (see, for example, *arthritis*; *bone tumour*; *developmental dysplasia of the hip*; *scoliosis*; *talipes*). A painful limp may be due to a fracture or disease of the leg bones (*tibia*, *fibula*, or *femur*). Children may develop *knock-knee* or *bowleg*; *synovitis* of the hip and *Perthes' disease* are also common. Adolescents may develop a painful limp due to a slipped epiphysis (see *femoral epiphysis, slipped*). Abnormal gait may also be caused by neurological disorders such as *stroke* (commonly causing *hemiplegia*), *multiple sclerosis*, *parkinsonism*, peripheral *neuritis*, various forms of *myelitis*, and *chorea*. *Ménière's disease* may cause severe loss of balance and instability.

walking aids

Equipment such as sticks, crutches and frames for increasing the mobility of people who have problems walking.

walking, delayed

Most children start to walk by around 15 months of age. Delayed walking may be suspected if the child is unable to walk unassisted by the age of 18 months (see *developmental delay*).

warfarin

An *anticoagulant drug* used in the prevention and treatment of abnormal *blood clotting*. Warfarin is used to treat deep vein thrombosis (formation of a blood clot within the deep-lying veins of the leg; see *thrombosis, deep vein*), *pulmonary embolism* (a fragment of a blood clot in the bloodstream becoming lodged in the lungs), and people with *atrial fibrillation* (an abnormality of the heartbeat) who are at risk of an *embolism*. It is also prescribed to prevent emboli from developing on replacement heart valves (see *heart-valve surgery*).

A faster-acting anticoagulant, such as *heparin*, may also be prescribed for the first few days following a deep vein thrombosis or pulmonary embolism.

Warfarin may cause abnormal bleeding in different parts of the body, so regular blood tests are carried out to allow careful regulation of dosage. It may also cause nausea, diarrhoea, rash, and jaundice.

wart

A common, contagious, and harmless growth that occurs on the skin or mucous membranes. Only the topmost layer of skin is affected. An overgrowth of cells in this layer causes a visible lump to develop.

CAUSES AND TYPES

Warts are caused by the human papillomavirus, of which at least 100 different types are known. These cause different types of warts at various sites, such as

THE MECHANICS OF **WALKING**

Many different muscles take part in the walking process. They contract in a complex, rhythmic sequence in response to programmes of signals sent from the motor cortex in the brain. Feedback of information from the muscles and joints to the brain helps to ensure that the gait is smooth, steady, and coordinated.

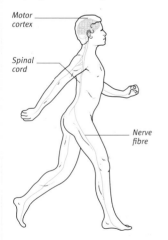

Motor cortex

Spinal cord

Nerve fibre

Route of the signals
The signals for walking originate in the motor cortex and are carried via the spinal cord and nerve fibres to muscles.

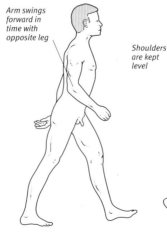

Arm swings forward in time with opposite leg

1 As the left foot touches the ground, the right arm swings forward and the right foot shifts on to tiptoe.

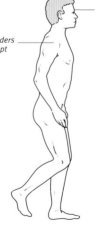

Shoulders are kept level

2 Once the left foot is fully planted on the ground and supporting the body, the right foot is raised.

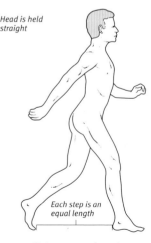

Head is held straight

Each step is an equal length

3 A sequence of muscle contractions advances the right leg, and the left arm swings forward.

W

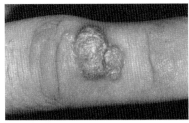

Common warts on finger
Warts often grow in crops. In time they disappear spontaneously, but they can be removed by freezing.

on the hands, feet (see *wart, plantar*), or genitals (see *warts, genital*). Flat warts are flesh-coloured; they are sometimes itchy lumps with flat tops that occur mainly on the wrists, backs of the hands, and the face.

TREATMENT
Many warts disappear in 6 to 12 months without treatment. Genital warts should be treated promptly, however. Common, flat, and plantar warts can sometimes be destroyed using a wart-removing liquid or special plaster. Several treatments may be needed, however, and sometimes the wart returns. Warts are commonly treated by *cryosurgery*.

wart, plantar

A hard, horny, and rough-surfaced area on the sole of the foot caused by a virus called a papillomavirus. Plantar warts, also known as verrucas, may occur singly or in clusters. The wart is flattened and forced into the skin and may cause discomfort or pain when walking. Infection can be acquired from contaminated floors in swimming pools and communal showers.

Many plantar warts disappear without treatment, but some persist for years or disappear for a short time and then reappear. They can be removed by *cryosurgery*, by applying plasters or gel containing salicylic acid, or by other chemical treatments.

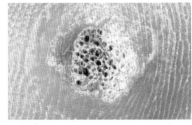

Typical plantar wart
This type of wart may need treatment; a doctor may treat it by paring it down with a scalpel and applying a corrosive paint.

warts, genital

Fleshy, painless, usually soft lumps that grow in and around the vagina, around the anus, and on the penis. Genital warts are transmitted by sexual contact, and they are caused by some forms of *human papillomavirus* (HPV). The warts appear from a few weeks to 18 months after infection. They may be removed by *cryosurgery* or the drug *podophyllin*, but they tend to recur.

Genital warts caused by to some types of human papillomavirus are linked with the development of cervical cancer (see *cervix, cancer of*).

wasp stings

See *insect stings*.

water

A simple compound that is essential for all life. Its molecular structure is H_2O (two atoms of hydrogen bonded to one of oxygen). Water is the most common substance in the body, accounting for about 99 per cent of all molecules, but a smaller percentage of total body weight. Approximately two-thirds of the body's water content is contained within cells, and the remaining third is extracellular (found, for example, in blood *plasma*, *lymph*, *cerebrospinal fluid*, and *tissue fluid*).

ROLE IN THE BODY
Water provides the medium in which all metabolic reactions take place (see *metabolism*), and transports substances around the body. The blood plasma carries water to all body tissues, and excess water from tissues for elimination via the *liver*, *kidneys*, *lungs*, and *skin*. The passage of water in the tissue fluid into and out of cells takes place by *osmosis*.

WATER BALANCE
Water is taken into the body in food and drink and is lost in *urine* and *faeces*, as exhaled water vapour, and by sweating (see *dehydration*). The amount of water excreted in urine is regulated by the kidneys. Extra water is needed to excrete excess amounts of substances, such as sugar or salt, in the blood.

In some disorders, such as *kidney failure* or *heart failure*, insufficient water is excreted in the urine, resulting in *oedema* (accumulation of water in body tissues).

water-borne infection

A disease caused by infective or parasitic organisms transmitted via water. Infections can be contracted if infected water is drunk, if it contaminates food, or if individuals swim or wade in it. World-

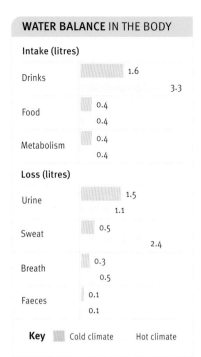

WATER BALANCE IN THE BODY

Intake (litres)

	Cold climate	Hot climate
Drinks	1.6	3.3
Food	0.4	0.4
Metabolism	0.4	0.4

Loss (litres)

	Cold climate	Hot climate
Urine	1.5	1.1
Sweat	0.5	2.4
Breath	0.3	0.5
Faeces	0.1	0.1

Key   Cold climate   Hot climate

wide, contamination of drinking water is an important mode of transmission for various diseases, including *hepatitis A*, many viral and bacterial causes of *diarrhoea*, *typhoid fever*, *cholera*, *amoebiasis*, and some types of *worm infestation*.

Swimming in polluted water should be avoided because, if swallowed, there is a risk of contracting disease. A form of *leptospirosis* is caused by contact with water contaminated by rats' urine. In tropical countries, there is also a risk of contracting *schistosomiasis* (bilharzia) – a serious disease caused by a fluke that can burrow through the swimmer's skin.

waterbrash

Sudden filling of the mouth with tasteless saliva. It is not to be confused with *gastro-oesophageal reflux disease*, in which the regurgitated fluid tastes sour. Waterbrash normally has other symptoms, such as abdominal pain before a meal, and usually indicates a disorder of the upper gastrointestinal tract.

Waterhouse–Friderichsen syndrome

A serious condition caused by infection of the bloodstream by bacteria of the meningococcus group. The main features are bleeding into the skin, low blood pressure, and *shock*. Without medical treatment, coma and death follow within

W

Water from any source that falls into the suspect or very suspect categories should be sterilized. Techniques include boiling, filtering, and chemical treatment.

Category	Developed countries	Developing countries
Usually safe	Tap water from public supply; rainwater; canned or bottled drinks; spring water	Canned or bottled drinks of well-known brands; rainwater
Suspect	Water direct from rivers, streams, lakes, ponds, canals, and wells	Tap water (cities); spring water
Very suspect	Obviously polluted water (i.e. cloudy in appearance or with an unpleasant smell)	Tap water (rural areas); water direct from rivers, streams, lakes, ponds, and canals

hours. The syndrome is often associated with *meningitis*, which affects the membranes covering the brain and spinal cord.

watering eye

An increase in volume of the tear film, usually producing epiphora (overflow of *tears*). It may be caused by excess tear production due to emotion, conjunctival or corneal irritation, or an obstruction to the channel that drains tears. (See also *lacrimal apparatus*.)

water intoxication

A condition that is caused by excessive water retention in the brain. The principal symptoms are headaches, dizziness, nausea, confusion, and, in severe cases, seizures and unconsciousness.

Various disorders can disrupt the water balance in the body, leading to accumulation of water in the tissues. Examples include *kidney failure*, liver *cirrhosis*, severe *heart failure*, diseases of the *adrenal glands*, and certain lung or ovarian tumours producing a substance similar to *ADH* (antidiuretic hormone). Water intoxication is also seen in association with the use of *Ecstasy* (MDMA), during which excessive amounts of water are drunk. There is also a risk of water intoxication after surgery, caused by increased ADH production.

water on the brain

A nonmedical term for *hydrocephalus*.

water on the knee

A popular term for accumulation of fluid in or around the knee joint. A common cause is *bursitis* (inflammation of a bursa, one of the fluid-filled sacs that cushion pressure points in the body). (See also *effusion, joint*.)

water retention

Accumulation of fluid in body tissues (see *oedema*).

water tablets

A nonmedical term for *diuretic drugs*.

wax bath

A type of *heat treatment* in which hot liquid wax is applied to a part of the body in order to relieve pain and stiffness in an inflamed or injured joint. Wax baths may be used to treat the hands of people with *rheumatoid arthritis*.

wax, ear

See *earwax*.

weakness

A term used to describe a lack of vigour or strength. This is a common symptom of a range of conditions, such as *anaemia*, *emotional problems*, and various disorders affecting the heart, nervous system, bones, joints, and muscles. When associated with emotional disorders, weakness may represent lack of desire or ambition, rather than loss of muscle strength.

More specifically, the term describes loss of power in particular muscle groups, which may be accompanied by muscle wasting and loss of sensation. (See also *paralysis*.)

weal

A raised bump on the skin that is paler than the adjacent tissue and may be surrounded by red inflammation. Weals are characteristic of *urticaria* (hives).

weaning

The gradual substitution of solid foods for milk or milk formula in an infant's diet (see *feeding, infant*).

webbing

A flap of skin, such as that which might occur between adjacent fingers or toes. Webbing is a common congenital (present from birth) abnormality that often runs in families and which may affect two or more digits. Mild webbing is completely harmless, but surgical correction may be performed for cosmetic reasons. In severe cases, adjacent digits may be completely fused (see *syndactyly*). Webbing of the neck is a feature of the condition *Turner's syndrome*.

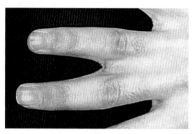

Webbing of the fingers
This curious feature is often an inherited trait, appearing in each of several generations of a family. Most cases are completely harmless and do not require treatment.

Wegener's granulomatosis

A rare disorder in which *granulomas* (nodular collections of abnormal cells), associated with areas of chronic tissue inflammation due to *vasculitis* (inflammation of the blood vessels) develop in the nasal passages, lungs, and kidneys. It is thought that Wegener's granulomatosis is an *autoimmune disorder* (in which the body's immune system attacks its own tissues).

SYMPTOMS
Principal symptoms include a bloody nasal discharge, coughing (which sometimes produces bloodstained sputum), breathing difficulty, chest pain, and blood in the urine. There may also be loss of appetite, weight loss, weakness, fatigue, and joint pains.

TREATMENT AND OUTLOOK
Treatment of the condition is with *immunosuppressant drugs*, such as *cyclophosphamide*, which are combined with *corticosteroids* to alleviate symptoms and attempt to bring about a remission.

With prompt treatment, most people recover completely within about a year, but *kidney failure* occasionally develops. Without treatment, complications may occur, including perforation of the nasal septum; inflammation of the eyes; rash, nodules, or ulcers on the skin; and damage to the heart, which may be fatal.

W

weight

The heaviness of a person. In children, weight is routinely used as an index of growth. In healthy adults, weight remains more or less stable if dietary energy intake matches energy expenditure (see *metabolism*). *Weight loss* or weight gain occurs if the net energy balance is disturbed.

WEIGHT ASSESSMENT

The standard method of assessing weight is to use the *body mass index* (BMI), obtained by dividing the weight in kilograms by the square of the height in metres. A BMI of less than 18.5 kg/m^2 is classed as underweight; 18.5–24.9 is classed as a healthy weight; 25–29.9 is classed as overweight; 30–39.9 is classed as obese; and a BMI over 40 is classed as very obese (see also the accompanying chart). These figures are general ones that apply to most healthy adults under the age of 60. They are not applicable to children; people over 60; people with chronic health problems; women who are pregnant or breast-feeding; or people with a high proportion of muscle, such as athletes.

The proportion and distribution of body fat is also important: people with too much fat and/or excessive fat around the waist are at increased risk of health problems, even if their BMI is in the healthy range. For average men aged 20–60 with no chronic health problems, body fat should account for about 8–22 per cent of total body weight, and the waist should be no larger than 94 cm. For average women aged 20–60 with no chronic health problems and who are not pregnant or breast-feeding, body fat should account for about 22–35 per cent of body weight, and the waist should be no larger than 81 cm.

In children, weight can be compared with standardized predictions for age, which differ according to the gender and race of a child. Such weight charts may be used to assess how well a child is thriving. Special BMI charts for children are also available but they require expert interpretation because a child's BMI may change rapidly, due to a growth spurt, for example.

WEIGHT AND HEALTH

At all ages, divergence from standard figures (either using BMI or body fat percentages) may have medical implications. If an individual is underweight, his or her *nutrition* may be inadequate as a result of a poor diet or disease; if an individual is significantly overweight, he or she is at increased risk of various health problems, such as *hypertension* (high blood pressure), *coronary artery disease*, *stroke*, and *diabetes mellitus*. (See also *obesity*).

weight loss

When there is a decrease in energy intake compared with energy expenditure, weight loss is likely to occur. The decrease may be the result of deliberate *weight reduction* or a change in diet or activity level. Weight loss may also result from fluid loss (for example, because of sweating in a hot climate) or it may be a symptom of a disorder. Any unexplained weight loss should always be investigated by a doctor.

LOSS OF APPETITE

Many diseases can disrupt the appetite to the extent that an individual loses the desire to eat, which in turn leads to weight loss. Loss of appetite may also be a sign of generalized ill health. *Depression* reduces a person's motivation to eat; *peptic ulcer* causes pain and, in some cases, food avoidance; and some kidney disorders cause loss of appetite due to the effects of *uraemia* (raised levels of the waste product urea in the blood). In *anorexia nervosa* and *bulimia*, complex psychological factors affect an individual's eating pattern, sometimes with dramatic results.

DIGESTIVE CAUSES

Digestive disorders, such as *gastroenteritis*, lead to weight loss as a result of vomiting or diarrhoea. Weight is also affected by cancer of the oesophagus (see *oesophagus, cancer of*) and *stomach cancer*. *Malabsorption* also affects weight.

METABOLIC CAUSES

Some disorders cause weight loss by increasing the rate of metabolic activity in cells. Examples are any type of *cancer*, chronic infection such as *tuberculosis*, and *hyperthyroidism* (overactivity of the thyroid gland). Untreated *diabetes mellitus* may also cause weight loss.

weight reduction

The process of losing excess body fat. A person who is severely overweight (see *obesity*) is at an increased risk of developing various illnesses, such as *diabetes mellitus*, *hypertension* (high blood pressure), and heart disease.

HOW IT IS DONE

The most efficient way to lose weight is to eat a healthy diet (see *nutrition*). This may involve reducing the intake of excess calories (those over the recommended daily limit), combined with regular exercise, both *aerobic* (fat-burning) and toning (muscle-building). Motivation, emotional support, and exploration of psychological factors affecting eating are also important for success.

WEIGHT/HEIGHT GRAPH FOR MEN AND WOMEN

To find out whether or not you are underweight, normal weight, or overweight, first find your height, then run your finger up to your present weight. People with a BMI of $18.5–24.9 \text{ kg/m}^2$ are considered to be a healthy weight; those whose BMI is less than 18.5 are underweight, those with a BMI over 25 are overweight.

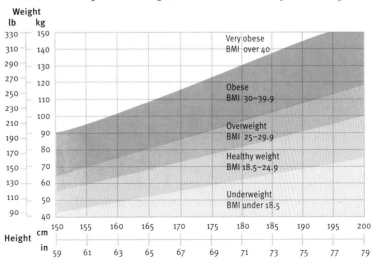

W

RECOMMENDATIONS FOR WEIGHT REDUCTION

- Cut down drastically on all visible fats, including butter, margarine, cream, and cooking oils, as well as the invisible fats that are present in pastries, biscuits, and cakes. Choose low-fat milk, cheeses, and yogurts.

- Choose lean cuts of meat and avoid processed meat such as salami. Grill or roast meat without adding fat instead of frying.

- Eat more boiled legumes (e.g. lentils and beans), which provide protein but contain very little fat.

- Avoid refined carbohydrates such as sugar (sucrose) as well as refined grain products such as white flour and white rice.

- Increase your consumption of unrefined carbohydrates. Eat wholemeal bread, whole-grain rice and cereals, fresh fruit, and plenty of vegetables.

- Reduce your intake of alcoholic drinks, which are high in calories.

DRUG AND OTHER TREATMENTS

In most circumstances, drugs play little part in a weight-loss programme. However, *orlistat* (an antiobesity drug) or appetite suppressants (such as *sibutramine* and *rimonabant*) may be useful adjuncts to a reduced diet in specific individuals who have a high *body mass index* (BMI). Surgery – such as wiring of the jaws or operations to reduce the capacity of the stomach or bypass part of the intestinal tract – may be considered for some people who are very obese (with a BMI over 40).

Weil's disease

Another name for *leptospirosis*.

welder's eye

Also known as arc eye, acute *conjunctivitis* and *keratopathy* (corneal damage) caused by the intense *ultraviolet light* emitted by an electric welding arc.

Werdnig–Hoffmann disease

A very rare inherited disorder of the *nervous system* that affects infants. Also known as infantile spinal muscular atrophy, Werdnig–Hoffmann disease is a type of *motor neuron disease*.

Marked floppiness and paralysis occur during the first few months, and affected children rarely survive beyond the age of three. There is no cure for the disease. Treatment aims to keep the affected infant as comfortable as possible.

Wernicke–Korsakoff syndrome

An uncommon brain disorder, almost always related to malnutrition, that occurs in chronic alcohol dependence. It may also occasionally occur in cancer. The syndrome results from deficiency of thiamine (see *vitamin B complex*), which affects the brain and nervous system.

SYMPTOMS

The disease has two stages: Wernicke's encephalopathy and Korsakoff's psychosis. Wernicke's encephalopathy usually develops suddenly and produces nystagmus (abnormal, jerky eye movements), ataxia (difficulty coordinating body movements), slowness, and confusion. Sufferers usually have signs of neuropathy (nerve damage), such as sensation loss, pins-and-needles, or impaired reflexes. The level of consciousness falls progressively and may lead to coma and death unless treated.

Korsakoff's psychosis may follow Wernicke's encephalopathy if treatment is not prompt. Symptoms consist of *amnesia*, apathy, and disorientation.

TREATMENT AND OUTLOOK

Wernicke's encephalopathy is an emergency. High doses of intravenous thiamine can reverse most symptoms, sometimes within hours. However, once the disease progresses to Korsakoff's psychosis, it is usually irreversible.

Wernicke's area

An area of the cerebral cortex in the brain that is involved in the interpretation of spoken and written language. Damage to Wernicke's area may result in *aphasia* (a complete loss of previously acquired language skills).

Wernicke's encephalopathy

See *Wernicke–Korsakoff syndrome*.

West Nile virus

A virus that is transmitted from infected animals or birds to humans by a mosquito bite. In most cases, there are either

CAUSE OF **WHIPLASH INJURY**

This injury to the neck section of the spine may occur when a car is subjected to a sudden violent force and the occupant's body is restrained in the seat but his or her head is not restrained by an appropriate head restraint.

Sudden acceleration
Here, there is a sudden force from behind (usually due to another vehicle's striking the rear of the car). As the body accelerates forwards, the head jerks violently backwards relative to the body, stretching and bending the neck; the head then rebounds forwards.

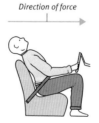

Direction of force

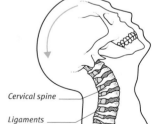

Cervical spine

Ligaments

Sudden deceleration
Here, there is a sudden violent force from the front towards the back of the vehicle, due, for example, to a collision with a tree. The seat belt restrains the body, but the head continues to move forwards, stretching the neck; the head then rebounds backwards.

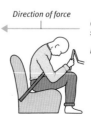

Direction of force

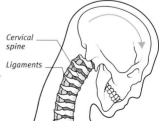

Cervical spine

Ligaments

W

no symptoms or there is a flulike illness. Rarely, a serious and potentially fatal illness, in which the virus infects the brain, can develop. The virus is found in Africa, Eastern Europe, West Asia, the Middle East, and, since 1999, the east coast of the USA.

wet dream

Ejaculation of semen during sleep. (See also *nocturnal emission*.)

wet gangrene

A type of *gangrene*.

wheelchair

A chair mounted on wheels used to provide mobility for a person unable to walk. Manual wheelchairs are designed so that the hand-rims can be easily gripped by a disabled person. They can also be pushed by a helper. Powered wheelchairs use batteries and are controlled electronically by finger or chin pressure, or by breath control.

wheeze

A high-pitched, whistling sound produced in the chest, usually on breathing out, that is caused by narrowing of the airways. It is a feature of the lung disorders *asthma*, *bronchitis*, *bronchiolitis*, and *pulmonary oedema* (the accumulation of fluid in the lungs). Inhalation of a foreign body may also be a cause. (See also *breathing difficulty*.)

whiplash injury

An injury to the soft tissues, *ligaments*, and spinal joints of the neck caused by a forcible and violent bending of the neck backwards (hyperextension) and then forwards (flexion), or vice versa. Such injury most commonly results from sudden acceleration or deceleration, as occurs in a car collision (see the illustrated box, left).

Damage to the spine usually involves minor *sprain* of a neck ligament or *subluxation* (partial dislocation) of a cervical joint. Occasionally, a ligament may rupture or a cervical vertebra may fracture (see *spinal injury*). Characteristically, pain and stiffness in the neck are much worse 24 hours after the injury.

Treatment of whiplash injury is with early mobilization and *analgesic drugs*, together with advice about posture. It may take a few weeks before full pain-free movement is possible. If these measures do not clear up the symptoms, *physiotherapy* may be recommended.

Whipple's disease

A rare disorder, also called intestinal lipodystrophy, that can affect many organs. Symptoms include *steatorrhoea* (the presence of fat in the faeces) as a result of *malabsorption*, abdominal pain, joint pains, swollen lymph nodes, progressive weight loss, anaemia, and fever. The heart, lungs, and brain can also be affected. The condition is most common in middle-aged men.

The cause is thought to be bacterial; affected tissues are found to contain macrophages (a type of scavenging cell) containing rod-shaped bacteria.

Treatment is with *antibiotic drugs* for at least a year. Dietary supplements are used to correct nutritional deficiencies occurring as a result of malabsorption.

Whipple's operation

A type of *pancreatectomy* in which the head of the pancreas and the loop of the duodenum (first section of the small intestine) are surgically removed.

whipworm infestation

Small, cylindrical whiplike worms that are 2.5–5 cm long and live in the human large intestine. Infestation occurs worldwide but is most common in the tropics. Light infestation causes no symptoms, but heavy infestation can cause abdominal pain, diarrhoea, and, sometimes, *anaemia*.

Diagnosis is through the identification of eggs in the faeces. Treatment is with *anthelmintic drugs*, such as *mebendazole*. A heavy infestation may require more than one course of treatment.

white blood cell

Also known as an leucocyte, a *blood cell* that contains a nucleus. Granulocytes, lymphocytes, and monocytes are three types of white blood cell that are involved in the production of antibodies and protection of the body against foreign substances as part of the *immune system*. (See also *red blood cell*.)

whitehead

A very common type of skin blemish (see *milia*).

white matter

Tissue in the nervous system composed of nerve fibres (*axons*). White matter makes up the bulk of the cerebrum (the two large hemispheres of the *brain*) and continues down into the *spinal cord*; its main role is to transmit nerve impulses. (See also *grey matter*.)

whitlow

An abscess on the fingertip or toe that causes the affected digit to swell and become extremely painful and sensitive to pressure and touch. A whitlow may be caused by the virus responsible for

LIFE-CYCLE OF WHIPWORM

Whipworm infestation (known medically as trichuriasis) occurs worldwide and is particularly common in the tropics. In the UK, whipworm infestation mainly affects immigrants and residents of psychiatric hospitals. Adult whipworms are 2.5 to 5 cm long. They may live in a person's intestine for up to 20 years. Most infestations do not cause symptoms.

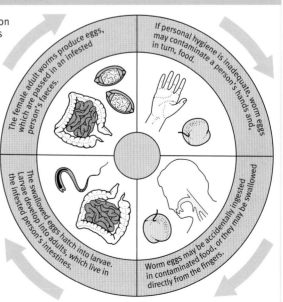

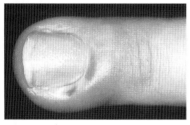

Herpetic whitlow
This extremely painful finger infection, caused in this case by the herpes simplex virus, may be helped by applying an antiviral ointment.

herpes simplex or it may be due to a bacterial infection. In some cases, pus needs to be drained from the abscess.

WHO

The commonly used abbreviation for the *World Health Organization*.

whooping cough

See *pertussis*.

will, living

See *living will*.

Wilms' tumour

A type of *kidney cancer*, also called nephroblastoma, that occurs mainly in children.

Wilson's disease

A rare, inherited disorder in which copper accumulates in the liver, resulting in conditions such as *hepatitis* and *cirrhosis*. Copper is slowly released into other body parts, damaging the brain, causing mild intellectual impairment, and leading to debilitating rigidity, tremor, and dementia. Symptoms of Wilson's disease usually appear in adolescence, but they can occur much earlier or later.

Lifelong treatment with *penicillamine* is necessary and, if begun soon enough, it can produce an improvement. If the disease is discovered before symptoms begin, the drug may prevent them.

wind

A common name for gas in the gastrointestinal tract, which may be expelled through the mouth (see *belching*) or passed through the anus (see *flatus*).

Babies often swallow air during feeding which, unless the baby is "winded", can accumulate in the stomach and cause discomfort.

windpipe

Another name for the *trachea*.

wiring of the jaws

Immobilization of the jaws by means of metal wires to allow a jaw fracture to heal or as part of treatment for *obesity*. When a fracture is being treated, the jaws are kept wired in a fixed position for about six weeks. For promoting weight loss, the jaws are wired for as long as a year. In both cases, the person is unable to chew and can take only a liquid or semi-liquid diet.

wisdom tooth

One of the four rearmost *teeth*, also known as third molars. The wisdom teeth normally erupt between the ages of 18 and 25 but often erupt later; in some people, one or more fails to develop or erupt. In many cases, wisdom teeth are unable to emerge fully from the gum as a result of overcrowding (see *impaction, dental*).

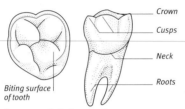

Crown
Cusps
Neck
Roots
Biting surface of tooth

Structure of wisdom tooth
Like other molars, each wisdom tooth has strong roots and a bulky crown with many cusps and an extensive grinding surface.

Wiskott-Aldrich syndrome

An inherited condition in which the function of the immune system is impaired and there is a low number of platelets (blood cells that are needed for clotting). The defect is inherited in an X-linked recessive manner (see *genetic disorders*). It causes disease in males; females may have no symptoms, but may pass the gene to their children.

Features may include recurrent infections (caused by impaired immunity), an increased tendency to bleed (due to the reduced number of platelets), and *eczema*. Symptoms first develop soon after birth or during the first year of life. Affected individuals also have an increased risk of developing cancers, such as *lymphoma* and *leukaemia*, usually in adolescence or early adulthood.

Treatment is aimed at relieving the symptoms of the condition.

witches' milk

A thin, white discharge from the nipple of a newborn infant, caused by maternal hormones that entered the fetus's circulation through the placenta. Witches' milk occurs quite commonly. It is usually accompanied by enlargement of one or both of the baby's breasts. The condition is harmless and usually disappears within a few weeks.

withdrawal

The process of retreating from society and from relationships with others; usually indicated by aloofness, lack of interest in social activities, preoccupation with one's own concerns, and difficulty in communicating.

The term is also applied to the psychological and physical symptoms that develop on discontinuing use of a substance on which a person is dependent (see *withdrawal syndrome*).

withdrawal bleeding

Vaginal blood loss that occurs when the level of *oestrogen* or *progesterone hormones* or *progestogen drugs* in the body drops suddenly.

The withdrawal bleeding that occurs at the end of each month's supply of combined *oral contraceptive pills* mimics menstruation but is usually shorter and lighter. Discontinuation of an oestrogen-only or progestogen-only preparation also produces bleeding, which may differ from normal menstruation in its amount and duration.

withdrawal method

See *coitus interruptus*.

withdrawal syndrome

Unpleasant mental and physical symptoms experienced when an individual stops using a drug on which he or she is dependent (see *drug dependence*). Withdrawal syndrome most commonly occurs in those with *alcohol dependence* or dependence on opioid *analgesic drugs*, in smokers, and in people who are addicted to *tranquillizers*, *amphetamines*, *cocaine*, *marijuana*, and *caffeine*.

ALCOHOL WITHDRAWAL
In an alcohol-dependent person, alcohol withdrawal symptoms start six to eight hours after cessation of intake and may last up to seven days. They include trembling of the hands, nausea, vomiting, sweating, cramps, anxiety, and, sometimes, seizures and visual *hallucinations*.

OPIOID WITHDRAWAL
Withdrawal symptoms from opioids start after eight to 12 hours, and may last for seven to ten days. Symptoms include restlessness, sweating, runny

W

eyes and nose, yawning, dilated pupils, diarrhoea, vomiting, abdominal cramps, loss of appetite, irritability, weakness, tremor, and depression.

TRANQUILLIZER WITHDRAWAL

Withdrawal symptoms from *barbiturate drugs* and *meprobamate* begin, after 12 to 24 hours, with tremors, anxiety, restlessness, and weakness, sometimes followed by *delirium*, hallucinations, and, occasionally, seizures. A period of prolonged sleep occurs three to eight days after onset. Withdrawal from *benzodiazepine drugs* may begin more slowly and can be serious, often resulting in depression, confusion, *agoraphobia* (a fear of open spaces and public places), and/or *psychosis*.

STOPPING SMOKING

Withdrawal symptoms from *nicotine* develop over 24 to 48 hours and include irritability, concentration problems, frustration, headaches, and anxiety.

WITHDRAWAL FROM OTHER DRUGS

Discontinuation of cocaine or amphetamines results in dizziness, lethargy, and extreme tiredness. Cocaine withdrawal may also lead to tremor, sweating, and severe depression. Withdrawal symptoms from marijuana include tremor, nausea, vomiting, diarrhoea, sweating, irritability, and sleep problems. Withdrawal from caffeine may lead to tiredness, headaches, and irritability.

TREATMENT

Severe withdrawal syndromes require medical treatment. Symptoms may be suppressed by giving the patient small quantities of the drug he or she had been taking. More commonly, a substitute drug is given, such as *methadone* for opioid drugs or a benzodiazepine drug for alcohol. The dose of the drug is then gradually reduced.

wobble board

A balancing board used during *physiotherapy* to improve muscle strength and coordination in the feet, ankles, and legs. A wobble board is sometimes used after an ankle sprain.

womb

See *uterus*.

word blindness

See *alexia*; *dyslexia*.

World Health Organization (WHO)

An international organization established in 1948 as an agency of the United Nations with responsibilities for international health matters and public health. The WHO headquarters are in Geneva, Switzerland.

The WHO has campaigned effectively against some infectious diseases, most notably smallpox, which was eradicated in 1980. Other functions include sponsoring medical research programmes, organizing national laboratories, and providing expert health advice and specific targets to its 192 member states.

worm infestation

Several worms, or their larvae, existing as parasites of humans. They may live in the intestines, blood, lymphatic system, bile ducts, or in organs such as the liver. In many cases, they cause few or no symptoms, but some cause chronic illness. The two main classes are: *roundworms* and *platyhelminths*, with subdivisions, cestodes (tapeworms) and trematodes (flukes).

Worm diseases occurring in developed countries include *threadworm infestation*, *ascariasis*, *whipworm infestation*, *toxocariasis*, liver-fluke infestation, and various *tapeworm infestations*. Those occurring in tropical regions include, in addition, *hookworm infestation*, *filariasis*, *guinea worm disease*, and *schistosomiasis*.

Worms may be acquired by eating undercooked, infected meat, contact with soil or water containing worm larvae, or accidental ingestion of worm eggs from soil contaminated by infected faeces. Most infestations can be easily eradicated with *anthelmintic drugs*.

wound

Damage to the skin and/or underlying tissues caused by an accident, violence, or surgery. Wounds in which the skin or mucous membrane is broken are called "open"; those in which they remain intact, for example bruises, are termed "closed". Wounds can be divided into these categories: incised wounds; abrasions (or grazes); *lacerations*; penetrating wounds; and *contusions* (see *Types of wounds* box, overleaf).

wound infection

Any type of *wound* is susceptible to the entry of bacteria; the resultant infection may delay healing, result in disability, and even cause death. Infection of a wound is indicated by redness, swelling, warmth, pain, and, sometimes, by the presence of pus or the formation of an *abscess*. Infection may spread locally, to adjacent organs or tissue, or to more distant parts of the body via the blood.

The type of infection depends on how the wound occurred. For example, a wound that has come into contact with soil can result in *tetanus*. Staphylococcal bacteria, including *MRSA*, are common causes of wound infection.

DRUGS TO TREAT **WORM INFESTATIONS**

Drugs such as those listed below are the main treatment for worm infestations. Usually just one or two doses are required but sometimes longer treatment is needed. Laxatives may also be given to aid expulsion of worms living in the intestines.

Infestation	Drug
Threadworm	Mebendazole, piperazine
Common roundworm (ascariasis)	Mebendazole, piperazine
Whipworm	Mebendazole
Hookworm	Mebendazole, albendazole
Strongyloidiasis	Tiabendazole, albendazole, ivermectin
Toxocariasis	Tiabendazole
Tapeworm	Niclosamide, praziquantel
Filariasis	Diethylcarbamazine, ivermectin
Schistosomiasis	Praziquantel

W

TYPES OF WOUNDS

Wounds can be divided into the following categories: incised wounds, in which the skin is cleanly cut (e.g. surgical incision); abrasion (or grazes), in which surface tissue is scraped away; lacerations, in which the skin is torn (e.g. animal bites); contusions, in which the underlying tissues are damaged by a blunt instrument; and penetrating wounds (e.g. stab or gunshot wounds).

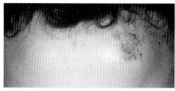

Abrasion
Abrasions usually result from sliding falls and may contain dirt. They should be carefully cleaned and dressed.

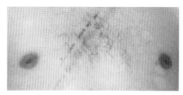

Contusion
Although the skin remains intact in this type of wound (caused, here, by a seat belt), there may be damage to the underlying tissues.

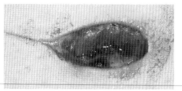

Penetration wound
A penetrating wound (here, a stab wound) may appear small, but the knife may have punctured organs deep in the body.

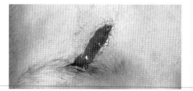

Laceration
Such wounds are usually cleaned and then left open to heal. Antibiotic and antitetanus treatment may be given.

Once infection is discovered, a sample of pus or blood may be taken and the patient is given an *antibiotic drug*. An abscess should be drained surgically.

wrinkle

Wrinkling is due to loss of skin elasticity and occurs naturally with aging. Premature wrinkling is usually caused by overexposure to sunlight and smoking. No treatment can restore skin elasticity permanently. However, some *vitamin A* derivatives are believed to reduce wrinkling. A *face-lift* smoothes out wrinkles by stretching the skin; the effects may last for up to 10 years. Injections of botulinum toxin (Botox) may also be used to temporarily reduce wrinkles.

wrist

The joint between the *hand* and the arm that allows the hand to be bent forward and backward relative to the arm and also to be moved side to side.

The wrist contains eight bones (known collectively as the carpus), arranged in two rows, one articulating with the forearm bones, and the other connecting to the bones of the palm. Tendons connect the forearm muscles to the fingers and thumb, and arteries and nerves supply the muscles, bones, and skin of the hand and fingers.

DISORDERS

Wrist injuries may lead to disability by limiting hand movement. A common injury in adults is *Colles' fracture*, in which the lower end of the radius is fractured and the hand is displaced backwards. In young children, similar displacement results from a fracture through the epiphysis (growing end) of the radius. A *sprain* can affect ligaments at the wrist joint, but most are not severe. (See also *carpal tunnel syndrome*; *osteoarthritis*; *tenosynovitis*; *wrist-drop*.)

wrist-drop

Inability to straighten the *wrist*, so that the back of the hand cannot be brought into line with the back of the forearm., causing weakness of grip.

Wrist-drop is caused by damage to the *radial nerve*, either by prolonged pressure in the armpit (see *crutch palsy*) or by fracture of the humerus (upper-arm bone; see *humerus, fracture of*).

Treatment involves holding the wrist straight. This may be achieved with a splint, but if damage to the radial nerve is permanent, the treatment is *arthrodesis* (surgical fusion) of the wrist bones.

writer's cramp

See *cramp, writer's*.

wry neck

Abnormal tilting and twisting of the head. It may be partly due to neck muscle injury or spasm (see *torticollis*).

STRUCTURE OF THE **WRIST**

The wrist is a complex joint that allows the hand to be bent forward and backward relative to the arm (through an angle of almost 180 degrees) and also moved side to side (through about 70 degrees).

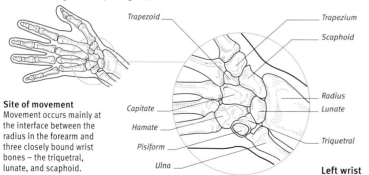

Site of movement
Movement occurs mainly at the interface between the radius in the forearm and three closely bound wrist bones – the triquetral, lunate, and scaphoid.

Trapezoid
Trapezium
Scaphoid
Capitate
Hamate
Pisiform
Ulna
Radius
Lunate
Triquetral

Left wrist

W

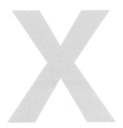

Xalacom

A brand-name drug containing latanoprost, a *prostaglandin drug*, and timolol, a *beta-blocker drug*. Xalacom is used as eye-drops to treat *glaucoma* (increased pressure of fluid in the eyeball).

Xalatan

A brand name for latanoprost, a *prostaglandin drug* that is used in the form of eye-drops to treat *glaucoma* (increased pressure of fluid in the eyeball).

xanthelasma

A yellowish deposit of fatty material in the skin around the eyes. Xanthelasmas are common in elderly people and are usually not significant. In younger people, however, they may be associated with *hyperlipidaemias* (excess fat in the blood). Xanthelasmas may be removed, if necessary, by a simple surgical procedure under a local anaesthetic. Any associated hyperlipidaemia must also be treated. (See also *xanthomatosis*.)

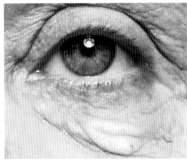

Appearance of xanthelasma
These fatty deposits around the eyes are common in elderly people but are usually of no more than cosmetic importance.

xanthine drugs

A group of *bronchodilator drugs* usually used for the long-term prevention of attacks of breathing difficulty, such as in *asthma* and chronic obstructive pulmonary disease (see *pulmonary disease, chronic obstructive*). Xanthine drugs may be given orally, or by intravenous infu-sion if the condition is severely exacerbated. *Aminophylline* and *theophylline* are common examples of xanthine drugs. Possible side effects of the drugs include headaches, nausea, and palpitations.

xanthoma

A yellowish deposit of fatty material in the skin, often on the elbow or buttock. Xanthomas may be associated with *hyperlipidaemias*, a group of disorders in which there are raised levels of fats in the blood (see *xanthomatosis*).

xanthomatosis

A condition in which deposits of yellowish, fatty material develop in various parts of the body, particularly in the skin, internal organs, corneas of the eyes, brain, and tendons. The deposits may occur only in the eyelids (see *xanthelasma*). A key feature of xanthomatosis is the tendency for fatty material to be deposited in the linings of blood vessels, leading to generalized *atherosclerosis*. Xanthomatosis is often associated with *hyperlipidaemias* (a group of disorders in which there are raised levels of fats in the blood).

Treatment aims to lower the levels of fats in the blood by means of a diet that is low in cholesterol and high in polyunsaturated fat, and by drug treatment.

X chromosome

A *sex chromosome*, of which every normal female body cell has a pair. Male body cells have one X and one *Y chromosome*; each sperm carries either an X or a Y chromosome. Abnormal genes that are located on X chromosomes result in *X-linked disorders*.

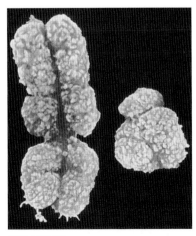

X chromosome
This is a coloured scanning electron microscope (SEM) view of the X chromosome (left), and the Y, which are also known as the sex chromosomes.

Xenical

A brand name for *orlistat*, a drug used in the treatment of severe *obesity*.

xenotransplantation

The transplantation of an organ (a heart or lung, for example) from one species into another species, such as the transplantation of pig organs into humans. Research into the *genetic engineering* of pig embryos is currently underway in order to produce animals with organs that will not be rejected by a human body following *transplant surgery*.

xeroderma pigmentosum

A rare, inherited skin disease. The skin is normal at birth, but *photosensitivity* (extreme sensitivity to sunlight) causes it to become dry, wrinkled, freckled, and prematurely aged by about the age of five. Noncancerous skin tumours and *skin cancers* also develop. Xeroderma pigmentosum is often accompanied by related eye problems, such as *photophobia* and *conjunctivitis*.

Treatment of the condition consists of protecting the skin from sunlight. Skin cancers are usually treated surgically or with *radiotherapy*.

xerophthalmia

An *eye* disorder in which deficiency of *vitamin A* causes the conjunctiva and cornea to become abnormally dry. Without treatment, xerophthalmia may progress to *keratomalacia*, a condition in which severe damage is caused to the cornea.

xerostomia

Abnormal dryness of the mouth, which can cause bad breath and may predispose the sufferer towards tooth decay (see *caries, dental*). Xerostomia is sometimes a symptom of *Sjögren's syndrome*. (See also *mouth, dry*.)

xipamide

A thiazide *diuretic* drug that is used to treat *oedema* (accumulation of fluid in the body tissues) and *hypertension* (high blood pressure). Side effects of xipamide may include dizziness and mild gastrointestinal disturbances.

xiphisternum

An alternative name for the *xiphoid process*, the small, leaf-shaped projection

X

USING **X-RAYS** TO LOOK AT THE BODY

X-rays are perhaps the most widely used method of imaging the body. When passed through body tissues on to photographic film, X-rays cast images of internal structures, allowing alterations in silhouette to be seen. Soft tissues do not show up as well as bone on X-rays, but, by using a contrast medium, they too can be visualized. New computer techniques produce even clearer, more detailed images, making X-ray an increasingly efficient diagnostic tool.

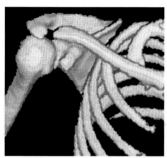

3-D CT scan
A computer can transform X-ray images of body slices into a three-dimensional image of part of the body.

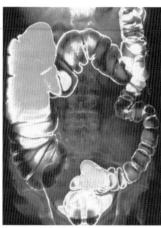

Barium X-ray
Introducing barium, which is opaque to X-rays, into the large intestine allows it to be visualized.

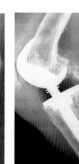

X-rays of knee joint
The X-ray on the left shows erosion of bone and cartilage. The parts of an artificial knee are seen in the X-ray on the right.

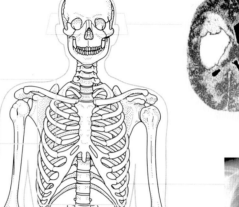

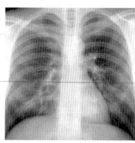

CT scan
Combined use of a computer and X-rays produces cross-sectional images. In this brain scan, the white area is a mass of blood (haematoma) caused by a stroke.

Chest X-ray
X-rays allow bones and internal organs to be imaged.

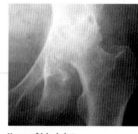

X-ray of hip joint
This X-ray of an osteoarthritic hip shows almost complete degeneration of the cartilage.

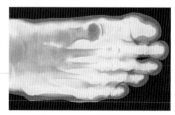

X-ray of foot
All the bones can be clearly seen in this X-ray of a healthy foot.

X

that hangs down from the body of the *sternum* (breastbone), forming the lowest of the sternum's three parts.

xiphoid process

Also known as the xiphisternum, the lowermost section of the *sternum* (breastbone). The xiphoid process is a small, leaf-shaped piece of tissue that projects downwards from the body of the sternum. The xiphoid process is initially composed of *cartilage* (connective tissue formed of collagen), which gradually ossifies throughout a person's life until it is completely replaced by bone. This section of the sternum does not articulate with any of the *ribs*.

X-linked disorders

Sex-linked *genetic disorders* in which the abnormal gene or genes (the causative factors) are located on the X chromosome. Almost all affected people are males. *Haemophilia*, *fragile X syndrome* and *colour vision deficiency* are examples of X-linked disorders.

X-rays

A form of electromagnetic radiation of short wavelength and high energy. X-rays are widely used in medicine for diagnosis because they can be used to image bones, organs, and internal tissues. They are also used in medicine for treatment, particularly of cancer.

HOW THEY WORK

X-rays are produced artificially by bombarding a heavy metal tungsten (or other such metal) target with electrons in a device known as an X-ray tube. Low

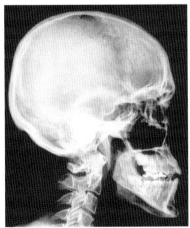

Skull X-ray
An X-ray of a healthy skull seen from the side. The very white area in the centre shows where the bones of the cranium are fused together.

doses of the X-rays that are emitted are passed through body tissue and form images on film or a fluorescent screen. The X-ray image, also called a radiograph or roentgenogram, shows the internal structure of the area being examined. Dense structures, such as bone, absorb X-rays well and appear white on an X-ray image. Soft tissues, such as muscle, absorb less well and appear grey.

SPECIAL X-RAY TECHNIQUES

Hollow or fluid-filled parts of the body often do not show up well on X-ray film unless they first have a contrast medium (a substance that is opaque to X-rays) introduced into them. Contrast-medium X-ray techniques are used to image the gallbladder (see *cholecystography*), bile ducts (see *cholangiography*), the urinary tract (see *urography*), the gastrointestinal tract (see *barium X-ray examinations*), blood vessels (see *angiography*; *venography*), and the spinal cord (see *myelography*).

X-rays can be used to obtain images of "slices" through an organ or part of the body by using a technique known as *tomography*. More detailed images of a body slice are produced by combining tomography with the capabilities of a computer (see *CT scanning*).

X-RAY SAFETY

Large doses of X-rays can be extremely hazardous, and even small doses carry some risk (see *radiation hazards*). Modern X-ray equipment and techniques produce high-quality images with the lowest possible radiation exposure to the patient. The risk of genetic damage can be minimized by using a lead shield to protect the patient's reproductive organs from X-rays. Radiographers and radiologists wear a *film badge* to monitor their exposure to radiation.

RADIOTHERAPY

Because X-rays can damage living cells, especially those that are dividing rapidly, high doses of radiation are often used in the treatment of cancer (see *radiotherapy*). (See also *imaging techniques*; *radiography*; *radiology*.)

X-rays, dental

See *dental X-ray*.

xylitol

A naturally occurring *carbohydrate* that is only partially absorbed by the body. Xylitol is sometimes used as a noncariogenic (does not cause dental caries) sweetener in confectionery and drinks. It is also used as a sweetener, in place of

sugar, by people with diabetes. Xylitol chewing gum has been shown to reduce recurrent ear infections in some children. Excess xylitol may lead to abdominal discomfort and flatulence.

Xylocaine

A brand name for lidocaine, a local anaesthetic (see *anaesthesia, local*) used to numb tissues before minor surgical procedures and as a *nerve block*.

xylometazoline

A *decongestant* drug that is used in the form of a spray or drops to relieve nasal congestion caused by a common *cold*, *sinusitis*, or hay fever (see *rhinitis, allergic*). Xylometazoline is also used as an ingredient of eye-drops in the treatment of allergic *conjunctivitis*.

Excessive use of xylometazoline may cause headache, palpitations, or drowsiness. Continuous use of the drug may cause nasal congestion to worsen when treatment is stopped.

X

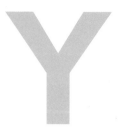

YAG laser

The abbreviation for yttrium–aluminium–garnet laser, a versatile laser that may be used in a range of treatments, including hair and tattoo removal, dentistry, *lithotripsy* (the breaking up of kidney stones), and the cutting of tissue, for example during *iridotomy*.

Yasmin

The brand name for a combined contraceptive pill (see *oral contraceptives*) that contains drospirenone (a progestogen drug) and ethinylestradiol (an oestrogen drug).

yawning

An involuntary act, or *reflex* action, that is usually associated with drowsiness or boredom. The mouth is opened wide and a slow, deep breath is taken. Yawning is accompanied by a momentary increase in the heart rate and, in many cases, watering of the eyes.

The purpose of yawning is unknown, but one theory suggests that it is triggered by raised levels of carbon dioxide in the blood; its purpose, therefore, could be to reduce carbon dioxide and increase oxygen in the blood.

yaws

An infectious disease that is found in poorer subtropical and tropical areas of the world. Yaws is caused by a form of *spirochaete* (a spiral-shaped bacterium) called TREPONEMA PERTENUE, which is similar to the bacterium that causes syphilis. Yaws is not, however, a sexually transmitted infection; it spreads principally in conditions in which there is poor hygiene. The infection is almost always acquired in childhood, and it mainly affects the skin and bones.

SYMPTOMS AND TREATMENT

The bacteria enter the body through abrasions in the skin. Three or four weeks after infection, a raspberry-like, itchy growth appears at the site of infection, sometimes preceded by fever and pains. The lesion (abnormal area of tissue) is

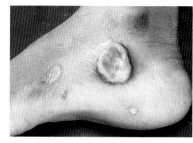

Yaws ulcer on leg
Yaws is an infection that mainly affects the skin and bones. Ulceration and tissue destruction may occur in advanced cases.

highly infectious; scratching the area spreads the infection and causes more growths to develop elsewhere.

Without treatment, the growths heal slowly over the course of about six months, but recurrence is common. In some untreated cases, widespread tissue loss eventually occurs. This may eventually lead to gross destruction of the skin, bones, and joints of the legs, nose, palate, and upper jaw.

Yaws can be cured by a single large dose of a *penicillin drug*, which is given by injection into muscle.

Y chromosome

A *sex chromosome* that is present in every normal male body cell. It is paired with an *X chromosome*. Males inherit the Y chromosome from their fathers. Every egg (from the mother) carries an X chromosome, but each sperm (from the father) may carry either a single X or a single Y chromosome. When *fertilization* (the union of an egg and a sperm cell) occurs, the combination of two X chromosomes creates a female offspring, while the combination of an X and a Y produces a male offspring.

Unlike the X chromosome, the Y chromosome carries little genetic material. Its principal function is to stimulate development of the *testes* in the male *embryo*. No significant diseases are related to Y chromosome abnormalities, but hairy ears is a trait thought to be determined by a Y-linked gene.

yeasts

Types of *fungi* in which the body of the fungus comprises individual cells that occur either singly, in pairs, or in longer chains. Certain yeasts can cause infections of the skin or mucous membranes. The most important of these disease-causing yeasts is CANDIDA ALBICANS, which causes *candidiasis* (thrush). Yeasts may

also cause *dandruff*, seborrhoeic *dermatitis*, and the nail condition *paronychia*, in which there is swelling of the nail folds.

Yellow Card system

A method of reporting adverse drug reactions (see *side effect*) in the UK. Doctors or pharmacists complete a Yellow Card if they suspect that an unwanted or unexpected symptom has occurred as a reaction to a prescribed drug (including vaccines), self medication, or herbal remedy. This information is collected and analysed centrally. The Yellow Card system is important for recognizing problems that were not identified during the testing phase of newly introduced drugs.

yellow fever

An infectious disease of short duration and variable severity that is caused by a virus transmitted by mosquitoes. In severe cases, the skin of the sufferer turns yellow due to *jaundice*, from which the name "yellow fever" is derived.

CAUSES

The infection may be spread from monkeys to humans in forest areas through various species of mosquito. In urban areas it can be transmitted from human to human by AEDES AEGYPTI mosquitoes.

INCIDENCE

Today, yellow fever is endemic in Central America, parts of South America, and a large area of Africa. The eradication of the infection-bearing mosquito from populated areas has greatly reduced the incidence of the condition.

SYMPTOMS

Yellow fever is characterized by a sudden onset of fever and headache, often with nausea and nosebleeds, which occurs three to six days after infection. Despite the high fever, the heart rate is very slow. In many cases, the affected person recovers quickly.

In serious cases, the fever is higher and there is severe headache and pain in the neck, back, and legs. Damage may occur rapidly in the liver and kidneys, causing jaundice and *kidney failure*. This may be followed by *meningitis*, severe agitation and delirium, leading to coma and death.

PREVENTION

Vaccination confers long-lasting immunity and should always be obtained before travel to affected areas. A single injection of the vaccine gives protection for at least 10 years; the vaccine is effective from 10 days after the injection.

Y

Infants under six months old should not be given the vaccine, and those aged six to nine months should only be vaccinated if there is an unavoidable risk of infection. People who are *immunocompromised* or who have had a severe allergic reaction to egg should also not be vaccinated. Pregnant women should obtain specific medical advice before being vaccinated. Reactions to the vaccine may include headache, fever, tiredness, rash, and muscle aches. However, severe reactions are rare.

DIAGNOSIS
During yellow fever epidemics, a diagnosis can be made by the symptoms. It can be confirmed by carrying out blood tests to isolate the causative virus or to find *antibodies* (proteins manufactured by the immune system) to the virus.

TREATMENT
No drug is effective against the yellow fever virus, and treatment is directed at maintaining the blood volume. Transfusion of fluids is often necessary.

Many patients recover in about three days and, in mild to moderate cases, complications are few. Relapses do not occur and one attack confers lifelong immunity. However, *dialysis* may be necessary if kidney failure develops. Despite treatment, yellow fever is fatal in some cases.

yellow nail syndrome

A condition in which the nails become thickened and yellow, or sometimes green; this is accompanied by swelling of the legs and *pleural effusion* (buildup of fluid around the lungs). Yellow nail syndrome is caused by a defect of lymphatic drainage (see *lymphatic system*).

Yersinia

A group of bacteria the includes the organism responsible for the *plague* (YERSINIA PESTIS). This organism is carried by fleas on rats, ground squirrels, and other rodents. It is transmitted from rodents to humans by bites from infected fleas. The organism can affect the *lymph nodes* resulting in large swellings, such as occurs in the bubonic form of plague. If the lungs are affected, the result is pneumonic plague; this can be transmitted from person to person if an infected individual spreads droplets in a cough.

Another form, YERSINIA ENTEROCOLITICA, can cause the development of *gastroenteritis*, particularly in young children, and *arthritis* and *septicaemia* (blood poisoning) in adults.

yield

The amount or quantity of a particular substance, such as an *enzyme* or *hormone*, that has been produced. For example, higher yields of *insulin* may be prepared for medical purposes using *genetic engineering* than through the natural production of the hormone in the pancreas of an animal.

yin and yang

The two opposing and interdependent principles that are fundamental to traditional *Chinese medicine* and philosophy. Yin is associated with the female, darkness, coldness, and quiescence, whereas yang embodies maleness, brightness, heat, and activity.

In a healthy body, yin and yang are in balance. Disorders are said to arise if one or other quality predominates; an excess of yin is said to cause conditions such as osteoarthritis, while an excess of yang results in inflammatory disorders. The concepts of yin and yang are also central to the dietary system known as *macrobiotics*.

yoga

A system of Hindu philosophy and physical discipline that is popular throughout the world. The main form of yoga practised in the West is hatha yoga. The follower adopts a series of poses, called asanas, to stimulate nerves and organs and to strengthen muscles, and performs a system of breathing control techniques called pranayama to relax the body and calm the mind. Popular forms of hatha yoga include Iyengar and ashtanga ("power yoga").

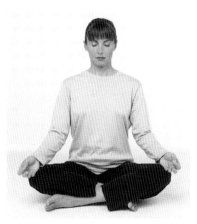

Yoga position
This woman is sitting in a loose lotus position, with her legs crossed and palms open. The position is used for relaxation and meditation.

The practice of yoga maintains flexibility, teaches physical and mental control, and is a *relaxation technique*.

Yoga should be practised only under the guidance of a qualified teacher. If yoga is attempted by people in poor health, or if it is practised incorrectly, it may pose certain health hazards, such as back disorders, high blood pressure, and *glaucoma* (raised pressure in the eye).

yohimbine

A naturally occurring *alkaloid* that dilates (widens) the pupil of the eye and also increases blood flow to the periphery of the body. Yohimbine has sometimes been used in the treatment of *erectile dysfunction* but newer, more effective treatments are generally recommended.

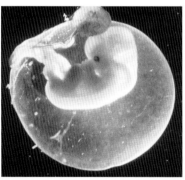

Yolk sac
This photograph is of an embryo, approximately six weeks old, surrounded by its amniotic sac. The remains of the yolk sac can be seen above its head.

yolk sac

The membranous sac, also called the vitelline sac, that is attached to the front of the *embryo* during the early stages of its existence. The yolk sac is believed to help transfer nutrients from the mother's bloodstream to the embryo. During fetal development, the yolk sac shrinks to form a narrow duct that passes through the *umbilicus*.

Young's syndrome

A form of *azoospermia* (absence of sperm in the semen) in which sperm production is normal, but the sperm ducts are obstructed. In Young's syndrome, azoospermia may sometimes be associated with *bronchiectasis* and *sinusitis*.

yttrium

A very rare metallic element that, in its radioactive form, is sometimes used in cancer therapy and to treat joints that are affected by arthritis.

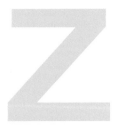

zafirlukast

A *leukotriene receptor antagonist* that is used in the prevention of *asthma*.

zanamivir

An *antiviral drug* used to treat infection with the *influenza* A and B viruses, particularly in people who are at a high risk of developing complications, such as those with *diabetes mellitus* or chronic chest problems. To be effective, the drug should be taken within 48 hours (36 hours in children) of the onset of influenza symptoms. Zanamivir may also sometimes be used preventively when influenza is circulating in the community. Possible side effects of the drug include nausea, vomiting, and diarrhoea. Occasionally, it may cause breathing problems or worsen asthma.

Zantac

A brand name for *ranitidine*, an H$_2$-receptor antagonist (see *ulcer-healing drugs*) used in the treatment of *peptic ulcer* and *gastro-oesophageal reflux disease*.

zidovudine

An *antiretroviral drug*, (formerly known as azidothymidine, or *AZT*) used in combination with other antiretroviral drugs to slow the progression of *AIDS*. Zidovudine was the first drug to be introduced to combat *HIV* infection. Antiretrovirals do not constitute a cure; their principal aim is to keep viral replication to as low a level as possible for as long as possible.

Possible side effects include *anaemia*, which may be severe enough to require a blood transfusion; nausea; loss of appetite; headache; and a reduced number of *white blood cells* in the blood.

ZIFT

See *zygote intrafallopian transfer*.

zinc

A *trace element* essential for normal growth, development of the reproductive organs, normal functioning of the prostate gland, manufacture of *proteins* and *nucleic acids*, and healing of wounds. Zinc also controls the activities of more than 100 enzymes and is involved in the functioning of the hormone *insulin*. Rich sources of zinc include lean meat, seafood, dried beans, wholemeal breads, and wholegrain cereals.

DEFICIENCY AND EXCESS

Zinc deficiency is rare. Most cases occur in people who are generally malnourished. Deficiency may also be due to any disorder that causes *malabsorption*; *acrodermatitis enteropathica* (a disorder of zinc absorption); or increased zinc requirements due to cell damage (for example, as a result of a burn).

Symptoms of deficiency include taste impairment and appetite loss; there may also be hair loss and inflammation of the skin, mouth, tongue, and eyelids. In children, zinc deficiency impairs growth and delays sexual development.

Prolonged excessive intake of zinc may interfere with the intestinal absorption of *iron* and *copper*, leading to a deficiency of these minerals.

MEDICAL USES

Zinc compounds, such as *zinc oxide*, are included in many preparations for treating skin and scalp disorders.

zinc oxide

An ingredient of many skin preparations that has a mild *astringent* action and a soothing effect. Zinc oxide is used for painful, itchy, or moist skin conditions and to ease pain due to haemorrhoids and insect bites or stings. It also blocks the sun's ultraviolet rays (see *sunscreens*).

Zollinger–Ellison syndrome

A rare condition characterized by severe and recurrent *peptic ulcers* in the stomach and the duodenum and jejunum (first and middle sections of the small intestine). It is caused by one or more gastrin-secreting tumours, which usually arise in the *pancreas* but occasionally develop in the stomach or duodenum. Gastrin stimulates production of large quantities of acid by the stomach, leading to ulceration. The high levels of acid in the digestive tract often also cause diarrhoea.

The tumours are often cancerous but are slow-growing. If possible, they are removed surgically. *Proton pump inhibitor* drugs are given to treat the ulcers.

zolmitriptan

A *serotonin agonist* that is used in the treatment of acute attacks of *migraine*.

SELECTED **ZOONOSES** (DISEASES CAUGHT FROM ANIMALS)

With the exception of fungal infections and mites caught from pets, all the diseases listed below are rare or unknown in the UK. Several may be caught from animals used as food (pigs and cows, for example), but such diseases occur mainly where food hygiene regulations and/or practices are lax. Rabies can be caught from various animals in addition to those listed (foxes, skunks, and mongooses, for example).

Animal	Disease	Animal	Disease
Bat	• Histoplasmosis • Rabies	Horse	• Glanders
Cat	• Toxoplasmosis • Cat-scratch fever • Fungal infections	Pig	• Trichinosis • Pork tapeworm • Brucellosis
Chicken	• Salmonella infection • Psittacosis	Rabbit	• Tularaemia
Cow	• Brucellosis • Beef tapeworm • Q fever • Cowpox	Rat	• Leptospirosis
Dog	• Rabies • Toxocariasis • Mite infestations • Fungal infections	Sheep	• Liver fluke • Anthrax

Z

TECHNIQUE OF **Z-PLASTY**

This relatively simple plastic surgery technique is carried out to revise unsightly scars or to relieve skin tension caused by scar contracture. It can be particularly useful for dealing with facial scars or scars that cross natural skin creases.

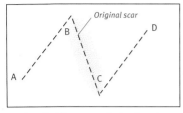

1 Three incisions are made, forming a Z. The central incision is made lengthwise through the scar.

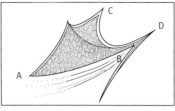

2 Two triangular flaps are developed by cutting skin away from underlying tissue, and the flaps are then transposed.

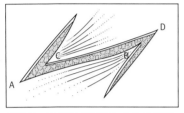

3 This manoeuvre creates a new Z, of which the central arm is at right angles to the original direction of the scar.

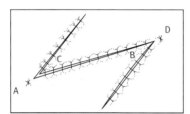

4 The flaps are sutured in place. With careful planning, the suture lines can be hidden in natural skin creases.

zolpidem

A drug used in the short-term treatment of *insomnia*. Zolpidem causes little hangover effect. Possible side effects include diarrhoea, nausea, and dizziness.

zona pellucida

The thick, transparent, noncellular layer that surrounds a developing egg cell in the ovarian follicle.

zoonosis

Any infectious or parasitic disease that affects animals and can be transmitted to humans. Zoonoses are usually caught from animals that are closely associated with humans. Examples include *toxocariasis*, *cat-scratch fever*, some *fungal infections*, *psittacosis*, *brucellosis*, *trichinosis*, and *leptospirosis*. *Rabies* can infect virtually any mammal, but dog bites are a common cause of zoonosis infection in humans worldwide.

Other zoonoses are transmitted from animals less obviously associated with humans, usually by insect vectors. For example, *yellow fever* is transmitted by mosquito bites. (See also *cats, diseases from*; *dogs, diseases from*; *insects and disease*; *rats, diseases from*.)

zopiclone

A drug that is used in the short-term treatment of *insomnia*. Zopiclone has a brief duration of action and causes little hangover effect. Because of the risk of dependence, zopiclone is intended for occasional use only.

Possible side effects of the drug include a bitter metallic taste, nausea, and a dry mouth.

Zovirax

A brand name for *aciclovir*, an *antiviral drug* used to treat viral infections such as herpes simplex, herpes zoster, and some cases of chickenpox.

Z-plasty

A technique that is used in *plastic surgery* to change the direction of a pre-existing scar in order for it to be hidden within the natural creases of the skin. Z-plasty is also used to relieve skin tension that occurs as a result of *contracture* of a scar. The technique is especially useful for revising unsightly scars on the face, and for releasing scarring across joints, such as on the fingers or in the armpits, that may restrict normal movement or cause deformity.

Zyban

A brand name for *amfebutamone*, a drug that is used, along with self-help measures, as an aid to stopping smoking.

zygomatic arch

The arch of bone, commonly known as the cheek bone, on either side of the *skull* just below the eye socket. The zygomatic arch is formed of the zygomatic and temporal bones.

zygote

The cell that is produced when a *sperm* fertilizes an *ovum* (egg). A zygote, which measures about 0.1 mm in diameter in humans, contains all the genetic material needed for a new individual. The zygote is surrounded by a thick, transparent, protein-rich layer known as the *zona pellucida*.

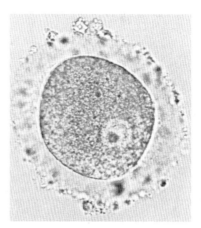

Appearance of a zygote
The photograph shows a human egg shortly after it has been fertilized by a sperm. The two circular areas at the centre of the image are the nuclei of the sperm and egg merging.

The zygote travels down one of the woman's *fallopian tubes*, dividing as it does so. After about a week, the mass of cells (now called a blastocyst) implants into the lining of the uterus, and the next stage of embryological growth begins. (See also *embryo*; *fertilization*.)

zygote intrafallopian transfer

A type of *in vitro fertilization*, also referred to as ZIFT, in which *ova* (eggs) are fertilized outside the body and returned to a *fallopian tube* rather than to the *uterus*.

Z

ACKNOWLEDGMENTS

The publisher would like to thank the following for their kind permission to reproduce their photographs:
(Page position abbreviations key: t=top, b=below, r=right, l=left, c=centre, a=above)

(Agency Abbreviation: SPL = Science Photo Library)
13: SPL/Dr. Zara/BSIP; **14:** Wellcome Photo Library (cb); **22:** SPL (ca), Dr P. Marazzi (cra); **25:** Wellcome Photo Library (cla); **26:** SPL/Nancy Hamilton (cr), Dr P. Marazzi (tr); **27:** Wellcome Photo Library; **28:** SPL/Astrid & Hanns-Frieder Michler (bcl), (bcr); **31:** Dr D.A.Burns (bc), (br); SPL/David Scharf (cl); **34:** SPL/Dr W. Crum, Dementia Research Group/Tim Beddow (br); **41:** Wellcome Photo Library; **48:** SPL/Lunagrafix (bc), Zephyr (br); **67:** SPL/Dr P. Marazzi (tl); **69:** Wellcome Photo Library (tr); **71:** SPL/CNRI; **76:** SPL/Eye of Science (bc); **77:** SPL/Dr P. Marazzi; **90:** SPL (cra), (br); Wellcome Photo Library (tr), (bc); **93:** SPL (ca); **102:** Wellcome Photo Library; **103:** Wellcome Photo Library (bl); **106:** Frank Meronk, Jr., M.D (tc), (ca); **108:** Wellcome Photo Library (tc); **109:** SPL/Jackie Lewin, Royal Free Hospital; **110:** Wellcome Photo Library /David Gregory & Debbie Marshall (tc); **114:** Corbis/Ariel Skelley (bl); **115:** SPL/Michael Abbey (cla); Wellcome Photo Library (cra); **117:** Wellcome Photo Library (car); **120:** SPL/Scott Camazine (bl), CNRI (bc), Simon Fraser/Neuroradiology Dept/Newcastle General Hospital (br); **122:** SPL/Simon Fraser (tr); **124:** SPL/Bates/Custom Medical Stock Photo (bc); **130:** SPL/BSIP Ducloux (cb); **132:** SPL/Francoise Sauze; **133:** SPL/Princess Margaret Rose Orthopaedic Hospital (bl); **137:** SPL/Dr. E. Walker (br); **137:** Wellcome Photo Library (bc); **139:** Mediscan (br), Mediscan (bc); **145:** SPL/Dr P. Marazzi; **146:** SPL/David McCarthy (cr); **149:** SPL/Sue Ford (cr); **151:** Wellcome Photo Library; **153:** Biofotos (cl); SPL/CNRI (cr), National Cancer Institute (tr); M.I.Walker (tl); **154:** Wellcome Photo Library; **158:** SPL (bc), Dr. E. Walker (cb); **160:** Wellcome Photo Library; **163:** SPL/BSIP/Villareal (cr); **169:** SPL/GCA (cl); **173:** Wellcome Photo Library /Dr T J McMaster (bc); **174:** SPL/Biophoto Associate (tcl); **176:** SPL/Martin Dohrn/Royal College of Surgeons (tc); **184:** Wellcome Photo Library (bl); **186:** Wellcome Photo Library (bl); **192:** SPL/David Parker (br); **197:** SPL/Simon Fraser (br); **201:** Wellcome Photo Library; **206:** SPL/Ohio Nuclear Corporation (cr); **210:** Keymed (Medical & Industrial Equipment) Ltd, Southend-on-Sea (crb); **220:** Mr Ian Beider B.D.S (U. Lond) (tl); SPL/George Bernard (ca), Ken Eward (tr); **223:** SPL/Dr P. Marazzi; **224:** SPL/CNRI; **230:** Kidneywise (br); SPL/Dr. E. Walker (tr); **238:** SPL/Dr P. Marazzi (cla); **241:** SPL/David M. Martin, M.D.; **243:** SPL/Hattie Young; **249:** Wellcome Photo Library; **257:** SPL/John Radcliffe Hospital; **258:** SPL (bc); **261:** SPL/Mehau Kulyk (bc); **263:** SPL/Edelmann (tr); **269:** SPL/CNRI (br); **281:** SPL/CNRI (bc); **287:** SPL/Dr P. Marazzi; **292:** SPL/Custom Medical Stock Photo (bl); **304:** SPL/D. Phillips (cl); **306:** SPL/Simon Fraser (cl); **318:** SPL/Eye of Science (cl); **322:** SPL (c), Princess Margaret Rose Orthopaedic Hospital (c); Wellcome Photo Library (clb); **327:** SPL/Dr P. Marazzi (tc); Wellcome Photo Library (tl); **330:** Wellcome Photo Library; **340:** Wellcome Photo Library (cl); **342:** SPL/Zephyr (cr); **346:** Wellcome Photo Library; **348:** SPL/Dr P. Marazzi (c); **358:** SPL/Astrid & Hanns-Frieder Michler (clb); **359:** Wellcome Institute Library, London; **364:** SPL/Dr Goran Bredberg (br); **366:** SPL (cb); **371:** SPL/Simon Fraser (tc), James Steveson (bl), St Bartholomew's Hospital (bcl); **372:** SPL (crb); **373:** Wellcome Photo Library (cb), (crb), (cbr); **380:** Mediscan (tc); **382:** SPL/Princess Margaret Rose Orthopaedic Hospital (c), (cr); **385:** SPL/David Scharf (cb); **386:** SPL/Dr P. Marazzi; **391:** Wellcome Photo Library (cr); **399:** SPL/Dr P. Marazzi (cr); **400:** SPL/Dr. Chris Hale; **405:** SPL (cr); **409:** SPL (tc), Camal, ISM (cr), Simon Fraser/Freeman Hospital, Newcastle Upon Tyne (bl), J. Leveille/Hotel-Dieu de Montreal (cl); **412:** SPL (br); **415:** SPL/BSIP VEM (bc), Dr P. Marazzi (crb); **417:** SPL/Stevie Grand; **419:** SPL/A.B. Dowsett (bc); **423:** SPL (c), Z.Binor/Custom Medical Stock Photo (cb), John Walsh (br); **429:** SPL/BSIP, Laurent, Meeus; **445:** Wellcome Photo Library; **450:** SPL (ca), Camal, ISM (c), J. Leveille/Hotel-Dieu de Montreal (cb); Sovereign/ISM (br), Zephyr (tc); **451:** SPL/Brad Nelson/Custom Medical Stock Photo (bl); **453:** SPL/CNRI (bl), Zephyr (bc); **454:** SPL/Dr P. Marazzi (bl), Princess Margaret Rose Orthopaedic Hospital (tl); **458:** SPL/CNRI (cr); **460:** Wellcome Photo Library (bcl), (bcr); **462:** SPL/Pascal Goetgheluck (ca); **462:** Wellcome Photo Library (br); **463:** Wellcome Photo Library (c); **470:** Wellcome Photo Library (br); **476:** SPL/Martin Dohrn/Royal College of Surgeons (bl); **478:** SPL/Custom Medical Stock Photo (c), Simon Fraser (cb); **479:** Wellcome Photo Library; **481:** Wellcome Photo Library (br); **485:** SPL/Dr Gopal Murti (cr); **487:** SPL/Bates/Custom Medical Stock Photo (c), (cr), Dr P. Marazzi (cl); **489:** SPL/John Radcliffe Hospital; **497:** Wellcome Photo Library; **507:** SPL/James Stevenson (tl); Wellcome Photo Library (tr); **513:** Wellcome Photo Library; **517:** Photo courtesy of Philips Medical Systems (tc); **519:** SPL; **542:** Wellcome Photo Library/Isabella Gavazzi (cr); **551:** SPL; **558:** SPL/Dr P. Marazzi (bc); **563:** SPL/Dr P. Marazzi (cr); **570:** SPL/Oscar Burriel (crb); **572:** SPL/Dr P. Marazzi (c); **573:** Wellcome Photo Library; **575:** SPL/Prof. P. Motta/Dept. of Anatomy/University "La Sapienza", Rome (cra), (car); **577:** SPL/Z. Binor/Custom Medical Stock Photo (bl); **578:** Wellcome Photo Library; **586:** Wellcome Photo Library; **595:** Wellcome Photo Library (tr); **597:** SPL/CNRI (c), David M. Martin, M.D (cl); **599:** SPL/CNRI; **603:** SPL/Dr Robert Friedland; **613:** SPL/David Scharf (tc); **614:** SPL/NIBSC; **615:** SPL (br); **617:** Wellcome Photo Library; **625:** SPL (bl); **626:** Paula Willett/Mediscan; **636:** SPL/James Stevenson (cla); **637:** Frank Meronk, Jr., M.D (tr); SPL/Paul Parker (tc); **641:** Wellcome Photo Library (cb); **646:** SPL/CNRI; **647:** Mediscan (br), (bra); **664:** SPL/Sue Ford (cb); **678:** SPL/Dr P. Marazzi (cra); **694:** SPL/Mike Devlin (bc), Dr P. Marazzi (tc); **695:** SPL (br); **698:** SPL (cla); **700:** Wellcome Photo Library (tr); **704:** SPL/John Walsh (bc); **705:** Mike Wyndham (cl); **710:** SPL/Dr P. Marazzi (tr), (c); **716:** SPL (br); **718:** SPL/Zephyr (cr); **719:** SPL/Sue Ford (bl), Mehau Kulyk (tl), Dr P. Marazzi (br); **722:** SPL/Kings College School of Medicine, Department of Surgery; **724:** Wellcome Photo Library (cra); **725:** SPL/James Stevenson (cr); **728:** SPL/Jim Stevenson; **730:** SPL/Omikron (bc); **731:** SPL/Tony McConnell; **732:** SPL/George Bernard (cla); **743:** SPL/James King-Holmes (bl); **746:** SPL/Alfred Pasieka (bl); **750:** SPL/John Radcliffe Hospital (cb); **751:** SPL/Dr P. Marazzi (br); **752:** SPL/Manfred Kage (br); **754:** Wellcome Photo Library (cr); **759:** SPL/Ed Reschke/Peter Arnold Inc. (bc); **761:** Mike Wyndham (cl); **763:** SPL (bl); **766:** SPL/Dr P. Marazzi; **768:** SPL (cra); **770:** SPL; **772:** SPL/John Durham (br); **775:** SPL (tc); **777:** SPL/John Radcliffe Hospital (tl); **782:** SPL/Alex Bartell (bc); **788:** SPL/Eye of Science (bl); **797:** SPL; **798:** SPL/CNRI (ca); **801:** SPL/CNRI (tl), David Parker (bl); **802:** SPL/James Stevenson (cb); **806:** Mike Wyndham (tl); **808:** SPL/Dr P. Marazzi (ca), Garry Watson (cla); Wellcome Photo Library (tl), (tc); **809:** SPL/Biophoto Associate (bc); Wellcome Photo Library (bl); **810:** SPL/Scott Camazine (cl), Du Cane Medical Imaging Ltd (cra), Mehau Kulyk (tl), (br), Dr P. Marazzi (crb), (bl), Zephyr (tr), (bcl); **811:** SPL/Alfred Pasieka; **812:** Wellcome Photo Library; **813:** SPL/Edelmann (cr); **815:** SPL/CC Studio (cr).

All other images © DK Images.
For further information see: **www.dkimages.com**